Breastfeeding

A GUIDE FOR THE MEDICAL PROFESSION

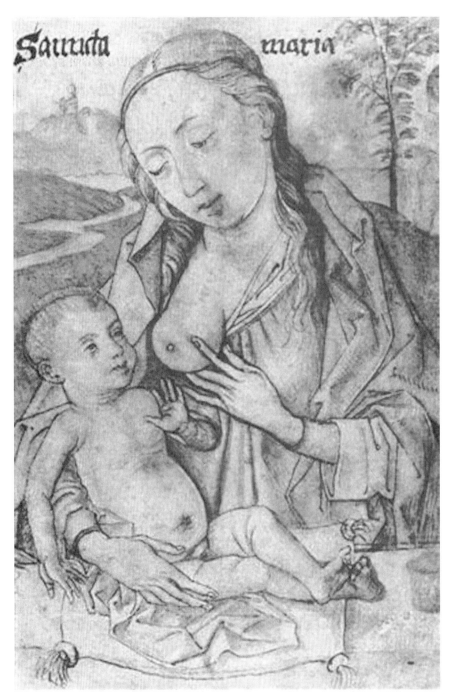

Madonna and Child, School of Bruges, Flemish, 15th century colored drawing. *(Reproduced with permission from Memorial Art Gallery of the University of Rochester.)*

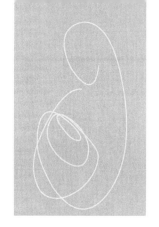

Breastfeeding

A GUIDE FOR THE MEDICAL PROFESSION

Eighth Edition

Ruth A. Lawrence, MD

Northumberland Trust Chair in Pediatrics
Distinguished Alumna Professor of Pediatrics, Obstetrics, and Gynecology
Department of Pediatrics
University of Rochester School of Medicine and Dentistry
Rochester, New York

Robert M. Lawrence, MD

Clinical Professor of Pediatrics
Pediatric Immunology, Rheumatology, and Infectious Diseases
Department of Pediatrics
University of Florida College of Medicine
Gainesville, Florida

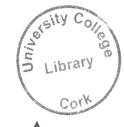

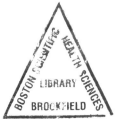
ELSEVIER

234702276

ELSEVIER

1600 John F. Kennedy Blvd.
Ste 1800
Philadelphia, PA 19103-2899

BREASTFEEDING: A GUIDE FOR THE MEDICAL PROFESSION, EIGHTH EDITION

ISBN: 978-0-323-35776-0

Notices

Knowledge and best practice in this field are constantly changing. As new research and experience broaden our understanding, changes in research methods, professional practices, or medical treatment may become necessary.

Practitioners and researchers must always rely on their own experience and knowledge in evaluating and using any information, methods, compounds, or experiments described herein. In using such information or methods they should be mindful of their own safety and the safety of others, including parties for whom they have a professional responsibility.

With respect to any drug or pharmaceutical products identified, readers are advised to check the most current information provided (i) on procedures featured or (ii) by the manufacturer of each product to be administered, to verify the recommended dose or formula, the method and duration of administration, and contraindications. It is the responsibility of practitioners, relying on their own experience and knowledge of their patients, to make diagnoses, to determine dosages and the best treatment for each individual patient, and to take all appropriate safety precautions.

To the fullest extent of the law, neither the Publisher nor the authors, contributors, or editors, assume any liability for any injury and/or damage to persons or property as a matter of products liability, negligence or otherwise, or from any use or operation of any methods, products, instructions, or ideas contained in the material herein.

Previous editions copyrighted 2011, 2005, 1999, 1994, 1989, 1985, 1980 by Mosby, an affiliate of Elsevier Inc.

Library of Congress Cataloging-in-Publication Data
Lawrence, Ruth A., date, author.
  Breastfeeding : a guide for the medical profession / Ruth A. Lawrence, Robert M. Lawrence. – Edition: 8.
    p. ; cm.
  Includes bibliographical references and index.
  ISBN 978-0-323-35776-0 (pbk. : alk. paper)
  I. Lawrence, Robert M. (Robert Michael), date, author. II. Title.
  [DNLM: 1. Breast Feeding. 2. Lactation. 3. Milk, Human. WS 125]
  RJ216
  649'.33–dc23
                                                                        2015032368

Executive Content Strategist: Kate Dimock
Content Development Specialist: Margaret Nelson
Publishing Services Manager: Patricia Tannian
Senior Project Manager: Sharon Corell
Book Designer: Ryan Cook

  Working together to grow libraries in developing countries

Printed in United States of America.

Last digit is the print number: 9 8 7 6 5 4 3 2

www.elsevier.com • www.bookaid.org

In loving memory of
John Charles Lawrence
March 5, 1966, to October 9, 2008
and
Robert Marshall Lawrence, MD
June 28, 1923, to August 13, 2005

— Ruth A. Lawrence

Sincerely dedicated to
all of the health professionals who continue to support women
in their efforts to breastfeed their children

— Robert M. Lawrence

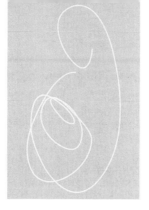

Foreword

The 5 years since the publication of the seventh edition of this excellent book have been a time of incredible advances in understanding several previously unknown physiologic and behavioral processes directly linked to or associated with breastfeeding and beautifully described in this new volume.

These findings change our view of the mother-infant relationship and signal an urgent need to completely review present perinatal care procedures. These new research results include the observation that, when an infant suckles from the breast, there is a large outpouring of 19 different gastrointestinal hormones, including cholecystokinin, gastrin, and insulin, in both mother and infant. Several of these hormones stimulate the growth of the baby's and the mother's intestinal villi, thus increasing the surface area for the absorption of additional calories with each feeding. The stimulus for these changes is touching the nipple of the mother or the inside of the infant's mouth. The stimulus in both infant and mother results in the release of oxytocin in the periventricular area of the brain, which leads to production of these hormones via the vagus nerve. These pathways were essential for survival thousands of years ago, when periods of famine were common, before the development of modern agriculture and the storage of grain.

The discovery of the additional significance of a mother's breast and chest to the infant comes from the studies of Swedish researchers who have shown that a normal infant, placed on the mother's chest, and covered with a light blanket, will warm or maintain body temperature as well as an infant warmed with elaborate, high-tech heating devices. The same researchers found that, when infants are skin-to-skin with their mothers for the first 90 minutes after birth, they hardly cry at all compared with infants who are dried, wrapped in a towel, and placed in a bassinet. In addition, the researchers demonstrated that if a newborn is left quietly on the mother's abdomen after birth he or she will, after about 30 minutes, gradually crawl up to the mother's breast, find the nipple, self-attach, and start to suckle on his or her own.

It would appear that each of these features—the crawling ability of the infant, the absence of crying when skin-to-skin with the mother, and the warming capabilities of the mother's chest—evolved genetically more than 400,000 years ago to help preserve the infant's life.

Research findings related to the 1991 Baby Friendly Hospital Initiative (BFHI) of WHO and UNICEF provided insight into an additional basic process. After the introduction of the BFHI, which emphasized mother-infant contact with an opportunity for suckling in the first 30 minutes after birth and mother-infant rooming-in throughout the hospital stay, there has been a significant drop in neonatal abandonment reported in maternity hospitals in Thailand, Costa Rica, the Philippines, and St. Petersburg, Russia.

A key to understanding this behavior is the observation that, if the lips of an infant touch the mother's nipple in the first half hour of life, the mother will decide to keep the infant in her room 100 minutes longer on the second and third days of hospitalization than a mother whose infant does not touch her nipple in the first 30 minutes. It appears that these remarkable changes in maternal behavior are probably related to increased brain oxytocin levels shortly after birth. These changes, in conjunction with known sensory, physiologic, immunologic, and behavioral mechanisms, attract the mother and infant to each other and start their attachment. As pointed out back in the fifth edition, a strong, affectionate bond is most likely to develop successfully with breastfeeding, in which close contact and interaction occur repeatedly when an infant wishes and at a pace that fits the needs and wishes of the mother and the infant, resulting in gratification for both. Thus breastfeeding plays a central role in the development of a strong mother-infant attachment when begun with contact immediately after birth, which in turn has been shown to be a simple maneuver to significantly increase the success of breastfeeding. All of these exciting findings provide further evidence of why breastfeeding has been so crucial in the past and deserves even strong support now.

In addition, the past few years have been associated with fundamental biochemical findings, including the importance of docosahexaenoic acid (DHA) in optimal brain development. All in all, the many new observations described in this eighth edition place milk and the process of breastfeeding in a key position in the development of many critical functions in human infants and their mothers. We salute the author for her special skill in bringing together these many unique and original observations in this new and most valuable book.

SUGGESTED READING

1. Christensson K, Cabrera T, Christensson E, et al: Separation distress call in the human neonate in the absence of maternal body contact. In Christensson K, editor: *Care of the newborn infant: satisfying the need for comfort and energy conservation [thesis]*, Stockholm, 1994, Karolinska Institute.
2. Christensson K, Siles C, Moreno L, et al: Temperature, metabolic adaptation and crying in healthy newborn cared for skin-to-skin or in a cot, *Acta Paediatr Scand* 81:488, 1992.
3. Uvnäs-Moberg K: The gastrointestinal tract in growth and reproduction, *Sci Am* 261:78, 1988. 2568686.
4. Widström AM, Ransjo-Arvidson AB, Christensson K, et al: Gastric suction in healthy newborn infants: effects on circulation and developing feeding behavior, *Acta Paediatr Scand* 76:566, 1987. 3630673.
5. Widström AM, Wahlberg V, Matthiesen AS, et al: Short-term effects of early suckling and touch of the nipple on maternal behavior, *Early Hum Dev* 21:153, 1990. 2311552.
6. Klaus M, Klaus P: Academy of Breastfeeding Medicine Founder's Lecture 2009: maternity care re-evaluated, *Breastfeed Med* 5(3):3, 2010. 20121428.

John H. Kennell (1922–2013)
Marshall J. Klaus

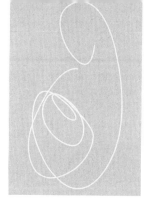

Preface

||||||||||||||||||||||||||||||||||||||||||||||||||||||||||||||

Almost five decades ago, work began on the first edition of this text. Much has changed in the field of human lactation and in the world at large. The trickle of scientific work on the subject in 1975 has swollen into a river overflowing its banks. The Lactation Study Center at the University of Rochester has more than 50,000 documents in its database that describe peer-reviewed scientific studies and reports, and there are thousands more unfiled documents that recount individual experience and anecdotal reports of events. The field has abandoned the dogmatic rules about breastfeeding that demanded rigid scheduling of hospitalized dyads. Thoughtful contemplation and recognition of the variability of the human condition are recognized as key. Well-trained, skilled clinicians recognize the value of flexibility and the need for individualized care. The Baby Friendly Hospital Initiative BFHI, which was conceived to set women free from rigid dicta requires specific protocols and policies. Mothers tell their doctors that they cannot breastfeed because there are too many rules, an impression created by overzealous teaching of too much detail. Medicine, in the era of managed care, has come forth with care guidelines for one disease or circumstance after another. The electronic record has made recording care a rigid series of boxes to check. It consumes inordinate amounts of time that could be spent with the patient but hopefully will not return us to the rigid mandates of the 1950s. The Academy of Breastfeeding Medicine, founded for the promotion and support of breastfeeding, is 20 years old. It was designed to provide physicians around the world and from every discipline a forum for scientific learning and discussion about breastfeeding and human lactation. Its members form a nucleus of medical professionals dedicated to the advancement of breastfeeding. In December, 1997, the American Academy of Pediatrics proclaimed that mothers should breastfeed for 6 months exclusively and then continue breastfeeding while introducing weaning foods through the first year and for as long thereafter as desired by mother and infant. The Section on Breastfeeding of the American Academy of Pediatrics reaffirmed that position in 2005 and again more strongly in 2010 statement. The AAP urged human milk for the premature infant in the reissued policy of 2010. The health care provider can promote these goals most effectively when armed with sufficient information. The AAP has provided the mandate that has driven progress.

The intent of this volume is to provide the basic tools of knowledge and experience that will enable a clinician to provide the thoughtful counseling and guidance to the breastfeeding family that is most applicable to that particular breastfeeding dyad and its circumstances, problems, and lifestyle. No protocol, however, should ever replace thinking.

As the field has become more complex, it is clear that one of the most difficult issues centers on infection in the mother or infant and sometimes both. Robert Michael Lawrence, MD, Clinical Professor of Pediatrics and Immunology at the University of Florida College of Medicine, has again produced the chapters on immunology and infectious disease, as well as Appendix F, to bring the most accurate information in these areas to these pages. He has also assisted in the editing of many other chapters. The drug chapter has been thoroughly revamped. It has been replaced with a chapter explaining drug pharmacology and physiology during lactation. Specific drug information is referenced in LACT-MED electronically available at the NIH website. The thousands of queries to the Lactation Study Center at the University of Rochester have served as a basis for new topics and new clinical discussions.

The eighth edition is secure in cyberspace. Gone are the days when cut and paste meant cut with scissors and paste with glue. A process that used to be simple is much more complicated, now requiring the expertise of computer wizards. David Lawrence (my son, Rob's brother) entered every chapter digitally and created the extensive tables and charts, keyboarding with the speed of sound from raw, handwritten manuscript. In my office, Jane Eggiman printed copy after copy. Adina Flynn, a born computer wizard, rescued fresh data from library archives, searching out the many citations, bibliographies, and elusive details. I thank all the lactation consultants and medical doctors who have called the center with their challenging clinical issues.

I continue to be grateful to Rosemary Disney (1923–2014) for the creation of the enduring breastfeeding symbol on the cover. I thank my friends and family who have tolerated my home and office in chaos with 23 piles of reprints, one for each chapter, spilling over the floor, along with boxes of reference books, pamphlets, and disks.

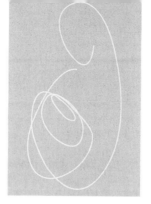

Contents

CHAPTER 1   *The Revolution in Infant Feeding* *1*

CHAPTER 2   *Anatomy of the Breast* *34*

CHAPTER 3   *Physiology of Lactation* *56*

CHAPTER 4   *Biochemistry of Human Milk* *91*

CHAPTER 5   *Host-Resistance Factors and Immunologic Significance of Human Milk* *146*

CHAPTER 6   *Psychological Impact of Breastfeeding* *194*

CHAPTER 7   *Benefits of Breastfeeding for Infants/Making an Informed Decision* *214*

CHAPTER 8   *Practical Management of the Mother-Infant Nursing Couple* *230*

CHAPTER 9   *Maternal Nutrition and Supplements for Mother and Infant* *285*

CHAPTER 10   *Weaning* *320*

CHAPTER 11   *Normal Growth, Failure to Thrive, and Obesity in Breastfed Infants* *338*

CHAPTER 12   *Medications, Herbal Preparations, and Natural Products in Breast Milk* *364*

CHAPTER 13   *Transmission of Infectious Diseases Through Breast Milk and Breastfeeding* *407*

CHAPTER 14   *Breastfeeding Infants with Problems* *483*

CHAPTER 15   *Premature Infants and Breastfeeding* *524*

CHAPTER 16   *Medical Complications of Mothers* *563*

CHAPTER 17   *Human Milk as a Prophylaxis* *633*

CHAPTER 18   *Employment and Away from Home Activities while Breastfeeding* *650*

CHAPTER 19   Induced Lactation and Relactation (Including Nursing an Adopted Baby) and Cross-Nursing 667

CHAPTER 20   Reproductive Function During Lactation 688

CHAPTER 21   The Collection and Storage of Human Milk and Human Milk Banking.....................712

CHAPTER 22   Breastfeeding Support Groups and Community Resources.......................................743

CHAPTER 23   Educating and Training the Medical Professional 754

Appendices

APPENDIX A   Composition of Human Milk 766

APPENDIX B   Normal Serum Values for Breastfed Infants 768

APPENDIX C   Herbals and Natural Products...770

APPENDIX D   Precautions and Breastfeeding Recommendations for Selected Maternal Infections.........776

APPENDIX E   Manual Expression of Breast Milk 792

APPENDIX F   The Storage of Human Milk 794

APPENDIX G   Measurements of Growth in Breastfed Infants 797

APPENDIX H   Organizations Interested in Supporting and Providing Materials for Breastfeeding.......803

APPENDIX I   Breastfeeding Health Supervision 808

APPENDIX J   Academy of Breastfeeding Medicine Protocols 1-21...817

    Protocol #1: Guidelines for Blood Glucose Monitoring and Treatment
        of Hypoglycemia in Term and Late-Preterm Neonates 817

    Protocol #2: Guidelines for Hospital Discharge of the Breastfeeding
        Term Newborn and Mother: "The Going Home Protocol" 825

    Protocol #3: Hospital Guidelines for the Use of Supplementary Feedings
        in the Healthy Term Breastfed Neonate 831

    Protocol #4: Mastitis 840

    Protocol #5: Peripartum Breastfeeding Management for the Healthy Mother
        and Infant at Term...845

    Protocol #6: Guideline on Co-Sleeping and Breastfeeding...851

    Protocol #7: Model Breastfeeding Policy..856

    Protocol #8: Human Milk Storage Information for Home Use for Healthy
        Full-Term Infants 861

Protocol #9: *Use of Galactogogues in Initiating or Augmenting Maternal Milk Supply*...864

Protocol #10: *Breastfeeding the Near-Term Infant (35-37 Weeks' Gestation)*.............869

Protocol #11: *Guidelines for the Evaluation and Management of Neonatal Ankyloglossia and Its Complications in the Breastfeeding Dyad*..........874

Protocol #12: *Transitioning the Breastfeeding/Breast-Milk-Fed Premature Infant from the Neonatal Intensive Care Unit to Home.*........................879

Protocol #13: *Contraception During Breastfeeding*...886

Protocol #14: *Breastfeeding-Friendly Physician's Office: Optimizing Care for Infants and Children* 897

Protocol #15: *Analgesia and Anesthesia for the Breastfeeding Mother* 901

Protocol #16: *Breastfeeding the Hypotonic Infant*...907

Protocol #17: *Guidelines for Breastfeeding Infants with Cleft Lip, Cleft Palate, or Cleft Lip and Palate*...913

Protocol #18: *Use of Antidepressants in Nursing Mothers*..919

Protocol #19: *Breastfeeding Promotion in the Prenatal Setting* 929

Protocol #20: *Engorgement*..933

Protocol #21: *Guidelines for Breastfeeding and Substance Use or Substance Use Disorder*...937

APPENDIX K   *Medical Education for Basic Proficiency in Breastfeeding*............................946

APPENDIX L   *Glossary* 949

TABLE 1-1   National Health Promotion and Disease Prevention Objectives

Mothers Breastfeeding Their Babies (Special Population Targets)	1998 Baseline (%)	2010 Target (%)
During early postpartum period		
Low-income mothers (WIC mothers)	56.8	75.0
Black mothers	45.0	75.0
Hispanic mothers	66.0	75.0
American Indian/Alaska Native mothers	1998 data not collected 1988 baseline: 47	75.0
At age 5-6 months		
Low-income mothers (WIC mothers)	18.9	50.0
Black mothers	19.0	50.0
Hispanic mothers	28.0	50.0
American Indian/Alaska Native mothers	1998 data not collected 1988 baseline: 28	50.0
At age 12 months		
Low-income mothers (WIC mothers)	12.1 (in 1999)	25.0
Black mothers	9.0	25.0
Hispanic mothers	19.0	25.0
American Indian/Alaska Native mothers	1998 data not collected	25.0

Healthy People 2010 is a statement of national opportunities. Although the federal government facilitated its development, it is not intended as a statement of federal standards or requirements. It is the product of a national effort involving 22 expert working groups, a consortium that has grown to include almost 300 national organizations and all the state health departments and the Institute of Medicine of the National Academy of Sciences, which helped the U.S. Public Health Service to manage the consortium, convene regional and national hearings, and receive testimony from more than 750 individuals and organizations. After extensive public review and comment involving more than 10,000 people, the objectives were revised and refined to produce this report.

From U.S. Department of Health and Human Services: *Healthy People 2010* [Conference Edition in Two Volumes], Washington, DC, January 2000.

exchange of scientific information about issues of human lactation, breastfeeding, and human milk is developing. The more detail that is obtained about the specific macro- and micronutrients in human milk, the clearer it becomes that human milk is precisely engineered for the human infant.[3] A clinician should not have to justify a recommendation for breastfeeding; instead, a pediatrician should have to justify replacement with a cow milk substitute. Harnessing the expanding stream of scientific information into a clinically applicable resource has been challenged by the need to identify reproducible, peer-reviewed scientific information and to cull the uncontrolled, poorly designed studies and reports even though they have appeared in print. Many scientists were unable to publish credible work because the best journals had no space for the increasing numbers. The journal *Breastfeeding Medicine* was created to fill this need in 2006.

The *Healthy People 2020* goals,* first published in 1978 and restated in 1989 and in 1999, recommend

that the nation increase the proportion of mothers who exclusively or partially breastfeed their babies in the early postpartum period to at least 75% and the proportion who continue breastfeeding until their babies are 5 to 6 months old to at least 50% (Table 1-1). Furthermore, at least 25% of babies should be breastfed at a year postpartum (Figure 1-1). A midcourse correction was developed by the Centers for Disease Control and Prevention (CDC) and the National Institutes of Health (NIH) in 2005 to add a 3-month goal of 50% breastfeeding. The health goals for 2020 are shown in Table 1-1. Focus groups, town meetings, and professional think tanks were working for several years to develop the new goals. The final draft can be found at http://www.womenshealth.gov/breastfeeding.

The report further states that special populations should be targeted (see Table 1-1) because breastfeeding is the optimal way of nurturing infants and simultaneously benefiting the lactating mother, and minority populations have continued to lag behind the majority in every category. Former Surgeon General of the United States C. Everett Koop stated in 1984, "We must identify and reduce the barriers which keep women from beginning or continuing to breastfeed their infants."[6]

*Healthy People 2000: National health promotion and disease prevention objectives, DHHS Pub. No. (PHS) 91-50213. Washington, DC, 1990, U.S. Department of Health and Human Services, Public Health Service, U.S. Government Printing Office.

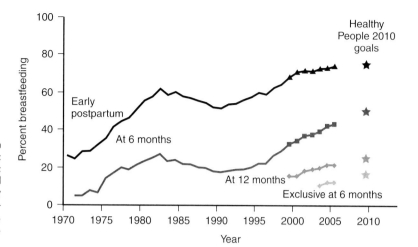

Figure 1-1. National trends in rate of breastfeeding. Data source: pre-1999, Ross Mothers Survey[2,4,5]; 1999-present, CDC, NIS. (Modified from Grummer-Strawn LM, Shealy KR: Progress in protecting, promoting, and supporting breastfeeding, *Breastfeeding Med* 4(Suppl 1):533, 2009.)

Former Surgeon General David Satcher developed the Health and Human Services Blueprint for Action on Breastfeeding in 2000, saying, "Breast-feeding is one of the most important contributions to infant health. In addition, breastfeeding improves maternal health and contributes economic benefits to the family, health care system, and work place."[7]

Each surgeon general has taken a strong and visible stand on breastfeeding. In 2011, the U.S. Department of Health and Human Services released "The Surgeon General's call to action to support breastfeeding." This report is available at http://www.surgeongeneral.gov/library/calls/breastfeeding/index.html (accessed 11 Dec 2014).

Another targeted need for the nation was public education about the subject.[8] To put breastfeeding in the mainstream and to classify it as normal behavior, education has to start with preschoolers and continue through the educational system. Courses in biology, nutrition, health, and human sexuality should include the breast and its functions.

New York State has taken a leadership position for education of its youth. In 1994, a curriculum from kindergarten through twelfth grade was jointly developed by the Department of Education and the Department of Health* and reviewed by teachers and school districts. The curriculum is not a separate course but provides recommendations about how to include age-appropriate information on breastfeeding and human lactation throughout the school years. The senior high-school materials are more detailed and are designed to be included in subject matter regarding reproduction and family life.

This commitment to policy for breastfeeding has been part of the Code for Infant Feeding of the World Health Assembly, described as the World Health Organization Code (WHO Code). The WHO Code seeks to protect developing countries from being inundated with formula products, which discourage breastfeeding, because infant survival in these countries depends on being nourished at the breast.[9–12]

Although the major countries of the world endorsed the WHO Code in 1981, the United States did not. Finally, on May 9, 1994, President Clinton supported the worldwide policy of the WHO International Code of Marketing of Breast Milk Substitutes by joining with the other member nations at the World Health Assembly in Geneva, signaling a tremendous policy shift. Despite many efforts by the United States, Italy, and Ireland to add weakening amendments, the Swaziland delegation, speaking for the African nations, voted to strengthen the resolution even more, and all amendments were dropped. One by one, all the countries, including the United States, agreed to Resolution 47.5, and it was ratified.[13]

The battle to control formula distribution worldwide has not been won. The pandemic of acquired immunodeficiency syndrome (AIDS) has provided a new reason to distribute formula to developing countries to stop the spread of human immunodeficiency virus (HIV) to infants from their HIV-positive mothers. Careful studies of the issues have proved that exclusive breastfeeding is protective for the first 6 months of life. It is the addition of herbal teas and other foods that irritate the gut and allow invasion by the virus.

Box 1-1 provides a summary of interventions presented at the Surgeon General's Workshop.[1]

---

*New York State Health Department: Breastfeeding: first step to good health—a breastfeeding education activity package for grades K-12. Albany, NY, 1995, NYS Health Research Inc.

A federally funded national conference held in 1994 in Washington, DC, came to the same conclusions as in 1984. A conference held in Washington, DC, sponsored by the Academy of Breastfeeding Medicine (ABM) and the Kellogg Foundation focused on a follow-up 25 years after the original Surgeon General's Workshop looked at disparity issues. Progress is illustrated in Figure 1-2.

Although these recommendations have been promoted since 1984, many hospitals and health care facilities have not achieved them.[14] As a result, United Nations Children's Fund (formerly United Nations International Children's Emergency Fund,

---

BOX 1-1. Key Elements for Promotion of Breastfeeding in the Continuum of Maternal and Infant Health Care

1. Primary care settings for women of childbearing age should have:
   - A supportive milieu for lactation
   - Educational opportunities (including availability of literature, personal counseling, and information about community resources) for learning about lactation and its advantages
   - Ready response to requests for further information
   - Continuity allowing for the exposure to, and development over time of, a positive attitude regarding lactation on the part of the recipient of care
2. Prenatal care settings should have:
   - A specific assessment at the first prenatal visit of the physical capability for, and emotional predisposition to, lactation. This assessment should include the potential role of the father of the child and other significant family members. An educational program about the advantages of, and ways of preparing for, lactation should continue throughout the pregnancy
   - Resource personnel—such as nutritionists/dietitians, social workers, public health nurses, La Leche League members, childbirth education groups—for assistance in preparing for lactation
   - Availability and utilization of culturally suitable patient education materials
   - An established mechanism for a predelivery visit to the newborn care provider to ensure initiation and maintenance of lactation
   - A means of communicating to the in-hospital team the infant-feeding plans developed during the prenatal course
3. In-hospital settings should have:
   - A policy to determine a patient's infant-feeding plan on admission or during labor
   - A family-centered orientation to childbirth, including the minimum use of intrapartum medications and anesthesia
   - A medical and nursing staff informed about, and supportive of, ways to facilitate the initiation and continuation of breastfeeding (including early mother-infant contact and ready access by the mother to her baby throughout the hospital stay)
   - The availability of individualized counseling and education by a specially trained breastfeeding coordinator to facilitate lactation for those planning to breastfeed and to counsel those who have not yet decided about their method of infant feeding

   - Ongoing in-service education about lactation and ways to support it. This program should be conducted by the breastfeeding coordinator for all relevant hospital staff
   - Proper space and equipment for breastfeeding in the postpartum and neonatal units. Attention should be given to the particular needs of women breastfeeding babies with special problems
   - The elimination of hospital practices/policies that have the effect of inhibiting the lactation process (e.g., rules separating mother and baby)
   - The elimination of standing orders that inhibit lactation (e.g., lactation suppressants, fixed feeding schedules, maternal medications)
   - Discharge planning that includes referral to community agencies to aid in the continuing support of the lactating mother. This referral is especially important for patients discharged early
   - A policy to limit the distribution of packages of free formula at discharge to only those mothers who are not lactating
   - The development of policies to support lactation throughout the hospital units (e.g., medicine, surgery, pediatrics, emergency room)
   - The provision of continued lactation support for those infants who must remain in the hospital after the mother's discharge
4. Postpartum ambulatory settings should have:
   - A capacity for telephone assistance to mothers experiencing problems with breastfeeding
   - A policy for telephone follow-up 1 to 3 days after discharge
   - A plan for an early follow-up visit (within first week after discharge)
   - The availability of lactation counseling as a means of preventing or solving lactation problems
   - Access to lay support resources for the mother
   - The presence of a supportive attitude by all staff
   - A policy to encourage bringing the infant to postpartum appointments
   - The availability of public-community-health nurse referral for those having problems with lactation
   - A mechanism for the smooth transition to pediatric care of the infant, including good communication between obstetric and pediatric care providers

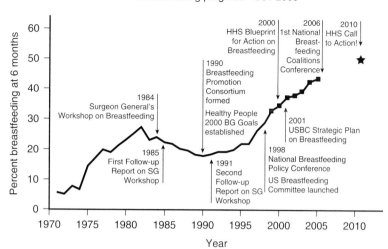

Breastfeeding progress: 1984-2009

Figure 1-2. Federal activities in support of breastfeeding (BF). *HHS,* U.S. Department of Health and Human Services; *SG,* surgeon general. (Modified from Grummer-Strawn LM, Shealy KR: Progress in protecting, promoting, and supporting breastfeeding, *Breastfeed Med* 4(Suppl 1):531, 2009.)

UNICEF) and WHO initiated the Baby Friendly Hospital Initiative, which has been implemented in developing countries with considerable success. Box 1-2 lists the 10 steps to becoming a designated Baby Friendly Hospital. A joint WHO/UNICEF statement, *Protecting, promoting,* and *supporting breastfeeding,* describes suggested actions for maternity services.[10]

BOX 1-2. Toward Becoming a Baby Friendly Hospital: 10 Steps to Successful Breastfeeding

Every facility providing maternity services and care for newborn infants should:
1. Have a written breastfeeding policy that is routinely communicated to all health care staff.
2. Train all health care staff in skills necessary to implement this policy.
3. Inform all pregnant women about the benefits and management of breastfeeding.
4. Help mothers initiate breastfeeding within a half hour of birth.
5. Show mothers how to breastfeed and how to maintain lactation even if they should be separated from their infants.
6. Give newborn infants no food or drink other than breast milk, unless medically indicated.
7. Practice rooming-in—allow mothers and infants to remain together—24 hours a day.
8. Encourage breastfeeding on demand.
9. Give no artificial teats or pacifiers (also called dummies or soothers) to breastfeeding infants.
10. Foster the establishment of breastfeeding support groups and refer mothers to them on discharge from the hospital or clinic.

In 1996, Evergreen Hospital in Kirkland, Washington, was the first Baby Friendly Hospital designated in the United States. This initiative has been reorganized and reestablished through Healthy Children, a not-for-profit organization that created Baby Friendly, USA. The program is slowly expanding. For certification for Baby Friendly, the hospital must provide evidence that it has met the 10 criteria (see Box 1-2) and must demonstrate its effectiveness to a visiting team of assessors. In 2014, hospitals in the United States with the Baby Friendly designation reached 200.

The History of Breastfeeding

The world scientific literature, predominantly from countries other than the United States, includes many tributes to human milk. Early writings on infant care in the 1800s and early 1900s pointed out the hazards of serious infection in bottle-fed infants. Mortality charts were clear on the difference in mortality risk between breastfed and bottle-fed infants.[15] Only in recent years have the reasons for this phenomenon been identified in terms comparable with those used to define other antiinfectious properties. The identification of specific immunoglobulins and determination of the specific influence of the pH and flora in the intestine of the breastfed infant are examples. It became clear that the infant receives systemic protection transplacentally and local intestinal tract protection orally via the colostrum and mature milk. The intestinal tract environment of a breastfed infant continues to afford protection against infection by influencing the bacterial flora until the infant is weaned. Breastfed infants also have fewer respiratory infections, occurrences of otitis media, gastrointestinal infections, and other illnesses. The immunologic protection afforded by specific antibodies such as respiratory syncytial virus and rotavirus also protects the infant from illness.

Refinement in the biochemistry of nutrition has afforded an opportunity to restudy the constituents of human milk. Attention to brain growth and neurologic development emphasizes the unique constituents of human milk that enhance the growth and development of the exclusively breastfed infant. Because the human brain doubles in size in the first year of life, the nutrients provided for brain growth are critical (see Chapter 7). A closer look at the amino acids in human milk has demonstrated clearly that the array is physiologically suited for the human newborn. Forced by legislation in the 1970s that mandated mass newborn screening for phenylalanine in all hospitals, physicians were faced with the problem of the newborn that had high phenylalanine or tyrosine levels. It became apparent that many traditional formulas provided an overload of these amino acids, which some infants were unable to tolerate even though they did not have phenylketonuria.

The mysteries and taboos about colostrum go back to the dawn of civilization.[8] Most ancient peoples let several days pass before putting the baby to the breast, with exact times and rituals varying from tribe to tribe. Other liquids were provided in the form of herbal teas; some were pharmacologically potent, and others had no nutritional or pharmacologic worth. Breastfeeding positions varied as well.[14] In most cultures, mothers held their infants while seated; however, Armenian and some Asian women would lean over the supine baby, resting on a bar that ran above the cradle for support (Figure 1-3). The infants were not lifted for the purpose of burping. Many groups carried infants on their backs and swung them into position frequently for feedings, a method that continues today. These infants are also not burped but remain semierect in the swaddling on the mother's back. The ritual of burping is actually a product of necessity in bottle-feeding because air is so easily swallowed.

Although modern women may be selectively chastised for abandoning breastfeeding because of the ready availability of prepared formulas, paraphernalia of bottles and rubber nipples, and ease of sterilization, this is not a new issue. Meticulous combing of civilized history reveals that almost every generation had to provide alternatives when the mother could not or would not nurse her infant.

Hammurabi's Code from about 1800 BC contained regulations on the practice of wet nursing, that is, nursing another woman's infant, often for

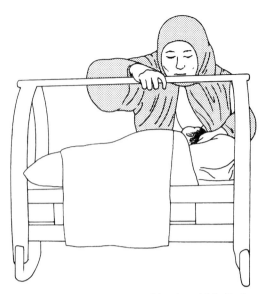

Figure 1-3. Armenian woman suckling her child. (Redrawn from Wickes IG: A history of infant feeding, *Arch Dis Child* 28:151, 1953.)

hire. Throughout Europe, spouted feeding cups have been found in the graves of infants dating from about 2000 BC.

Although ancient Egyptian feeding flasks are almost unknown, specimens of Greek origin are fairly common in infant burials. Paralleling the information about ancient feeding techniques is the problem of abandoned infants. Well-known biblical stories report such events, as do accounts from Rome during the time of the early popes. In fact, so many infants were abandoned that foundling homes were started. French foundling homes in the 1700s were staffed by wet nurses who were carefully selected and their lives and activities controlled to ensure adequate nourishment for the foundlings.

In Spartan times a woman, even if she was the wife of a king, was required to nurse her eldest son; plebeians were to nurse all their children.[16] Plutarch, an ancient scribe, reported that a second son of King Themistes inherited the kingdom of Sparta only because he was nursed with his mother's milk. The eldest son had been nursed by a stranger and therefore was rejected.

No known written works describe infant feeding from ancient times to the Renaissance.[17] In 1472, the first pediatric incunabulum, written by Paul Bagellardus, was printed in Padua, Italy. It described the characteristics of a good wet nurse and provided counseling about hiccups, diarrhea, and vomiting. Thomas Moffat (1584) wrote of the medicinal and therapeutic use of human milk for men and women of "riper years, fallen by age or by sickness into compositions." His writings referred to the milk of the ass as being the best substitute for human milk at any age when nourishment was an issue. The milk of an ass is low in solids compared with that of most species, low in fat and protein, and high in lactose.

From AD 1500 to 1700, wealthy English women did not nurse their infants, according to Fildes,[18] who laboriously and meticulously reviewed infant feeding history in Great Britain. Although breastfeeding was well recognized as a means of delaying another pregnancy, these women preferred to bear anywhere from 12 to 20 babies than to breastfeed them.[19] They had a notion that breastfeeding spoiled their figures and made them old before their time. Husbands had much to say about how the infants were fed. Wet nurses were replaced by feeding cereal or bread gruel from a spoon. The death rate in foundling homes from this practice approached 100%.

The Dowager Countess of Lincoln wrote on "the duty of nursing, due by mothers to their children" in 1662.[20] She had borne 18 children, all fed by wet nurses; only one survived. When her son's wife bore a child and nursed it, the countess saw the error of her ways. She cited the biblical example of Eve, who breastfed Cain, Abel, and Seth. She also noted that Job 39:16 states that to withhold a full breast is to be more savage than dragons and more cruel than ostriches to their little ones. The noblewoman concluded her appeal to women to avoid her mistakes: "Be not so unnatural as to thrust away your own children; be not so hardy as to venture a tender babe to a less tender breast; be not accessory to that disorder of causing a poorer woman to banish her own infant for the entertaining of a richer woman's child, as it were bidding her to unlove her own to love yours."

Toward the end of the eighteenth century in England, the trend of wet nursing and artificial feeding changed, partially because medical writers drew attention to health and well-being and mothers made more decisions about feeding their young.

In eighteenth-century France, both before and during the revolution that swept Louis XVI from the throne and brought Napoleon to power, infant feeding included maternal nursing, wet nursing, artificial feeding with the milk of animals, and feeding of pap and panada.[7] Panada is from the French *panade*, meaning bread, and means a food consisting of bread, water or other liquid, and seasoning and boiled to the consistency of pulp (Figure 1-4). The majority of infants born to wealthy and middle-income women, especially in Paris, were placed with wet nurses. In 1718, Dionis wrote, "Today not only ladies of nobility, but yet the rich and the wives of the least of the artisans have lost the custom of nursing their infants." As early as

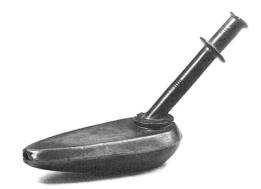

Figure 1-4. Pewter pap spoon, circa AD 1800. Thin pap, a mixture of bread and water, was placed in bowl. Tip of bowl was placed in child's mouth. Flow could be controlled by placing finger over open end of hollow handle. If contents were not taken as rapidly as desired, one could blow down on handle.

1705, laws controlling wet nursing required wet nurses to register, forbade them to nurse more than two infants in addition to their own, and stipulated that a crib should be available for each infant, to prevent the nurse from taking a baby to bed and chancing suffocation.[21] On the birth of the Prince of Wales (later George IV) in 1762, it was officially announced: wet nurse, Mrs. Scott; dry nurse, Mrs. Chapman; rockers, Jane Simpson and Catherine Johnson.[17]

A more extensive historical review would reveal other examples of social problems in achieving adequate care of infants.[22] Long before our modern society, some women failed to accept their biologic role as nursing mothers, and society failed to provide adequate support for nursing mothers (Figure 1-5).* Breastfeeding was more common and of longer duration in stable eras and rarer in periods of "social dazzle" and lowered moral standards. Urban mothers have had greater access to alternatives, and rural women have had to continue to breastfeed in greater numbers.[12]

In the 1920s, women were encouraged to raise their infants scientifically. "Raising by the book" was commonplace. The U.S. government published *Infant Care*, referred to as the "good book," which was the bible of child rearing read by women from all walks of life. It emphasized cod liver oil, orange juice, and artificial feeding. A quote from *Parents* magazine in 1938 reflects the attitude of women's magazines in general, undermining even the staunchest breastfeeders: "You hope to nurse him, but there are an alarming number of young mothers today who are unable to breastfeed their

---

*The National Convention of France of 1793 passed laws to provide relief for infants of indigent families. The provisions are quite similar to those in our present-day welfare programs.[23]

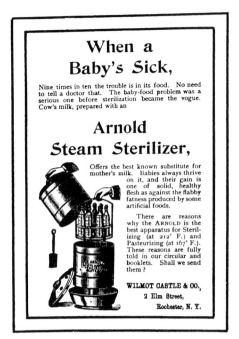

Figure 1-5. Arnold Steam Sterilizer advertisement. (From *N Y Med J* June 22, 1895.)

babies and you may be one of them."[24] Apple detailed the transition from breastfeeding to raising children scientifically, by the book, and precisely as the doctor prescribes.[25]

There are encouraging trends, however. The acceptance or rejection of breastfeeding is being influenced in the Western world to a greater degree by the knowledge of the benefits of human milk and breastfeeding. Cultural rejection, negative attitudes, and lack of support from health professionals are being replaced by well-educated women's interest in child rearing and preparation for childbirth.[26] This has created a system that encourages a prospective mother to consider the options for herself and her infant.[27–29] The attitude in the Western world toward the female breast as a sex object to the exclusion of its ability to nurture has influenced young mothers in particular not to breastfeed. The emancipation of women, which began in the 1920s, was symbolized by short hair, short skirts, contraceptives, cigarettes, and bottle-feeding. In the second half of the twentieth century, women sought to be well informed, and many wanted the right to choose how they fed their infants.

The first action began in the 1940s when Edith Jackson, MD, of Yale University School of Medicine and the Grace-New Haven Hospital was awarded a federal grant to establish the First Rooming-In Unit in the United States. This project included the first program to prepare women for childbirth modeled after the British obstetrician Grantly Dick-Read's *Child Birth Without Fear*. This

was developed with the Department of Obstetrics to reduce maternal medication during birth and keep mother and baby alert and together. Of course, it included breastfeeding. Trainees from this program in Pediatrics and Obstetrics spread across the country starting programs elsewhere. Mothers chimed in when La Leche League was organized in the late 1950s. Professional organizations such as the AAP, American College of Obstetrics and Gynecology (ACOG), and American Academy of Family Practice (AAFP) were slow to speak out as they wrestled with the grip the formula companies had on medical education.

The great success of the mother-to-mother program of the La Leche League and other women's support groups in helping women breastfeed or, as with International Childbirth Education Association (ICEA), in helping women plan and participate in childbirth, is an example of the power of social relationships.[30] Raphael[31] described the doula as a "friend from across the street" who came by at the birth of a new baby to support the mother. She would "mother the mother." The doula is now known as a key person for lactation support, especially in the first critical days and weeks after delivery.

Bryant[32] explored the social networks in her study of the impact of kin, friend, and neighbor networks on infant-feeding practices in Cuban, Puerto Rican, and Anglo families in Florida. She found that these networks strongly influenced decisions about breastfeeding, bottle-feeding, use of supplements, and introduction of solid foods. Network members' advice and encouragement contributed to a successful lactation experience. The impact of the health care professional is inversely proportional to the distance of the mother from her network. The health care worker must work within the cultural norms for the network. For individuals isolated from their cultural roots, the health care system may have to provide more support and encouragement to ensure lactation success and adherence to health care guidelines.[33]

The trend in infant feeding among mothers who participated in the Women, Infants, and Children (WIC) program in the late 1970s and early 1980s was analyzed separately by Martinez and Stahl[34,35] from the data collected by questionnaires mailed quarterly as part of the Ross Laboratories Mothers Survey. The responses represented 4.8% of the total births in the United States in 1977 and 14.1% of the total births in the United States in 1980. WIC participants in 1977, including those who supplemented with formula or cow milk, were breastfeeding in the hospital in 33.6% of cases. A steady and significant increase occurred in the frequency of breastfeeding; it rose to 40.4% in 1980 ($p < 0.5$). WIC data continue to be collected, and the trends have paralleled other groups.

The Food and Consumer Service (FCS) of the U.S. Department of Agriculture (USDA) entered into a cooperative agreement with Best Start, a not-for-profit social marketing organization that promoted breastfeeding to develop a WIC breast-feeding promotion project that was national in scope and implemented at the state level. The project consisted of six components: social marketing research, a media campaign, a staff support kit, a breastfeeding resource guide, a training conference, and continuing education and technical assistance. With an annual $8 million budget for WIC, the project's goals are to increase the initiation and duration of breastfeeding among clients of WIC and to expand public acceptance and support of breastfeeding. Breastfeeding women are favored in the WIC priority system when benefits are limited; they can continue in the program for a year, but those who do not breastfeed are limited to 6 months. All pregnant participants of WIC are encouraged to breastfeed.

Montgomery and Splett[36] reported the economic benefits of breastfeeding infants for mothers enrolled in WIC. Comparing the costs of the WIC program and Medicaid for food and health care in Colorado, administrative and health care costs for a formula-fed infant minus the rebate for the first 180 days of life were $273 higher than those for the breastfed infant. These calculations did not include the pharmacy costs for illness. When these figures were translated to large WIC programs in high-cost areas (e.g., New York City, Los Angeles) and multiplied by millions of WIC participants, the savings from breastfeeding were substantial (Table 1-2). If the goal of 75% breastfeeding women by the year 2010 had been realized among WIC recipients, the cost savings could have been at least $4 million a month for the WIC program.[36] Since 2000, WIC programs have energetically promoted breastfeeding, but the street value of the package for bottle-feeders has been popular. A new WIC package has been developed and slowly supported through the system. It increased the food allowance for lactating women. Progress continues slowly.

The WIC program, through the extensive actions of the directors and staff, has increased the numbers of WIC mothers choosing to breastfeed. Many programs have hired and trained peer support mothers with breastfeeding experience to help other clients.

Frequency of Breastfeeding

Data collected in the 1970s in the Ross Laboratories Mothers Survey MR77-48, which included 10,000 mothers, revealed a general trend toward breastfeeding.[37] In 1975, 33% of the mothers started out breastfeeding, and 15% were still breastfeeding at 5 to 6 months. In 1977, 43% of the

TABLE 1-2	Percentage of Breastfeeding among WIC Participants 1977 to 2002	
Year	In Hospital (%)	At 6 Months of Age (%)
1977	33.6	12.5
1978	34.5	9.7
1979	37.0	11.2
1980	40.4	13.1
1981	39.9	13.7
1982	45.3	16.1
1983	38.9	11.5
1984	39.1	11.9
1985	40.1	11.7
1986	38.0	10.7
1987	37.3	10.6
1988	35.3	9.2
1989	34.2	8.4
1990	33.7	8.2
1991	36.9	9.0
1992	38.8	10.1
1993	41.6	10.8
1994	44.3	11.6
1995	46.6	12.7
1996	46.6	12.9
1997	50.4	16.5
1998	56.8	18.9
1999	56.1	19.9
2000	56.8	20.1
2001	58.2	20.8
2002	58.8	22.1

Data collected from Martinez GA, Stahle DA: The recent trend in milkfeeding among WIC infants, *Am J Public Health* 72:68, 1982; Ryan AS, Rush D, Krieger FW: Recent declines in breastfeeding in the United States, 1984 through 1989, *Pediatrics* 88:719, 1991; Krieger FW: A review of breastfeeding trends. Presented at the Editor's Conference, New York, September 1992; Ross Laboratories Mothers Survey, unpublished data, Columbus, Ohio, 1992; Mothers Survey, Ross Products Division, Abbott Laboratories, unpublished data, 1998; Ryan AS: The resurgence of breastfeeding in the United States, *Pediatrics* 99:2, 1997 (electronic article); Mothers Survey, Ross Products Division, and Abbott Laboratories—Breastfeeding Trends 2002.

mothers left the hospital breastfeeding, and 20% were still breastfeeding at 5 to 6 months. Other studies have shown a regional variation, with a higher percentage of mothers breastfeeding on the West Coast than in the East.

A continuation of the study of milk-feeding patterns in 1981 in the United States by Martinez and Dodd[34] showed a sustained trend toward breastfeeding in 55% of the 51,537 new mothers contacted by mail. Although mothers who breastfeed continue to be more highly educated and have a higher income, the greatest increase in breastfeeding occurred among women with less education. From

1971 to 1981, breastfeeding in the hospital more than doubled (from 24.7% to 57.6%), with an average rate of gain of 8.8%. For infants 2 months old, breastfeeding more than tripled (from 13.9% to 44.2%) in this 10-year period (Table 1-3).

The National Natality Surveys (NNS) conducted by the CDC in 1969 and 1980 included questions for married women about infant-feeding practices after birth.[38,39] Questionnaires were mailed at 3 and 6 months postpartum. In 1969, 19% of white women and 9% of black women were exclusively breastfeeding. The highest rate was among white women up to 34 years old, with three to six children. In 1980, 51% of white women and 25% of black women were exclusively breastfeeding, and they were more highly educated and primiparous.[39]

The Ross surveys continue, and 725,000 surveys are mailed annually. The results have documented the persistent decline in the number of women initially breastfeeding, from a high in 1982 of 61.9% to an apparent low in 1991 of 51%, with the decline finally involving all categories of women, including those with higher socioeconomic status and higher education.

The Mothers Survey included 1.4 million questionnaires mailed in 2001, and this time two categories of questions were asked: any amount of breastfeeding and exclusive breastfeeding. Record high levels of any breastfeeding were reported: 69.5% initiation rate and 32.5% at 6 months postpartum with increases across all sociodemographic groups. The greatest increases were among young mothers (older than 20 years of age), the less educated, primiparous mothers, and those employed at the time of the survey. Mothers who practiced exclusive breastfeeding at hospital discharge (46.2%) and at 6 months (17.2%) were older and better educated.[29]

The CDC took an active role in gathering breastfeeding data in 1988 and gradually established a system for monitoring progress. The Breastfeeding Report Card was established, and the CDC's Maternity Practices in Infant Nutrition and Care (MPINC) survey assesses and scores how well maternity care practices at hospitals and birth centers support breastfeeding on a scale of 0 to 100—the higher the score, the better the practices. The national average from 2009 to 2011 increased from 65 to 70. The number of babies born in Baby Friendly Hospitals increased from less than 2% in 2008 to 6% in 2012.

Ethnic Factors

The Pediatric Nutrition Surveillance System (PedNSS) is a child-based public health surveillance system that monitors the nutritional status of low-income children in federally funded maternal and child health programs. The process begins in the clinic, it aggregates at the state level, and the data are submitted to the CDC for analysis. In 2001, 39 states, the District of Columbia, Puerto Rico, American Samoa, and six tribal governments participated, representing 5 million children from birth to 5 years of age; 37% of findings were from children younger than 1 year old from the six major ethnic groups.

In 2001, PedNSS reported 50.9% of children were ever breastfed, 20.8% were breastfed for at least 6 months, and 13.6% were breastfed for at least 12 months (Figure 1-6). Breastfeeding rates improved 45% from the 1992 rate of 34.9% across all racial and ethnic groups. The CDC has continued to monitor breastfeeding rates and issued a breastfeeding report card in 2007; 73.8% of infants born in 2004 were ever breastfed, and only 41.5% were still breastfeeding at 6 months and 20.9% at 12 months. Exclusive breastfeeding was 30.5% at 3 months and 11.3% at 6 months. Tables 1-4 and 1-5 show the states that have met the 2010 breastfeeding objectives.[9]

International trends are difficult to summarize because definitions vary and population assessments may be more or less complete. In an effort to improve reporting and implement its global strategy, WHO has prepared a tool for assessing national practices, policies, and programs entitled, "Infant and Young Child Feeding in 2003." It is detailed and extensive and is available at http://www.who.int/nutrition/publications/infantfeeding/9241562218/en/.[9]

Breastfeeding practices in developing countries have been improving since 1990, according to population reports. The level of exclusive breastfeeding in the first 3 months increased 10% in 35 countries predominantly because mothers stopped the introduction of nonmilk foods so early. Malawi improved 59% in exclusive breastfeeding. The trend is to delay complementary foods until 6 months as recommended by WHO (Table 1-6). Still, exclusive breastfeeding dropped in Jordan, Benin, Turkey, Niger, and Rwanda. Surveys have continued to confirm the impact of breastfeeding on child survival. With other factors accounted for, an infant is four times more likely to die if a mother stops any breastfeeding at 2 to 3 months of age than an infant who continues to breastfeed. At 9 to 12 months, if the infant is not breastfed, the risk of death is 2.3 times greater (Figure 1-7).

Almost all infants in developing countries are at least partially breastfed in the first 3 months. In 56 countries, one third of infants are exclusively breastfed for 4 months. Breastfeeding to age 2 years with appropriate complementary feeding after 6 months contributes to good nutrition and the prevention of diarrhea. At 12 to 15 months, 78% are

TABLE 1-3 Summary of Federally Funded Datasets Assessing Breastfeeding Outcomes of Individuals

	Methods	Format	Timing of Data Collection	Languages Conducted	Year Last Conducted	Frequency	Nationally Representative
ECLS-B	Longitudinal study with cross-sectional assessment of breastfeeding status	In-person, computer assisted interviews +self-administered questionnaires	BF questions on 9 mo pp survey	English, Spanish, others if translator available	Ongoing with children born in 2001	Not previously conducted	Yes
IFPSII	Longitudinal	One brief telephone interview, multiple mailed questionnaires	Data collected prenatally, just after birth, 3 wk pp and 2, 3, 4, 5, 6, 7, 9, 10, 12 mo pp	English	2007	Previously conducted in 1993/1994	No, consumer opinion panel
NHANES	Cross-sectional	In-person	Variable, asked for each child ≤6 yr	English, Spanish, translator used for other languages	Ongoing	Biennial	Yes
NIS	Cross-sectional	Telephone interview for parents, mailed survey to MDs	19-35 mo pp	English, Spanish, others (1.7%) via AT&T language line	Ongoing	Annual	Yes
NSCH	Cross-sectional	Telephone	≤6 yr	English, Spanish, others via AT&T language line	2007	Every 4 yrs	Yes
NSECH	Cross-sectional	Telephone interview	4-35 mo pp	English and Spanish	2000	One time survey	Yes
NSFG	Cross-sectional	In-person	Variable, asked for each child ≤18 yr	English	Ongoing	Annual	Yes
PedNSS*	Program-based surveillance	Utilized predominantly (86%) WIC data	Variable, assesses BF practices through 24 mo	English, Spanish, other languages spoken in WIC offices	Ongoing	Annual	No, reflects predominantly WIC participants from PedNSS contributors (approx 40 states, Washington DC, Puerto Rico, and 5 tribal governments)
PNSS*	Program-based surveillance	Utilizes predominantly (99%) WIC program data	2-5 mo pp	English, Spanish, other languages spoken in WIC offices	Ongoing	Annual	No, reflects WIC participants from PNSS contributors (approx 26 states, 5 tribal governments, 1 U.S. territory)
PRAMS	Cross-sectional	Predominantly mail, telephone follow-up with nonresponders	Surveyed approximately 2-6 mo pp	English and Spanish	Ongoing	Annual	Random sample in 37 participating states
WPPC	Cross-sectional	Utilizes WIC program data	6-13 mo pp	English, Spanish, and other languages spoken in WIC offices	2006†	Biennial	No, reflects WIC population

BF, Breastfeeding; ECLS-B, Early Childhood Longitudinal Survey, Birth Cohort; IFPSII, Infant Feeding Practices Survey II; NHANES, National Health and Nutrition Examination Survey 2007; NIS, National Immunization Survey 2006; NSCH, National Survey of Children's Health 2007; NSECH, National Survey of Early Childhood Health; NSFG, National Survey of Family Growth; PedNSS, Pediatric Nutrition Surveillance System; PNSS, Pregnancy Nutrition Surveillance System; pp, postpartum; PRAMS, Pregnancy Risk Assessment Monitoring System; WPPC, WIC Participant and Program Characteristics 2006.
*Breastfeeding data collection optional in PNSS and PedNSS.
†Most recent report.

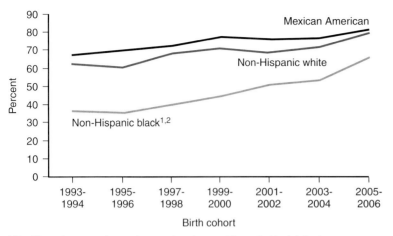

[1]Significant increase in trends over time for non-Hispanic black infants.
[2]Non-Hispanic black infants are significantly different from non-Hispanic white and Mexican-American infants in each birth cohort.

Figure 1-6. Percentage of infants who were ever breastfed by birth cohort and race-ethnicity: United States, 1993 to 2006. (From Mc-Dowell MM, Wang CY, Kennedy-Stephenson J: Breastfeeding in the United States: findings from the National Health and Nutrition Examination Surveys, 1999-2006, *NCHS Data Brief* April(5):1–8, 2008.)

TABLE 1-4	Breastfeeding Rates by State—2004				
Outcome Indicators					
Breastfeeding Rates (%)					
State	**Ever Breastfed**	**Breastfeeding at 6 Months**	**Breastfeeding at 12 Months**	**Exclusive Breastfeeding at 3 Months**	**Exclusive Breastfeeding at 6 Months**
U.S. National	73.8	41.5	20.9	30.5	11.3
Alabama	52.1	25.4	11.5	19.3	4.9
Alaska	**84.8**	**60.9**	**31.8**	**47.2**	**24.3**
Arizona	83.5	46.5	23.4	38.8	14.3
Arkansas	59.2	23.2	8.5	15.8	6.2
California	**83.8**	**52.9**	**30.4**	38.7	**17.4**
Colorado	**85.9**	42.0	23.6	36.2	10.8
Connecticut	**79.5**	44.6	23.7	35.6	10.1
Delaware	63.6	35.7	14.6	26.3	11.4
Dist. of Columbia	68.0	40.0	21.4	27.8	9.8
Florida	**77.9**	37.5	15.6	27.8	9.1
Georgia	68.2	38.0	16.8	25.6	11.0
Hawaii	**81.0**	**50.5**	**35.5**	37.8	15.8
Idaho	**85.9**	49.0	22.6	38.7	10.3
Illinois	72.5	40.9	17.6	31.6	10.0
Indiana	64.7	34.6	18.0	28.3	10.4
Iowa	74.2	44.9	20.0	37.6	11.6
Kansas	74.4	42.2	16.9	30.0	9.2
Kentucky	59.1	26.4	14.4	25.3	7.5
Louisiana	50.7	19.2	8.3	15.2	2.8
Maine	**76.3**	46.6	**27.6**	**42.1**	15.9
Maryland	71.0	40.2	21.2	32.1	8.6
Massachusetts	72.4	42.1	19.0	32.7	11.9
Michigan	63.4	36.4	18.6	27.4	8.3
Minnesota	**80.9**	46.5	23.8	33.9	16.1
Mississippi	50.2	23.3	8.2	19.0	8.0

Continued

TABLE 1-4	Breastfeeding Rates by State—2004—cont'd				
			Outcome Indicators		
			Breastfeeding Rates (%)		
State	Ever Breastfed	Breastfeeding at 6 Months	Breastfeeding at 12 Months	Exclusive Breastfeeding at 3 Months	Exclusive Breastfeeding at 6 Months
Missouri	67.3	32.5	15.8	26.6	7.4
Montana	**87.7**	**53.8**	**28.8**	**50.9**	**18.3**
Nebraska	**79.3**	47.6	21.8	31.7	9.8
Nevada	**79.7**	45.6	21.9	31.9	10.3
New Hampshire	73.7	48.7	27.5	34.3	13.6
New Jersey	69.8	45.1	19.4	27.0	11.8
New Mexico	**80.7**	41.2	21.1	32.9	14.3
New York	73.8	**50.0**	**26.9**	26.0	11.4
North Carolina	72.0	34.2	18.3	23.0	6.9
North Dakota	73.1	45.1	19.5	39.4	15.4
Ohio	59.6	33.3	12.9	27.2	9.8
Oklahoma	67.1	29.6	12.7	23.0	10.6
Oregon	**88.3**	**56.4**	**33.5**	**41.5**	**19.9**
Pennsylvania	66.6	35.2	16.8	27.1	8.0
Rhode Island	69.1	31.2	14.0	31.2	9.5
South Carolina	67.4	30.0	11.1	26.6	5.4
South Dakota	71.1	40.5	23.4	32.2	12.2
Tennessee	71.2	32.6	16.6	26.7	11.9
Texas	**75.4**	37.3	18.7	25.2	7.1
Utah	**84.5**	**55.6**	**28.1**	39.8	10.2
Vermont	**85.2**	**55.3**	**34.1**	47.3	15.9
Virginia	**79.1**	49.8	**25.6**	32.6	13.4
Washington	**88.4**	**56.6**	**32.3**	**49.6**	**22.5**
West Virginia	59.3	26.8	14.0	21.3	5.2
Wisconsin	72.1	39.6	19.0	32.5	13.4
Wyoming	**80.5**	42.9	18.5	36.2	11.4

Note: Numbers in bold are those that have met the *Healthy People 2010* goal.
From Centers for Disease Control and Prevention: *National immunization survey, 2004 births*, Washington, DC, 2007, U.S. Department of Health and Human Services. CDC: MMWR 56(30):760–763, 2007

breastfeeding and by 24 months only 45%. Mothers in sub-Saharan Africa and Asia are almost twice as likely to continue breastfeeding through the second year, as are those in other developing regions (Tables 1-7 through 1-9).

Demographic Factors

The demographic factors associated with a higher incidence of breastfeeding have remained the same since the low point in the 1970s.[25] The rate for well-educated, higher socioeconomic status families was more than 80% initiation at birth in 2002 (Table 1-10). In 2002, 45.8% of the infants in this

group were still breastfeeding at 5 to 6 months of age and older with an average of all groups at 5 to 6 months of 32.5%. The rate among black women was 21.9% and among participants of WIC only 20.8% at 6 months, an increase in all groups.

Study after study has confirmed the relationship of breastfeeding to education, social status, marriage, and other demographic factors. The well-educated, well-to-do groups of all races breastfeed. In a study by Wright et al.[17] of 1112 healthy infants in a health maintenance organization (HMO) in Arizona, 70% were breastfed with a mean duration of almost 7 months. Education and marriage were associated with breastfeeding. Maternal employment

TABLE 1-5 Impact of Baby-Friendly Facilities, Lactation Support, and State Legislation

Process indicators

State	Percentage of Live Births Occurring at Facilities Designated as Baby Friendly (BFHI)	Number of IBCLCs per 1000 Live Births, 2007	Number of La Leche League Groups per 1000 Live Births	Number of State Health Dept. FTEs Dedicated to Breastfeeding	State Legislation about Breastfeeding in Public Places	State Legislation about Lactation and Employment	Presence of an Active Statewide Breastfeeding Coalition	Presence of Statewide Breastfeeding Coalition Web Site
U.S. National	3.31	2.12	0.35	80.66	46	15	42	33
Alabama	0	1.90	0.23	2.00	Yes	No	Yes	Yes
Alaska	0	5.83	0.96	0.25	Yes	No	Yes	Yes
Arizona	0	1.31	0.25	1.50	Yes	No	Yes	Yes
Arkansas	0	1.68	0.23	3.50	Yes	No	Yes	Yes
California	3.28	1.66	0.21	8.50	Yes	Yes	Yes	Yes
Colorado	2.13	2.00	0.45	0.88	Yes	No	Yes	Yes
Connecticut	12.44	3.76	0.67	1.00	Yes	Yes	Yes	Yes
Delaware	0	2.92	0.25	2.00	Yes	No	Yes	Yes
District of Columbia	0	1.14	0.09	1.00	No	No	Yes	Yes
Florida	1.80	1.56	0.24	1.00	Yes	No	No	No
Georgia	0	1.73	0.20	2.00	Yes	Yes	Yes	Yes
Hawaii	10.46	2.51	0.22	0.50	Yes	Yes	Yes	Yes
Idaho	6.10	1.95	0.43	1.00	No	No	No	No
Illinois	1.49	2.04	0.34	2.00	Yes	Yes	Yes	No
Indiana	2.39	2.44	0.32	1.75	Yes	No	Yes	Yes
Iowa	0	2.01	0.33	0.50	Yes	No	Yes	No
Kansas	0	2.23	0.60	1.00	Yes	No	No	No
Kentucky	5.69	1.95	0.30	2.50	Yes	No	Yes	No
Louisiana	0	1.41	0.23	2.00	Yes	No	Yes	No
Maine	17.37	5.31	0.71	1.00	Yes	No	Yes	No
Maryland	0	3.08	0.35	1.05	Yes	No	Yes	Yes
Massachusetts	2.83	4.45	0.61	1.33	No	No	Yes	Yes
Michigan	0	1.96	0.49	2.00	Yes	No	Yes	Yes
Minnesota	0	2.54	0.49	1.00	Yes	Yes	Yes	No
Mississippi	0	1.39	0.21	2.00	Yes	No	Yes	Yes
Missouri	0	1.92	0.50	1.00	Yes	No	No	No

State								
Montana	0.34	1.98	0.60	1.00	Yes	No	Yes	Yes
Nebraska	13.54	1.61	0.76	0.50	No	No	No	No
Nevada	0	0.91	0.21	2.00	Yes	No	Yes	Yes
New Hampshire	5.73	5.68	0.49	1.00	Yes	No	Yes	Yes
New Jersey	0	2.16	0.40	2.00	Yes	No	Yes	Yes
New Mexico	0	2.01	0.38	1.00	Yes	Yes	Yes	Yes
New York	1.01	2.18	0.31	2.50	Yes	Yes	Yes	No
North Carolina	0	2.82	0.45	2.00	Yes	No	Yes	Yes
North Dakota	0	1.43	0.36	1.00	No	No	Yes	Yes
Ohio	2.36	2.71	0.43	1.00	Yes	No	No	No
Oklahoma	0	1.70	0.33	2.00	Yes	Yes	Yes	No
Oregon	6.37	4.48	0.37	1.20	Yes	Yes	Yes	Yes
Pennsylvania	0.21	2.26	0.32	2.00	Yes	No	Yes	Yes
Rhode Island	9.69	3.86	0.32	1.00	Yes	Yes	Yes	Yes
South Carolina	0	1.56	0.28	1.00	Yes	No	Yes	Yes
South Dakota	0	2.01	0.09	1.00	Yes	No	Yes	Yes
Tennessee	0.46	1.84	0.20	1.00	Yes	Yes	No	No
Texas	0	1.28	0.18	5.00	Yes	Yes	Yes	Yes
Utah	0	1.20	0.21	1.20	Yes	No	Yes	Yes
Vermont	3.77	8.96	1.54	1.00	Yes	No	Yes	Yes
Virginia	0	2.96	0.52	1.00	Yes	Yes	Yes	Yes
Washington	8.97	4.15	0.59	1.00	Yes	Yes	Yes	Yes
West Virginia	0	2.54	0.05	1.00	Yes	No	No	No
Wisconsin	9.10	2.58	0.55	1.00	Yes	No	No	No
Wyoming	0	2.07	0.69	2.00	Yes	No	No	No

FTEs, Full-time equivalents; IBCLC, International Board of Certified Lactation Consultants.

TABLE 1-6 Trends in Exclusive Breastfeeding Internationally

Country Groups	Percentage of Children (2000-2006) Who Are Exclusively Breastfed (<6 Months)	Percentage of Children (2000-2006) Who Are Breastfed with Complementary Food (6-9 Months)	Percentage of Children (2000-2006) Who Are Still Breastfeeding (20-23 Months)
Central and Eastern Europe, Commonwealth of Independent States	19	44	23
Developing countries	38	56	40
East Asia and Pacific	43	45	27
Eastern and Southern Africa	39	71	56
Industrialized countries	–	–	–
Latin America and Caribbean	–	–	–
Least developed countries	35	64	63
Middle East and North Africa	28	57	25
South Asia	45	55	–
Sub-Saharan Africa	30	67	50
Western and Central Africa	21	63	46
World	38	56	39

World Health Organization Population Reports, Geneva, 2004.

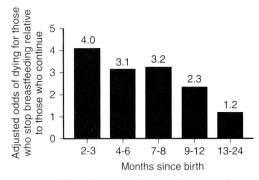

Figure 1-7. Effect of stopping breastfeeding on infant and child mortality. (Figure 2 from Zlidar VM, Gardner R, Rutstein SO, et al: *New survey findings: the reproductive revolution continues, Population Reports,* Series M, No 17, Baltimore, The Johns Hopkins Bloomberg School of Public Health, The INFO Project, Spring 2003; Rutstein S: *Effect of birth intervals on mortality and health,* Calverton, Maryland, Measure/DHS+, Macro International, Inc.)

TABLE 1-7 WHO Statistics 2009 by Resources. Infants Exclusively Breastfed for First 6 Months

Country	Access to Clean Water (%)	Adult Obesity (%)	Gross Domestic Product (%)	Breastfed Exclusively for 6 Months (%)
Afghanistan	22	4.6	9.2	?
Brazil	91	11.1	7.5	39.8
Bangladesh	85	0.7	3.2	47
Belarus	100	9.7	6.4	9
Cameroon	70	8.2	4.6	21.2
Canada	100	22.9	10.0	17
Congo	71	7.5	2.1	19.1
Cuba	91	11.8	7.7	26.4
Egypt	98	46.6	6.3	46.8
India	89	2.0	3.6	46.4
Malawi	72	1.0	12.9	56.7
Peru	84	12.0	4.4	63.9
United Kingdom	100	22.9	8.2	1.0
United States	99	32.1	15.3	11.9

outside the home and ethnicity (being Hispanic rather than white) were related to higher rates of bottle-feeding. The authors suggest that effects of ethnicity are independent of those of education. New immigrants who would have breastfed in their homeland tend to bottle-feed in the United States because they think this practice is "American."

Impoverished mothers choose to bottle-feed not because they are working; statistics show they are staying home and bottle-feeding. When mothers were interviewed about their infant feeding choice at a prenatal WIC clinic, they knew mother's milk was best.[39] They said it was too difficult to breastfeed and there were too many rules. In the classes on breastfeeding given by lactation experts, the instructions on preparing the breasts and diet rules were overwhelming. The mothers said if their physician would tell them breastfeeding was important, they would do it for as long as the physician said.[15] Mothers trusted their physician's advice and were more successful at breastfeeding if the physician was supportive and expressed his or her views.[6,41]

TABLE 1-8	WHO Statistics 2009 by Region and Income

	Exclusive Breastfeeding at 6 Months (%)
WHO regions	
Africa	29.5
Americas	30.3
South East Asia	43.2
European	17.7
Eastern Mediterranean	34.2
Income group	
Low	32.1
Lower middle	40.8
Upper middle	29.1
High	12.1
Global	34.8

World Health Statistics 2009, Geneva, Switzerland, 2009, WHO Press.

Duration of Breastfeeding

A sharp decline in breastfeeding occurs by age 6 months. Overall, 21.7% of infants were breastfed at 6 months in 1996, 41.5% in 2007 (a 50% improvement), and 47.2% in 2012 (Figures 1-8 and 1-9).

The two types of breastfeeding, as Newton[42] pointed out, are *unrestricted* and *token*. Unrestricted breastfeeding usually means that the infant is put to the breast immediately after delivery and breastfed on demand thereafter, without rules or limitations. There may be 10 or 12 feedings per day in the early weeks, with the number gradually decreasing over the first year of life. Breast milk continues to be a major source of nourishment during infancy.

TABLE 1-9	Breastfeeding to 24 Months of Age, 1990 to 2001, by Country

Region, Country, and Year	Percentage of Infants of Age					
	0-3 Months			6-9 Months Complemented‡ (%)	12-15 Months Continued BF§	20-23 Months Continued BF‖ (%)
	Not BF	Exclusive* (%)	Predominant† (%)			
Sub-Saharan Africa						
Benin 2001	2	47	23	64	94	60
Burkina Faso 1998-1999	1	5	88	49	96	86
Cameroon 1998	3	16	55	71	85	30
Cape Verde 1998	2	57	15	64	60	NA
Central African Rep. 1994-1995	1	4	63	93	96	54
Chad 1995-1996	3	2	82	71	91	63
Comoros 1996	3	5	48	86	80	44
Côte d'Ivoire 1998-1999	2	4	77	63	94	55
Eritrea 1995	1	65	28	45	91	60
Ethiopia 2000	1	62	20	42	94	77
Gabon 2000	13	7	28	62	44	8
Ghana 1998	1	36	48	63	97	57
Guinea 1999	2	12	68	27	95	73
Kenya 1998	1	17	33	88	89	54
Madagascar 1997	2	61	25	88	90	49
Malawi 2000	2	62	15	92	97	72
Mali 2001	2	28	62	32	93	65
Mozambique 1997	4	38	37	83	94	59
Namibia 1992	2	22	52	66	75	27
Niger 1998	2	1	86	71	95	48
Nigeria 1990	4	1	60	51	87	44
Rwanda 2000	2	88	2	75	93	61
South Africa 1998	16	10	15	62	68	33
Senegal 1997	2	14	63	62	90	50
Tanzania 1999	2	40	39	63	90	49
Togo 1998	3	15	54	88	96	77

Continued

TABLE 1-9 Breastfeeding to 24 Months of Age, 1990 to 2001, by Country—cont'd

Region, Country, and Year	Percentage of Infants of Age					
	0-3 Months			6-9 Months Complemented‡ (%)	12-15 Months Continued BF§	20-23 Months Continued BF‖ (%)
	Not BF	Exclusive* (%)	Predominant† (%)			
Uganda 2000-2001	2	74	5	73	88	44
Zambia 1996	3	25	45	93	94	43
Zimbabwe 1999	3	39	26	90	95	37
Median	2	22	45	66	93	54
Mean (unweighted)	3	29	43	68	88	53
Near East and North Africa						
Egypt 2000	4	66	18	64	79	30
Jordan 1997	6	15	32	63	42	12
Mauritania 2000-2001	1	28	38	62	88	52
Morocco 1992	6	62	15	35	63	19
Turkey 1998	7	9	50	33	51	21
Yemen 1997	8	22	30	51	59	37
Median	6	25	31	57	61	25
Mean (unweighted)	5	34	30	51	64	29
Asia						
Bangladesh 1999-2000	1	53	18	59	94	86
Cambodia 2000	2	14	71	71	87	54
India 1998-1999	2	55	25	34	88	69
Indonesia 1997	3	52	8	81	86	66
Nepal 2001	1	78	10	66	98	85
Pakistan 1990-1991	5	25	41	29	78	51
Philippines 1998	18	48	11	58	48	23
Vietnam 1997	4	25	39	84	80	23
Median	3	50	22	63	87	60
Mean (unweighted)	4	44	28	60	82	57
Latin America and Caribbean						
Belize 1999	10	24	24	54	NA	23
Bolivia 1998	2	60	10	70	76	31
Brazil 1996	15	40	15	30	33	17
Colombia 2000	6	33	15	60	49	23
Dominican Rep. 1996	12	26	15	38	31	8
Ecuador 1999	6	42	23	70	60	25
El Salvador 1998	7	21	28	77	65	40
Guatemala 1998-1999	5	45	27	61	83	45
Haiti 2000	4	31	26	74	79	27
Honduras 2001	8	43	16	61	76	34
Nicaragua 2001	5	39	15	67	62	36
Paraguay 1995-1996‖	8	7	59	59	40	15
Peru 2000	1	72	9	75	83	46
Median	6	39	16	61	64	27
Mean (unweighted)	7	37	22	61	61	28
Eastern Europe and Central Asia						
Armenia 2000	6	44	29	51	29	13
Azerbaijan 2001	5	NA	NA	NA	NA	NA
Kazakhstan 1999	1	47	38	64	61	18
Kyrgyz Rep. 1995	5	30	45	55	73	18

Continued

TABLE 1-9	Breastfeeding to 24 Months of Age, 1990 to 2001, by Country—cont'd					
	Percentage of Infants of Age					
	0-3 Months			**6-9 Months**	**12-15 Months**	**20-23 Months**
Region, Country, and Year	**Not BF**	**Exclusive* (%)**	**Predominant[†] (%)**	**Complemented[‡] (%)**	**Continued BF[§]**	**Continued BF[‖] (%)**
Turkmenistan 2000	5	16	68	70	76	27
Uzbekistan 1996	5	4	60	57	64	34
Median	5	30	45	57	64	18
Mean (unweighted)	4	28	48	59	60	22
All developing countries						
Median	3	29	28	63	87	45
Mean (unweighted)	4	34	35	64	79	45

BF, Breastfeeding; *NA,* not available.

Breastfeeding is considered exclusive when a child receives no food or liquid other than breast milk. Predominant breastfeeding is defined as infrequent feedings of vitamins, minerals, water, juice, or ritualistic feedings in addition to breast milk. No food-based fluids other than fruit juice or sugar water are allowed under this definition (Labbok[40] and World Health Organization.[14] Population Reports).

*Exclusive: breast milk only.
[†]Predominant: breast milk and water and other nonmilk liquids.
[‡]Complemented: breast milk and solid or semisolid foods.
[§]Continued: any breastfeeding, independent of type of supplements.
[‖]Data NA for 1998 survey.

TABLE 1-10	Distribution of Select Characteristics among Participants in the IFPS II and among Participants in the NSFG (Cycle 6), 2002 (in the USA)	
Characteristic	**Percentage of IFPS II Sample (Mothers of Infants Born in 2005) (N = 3033)***	**Percentage of NSFG Sample (Mothers of Infants Born in 1998-2000) (N = 1415)[†]**
Age		
18-24 yr[‡]	23.3	32.6
25-34 yr	61.4	54.9
35-43 yr	15.3	12.4
Marital status		
Married or cohabiting[§]	79.1	79.5
Other	20.9	20.5
Education		
High school or less[‡]	21.0	47.5
Some college	40.2	27.8
College graduate	38.8	24.7
Income		
<185% of FPL[‡]	41.9	45.2
185-349% of FPL	35.8	27.4
>350% of FPL	22.3	27.4
Employment status (prenatal)		
Employed[‡]	66.3	61.2
Not employed	33.7	38.8
Parity		
1[‡]	29.2	25.3
2	40.9	39.7
≥3	29.9	35.0
Race/ethnicity		
White[‡]	84.4	61.5
Black	4.9	14.1

Continued

distinct correlation between the time of weaning and the behavior of the tribes.[46] In tribes in which weaning was delayed, the culture was peaceful. In contrast, tribes that abruptly weaned their infants at 6 months of age and practiced other rigid disciplinary practices were warlike.

When weaning practices were evaluated among 945 women in Guinea-Bissau, West Africa, the data revealed that all infants had been breastfed for at least 18 months. Among the reasons for terminating breastfeeding were that the child became ill, the mother became ill, or the mother became pregnant. By 23 months, weaning occurred because the infant was healthy and old enough.[47] Although there are few studies since the 1980s focusing on the reasons why women wean early, a study by Schwartz et al.[28] of women in Michigan and Nebraska revealed that the reasons for weaning are similar. They reported a prospective cohort study of 946 women over the first 12 weeks postpartum. The demographic features were similar to older studies. Women older than 30 years with a bachelor's degree were most likely to continue breastfeeding throughout the study. In the first 3 weeks, "not enough milk" was the most common reason to stop, and after 4 weeks the most common reason was a "return to work." (Table 1-11).

In a study by Ramos and Almeida[48] in a baby-friendly maternity hospital in Brazil, 24 mothers who weaned their infants by 4 months were interviewed in depth. The reasons for weaning were similar to studies from decades before: weak or little milk, problems with breasts (sore nipples), lack of experience, disparity between needs of mother and needs of the baby, and work. Earlier, House et al. described a sense of isolation and solitude on the part of the mother and need for support from health care providers and society in general.[49] They concluded that breastfeeding should be treated as an act to be learned by women and protected by society. These studies point out the pivotal role for the pediatrician in the successful maintenance of lactation and the importance of the postpartum environment[10,49] (Tables 1-12 and 1-13).

The positive and negative emotional and physical experiences of 152 long-term breastfeeding American and Canadian women were reported by Reamer and Sugarman.[22] This sample of mothers was randomly selected from 1038 women who responded to a request for volunteers in a La Leche League newsletter. All answered the eight-page questionnaire, which had 51 short-answer and 52 free-response questions. The respondents were older, better educated, predominantly white, and had belonged to the league at some time. The average age was 29.4 years, age at first child was 25, 77% had more than 1 year of college, and 44% had 4 or more years of college. Far fewer were employed than the national average (13% full or part time versus 34% nationally). The average weaning age for the 339 children represented by this study was 18 months, with a range of 3 weeks to 5 years. At the time of the study, 136 children were still being breastfed. Two mothers thought there were no positive effects of prolonged nursing of their children, but others offered more than one perceived positive consequence (Table 1-14). Emotional security, happiness, mutual love, and future independence were the key positive outcomes of long-term nursing in the mothers' views. Good health was mentioned by 22%.

When asked to list the negative aspects of nursing longer than 6 months, 47% of mothers said there were none at 6 months, but only 26% of mothers had no negative feelings about nursing past 12 months. Perceived social hostility was the major negative effect, reported by 24% of mothers at 6 months and by 42% at 12 months (Table 1-15). Ninety percent felt there were no negative effects for the children. The social stigma has driven many well-educated, caring, dedicated mothers to conceal nursing, called "closet nursing." Unfortunately, this leads physicians and the public alike to think that breastfeeding in the United States terminates by 6 months of age.

Impact of Commercial Discharge Packs

Several studies have evaluated whether commercial discharge packs result in diminished breastfeeding duration. Unfortunately, none of the studies was so well randomized and controlled that the answer was clear. The studies that did mention use of bottles in the hospital noted a stronger correlation between bottle use and diminished duration of breastfeeding.[13] What had not been measured was the impact of office prenatal formula advertising on breastfeeding. In a study by Howard et al.[45] of 547 women randomized to receive formula company gift packs or specially designed educational packs at their first prenatal visit, feeding method was recorded at delivery. The 294 women who chose to breastfeed were interviewed at 2, 6, 12, and 24 weeks postpartum. Women who received the commercial pack were more likely to discontinue breastfeeding by 2 weeks. Among women who had indefinite goals of breastfeeding for less than 12 weeks, exclusive, full, and overall breastfeeding duration were shortened.

In New York State, regulations regarding breastfeeding support instituted in July 1984, among other things, disallowed discharge packs to breastfeeding women unless requested by the mother or

TABLE 1-11 Percentage of Mothers Who Indicated That Specified Reasons Were Important in Their Decision to Stop Breastfeeding, According to Infants' Age at Weaning

Reasons Cited as Important	Infants' Age When Breastfeeding Was Completely Stopped (mo)					Average
	<1	1-2	3-5	6-8	≥9	
Lactational factor						
My baby had trouble sucking or latching on*	53.7	27.1	11.0	2.6	1.5	19.2
My nipples were sore, cracked, or bleeding*	36.8	23.2	7.2	5.7	4.2	15.4
My breasts were overfull or engorged*	23.9	12.3	4.8	1.6	1.2	8.8
My breasts were infected or abscessed*	8.1	5.7	3.1	3.1	3.1	4.6
My breasts leaked too much*	14.1	8.0	3.8	1.6	1.9	5.9
Breastfeeding was too painful*	29.3	15.8	3.4	3.7	4.2	11.3
Psychosocial factor						
Breastfeeding was too tiring*	19.8	17.2	11.0	7.8	5.3	12.2
Breastfeeding was too inconvenient*	20.4	22.4	18.6	12.5	4.2	15.6
I wanted to be able to leave my baby for several hours at a time*	11.2	24.1	18.2	15.6	7.3	15.3
I had too many household duties*	12.6	14.0	9.6	5.2	3.8	9.0
I wanted or needed someone else to feed my baby*	16.4	23.2	21.0	17.2	6.1	16.8
Someone else wanted to feed the baby*	13.5	15.5	12.0	5.7	3.4	10.0
I did not want to breastfeed in public*	14.9	18.6	15.1	4.7	4.6	11.6
Nutritional factor						
Breast milk alone did not satisfy my baby	49.7	55.6	49.1	49.5	43.5	49.5
I thought that my baby was not gaining enough weight*	23.0	18.3	11.0	14.1	8.4	15.0
A health professional said my baby was not gaining enough weight*	19.8	15.2	8.6	9.9	5.0	11.7
I had trouble getting the milk flow to start*	41.4	23.2	19.6	14.6	5.7	20.9
I didn't have enough milk*	51.7	52.2	54.0	43.8	26.0	45.5
Lifestyle factor						
I did not like breastfeeding*	16.4	10.9	6.2	3.1	1.9	7.7
I wanted to go on a weight-loss diet	6.6	7.2	10.3	10.9	6.5	8.3
I wanted to go back to my usual diet	5.5	9.5	7.2	5.2	5.0	6.5
I wanted to smoke again or more than I did while breastfeeding*	6.0	5.2	3.4	1.0	0.8	3.3
I wanted my body back to myself*	8.9	13.2	16.8	18.8	15.7	14.7
Medical factor						
My baby became sick and could not breastfeed*	9.5	7.4	5.5	6.3	1.9	6.1
I was sick or had to take medicine*	14.4	16.3	14.8	12.5	8.0	13.2
I was not present to feed my baby for reasons other than work	3.2	6.9	5.2	5.2	2.7	4.6
I became pregnant or wanted to become pregnant again*	1.7	3.4	3.4	6.8	12.2	5.5
Milk-pumping factor						
I could not or did not want to pump or breastfeed at work*	11.2	22.4	21.3	13.5	4.6	14.6
Pumping milk no longer seemed worth the effort that it required*	16.7	21.2	23.7	17.7	11.5	18.2
Infant's self-weaning factor						
My baby began to bite*	5.2	5.7	13.4	38.5	31.7	18.9
My baby lost interest in nursing or began to wean himself or herself*	13.2	19.7	33.1	47.9	47.3	32.2
My baby was old enough that the difference between breast milk and formula no longer mattered*	5.2	11.4	16.5	26.6	28.2	17.6

*$p<0.01$ for association between each reason and weaning age after adjustments for maternal age, marital status, parity, education, poverty, WIC participation, race, and region.

From Li R, Fein SB, Chen J, et al: Why mothers stop breastfeeding: mothers' self reported reasons for stopping during the first year, *Pediatrics* 122:S69–S76, 2008.

prescribed by the physician. A mother who requests such a pack is usually at high risk for early termination of lactation in most investigators' experience. Giving such a packet to a vulnerable mother (young, less educated, single, poor support system) may be a message not unlike *Parents* magazine circa 1938: "You may be one of them" (i.e., those who fail).[25]

TABLE 1-12 Selected Demographic Characteristics Associated with Duration of Breastfeeding*

	Group 1: Never Breastfed (n=12)	Group 2: Breastfed ≤7 Days (n=22)	Group 3: Breastfed >7 Days (n=153)
Black	9 (75%)	10 (46%)	57 (37%)
		$\chi^2=6.81$; df=2; $p=0.03$	
Mean years of education	11.3	13.5	14.9
		$F=10.14$; df=2; $p=0.0001$	
Mean age	23.3	26.7	27.9
		$F=4.57$; df=2; $p=0.01$	
Married	2 (17%)	16 (73%)	124 (81%)
		$\chi^2=25.37$; df=2; $p=0.001$	
<$10,000 income	6/10 (60%)	3/19 (16%)	15/143 (10%)
		$\chi^2=27.02$; df=6; $p=0.001$	
First pregnancy	5 (42%)	9 (41%)	53 (35%)
		$\chi^2=0.52$; df=2; $p=0.77$	

*See Table 1-9 for explanation.

TABLE 1-13 Probability of Early Cessation by Selected Prenatal and Postpartum Characteristics among Women Initiating Breastfeeding

	Probability	Odds Ratio (95% Confidence Interval)
Prenatal characteristics		
Confidence in ability		
Low (n=47)	0.28*	5.05 (1.99, 6.42)
High (n=128)	0.07*	
Certainty of decision		
Low (n=21)	0.33†	4.86 (1.68, 14.01)
High (n=150)	0.09†	
Postpartum characteristics		
Timing of first breastfeeding		
Late (n=92)	0.18‡	3.44 (1.21, 9.87)
Early (n=81)	0.06‡	
Baby's daytime location		
Nursery (n=23)	0.26§	3.00 (1.03, 8.71)
Mother's room (n=152)	0.11§	

Early cessation is defined as breastfeeding for 7 days or less. The confidence scale was dichotomized to reflect less confident (raw scores 1-3) and more confident (raw scores 4-6).
*$\chi^2=13.31$; df=1; $p<0.001$.
†$\chi^2=9.85$; df=1; $p<0.01$.
‡$\chi^2=5.88$; df=1; $p<0.02$.
§$\chi^2=4.40$; df=1; $p<0.05$.
Modified from Buxton KE, Gielen AC, Faden RR, et al: Women intending to breastfeed: predictors of early infant feeding experiences, *Am J Prev Med* 7:101, 1991.

A significant plank in the Baby Friendly ten steps is the banning of commercial discharge packs or supplies. This is strengthened by the requirement that the hospital pay market price for the formula it uses, in order to meet Baby Friendly Requirements.

TABLE 1-14 Positive Consequences of Long-Term Nursing as Perceived by the Mother

Perceived Consequences	Mothers (n=130)	%*
Positive emotional effect on child; child is more secure	65	50.0
Better physical health (fewer allergies)	29	22.3
Child is loving, friendly, cheerier	27	20.8
Child can separate more easily; relative independence achieved with less stress	22	16.9
Enhanced maternal sensitivity	19	14.6
Close relationship of mother and child	18	13.8
Positive influence or education for older siblings	11	8.5
Child easily comforted during crisis, pain, or teething	10	8.0
Broad, all-encompassing positive effect	6	4.6
Incidental positive consequences	13	10.4
No positive effects perceived	2	1.5

*Mothers could give multiple responses; thus percentages add up to more than 100%.
From Reamer SB, Sugarman M: Breastfeeding beyond six months: mothers' perceptions of the positive and negative consequences, *J Trop Pediatr* 33:93, 1987.

The real problem is inadequate counseling about breastfeeding and a system to support the mother who needs it. Baby Friendly addresses the counseling and support in the hospital but has yet to develop a substantial support system following discharge. WIC and other programs are making an effort to provide these services.

A force that is difficult to measure is the public advertising of infant formula, a direct violation of

TABLE 1-15 Mothers' Responses to the Question, "What Do You Think Are the Negative Aspects of Nursing Past 6 Months (Past 1 Year)?"

Negative Aspects Listed by Mothers	Past 6 Months (Total Responses = 132)		Past 12 Months (Total Responses = 133)	
	No.	(%)	No.	(%)
Mother states there are no negative aspects	62	47.1	35	26.4
Social stigma; negative attitudes of others	32	24.3	56	41.9
Mother's activities are restricted	19	14.7	9	6.6
Baby is less discreet; embarrassing in public	3	2.2	13	9.6
Tiredness	7	5.1	3	2.2
Breastfeeding mother has special concerns	1	0.7	5	3.7
Intrudes upon life with husband	1	0.7	4	2.9
Breast discomfort/leaking, soreness	2	1.5	1	0.7
Sex life interrupted; less interest in sex	2	1.5	2	1.5
Mother believes she should ignore negative aspects	2	1.5	1	0.7
Intrudes upon mother's time with siblings	0	–	1	0.7
Baby care, not nursing, causes negative aspects	0	–	1	0.7

From Reamer SB, Sugarman M: Breastfeeding beyond six months: mothers' perceptions of the positive and negative consequences, *J Trop Pediatr* 33:93, 1987.

TABLE 1-16 Savings and Costs Associated with Improved Breastfeeding from a Societal Perspective

Perspective	Savings	Costs
Infant and parent	Infant formula; physician copays; prescription copays; hospital deductible; over-the-counter medications; transportation costs; lost wages or sick child care; decreased quality of life associated with permanent sequelae of illnesses, e.g., hearing loss, short bowel; reduced intelligence quotient	Food intake of breastfeeding mother; breast pump; human breast milk storage
Employer	Less employee absence; less lost productivity; lower insurance premiums; less employee turnover; less employee recruitment	Breastfeeding room with breast pump and refrigerator; promotion of lactation program; work schedule flexibility
Payer	Fewer physician fees (minus copays); specialty referrals (minus copays); emergency room/urgent care visits (minus copays); prescriptions (minus copays); hospitalization (minus deductible); laboratory procedures; increased provider availability caused by lower visit rate of infants	Lactation consultant referrals; provider time used for breastfeeding counseling and management
Federal and state governments	Formula purchase for WIC program; medical care for children in Medicaid; worker productivity and global competition	Legislative or program costs to promote a breastfeeding-friendly culture

Breastfeeding has broad social and economic implications. Insufficient breastfeeding is expensive for the U.S. government, which finances infant nutrition through the Women, Infants, and Children (WIC) program and infant health care through the Medicaid program. Compared with formula-fed infants, infants enrolled in WIC who were breastfed saved $478 each month in WIC costs and Medicaid expenditures during the first 6 months of life. Other costs, equally important but more difficult to measure, also must be considered, including long-term health concerns.
From Bell TM, Bennett DM: The economic impact of breastfeeding, *Pediatr Clin North Am* 48:253–262, 2001.

the letter and the intent of the WHO Code (see earlier discussion). Some formula companies have television advertisements that include a subliminal message that their product is equal to breastfeeding.[50] Furthermore, when the message says, "Just ask your doctor," it implies that physicians agree. Sending free samples and coupons aimed at a vulnerable woman 2 to 4 weeks postpartum, when she is likely fatigued and overwhelmed, can undermine the confidence of even a dedicated breastfeeding mother. In addition to the pregnant woman or new mother, the audience consists of the world of television viewers. The daily repetition of the message that bottle-feeding is just as good as breastfeeding cemented the national image that it is "American" to bottle-feed (Table 1-16).[3]

Infants in Latin America were less likely to be breastfed than infants in Africa and Asia, and the duration was 6 months compared with 12 months or more in Asia and Africa. A significant increase in the Latin American rates resulted after an aggressive breastfeeding promotion program (PROALMA) was initiated and supported by various governments.[52,53]

A number of hospital routines were found to be potentially detrimental to breastfeeding. These included interruption of mother-infant contact, supplementation, and restricted feedings. The AAP and the ABM have both prepared guidelines for hospital management to promote breastfeeding.

Attitudes of Health Care Professionals

A 1980 survey of physicians' and nurses' medical and educational practices regarding breastfeeding was published when breastfeeding was at its zenith. A follow-up survey was completed in the summer of 1991, after several years of decline. A comparison of the results of these two surveys showed little change in the current practices of health care professionals regarding breastfeeding, their attitudes toward breastfeeding, and who among them they believed to be primarily responsible for managing breastfeeding and supporting breastfeeding mothers. Twenty years later, attitudes among professionals are very supportive.

In terms of responsibility for managing breastfeeding mothers and infants, more than 80% of pediatricians believed that medical encouragement or support of breastfeeding was primarily a responsibility of the infant's physician. Approximately two thirds of family practitioners thought that both the mother's physician and the infant's physician were responsible.

The respondents viewed the mother's employment as the main reason for the decline in breastfeeding.[54] Most obstetricians have always supported breastfeeding according to Queenan,[53] an active advocate of breastfeeding, but some have appeared to be neutral. He stated that mothers should be informed of the strikingly valuable health benefits of breastfeeding so the mother can make an informed choice; "It's your gift to the mother and it's her gift to her baby."[53] A follow-up study of pediatricians' attitudes and practices regarding breastfeeding in 1995 versus 2004, reported by Feldman-Winter et al.,[55] was included in the periodic Surveys of Fellows of the AAP. Fewer responses were received—875 (53.5%) compared to 1132 (70.7%)—in 1995. Feeding practices for their own children showed an increase in breastfeeding from 37% to 72% in 2004.

Morbidity and Mortality Studies in Breastfed and Artificially Fed Infants

Assessing the mortality rate of breastfed infants compared with bottle-fed infants is difficult today because many breastfed infants also receive supplements of formula and solid foods. The risk of death in the first year of life diminished in developed countries in the twentieth century following the advent of antibiotics, additional immunizations, and many other advances in pediatric care.[56] Data from previous decades and other nations do show a significant difference, however.[15] Knodel[57] presented a complete table, including rates from cities in Germany, France, England, Holland, and the United States (Table 1-17). The mortality rate among breastfed infants is clearly lower than that among bottle-fed infants. Knodel[57] pointed out that early neonatal deaths, in the first week or so of life, were excluded. In the early twentieth century, posters that urged mothers to breastfeed that were part of the National Campaign to lower infant mortality rates were displayed everywhere by the health department without fear of inducing guilt in mothers. According to Wolf, the language was direct: "To lessen baby death let us have more mothers breastfeed"; "For your baby's sake, nurse it." Little has changed in a century.[17]

Woodbury[58] reported the trends in infant feeding (Figure 1-11) and in another study in 1922 reported mortality rates of infants by type of feeding. Mortality rate is lower at all ages for breastfed infants. Overwhelming evidence of the impact of human milk on mortality rate is displayed in the widely publicized statistics currently available on third world countries, where infant formulas have replaced human milk. The death rate is higher, malnutrition starts earlier and is more severe, and the incidence of infection is greater in formula-fed infants (Figures 1-12 and 1-13). Data from the work of Scrimshaw et al.[29] show a mortality rate of 950 of 1000 live births in artificially fed infants and 120 of 1000 in breastfed infants. The data were collected in Punjab villages from 1955 through 1959. The deaths were predominantly caused by diarrheal disease. The Pan American Health Organization has reported similar correlations among malnutrition, infection, and mortality. In the work by Puffer and Serrano[52] in 1973 in São Paulo, death rates among breastfed infants and proportions from diarrheal disease and malnutrition were also lower than among bottle-fed infants.

The incidence of illness or morbidity among artificially fed infants in third world countries is as dramatic as the mortality rate. Observations of

TABLE 1-17	Mortality Rates and Survivorship to Age 1 Year in Breastfed and Artificially Fed Infants*					
		Mortality Rate (per 1000)		Survivors to Age 1 yr (per 1000)		
Study Area	Date	Breastfed	Artificially Fed	Breastfed	Artificially Fed	Difference
Berlin, Germany	1895-1896	57	376	943	624	319
Bremen, Germany	1905	68	379	932	621	311
Hanover, Germany	1912	96	296	904	704	200
Boston, Mass.	1911	30	212	970	788	182
Eight U.S. cities[†]	1911-1916	76	255	924	745	179
Paris, France	1900	140	310	860	690	170
Cologne, Germany	1908-1909	73	241	927	759	168
Amsterdam, Holland	1904	144	304	856	696	160
Liverpool, England	1905	84	134	916	866	144
Eight U.S. cities[‡]	1911-1916	76	215	924	785	139
Derby, England	1900-1903	70	198	930	802	128
Chicago, Ill.	1924-1929	2	84	998	916	82
Liverpool, England	1936-1942	10	57	990	943	47
Great Britain	1946-1947	9	18	991	982	9

*Most of these rates do not include deaths in the first few days or weeks of life; mortality rate is therefore underestimated and survival rate overestimated. Only the rates for the eight U.S. cities in 1911 to 1916 represent mortality rate from birth; deaths that occurred before any feeding are proportionally allocated to the two feeding categories. The rates for Berlin, Bremen, Hanover, Cologne, and the eight U.S. cities were derived by applying life table techniques to mortality rates given by single months of age.
[†]Comparison of breastfed infants with infants artificially fed from birth.
[‡]Comparison of breastfed infants with all infants artificially fed in the period of observation.
From Knodel J: Breastfeeding and population growth. *Science* 198:1111, 1977. Copyright © 1977 by the American Association for the Advancement of Science.

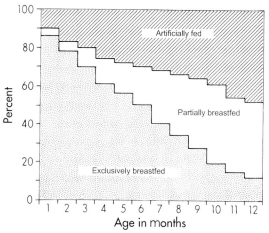

Figure 1-11. Percentage of infants who were breastfed, partially breastfed, and artificially fed by age in months. (Modified from Woodbury RM: The relation between breast and artificial feeding and infant mortality, *Am J Hyg* 2:668, 1922.)

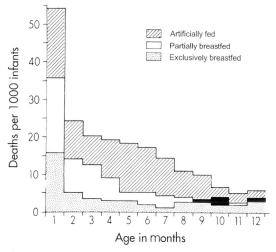

Figure 1-12. Death rate per 1000 infants by type of feeding and age in months. (Modified from Woodbury RM: The relation between breast and artificial feeding and infant mortality, *Am J Hyg* 2:668, 1922.)

Arab villages in Israel showed hospitalization rates vary with method of feeding. Only 0.5% of breastfed infants required hospitalization; infants who were breastfed more than 3 months but less than 6 months had a 2.9% hospitalization rate, and infants who were bottle-fed had a 24.8% rate. This is a 50-fold difference.

There is a bias against bottle-feeding, because sicker, smaller infants are bottle-fed. Infants who

die are weaned early by death. The benefits of breastfeeding are enhanced by these confounding variables. Habicht et al.[23] point out that had there been no breastfeeding in the sample, twice as many infants would have died after the first week of life. In 1968, Hill[60] articulated what many physicians believed: "Formula feeding has become so simple, safe, uniformly successful that breastfeeding no

The message on breast-feeding isn't new

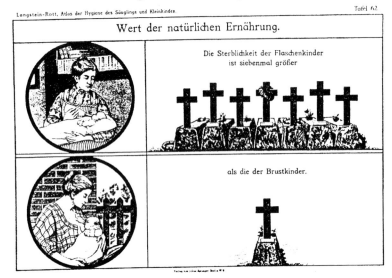

Langstein-Rott, Atlas der Hygiene des Säuglings und Kleinkindes. Tafel 62.

Wert der natürlichen Ernährung.

Die Sterblichkeit der Flaschenkinder
ist siebenmal größer

als die der Brustkinder.

Verlag von Julius Springer, Berlin W. 9

Figure 1-13. "Value of Natural Feeding" poster used in 1918 to educate parents. Text explains that the mortality rate of bottle-fed infants (Flaschenkinder) is seven times higher than that of breastfed infants (Brustkinder). (From Langstein R: *Atlas der Hygiene des Sauglings und Kleinkindes*, Berlin, 1918, Springer-Verlag.)

longer seems worth the bother." This statement ignores the protective qualities of human milk, not only in the third world but in industrialized nations as well. It neglects the immunologic protection.

Evidence for protection by breastfeeding against infant death from infectious diseases in Brazil in 1987 is even more persuasive, as noted in a carefully controlled study by Victora et al.[16,61,62] Compared with infants who were breastfed without supplementation, those who were completely bottle-fed had a relative risk 14.2-times greater for death from diarrhea and a relative risk 3.6 times greater for death from respiratory infection. Partial breastfeeding was less protective. Formula and cow milk were equally hazardous. The greatest risk from diarrhea was in the first 2 months of life.

Demonstrating the differences in morbidity between breastfed and bottle-fed infants has become even more complex in industrialized countries since the resurgence of breastfeeding. Among the confounding variables are the inherent differences between mothers who choose to breastfeed and those who choose to bottle-feed. Although many investigators have recognized the necessity of controlling these variables, none has succeeded totally because an unavoidable factor of self-selection makes random assignment of infants impossible. There is a one-way flow of infants from the breastfed group to the bottle-fed group because a baby may change from breast to bottle but rarely from bottle to breast. Documenting breastfeeding practices is difficult when the possibility exists that some bottle-feedings are included or that solid foods have been introduced.

Differences between breastfed and bottle-fed infants in the incidence of morbidity associated with diarrhea, respiratory infections, otitis media, and pneumonia are documented. The relationship between breastfeeding versus bottle-feeding and respiratory illness in the first year of life among nearly 2000 cohort children was reported by Watkins et al.[63] in England. There was a significant advantage to breastfeeding. Mothers who smoked were less likely to breastfeed, but even when smoking was considered, the breastfeeding advantage remained. A number of well-controlled studies of industrialized countries have shown at least a two-fold relative risk of respiratory infection with bottle-feeding and that the infections breastfed infants do experience are usually less severe.[64] A meta-analysis by Bachrach et al.[65] in 2003 revealed that "among generally healthy infants in developed nations, more than a tripling in severe respiratory tract illnesses resulting in hospitalizations was noted for infants who were not breastfed compared with those who were exclusively breastfed for 4 months."

When Victora presented his studies of the impact of early weaning on infection and disease at a workshop held by the Pontifical Academy of Sciences and The Royal Society,[66] he stated that a 40% reduction in nonbreastfeeding would prevent up to 15% of diarrhea deaths and 7% of pneumonia deaths. He noted that even the introduction of water or herbal teas to a previously exclusively breastfed infant increases morbidity and mortality rates. Figures 1-14 and 1-15 illustrate the relative risks of pneumonia and otitis media.

Breastfeeding was associated with a higher level of parental education, but controlling for that

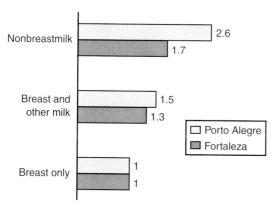

Figure 1-14. Risk of pneumonia (odds ratio for incidence) in children under 2 years of age at two Brazilian sites, Porto Alegre and Fortaleza, in 1993 to 1995 according to type of milk. (Modified from Victora CG: Infection and disease: the impact of early weaning, *Food Nutr Bull* 17:390, 1996.)

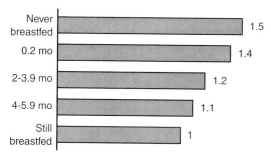

Figure 1-15. Risk of otitis media (odds ratio for incidence in last month) in infants 6 months of age in Brazil in 1993 and 1994 according to duration of breastfeeding. (Modified from Victora CG: Infection and disease: the impact of early weaning, *Food Nutr Bull* 17:390, 1996.)

factor, the difference in the morbidity rate is even more significant.[62]

In the United States, diarrheal disease is uncommon in breastfed infants, and the treatment is usually to continue to breastfeed.[2] Similarly, breastfed infants have fewer episodes of respiratory illness and otitis media. When afflicted with such febrile illnesses, the breastfed infant does not become dehydrated and rapidly toxic.[51]

The issue is not as clear in other Western countries because of the associated variables among those who bottle-feed infants, that is, young mothers with low socioeconomic status and less education and small, sick infants who are more likely to be bottle-fed.

Despite the clear-cut data on mortality and morbidity rates from past generations and from cultures seemingly remote from industrialized and medically sophisticated societies, pediatricians had discounted any but the psychologic advantages of breastfeeding for many years.[67] The current increase in illness in young infants in daycare

centers is providing a new study group. To date, breastfeeding appears to be protective for the few children whose mothers continue to nurse them while in daycare.

In the third millennium, adequate consumption of human milk as an infant and toddler is still a powerful guarantor of health and long life. Pediatricians must recognize that failure to consume sufficient human milk carries vital implications for public health.[68] There is abundant literature confirming the impact of breastfeeding on outcomes in infancy. The report by the AHRQ[69] has collected and reviewed all of the literature for the past decade and confirmed the impact of breastfeeding on infant mortality and morbidity (Table 1-18).

Evidence of the long-term effects of breastfeeding published by WHO from systematic reviews and meta-analyses from the world literature also confirmed the value of breastfeeding. It reported lower mean blood pressure and total cholesterol, as well as higher performance in intelligence tests. The prevalence of overweight and obesity as well as type 2 diabetes was also noted to be lower when an infant was breastfed.

Sudden Infant Death Syndrome and Other Issues

Recent interest in sudden infant death syndrome (SIDS) has generated several studies investigating the position in which the infant is put down in the crib and the occurrence of SIDS.[21,66,70] The New Zealand Cot Death Study showed the prone sleeping position to be a greater risk, but not greater than the risk for not being breastfed.[54] Other investigators have shown the importance of breastfeeding as a risk-lowering factor.[21] Although breastfeeding does not eliminate SIDS, its incidence is lower among breastfed infants.

No single consistent factor has been a predictor of SIDS.[21] Prone sleeping has continued to be a cofactor in studies, but maternal smoking is a relative causative factor as well. Breastfeeding has been shown to be the strongest protection. Infants of smokers who breastfeed and sleep supine have a reduced risk for SIDS. Several studies confirmed a reduced risk while breastfeeding, and one study linked the effect to a dose response of the amount of breastfeeding. The National Maternal and Infant Health Survey of 100,000 births and 6000 deaths of infants born in 1988 and 1989 was analyzed using a consistent "dosage definition" of breastfeeding while controlling for major confounding factors. These factors included birth weight; maternal age, race, and education; smoking; prenatal cocaine use; lack of private insurance; household smoking;

TABLE 1-18   Illness, Disease, and Development with Feeding Measure and Risk Ratio Range

	Feeding Measure	Risk Ratio Range*	Reference(s)
Common illnesses			
Acute diarrhea	Breastfed <3 mo	6.10 (4.1-9.0)	Victoria and Barros (2000)
Lower respiratory tract infections	Breastfed <4 mo/sharing bedroom	3.29 (1.8-6.0)	Wright et al. (1989)
Pneumonia	No breastfeeding	16.7 (7.7, 36.0)	César et al. (1999)
Ear infections (recurring vs. acute)	Breastfed <6 mo	1.61 (1.27, 1.79)*	Duncan et al. (1993)
Asthma	Breastfed <4 mo	1.25 (1.02, 1.52)	Oddy et al. (1999)
Atopy	Breastfed <4 mo	1.30 (1.04, 1.61)	Oddy et al. (1999)
Less common illnesses			
Necrotizing enterocolitis	39% formula fed/7% breastfed	4.50 (3.00, 6.00)*	Lucas and Cole (1990)
Urinary tract infections	Never breastfed	1.62 (1.35, 1.78)*	Mårild et al. (1990, 1989) and Pisacane et al. (1992)
Insulin-dependent diabetes mellitus	Breastfed <4 mo	1.63 (1.22, 2.17)	Fort et al. (1986)
Acute lymphoblastic leukemia	Never breastfed	1.21 (1.09, 1.30)*	Shu et al. (1999)
Sudden infant death syndrome	Current infant formula-feeding	1.35 (1.09, 1.54)*	Ford et al. (1993)
Cholera	Not breastfeeding	1.70 (p <0.0001)*	Clemens et al. (1990)
Immunologic diseases			
Celiac disease	Breastfed <3 mo	1.63 (1.36, 1.79)*	Falth-Magnusson et al. (1996) and Peters et al. (1996)
Crohn's disease	Lack of breastfeeding	1.90 (1.50, 3.60)	Corrao et al. (1998) and Koletzko et al. (1989)
Ulcerative colitis	Lack of breastfeeding	1.50 (1.10, 2.10)	Corrao et al. (1998) and Koletzko et al. (1991)
Juvenile rheumatoid arthritis	Lack of breastfeeding	1.60 (1.19, 1.80)	Mason et al. (1995)
Multiple sclerosis	Breastfed <7 mo	1.62 (1.26, 1.81)	Pisacane et al. (1994)
Development			
Cognitive development in preterm	Lack of breastfeeding	↓ Mean IQ of 8.3 pts*	Lucas et al. (1992)
Cardiovascular disease	Lack of breastfeeding	↑ Mean total cholesterol*	Bergstrom et al. (1995)
Metabolic development	Lack of breastfeeding	↑ ApoB values*	Bergstrom et al. (1995)
Obesity	Breastfed <6 mo	1.25 (1.02, 1.43)	von Kries et al. (1999)

ApoB, Apolipoprotein B.

  *The risk ratios have been adjusted to reflect a level of risk of infant formula rather than protection of breast milk. This was done to ensure consistency of results. Some results are given as *p* value or other measurement effect.

  From Oddy W: The impact of breastmilk on infant and child health, *Breastfeeding Rev* 10:5, 2002.

daycare; and household size. In 7102 control subjects, 499 SIDS deaths and 584 non-SIDS deaths occurred. Fredrickson et al.[15a] reported that "the risk of SIDS for black infants increased by 1.19 for every month of not breastfeeding, and 2.13 for every month of not exclusively breastfeeding. Among white infants, the risk increased by 1.19 and 2.0 times, respectively. These associations remained even when deaths within the first month of life were excluded. A similar protective association existed for non-SIDS deaths."

The Committee on SIDS of the AAP then recommended pacifiers for all children. Recognizing the early use of pacifiers as a risk factor for early discontinuance of breastfeeding, the AAP recommended that breastfeeding infants not be given a pacifier until 2 weeks of age. It has resulted in an excessive use of pacifiers in all infants. A decrease in SIDS has not been reported.

Sleep patterns of infants have been the subject of much study.[21] In the early weeks of life, infants have rapid eye movement (REM) sleep, active body movements, and rapid, irregular heart and respiratory rates. At about 2 to 3 months of age, they begin to increase the proportion of quiet sleep, which coincides with the peak incidence of SIDS. When breastfeeding decreased, the advantage of co-sleeping seemed to diminish. Child care became very organized and focused on encouraging the infant to sleep alone and through the night. Only in about the last century have Western industrialized societies considered breastfeeding and infant sleep location to be separate issues. McKenna and Bernstraw[40] and Mosko[71] describe the physiologic benefits to infants sleeping in proximity to their caregivers. They have documented the physiologic changes infants experience as they move from a solitary sleep environment to co-sleeping. They monitored a group of mother-infant pairs in the sleep laboratory, using each pair as their own control (i.e., co-sleeping and sleeping separately). Infants moved from one stage of sleep to the other more frequently when co-sleeping than when sleeping alone, even when briefly waking and increasing their heart and respiratory rates. The authors commented that modern technology, including baby monitors, breathing teddy bears, and other gadgets, has replaced traditional co-sleeping.[71] Accidental suffocation and strangulation in bed has increased four times since 1984 in spite of the back to sleep program and the introduction of pacifiers that were predicted to reduce SIDS. In 2012, the Committee on SIDS of the AAP[2] issued an update of their recommendations regarding the avoidance of SIDS. The most significant issue for breastfeeding families and their physicians is the strong prohibition of bed sharing. The leading modifiable risk factors for SIDS are smoking, infant sleeping prone, formula feeding, baby sleeping unattended, and poverty. Sofas and soft sleep surfaces and sleeping in lounge chairs and rockers are great risks, as well as parental use of alcohol and drugs.

Bed sharing has been publicized and promoted as the solution to SIDS. The practice of bed sharing was analyzed in 2014 by Blair et al.[24] who demonstrated the risk of bed sharing was with an impaired caretaker and a premature infant. They showed that sleeping on a sofa was more dangerous. An evidence-based infant sleep recommendation was reported by Bartwick and Smith[72] that reviewed the world literature on risky behavior regarding infant sleep. They concluded that efforts need to be focused on impaired caregivers, lack of breastfeeding, and risky surfaces such as sofas, lounge chairs, and rockers to make the greatest difference in the incidence of SIDS.

The Mammary Gland and Science

Newer additions to the laboratory have permitted rapid advances in the understanding of the mammary gland, especially actions of hormones and enzymes.[19] The "knock-out mouse" is a concept of using mice in which DNA (deoxyribonucleic acid) has been altered to "knock out" a specific gene that controls a specific hormone, such as one important to lactation. Observations of growth and development in these animals provide new insights into the physiology of the mammary gland. In evolutionary biology, lactogenesis is one of the most important functions for the survival of the species. Advances in molecular biology have provided biologists with a better understanding of the mechanisms that produce milk and its specific nutrient constituents. Mammary epithelial cells secrete milk. In an innovative experimental model, mammary epithelial cells are cultured in a petri dish and form a mammosphere, a micromodel of the mammary gland. The advantage of bioengineering the mammary gland, initially focused on the dairy species, is to advance our knowledge and understanding of human lactation in the laboratory so that more women may nurse their infants successfully.[6]

Support for the Breastfeeding Women of the World

On May 12, 1995, His Holiness John Paul II* granted a Solemn Papal Audience in the Apostolic Palace of the Vatican to the participants of the Working Group on Breastfeeding: Science and Society.[66] In response to the group report, the Holy Father pronounced the following discourse (in part):

> The advantages of breastfeeding for the infant and the mother include two major benefits to the child: proper nourishment and protection against disease. This natural way of feeding can create a bond of love and security between mother and child and enable the child to assert its presence as a person through interaction with the mother. Responsible international agencies are calling on governments to ensure that women are enabled to breastfeed their children for four to six months from birth and to continue this practice, supplemented by other appropriate foods, up to the second year of life and beyond.[66]

A National Campaign to Promote Breastfeeding

In an attempt to capture the attention of the American public and improve the national statistics on breastfeeding initiation and duration, the Office of Women's Health (OWH) and the USBC

---

*John Paul II was proclaimed a Saint by rigorous due process in Rome in April 2014.

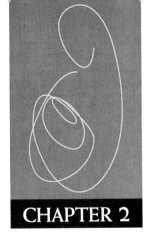

CHAPTER 2

Anatomy of the Breast

‖‖‖

Gross Anatomy

The mammary gland, as the breast is medically termed, received its name from *mamma*, the Latin word for breast. The human mammary gland is the only organ that is not fully developed at birth. It experiences dramatic changes in size, shape, and function from birth through pregnancy, lactation, and ultimately involution. Mediated by large changes in gene expression, there are drastic changes in composition, architecture, and function during the life cycle of the human mammary gland. The gland only reaches full maturity when pregnancy occurs. This is the most significant stage of the breast because of the very high metabolic demand that utilizes 25% of the maternal energy intake. Pregnancy and lactation create permanent breast changes that provide a protective, yet not well understood, effect against breast malignancy. The gland undergoes three major phases of growth and development before pregnancy and lactation: in utero, during the first 2 years of life, and at puberty.

Embryonic Development

The milk streak appears in the fourth week, when the embryo is 2.5 mm long. It becomes the milk line, or ridge, during the fifth week (2.5 to 5.5 mm). Mammary glands begin to develop in the 6-week-old embryo, continuing their proliferation until milk ducts are developed by the time of birth[32] (Tables 2-1 and 2-2). Embryologically, the mammary glands develop as ingrowths of the ectoderm into the underlying mesodermal tissue.[17] In the human embryo, a thickened, raised area of the ectoderm can be recognized in the region of

the future gland at the end of the fourth week of pregnancy. The thickened ectoderm becomes depressed into the underlying mesoderm, the surface of the mammary area soon becomes flat, and it finally sinks below the level of the surrounding epidermis. The mesoderm in contact with the ingrowth of the ectoderm is compressed, and its elements become arranged in concentric layers, which at a later stage give rise to the gland's stroma. The ingrowing mass of ectodermal cells soon becomes pouch or pear shaped and then grows out into the surrounding mesoderm as a number of solid processes that represent the gland's future ducts. These processes, by dividing and branching, give rise to the future lobes and lobules and, much later, to the alveoli.

By 16 weeks' gestation, the branching stage has produced 15 to 25 epithelial strips or solid cords in the subcutaneous tissue that represent future secretory alveoli. The smooth musculature of nipple and areola are developed. By apoptosis of the central epithelial cells, branching and canalization continue. By 32 weeks' gestation the primary milk ducts appear and the mammary vascular system is completely developed. At this time, the secondary mammary anlage (primordium) develops. The secondary mammary anlage then develops with elements of hair follicles, sebaceous glands, and sweat glands, along with the Montgomery glands, around the alveoli. Mesenchymal cells differentiate into the smooth muscle of the nipple and areola between 12 and 16 weeks' gestation.[26] Thus far, development is independent of hormone stimulation. By 28 weeks' gestation, placental sex hormones enter the fetal circulation and induce canalization in the fetus.[26]

The lumina develop in the outgrowths, forming the lactiferous ducts and their branches. The lactiferous ducts open into a shallow epithelial depression

TABLE 2-1 Embryonic Timetable of Breast Development in the Human

Age of Embryo (wk)	Crown-Rump Length of Embryo (mean)	Developmental Stage
4	2.5 mm	Mammary streak
5	2.5-5.5 mm	Milk line, or milk ridge
6	5.5-11 mm	Parenchymal cells proliferate
7-8	11-25 mm	Mammary disk progresses to globular stage
9	25-30 mm	Cone stage: Inward growth of parenchyma
10-12	30-68 mm	Epithelial buds sprout from invading parenchyma
12-13	68 mm to 5 cm	Indentation buds become lobular with notching at epithelial-stromal border
15	10 cm	Buds branch into 15-25 epithelial strips
20-24	20 cm	Solid cords canalize by desquamation and lysis
24-32	30 cm	Further canalization
32-40	35-50 cm	Lobular-alveolar development

Data from Russo J, Russo IH: Development of the human mammary gland. In Neville MC, Daniel CW, editors: *The mammary gland*, New York, 1987, Plenum.

TABLE 2-2 Stages of Mammary Development

Developmental Stage	Hormonal Regulation	Local Factors	Description
Embryogenesis	???	Fat pad necessary for ductal extension	Epithelial bud develops in 18- to 19-week fetus, extending a short distance into mammary fat pad with blind ducts that become canalized; some milk secretion may be present at birth
Pubertal development before onset of menses	Estrogen, GH	IGF-1, HGF, TGF-β, ???	Ductal extension into the mammary fat pad; branching morphogenesis
After onset of menses	Estrogen, progesterone, PRL?		Lobular development with formation of terminal duct lobular unit
Development in pregnancy	Progesterone, PRL, placental lactogen	HER, ???	Alveolus formation; partial cellular differentiation
Transition: lactogenesis	Progesterone withdrawal, PRL, glucocorticoid	Unknown	Onset of milk secretion: stage I, midpregnancy; stage II, parturition
Lactation	PRL, oxytocin	FIL, stretch	Ongoing milk secretion, milk ejection
Involution	Withdrawal of prolactin	Milk stasis (FIL??)	Alveolar epithelium undergoes apoptosis and remodeling and gland reverts to prepregnant state

? and ??, Possibly; *???,* unknown; *FIL,* Feedback inhibitor of lactation; *GH,* growth hormone; *HER,* herregulin; *HGF,* human growth factor; *IGF-1,* insulin-like growth factor-1; *PRL,* prolactin; *TGF-β,* transforming growth factor-β.
From Neville MC: Breastfeeding, part I: the evidence for breastfeeding. Anatomy and physiology of lactation, *Pediatr Clin North Am* 48:13, 2001.

known as the mammary pit. The pit becomes elevated as a result of the mesenchymal proliferation forming the nipple and areola. An inverted nipple is a result of the failure of the pit to elevate.[3] A lumen is formed in each part of the branching system of cellular processes after 32 weeks' gestation. Near term, about 15 to 25 mammary ducts form the fetal mammary gland (Figure 2-1). Duct and sebaceous glands coalesce near the epidermis. Parenchymal differentiation occurs with the development of lobular-alveolar structures that contain colostrum. This change occurs at 32 to 40 weeks and is called the end-vesicle stage.

Fetal and Prepubertal Development

The mammary glands of male and female fetuses of 13 to 40 weeks' gestation were studied ultrastructurally by Tobon and Salazar.[43] This work confirms morphologic developments in the fetal breast tissue in response to hormonal stimuli that are similar to

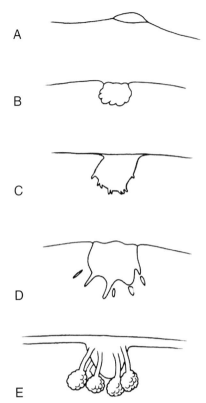

Figure 2-1. Evolution of nipple. **A,** Thickening of epidermis with formation of primary bud. **B,** Growth of bud into mesenchyma. **C,** Formation of solid secondary buds. **D,** Formation of mammary pit and vacuolation of buds to form epithelial-lined ducts. **E,** Lactiferous ducts proliferate. Areola is formed. Nipple is inverted initially. (Modified from Weatherly-White RCA: *Plastic surgery of the female breast,* Hagerstown, Md., 1980, Harper & Row.)

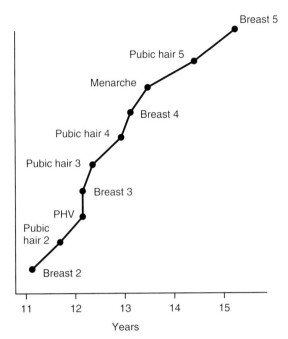

Figure 2-2. Pubertal development in the female. The sequence and mean ages of pubertal events in females, adapted from the data of Marshall and Tanner. *PHV,* Peak height velocity. (From Root AW: Endocrinology of puberty, *J Pediatr* 83:1, 1973.)

those in the maternal breast. The Golgi system and abundant reticula with dilated cisternae filled with fine granular material are present in the cellular structure. Abundant mitochondria and lipid droplets are observed. Proliferation and conditioning of the epithelial cells are evident, and, in the last trimester, microvilli along the ductal lumen are accompanied by large cytoplasmic protrusions (see Table 2-2).

Study of the ultrastructure of the fetal breast may help in understanding the functional lactating breast. The secretion of a fluid resembling milk may take place at birth as a result of maternal hormones that have passed across the placenta into the fetal circulation. The lactiferous sinuses appear before birth as swellings of the developing ducts.

An extensive anatomic and histologic study of the human infant breast revealed an epithelial differentiation that followed a chronologic pattern, starting with secretory changes and apparently going through a period of apocrine metaplasia before the postsecretory changes and involution.[2] The embryonic fat probably plays a role in growth

and morphogenesis of the ductal system. No distinguishing features were found between the breasts of female and male infants,[2] however.

The terminal end buds, lateral buds, and lobules of three to five alveolar buds predominate in prepubertal tissue. Lobules of alveolar buds and lobules of up to 60 ductules predominate in pubertal females. In prepuberty, these epithelium-lined ducts will bud out to form alveoli when stimulated by hormones of menarche (see Figure 2-1).

The breast is made up of glandular tissue, supporting connective tissue, and protective fatty tissue. Immediately after birth, the newborn's breast may even be swollen and secreting a small amount of milk, often termed witch's milk. This phenomenon, common among both male and female infants, is caused by the stimulation of the infant's mammary glands by the same hormones produced by the placenta to prepare the mother's breast for lactation. This secretory activity subsides within 3 to 4 weeks, and then the mammary glands are inactive until shortly before the onset of puberty, when hormones begin to stimulate growth again. During childhood (prepuberty), the gland merely keeps pace with physical growth[42] (Figures 2-2 and 2-3).

The molecular biology of mammary gland development depends on a combination of systemic mammotropic hormones plus local cell-to-cell interactions.[42] A variety of growth factors mediate the local cell interactions. These factors

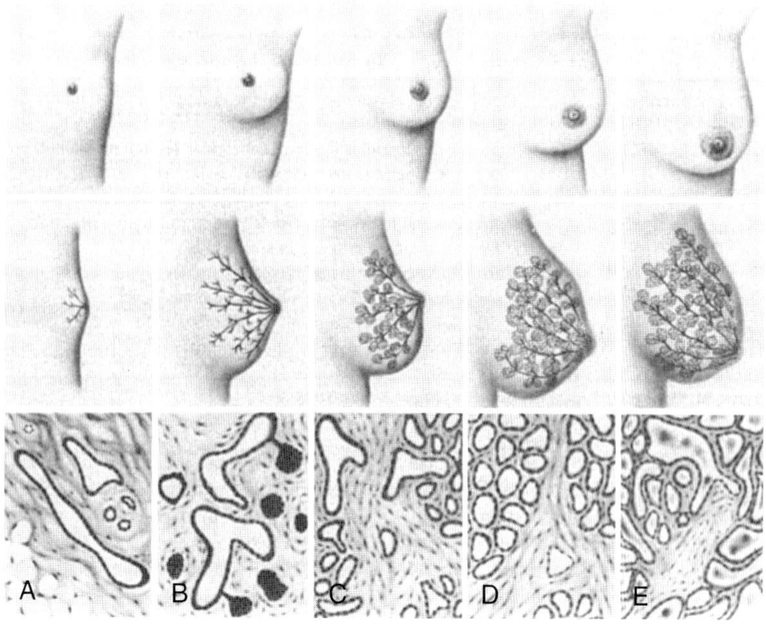

Figure 2-3. Female breast from infancy to lactation with corresponding cross section and duct structure. **A, B,** and **C,** Gradual development of well-differentiated ductular and peripheral lobular-alveolar system. **D,** Ductular sprouting and intensified peripheral lobular-alveolar development in pregnancy. Glandular luminal cells begin actively synthesizing milk fat and proteins near term; only small amounts are released into lumen. **E,** With postpartum withdrawal of luteal and placental sex steroids and placental lactogen, prolactin is able to induce full secretory activity of alveolar cells and release of milk into alveoli and smaller ducts.

include the epidermal growth factor (EGF), transforming growth factor-β (TGF-β), fibroblast growth factor (FGF), and the *Wnt* gene families. In the developing breast these factors are thought to act in concert with systemic hormones.[19]

In a longitudinal cohort of 6 to 8 years of age, girls were followed from 2004 to 2011 in three geographic areas in the United States. Using Tanner staging, the age at onset of breast maturation was documented. Stage 2 onset varied by race/ethnicity, BMI at baseline, and site. Mean onset was 8.8, 9.3, 9.7, and 9.7 years for black, Hispanic, white and non-Hispanic, and Asian, respectively. The greater the BMI, the younger the age of maturation. This study confirmed earlier maturation in girls in the last decade.

Pubertal Development

Puberty stimulates rapid breast growth activated by ovulation and establishment of menses. The development of the human breast involves two distinct processes: organogenesis and milk production.[7] Organogenesis involves ductal and lobular growth and begins before and continues through puberty, resulting in growth of the breast parenchyma with its surrounding fat pad. When a girl is between 10 and 12 years of age, just before puberty, the ductal tree extends and generates its branching pattern, lengthening the existing ducts, dichotomously branching the growing ductal tips, and monopodially branching, with the growth of the lateral buds at the sides of the ducts[18] (Tables 2-2 and 2-3).

TABLE 2-3		Phases of Breast Development
Phase	**Age (yr)**	**Developmental Characteristics**
I	Puberty	Preadolescent elevation of nipple with no palpable glandular tissue or areolar pigmentation
II	11.1 ± 1.1	Presence of glandular tissue in subareolar region; nipple and breast project as single mound from chest wall
III	12.2 ± 1.09	Increase in amount of readily palpable glandular tissue, with enlargement of breast and increased diameter and pigmentation of areola; contour of breast and nipple remains in single plane
IV	13.1 ± 1.15	Enlargement of areola and increased areolar pigmentation; nipple and areola form secondary mound above breast level
V	15.3 ± 1.7	Final adolescent development of smooth contour with no projection of areola and nipple

Modified from Tanner JM: *Wachstun und Reifung des Menschen*, Stuttgart, 1962, Thieme-Verlag.

During this period of rapid growth, the ducts can develop bulbous terminal end buds. The formation of alveolar buds begins within a year or two of the onset of menses.[15] During the menstrual cycle, the breast changes, beginning with the follicular phase of days 3 to 14. The stroma becomes less dense. Lumina expansion takes place in the ducts.

Occasionally mitosis occurs, but no secretion has been seen. In days 15 to 28, or the luteal phase, the density of the stroma progresses, and the ducts have a lumen and some secretion. From days 26 to 28 epithelial cells are reduced as apoptosis occurs, and blood flow is greatest in midcycle.[40] The sprouting of new alveolar buds continues for several years, producing alveolar lobes.[32] Mammary stem cell (MaSC) populations from the basal ductal layer are driven by the ovarian hormonal circuit, and changes in epitheal and stromal development result. The mammary mini-remodeling with each cycle does not fully regress at the end of the cycle.

Anatomic Location

The breast is located in the superficial fascia between the second rib and sixth intercostal cartilage and upon the deep pectoral fascia that is superficial to the pectoralis major muscle.[19] It tends to overlap this muscle inferiorly to become superficial to the external oblique and serratus anterior muscles. The loose connective tissue between the breast and deep fascia forms the "submammary space," which allows some movement.[23] It measures 10 to 12 cm in diameter. It is located horizontally from the parasternal to midaxillary line. The central thickness of the breast is 5 to 7 cm (Figure 2-4).

At puberty, the breasts of a girl enlarge to their adult size, with the left frequently slightly larger than the right.[46] In a nonpregnant woman the mature breast weighs approximately 200 g. During pregnancy, breast size and weight increase; thus when a pregnant woman is near term, the breast weighs 400 to 600 g. During lactation the breast weighs 600 to 800 g (see Figure 2-3).

The shape of breasts varies from woman to woman, just as body build and facial characteristics do. Genetic, racial, and dietary variations may be associated with discoidal, hemispheric, pear-shaped, or conical forms.[23] Typically, the breast is dome-shaped or conic in adolescence, becoming more hemispheric and finally pendulous in a parous woman. Mammary glandular tissue projects somewhat into the axillary region. This is known as the tail of Spence (Figure 2-5). Mammary tissue in the axilla, which is connected to the central duct system, becomes more obvious during pregnancy and produces milk during lactation, when it may cause various symptoms (see Chapter 8).[1] The tail of Spence is distinguished from a supernumerary gland because it connects to the normal duct system. Occasionally, in normal women, small masses of breast tissue may grow through the deep fascia to the muscle below. This may explain some pain distribution when the breast is engorged.

The three major structures of the breast are skin, subcutaneous tissue, and corpus mammae. The corpus mammae is the breast mass that remains after freeing the breast from the deep attachments and

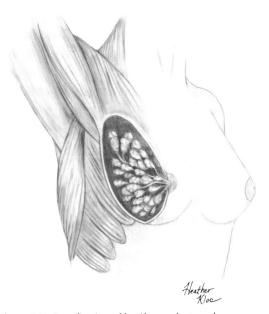

Figure 2-5. Ramification of lactiferous ducts and mammary tissue. Ducts extend onto upper medial aspect of arm, to midline, and into epigastrium. Composite drawing from mammographic studies. (Modified from Hicken NF: Mastectomy: pathologic study demonstrating why most mastectomies result in incomplete removal of the mammary gland, *Arch Surg* 40:6, 1940.)

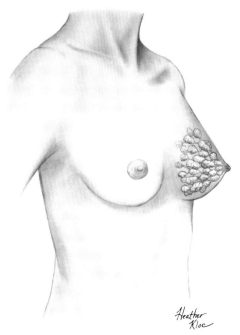

Figure 2-4. Mammary gland in longitudinal cross section showing mature, nonlactating duct system.

removing the skin, subcutaneous connective tissue, and adipose tissue.

The breasts of an adult woman are always paired and develop from a line of glandular tissue found in the fetus and known as the milk line. This milk streak, or galactic band, develops from the axilla to the groin during the fifth week of embryonic life.[26] In the thoracic region, the band develops into a ridge, and the rest of the band regresses (Figure 2-6).

Abnormalities

In some women, additional residual tissue of the galactic band remains as mammary tissue, which can develop anywhere along this line. Hypermastia is the presence of accessory mammary glands, which are phylogenic remnants of the embryonic mammary ridge resulting from incomplete regression or dispersion of the primitive galactic band (see Figure 2-6). Because of this origin, accessory nipples and glandular tissue may be found along these lines, which extend from the clavicular to the inguinal regions. Occasionally, supernumerary glands are found in the urogenital region, on the

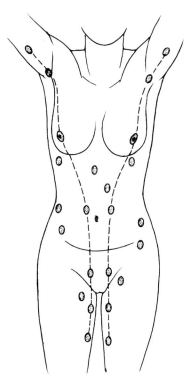

Figure 2-6. Sites of supernumerary nipples along milk line. Ectopic nipples, areolae, or breast tissue can develop from groin to axilla and upper inner arm. They can lactate or undergo malignant change. (Modified from Weatherly-White RCA: *Plastic surgery of the female breast*, Hagerstown, Md., 1980, Harper & Row.)

buttocks, or on the back.[47] The glands are derived from the ectoderm, whereas the connective tissue stroma is mesodermal in origin.

The accessory tissue may involve the corpus mammae, the areola, and the nipple.[27] Hypermastia occurs in 2% to 6% of women. The response of hypermastia to pregnancy and lactation depends on the tissue present.

Box 2-1 defines other selected breast abnormalities. Symmastia is a webbing across the midline between the breasts, which are usually symmetric.[3] A more common variation is the presternal confluence representing blending of breast tissue associated with large breasts. These abnormalities are ectodermal in origin and have many variations, from an empty skin web to the presence of significant glandular tissue. Little is known about their function, but several procedures exist for their surgical amelioration.[3]

Congenital absence of the breast is called amastia, which is rare. When a nipple is present but no breast tissue, the condition is called amazia. Another term for this condition when it occurs in addition to a normal breast is hyperthelia.

Some have suggested a relationship between polythelia (supernumerary nipple) and renal defect. Polythelia has also been associated with renal agenesis, renal cell carcinoma, obstructive disease, and supernumerary kidneys.[29] Others have described associations with congenital cardiac anomalies, pyloric stenosis, ear abnormalities, and arthrogryposis multiplex congenita.[3] After careful study of 65 patients with a supernumerary nipple, Hersh et al.[15] found 7 individuals (11%) who had significant renal lesions, somewhat less than the incidence reported originally. Apparently no association exists in black patients.

Poland syndrome, first described in 1841 (Box 2-2), includes absence of the pectoral muscle, chest wall deformity, and breast anomalies.[26] It is now known also to include symbrachydactyly, with hypoplasia of the middle phalanges and central skin webbing. Breast hypoplasia is underdevelopment of the breast. Although 90%

BOX 2-1. Breast Abnormalities

- **Accessory breast**: Any tissue outside the two major glands
- **Amastia**: Congenital absence of breast and nipple
- **Amazia**: Nipple without breast tissue
- **Hyperadenia**: Mammary tissue without nipple
- **Hypoplasia**: Underdevelopment of breast
- **Polythelia**: Supernumerary nipple(s) (also hyperthelia)
- **Symmastia**: Webbing between breasts

> **BOX 2-2. Types of Breast Hypoplasia, Hyperplasia, and Acquired Abnormalities**
>
> - Unilateral hypoplasia, contralateral breast normal
> - Bilateral hypoplasia with asymmetry
> - Unilateral hyperplasia, contralateral breast normal
> - Bilateral hyperplasia with asymmetry
> - Unilateral hypoplasia, contralateral breast hyperplasia
> - Unilateral hypoplasia of breast, thorax, and pectoral muscles (Poland syndrome)
> - Acquired abnormalities caused by trauma, burns, radiation treatment for hemangioma or intrathoracic disease, chest tube insertion in infancy, and preadolescent biopsy

of cases of breast hypoplasia are associated with hypoplasia of the pectoral muscles, 92% of women with pectoral muscle abnormalities have normal breasts. Box 2-2 lists types of breast hypoplasia, hyperplasia (overdevelopment), and acquired breast abnormalities.

Hyperadenia is the presence of mammary tissue without nipples. The swelling and secretion of this tissue may produce pain during lactation. Occasionally, aberrant breast tissue can cause discomfort or embarrassment in adolescence and during menses, especially when located in the axilla.[16] Mammographic features of normal accessory axillary breast tissue were reviewed by Adler et al.[1] in 13 women who were diagnosed on routine mammography. Seven of these women had a mass or fullness on physical examination; one was seen postpartum because of pain; nine were asymptomatic. They ranged in age from 31 to 67 years. On radiographics, the accessory tissue resembled the rest of the normal glandular tissue but was separate from it. It occurred on the right in 11 of the 13 women. The accessory tissue was recognized as a normal developmental variant, distinguishable from the frequent axillary tail of Spence, which represents a direct extension from the outer margin of the main mass of glandular tissue.

On mammography, accessory tissue is best visualized on oblique and exaggerated craniocaudal views and by ultrasound. In rare cases, it may be appropriate to remove the tissue surgically, a treatment well known to experienced plastic surgeons. If treatment is not initiated before pregnancy and lactation in these women, pain and swelling will be intensified and may progress to mastitis or the necessity to terminate lactation.

Apart from physiologic variations, other conditions of abnormal anatomy include hypomastia (abnormally small breasts), hypertrophy, and inequality.

Acquired Abnormalities

The most common cause of acquired breast abnormality is iatrogenic and is most commonly caused by chest wall trauma in premature infants when chest tubes are inserted. Biopsy in prepubertal girls may remove vital tissues. Cutaneous burns to the chest wall may result in scaring and breast deformity. Such findings do not automatically prevent breastfeeding. The lactation center at the University of Rochester has been consulted about several such women who have been able to breastfeed with assistance and encouragement in spite of scarring and seeming deformity.

Corpus Mammae

The mammary gland is an orderly conglomeration of a variable number of independent glands. It undergoes a series of changes that can be divided into developmental and differentiation phases. Surgical dissection of many postoperative specimens has contributed more precise information about the anatomic structure of the breast. The ramifications of the lactiferous ducts and stroma were carefully studied by Weatherly-White,[47] who reported that in 95% of women the ducts ascend into the axilla, occasionally following the brachial plexus and axillary vessels into the apex of the axilla. Ducts are found in the epigastric region in 15% of women. In rare cases, ducts cross the midline (see Figure 2-6).

The morphology of the corpus mammae includes two major divisions, the parenchyma and the stroma.[1] The parenchyma includes the ductular-lobular-alveolar structures. It is composed of the alveolar gland with treelike ductular branching alveoli, which are approximately 0.12 mm in diameter. The ducts are approximately 2 mm in diameter. The lobi, which are arranged like spokes converging on the central nipple, are 15 to 25 in number. Each lobus is divided again into 20 to 40 lobuli, and each lobulus is again subdivided into 10 to 100 alveoli, or tubulosaccular secretory units. The stroma includes the connective tissue, fat tissue, blood vessels, nerves, and lymphatics.[19]

The mass of tissue in the breast consists of the tubuloalveolar glands embedded in fat (the adipose tissue), giving the gland its smooth, rounded contour. The mammary fat pad is essential for the proliferation and differentiation of the mammary epithelium, providing the necessary space, support, and local control for duct elongation and, ultimately, lobuloalveolar proliferation. Each gland forms a lobe of the breast, and the lobes are separated by connective tissue septa. These septa attach to the skin. Each tubuloalveolar gland opens into a lactiferous duct, which leads into a more elastic duct. A slight constriction occurs before the duct opens onto the surface of the nipple (Figure 2-7). Extension of ducts within the fat pad is orderly. The fat pad is critical to the development of the arborization.[24] Fat is distributed throughout the gland buffering the alveolae and ducts. An inhibitory zone into which other ducts cannot penetrate exists around each duct, and development does not normally proceed beyond the duct end-bud stage before puberty.[2]

Nipple and Areola

The skin of the breast includes the nipple, areola, and general skin. The skin is the thin, flexible, elastic cover of the breast and is adherent to the fat-laden subcutaneous tissue. It contains hair, sebaceous glands, and apocrine sweat glands. The nipple, or papilla mammae, is a conic elevation located in the center of the areola at about the fourth intercostal space, slightly below the midpoint of the breast. Although very different in size, the nipples and areolae of women and men are qualitatively identical.[21] The nipple contains 23 to 27 milk ducts on average, with a range of 11 to 48. Each of the tubuloalveolar glands that make up the breast opens onto the nipple by a separate opening. The precise anatomy of the nipple has drawn little attention since the work of Sir Ashley Cooper in 1839.[20] Cancer scientists are exploring the anatomy of the breast in detail to determine how cancers grow and how they spread, not to determine how the breast functions. Studies of autopsies and breasts removed for cancer in young vital women are used.[33] Data from mastectomy breasts have shown that collecting duct numbers

in the nipple averaging 25 to 27 are greater in number than the number of nipple duct openings (6 to 8) identifiable on the nipple surface. A 3-D model of the nipple from a mastectomy specimen showed three distinct populations of ducts. The largest lobe was 23% of breast volume. Half the breast was drained by three ducts and 75% by the six largest ducts. Eight small ducts drained about 1.6% of the breast volume. Seven ducts the authors called type A maintained a wide lumen up to the skin surface, 20 ducts (type B) tapered to a minute lumen in the vicinity of the skin on the apex of the nipple, and a minor duct population (type C) arose around the base of the nipple. These distinctions are not distinguishable on microscopic examination except for type C ducts.[12] Using similar 3-D technology, Rusby et al.[33] sought clinical relevance for diagnostic techniques by accessing by cannulation of the ducts. They describe a central duct bundle narrowing to form a "waist" as the ducts enter the breast parenchyma. In a single sample 29 ducts arose from 15 orifices. At skin level, ducts are narrow, becoming larger deeper within the nipple. Many ducts share a few common openings, confirming the apparent discrepancy between number of ducts and number of orifices. Duct diameter does not predict the penetrance of the duct deeper into the breast. Rusby et al.[33] demonstrated that a shared opening of many ducts on the surface of the nipple and the narrow caliber of the ducts closest to the nipple lip changes the clinical interpretation of ductography, ductal lavage, and ductoscopy. In early anatomic studies of the breast, which were done on autopsy specimens, the duct system was identified by pushing dye into the duct under pressure.[6] The duct, being elastic, stretched to suggest ductal sinuses leading to the impression—the ducts had sinuses that collected milk in the areola. This has been shown to be incorrect.[45]

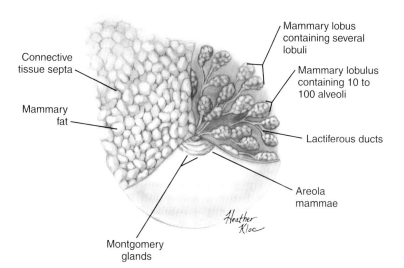

Figure 2-7. Morphology of mature breast with dissection to reveal mammary fat and duct system.

The nipple also contains smooth muscle fibers and is richly innervated with sensory nerve endings and Meissner corpuscles in the dermal papillae; it is well supplied with sebaceous and apocrine sweat glands but no hair.

The nipple is surrounded by the areola, or areola mammae, a circular pigmented area. It is usually faintly darker before pregnancy, becoming reddish brown during pregnancy, and always maintaining some darker pigmentation thereafter. The average areola measures 15 to 16 mm in diameter, although the range is great, enlarging during pregnancy and lactation.[20] The pigmentation results from many melanocytes distributed throughout the skin and glands. The understructure of the epidermis of the areola is not as elaborate as that of the nipple but is intermediate to that of the surrounding skin. The nipple and areola are extremely elastic.

Little or no true lobuloalveolar development occurs before the first pregnancy. A framework is laid down, within which the specialized secretory cells will proliferate (Figure 2-8).[6] The framework forms a vital part of the gland's overall developmental course, and maldevelopment or trauma during fetal or juvenile life can seriously reduce the size and secretory potential of the mature gland.

Montgomery tubercles, containing the ductular openings of sebaceous and lactiferous glands, are present in the areola,[39] as are sweat glands and smaller, free sebaceous glands. The Montgomery glands become enlarged and look like small pimples during pregnancy and lactation (Figure 2-9). They secrete a substance that lubricates and protects the nipples and areolae during pregnancy and lactation. A small amount of milk is also secreted from these tubercles. After lactation, these glands recede again to their former unobtrusive state.

Light microscopy has shown that Morgagni was correct in 1719 when he first described the 12 to 20 areolar glands and noted them to be sebaceous and to include lactiferous structures as well. Building on the original work, in 1837 Montgomery prepared a more detailed treatise on the tubercle itself and named it after himself. Serial sections of 35 tubercles also showed that lactiferous ducts from the deeper breast parenchyma ascended into the sebaceous glands of the tubercle (see Figure 2-9).[39] The sebaceous gland itself was no different from those of the skin or those associated with the terminal lactiferous ducts of the nipple. The mammary duct was lined with two layers of cuboidal to columnar cells. They arose from the underlying mammary lobules through the subcutaneous tissues and into the region of the sebaceous gland. The terminal portion of the mammary duct in some cases joined the duct to the sebaceous gland and in other cases opened separately but close to it. The ducts appear to be a miniature of the major mammary system. Sebaceous and mammary ductal components underlie the areolar tubercle.[20]

The areola and nipple are darker than the rest of the breast, ranging from light pink in fair-skinned

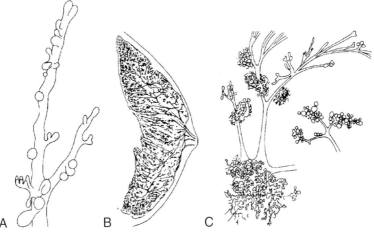

Figure 2-8. A, Duct end from a 15-year-old nulligravida adolescent on second day of menstruation showing typical form of puberty: a coarsely diversified system of thick, mostly well-filled ducts with round, often ball-shaped or half-ball-shaped ends. Note use of connective tissue as guiding tracts, circumvention of fat tissue, and paucity of secretory alveoli. B, Sagittal section through milk gland of a nulligravida 19-year-old woman between menses (died of skull fracture). Note massive body of connective tissue without preserved lobes of fatty tissue and richness of connective tissue with respective richness of parenchyma. Note also the distribution of larger ducts in superficial parallel connective tissue septum of former subcutaneous fat tissue and smaller ducts in vertical septa. Thin section; drawing with Busch magnifying glasses. C, Gland of a nulligravida 19-year-old woman (part of a 4-mm-thick section). Bushy short sprout and duct build long sprout, with the latter in acute angled bifurcation, often lying very close to each other. This demonstrates development of ductal and secretory elements during menstrual cycle; however, connective tissue and fat are predominant. (From Dabelow A: Die Milchdrüse. In *Handbuch der Mikroskopischen Anatomie des Menschen*, vol 3, part 3, Berlin, 1957, Springer-Verlag.)

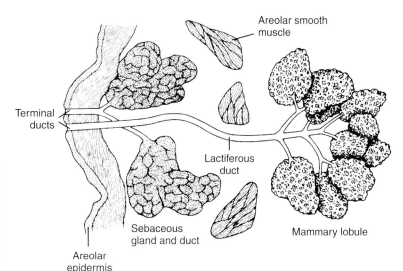

Figure 2-9. Tubercle of Montgomery and underlying structures. Lactiferous duct may join sebaceous gland ducts and terminate at common opening in areolar epidermis as shown. (Modified from Smith DM, Peters TG, Donegan WL: Montgomery's areolar tubercle: a light microscopic study, *Arch Pathol Lab Med* 106:62, 1982.)

women to dark brown in others. The areola's darker color may be a visual signal to newborns so that they will close their mouth on the areola, not on the nipple alone, to obtain milk. Nipple erection is induced by tactile, sensory, and autonomic sympathetic stimuli. The corium (dermis) of the areola lacks fat but contains smooth muscle and collagenous and elastic connective tissue fibers in radial and circular arrangements. The dermis of the nipple and the areola contains many multibranched, free nerve fiber endings. Local venostasis and hyperemia occur to enhance the process of erection of the nipple because the nipple and areola are rich in arteriovenous anastomoses. The glabrous skin of the nipple is wrinkled, containing large papillae of the corium.

Each nipple contains 15 to 25 lactiferous ducts surrounded by fibromuscular tissue[12] (Figures 2-10 through 2-13). This number has often been challenged but was finally confirmed by Taneri et al.[41] and also Rusby et al.[33] to be a mean of 23. These ducts end as small orifices near the tip of the nipple. Within the nipple, the lactiferous ducts may merge. The ductular orifices, therefore, are sometimes fewer in number than the respective breast lobi. The ampullae function as temporary milk containers during a feeding but contain only epithelial debris in the nonlactating state. The use of ultrasound imagery of the contralateral breast while the infant is nursing on the other breast or the other breast is being pumped has shown that the profound elasticity of the ductal system allows for an acute increase in milk duct diameter during let-down and milk production (see Figure 2-10). Contrary to the sketches of the breast in many professional and lay journals, the ducts do not form sinuses just before the nipple.[13] The concept of lactiferous

sinuses was described when postmortem specimens were injected with solidifying liquid under pressure causing a ballooning of the duct. The lining of the infundibular and ampullar parts of the lactiferous ducts consists of an 8- to 10-cell layered squamous epithelium. The bulk of the nipple is composed of smooth musculature, which represents a closing mechanism for the milk ducts of the nipple. The milk ducts in the nipple are embedded in stretchable and mobile connective tissue. The inner longitudinal muscular arrangements and the outer, more circular and radial arrangements do not obstruct the milk

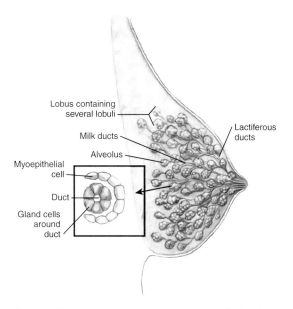

Figure 2-10. Simplified schematic drawing of duct system with cross section of myoepithelial cells around duct opening. Myoepithelial cells contract to eject milk.

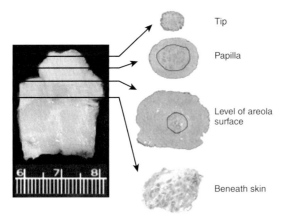

Tip

Papilla

Level of areola surface

Beneath skin

Figure 2-11. Photograph of a sagittal section through a nipple with coronal block sections from a different nipple. The sagittal section illustrates the approximate location of tissue sections. Block sections from a coronally sectioned nipple show differences in morphology with depth. The duct bundle is outlined in black. The beginnings of the waist can be seen at the level of the areola. (From Rushby J, et al: Breast duct anatomy in the human nipple: 3-dimensional patterns and clinical implications, *Breast Cancer Res Treat* 106:171, 2006.)

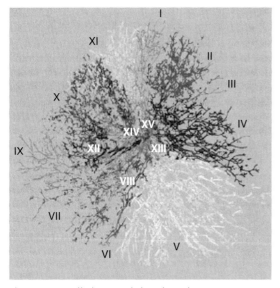

Figure 2-12. All ducts and their branches in an autopsy breast, viewed en face. Each Roman numeral refers to a different independent duct system. (From Going JJ, Moffat DF: Escaping from flatland: clinical and biological aspects of human mammary duct anatomy in three dimensions, *J Pathology* 203:538, 2004.)

ducts. Tangential fibers also branch off from the more circular muscular fibers of the nipple bases to the outer circular muscular range.

The functions of the muscular fibroelastic system of the areola and nipple include decreasing the surface area of the areola, producing nipple erection, and emptying the swollen ducts during

nursing. When the nipple erects because of tactile, thermal, or sexual stimulation, the system causes the nipple to become smaller, firmer, everted, and more prominent.[30]

The mammary tissues are enveloped by the superficial pectoral fascia, and the breast is fixed by fibrous bands to the overlying skin and the underlying pectoral fascia, which are known as ligaments of Cooper. The glandular part of the breast is surrounded by a fat layer that seldom extends beyond the lower border of the pectoralis major muscle. The breast is attached to the muscles between the ribs, the clavicle, and the bones of the upper arm near the shoulder. The breast itself contains no supporting muscles and relies on ligaments to sustain its shape. The measurement of the glandular tissue compared to the amount of intermingling fat tissue has been estimated by Ramsey et al.[31] using ultrasound in 21 lactating white women. The ratio was variable, ranging from 50% to 100% of the breast, proving again that size of the breast does not predict milk production. Ethnicity has little impact on breast size and production but the density of the breast is measurably less in Asian women than white or black women according to work by Chen et al.[4] (Figures 2-14 and 2-15).

Blood Supply

The blood supply to the breast is from branches of the intercostal arteries and the perforating branches of the internal thoracic artery; the third, fourth, and fifth are usually most prominent. The major blood supply to the breast is provided by the internal mammary artery and the lateral thoracic artery. A small supply is obtained from the intercostal arteries and the arterial branches of the axillary and subclavian arteries, but this contribution is minimal; 60% of the total breast tissue, especially the medial and central part, receives blood from the internal mammary artery. All the mammary branches of this artery lead transversely to the nipple and anastomoses, with branches coming from the lateral thoracic artery.[40] Anastomoses with intercostal arteries are less common, but the blood supply to the nipple is extensive and close to the surface, contributing to the richer color. Many areas of the breast are supplied by two or three arterial sources (Figure 2-16).

The venous supply parallels the arterial supply and bears similar names. The veins drain the breast and enter the fascia, muscle layers, and intercostal spaces at the same point. The veins end in the internal thoracic and the axillary veins. Some veins may reach the external jugular vein. The veins create an anastomotic circle around the base of the papilla, called the circulus venosis.[40] Individual variation is common.

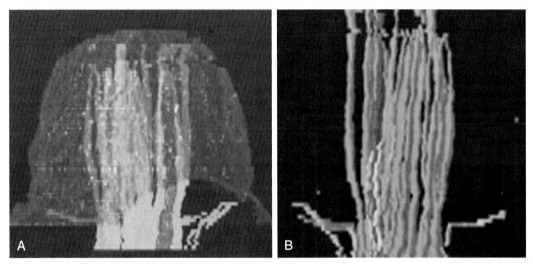

Figure 2-13. Digital model of nipple duct anatomy. **A,** Relationship of nipple duct bundle *(inner fibers)* to skin of the papilla *(outer film).* **B,** Lateral view of duct bundle. Seven ducts of varying caliber extend up to the surface of the nipple (population A); 20 other ducts (population B) diminish in caliber and terminate 0.8 to 1.0 mm beneath the surface, close to skin appendages. Seven accessory ducts (population C) are shown as short fibers at base. (From Going JJ, Moffat DF: Escaping from flatland: clinical and biological aspects of human mammary duct anatomy in three dimensions, *J Pathology* 203:538, 2004.)

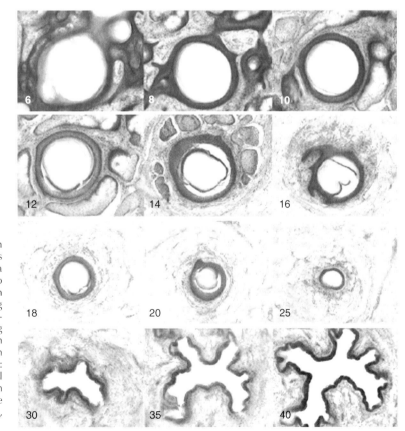

Figure 2-14. A typical "population A" nipple duct: selected sections between 6 and 40. The duct has a wide, funnel-shaped opening onto the surface of the nipple. The lumen tapers moderately before opening out into the characteristically convoluted profile of the collecting ducts in the nipple. The lumen is plugged by keratin in section 20.[17] (From Going JJ, Moffat DF: Escaping from flatland: clinical and biological aspects of human mammary duct anatomy in three dimensions, *J Pathology* 203:544, 2004.)

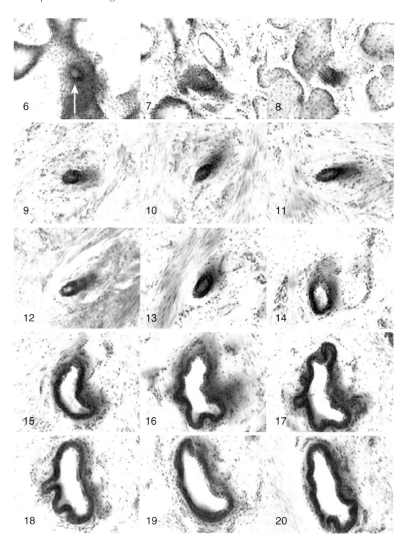

Figure 2-15. A typical "population B" nipple duct: consecutive serial sections from 6 to 20. The duct takes origin from the deep aspect of the nipple epidermis in close proximity to skin appendages *(arrow, section 6, top left)*. It retains a minute lumen over about eight sections (800 μm) before the lumen begins to widen in sections 14 to 20. Such a duct will be difficult to cannulate.

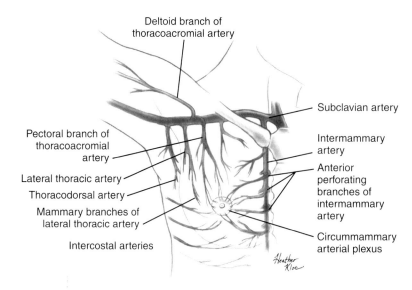

Figure 2-16. Blood supply to mammary gland. Major blood supply is from anterior perforating branches of internal mammary artery.

Lymphatic Drainage

The lymphatic drainage of the breast has been the subject of considerable study because of the frequency of breast cancer, but it has significance for lactating breasts as well. The lymphatic drainage can be extensive. The main drainage is to axillary nodes and to the parasternal nodes along the internal thoracic artery inside the thoracic cavity. The lymphatics of the breast originate in the lymph capillaries of the mammary connective tissue, which surrounds the mammary structures, and drain through the deep substance of the breast. The subepithelial or papillary plexus of the lymphatics of the breast is confluent with the subepithelial lymphatics over the surface of the body. These valveless lymphatics communicate with subdermal lymphatic vessels and merge with the subareolar plexus.[26]

The lymph drainage of the breast consists of the superficial or cutaneous section, the areola, and the glandular or deep-tissue section. More than 75% of the lymph from the breast goes to the axillary nodes. Other points of drainage are to pectoral nodes between the pectoralis major and minor muscles and to the subclavicular nodes in the neck deep to the clavicle. Flow from the deep subcutaneous and intramammary lymphatic vessels travels centrifugally toward the axilla and the internal mammary lymph nodes. The recent physiologic studies have disproved the former hypothesis of centripetal flow toward the subareolar plexus; 97% of lymph flow is into the axillary nodes.[26] Some transmammary lymph drainage occurs to the opposite breast as well as to subdiaphragmatic lymphatics that lead ultimately to the liver and intraabdominal nodes (Figure 2-17). There

has been minimal study of lymphatic drainage of the lactating breast in spite of its importance in engorgement and mastitis.

Innervation

The nerves of the breast are from branches of the fourth, fifth, and sixth intercostal nerves and consist of sensory fibers innervating the smooth muscles in the nipple and blood vessels. The sensory innervation of the nipple and areola is extensive and consists of both autonomic and sensory nerves. A detailed anatomic and clinical study of the nipple-areola complex showed that it is innervated from the lateral cutaneous branch of the fourth intercostal nerve, which penetrates the posterior aspect of the breast at the intersection of the fourth intercostal space and the pectoralis major muscle (4 o'clock on the left breast and 8 o'clock on the right breast).[8] The nerve divides into five fasciculi, one central to the nipple, two upper, and two lower branches (always at 5 and 7 o'clock, left and right side, respectively) (Figures 2-18 and 2-19).

The innervation of the corpus mammae is minimal by comparison and predominantly autonomic. No parasympathetic or cholinergic fibers supply any part of the breast. No ganglia are found in mammary tissue. Norepinephrine-containing nerve fibers are abundant among the smooth muscle cells of the nipple and at the interface between the media and adventitia of the breast arteries. Physiologic observations demonstrate that the efferent nerves to these structures are sympathetic adrenergic.

The majority of the mammary nerves follow the arteries and arterioles and supply these structures. A few fibers from the perivascular networks course

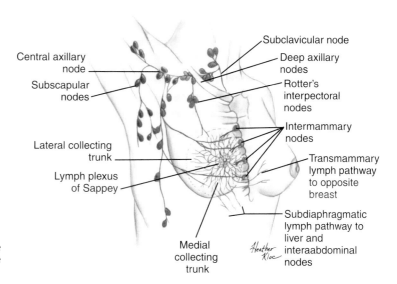

Figure 2-17. Lymphatic drainage of mammary gland. Major drainage is toward axilla.

Central axillary node

Subscapular nodes

Lateral collecting trunk

Lymph plexus of Sappey

Medial collecting trunk

Subclavicular node

Deep axillary nodes

Rotter's interpectoral nodes

Intermammary nodes

Transmammary lymph pathway to opposite breast

Subdiaphragmatic lymph pathway to liver and interaabdominal nodes

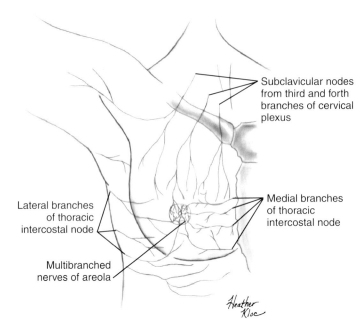

Subclavicular nodes
from third and forth
branches of cervical
plexus

Medial branches
of thoracic
intercostal node

Lateral branches
of thoracic
intercostal node

Multibranched
nerves of areola

Figure 2-18. Innervation of mammary gland. Supraclavicular nerves and lateral and medial branches of intercostal nerves provide sensory innervation. Sympathetic and motor nerves are provided by supracervical and intercostal nerves.

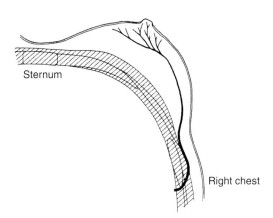

Sternum

Right chest

Figure 2-19. Cross section of nerve supply of breast and nipple. Cutaneous nerves run close to deep fascia before turning outward toward skin.

along the walls of the ducts. They may correspond to sensory fibers for sensing milk pressure. No innervation of mammary myoepithelial cells has been identified. It can, therefore, be concluded that secretory activities of the acinar epithelium depend on hormonal stimulation, such as that of oxytocin and other hormones, and are not stimulated via the nervous system directly. The nipple and areola are reportedly always innervated by the anterior and lateral cutaneous branches of the third to fifth intercostal nerves,[38] which lie along the ducts to the nipple.

Stimulation of the sensory nerve fibers or sensory receptors does induce the release of adenohypophyseal prolactin and neurohypophyseal oxytocin via an afferent sensory reflex pathway whereby stimuli reach the hypothalamus. Sympathetic mammary stimulation causes the contraction of the small myoepithelial cells of the areola and the nipple. The locally released norepinephrine induces stimulation of the myoepithelial adrenergic receptors, causing muscular relaxation. In the absence of parasympathetic activity, a minor physiologic catecholamine inhibitory effect on the mammary myoepithelium may exist. This is overcome by oxytocin release during suckling, inducing myoepithelial contraction.

The supraclavicular nerves supply the sensory fibers for innervation of the upper cutaneous parts of the breast. Branches of the intercostal nerves provide the major sensory innervation of the mammary gland. The sympathetic sensory and motor fibers are derived from the supraclavicular and intercostal nerves, respectively. Sympathetic fibers run only along the mammary gland—supplying arteries to innervate the glandular body. There is relatively restricted innervation to the epidermal parts of the nipple and areola, leading to lack of superficial sensory acuity.

Courtiss and Goldwyn[5] measured breast sensation in a large number of women using a device that emitted a variable current producing a burning sensation when the threshold was exceeded. The areola was shown to be the most sensitive and the nipple the least sensitive, with the skin of the breast intermediate. The nipple and areola are sparsely innervated with neural elements at the base of the nipple and almost none in the areola.[10] A study of lactating women showed marked increase in areola and nipple sensitivity within 24 hours of birth.[29]

After 1 to 6 months of breastfeeding, women were noted to have minimal two-point discrimination of the skin of the breast.[10] Thus the skin in these areas responds only to major stimuli, such as sucking. The relatively large number of dermal nerve endings provides a high mammary responsiveness toward stimuli for elicitation of the sucking reflex. The neuroreflex induces adequate release of both prolactin and oxytocin. It appears that, in addition to the hormonal actions, breast nerves can also influence the mammary blood supply and milk secretion. Abnormalities of sensory or autonomic nerve distributions in the areola and nipple, therefore, could impair adequate lactation, especially in the functioning of the let-down reflex and the secretion of prolactin and oxytocin.

In summary, the somatic sensory cutaneous nerve supply of the breast includes the supraclavicular nerves and the thoracic intercostal nerves. The autonomic motor nerve supply of the breast is derived from the sympathetic fibers of the intercostal nerves, which supply the smooth musculature of the areola and the nipple. The autonomic supply is also derived from sympathetic fibers of the accompanying arteries, which innervate the smooth musculature of the inner glandular blood vessel walls to produce constriction. The nerve supply to the area of the areola and the nipple includes free sensory nerve endings, tactile corpuscles to the papillae of the corium of the nipple and areola, and the fibers around the larger lactiferous duct and in the dermis of the areola and peripheral breast. All cutaneous nerves run radially to the glandular body toward the nipple. The nerve supply to the inner gland is sparse and contains only sympathetic nerves accompanying blood vessels (see Figure 2-19). Twenty-four hours postpartum, the nipple and areola sensitivity is markedly heightened but decreases in the next few days. The skin of the breast, areola, and nipple showed reduced two-point discrimination when lactation is well established. Clinical evidence supports the observation of limited nerve distribution in the breast.[14]

Microscopic Anatomy

After many decades of neglect since the phylogenic studies of the mammary gland in the 1800s and early 1900s, the mammary gland has become one of the most studied organs because of its usefulness as a tool in developmental biology, biochemistry, endocrinology and biology, histology, oncology, toxicology, virology, and molecular biology.[37] No cell can exist independent of its surrounding cells. All cells have relations with neighboring cells and with cells at distant sites. The interactions of the epithelial parenchyma and mesenchymal stroma are most important in primary and secondary induction in organogenesis. The microstructure of nonlactating mature breasts varies with age, the phase of the menstrual cycle, pregnancy, and lactation. The ducts are lined with columnar epithelium of two cells thick in larger ducts and single layers in the smaller ones. Myoepithelial cells are numerous, creating a distinct layer around ducts and potential alveola.[37]

The mammary gland consists of a branching system of excretory ducts embedded in connective tissue.[11] The gland is composed of two layers of epithelial cells: luminal epithelium and basal layer epithelium, along with a few basal (stem) cells. The whole structure is surrounded by a basement membrane. In the ducts, elongated myoepithelial cells make up a continuous sheath. The luminal cell interaction with the extracellular matrix is mediated by the myoepithelium.

The integrity of the normal mammary gland is maintained by several adhesion systems.[11] The mammary gland is composed of epithelial parenchyma and two types of mesenchymal stroma: dense mammary mesenchyma and fatty stroma. The dense mammary mesenchyma is present in the embryonic stage, in end buds of puberty, and in cancers. It determines mammary epithelium and fixes the ability of the epithelium to interact with the fatty stroma. The fatty stroma is essential for typical mammary gland morphogenesis.[37]

The two types of mammary stroma synthesize different extracellular matrix proteins. Dense mesenchyma makes fibronectin and tenascin. Fatty stroma makes laminin, proteoglycans, and fibronectin.

In their structure and mode of development, the mammary glands somewhat resemble the sweat glands.[9] During embryonic life, their differentiation is similar in the two sexes. Male humans experience little additional development postnatally. Female humans, in contrast, experience extensive structural change paralleling age and the functional state of the reproductive system.

Vogel et al.[45] studied histologic changes in the normal human mammary gland in association with the menstrual cycle. They describe five phases: proliferative (days 3 to 7), follicular phase of differentiation (days 8 to 14), luteal phase of differentiation (days 15 to 20), secretory (days 21 to 27), and menstrual (days 28 to 2). Table 2-4 outlines the morphologic criteria for these phases. These findings illustrate the correlation of morphologic response to hormonal stimulus of the mammary gland during normal cycling.

The greatest development in girls is reached by the twentieth year. Gradual changes are correlated with the menstrual cycle, and major changes

TABLE 2-4 Morphologic Criteria for Phase Assignment in Menstrual Cycle

Phase	Stroma	Lumen	Cell Types	Epithelium			Active Secretion
				Orientation of Epithelial Cells	Mitoses		
Phase I (days 3-7)	Dense, cellular	Tight	Single predominant pale eosinophilic cell	No stratification apparent	Present, average 4/10 HPF		None
Phase II (days 8-14)	Dense, cellular-collagenous	Defined	1. Luminal columnar basophilic cell 2. Intermediate pale cell 3. Basal clear cell with hyperchromatic nucleus (myoepithelial)	Radial around lumen	Rare		None
Phase III (days 15-20)	Loose, broken	Open with some secretion	1. Luminal basophilic cell 2. Intermediate pale cell 3. Prominent vacuolization of basal clear cell (myoepithelial)	Radial around lumen	Absent		None
Phase IV (days 21-27)	Loose, edematous	Open with secretion	1. Luminal basophilic cell 2. Intermediate pale cell 3. Prominent vacuolization of basal clear cell (myoepithelial)	Radial around lumen	Absent		Active apocrine secretion from luminal cell
Phase V (days 28-2)	Dense, cellular	Distended with secretion	1. Luminal basophilic cell with scant cytoplasm 2. Extensive vacuolization of basal cells	Radial around lumen	Absent		Rare

HPF, High-powered field.
Modified from Vogel PM, Georgiade NG, Fetter BF, et al.: The correlation of histologic changes in the human breast with the menstrual cycle, *Am J Pathol* 104:23, 1981.

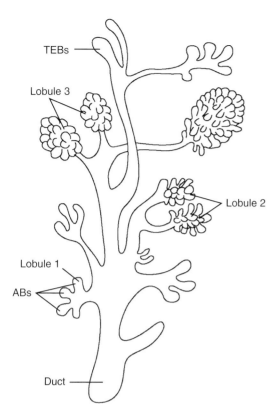

TEBs

Lobule 3

Lobule 2

Lobule 1

ABs

Duct

Figure 2-20. Schematic representation depicting various topographic compartments of human mammary gland: terminal end buds (TEBs); alveolar buds (ABs); lobules types 1, 2, and 3; and ducts. (Modified from Russo J, Russo IH: Development of human mammary gland. In Neville MC, Daniel CW, editors: *The mammary gland*. New York, 1987, Plenum.)

accompany pregnancy and lactation[34,36] (see Figure 2-8).

Russo and Russo[35] describe the development of the mammary gland as "an asynchronous process of progressive invasion of the mammary stroma by a parenchyma composed of ductal elements in which the advancing ends are the club-shaped terminal end buds (TEBs) that progressively differentiate into alveolar buds (ABs) or regress to terminal ducts (TDs)" (Figure 2-20).

Mature Mammary Gland

The mammary gland is a compound tubuloalveolar gland containing 15 to 25 irregular lobes radiating from the nipple. Each lobe has a lactiferous duct (2 to 4 mm in diameter) lined by stratified squamous epithelium. The duct opens on the nipple and has an irregular angular outline. Beneath the areola, each duct finally emerges at the end of the nipple as a 0.4- to 0.7-mm opening. Each lobe is subdivided into lobules of various orders; the smallest are

elongated tubules, the alveolar ducts, covered by small saccular evaginations, the alveoli. The interlobular connective tissue is dense; however, it is more cellular, has fewer collagenous fibers, and contains almost no fat. Greater distensibility is permitted by the looser connective tissue.

The ducts and ductules of mature women consist chiefly of two cell types: the inner lining of epithelial cells and the outer lining of myoepithelial cells. A basement membrane separates these structures from the stroma. Histochemical and immunocytochemical reagents can distinguish these elements, their positions, and their infrastructures. Rudland[32] has reported on the histochemical organization and cellular composition of ductal buds in the developing human breast. This work suggests that cytochemical intermediates occur between epithelial and myoepithelial cells. The undifferentiated peripheral cap cells may be transitional forms of the cortical epithelial cells that will line the lumina and of the myoepithelial cells of the subtending duct.

Transforming growth factors (TGF-β1, 2, and 3) are potent inhibitors of cell proliferation but play an important role in mammary gland development. They exhibit overlapping patterns of expression within the epithelium of the developing gland. TGF-β3 is detected in the myoepithelial progenitor cells of the growing end buds and the myoepithelial cells in the mature duct.[28]

The secretory portions of the gland, the alveolar ducts and the alveoli, have cuboidal or low-columnar secretory cells, resting on basal laminae and myoepithelial cells. These myoepithelial cells enclose the alveoli in a loosely meshed network with their many starlike branchings. The myoepithelial cells are stimulated by oxytocin and sex steroids. The presence of myoepithelial cells has been used as evidence that the mammary gland is related to the sweat gland.

In the at rest phase, epithelial structures consist of the ducts and their branches. The presence of a few alveoli budding from the ends of ducts is still under investigation. This variance may be caused by the effect of the menstrual cycle. The swelling and engorgement accompanying the menstrual cycle are associated with hyperemia and some edema of the connective tissue. Most significant is that the gland does not have a single duct but many. Each lobe is a separate compound alveolar gland in which primary ducts join into larger and larger ducts. These ducts drain into a lactiferous duct. Each lactiferous duct drains separately at the tip of the nipple.

The epidermis of the nipple and areola is invaded by unusually long dermal papillae in which capillaries richly vascularize the surface and impact the richer hue. Bundles of smooth muscle, placed longitudinally along the lactiferous ducts and circumferentially within the nipple and at its base, permit the erection of the nipple. In the areola are the areolar Montgomery glands, which are intermediate in their microscopic structure between sweat glands and true mammary glands. The periphery of the areola also has sweat glands and sebaceous glands (see Figure 2-9).

Mammary Gland in Pregnancy

Although mini-remodeling of the breast occurs at each menstrual cycle, it is not until pregnancy that complete remodeling occurs. It is transformed into a mature functional organ. The MaSC population is activated by the ovarian hormonal circuit. The levels of estrogen, progesterone, and prolactin are increased. Other hormones and growth factors regulate the mammary expansion.

The first 3 to 4 weeks of pregnancy has marked ductular sprouting with some branching and lobular formation, stimulated by estrogenic release. By 5 to 8 weeks, the breast changes are physically notable with dilation of the superficial veins, heaviness, and increased pigmentation of the nipple and areola. Changes in levels of circulating hormones result in profound changes in the ductular-lobular-alveolar growth during pregnancy (Figure 2-21). During the first trimester, growth and branching from the terminal portion of the duct system into the adipose tissue is rapid.[43] As the epithelial structures proliferate, the adipose tissue seems to diminish. During this time, increasing infiltration of the interstitial tissue

occurs with lymphocytes, plasma cells, and eosinophils. The rate of hyperplasia levels off. In the last trimester, any enlargement is the result of parenchymal cell growth and distention of the alveoli with early colostrum, which is rich in protein and relatively low in lipid. Fat droplets gradually accumulate in the secretory alveolar cells. The interlobular connective tissue is noticeably decreased, and alveolar proliferation is extensive. In experimental studies, these effects can be duplicated when estrogen and progesterone stimulate a release of prolactin-inhibiting factor (PIF). Prolactin is released in humans during pregnancy, thus stimulating epithelial growth and secretion. Prolactin levels increase over time during pregnancy.

Pregnancy induced changes are important clinical observations usually completed by 22 weeks. The size varies markedly. Although important, breast size during pregnancy is not an accurate indicator of lactation potential. The lactation potential of women who deliver prematurely may be diminished and result in delayed secretory initiation.

The histologic appearance of the gland varies. The functional state appears to vary from dilated, thin-walled lumen to narrow-lumened, thick-walled glandular tissue. Epithelial cells vary, being flat to low columnar in shape with indistinct boundaries. Some cells protrude into the lumen of the alveoli; others are short and smooth. The lumen of the alveolus is crowded with fine granular material and lipid droplets similar to those protruding from the cells. The mammary alveoli but not the

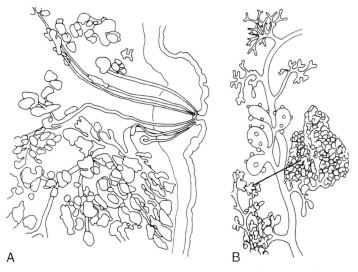

A   B

Figure 2-21. **A,** Milk gland of 21-year-old primigravida woman in second month of pregnancy. Development of small lobes has protruded almost to mammilla. Very regular development is shown over whole range of this thick section. Natural dimensions: 2.6 × 2.1 cm. **B,** Milk gland of same 21-year-old primigravida woman. Note very different forms of sprouting. Partly atypical sprouts above diagonal line are composed from same section; bifurcations below line are in natural position. Alveoli are beginning to resemble mature gland. (From Dabelow A: Die Milchdrüse. In *Handbuch der Mikroskopischen Anatomie des Menschen*, vol 3, part 3, Berlin, 1957, Springer-Verlag.)

milk ducts lose the superficial layer of cells in the second trimester. The monolayer differentiates into a cell layer that accumulates eosinophilic cells, plasma cells, and leukocytes around the alveoli. Lymphocytes, round cells, and desquamated phagocytic alveolar cells are also found in the lumen. The resting breast consists of ductal epithelial tissue with a fibrous stroma. The duct wall is lined with layers of epithelial cells. The inner layer encapsulates the ductal lumen, which is made up of cuboidal epithelial cells, some of which can actually further differentiate into milk secretory cells (lactocytes) during lactation. The outer layer, or basal layer, is made up of contractile myoepithelial cells that encircle the luminal layer and behave like smooth muscle cells (see Figure 2-21). The basal layer lies on the basement membrane and is believed to contain MaSCs.

More recent studies have identified stem cells in the breast that are related to the breast's ability to expand and regress repeatedly throughout adult life. The presence of self-renewing bipotent MaSCs as well as unipotent progenitors have been identified in the resting epithelium. Most of the observations have been made in mice whose mammary stroma differ. Human mammary stroma is highly dense fibrous connective tissue which embeds in the adipose tissue. The intralobular stroma consists of mesenchymal cells. These cells are very responsive to the hormonal microenvironmental cues. They initiate and promote the various stages of mammary development as they interact with the mammary epithelium. The cellular hierarchy of the lactating breast is found in the milk itself. It includes early stage stem cells and more differentiated myoepithelial and milk secreting cells.

By the end of pregnancy, lobular, highly branched epithelial tissue separated by some fibrous stroma is the predominant structure. Secretory differentiation has occurred in some luminal cells of the alveoli. Fat globules are visible with the cells, and alveoli are formed at the end of the duct termini, which contain the lactocytes. The lactocyte is a cuboidal polarized cell. Polarization promotes the movement of milk toward the lumen. The milk moves through the duct containing the biochemical factors secreted by lactocytes and some cells from the epithelium.

Lactating Mammary Gland

The lactating mammary gland is characterized by a large number of alveoli (Figure 2-22). The alveoli of the lactating gland are made up of cuboidal epithelial and myoepithelial cells.[34] Only a small amount of connective tissue separates the neighboring alveoli. Under special preparations, lipid can be seen as

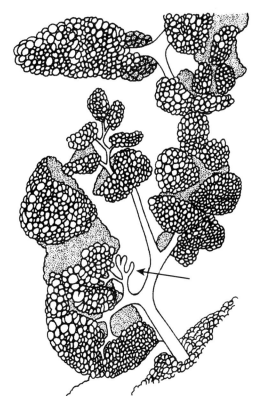

Figure 2-22. Part of a mammary gland with significant milk obstruction in a 26-year-old woman who died from food poisoning after ingesting spoiled fish 3 weeks postpartum and who had not breastfed for 48 hours before death. In upper half, formed duct and lobes are located on alternating sides. This form results from different development of two parts of a dichotomized bifurcation: one takes over production of small lobes, while the other continues the stem. Thick section; very primitive, undeveloped sprouts (arrow). (From Dabelow A: Die Milchdrüse. In *Handbuch der Mikroskopischen Anatomie des Menschen*, vol 3, part 3, Berlin, 1957, Springer-Verlag.)

small droplets within the cells. These droplets become larger and are discharged into the lumen.

The functioning of the mammary gland depends on the interplay of multiple and complex nervous system and endocrine factors.[44] Some factors are involved in the development of the mammary glands to a functional state (mammogenesis), others in the establishment of milk secretion (lactogenesis), and others in the maintenance of lactation (galactopoiesis).[43]

The division and differentiation of mammary epithelial cells and presecretory alveolar cells into secretory milk-releasing alveolar cells take place in the third trimester. Stimulation of ribonucleic acid (RNA) synthesis promotes galactopoiesis and apocrine milk secretion into the alveoli. The deoxyribonucleic acid (DNA) and RNA content of the cellular nuclei increases during pregnancy and is highest at lactation (see Figure 2-3).

The former concepts of mammary gland secretion indicated that the mode of release was apocrine secretion. Apocrine secretion is the process by which the cell undergoes partial disintegration. A fat-filled portion projects into the lumen; the fat globule constricts at the base; and the cell replaces itself. Electron microscopy has shown that the cell has two distinct secretory products, formed and released by different mechanisms. The protein constituents of milk are formed and released identically to those of other protein-secreting glands, classified as merocrine glands. Secretory materials are passed out through the cell apex without appreciable loss of cytoplasm in merocrine glands.

The fatty components of milk arise as lipid droplets free in the cytoplasmic matrix. The droplets increase in size and move into the apex of the cell. They project into the lumen, covered by a thin layer of cytoplasm. The droplets are ultimately cast off, enveloped by a detached portion of the cell membrane and a thin rim of subjacent cytoplasm (see Figure 2-3 and Chapter 3 for further discussion).

The ultrastructure of the human mammary gland during lactogenesis was studied by Tobon and Salazar,[43] who reviewed surgical specimens from seven lactating women 1 day to 5½ months postpartum. They noted widespread hypertrophy and hyperplasia of the acini accompanied by dilatation and engorgement of the lumen by milk. The vascular channels were engorged. The lactogenic epithelial cells had rich cytoplasm, prominent layers of reticulum, and enlarged oval mitochondria. The Golgi apparatus was hypertrophied. The myoepithelium was stretched and thinned to contain the filled acini.

The ratio of glandular tissue to fat tissue changes during lactation from a 1:1 ration in the nonlactating breast to 2:1 during lactation.

The least well studied and, therefore, understood is the adipose cell, which has been recognized as important by Geddes.[10] Adipocytes have been observed to be transformed into lactocytes during pregnancy by Morroni et al.[22] using the mouse model. They then returned to adipocytes during the involuntary phase. Breast milk contains a cellular hierarchy from early stage stem cells with embryonic-like features and multilineage differentiation potential to MaSCs from the resting breasts, cells with progenitor characteristics to the mature myoepithelial and milk secreting cells (see Figure 2-3 and Chapter 3 for further discussion).

Not all alveoli are at the same development stage; there are some nonfunctioning ducts at any given time during lactation. The signaling cascade that influences alveoli is development and differentiation patterns between different lobules. The role of vascularization may be significant in the functional heterogeneity of the lactating breast.

Postlactation Regression of Mammary Gland

If milk is not removed from the breast, the glands become greatly distended and milk production gradually ceases. Part of the decrease results from the lack of stimulation of sucking, which initiates the neurohormonal reflex for maintenance of prolactin secretion. Perhaps a stronger effect is the engorgement of the breast with compression of blood vessels, causing diminished flow. The diminished blood flow results in decreased oxytocin to the myoepithelium. The alveoli are greatly distended and the epithelium flattened. The secretion remaining in the alveolar spaces and ducts is absorbed. The alveoli gradually collapse, with an increase in perialveolar connective tissue. The glandular elements gradually return to the at rest state. Adipose tissue and macrophages increase. The gland does not return completely to the prepregnancy state in that the alveoli formed do not totally involute. Some appear as scattered, solid cords of epithelial cells.

Microscopically, increased autophagic and heterophagic processes occur in the first few days after weaning. Lysosomal enzymes increase, whereas nonlysosomal enzymes decrease. The gland undergoes alveolar epithelium apoptosis and remodeling, reverting back to the prepregnant state with the loss of prolactin.

Although the process of regression has been studied carefully in animals, little study has been done in humans. Slow weaning, which usually takes 3 months, probably has a very different timetable from abrupt weaning, in which marked involution has been intense and rapid over days or weeks. At the conclusion of weaning or involution the breast returns to a resting or nonlactating state. The structure and morphology is not the same as it was in the nulliparous stage. Some lobular structures remain in the parous gland. Some partially differentiated epithelial cells escape the involution and act as "memory precursor cells" in the next pregnancy. The cell types that actually phagocytose the apoptotic epithelial cells are still unsettled (nonhuman research on the subject varies). Apoptotic cells may be phagocytosed by neighboring nonhematopoietic cells. The mechanisms through which involution is initiated and the gene networks involved remain under investigation.

REFERENCES

1. Adler DD, Rebner M, Pennes DR: Accessory breast tissue in the axilla: mammographic appearance, *Radiology* 163:709, 1987.
2. Anbazhagan R, Bartek P, Monaghan P, et al: Growth and development of the human infant breast, *Am J Anat* 192:407, 1991.

3. Bland KI, Romnell LJ: Congenital and acquired disturbances of breast development and growth. In Bland KI, Copeland EM III, editors: *The breast: comprehensive management of benign and malignant diseases*, Philadelphia, Pa., 1991, WB Saunders.
4. Chen Z, Wu AH, Gaudermann WJ, et al: Does mammographic density reflect ethnic differences in breast cancer incidence rates? *Am J Epidemiol* 159:140–147, 2004.
5. Courtiss EH, Goldwyn RM: Breast sensation before and after plastic surgery, *Plast Reconstr Surg* 58:1, 1976.
6. Dabelow A: Die Milchdrüse. In *Handbuch der Mikroskopischen Anatomie des Menschen*, vol III, part 3, Berlin, 1957, Springer-Verlag.
7. Egan RL: Breast embryology, anatomy, and physiology. In *Breast imaging: diagnosis and morphology of breast diseases*, Philadelphia, Pa., 1988, WB Saunders.
8. Farina MA, Newby BG, Alani HM: Innervation of the nipple-areolar complex, *Plast Reconstr Surg* 66:497, 1980.
9. Fawcett DW: *Bloom and Fawcett: a textbook on histology*, ed 11, Philadelphia, Pa., 1986, WB Saunders.
10. Geddes DT: Gross anatomy of the lactating breast. In Hale TW, Hartmann PE, editors: *Textbook of human lactation*, Amarillo, Tex., 2007, Hale Publishing.
11. Glukhova M, Koteliansky V, Sastre X, et al: Adhesion systems in normal breast and in invasive breast carcinoma, *Am J Pathol* 146:706, 1995.
12. Going JJ, Moffat D: Escaping from flatland: clinical and biological aspects of human mammary duct anatomy in three dimensions, *J Pathol* 203:538–544, 2004.
13. Hartmann PE, Cregan MD, Ramsay DT, et al: Physiology of lactation in preterm mothers: initiation and maintenance, *Pediatr Ann* 32:351, 2003.
14. Hassiotou F, Geddes D: Anatomy of the human mammary gland: current status of knowledge, *Clin Anat* 26:29–48, 2013.
15. Hersh JH, Bloom AS, Cromer AO, et al: Does a supernumerary nipple/renal field defect exist? *Am J Dis Child* 141:989, 1987.
16. Kaye BL: Axillary breasts: a significant esthetic deformity, *Plast Reconstr Surg* 53:61, 1974.
17. Knight CH, Peaker M: Development of the mammary gland: symposium report no 19. *J Reprod Fertil* 65:521, 1982.
18. Kreipe RE: Normal somatic adolescent growth and development, *J Pediatr* 83:1, 1973.
19. Larson BL, editor: *Lactation*, Ames, 1985, Iowa State University Press.
20. Love SM, Barsky SH: Anatomy of the nipple and breast ducts revisited, *Cancer* 104:947, 2004.
21. Montagna W, Macpherson EE: Some neglected aspects of the anatomy of human breasts, *J Invest Dermatol* 63:10, 1974.
22. Morroni M, Giordano A, Zingarett MC, et al: Reversible transdifferentiation of secretory epithelial cells into adipocytes in the mammary gland, *Proc Natl Acad Sci U S A* 101:16801–16806, 2004.
23. Netter FH: *Atlas of human anatomy*, Summit, N.J., 1990, Ciba-Geigy.
24. Neville MC: Breastfeeding. Part I: the evidence for breastfeeding. Anatomy and physiology of lactation, *Pediatr Clin North Am* 48:13, 2001.
25. Nickell WB, Skelton J: Breast fat and fallacies: more than 100 years of anatomical fantasy, *J Hum Lact* 21 (2):126–130, 2005.
26. Osbourne MP: Breast development and anatomy. In Harris JR, Lippman ME, Morrow M, Hellman S, editors: *Diseases of the breast*, Philadelphia, Pa., 1996, Lippincott-Raven.
27. Pellegrin JR, Wagner RF Jr: Polythelia and associated conditions, *Am Fam Physician* 28:129, 1983.
28. Pierce DF Jr, Johnson MD, Matsui Y, et al: Inhibition of mammary duct development but not alveolar outgrowth during pregnancy in transgenic mice expressing active TGF-b1, *Genes Dev* 7:2308, 1993.
29. Rahbar F: Clinical significance of supernumerary nipples in black neonates, *Clin Pediatr* 21:46, 1983.
30. Ramsey DT, Kent JC, Owens RA, et al: Ultrasound imaging of the milk ejection in the breast of the lactating women, *Pediatrics* 113:361–367, 2004.
31. Ramsey DT, Kent JC, Hartman RL, et al: Anatomy of the lactating human breast redefined with ultrasound Imaging, *J Anat* 206:525–534, 2005.
32. Rudland PS: Histochemical organization and cellular composition of ductal buds in developing human breast: evidence of cytochemical intermediates between epithelial and myoepithelial cells, *J Histochem Cytochem* 39:1471, 1991.
33. Rusby JE, Brachtel EF, Michaelson JS, et al: Breast duct anatomy in the human nipple: three-dimensional patterns and clinical implications, *Breast Cancer Res Treat* 106:171, 2007.
34. Russo J, Russo IH: Development of human mammary gland. In Neville MC, Daniel CW, editors: *The mammary gland*, New York, N.Y., 1987, Plenum.
35. Russo IH, Russo J: Progestagens and mammary gland development: differentiation versus carcinogenesis, *Acta Endocrinol* 125:7, 1991.
36. Russo J, Russo IH: *Molecular basis of breast cancer prevention and treatment*, New York, 2004, Springer.
37. Sakakura T: New aspects of stroma-parenchyma relations in mammary gland differentiation, *Int Rev Cytol* 125:165, 1991.
38. Schlenz I, Kuzbarir R, Gruber H, et al: The sensitivity of the nipple-areola complex: an anatomic study, *Plast Reconstr Surg* 105:905–909, 2000.
39. Smith DM, Peters TG, Donegan WL: Montgomery's areolar tubercle, *Arch Pathol Lab Med* 106:60, 1982.
40. Standrings S: Chestwall and breast, *Gray's anatomy*, ed 40, London, 2008, Churchill Livingstone.
41. Taneri F, Kurukahvecioglu O, Akyurek N, et al: Microanatomy of milk ducts in the nipple, *Eur Surg Res* 38:545–549, 2006.
42. Tanner JM: *Wachstun und Reifung des Menschen*, Stuttgart, 1962, Thieme-Verlag.
43. Tobon H, Salazar H: Ultrastructure of the human mammary gland. I. Development of the fetal gland throughout gestation, *J Clin Endocrinol Metab* 39:443, 1974.
44. Tobon H, Salazar H: Ultrastructure of the human mammary gland. II. Postpartum lactogenesis, *J Clin Endocrinol Metab* 40:834, 1975.
45. Vogel PM, Georgiade NG, Fetter BF, et al: The correlation of histologic changes in the human breast with the menstrual cycle, *Am J Pathol* 104:23, 1981.
46. Vorherr H: *The breast: morphology, physiology, and lactation*, New York, N.Y., 1974, Academic Press.
47. Weatherly-White RCA: *Plastic surgery of the female breast*, Hagerstown, Md., 1980, Harper & Row.

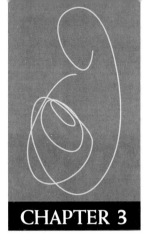

CHAPTER 3

Physiology of Lactation

|||||||||||||||||||||||||||||||||||||||||||||||||||||||||||||||||||||

Lactation is the physiologic completion of the reproductive cycle.[*,23,53,62,63,66,103] Human infants at birth are the most immature and dependent of all mammals, except for marsupials. The marsupial joey is promptly attached to the teat of a mammary gland in an external pouch. The gland changes as the offspring develops, and the joey remains there until able to survive outside the pouch. In humans, throughout pregnancy the breast develops and prepares to take over the role of fully nourishing the infant when the placenta is expelled.

There are two stages in the initiation of lactation: secretory differentiation and secretory activation. Pang and Hartman[66] said it best: "Secretory differentiation represents the stage of pregnancy when the mammary epithelial cells differentiate into lactocytes with the capacity to synthesize unique milk constituents such as lactose." They further explain that this requires the presence of a "lactogenic hormone complex." This complex of reproductive hormones includes estrogen, progesterone, prolactin, and some other metabolic hormones. Secretory activation, they note, is the initiation of copious milk secretion associated with major changes in the concentrations of many milk constituents. With the withdrawal of progesterone, secretory activation is triggered. This requires prolactin as well as insulin and cortisol.

The breast is prepared for full lactation from 16 weeks' gestation without any active intervention from the mother. It is kept inactive by a balance of inhibiting hormones that suppress target cell response. In the first few hours and days postpartum, the breast responds to changes in the hormonal milieu and to the stimulus of the newborn infant's suckling to produce and release milk.[50,59,61,63] The existence of mammary stem cells has been speculated because the mammary gland has been regenerated by transplanting epithelial fragments in mice.

Transplanted cells contributed to both luminal and myoepithelial lineages. From these were generated functional lobuloalveolar units during pregnancy. The cells had self-renewing properties. The serial transplantations of Shackleton et al.[78] have established that single cells are multipotent and self-renewing and can generate a functional mammary gland. The potential for further understanding of the mammary gland is unlimited.

The energy expenditure during lactation has suggested an efficiency of human milk synthesis greater than the 80% value previously hypothesized by investigators. From work in Gambian women and extensive review of other studies, Frigerio et al.[25] suggest that the energy cost of human lactation is minimal and the process functions at 95% efficiency.

This chapter provides a review of the physiologic adaptation of the mammary gland to its role in infant survival. Several major reviews that include substantial bibliographies for readers who need the detailed reports of the original investigators are referenced. Newer scientific techniques in the study of human lactation provide more precise, more detailed, and more integrated data on which the clinician can base a physiologic approach to lactation management.

Box 3-1 lists the abbreviations for the hormones that are involved in lactation and are discussed in this chapter.[*]

Apoptosis in the Mammary Gland

Epithelial apoptosis has a key role in the development and function of the mammary gland. It begins with the formation of the ducts in the embryonic

---

[*]13,14,16,44,54,92

BOX 3-1. Hormone Abbreviations

Adrenocorticotropic hormone	ACTH
Epidermal growth factor	EGF
Feedback inhibitor of lactation	FIL
Follicle-stimulating hormone	FSH
Growth hormone (human growth hormone)	GH (hGH)
Heregulin	HER
Human growth factor	hGF, HGF
Human placental lactogen	hPL
Insulin-like growth factor-1	IGF-1
Prolactin	PRL
Prolactin-inhibiting factor	PIF
Thyroid-stimulating hormone	TSH
Thyrotropin-releasing hormone	TRH
Transforming growth factor beta	TGF-β

phase and occurs again at puberty and with a stage of menses. Regulated apoptosis occurs at several stages of mammary development. In the embryo, epithelial buds emerge from ectoderm into mammary mesenchyme, which is the origin of the ductal tree. When the ducts later hollow out in puberty, extensive apoptosis occurs within the terminal bud.[27]

Deregulated apoptosis contributes to the malignant progression in the genesis of breast cancer. Research in apoptosis continues because it may lead to new cancer treatments, but the knowledge itself will be valuable.

When suckling ceases during weaning, the alveolar component of the gland involutes by both apoptosis and tissue remodeling, which rebuilds the gland to the prepregnancy state.

Much is being learned about mammary development and function through the intense study of the breast as an experimental system. The use of novel "knockout" mouse models has been employed to study nursing failure. The apoptosis control mechanism from the angle of the signaling pathways has been studied. Further work at the level of the cell is underway, including extensive genetic analysis.[27]

Hormonal Control of Lactation

In contrast to most organs, which are fully developed at birth, the mammary gland undergoes most of its morphogenesis postnatally, in adolescence, and in adulthood.[57] Lactation is an integral part of the reproductive cycle of all mammals, including humans. The hormonal control of lactation can be described in relation to the five major stages in the development of the mammary gland: (1) embryogenesis; (2) mammogenesis, or mammary growth; (3) lactogenesis, or initiation of milk secretion; (4) lactation (stage III lactogenesis), or full milk secretion; and (5) involution (Table 3-1).[57]

Current terminology divides lactogenesis into two stages.[32] Stage I takes place during pregnancy when the gland is sufficiently developed to actually produce milk. It begins about midpregnancy (approximately 16 weeks). It can be identified by measuring the levels of plasma lactose and α-lactalbumin.[2] Should the mother deliver at this point, milk would be produced. Some mothers can express

TABLE 3-1   Stages of Mammary Development*

Developmental Stage	Hormonal Regulation	Local Factors	Description
Embryogenesis	?	Fat pad necessary for ductal extension	Epithelial bud develops in 18- to-19-week-old fetus, extending short distance into mammary fat pad with blind ducts that become canalized; some milk secretion may be present at birth
Puberty Before onset of menses After onset of menses Mammogenesis	Estrogen, GH Estrogen, progesterone ? PRL	IGF-1, hGF, TGF-β, ? others	Ductal extension into mammary pad; branching morphogenesis Lobular development with formation of terminal duct lobular unit (TDLU) Anatomic development
Pregnancy	Progesterone, PRL, hPL	HER, ? others	Alveolus formation; partial cellular differentiation
Lactogenesis	Progesterone withdrawal, PRL, glucocorticoid	Not known	Onset of milk secretion Stage I: midpregnancy Stage II: parturition
Lactation	PRL, oxytocin	FIL	Ongoing milk secretion
Involution	PRL withdrawal	Milk stasis, ? FIL	Alveolar epithelium undergoes apoptosis and remodeling; gland reverts to prepregnant state

*See Box 3-1 for abbreviations.

Modified from Neville MC: Mammary gland biology and lactation: a short course. Presented at biannual meeting of the International Society for Research on Human Milk and Lactation, Plymouth, Mass., 1997.

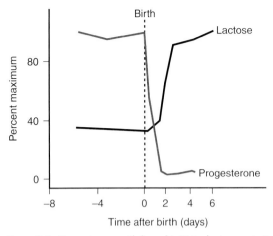

Figure 3-1. Progesterone withdrawal initiates lactogenesis II in women. The increase in lactose concentrations associated with increased synthesis of milk components coincides with a rapid decrease in progesterone concentration when the placenta is removed at parturition. (From Czan KC, Henderson JJ, Kent JC, et al: Hormonal control of the lactation cycle. In Hale TW, Hartmann PE, editors: *Textbook of human lactation*, Amarillo, Tex., 2007, Hale Publishing LP.)

colostrum during this time. As the pregnancy proceeds, milk production is inhibited by high levels of circulating progesterone in most mammals and estrogen as well in humans.

Stage II of lactogenesis is the onset of copious milk production at delivery. In all mammals, it is associated with the drop in progesterone levels (Figure 3-1). This drop occurs to herald delivery in some species so that milk is copious when the young are born. In humans, these levels drop during the first 4 days postpartum, which is reflected by the milk "coming in" during this time. The drop in progesterone is accompanied by the transformation of the mammary epithelium to produce volumes of milk by the fifth day. This change includes a change in permeability of the paracellular pathway and changes in secretion of protective factors (i.e., lactoferrin, immunoglobulins), as well as increases in all milk components that parallel increased glucose production.

During the next 10 days, the composition of the milk slowly changes to mature milk. Composition then changes slowly over the months of full exclusive breastfeeding.

Embryogenesis

Embryogenesis begins with the mammary band, which develops about the 35th embryonic day and progresses to a bud at the 49th day (see Chapter 2). Ducts continue to elongate to form a mammary sprout, which invades the fat pad, branches, and canalizes, forming the rudimentary

mammary ductal system present at birth. After birth, growth of this set of small branching ducts parallels the child's linear growth but remains limited, probably controlled by growth hormone (GH) before onset of ovarian activity.

Under the influence of sex steroids, especially the estrogens, the mammary glandular epithelium proliferates, becoming multilayered. Buds and papillae then form. The growth of the mammary gland is a gradual process that starts during puberty. The process depends on pituitary hormones. Lobuloalveolar development and ductal proliferation also depend on an intact pituitary gland.

The following six well-documented factors help explain the organization of mammary growth. Much of this work has resulted since the availability of "knockout" studies in mice and associated techniques.

1. Mammary ducts must grow into an adipose tissue pad if morphogenesis is to continue. Only adipose stroma supports ductal elongation. The mammary epithelium is closely associated with the adipocyte-containing stroma in all phases of development. In midgestation during human fetal development, a fat pad is laid down as a separate condensation of mesenchyma. Rudimentary ducts expand into the fat pad but do not progress.[57] At puberty, the ducts elongate to fill the entire fat pad, terminating growth as they reach the margins of the fat pad.
2. Estrogen is essential to mammary growth.[100] Ductal growth does not occur in the absence of ovaries but can be stimulated when estrogen is provided. In the ovariectomized (oophorectomized) mouse, an estrogen pellet placed in the mammary tissue stimulates growth in that gland but not in the opposite gland. When the estrogen receptor is "knocked out" in the mouse, no mammary development occurs. The increase in estrogen at puberty results in mammary development. Although estrogen is essential, it is not adequate alone.[6]
3. The exact location of the estrogen receptors in human breasts is unclear. Estrogen receptors are not in the proliferating cells and have not been located in the stroma. Cells with estrogen receptors, however, secrete a paracrine factor that is responsible for the proliferation of ductal cells. This paracrine factor may hold the key to understanding both normal and abnormal breast development.
4. In addition to estrogen, the pituitary gland is necessary for breast development. Kleinberg[39] has identified GH as important to pubertal development and development of the terminal end buds in the breast. Prolactin could not replace GH in these experiments, but insulin-like

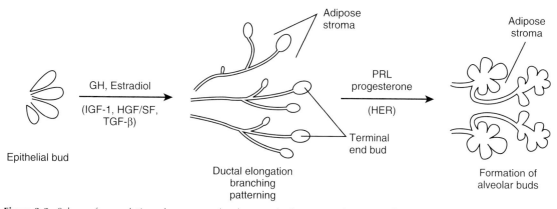

Figure 3-2. Scheme for regulation of mammary development in the mouse. (From Neville MC: Mammary gland biology and lactation: a short course. Presented at the annual meeting of the International Society for Research on Human Milk and Lactation, Plymouth, Mass., 1997.)

growth factor-1 (IGF-1) could. It is produced in the stromal compartment of the mammary gland under stimulation by GH, and together with estradiol from the ovaries, IGF-1 brings about ductal development at puberty.

5. Transforming growth factor beta (TGF-β) maintains the spacing of the mammary ducts as they branch and elongate.[57] These ducts exhibit unique behavior during growth, turning away to avoid other ducts and end buds. This avoidance behavior accounts for the orderly development of the duct system in the breast and the absence of ductal entanglements. This pattern provides ample space between ducts for later development of alveoli. TGF-β has been identified as the negative regulator and is found in many tissues, including breast tissue produced by an epithelial element. The pattern formation in ductal development depends on the localized expression of TGF-β.[18]

6. Progesterone secretion brings about the side branching of the mammary ducts.[35] The presence of progesterone receptors in the epithelial cells has been confirmed by studies in knockout mice in which mammary glands develop to the ductal stage but not to alveolar morphogenesis. Ormandy et al.[66] established that prolactin is necessary for full alveolar development through prolactin receptor studies in knockout mice in which mammary glands do not develop beyond the ductal stage. This was further confirmed in murine mammary cultures in which full development of the alveoli depends on prolactin. Further, when prolactin is withdrawn, apoptosis of the alveolar cells occurs.[95]

The coordination of epithelial and stromal activity in the mammary gland is complex. Hepatocyte growth and scatter factor has been associated with the process during puberty.[64] Another growth factor, heregulin, a member of the epidermal growth factor (EGF) family, has been identified in the stroma of mammary ducts during pregnancy.

Neville[57] has diagrammed the regulation of mammary development (Figure 3-2). She notes that the concentrations of estrogen, progesterone, and lactogenic hormone in the form of prolactin or placental lactogen (PL) greatly increase, enhance alveolar development, and result in the differentiation of alveolar cells. Although many investigators have contributed pieces to the puzzle of mammogenesis, Neville succeeded in creating the current visualization.[57]

Mammogenesis: Mammary Growth

PREPUBERTAL GROWTH

Mammogenesis occurs in two phases as the gland responds to the hormones of puberty and later of pregnancy.[54] During the prepubertal phase, the primary and secondary ducts that develop in the fetus in utero continue to grow in both boys and girls in proportion to growth in general. Shortly before puberty, a more rapid expansion of the duct system begins in girls. The growth of the duct system seems to depend predominantly on estrogen and does not occur in the absence of ovaries. The complete growth of the alveoli requires stimulation by progesterone as well.

Studies of hypophysectomized animals have shown failure of full mammary growth even with adequate estrogen and progesterone. Secretion of prolactin and somatotropin by the pituitary gland results in mammary growth. Adrenocorticotropic hormone (ACTH) and thyroid-stimulating hormone (TSH) acting on the adrenal and thyroid glands also play a minor role in the growth of the mammary gland.

Growth and development during organogenesis involve the interaction of cells with extracellular matrices and neighboring cells.[76] Necropsy breast specimens from six male and eight female infants ranging in age from 1 day to 9 months were studied to determine the process of organogenesis in humans.[1] Integrins were expressed in a pattern that correlates with morphologic and functional differentiation of the normal mammary gland. Integrins are transmembrane glycoproteins that form receptors for extracellular matrix proteins, such as fibronectin, laminin, and collagen. Integrins are widely expressed in normal tissue and are considered critical to the control of cell growth and differentiation. This suggests integrin involvement in the functional characterization of the adhesion molecules in the breast.

PUBERTAL GROWTH

When the hypophyseal-ovarian-uterine cycle is established, a new phase of mammary growth, which includes extensive branching of the system of ducts and proliferation and canalization of the lobuloalveolar units at the distal tips of the branches, begins. Organization of the stromal connective tissue forms the interlobular septa. The ducts, ductules (terminal intralobular ducts), and alveolar structures are formed by double layers of cells. One layer, the epithelial cells, circumscribes the lumen. The second layer, the myoepithelial cells, surrounds the inner epithelial cells and is bordered by a basement lamina.

MENSTRUAL CYCLE GROWTH

The cyclic changes of the adult mammary gland can be associated with the menstrual cycle and the hormonal changes that control that cycle. Estrogens stimulate parenchymal proliferation, with formation of epithelial sprouts. This hyperplasia continues into the secretory phase of the cycle. Anatomically, when the corpus luteum provides increased amounts of estrogens and progesterone, there is lobular edema, thickening of the epithelial basal membrane, and secretory material in the alveolar lumen. Lymphoid and plasma cells infiltrate the stroma. Clinically, mammary blood flow increases in this luteal phase. This increased flow is experienced by women as fullness, heaviness, and turgescence. The breast may become nodular because of interlobular edema and ductular-acinar growth.

After onset of menstruation and reduction of sex steroid levels, milk-secretory prolactin action is limited. Postmenstrual changes occur rapidly, with degeneration of glandular cells and proliferation tissue, loss of edema, and decrease in breast size. The ovulatory cycle actually enhances mammary growth in the early years of menstruation (until

about age 30 years) because the postmenstrual regression of the glandular-alveolar growth after each cycle is not complete. These changes of ductal and lobular proliferation, which occur during the follicular phase before ovulation, continue in the luteal phase and regress after the menstrual phase, exemplifying the sensitivity of this target organ to variations in the balance of hormones.

Fowler et al.[21] measured cyclic changes in composition and volume of the breast during the menstrual cycle using nuclear magnetic resonance T1-weighted imaging. The T1 relaxation time (spin-lattice T1 relaxation) is a measure of the rate of energy loss from tissues after T1 excitation. This energy loss depends on the biophysical environment of the excited protons. A short T1, therefore, indicates the presence of lipids and organic structures that bind water tightly. A longer T1 occurs with greater hydration and with the greatest amount of cellular water. This study revealed the lowest total breast volume and parenchymal volume. T1 and water content occurred between days 6 and 15 of the cycle. Between days 16 and 28, T1 rose sharply and it peaked on the 25th day. The rise in parenchymal volume in the second half of the cycle resulted from not only increased tissue water but also from growth and increased tissue fluid, according to Fowler et al.[21]

Growth During Pregnancy

Hormonal influences on the breast cause profound changes during pregnancy (Figures 3-3 and 3-4). Early in pregnancy, a marked increase in ductular sprouting, branching, and lobular formation is evoked by luteal and placental hormones.[99] PL, prolactin, and chorionic gonadotropin have been identified as contributors to the accelerated growth (Figure 3-4). The dichorionic ductular sprouting has been attributed to estrogen and lobular formation to progesterone.

Prolactin is essential for complete lobular-alveolar development of the gland. Almost complete growth of the mammary lobular-alveolar system can be obtained experimentally in the hypophysectomized-adrenalectomized rat if the animal receives estrogen, progesterone, and prolactin.[42] Prolactin, as with other protein hormones, exerts its effect through receptors for the initiation of milk secretion located on the alveolar cell surfaces. The induction of milk synthesis requires insulin-induced cell division and the presence of cortisol. Prolactin is secreted by the pituitary, which is negatively controlled by prolactin-inhibiting factor (PIF) from the hypothalamus.[42]

From the third month of gestation, secretory material that resembles colostrum appears in the acini. Prolactin from the anterior pituitary gland

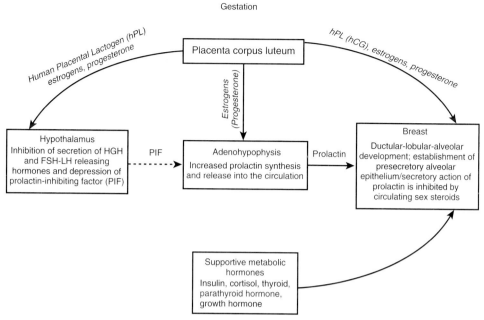

Figure 3-3. Hormonal preparation of breast during pregnancy for lactation. (Modified from Vorherr H: *The breast: morphology, physiology and lactation*, New York, 1974, Academic Press.)

stimulates the glandular production of colostrum. By the second trimester, PL begins to stimulate the secretion of colostrum. A mother who delivers after 16 weeks' gestation will secrete colostrum, even though she has had a nonviable infant. This demonstrates the effectiveness of hormonal stimulation on lactation.

An estrogen-mediated increase in prolactin secretion in pregnancy may produce as much as a tenfold to twentyfold increase in plasma prolactin. This effect may be partially controlled by lactogen from the placenta, which inhibits the production of prolactin. Hormonal regulation of the growth and proliferation of the mammary gland cells has been carefully studied in many species.

Studies of mice in which receptors for each of the hormones have been ablated demonstrate that progesterone and prolactin (or possibly placenta lactogen) are key to alveolar development in pregnancy. The major inhibitor of milk production during pregnancy has been shown to be progesterone.[35]

A complex sequence of events, governed by hormonal action, prepares the breast for lactation (see Figure 3-3). During pregnancy, 17β-Estradiol stimulates the ductal system of epithelial cells to elongate. In contrast to puberty, however, when estrogens appear to directly and indirectly stimulate breast development, estrogens have no indispensable role in mammary development during pregnancy except as a prolactin potentiator: according to Neville,[54] when estrogen levels are low in pregnancy, the breast still develops.

Estrogen levels are normally high in pregnancy, but not for mammogenesis. Induced lactation in the cow is dependably reproduced with 7 days of estrogen and progesterone treatment. Progesterone, in turn, induces the specific epithelial cells of the tubular invaginations to produce distinct ducts, which branch from the main tubules.[35]

The end result of the combined actions of estrogen and progesterone is a richly branched arborization of the gland. Highly differentiated secretory alveolar cells develop at the ends of these ducts under the influence of prolactin (Figure 3-5).

Serum growth factor, which is present in normal human serum, and insulin can stimulate the stem cells of the gland to proliferate. These dividing cells are further directed to the formation of alveoli by corticosteroid hormones. At least two types of cells are identified in the epithelial layer of the gland: stem cells and secretory alveolar cells. At this point in the pregnancy, prolactin influences the production of the constituents of milk.

TGF-β influences pattern formation in the developing mammary gland and may negatively regulate ductal growth as well.[18] The pattern of mammary ductal development varies widely among species and is a function of both genotype and hormonal status. Normal human breast cells secrete TGF-β and are themselves inhibited by it, suggesting an autoregulatory feedback circuit that may be modulated by estradiol. Growth and patterning of the ductal tree are regulated in part by TGF-β operating through an autocrine feedback mechanism

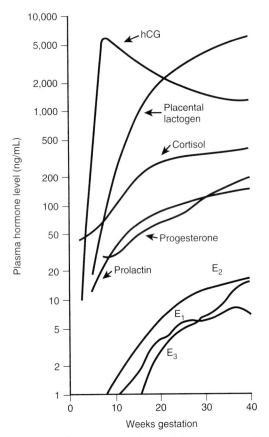

Figure 3-4. Plasma hormone levels during pregnancy. *E1*, estrone; *E2*, estradiol; *E3*, estriol; *hCG*, human chorionic gonadotropin. (From Neville MC, Morton J, Umemura S: The evidence for breastfeeding, *Pediatr Clin North Am* 48:42, 2001.)

and by paracrine circuits associated with epithelial-stromal interactions.[18]

The high circulating levels of prolactin in pregnancy are not associated with milk production partly because of the progesterone antagonism of the stimulatory action of prolactin on casein messenger ribonucleic acid (mRNA) synthesis. During late pregnancy, the lactogenic receptors, which have similar affinities for both prolactin and human placental lactogen (hPL), are predominantly occupied by hPL. High doses of estradiol impair the incorporation of prolactin into milk secretory cells.

Prolactin is prevented from exerting its effect on milk excretion by the elevated levels of progesterone. Following the drop in progesterone and estrogen at delivery, copious milk secretion begins. The key hormone requirements for lactation to begin are prolactin, insulin, and hydrocortisone. A high level of plasma prolactin is essential to lactogenesis in humans as well. There is a question as to whether it is a surge in prolactin that is necessary for lactogenesis at parturition. Prolactin levels are now described as biphasic in humans for the initiation of lactogenesis at birth.[56] Prolactin stabilizes and

promotes transcription of casein mRNA and stimulates synthesis of a lactalbumin that is the regulatory protein of the lactose-synthetase enzyme system.[65] Prolactin further increases the lipoprotein lipase activity in the mammary gland. Prolactin exists in three heterogenic forms of varying biologic activity. The monomer is in greatest quantity and is the most active form.

Lactogenesis: Initiation of Milk Secretion

Stage I lactogenesis starts approximately 12 weeks before parturition and is heralded by significant increases in lactose, total proteins, and immunoglobulin and by decreases in sodium and chloride, and the gathering of substrate for milk production. The composition of prepartum secretion is fairly constant until delivery, as monitored by the milk protein α-lactalbumin.

Lactogenesis is initiated in the postpartum period by a fall in plasma progesterone, but prolactin levels remain high (Figure 3-6). The initiation of the process does not depend on suckling by the infant until the third or fourth day, when the secretion declines if milk is not removed from the breast.[98]

Stage II lactogenesis includes the increase in blood flow and oxygen and glucose uptake as well as the sharp increase in citrate concentration, considered a reliable marker for lactogenesis stage II. Stage II at 2 to 3 days postpartum begins clinically when the secretion of milk is copious and biochemically when plasma α-lactalbumin levels peak (paralleling the period when "the milk comes in"). The major changes in milk composition continue for 10 days, when "mature milk" is established. The establishment of the mature milk supply, once called galactopoiesis, is now referred to as stage III of lactogenesis (Figures 19-2 to 19-4 and 3-6).[98,99]

The profound changes in milk composition have been established for the period of transition to mature milk in relationship to increase in milk volume.[55] Detailed studies of successfully lactating women were performed by Neville et al.,[58] who report that a significant fall in sodium, chloride, and protein and a rise in lactose precede the major increase in milk volume during early lactogenesis. At 46 to 96 hours postpartum, copious milk production is accompanied by an increase in citrate, glucose, free phosphate, and calcium concentrations and a decrease in pH.

The breast, one of the most complex endocrine target organs, has been prepared during pregnancy and responds to the release of prolactin by producing the constituents of milk (see Figure 3-5). The

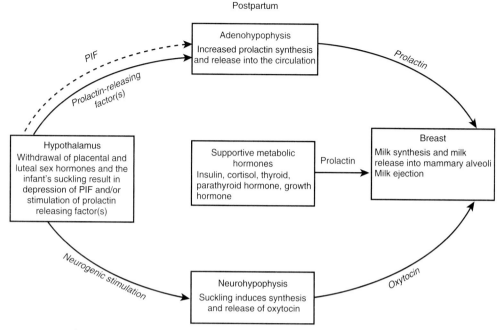

Postpartum

Figure 3-5. Hormonal preparation of breast for lactation postpartum. *PIF,* prolactin-inhibitory factor. (Modified from Vorherr H: *The breast: morphology, physiology and lactation,* New York, 1974, Academic Press.)

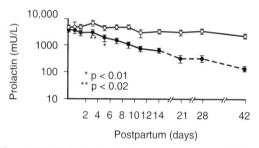

Figure 3-6. Prolactin levels in the postpartum period in women who are lactating *(open circles)* and nonlactating *(dots)*. Levels in lactating women vary with intensity of suckling. (From Neville MC, Morton J, Umemora S: The evidence for breastfeeding, *Pediatr Clin North Am* 48:44, 2001.)

lactogenic effects of prolactin are modulated by the complex interplay of pituitary, ovarian, thyroid, adrenal, and pancreatic hormones (Figure 3-7).

Prolactin

Stricker and Grueter[86] discovered the pituitary hormone prolactin in 1928. They observed that extracts of the pituitary gland induced lactation in rabbits.

Human prolactin is a significant hormone in pregnancy and lactation.[22] Prolactin also has a range of actions in various species that is greater than any other known hormone. Prolactin has been identified in many animal species whether they nurse their young or not. Because of the original

association with lactation, the term describes its action, "support or stimulation of lactation." Prolactin, however, has been shown to control nonlactating responses in other species and has been identified with more than 300 different physiologic processes, unrelated to lactation. Study of prolactin was hampered until 1970, when it became possible to separate prolactin from human growth hormone (hGH) and to isolate and characterize prolactin from human pituitary glands.

Before 1971, hGH and prolactin in humans were considered the same hormone. Until 1971, in fact, it was thought that prolactin did not exist in humans. However, hGH is present in the human pituitary gland in an amount 100 times that of prolactin.[43]

Although prolactin is secreted by the anterior pituitary gland, the brain is exposed to it. Prolactin is found in the cerebrospinal fluid and may even be produced by neurons in the portal vessels of the hypothalamus. Prolactin increases the activity of tuberoinfundibular neurons, which control dopamine.[96]

Prolactin, the lactogenic hormone, is essential for glucocorticoid stimulation of the milk-protein genes.[84] Little is known about the biochemical pathway of action of this important polypeptide hormone, which is required for both morphogenesis and expression of functional differentiation of the parenchyma of the breast (see Figures 3-8 and 3-9).[3]

Synthesis and secretion is not restricted to the anterior pituitary gland, but includes multiple sites

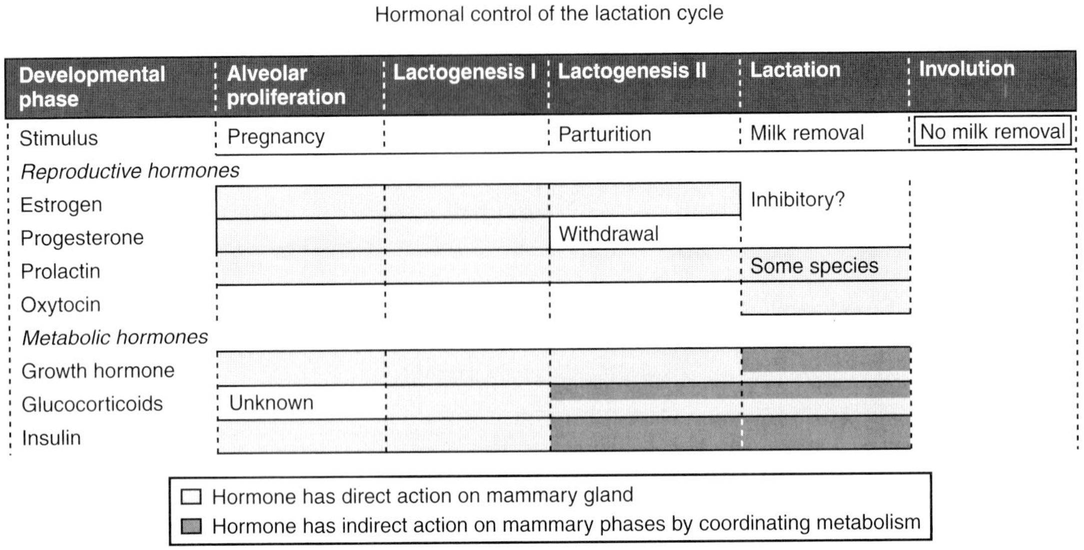

Hormonal control of the lactation cycle

Developmental phase	Alveolar proliferation	Lactogenesis I	Lactogenesis II	Lactation	Involution
Stimulus	Pregnancy		Parturition	Milk removal	No milk removal
Reproductive hormones					
Estrogen				Inhibitory?	
Progesterone			Withdrawal		
Prolactin				Some species	
Oxytocin					
Metabolic hormones					
Growth hormone					
Glucocorticoids	Unknown				
Insulin					

☐ Hormone has direct action on mammary gland
■ Hormone has indirect action on mammary phases by coordinating metabolism

Figure 3-7. Hormonal action necessary for phases of the lactation cycle. (From Czank C, Henderson JJ, Kent JC, et al: Hormonal control of lactation cycle. In Hale TW, Hartmann PE, editors: *Textbook of human lactation*, Amarillo, Tex., 2007, Hale Publishing LP, p 91.)

in the brain (cerebral cortex, hippocampus, amygdala, cerebellum, brainstem, and spinal cord). It is also produced in the placenta, amnion, decidua, and uterus. Evidence suggests that lymphocytes from the immune system, thymus, and spleen release bioactive prolactin. Prolactin is found in epithelial cells of the lactating mammary gland and the milk itself. Prolactin reaches the milk by crossing the mammary epithelial cell basement membrane, attaches to a specific prolactin binding protein, and ultimately moves by exostosis through the apical membranes into the alveolar lumen. Prolactin mRNA in milk contains more prolactin variants than serum. Milk prolactin participates in the maturation of the neuroendocrine and immune systems.

The information generated by the use of knockout mice with prolactin knockouts or prolactin receptor knockouts has refined the understanding of mammary morphogenesis and subsequent lactogenesis.[16] It has been confirmed that prolactin does not operate alone but depends on estrogen, progesterone, and glucocorticoids, as well as insulin, thyroid hormone, parathyroid hormone, and even oxytocin. Prolactin also stimulates uptake of some amino acids, uptake of glucose, and synthesis of milk sugar and milk fats (see Figure 3-7).[23]

Plasma prolactin varies in relation to psychosocial stress. Utilizing four different real-life stress studies in a longitudinal design, Theorell[89] found that changing situations associated with passive coping are accompanied by increased plasma prolactin levels. Changing situations associated with active coping are associated with unchanged or even lowered prolactin levels. The regulation of plasma prolactin is part of a dopaminergic system (see the list of pharmacologic suppressors in the next section).

In vitro, prolactin stimulates the synthesis of the mRNA of specific milk proteins by binding to membrane receptors of the mammary epithelial cells. Prolactin has been demonstrated to penetrate the cytoplasm of these cells and even their nuclei. These specific actions in the gland require the presence of extracellular calcium ions. Some prolactin actually appears in the milk substrate itself, the functional significance of which is uncertain, although it is thought to influence fluid and ion absorption from the neonatal jejunum.

The effect of the stimulation of protein synthesis by allowing the expression of milk protein genes is not a direct effect of the hormone, but rather the consequence of the activation of sodium/potassium adenosinetriphosphatase (Na/K ATPase) in the plasma membrane.[16] The intracellular concentration of potassium is kept high and that of sodium low compared with the concentrations in extracellular fluid. As a result, the Na/K ratio is high both in the milk and in the intracellular fluid. Further action of prolactin has been identified in the development of the immune system in the mammary gland and, possibly more directly, in the lymphoid tissue. In conjunction with estrogen and progesterone, prolactin attracts and retains immunoglobulin A (IgA) immunoblasts from the gut-associated lymphoid tissue for the development of the immune system for the mammary gland. A very sensitive bioassay has been developed using the in vitro biologic effect of prolactin to stimulate the growth of cell cultures for malignant niobium rat lymphomas.

TABLE 3-2	Prolactin Levels*	
	Range (ng/mL)	Average (ng/mL)
Males and prepubertal and postmenopausal females	2-8	-
Females' menstrual life	8-14	10
Term pregnancy	200-500	200
Amniotic fluid	Up to 10,000	-
Lactating women	**Response to breastfeeding**	
First 10 days	Baseline 200	Rise to 400
10-90 days	60-110	70-220
90-180 days	50	100
180 days to 1 year	30-40	45-80

*Collation of values from multiple studies and sources.

The baseline levels of prolactin are essentially the same in normal male and female humans (Table 3-2). Moreover, both men and women experience a rise in prolactin levels during sleep.[84] There is also a normal diurnal variation in levels in both men and women. At puberty, the increase in estrogens causes a slight but measurable increase in prolactin. Prolactin increases during the proliferative phase of the menstrual cycle but not during the secretory phase. A number of factors, including some that are significant for the nursing mother, such as psychogenic influence and stress, increase prolactin levels. Anesthesia, surgery, exercise, nipple stimulation, and sexual intercourse also produce increased amounts in both lactating and nonlactating women. Prolactin levels increase as serum osmolality increases.

Although prolactin levels in maternal serum are well established, less is known about prolactin levels in the milk and their role in the newborn. Prolactin in milk is known to be biologically potent and is absorbed by the newborn. In the intestine, prolactin influences fluid, sodium, potassium, and calcium transport. Prolactin content is highest in the early transitional milk just after the colostrum in the first postpartum week (levels of 43.1 ± 4 ng/mL). Levels drop to 11.0 ± 1.4 ng/mL in mature milk over time until approximately 40 weeks postpartum.[16]

Prolactin-Inhibiting Factor

PIF controls the secretion of prolactin from the hypothalamus. Prolactin is unusual among the pituitary hormones because it is inhibited by a hypothalamic substance. Catecholamine levels in the hypothalamus control the inhibiting factor, which is poured into the circulation as a result of dopaminergic impulses. Drugs and events that decrease catecholamines also decrease the inhibiting factor, causing a rise in prolactin. Dopamine itself can act directly on the pituitary gland to decrease prolactin secretion. Agents that increase prolactin by decreasing catecholamines, and thus the PIF level include the phenothiazines and reserpine.

Thyrotropin-releasing hormone (TRH) is a strong stimulator of prolactin secretion, but its physiologic role is not clear, because thyrotropin levels do not rise during normal nursing. In the postpartum period, a dose of TRH will cause a marked increase in prolactin. Even a nonnursing postpartum mother will experience engorgement and milk release when stimulated with TRH. Ergot, which is frequently prescribed for postpartum patients, inhibits prolactin secretion either by direct inhibition or by its effect on the hypothalamus.

Prolactin response to breast stimulation in lactating women is not mediated by endogenous opioids. Neither baseline nor stimulated prolactin values were affected by naloxone.[9]

The following factors affect prolactin release in normal humans:

- Physiologic stimuli
- Nursing in postpartum women: breast stimulation
- Sleep
- Stress
- Sexual intercourse
- Pregnancy
- Pharmacologic stimuli
- Neuroleptic drugs
- TRH
- Metoclopramide (procainamide derivative)
- Estrogens
- Hypoglycemia
- Phenothiazines, butyrophenones
- Norepinephrine
- Histamine
- Acetylcholine
- Pharmacologic suppressors
- Apomorphine, bromocriptine, cabergoline
- L-Dopa
- Ergot preparations (2-Br-α-ergocryptine)
- Clomiphene citrate
- Large amounts of pyridoxine
- Monoamine oxidase inhibitors
- Pramipexole
- Prostaglandins E and F2α
- Ropinirole, rotigotine, selegiline

In pregnancy, prolactin levels begin to rise in the first trimester and continue to rise throughout gestation. In a nonnursing mother, prolactin levels drop to normal in 2 weeks, independent of therapy to suppress lactation.

At delivery, with the expulsion of the placenta, levels of PL, estrogens, and progesterone abruptly decline (Figure 3-8 and 3-9).

PL disappears within hours.[55] Progesterone drops over several days, and estrogens fall to baseline levels in 5 to 6 days (see Figures 3-6 and 19-2 to 19-4). Prolactin in nonlactating women requires 14 days to reach baseline. Progesterone is considered the key inhibiting hormone, and decline in plasma progesterone levels is considered the lactogenic trigger for stage II lactogenesis.[51] However, progesterone does not inhibit established lactation because breast tissue does not contain progesterone-binding sites. Estrogens enhance the effect of prolactin on mammogenesis but antagonize prolactin by inhibiting secretion of milk. After delivery, there are low estrogen and high prolactin levels. Suckling provides a continued stimulus for prolactin release. If prolactin, essential for lactation, is diminished by hypophysectomy or medication, lactation ceases. Baseline prolactin levels do eventually diminish to more normal levels months after parturition, although lactation may continue.[37]

The surge in prolactin over baseline levels, however, is critical to milk production, not the baseline levels (Figures 3-6, 3-10, and 3-11). Although prolactin is necessary for milk secretion, the volume of milk secreted is not directly related to the concentration of prolactin in the plasma. Local mechanisms within the mammary gland that depend on the amount of milk removed by the infant are responsible for the day-to-day regulation of milk volume.[84] Suckling stimulates the release of adenohypophyseal prolactin and neurohypophyseal oxytocin. These

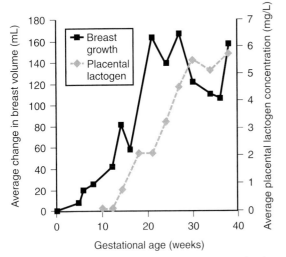

Figure 3-8. Breast growth and placental growth are closely associated. (Modified from Cox DB, Kent JC, Casey TM, et al: Breast growth, *Exp Physiol* 84:421-434, 1999.)

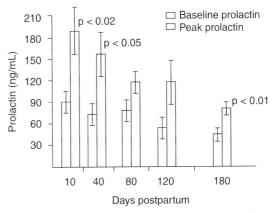

Figure 3-10. Prolactin levels after suckling. (From Battin DA, Marrs RP, Fleiss PM, et al: Effect of suckling on serum prolactin, luteinizing hormone, follicle-stimulating hormone, and estradiol during prolonged lactation, *Obstet Gynecol* 65:785, 1985.)

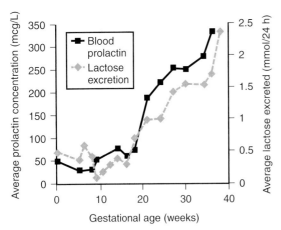

Figure 3-9. Relationship between lactose excretion into urine and prolactin concentration in the blood during pregnancy. (Modified from Cox DB, Kent JC, Casey TM, et al: Breast growth, *Exp Physiol* 84:421-434, 1999.)

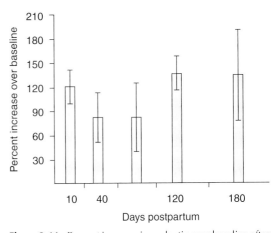

Figure 3-11. Percent increase in prolactin over baseline after suckling. (From Battin DA, Marrs RP, Fleiss PM, et al: Effect of suckling on serum prolactin, luteinizing hormone, follicle-stimulating hormone, and estradiol during prolonged lactation, *Obstet Gynecol* 65:785, 1985.)

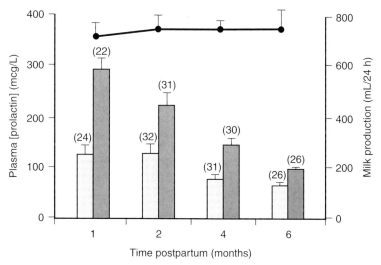

Figure 3-12. Immunoreactive prolactin determined in plasma samples collected from 11 mothers (at 1, 2, and 4 months) and from nine mothers (at 6 months), immediately before suckling (□) and 45 minutes after the commencement of suckling (•). Number of observations is shown in parenthesis. Twenty-four hour milk production (mL/24 h) of the same mothers determined by test weighing. Results are mean values+SEM. (From Cox DB, Owens RH, Hartman PE: Prolactin and milk synthesis in women, *Exp Physiol* 81:1007–1020, 1996.)

hormones stimulate milk synthesis and production of milk-ejection metabolic hormones, which are also necessary in the process of milk synthesis.[51] Thus suckling, emptying the breast, and receiving adequate precursor nutrients are essential to effective lactation (Figures 3-12 and 3-13).

When milk is not removed, secretion ceases in a few days, and the composition of the mammary secretion returns to a colostrum-like fluid. When the composition of the breast secretion of breastfeeding and nonbreastfeeding women was followed

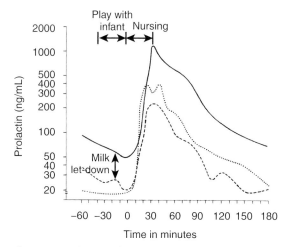

Figure 3-13. Plasma prolactin measured by radioimmunoassay before, during, and after a period of nursing in three mothers, 22 to 26 days postpartum. Prolactin levels rose with suckling and not with infant contact. (Modified from Josimovich JB, Reynolds M, Cobo E: Lactogenic hormones, fetal nutrition, and lactation. In Josimovich JB, Reynolds M, Cobo E, editors: *Problems of human reproduction,* vol 2, New York, 1974, John Wiley & Sons.)

by Kulski and Hartmann,[41] it was the same for 3 to 4 days. Thereafter, the sodium and chloride concentrations in the nonbreastfeeding women increased rapidly.

The regulation of milk production in full lactation is based primarily on infant demand.[60] Maternal nutrition, age, body composition, and parity have only secondary impact. Suckling is a powerful stimulus to prolactin synthesis and secretion, and prolactin is necessary for milk secretion.[89] The pulsatile nature of prolactin secretion makes it difficult to measure over time. Milk yield is not directly correlated to prolactin levels.

Two local mechanisms have been associated with milk volume control. An inhibitor of milk secretion builds up as milk accumulates. The actual volume of milk secreted may be reduced if the breast is not drained adequately. Distention or stretching of the alveoli also affects production and secretion of milk. Evidence indicates that a proteinaceous factor in milk itself actually inhibits milk production and is associated with residual milk in the breast. This has been identified as a feedback inhibitor of lactation (FIL).

It has been assumed that prolactin levels control the rate of milk synthesis. When 24-hour milk production was measured by Cox et al.,[13] however, the results were different. The short-term rates of milk synthesis (i.e., between feeds) and the concentration of prolactin in the blood and in the milk were measured from 1 to 6 months in 11 women. The 24-hour milk production remained constant (708 ± 54.7 g per 24 hours at 1 month and 742 ± 79.4 g per 24 hours at 6 months). Marked variation in short-term milk synthesis between breasts was observed. The baseline and suckling-stimulated prolactin levels declined over time but the peak over base remained. The concentration of prolactin in milk was related to the fullness of the breasts, being highest when the breasts were full. Cox et al.[13] found no relationship between the concentration of prolactin in the plasma and the rate of milk synthesis in either the short or long term.

Evidence indicates that a proteinaceous factor in milk itself actually inhibits milk production and is associated with residual milk in the breast. This has been identified as a FIL. Prolactin circadian rhythm persists throughout lactation. Prolactin levels are notably higher at night than during the day, despite greater nursing times during the day. The highest levels in the study by Stern and Reichlin[84] were when the least nursing occurred.

The most effective and specific stimulus to prolactin release is nursing. The stimulation is a result of nipple or breast manipulation, especially suckling, not a psychologic effect of the presence of the infant (see Figures 3-13 and 3-14). The prolactin-release reflex during nipple stimulation is suppressed in some adult women, being evidenced only during pregnancy and lactation.[48]

During human pregnancy, when serum prolactin rises steadily to 150 to 200 ng/mL at term, there is a brief drop in levels hours before delivery and then a rise again as soon as the neonate is suckled.[46,48] The response to nipple stimulation can be abolished by applying local anesthetic.[53] On the other hand, trauma or surgery to the chest wall can initiate a prolactin rise and, in some reported cases, milk production.

Although it was initially reported that the high levels of prolactin measured in the first days and weeks of lactation dwindled to normal baseline by 6 months and showed no response to suckling stimulus, later studies clearly showed a different picture with more sensitive assays.[46] Prolactin does not drop to normal, but further stimulus causes a doubling of levels over baseline at all stages of lactation through the second year (see Table 3-2).

Acute prolactin and oxytocin responses were measured by Zinaman et al.,[104] who compared various mechanical pumping devices with manual expression and infant suckling. Prolactin response to mechanical expression in quantity and duration depended on the device used, with a full-size pulsatile electric pump eliciting the greatest response. This compared equally with infant suckling. There was no difference seen in oxytocin response with various devices. These data confirm that results in studies of milk production and release in humans also depend on the equipment used to stimulate the breast.[104] Eight fully lactating women were followed through the first 6 months postpartum at 10, 40, 80, 120, and 180 days, recording serum prolactin, luteinizing hormone, follicle-stimulating hormone, and estradiol (zero time only) obtained just before the initiation of suckling and during the next 120 minutes.[3] Samples were obtained at 0, +15, +30, +60, and +120 minutes. Prolactin levels were high the first 10 days (90.1 ng/mL) but slowly declined over 180 days (44.3 ng/mL). The stimulus of suckling doubled the baseline values. Mean estradiol levels were low at 10 days (7.2 pg/mL), then gradually rose to a mean of 47.3 pg/mL at 180 days

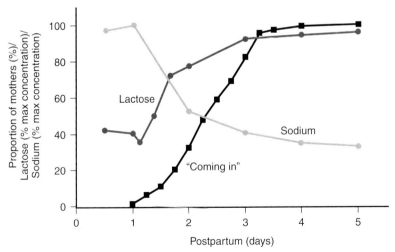

Figure 3-14. The sense of milk coming in. Secretory activation precedes the sense of milk "coming in." The distribution of the times when women first sensed the "coming in" of milk after normal delivery is compared with the changes in lactose and sodium concentrations of breast milk over the first postpartum days. The number of women for each time point was expressed as a cumulative percentage of the total number (*n* = 107) of women. Lactose and sodium concentrations obtained from left and right breasts for each woman were averaged and presented as percentages of the maximum lactose and sodium concentrations over the 5 days. (From Pang WW, Hartman PL: Initiation of human lactation: secretory differentiation and secretory activation, *J Mammary Gland Biol* 12:211–221, 2007.)

postpartum in the subjects whose menses had resumed. In the amenorrheic subjects the estradiol levels remained low (4.25 pg/mL), whereas baseline prolactin remained high (63.6 ng/mL). The subjects were breastfeeding on demand, averaging 11 feedings (range 8 to 16) per day at 10 days and 8 feedings (range 5 to 12) at 120 and 180 days. All infants had stopped one night feeding, and two infants had started some solids between the third and fourth months.

When specific binding sites for prolactin were looked for in the tammar wallaby, many sites were demonstrated in the lactating mammary gland but not the inactive gland. Mammary prolactin receptors were also identified in the rabbit. Thus the increased binding capacity would enhance tissue responsiveness, which may explain the maintenance of full lactation in the face of falling concentrations of prolactin. Prolactin also plays a critical role in increasing maternal bile secretory function postpartum.[48]

Human Placental Lactogen and Human Growth Hormone

Three main hormones are recognized in the lactogenic process: hPL, hGH, and prolactin. The progressive rise in prolactin during pregnancy parallels the rise in hPL, becoming measurable at 6 weeks' gestation and increasing to 6000 ng/mL at term (see Figure 3-4). This parallel action contributed to the belief that prolactin and hPL were the same. Although the principal function of hPL and prolactin in humans is a lactogenic one, no lactation ordinarily appears before delivery,[81] although some women report being able to express a few drops of colostrum.

First described in 1962, hPL has been studied more than lactogens from any other species.[53] Extensive immunologic and structural homology exists between hGH and hPL, which probably explains their similar biologic activities. Concentrations of hPL increase steadily during gestation and decrease abruptly with the delivery of the placenta. A large-molecular-weight substance, hPL is derived from the chorion. Receptor sites that bind lactogen also bind protein and hGH.[94] hPL has been associated with mobilization of free fatty acid and inhibition of peripheral glucose utilization and lactogenic action.

hGH is secreted from the anterior pituitary eosinophilic cells. These cells have been identified by staining techniques that distinguish them from those that produce prolactin. Toward the end of pregnancy, the cells that produce prolactin are noticeably more numerous, whereas those that produce hGH are "crowded out." The role of hGH in the maintenance of lactation is poorly defined and may be synergistic with prolactin and glucocorticoids.

Prolactin, hGH, PL, and chorionic somatotropin form a family of polypeptide hormones from the same ancestral gene, even though prolactin and hGH are produced by the pituitary and PL and chorionic somatotropin by the placenta.[100] The suckling stimulus in postpartum lactation causes a rapid increase in serum hGH and prolactin. hGH and prolactin evolve from the same precursor, and, although the hormones are distinct, the acute interruption of hGH secretion does not interfere with the milk secretion.

The possible role of TSH as a physiologic prolactin-releasing factor has been disproved by Gehlbach et al.,[26] who state that TSH is not responsible for the brisk release of prolactin with suckling. Normal lactation is possible in women with ateliotic dwarfism in the absence of detectable quantities of hGH. For any hormone to exert its biologic effects, however, specific receptors for the hormone must be present in the target tissue. Changes in serum concentration have no effect if receptors are not present in the mammary gland to bind the hormone.

Oxytocin was the first hormone studied in relation to breastfeeding and to the let-down reflex. Studies first explored its role in the initiation and progression of labor. Because it was measurable, isolated in the laboratory, and finally manufactured synthetically, our knowledge of oxytocin was more extensive than it was for prolactin until the last two decades.

Oxytocin is not just a female hormone; it is produced by both male and female humans, and it is increased not just during reproduction in women. It is now credited with producing increased responsiveness to receptivity, closeness, openness to relationships, and nurturing. The oxytocin circulating during breastfeeding has been credited with producing calm, lack of stress, and an enhanced ability to interact with infants. The calm and connectedness system is part of a system of nerves and hormones that together trigger these effects.

Oxytocin is a polypeptide found in all mammalian species and works though a mechanism through which it activates receptors on the outer surface of the cell membrane.[19] Oxytocin is produced in the supraoptic and paraventricular nuclei of the hypothalamus. Receptors have been identified for oxytocin in the uterus and the breast as well as the brain. It acts via the bloodstream and as a signaling substance in the nervous system. Substances that act to stimulate the release of oxytocin include serotonin, dopamine, noradrenaline, and glutamate. Other substances, such as opiates, enkephalin, and β-endorphin, inhibit its release. Spinal anesthesia has been associated with the inhibition of oxytocin release after childbirth.[37] Estrogen can increase the number of receptors and stimulate the production of oxytocin. The release of oxytocin by repetitive soothing touches or when given via injection produces a calming reaction and lowers blood pressure and pulse rate. Uvnäs Moberg[91] has studied oxytocin extensively and calls it the hormone of calm, love, and healing.

Stage III Lactogenesis (Galactopoiesis): Maintenance of Established Lactation

Early studies in the past 100 years established that milk was synthesized in the mammary gland from substances removed from the maternal arterial blood supply. Then it was confirmed that milk ejection was the removal of stored milk and not from the rapid synthesis of milk. The enzymes and hormones involved have been identified. Understanding the molecular biochemistry and physiology of the gland has revealed the details of the production of milk. A number of genes encode for components that are part of the intricate signaling pathways. Complex interactions of signaling molecules with epigenetic factors interact at the level of gene expression. Intracellular signaling is basic to understanding normal human mammary development.

The basic features of milk production are the identification of the cell surface and intracellular receptors for extra cellular signals (12 hormones autocrine and paracrine factors according to Martin and Czank).[52] Chain reactions convey the signal to

a site of action. A class of compounds that regulate gene expression depend on modification to their structures and the nature of their binding to the genetic material.

The maintenance of established milk secretion, originally called galactopoiesis, is now labeled stage III lactogenesis, or simply lactation. An intact hypothalamic-pituitary axis regulating prolactin and oxytocin levels is essential to the initiation and maintenance of lactation.[38] The process of lactation requires milk synthesis and milk release into the alveoli and the lactiferous sinuses. When the milk is not removed, the increased pressure lessens capillary blood flow and inhibits the lactation process. Lack of sucking stimulation means lack of prolactin release from the pituitary gland. Basal prolactin levels that are enhanced by the spurts that result from sucking are necessary to maintain lactation in the first postpartum weeks. Without oxytocin, however, a pregnancy can be carried to term, but the woman will fail to lactate because she will fail to let-down.

Sensory nerve endings, located mainly in the areola and nipple, are stimulated by suckling. The afferent neural reflex pathway, via the spinal cord to the mesencephalon and then to the hypothalamus, produces secretion and release of prolactin and oxytocin. Hypothalamic suppression of earlier PIF secretion causes adrenohypophyseal prolactin release. When prolactin is released into the circulation, it stimulates milk synthesis and secretion. A conditioned milk ejection can occur in lactating women without a concomitant release of prolactin, so that indeed the releases are independent, which may be significant in treating apparent lactation failure (Figure 3-15).

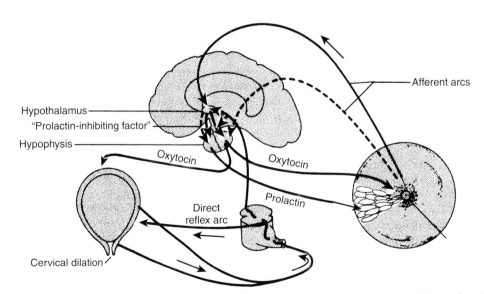

Figure 3-15. Neuroendocrine control of milk ejection. (Modified from Vorherr H: *The breast: morphology, physiology and lactation*, New York, 1974, Academic Press.)

Hormonal Regulation of Prolactin and Oxytocin

The release of prolactin is inhibited by PIF.[44] The PIF has not been described but is closely associated with dopamine. There is also evidence of either serotonin release of prolactin or catecholamine-serotonin control of prolactin release. TSH has also been shown to stimulate the release of prolactin. The amount of prolactin is proportional to the amount of nipple stimulation during early stages of lactation after the first 4 days. Milk synthesis proceeds for the first 4 days whether or not the breast is stimulated. At this time, prolactin levels are the same for lactators and nonlactators[56] (Figure 3-16).

Although both oxytocin and prolactin release are stimulated by nipple stimulation, some oxytocin is released by other sensory pathways, such as visual, tactile, olfactory, and auditory.[60] Thus a woman may release milk on seeing, touching, hearing, smelling, or thinking about her infant. Prolactin, however, is released only on nipple stimulation so that milk production is not initiated by other sensory pathways. Oxytocin is also released under physical stress, such as pain, exercise, cold, heat, changes in plasma osmolality, or hypovolemia, but these responses are blunted or reversed during lactation.[15,60]

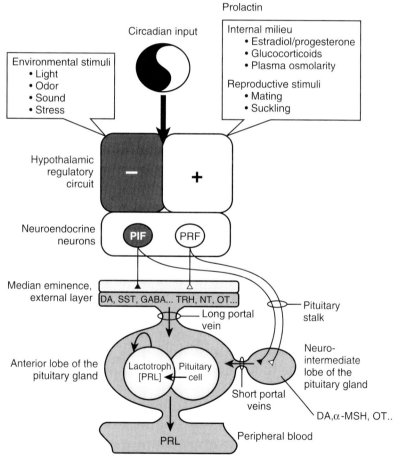

Figure 3-16. An overview of the regulation of prolactin secretion. Prolactin secretion is paced by a light-entrained circadian rhythm, which is modified by environmental input, with the internal milieu and reproductive stimuli affecting the inhibitory or stimulatory elements of the hypothalamic regulatory circuit. The final common pathways of the central stimulatory and inhibitory control of prolactin secretion are the neuroendocrine neurons producing prolactin-inhibiting factors (PIF), such as dopamine (DA), somatostatin (SST), and γ-aminobutyric acid (GABA), or prolactin-releasing factors (PRF), such as thyrotropin-releasing hormone (TRH), oxytocin (OT), and neurotensin (NT). PIF and PRF from the neuroendocrine neurons can be released either at the median eminence into the long portal veins or at the neurointermediate lobe, which is connected to the anterior lobe of the pituitary gland by the short portal vessels. Thus lactotrophs are regulated by bloodborne agents of central nervous system or pituitary origin (α-melanocyte stimulating hormone) delivered to the anterior lobe by the long or short portal veins. Lactotrophs are also influenced by PRF and PIF released from neighboring cells (paracrine regulation) or from the lactotrophs themselves (autocrine regulation). (From Freeman ME, Kanyicska B, Lerant A, Nagy G: Prolactin: structure, function and regulation of secretion, *Physiol Rev* 80:1523–1630, 2000.)

When suckling occurs, oxytocin is released.[12] It enters the circulation and rapidly causes ejection of milk from alveoli and smaller milk ducts into larger lactiferous ducts and sinuses. This is the pathway of the let-down, or ejection, reflex. Oxytocin also causes contraction of the myometrium and involution of the uterus (Figure 3-17).

The polypeptide oxytocin is a messenger molecule with diverse physiologic actions as well as modes of delivery to its target sites. Oxytocin exerts effects as a hormone carried by the systemic circulation to distant targets in the uterus and the breast.[15] Oxytocin also serves as a hypophysiotropic factor, released from nerve terminals in the median eminence into the pituitary portal vasculature to affect anterior pituitary secretion. Its action here is as a peptidergic neurotransmitter or neuromodulator within the central nervous system, influencing a variety of neuroendocrine, behavioral, and autonomic functions. Its well-known role is related to reproduction and lactation, but it has other, less well explored physical and metabolic roles.[15]

After suckling is initiated, the oxytocin response is transient and intermittent rather than sustained.

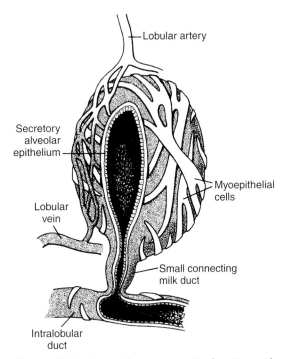

Figure 3-17. Fundamental mammary unit at lactation, with arrangement of secretory alveoli, myoepithelial cells, and vasculature. The secretory alveolar epithelium is monolayered, and the epithelial lining of milk ducts consists of two layers. Between bases of glandular epithelial cells and tunica propria, starlike myoepithelial mammary cells surround alveolus in a basketlike arrangement. (Modified from Vorherr H: *The breast: morphology, physiology and lactation,* New York, 1974, Academic Press.)

Plasma levels often return to basal between milk ejections, even though suckling continues. Ejection can be measured by placing a microcatheter in the mammary duct or can be noted subjectively by the mother as tingling or turgescence. The contractions last about 1 minute, with about 4 to 10 occurring in a 10-minute period. Corresponding pulses of oxytocin can be measured in the maternal bloodstream. The controls of oxytocin release are complex and are extensively described by Crowley and Armstrong.[15] That centrally released oxytocin is in control of the milk-ejection reflex was established in 1981 by Freund-Mercier and Richard.[24] They demonstrated in rats that intracerebroventricular administration of oxytocin greatly increased the frequency and amplitude of pulsatile oxytocin release during suckling. Administration of oxytocin antagonists produced the opposite effect and suppressed responses.[24]

The human pituitary has an excessive storage capacity and contains 3000 to 9000 mU of oxytocin, but the reflex milk ejection involves the release of only 50 to 100 mU.[101] Except in extreme cases (Sheenan syndrome), hormone depletion is rarely an issue, but hormone release and target-organ sensitivity are. Opiate and β-endorphin released during stress are known to block stimulus-secretion coupling by dissociating electrical activity at the terminal. This inhibition is naloxone reversible.

The mammary gland, from platypus to human, has an identical fine structure consisting of alveolar tissue that has increased its surface area 10,000-fold during gestation compared with the size of the gland.[47] It continuously produces milk throughout lactation, but the most complex issue is the release of milk. Because of the substantial surface tension forces opposing the movement of fluid in the small ducts, simple suction applied by suckling is relatively ineffective, especially in early lactation. Thus the alveolus is enveloped in a basketlike network of myoepithelial cells that respond to oxytocin by contracting and expelling the milk into larger and larger ductules until it can be removed by the infant (see Figure 3-17). This is a classic example of a neuroendocrine reflex, a process that is remarkably uniform in all mammals.[61]

Changes in Breast Hemodynamics in Breastfeeding Mothers

The tissue concentrations of oxyhemoglobin, deoxyhemoglobin, and total hemoglobin and the hemoglobin oxygen saturation while breastfeeding have been measured by near infrared time resolved spectroscopy because it is a noninvasive method of assessment during breastfeeding.[63] When both the breast being suckled and the contralateral breast were measured, both sides showed a significant decrease compared with the presuckling values. During the breastfeeding, values from both breasts fluctuated cyclically. Thus it was documented that blood volume decreases and fluctuates during breastfeeding as does oxygenation. The investigators speculate that this is a result of changes in pressure and resistance in blood vessels accompanying the milk-ejection reflex.[63]

Milk ejection involves both neural and endocrinologic stimulation and response. A neural afferent pathway and an endocrinologic efferent pathway are required.[53]

The ejection reflex depends on receptors located in the canalicular system of the breast. When the canaliculi are dilated or stretched, the reflex release of oxytocin is triggered. Tactile receptors for both oxytocin and reflex prolactin release are in the nipple. Neither the negative and positive pressures exerted by suckling nor the thermal changes trigger the milk-ejection reflex. Negative pressures have a minor effect, but tactile stimulation is the most important factor in milk ejection.

Studies in tactile stimulation show changes in sensitivity at puberty, during the menstrual cycle, and at parturition.[74] No difference exists in sensitivity between the sexes before puberty. In girls, tactile sensitivity increases after puberty and is increased at midcycle and during menstruation. (Midcycle peak is absent in women taking oral contraceptives, probably due to the suppression of ovulation.) Dramatic changes occur within 24 hours of delivery after several weeks of complete insensitivity. The nipple is the most sensitive area to both touch and pain, followed by the areola; the least sensitive area is the cutaneous breast tissue. The increased sensitivity of the breast continues several days postpartum, even when a woman does not breastfeed. Estrogen treatment suppresses the induction of prolactin release on nipple stimulation; on withdrawal of estrogen the prolactin response returns. Increased tactile sensitivity may be the key event activating the suckling-induced release of oxytocin and prolactin at delivery (Figures 3-18 and 3-19).

The clinical study of oxytocin challenge tests for use in measuring the viability of the fetus has led to the study of breast stimulus on the uterus. Numerous studies have confirmed that oxytocin levels rise significantly during nipple stimulation, with short bursts of oxytocin during accompanying uterine contractions.[10] When the effect of breast stimulation on prostaglandin secretion was tested at 38 to 40 weeks' gestation, uterine contractions occurred and prostaglandin metabolite levels increased in all cases. Shalev et al.[79] suggest that the principal action of oxytocin is to stimulate prostaglandin synthesis in uterine tissues, which then becomes the primary cause of the uterine contractions.

The oxytocin-binding sites are located within the basement membrane of the mammary alveolus and along the interlobular ducts. A gradual tenfold increase occurs in the concentration of oxytocin receptor sites in the mammary gland during pregnancy.[47] This contrasts sharply with the sudden fortyfold increase in oxytocin receptors in the uterus in the hours before delivery that then rapidly disappear. These changes in receptor availability may be why copious milk does not occur until shortly after delivery, because oxytocin first facilitates delivery and then promotes milk ejection sequentially. When the increase in intramammary pressure obtained with varying doses of oxytocin in nonpregnant, pregnant, and lactating women was recorded by Caldeyro-Barcia, the amount of oxytocin required for a response dropped from 1000 mU in nonpregnancy to about 1 mU in late pregnancy and to 0.5 mU in lactation (see Figure 3-19).[51] The maximum intramammary

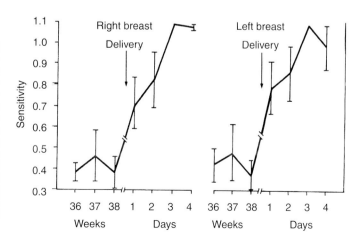

Figure 3-18. Changes in tactile sensitivity of cutaneous breast tissue in perinatal period. Sensitivity was calculated from two-point discrimination according to the formula K − log(e). K is an arbitrary figure employed to portray a low two-point discrimination value as peak of sensitivity. Dramatic increase in tactile sensitivity at delivery enhances response to suckling of newborn. (From Robinson JE, Short RV: Changes in breast sensitivity at puberty, during the menstrual cycle, and at parturition, Br Med J 1:1188, 1977.)

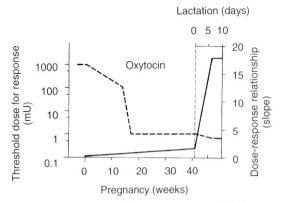

Figure 3-19. Sensitivity of human mammary epithelium to oxytocin during pregnancy and lactation. Scale at left shows threshold dose necessary to evoke increase in intramammary pressure; scale at right shows maximum intramammary pressure obtained. (Modified from Caldeyro-Barcia R: Milk ejection in women. In Reynolds M, Folley SJ, editors: *Lactogenesis: the initiation of milk secretion at parturition,* Philadelphia, 1969, University of Pennsylvania Press.)

pressure that could be evoked increased from 1 mm Hg early in pregnancy to a peak of 10 mm Hg at 5 days postpartum. Caldeyro-Barcia suggests that not only the sensitivity of the myoepithelial cells but the number of receptor sites also increases during pregnancy.

Conflicting information exists regarding the exact nature of the release of oxytocin from the pituitary. The dose-response curve of the mammary gland has a very limited dynamic range, so that a bolus of 0.1 mU oxytocin (0.2 mg) given intravenously to a lactating rat fails to change intramammary pressure. An injection of 1 mU evokes an increase in pressure that begins after a delay of 10 seconds and peaks in 15 seconds at 8 to 10 mm Hg. A bolus has greater effect than a slow push, suggesting that a pulsatile pattern of hormone release would be the most effective way of utilizing oxytocin to produce milk ejection.[48]

Plasma oxytocin levels measured by Lucas et al.[50] with continuous sampling every 20 seconds revealed the hormone was released in surges and persisted in the circulation for less than 1 minute. The multiparas had a greater total response than primiparas, but with no difference between early (1 to 3 days postpartum) and late (5 to 7 days). When a similar study was done by Dawood et al.,[19] collecting samples only every 3 minutes, no pulsing was identified. Oxytocin was measurable within 2 minutes of suckling, peaked at 10 minutes, and had a bimodal curve dropping to a mean at 20 minutes, comparable with that before suckling, which followed the burping and changing of breasts at approximately 15 minutes. A secondary peak occurred at 25 minutes. They found maximum response of intramammary pressures at the fifth to

seventh day. McNeilly et al. measured release of oxytocin in response to suckling in early and established lactation, drawing samples every 30 seconds. A catheter for blood sampling was placed in the forearm 40 minutes before lactation. Oxytocin levels increased 3 to 10 minutes before suckling in response to the baby crying or becoming restless or the mother preparing herself to feed. There was no prolactin response until suckling began.

Most results clearly showed response before tactile stimuli and then a second surge in response to suckling. The levels were pulsatile during suckling and not related to milk volume, prolactin response, or parity of the mother.

Significant elevations of the maternal oxytocin level occur at 15, 30, and 45 minutes after delivery when the infant is put skin to skin, compared with levels just before delivery during expulsion of the placenta.[62] Levels return to baseline after 60 minutes if the infant does not suckle. When oxytocin levels were measured after initiating breast stimulation with a mechanical breast pump in early lactation (10 to 90 days), midlactation (90 to 190 days), and late lactation (180 days to 12 months), baseline levels were similar in all three periods. The stimulated plasma oxytocin levels were greater in early than late lactation, but there was always a response. Thus the oxytocin secretory reflex appears to continue for at least the first year of lactation.

The release of oxytocin by neurohypophyseal responses during lactation has been evoked both by the infant's suckling and by mechanical dilatation of the mammary ducts. This release of oxytocin was demonstrated to be independent of vasopressin release. Conversely, further study[43,44] demonstrated that there could be stimulation of vasopressin release independent of oxytocin release.

When the levels of hGH, vasopressin, prolactin, calcitonin, gastrin, insulin, epinephrine, norepinephrine, and dopamine were measured in six lactating women during breastfeeding, Widstrom et al.[102] confirmed the rise in prolactin and demonstrated the progressive increase in insulin that may be secondary to prolactin rise and may participate in stimulating milk production. Gastrin level decreased, and there were no consistent findings for calcitonin, hGH, norepinephrine, or epinephrine and no change in dopamine and vasopressin. Vagally stimulated release of insulin and gastrin is antagonized when the tone of the sympathetic nervous system is increased, such as during stress, pain, or anxiety. Increased insulin also is known to stimulate the synthesis of casein and lactalbumin and thus, secondarily, milk production. It should be advantageous to breastfeed after a meal rather than before (practically, many mothers eat while feeding the infant).

Human myoepithelium, the effector tissue, is specifically stimulated by oxytocin, and this sensitivity and specificity increase throughout pregnancy. Suckling can induce milk secretion, which is under control of the adenohypophysis. In this case, oxytocin released by the neurohypophysis because of the suckling stimulus would cause both milk ejection and release of the anterior pituitary hormones responsible for milk secretion.[59] This is probably the mechanism behind relactation and induced lactation in a woman who has never been pregnant. Mammary growth and lactogenesis may be induced by suckling, massage, and breast stimulation in many species.

Oxytocin responsivity in human mothers was studied by Light et al.[43] Responses are well documented in animal models and include facilitating maternal behavior, reducing blood pressure, and reducing stress responses. The relationship of oxytocin responsivity to blood pressure in breastfeeding mothers was compared to bottle feeding mothers. The breastfeeding mothers had higher oxytocin levels but lower blood pressure while feeding, especially during stress. The authors concluded that oxytocin has antistress and blood pressure lowering effects.[43]

Alcohol has a dose-related effect on the central nervous system in inhibiting milk ejection. When intramammary pressure was measured in response to suckling by the infant while the mother received measured doses of alcohol, milk ejection was inhibited in a dose-dependent manner.[9] Doses to a maximum of 0.45 g per kilogram of body weight (blood alcohol less than 0.1%), however, had no effect on intramammary pressure. Mechanical breast stimulation for 10 minutes and concomitant administration of intravenous fluid containing normal saline, naloxone, ethanol, or a combination of ethanol and naloxone were initiated in normal nonlactating women on day 22 of the regular menstrual cycle.[11] Plasma oxytocin levels rose twofold, with breast stimulation peaking at 10 minutes. Responses were unchanged by naloxone but were completely abolished by alcohol taken orally (approximately 110 mL of whiskey). Naloxone partially reversed the inhibiting effects of ethanol. The authors concluded that naloxone-sensitive endogenous opioids do not appear to be involved in the control of the oxytocin rise induced by breast stimulation and that opioid peptides are partly involved in the alcohol action.[11] Alcohol has been used in obstetrics to suppress premature labor in humans.

In a study of women who had received oxytocin for stimulus during labor or postpartum for control of bleeding and/or epidural analgesia compared with women who were untreated, plasma oxytocin and prolactin concentrations were measured during suckling on the second day postpartum. All subjects showed a pulsatile oxytocin pattern during the first 10 minutes of breastfeeding. When women received both oxytocin and an epidural, the median oxytocin levels were the lowest. The more oxytocin they had received, the lower their endogenous oxytocin. A significant rise of prolactin occurred after 20 minutes in all women except those who had oxytocin, in whom the levels rose in 10 minutes. The rise in prolactin between 0 and 20 minutes correlated significantly with the median oxytocin and prolactin levels. Thus oxytocin infusion was observed to decrease endogenous oxytocin release dose dependently and facilitated the release of prolactin. Epidural analgesia, when combined with oxytocin, resulted in lowered endogenous oxytocin levels. The length of the breastfeeding session was increased by the prolactin levels; that is, the longer the mother breastfed the higher the levels.

Epidural anesthesia has been demonstrated to inhibit the release of oxytocin during labor into the circulation and the brain of sheep and cows. As a consequence, maternal behavior and bonding to the young are inhibited.[37]

In this study, in the women who received only an epidural, oxytocin levels matched controls. But other studies have shown that epidurals decrease oxytocin levels.

Normal, alert newborns have been observed to "crawl" to the nipple and latch on unassisted when placed on the maternal abdomen following a normal delivery and the clamping and severing of the umbilical cord.[73]

Suckling brings about functional changes in the offspring. An infant who sucks on an artificial nipple quickly decreases the amount of body movement, increases mouth activity, and decreases crying. The suckling experience may affect infant behavior and mother-infant interaction. Nonnutritive suckling is observed in many species. In the human infant, nutritive sucking is shown to be a continuous stream of regular sucks with few, if any, pauses. Nonnutritive sucking has bursts of activity alternating with no sucking. Suckling can be altered by extraneous aural, visual, or olfactory stimuli. Response of breasts to different stimulation patterns of an electric breast pump was measured by Kent et al.[38] When cycles were 45 per minute, let-down occurred in 147 ± 13 seconds. In response to breastfeeding, let-down occurred after 56 ± 4 seconds. Volume was a reflection of negative pressure or vacuum applied but not the time for milk ejection.[38]

Understanding the Myth of "Milk Coming In"

Much of lactation physiology in the human has been based on research done in the bovine and other mammals. This has led to some misinterpretation of human data. An important understanding is that in humans secretory activation occurs after parturition rather than before. Only a small volume of colostrum is available during the first 24 to 48 hours after birth. Today, in newborn nurseries, fixation on technology and measurements have led to determination of blood sugars and strict attention to intake. Human newborns are born with significant stores of energy in body fat and mobilize adequate energy from these sources. This suggests that the concentration of antibodies in the colostrum provides adequate surface protection for the gastrointestinal tract and the respiratory tree. This represents colostrum already secreted in the ducts and not the rapid synthesis and secretion of milk. Thus the awaiting of milk "coming in" has been reported in the first 96 hours. Many women do not experience a sudden change, but a gradual one. When the timing of "milk coming in" is compared with the actual physiologic measurements of increase in lactose and the decrease in sodium, it is noted to lag behind these markers (see Figure 3-4). It is thought[71] that the sensation of "milk coming in" is an "overshoot" seen more commonly in primiparas. The milk supply then has to downregulate to match the infant's needs. Physiologically, it is not a documentable event.

During active lactation the storage time of milk in the alveoli and ducts is about an hour in the human, but much longer in some other species, such as rabbits and sea mammals (to a maximum of 4 days). It is important to point out that the ejection reflex (see Figure 3-15) has been illustrated to imply that there is rapid synthesis and secretion with activation of both oxytocin and prolactin simultaneously. That is not the case. Secretory differentiation is independent of birth; secretory activation is closely associated with birth (see Figures 3-5 and 3-6). Progesterone drop in humans is associated with the delivery of the placenta; therefore, it is after delivery that secretory activation begins, approximately 30 to 40 hours after delivery.[77]

Maternal Effects of Suckling

Effects of suckling on the mother include the stimulation of afferent nerves for the removal of milk.[45] Reduction in sucking stimulus produces a reduction in prolactin and in milk synthesis.[59] The lactating glands adjust the milk supply to demand, probably as a result of both a local and an endocrinologic mechanism. Variations in milk secretion are rapidly reflected in anatomic changes in the mammary gland. Mammary tissue shows regression after the first week or so, if unstimulated. Tissue regression proceeds at a rate parallel to the demand for secretory tissue. Thus when a suckling infant signals needs, the breast will respond[75] (Figure 3-20).

Effects on maternal behavior have been attributed to lactation. Maternal behavior is more easily defined in many other species, in which early nursing is initiated by the mother, who stimulates the neonate to suckle by grooming. She then presents her mammary gland to the offspring so that the nipple is located with minimal effort. All species of lactating females have a lessened response to stress. In humans, however, nursing behavior has a strong voluntary nature. When lactating women were stressed with graded treadmill exercise, significant decreases in plasma levels of ACTH, cortisol, and epinephrine were observed compared with a matched group of nonlactating women.[8] Plasma glucose levels did not increase in either group. Oxytocin pulse in the plasma in response to suckling was also accompanied by a decrease in plasma ACTH and cortisol in the lactating women.

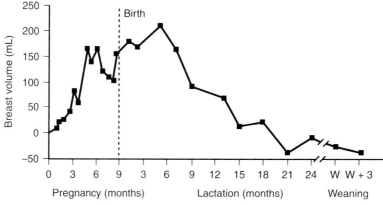

Figure 3-20. Average change in breast volume during pregnancy, lactation, and after weaning (w) compared to preconception breast volume. (From Kent JC, Mitoulas L, Cox DB, et al: Breast volume and milk production during extended lactation, *Exp Physiol* 84:435–447, 1999.)

Oxytocin administered intraventricularly to virgin rats induces maternal behavior. Local infusion of oxytocin antagonists to appropriate regions of the hypothalamus during parturition blocked the dams from pup retrieval, a measure of maternal behavior in rats. Similar observations have been made in sheep.[71] The neurophysical mechanism is under study in humans. Oxytocin promotes the development of human maternal behavior and mother-infant bonding.[70] Some effects of oxytocin in the nipple and mammary gland appear to be caused by peptides released in the nipple from axon collaterals of somatosensory afferent nerves. Oxytocin is also present in neurons projecting to many areas in the brain and exerts many central actions. In addition to maternal behavior, oxytocin causes more nonspecific behavior changes, such as sedation or antistress effects, and optimizes transfer of energy to the mammary gland.[70]

Investigations of the agile wallaby, Macropus agilis, have revealed the let-down reflex because this species displays concurrent asynchronous lactation. The young, weighing 35 g, attach to the teat at birth. The lactating gland continues to grow for 200 days, increasing tenfold in size. At 200 to 220 days, weighing 2500 g, the young first leaves the pouch. Twenty-six days later a second young is born, although the older one continues to suckle intermittently for another 160 days at the original teat. The second young attaches to an unused nipple, which begins to develop, displaying complete autonomy. Measurements of oxytocin during the initial lactation show an increase in intraductal pressure response with a decline in sensitivity over time. This permits milk ejection in response to a small release of oxytocin to be confined to the mammary gland to which the neonate is continuously attached. The release of large quantities of oxytocin in response to the suckling of the juvenile would cause release in both glands.

Mammals have thus evolved diverse strategies for survival. Tandem nursing in the human has not been as carefully studied, but, although the milk reverts to colostrum at the birth of the new infant, no known change occurs in let-down.

The spinothalamic tract is the most likely of the possible spinal and brainstem pathways by which the suckling stimulus reaches the forebrain. The areas of the forebrain influenced by the suckling stimulus include the hypothalamic structures that mediate oxytocin and prolactin release. The inhibition of milk ejection by visual and auditory stimuli, pinealectomy, and ventrolateral midbrain lesions in lactating rats has been studied to define further the neurohormonal pathways. In these experiments, the pineal gland appeared to mediate an inhibitory visual reflex on both oxytocin release and milk ejection.[30]

A mechanism consisting of smooth muscle and elastic fibers acting as a sphincter at the end of the ducts in the nipple appears to prevent most unwanted loss of milk. Sympathetic control does not appear to be present in humans, although it is demonstrable in most other species.

As the end of pregnancy approaches, the breast is prepared to respond to the suckling offspring.[73] In humans, this is evidenced by increased sensitivity of the breast to tactile stimulation; increased responsiveness of the ductules to oxytocin, thus preparing to eject the milk; and increased response of the breast to signaling the release of prolactin to stimulate milk production. The signal for lactation occurs when the placenta is removed and the end organs in the breast can fully respond to the surge of prolactin resulting from suckling.[92]

Concentrations of Oxytocin in Milk

Human milk samples obtained by manual expression daily from the first to the fifth postpartum day were collected immediately before and after a feeding as well as 2 hours after nursing.[88] The baseline mean oxytocin concentrations were 3.3 to 4.7 mg/mL, increasing significantly with nursing. Oxytocin in milk is fairly stable compared with that in maternal serum, which is inactivated by oxytocinase in plasma, liver, and kidney. When oxytocin was administered to rat dams, it was also found in the suckling offspring's gastric contents, where it is stable in acid. Some is absorbed into the neonatal blood, where it is unstable. Levels of oxytocin in neonatal serum are produced predominantly by the neonate itself. Whether oxytocin has a physiologic role on the gut or other hormones is unknown.

Role of Prostaglandins as Milk Ejectors

Because prostaglandins have many physiologic effects and are known to increase mammary duct pressure, Toppozada et al.[90] investigated their role as milk ejectors.[62] Comparison was made among three treatments: intravenous (IV) injections of oxytocin, prostaglandin (PG) E2 (PGE2), and 16-phenoxy-PGE2 given to one group of women on the third to sixth day postpartum; IV oxytocin, 15-methyl-PGF2α, and PGF2α tromethamine salt to a second group; and oxytocin and PGF intranasally to a third group. All combinations had some effect, with the IV route having a shorter latency period than the intranasal. PGF2α, the more potent of the prostaglandin preparations, was more potent via the nasal route than oxytocin nasally. The response lasted 25 minutes after intranasal instillation of 400 mg. PGE2 and PGF2α, orally administered, reduce prolactin levels and appear to be successful in suppressing lactation in the immediate postpartum period when given in large doses of 2 to 4 mg or in multiple doses to a maximum of 10 times greater. Although they are produced in larger quantities by the mammary gland in vitro and in vivo, the role of prostaglandins is still not clear, because these studies[90] are in conflict with previous results by Vorherr.[99] The practical application of this in-lactation failure has not been reported.

Milk-borne prostaglandins clearly survive in the environment of the infant's gastrointestinal tract and are delivered in an active form to peripheral organs. The significance of this remains under investigation.[40]

Production of Hormones by the Mammary Gland

Hormones synthesized by the mammary gland may have endocrine, autocrine, or paracrine effects within the mother. The chemical mediators known to be synthesized by the mammary gland are EGF, progesterone, prolactin, estrogens, and relaxin. Other hormones are transported to the gland.[68] These bioactive agents could have multiple roles in both mother and recipient infant. Insulin-like growth factors are found in high concentration in colostrum and at lower levels in mature milk. Milk factors other than nutrients are thought to control specific developmental processes in the infant. Because infants survive and grow on formula, this latter point is difficult to prove. Actions of milk regulatory substances are much more important in at-risk infants than in full-term infants.

Feedback Inhibitor of Lactation

The mammary gland is unique because, as an exocrine gland, it stores its secretion extracellularly. Storage within the gland's lumen suggests a local level of control on the rate of secretion.[57]

As stated earlier, milk is produced as long as it is removed from the mammary gland. Further, prolactin and oxytocin are responsible for the production and release of milk, allowing the infant to extract milk by suckling. The rate of milk secretion may differ between breasts if one breast is suckled more frequently or for a longer time. When lactating goats have an extra daily milking, the secretory rate is increased even if the milk is immediately replaced with an inert solution to maintain the gland's

distention. The dilution of stored milk in the gland with an inert isotonic solution results in increased milk secretion, suggesting the dilution of a chemical inhibitor.

Identification of a factor that is produced and functions at the mammary level, FIL, has evolved from multiple studies.[72] Wilde et al.[103] described autocrine regulation of milk secretion by a previously unknown protein in the milk. When this active whey protein, a FIL, was isolated and injected into the mammary gland of lactating goats, milk secretion was decreased temporarily. Similar work by Prentice et al.[72] confirmed the presence of FIL in humans. FIL is able to exert reversible concentration-dependent autocrine inhibition on milk secretion in the lactating gland. It controls secretion of all milk constituents simultaneously; that is, it affects secretion, not composition.

The search for the mechanism that explains regulation of milk supply continues. When goats were studied, it was noted that when milk accumulated in the mammary gland, production decreased. When the milk was removed and replaced with isotonic sucrose solution to volume, the rate of milk produced increased. This finding supports the concept that it is a compound in the milk and not distention of the mammary gland that regulates synthesis. This factor, FIL, is an autocrine mechanism.

FIL cannot be the sole control of milk synthesis, or removal of milk would not stimulate milk production (see Figure 3-20). Cregan and Hartmann speculate that the mechanism of local control of milk synthesis is related to the filling/emptying cycle of the alveoli.[14] Milk accumulation changes the morphology of the lactocytes lining the alveoli. When the luminal volume of mammospheres increased, according to St. Reuli and Edwards, it altered the interaction of the lactocytes with the basement membrane inhibiting prolactin receptors and further milk synthesis.[83]

Maternal Adaptation to Lactation

The hormonal trigger for lactogenesis is a decrease in progesterone while prolactin levels are maintained. Postpartum prolactin levels are comparable in breastfeeding and nonbreastfeeding women for a few days (see Figures 19-2 to 19-4 and Figure 3-6). Thus the basic process occurs regardless of whether breastfeeding is initiated. The mammary epithelium must be adequately prepared by the hormones of pregnancy to respond by synthesizing milk.

Each mammalian species has evolved its own lactational strategies to meet the nutritional needs of its offspring, with influences from both genetic and environmental forces. The endocrine signals promote mammary development, inhibit milk production during gestation, and then promote development of enhanced metabolic and transport functions in adipose tissue, visceral organs, and reproductive organs.[67] Lactational adaptations of adipose tissue metabolism have been recognized in all species and may be most dramatic in seals, hibernating bears, and whales, who produce fat-rich milk from their fat stores while fasting. Lactation results in profound changes in adipose tissue metabolism to provide energy stores, modulate mammary development, affect appetite, and influence the immune system function.[93]

The substantial adaptation of the maternal intestine during lactation is the large increase in its size and complexity, which ensures adequate absorption of nutrients to meet the increased energy demand.[28] A corresponding increase occurs in liver and heart performance. In addition to extra fat demands, calcium concentration must be sufficient to maintain maternal stores while providing for the demands of milk synthesis, which are greater than those of pregnancy.[34] The estimated calcium requirement is 12 mg/kg per day in humans. The elevation in plasma dihydroxycholecalciferol, or 1,25-(OH)2D3, during late gestation continues during early lactation. As lactation progresses beyond 3 months, plasma 1,25-(OH)2D3 levels decline. This results in decreased calcium absorption, which is offset by greater maternal bone losses and reduced urinary calcium. Glucose requirements during lactation require major adjustments in glucose production and utilization in the maternal liver, adipose tissue, bone, muscle, and other tissues. Adaptation of folic acid metabolism is equally important, although less well studied.[67]

The mechanisms by which early pregnancy and lactation decrease the incidence of breast cancer are unclear. Close examination of the more differentiated mammary cell, which is less susceptible to the loss of growth regulation, is a next step, along with inspection of mucin, a glycoprotein and normal differentiation antigen expressed in both milk fat globules and mammary tumors.

Delay in the Onset of Lactogenesis

Clinically, it has been observed that delayed lactogenesis occurs in women who have diabetes, are stressed during delivery, and occasionally experience retained placenta. When signs of lactogenesis are absent in the first 72 hours, a cause should be sought. In women with diabetes, extra effort should be made to ensure that the process goes well with good hydration, adequate dietary intake, insulin control, and attention to detail. A study of the impact of cesarean delivery on lactogenesis II found that early pumping did not help and may have interfered with the volume of milk produced.[7] After stressful deliveries, it may be necessary to initiate pumping if the infant is unable to adequately stimulate the breast, but this needs further study. Again, close monitoring is essential before discharge. Retained placenta is discussed in Chapter 16. The treatment, dilatation and curettage, is definitive and dramatically therapeutic.

Anticipating problems and identifying early signals of faltering are key to ultimately improving lactogenesis.

Synthesis of Human Milk

Computerized breast measurement (CBM) was developed by Hartmann et al.[32] because of the inaccuracy of the established methods for measuring milk synthesis. The three other techniques utilized are (1) weighing either the infant or the mother before and after every feeding for 24 hours; (2) isotope dilution used to estimate production over a 4- or 7-day period; and (3) breast expression in which a mother removes milk from breasts (this technique does not reflect the effect of the infant on milk production by suckling). CBM is designed to measure short-term rates of milk synthesis. This technique allows the appetite of the infant to dictate the amount of milk removed from the breast while also being able to measure the residual (Figure 3-21).

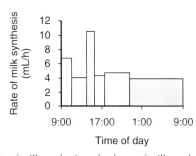 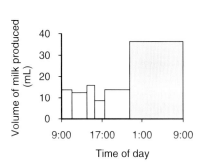

Figure 3-21. Rate of milk synthesis and volume of milk produced in one breast by an exclusively expressing mother over a 24-hour period. The shaded columns indicate the overnight period that had the lowest rate of milk synthesis but the highest volume expressed. (From Cregan MD, Hartmann PE: Computerized breast measurement from conception to weaning: clinical implications, *J Hum Lact* 15:89, 1999.)

CBM measures changes in breast volume without interfering with the infant's pattern of breastfeeding. CBM allows not only measurement of change in breast volume and volume of milk removed during a feeding but four additional parameters.

The first is the short-term rate of milk synthesis (S) between breastfeedings. The calculation takes the increase in breast volume from the end of one feeding (V_{B1}) to the beginning of the next (V_{B2}), divided by the time between these two measurements (T).

$$S = \frac{V_{B2} - V_{B1}}{T}$$

The second measures storage capacity (SC), which is defined by the authors as the maximum breast volume (V_{max}) minus the minimum breast volume (V_{min}) observed over a 24-hour period (see Figure 3-21).

$$SC = V_{max} - V_{min}$$

The third measurement is the degree of fullness (F), which is the ratio of any particular breast volume (V_B) divided by the storage capacity of the breast (SC).

$$F = \frac{V_B}{SC}$$

The range is from 1 when the breast is full to 0 when it is at minimum volume in a 24-hour period.

In addition, this CBM technology can be used to measure the increase in breast volume during pregnancy, thus measuring breast growth and breast involution after peak lactation.

The storage capacity was measured by Daly et al.[17] and varied from 80 to 600 mL. The rate of milk synthesis was minimal when the breast was full and maximum when the breast was emptied.

The function of the mammary gland is unique in that it produces a substance that makes tremendous demands on the maternal system without producing any physiologic advantage to the maternal organism. Because lactation is anticipated, the body prepares the breast anatomically and physiologically.[82] When lactation begins, the mother's metabolism changes greatly. The blood supply is redistributed, and the demand for nutrients increases, which requires an increased metabolic rate to accommodate their production. The mammary gland may need to produce milk at the metabolic expense of other organs. The supply of materials to the lactating breast for milk production and energy metabolism requires extensive cardiovascular changes in the mother. There is increased mammary blood flow, increased blood flow into the gastrointestinal tract and liver, and a high cardiac output. The mammary blood flow, cardiac output, and milk secretion are suckling dependent. Suckling induces the release of anterior pituitary hormones that act directly on breast tissue.

Milk is isosmotic with plasma in all species.[44] Human milk differs from many other milks in that the concentration of major monovalent ions is lower and that of lactose is higher; in other milks, the higher the ions, the lower the lactose, and vice versa. Many disparities in the intermediary metabolism among species of animals can be linked to evolutionary adaptations involving the digestive process.[43] Nonruminants rely on glucose, derived from carbohydrate in the diet. Ruminants, because of extensive fermentation in the rumen, absorb little glucose. The microbial fermentation products, which include acetate, propionate, and butyrate, play a significant part as energy and carbon sources for tissue metabolism. Amino acids are primary substitutes for glucose in ruminants.[44]

The biosynthesis of milk involves a cellular site where the metabolic processes occur. The epithelial cells of the gland contain stem cells and highly differentiated secretory alveolar cells at the terminal ducts. The stem cells are stimulated by hGH and insulin. Prolactin synergizes the insulin effect to stimulate the cells to secretory activity.

Prolactin binds to specific prolactin receptors on the surface of the lactocytes. There is a lactogenic signaling pathway which creates the switching on of the transcription of genes. These genes regulate the secretion of milk proteins, including casein and lactalbumin. The prolactin receptor is part of the cytokine receptor family. These are activated at the onset of pregnancy and lactogenesis. The binding of prolactin to the site triggers the kinase and the chain of reactions of phosphoration and activation of transcription[16] (Figure 3-22).

The cells of the acini and smaller milk ducts are active in milk synthesis and milk secretion into the alveoli and smaller milk ducts. Most milk is synthesized during the process of suckling; its production is stimulated by prolactin. Cortisol plasma levels are increased during suckling as well. The secretory cells are cuboidal, changing to a cylindrical shape just before milk secretion, while cellular water uptake is increased. The cell's single nucleus is at the base in the dormant cell but migrates to the apex just before milk secretion.

The differentiated structure of the functional cell is acquired gradually during pregnancy, differing little from species to species. Very early in lactation, mammary cells show active synthesis and secretion of proteins and fat. The cells are polarized with abundant rough endoplasmic reticulum and Golgi dictyosomes above the nucleus, which is smooth and rounded with many mitochondria.

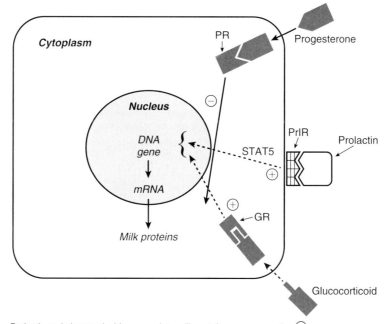

Prolactin and glucocorticoids up-regulate milk protein gene expression ⊕
Progesterone inhibits milk protein expression during pregnancy ⊖
PR = progesterone receptor, PrlR = prolactin receptor, GR = glucocorticoid receptor

Figure 3-22. Intracellular hormonal signaling in the lactocyte during lactation. (Adapted from Mercier and Gaye: Chapter 7. In Mepham TB, editor: *Biochemistry of lactation*, New York, 1983, Elsevier.)

The apical surface has microvilli, and the basal surface is extensively convoluted for the active transport of materials from the bloodstream into the cell. Fat droplets are in the cytoplasm and bulging at the membrane. Proteins, lactose, calcium, phosphate, and citrate are packaged into secretory vesicles and pass into the lumen of the alveolus by exocytosis.

The cytoplasm is finely granular in the resting phase but striated as milk secretion begins. As secretion commences, the enlarged cell with its thickened apical membrane becomes clublike in shape. The tip pinches off, leaving the cell intact. The protein is thus free in the secreted solution, retaining a cap of membrane (Figure 3-23).

Function of Cellular Components of the Lactating Breast

The schema of the mammary secretory cell is represented in Figures 3-24 and 3-25.

NUCLEUS

The nucleus is essential to the duplication of genetic material and the transcription of the genetic code.[97] The nucleus is also considered a regulatory organelle

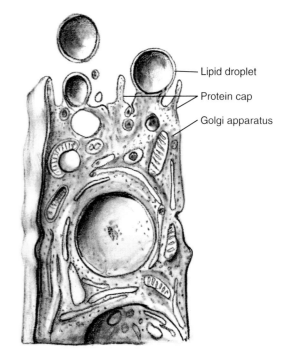

Figure 3-23. Apocrine secretory mechanism for lipids, proteins, and lactose in milk.

in cell metabolism, transmitting the design of the cell's enzymatic profile. The DNA and RNA content of the cellular nuclei increases during pregnancy and is highest during lactation.

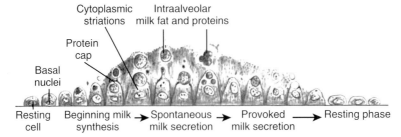

Figure 3-24. Diagram of cycle of secretory cells from resting stage to secretion and return to resting stage. (Modified from Vorherr H: *The breast: morphology, physiology and lactation,* New York, 1974, Academic Press.)

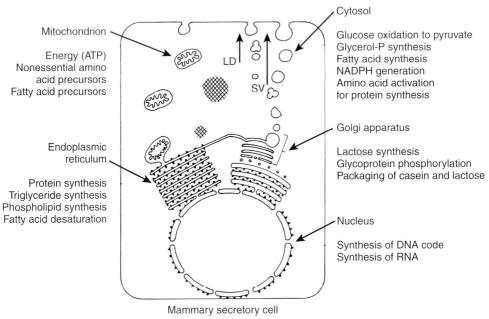

Figure 3-25. Schema of cytologic and biochemical interrelationships of secretory cell of mammary gland. *LD,* Lipid droplet; *SV,* secretory vesicle.

CYTOSOL

The cytosol, which consists of the cytoplasm minus the mitochondrial and microsomal fractions, is also called the particle-free supernatant. The cytosol contains enzymes that involve key intermediates and cofactors essential to the process of milk synthesis.

MITOCHONDRIAL PROLIFERATION

The alveolar cell population of the mammary gland must have a greatly expanded oxidative capacity during lactation. It is supplied by an increase in size and function of the cell's mitochondrial population. Mitochondria are increased in the epithelial cell at the onset of the lactation process. Mitochondrial proliferation has been observed in all cells with a high metabolic rate and high oxygen utilization.

During the presecretory differentiation phase in late pregnancy and early lactation, each mito-chondrion undergoes a type of differentiation in which the inner membrane and matrix expand greatly. As with other cells, the mitochondria are key to the respiratory activity of the cell. Mito-chondria control some cellular metabolism through differential permeability to certain anions. The cit-rate in the mitochondria is a major source of carbon for fatty acid biosynthesis. Mitochondria also supply the carbon for synthesis of nonessential amino acids.

MICROSOMAL FRACTION

The microsomal fraction of the cell, which includes the Golgi apparatus, the endoplasmic reticulum, and the cell membranes, is involved in lipid synthe-sis. The role of the microsomal fraction is also to assemble the constituent parts (e.g., amino acids, glucose, fatty acids) into the final products of pro-tein, carbohydrate, and fat for secretion.

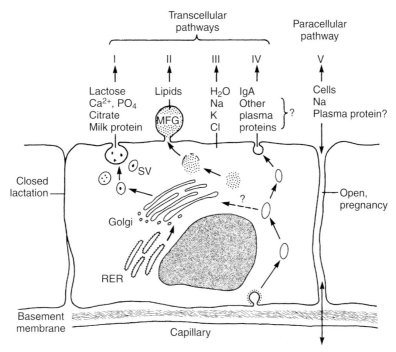

Figure 3-26. Pathways for milk synthesis and secretion into mammary alveolus. **I,** Exocytosis of milk protein and lactose in Golgi-derived secretory vesicles. **II,** Milk fat secretion via milk fat globule. **III,** Secretion of ions and water across apical membrane. **IV,** Pinocytosis-exocytosis of immunoglobulins. **V,** Paracellular pathway for plasma components and leukocytes. *MFG,* Milk fat globule; *RER*; rough endoplasmic reticulum; *SV,* secretory vesicle. (Modified from Neville MC: The physiological basis of milk secretion. Part I. Basic physiology, *Ann NY Acad Sci* 586:1, 1990.)

INTERMEDIARY METABOLISM OF MAMMARY GLAND

The pathways identified for milk synthesis and secretion in the mammary alveolus, as described by Neville et al.,[50] include four major transcellular pathways and one paracellular pathway (Figure 3-26):

1. Exocytosis of milk protein and lactose in Golgi-derived secretory vesicles
2. Milk fat secretion via the milk fat globule
3. Secretion of ions and water across the apical membrane
4. Pinocytosis-exocytosis of immunoglobulins
5. Paracellular pathway for plasma components and leukocytes

CARBOHYDRATES

The major carbohydrate for most species is lactose, a disaccharide found only in milk. In addition to lactose, more than 50 oligosaccharides of different structures have been identified in human milk. One of the most important is glucose.

Glucose metabolism has a key function in milk production.[4] Glucose serves as the main source of energy for other reactions as well as a critical source of carbon. Glucose is critical to the volume of milk produced and is used in the production of lactose. The synthesis of

lactose combines glucose and galactose, the latter originating from glucose-6-phosphate.[33]

Lactose synthesis is carried out by the following equations

$$UDP - galactose + N - acetylglucosamine \rightarrow N - acetyllactosamine + UDP$$

$$(3\text{-}1)$$

$$UDP - galactose + glucose \rightarrow lactose + UDP \quad (3\text{-}2)$$

UDP is uridine diphosphogalactose. The catalyst in the first equation is a galactosyl transferase, N-acetyllactosamine synthetase. The reaction is activated by metal ions that bind to the galactosyltransferase.

Most of the intracellular glucose is derived from blood sugar. A specific whey protein, α-lactalbumin, catalyzes the lactose synthesis. It is a rate-limiting enzyme, which is inhibited by progesterone during pregnancy. In the absence of α-lactalbumin, little lactose is present. With the drop in progesterone and estrogen levels after the removal of the placenta at delivery, prolactin increases. The synthesis of α-lactalbumin becomes greater, and large amounts of lactose are produced from glucose. Progesterone regulates the onset of lactose synthesis, causing the initiation of production just as the infant is in need of nutrition.

Because lactose is synthesized only from glucose, maternal glucose utilization is increased by 30% in full lactation.[59]

Various aspects of lactose synthesis continue to be vigorously investigated.[33] The molecular mechanism of lactose synthesis is activated by metal ions, manganese (Mn), and calcium (Ca). Lactose synthesis takes place within the Golgi apparatus (see Figure 3-26). The onset of copious milk secretion depends on rapid increase of lactose synthesis. Lactose synthetase performs the rate-limiting step in lactose synthesis, which is one of the few anabolic reactions involving glucose itself rather than a phosphorylated derivative.[5] Although progesterone, thyroxine, and lactogenic hormones are important in controlling synthesis, it is not known how they act in this system. The areas available for investigation about lactose synthesis remain vast.

FAT

Fat synthesis takes place in the endoplasmic reticulum. The alveolar cells are able to synthesize short-chain fatty acids, which are derived predominantly from acetate. Long-chain fatty acids, derived chiefly from blood plasma, are used in milk fat. Triglycerides are utilized from the plasma, as well as synthesized from intracellular glucose oxidized via the pentose pathway. Synthesis of fat from carbohydrate plays a predominant role in fat production in human milk.[36]

Two enzymes, lipoprotein lipase and palmitoyl-coenzyme A (CoA) L-glycerol-3-phosphate palmitoyl transferase, increase greatly after delivery. The lipase acts at the walls of the capillaries to catalyze the lipolysis and uptake of glycerol into the epithelial cells. The transferase catalyzes the process of synthesizing glycerides to triglycerides. It is believed that the marked increase of the lipase and transferase is stimulated by prolactin. Hormonal control of the glycerol precursors and the enzymatic release of fatty acids, leading to the formation of triglycerides, have been associated not only with prolactin but also with insulin, which stimulates the uptake of glucose into the mammary cells.

Esterification of fatty acids also takes place in the endoplasmic reticulum. The triglycerides subsequently accumulate into fat droplets in several cisternae. The small droplets sit on the base of the cell and coalesce to large droplets that move toward the apex of the cell. The fat droplets are engulfed in the apical membrane and project into the alveolar lumen. The discharge of fat droplets involves the bulging of the cell apex to envelop the fat globules, protein, and a small amount of cytoplasm; with the pinching off, the globule becomes detached into the lumen. The membrane of the fat globule contains all the normal plasma enzymes. The fat droplets contain predominantly polar lipid and phosphatidyl choline.

Fatty acid synthesis involves a source of substrates and associated enzymes for their conversion to acetyl-CoA and reduced nicotinamide-adenine dinucleotide phosphate in the cytoplasm of the cell and the conversion of acetyl-CoA to malonyl-CoA. The newly synthesized fatty acid is then released from the fatty acid-synthetase complex.

The milk-fat-globule membrane in human milk serves several roles. A layer of amphophilic (bipolar) substances at the globule/skim milk interface is required for the maintenance of emulsion stability of the fat globules.[36] This physiochemical fact applies to all emulsions and to the fat globules in the milk of all species. The globules and the milk-fat-globule membrane are compartments within the emulsion component of milk. Once in place, the components of the milk-fat-globule membrane, which is the oil-water interfacial compartment, are more or less firmly held in place by a variety of chemical and electrical forces. The stabilizing membrane acts as a reactive barrier on the interface between the globule and milk serum.[36] It is rate controlling for the binding of enzymes and trace elements, the controlled release of the products of lipolysis, the transfer of polar materials into milk serum, the maintenance of emulsion stability by the prevention of globule fission, and the availability of fatty acids and cholesterol for micellar absorption in the small intestine. All these interactions are dynamic. The envelopment mechanism involves rapid turnover of the plasma membrane lipids and proteins during milk production.

Study of RNA sequencing of the human fat layer transcription resulted in distinct gene expression profiles in all stages of lactation, colostral, transitional, and mature milk production. The contribution of maternal physiology to problems with lactation is just being explored. It is known that human milk fat globules, by enveloping cell contents as they are secreted into milk, are great sources of mammary cell RNA. Strong modulation of key genes is involved in lactose synthesis and insulin signaling. Protein tyrosine phosphatase is thought to serve as a biomarker linking insulin resistance to insufficient milk supply. The methodology is just being developed to research the physiologic contributions of suboptimal lactation.[42]

PROTEIN

Most proteins in milk are formed from free amino acids in the secretory cells of the mammary gland. The definitive data confirming the origin of milk proteins have been accumulated since 1980. The vast majority of proteins present in normal milk are specific to mammary secretions and are not identified in any quantity elsewhere in nature.[43]

The formation of milk protein and mammary enzymes is induced by prolactin and further stimulated by insulin and cortisol. De novo synthesis of protein uses both essential and nonessential plasma amino acids. Nuclear RNA, induced by prolactin, stimulates synthesis of mRNA and transfer RNA (tRNA). The mRNA conveys the genetic information to the protein-synthesizing centers of the cells. The tRNA interprets the message to assemble the amino acids in the appropriate sequence of polypeptide chains of the specific milk proteins. The newly synthesized proteins are secreted into the milk during lactation. Casein, α-lactalbumin, and β-lactoglobulin from plasma amino acids are synthesized on the ribosomes of the endoplasmic reticulum, where they are condensed and appear as visible secretory granules moving toward the cellular apex.

After some processing, the proteins pass to the Golgi complex, where they are further glycosylated and phosphorylated and then placed in secretory vesicles for export[54]; α-lactalbumin, a protein necessary for lactose synthesis by the enzyme galactosyltransferase, is among the proteins synthesized in the mammary gland. Lactose is synthesized within the trans-Golgi complex and secreted together with the major milk proteins. The casein micelle is formed with calcium within the Golgi compartment, which presents a high concentration of calcium, phosphate, and protein via the milk. Most of the casein is bound in this manner. This pathway I (see Figure 3-26) begins in the rough endoplasmic reticulum, where the proteins are inserted through the membrane into the lumen by exocytosis.[54]

The Golgi membrane is impermeable to lactose; thus the sugar is osmotically active. Water is drawn into the Golgi apparatus.[67] Casein micelle formation begins in the terminal Golgi vesicles, adding calcium in the secretory vesicle. These secretory vesicles move to the plasma membrane and through exocytosis extrude their contents into the alveolar lumen.[49]

Human casein micelles are smaller in size (30 to 75 nm in diameter) than bovine casein (600 nm). Human milk contains only β-casein. Only 6% of calcium in human milk is bound to casein, compared with 65% in bovine milk. The gene for human β-casein has been cloned and sequenced.[67]

Some merocrine secretion also occurs, in which proteins and other cellular constituents are secreted, leaving the cell membrane intact. Protein caps, or signets, protruding into alveolar lumen, have been described on the outside of the apical

TABLE 3-3	Alveolar Epithelial Membrane Permeability	
Cell ↔ Alveolar Lumen	**Cell → Alveolar Lumen**
Glucose	Lactose
Water	Sucrose
Sodium	Citrate
Potassium	Proteins
Chloride	Fat
Iodine	Calcium
Sulfate	Phosphate

membrane. Protein and lactose secreted into the lumen cannot be reabsorbed (Table 3-3).

The synthesis of proteins in the mammary gland follows the general pathway of all proteins under genetic control. Induction of synthesis is under hormonal control. This process involves synthesis from amino acids through the detailed system controlled by RNA and under genetic control of DNA. Glucocorticoid is required for the expression of the casein gene in the presence of prolactin. Cortisol is the limiting factor for casein gene expression.[28] Shennan[88] has reviewed the mechanisms of mammary gland ion transport.

IONS AND WATER

Sodium, potassium, chloride, magnesium, calcium, phosphate, sulfate, and citrate pass through the membrane of the alveolar cell in both directions.[58] Water also passes in both directions, predominantly from the alveolar cells but also from the interstitial fluid. Plasma water passage depends on the amount of intracellular glucose available for lactose. The aqueous phase of milk is isosmotic to plasma. The major osmole of the aqueous phase of milk is lactose. The concentrations of sodium and chloride are less than those in plasma.

Human milk differs from that of many other species in that the monovalent ions are in low concentration and lactose is in high concentration.[45] The osmolarity is the same, that is, isosmotic with plasma; thus the higher the lactose, the lower the ions. It is presumed that the intracellular concentration of potassium is held high and that of sodium low by a pump on the basal membrane. The sodium and potassium ions are distributed according to the electrical potential gradient.[58] Milk is electrically positive compared with intracellular fluid. The sodium/potassium ratio is 1:3 in both milk and intracellular fluid. Vorherr[98,99] thinks that lactose secretion is responsible for the potential difference across the apical membrane, thus keeping sodium and potassium ion concentration low.

The variation among species in the concentration of lactose and ions is caused by the rate of lactose synthesis, the permeability of the membrane, and the number of fixed negative charges on the membrane. The potential difference is higher in the human mammary gland than in any other species evaluated to date.

The relationship between infrastructure and function in the mammary gland changes from pregnancy to lactation. The junction between alveolar cells has attracted much interest. Cell junctions do not merely hold cells together but enable epithelia to function as permeable barriers, allowing communication between cells and coordination of activities. The three functions of cell junctions are adhesion, occlusion, and communication, which are carried out by desmosomes, tight junctions, and gap junctions, respectively. Changes in tight junctions may provide the basis for a reduction in permeability between cells. For instance, at the initiation of lactation, a tight junction changing from "leaky" to very tight blocks the paracellular movement of lactose and ions. This requires transport across cells of these materials and the maintenance of control of high intracellular potassium and low intracellular sodium concentrations.[20]

Citrate is thought to be the harbinger of lactogenesis. Citrate plays a central role in the metabolism of all cells, but its significance and mode of secretion remain unknown.[69] In the final stages of lactogenesis in ruminants, the previously quiescent epithelial cells suddenly start to secrete large quantities of protein, fat, and carbohydrates. The exact lactogenic trigger is unknown, although significant hormonal changes occur. In women, the onset of copious milk secretion does not begin until 3 to 4 days postpartum. Significantly, citrate levels are low at delivery and rise quickly, reaching a peak on day 4.[69] In cows and goats, copious production occurs at delivery, and the citrate levels begin to rise, increasing 10 to 100 times the baseline values.

Citrate is the main buffer system of milk.[58] It is formed within the secretory cell, but how it is secreted into the milk is not clear. Citrate and lactose may be secreted by a similar route. After dilution of milk in the gland with isosmotic lactose, the equilibrium is restored across the apical membrane in experimental models by the entrance of sodium, potassium, and chloride into the milk. No citrate, calcium, or protein enters in excess of the normal secretion rate. Inorganic phosphate is the other major buffer system, but how it is secreted is also unknown.

Calcium, much of which is bound to casein, enters the Golgi apparatus, where it is essentially trapped with casein in the micelle, and then enters the alveolar milk by unidirectional flow.

The mammary gland is unusual among exocrine glands because the rate of secretion slows and some secretion can be stored in its ducts.[80] Direct neural control of secretion is lacking. The parenchyma of the gland also consists of ductal tissue in addition to secretory tissue. The ductal cells, however, are impermeable to the major milk ions during lactation, so in contrast to the ductal cells of other exocrine glands (e.g., sweat, salivary) they cannot modify the secretion.

A comparison of the levels of various constituents of the milk with corresponding plasma levels demonstrates the mechanism partly responsible for that difference in levels (see Table 4-18).

MILK ENZYMES

Some milk enzymes enter the alveolar milk from the mammary blood capillaries via the intercellular fluid. Others come from the breakdown of the mammary secretory cells. The milk enzymes, xanthine oxidase, aldolase, and alkaline phosphatase, are contained in the fat globule, membrane, and milk serum. The most significant enzyme, lipase, splits triglycerides.

Human milk contains both proteolytic enzymes and protease inhibitors.[29] Amylase facilitates digestion of polysaccharides by the infant. Sulfhydryl oxidase catalyzes oxidation of sulfhydryl groups. Glutathione peroxidase facilitates the delivery of selenium to the infant. Lysozyme and peroxidase are bactericidal.

CELLULAR COMPONENTS

Human milk has been called a "live fluid" by many and "white blood" in many ancient rites. Breast milk contains up to 4000 cells/mL, which have been identified with leukocytes and enter the milk via the paracellular pathway, pathway V.[97] The cell number is particularly high in colostrum. The cells in greatest number are the macrophages, which secrete lysozyme and lactoferrin. Lymphocytes, neutrophils, and epithelial cells are also present. Lymphocytes produce IgA and interferon.

Macrophages constitute a major cellular component in milk compared with levels in blood and can survive under conditions simulating the infant's gastrointestinal tract.[31] Because they release secretory IgA in association with phagocytosis, it is thought they play a role in host defense. Macrophage colony-stimulating factor in human milk and mammary gland epithelial cells are thought to be responsible for expansion of the macrophages in milk.

Involution: Weaning and Apoptosis

During weaning, significant increases in milk protein, chloride, and sodium concentrations and a decrease in lactose occur when milk volumes fall below 400 mL per day. Glucose and magnesium levels are unchanged.[57] This suggests that volume is regulated differently during weaning than during lactogenesis. No sentinel substance is a reliable predictor of volume in all stages, but normal ranges of milk components during full lactation are sodium, 3 to 18 mmol/L; chloride, 8 to 24 mmol/L; protein, 8 to 23 g/L; and lactose, 140 to 230 mmol/L. Values outside these ranges suggest mastitis or weaning. During gradual weaning, between 6 and 15 months postpartum, glucose, citrate, phosphate, and calcium levels decrease, whereas lipid, potassium, and magnesium increase.[63]

Postlactational involution of the mammary gland is characterized by two distinct physiologic processes.[51] First, secretory epithelial cells undergo apoptosis and programmed cell death. Second, the mammary gland's basement membrane undergoes proteolytic degradation. Apoptosis is almost absent during lactation but develops within 2 days of involution. In the initial phase of involution, apoptosis of fully differentiated mammary epithelial cells occurs without visible degradation of the extracellular matrix. The second phase consists of extracellular remodeling and altered mesenchymal-epithelial interactions followed by apoptosis of cells no longer differentiating.[85] During postlactational mammary gland involution, most mammary epithelium dies and is reabsorbed.

In experimental models, apoptosis has been studied at weaning by using animals, removing the pups from the breast and studying the biochemical and genetic markers. Regulation of apoptosis during mammary gland involution is multifunctional. Forced weaning is used as a tool to accelerate and synchronize the involution process, thus allowing biochemical analysis. Apoptosis phenotypes resulting from specific gene deletions have been identified when these animal mothers are unable to nurse their pups.

When suckling ceases after lactation, the alveolar component of the gland involutes through a process that involves both apoptosis and tissue remodeling, which reconstructs the gland to the prepregnancy state. In situations of forced weaning, two phases occur. An initial apoptotic phase begins within 12 hours and persists for about 72 hours. The second phase involves further apoptosis, matrix degradation, and gland remodeling.

The first phase of involution before apoptosis is reversible and lactation can be reinstated within 2 days. During this time, milk accumulates within the alveolar lumen, and the level of lactogenic hormones drop. The initiation of apoptosis and the degradation of nuclear DNA into fragments is the best understood phase of the process. The second phase begins in which the gland remodeling takes place. The old connective tissue and the basement membrane are removed, then the ductal component is reformed. Apoptosis continues through this phase. High levels of tissue inhibitors of metalloproteinases are expressed, preventing excess matrix metalloproteinase activity.[27]

Significant advances have been made in the knowledge of signaling pathways that regulate epithelial cell apoptosis in the first phase. The precise nature of the triggers for apoptosis and the ultimate perpetrators of cell death are unknown. The available information suggests a complex network of signal transduction pathways that control apoptosis in the involuting mammary gland.[87]

Summary

In humans, lactogenesis occurs slowly over the first few days postpartum as progesterone levels drop. Women experience "milk coming in" as a feeling of fullness between 40 and 72 hours postpartum, usually corresponding to the degree of parity, with multiparas sensing this more quickly than primiparas. The physiologic explanation of the increase in milk volume, however, suggests that the sensation of "milk coming in" is not "normal" but a sign of over shooting the mark. Some women do not sense this special fullness but are excellent milk producers. Volume of milk increases over time for the first 2 weeks, starting at less than 100 mL per day and increasing to about 600 mL per day at 96 hours (Figure 3-27). This parallels the rise in citrate production, reflecting the metabolic activity of the mammary gland. Lactose, sodium chloride, and protein rise promptly, stabilizing at 24 hours and reflecting the closure of the pericellular pathway, which results in a decrease in direct flux into the milk. This suggests a two-step process of junctional closure followed by onset of secretory activity.

The changes in permeability of the tight junctions; rate of synthesis of lactose, lipids, and nutrient proteins; transport of glucose into the alveolar cells; transcytosis of secretory IgA; movement of immune cells into the alveolar lumen; and secretion of lactoferrin represent the distinct metabolic and cellular modifications. Neville[56] states, "The temporal sequence of these

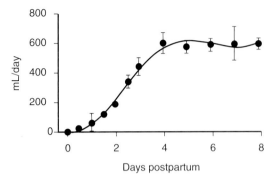

Figure 3-27. Milk volumes during first week postpartum. Mean values from 12 multiparous white women who test-weighed their infants before and after every feeding for first 7 days postpartum. Redrawn from Neville MC: Determinants of milk volume and composition. In Jensen RG, editor: *Handbook of milk composition,* San Diego, 1995, Academic Press.

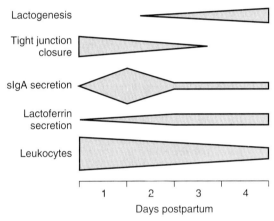

Figure 3-28. Summary model for temporal sequence of changes in mammary gland function during lactogenesis in women. From Neville MC: Determinants of milk volume and composition. In Jensen RG, editor: *Handbook of milk composition,* San Diego, 1995, Academic Press.

changes as they occur during lactogenesis suggests that they are either independently regulated or form part of an orderly cascade of temporally separate events." Figure 3-28 graphically illustrates these changes.

The use of new molecular techniques and the use of mutant animals with transgenic technology have advanced the understanding of human milk and the physiology of lactation. The regulation of mammary gland development has been demonstrated to depend not only on various hormones but their receptors, the signaling proteins such as protein kinases and transcription factors, as well as DNA binding proteins. The field is advancing rapidly. Signaling pathways are being identified and target genes of many regulatory pathways are being sought.

REFERENCES

1. Anbazhagan R, Bartek J, Stamp G, et al: Expression of integrin subunits in the human infant breast correlates with morphogenesis and differentiation, *J Pathol* 176:227, 1995.
2. Arthur PG, Hartmann PE, Smith M: Measurement of the milk intake of breastfed infants, *J Pediatr Gastroenterol Nutr* 6:419, 1989.
3. Banerjee MR, Menon RS: Synergistic actions of glucocorticoid and prolactin in murine milk-protein gene expression. In Rillema JA, editor: *Action of prolactin on molecular processes,* Boca Raton, Fla., 1987, CRC Press, pp 121–133.
4. Battin DA, Marrs RP, Fleiss PM, et al: Effect of suckling on serum prolactin, luteinizing hormone, follicle-stimulating hormone, and estradiol during prolonged lactation, *Obstet Gynecol* 65:785, 1985.
5. Bell AW, Bauman DE: Adaptations of glucose metabolism during pregnancy and lactation, *J Mammary Gland Biol Neoplasia* 2:265, 1997.
6. Bochinfuso WP, Korach KS: Mammary gland development and tumorigenesis in estrogen receptor knockout mice, *J Mammary Gland Biol Neoplasia* 2:323, 1997.
7. Chapman DJ, Young S, Ferris AM, et al: Impact of breast pumping on lactogenesis stage II after caesarean delivery: a randomized clinical trial, *Pediatrics* 107:2001, e94.
8. Chiodera P, Salvarani C, Bacchi-Modena A, et al: Relationship between plasma profiles of oxytocin and adrenocorticotropic hormone during suckling or breast stimulation in women, *Horm Res* 35:119, 1991.
9. Cholst IN, Wardlaw SL, Newman CB, et al: Prolactin response to breast stimulation in lactating women is not mediated by endogenous opioids, *Am J Obstet Gynecol* 150:558, 1984.
10. Christensson K, Nilsson BA, Stocks S, et al: Effect of nipple stimulation on uterine activity and on plasma levels of oxytocin in full term, healthy, pregnant women, *Acta Obstet Gynecol Scand* 68:205, 1989.
11. Coiro V, Alboni A, Gramellini D, et al: Inhibition by ethanol of the oxytocin response to breast stimulation in normal women and the role of endogenous opioids, *Acta Endocrinol* 126:213, 1992.
12. Cowie AT, Forsyth IA, Hart IC: Hormonal control of lactation. In Gross F, Grumbach MM, Labhart A, et al, editors: *Monographs on endocrinology,* vol 15, New York, 1980, Springer-Verlag.
13. Cox DB, Owens RA, Hartmann PE: Blood and milk prolactin and the rate of milk synthesis in women, *Exp Physiol* 81:1007–1020, 1996.
14. Cregan MD, Hartmann PE: Computerized breast measurement from conception to weaning: clinical implications, *J Hum Lact* 15:89, 1999.
15. Crowley WR, Armstrong WE: Neurochemical regulation of oxytocin secretion in lactation, *Endocr Rev* 13:33, 1992.
16. Czank C, Henderson JJ, Kent JC, et al: Hormonal control of the lactation cycle. In Hale TW, Hartmann PE, editors: *Hale and Hartmann's textbook of human lactation,* Amarillo, Tex., 2007, Hale Publishing LP, pp 89–111.
17. Daly SEJ, Owens RA, Hartmann PE: The short-term synthesis and infant-regulated removal of milk in lactating women, *Exp Physiol* 78:209, 1993.
18. Daniel CW, Robinson S, Silberstein GB: The role of TGF-α in faltering and growth of the mammary ductal tree, *J Mammary Gland Biol Neoplasia* 1:331, 1996.
19. Dawood MY, Khan-Dawood FS, Wahi RS, et al: Oxytocin release and plasma anterior pituitary and gonadal hormones in women during lactation, *J Clin Endocrinol Metab* 52:678, 1981.
20. Falconer IR, Rowe JM: Effect of prolactin on sodium and potassium concentration in the mammary alveolar tissue, *Endocrinology* 101:181, 1977.

21. Fowler PA, Casey CE, Cameron GG, et al: Cyclic changes in composition and volume of the breast during the menstrual cycle, measured by magnetic resonance imaging, *Br J Obstet Gynaecol* 97:595, 1990.

22. Frantz AG: Prolactin, *N Engl J Med* 298:201, 1978.

23. Freeman ME, Kanyicska B, Lerant A, et al: Prolactin: structure, function and regulation of secretion, *Physiol Rev* 80 (4):1523–1631, 2000.

24. Freund-Mercier MJ, Richard P: Excitatory effects of intraventricular injections of oxytocin on the milk ejection reflex in the rat, *J Physiol* 352:447, 1984.

25. Frigerio C, Schutz Y, Prentice A, et al: Is human lactation a particularly efficient process? *Eur J Clin Nutr* 45:459, 1991.

26. Gehlbach DL, Bayliss P, Rosa C: Prolactin and thyrotropin responses to nursing during the early puerperium, *J Reprod Med* 34:295, 1989.

27. Green KA, Streuli CH: Apoptosis regulation in the mammary gland: a review, *Cell Mol Life Sci* 61: 1867–1883, 2004.

28. Hammond KA: Adaptation of the maternal intestine during lactation, *J Mammary Gland Biol Neoplasia* 2:243, 1997.

29. Hamosh M: Enzymes in milk: their function in the mammary gland, in milk and in the infant. In Hanson LA, editor: *Biology of human milk, Nestle´ nutrition workshop series,* vol 15, Philadelphia, 1988, Lippincott William & Wilkins, p 45.

30. Hansen S, Gummesson BM: Participation of the lateral midbrain tegmentum in the neuroendocrine control of sexual behavior and lactation in the rat, *Brain Res* 251:319, 1982.

31. Hara T, Irie K, Saito S, et al: Identification of macrophage colony-stimulating factor in human milk and mammary gland epithelial cells, *Pediatr Res* 37:437, 1995.

32. Hartmann PE, Saint L: Measurement of milk yield in women, *J Pediatr Gastroenterol Nutr* 3:270, 1984.

33. Healy DL, Rattigan S, Hartmann PE, et al: Prolactin in human milk: correlation with lactose, total protein, and α-lactalbumin levels, *Am J Physiol* 238(Endocrinol Metab 1): E83, 1980.

34. Horst RL, Goff JP, Reinhardt TA: Calcium and vitamin D metabolism during lactation, *J Mammary Gland Biol Neoplasia* 2:253, 1997.

35. Humphreys RC, Lydon J, O'Malley BW, et al: Mammary gland development is mediated by both stromal and epithelial progesterone receptors, *Mol Endocrinol* 11:801, 1997.

36. Jensen RG: *The lipids of human milk,* Boca Raton, Fla., 1989, CRC Press.

37. Jonas W, Johansson LM, Nissen E, et al: Effects of intrapartum oxytocin administration and epidural analgesia on the concentration of plasma oxytocin and prolactin, in response of sucking during the second day postpartum, *Breastfeed Med* 4:71–81, 2009.

38. Kent JC, Ramsay DT, Doherty D: Response of breasts to different stimulation patterns of an electric breast pump, *J Hum Lact* 19:179, 2003.

39. Kleinberg DL: Early mammary development: growth hormone and IGF-1, *Mammary Gland Biol Neoplasia* 2:49, 1997.

40. Koldovsky O, Bedrick A, Rao R: Role of milk-borne prostaglandins and epidermal growth factor for the suckling mammal, *J Am Coll Nutr* 10:17, 1991.

41. Kulski JK, Hartmann PE: Changes in human milk composition during the initiation of lactation, *Aust J Exp Biol Med* 59:101, 1981.

42. Kwa HG, Bulbrook RD, Wang DY: An overall perspective on the role of prolactin in the breast. In Nagasawa H, editor: *Prolactin and lesions in breast, uterus and prostate,* Boca Raton, Fla., 1989, CRC Press.

43. Larson BL, editor: *Lactation, vol. 4. The mammary gland/human lactation/milk synthesis,* New York, 1978, Academic Press.

44. Larson BL, Smith VR, editors: *Lactation, vol. 2. Biosynthesis and secretion of milk/diseases,* New York, 1974, Academic Press.

45. Larson BL, Smith VR, editors: *Lactation, vol. 3. Nutrition and biochemistry of milk/maintenance,* New York, 1974, Academic Press.

46. Leake RD, Waters CB, Rubin RT, et al: Oxytocin and prolactin responses in long-term breastfeeding, *Obstet Gynecol* 62:565, 1983.

47. Lincoln DW, Paisley AC: Neuroendocrine control of milk ejection, *J Reprod Fertil* 65:571, 1982.

48. Liu Y, Hyde JF, Vore M: Prolactin regulates maternal bile secretory function postpartum, *J Pharmacol Exp Ther* 261:560, 1992.

49. Lönnerdal B, Atkinson S: Nitrogenous components of milk and human milk proteins. In Jensen RG, editor: *Handbook of milk composition,* San Diego, 1995, Academic Press.

50. Lucas A, Drewett RB, Mitchell MD: Breastfeeding and plasma oxytocin concentrations, *Br Med J* 281:834, 1980.

51. Lund LR, Rømer J, Thomasset N, et al: Two distinct phases of apoptosis in mammary gland involution: proteinase-independent and -dependent pathways, *Development* 122:181, 1996.

52. Martin T, Czank C: Molecular aspects of mammary gland development. In Hale TW, Hartmann PE, editors: *Textbook of human lactation,* Amarillo, Tex., 2007, Hale Publishing.

53. Meites J: Neuroendocrinology of lactation, *J Invest Dermatol* 63:119, 1974.

54. Neville MC: The physiological basis of milk secretion. Part I. Basic physiology, *Ann N Y Acad Sci* 586:1, 1990.

55. Neville MC: Determinants of milk volume and composition. A. Lactogenesis in women: a cascade of events revealed by milk composition. In Jensen RG, editor: *Handbook of milk composition,* San Diego, 1995, Academic Press.

56. Neville MC: Anatomy and physiology of lactation. Breastfeeding. Part I, *Pediatr Clin North Am* 48:35, 2001.

57. Neville MC: Mammary gland biology and lactation: a short course. Presented at biannual meeting of the International Society for Research on Human Milk and Lactation, Plymouth, Mass., 1997.

58. Neville MC, Allen JC, Archer PC, et al: Studies in human lactation: milk volume and nutrient composition during weaning and lactogenesis, *Am J Clin Nutr* 54:81, 1991.

59. Newton N: The relation of the milk-ejection reflex to the ability to breastfeed, *Ann N Y Acad Sci* 652:484, 1992.

60. Newton N: The quantitative effect of oxytocin (Pitocin) on human milk yield, *Ann N Y Acad Sci* 652:481, 1992.

61. Newton M, Newton NR: The let-down reflex in human lactation, *J Pediatr* 33:698–704, 1948.

62. Nissen E, Lilja G, Widström A-M, et al: Elevation of oxytocin levels early postpartum in women, *Acta Obstet Gynecol Scand* 74:530, 1995.

63. Ogawa K, Kusaka T, Tanimoto K, et al: Changes in breast hemodynamics in breastfeeding mothers, *J Hum Lact* 24:415–421, 2008.

64. Ormandy CJ, Binart N, Kelly PA: Mammary gland development in prolactin receptor knockout mice, *J Mammary Gland Biol Neoplasia* 2:355, 1997.

65. Ostrom KM: A review of the hormone prolactin during lactation: progress in food and nutrition, *Science* 14:1, 1990.

66. Pang WW, Hartmann PE: Initiation of human lactation: secretory differentiation and secretory activation, *J Mammary Gland Biol Neoplasia* 12:211–221, 2007.

67. Patton S, Neville MC: Introduction: maternal adaptation to lactation, *J Mammary Gland Biol Neoplasia* 2:201, 1997.

68. Peaker M: Production of hormones by the mammary gland: short review, *Endocr Regul* 25:10, 1991.

69. Peaker M, Linzell JL: Citrate in milk: a harbinger of lactogenesis, *Nature* 253:464, 1975.

70. Pederson CA: Oxytocin control of maternal behavior, *Ann N Y Acad Med* 807:126, 1997.

71. Pederson CA, Caldwell JD, Walker C, et al: Oxytocin activates the postpartum onset of rat maternal behavior in the ventral, tegmental and medial preoptic areas, *Behav Neurosci* 108:1163, 1994.

72. Prentice A, Addey CVP, Wilde CJ: Evidence for local feedback control of human milk secretion, *Biochem Soc Trans* 17:122, 1989.
73. Richard L, Alade MO: Effect of delivery room routines on success of first breast-feed, *Lancet* 336:1105, 1990.
74. Robinson JE, Short RV: Changes in breast sensitivity at puberty, during the menstrual cycle, and at parturition, *Br Med J* 1:1188, 1977.
75. Robyn C, Meuris S: Pituitary prolactin, lactational performance and puerperal infertility, *Semin Perinatol* 6:254, 1982.
76. Rosen JM, Humphreys R, Krnacik S, et al: The regulation of mammary gland development by hormones, growth factors and oncogenes, *Prog Clin Biol Res* 387:95, 1994.
77. Saint L, Smith M, Hartmann PE: The yield and nutrient content of colostrum and milk of women from giving birth to 1 month postpartum, *Br J Nutr* 52:87–95, 1984.
78. Shackleton M, Vaillant F, Simpson KL, et al: Generation of a functional mammary gland from a single stem cell, *Nature* 439:84–88, 2006 (Letter).
79. Shalev E, Weiner E, Tzabari A, et al: Breast stimulation in late pregnancy, *Gynecol Obstet Invest* 29:125, 1990.
80. Shennan DB: Mechanisms of mammary gland ion transport, *Comp Biochem Physiol* 97A:317, 1990.
81. Sherwood LM: Human prolactin, *N Engl J Med* 284:774, 1971.
82. Smith VR: *Lactation, vol. 1. The mammary gland/development and maintenance*, New York, 1974, Academic Press.
83. St Reuli CH, Edwards GM: Control of normal mammary epithelial phenotype by integrins, *J Mammary Gland Biol Neoplasia* 3:151, 1998.
84. Stern JM, Reichlin S: Prolactin circadian rhythm persists throughout lactation in women, *Neuroendocrinology* 51:31, 1990.
85. Strange R, Li F, Saurer S, et al: Apoptotic cell death and tissue remodeling during mouse mammary gland involution, *Development* 115:49, 1992.
86. Stricker P, Grueter R: Action du lobe du lobe anterieur de l'hypophyse sur la monte laiteusze, *C R Soc Biol* 99:1978, 1928.
87. Sutherland KD, Lindeman GL, Visvader JE: *J Mammary Gland Biol Neoplasia* 12:15–23, 2007.
88. Takeda S, Kuwabara Y, Mizuno M: Concentrations and origin of oxytocin in breast milk, *Endocrinol Jpn* 33:821, 1986.
89. Theorell T: Prolactin: a hormone that mirrors passiveness in crisis situations, *Integr Physiol Behav Sci* 27:32, 1992.
90. Toppozada MK, El-Rahman HA, Soliman AY: Prostaglandins as milk ejectors: the nose as a new route of administration. In Samuelson B, Paoletti R, Rawell P, editors: *Advances in prostaglandin, thromboxane, and leukotriene research*, vol 12, New York, 1983, Raven.
91. Uvnäs-Moberg K: *The oxytocin factor: tapping the hormone of calm, love and healing*, Cambridge, Mass., 2003, Da Capo Press.
92. Uvnäs-Moberg K, Eriksson M: Breastfeeding: physiological, endocrine and behavioral adaptations caused by oxytocin and local neurogenic activity in the nipple and mammary gland, *Acta Paediatr* 85:525, 1996.
93. Vernon RG, Pond CM: Adaptations of maternal adipose tissue to lactation, *J Mammary Gland Biol Neoplasia* 2:231, 1997.
94. Vigneri R, Squatrito S, Pezzino V, et al: Spontaneous fluctuations of human placental lactogen during normal pregnancy, *J Clin Endocrinol Metab* 40:506, 1975.
95. Vonderhaar BK, Bremel RD: Prolactin, growth hormone, and placental lactogen, *J Mammary Gland Biol Neoplasia* 2:1, 1997.
96. Voogt JL: Actions of prolactin in the brain. In Rillema JA, editor: *Actions of prolactin on molecular processes*, Boca Raton, Fla., 1987, CRC Press, pp 27–40.
97. Vorherr H: *The breast: morphology, physiology and lactation*, New York, 1974, Academic Press.
98. Vorherr H: Human lactation and breastfeeding. In Larson BL, editor: *Lactation. The mammary gland/human lactation/milk synthesis*, vol 4, New York, 1978, Academic Press.
99. Vorherr H: Hormonal and biochemical changes of pituitary and breast during pregnancy. In Vorherr H, editor: Human lactation, *Semin Perinatol*, vol 3, 1979, p 193.
100. Wehrenberg WB, Gaillard RC: Neuroendocrine mechanisms regulating growth hormone and prolactin secretion during lactation, *Endocrinology* 124:464, 1989.
101. Weitzman RE, Leake RD, Rubin RT, et al: The effect of nursing on neurohypophyseal hormone and prolactin secretion in human subjects, *J Clin Endocrinol Metab* 51:836, 1980.
102. Widstrom AM, Winberg J, Werner S, et al: Suckling in lactating women stimulates the secretion of insulin and prolactin without concomitant effects on gastrin, growth hormone, calcitonin, vasopressin, or catecholamines, *Early Hum Dev* 10:115, 1984.
103. Wilde CJ, Addey CVP, Boddy LM, et al: Autocrine regulation of milk secretion by a protein in milk, *Biochem J* 305:51, 1995.
104. Zinaman MJ, Hughes V, Queenan JT, et al: Acute prolactin and oxytocin responses and milk yield to infant suckling and artificial methods of expression in lactating women, *Pediatrics* 89:437, 1992.

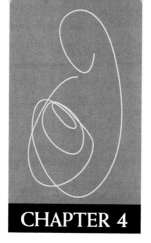

CHAPTER 4

Biochemistry of Human Milk

Human milk was considered a heavenly elixir, a living fluid. It was not until the end of the eighteenth century that chemical methods became available to decipher the content of milk. The biochemistry of human milk encompasses a mammoth supply of scientific data and information, most of which has been generated since 1970. Each report or study adds a tiny piece to the complex puzzle of the nutrients that make up human milk. The answers to some questions still elude us. A question as simple as the volume of milk consumed at a feeding remains a scientific challenge. The methodology must be accurate, reproducible, noninvasive, and suitable for home use night or day and must not interrupt breastfeeding. The precision analysis available for measuring the concentration of the most minuscule of elements, however, is remarkably accurate and reproducible in the laboratory. Milk has been demystified by laboratory chemistry.[121]

Advances in analytic methods bring greater sensitivity, resolving power, and speed to the analysis of milk composition. Previously unknown and unrecognized compounds have been detected. We now know milk provides both nutrients and nonnutritive signals to the neonate. With few exceptions, all milks contain the nutrients for physical growth and development. When the offspring develops rapidly, the milk is nutrient dense; when it develops slowly, the milk is more dilute. All milks contain fat, carbohydrates, and proteins, as well as minerals, vitamins, and other nutrients. The organization of milk composition includes lipids in emulsified globules coated with a membrane, colloidal dispersions of proteins as micelles, and the remainder as a true solution.[113] At no other time in life is a single food adequate as the sole source of nutrition.

The discussion in this chapter is limited to information perceived as immediately useful to the clinician. Considerable detail and species variability are overlooked to help focus attention on details directly influencing management. Extensive and exhaustive reviews are referenced to provide the reader with easy access to greater detail and validation of the general conclusions reported here.

Human milk is not a uniform body fluid but a secretion of the mammary gland of changing composition (Figure 4-1). The first drops at the beginning of a feeding differ from the last drops. Colostrum differs from transitional and mature milks. Milk changes with the time of day and as time goes by. As concentrations of protein, fat, carbohydrates, minerals, and cells differ, physical properties such as osmolarity and pH change. The impact of changing composition on the physiology of the infant gut is beginning to be appreciated. Many constituents have dual roles, not only nutrition but infection protection, immunity, or a host of other effects.

The more than 200 constituents of milk include a tremendous array of molecules, descriptions of which continue to be refined as qualitative and quantitative laboratory techniques are perfected. Resolution of lipid chemicals has advanced dramatically in recent years, but new carbohydrates and proteins have been identified as well. Some of the compounds identified may well be intermediary products in the process that occurs within the mammary cells and may be only incidental in the final product.[148] Milk includes true solutions, colloids, membranes, membrane-bound globules, and living cells.

Human and bovine milks are known in the greatest detail; however, much information exists about the milk of rats and mice, as well as five other species: the water buffalo, goat, sheep, horse, and pig.

Formula vs. human milk

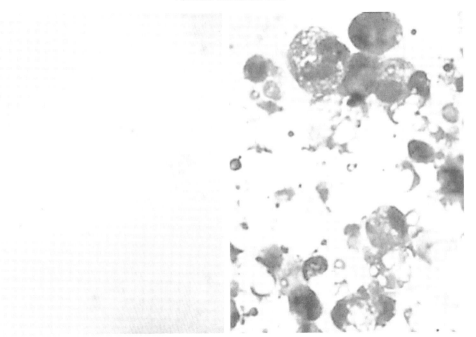

Figure 4-1. A comparison of formula *(left)* and human milk *(right)*. Human milk is a dynamic colloidal solution of perfect nutrients and growth factors for the infant. Formula is a totally homogenized solution of nutrient chemicals. (Courtesy of Nancy Wight MD, San Diego, Calif.)

TABLE 4-1	Composition of Milks Obtained from Different Mammals and Growth Rate of Their Offspring				
		Content of Milk (%)			
Species	**Days Required to Double Birth Weight**	**Fat**	**Protein**	**Lactose**	**Ash**
Human	180	3.8	0.9	7.0	0.2
Horse	60	1.9	2.5	6.2	0.5
Cow	47	3.7	3.4	4.8	0.7
Reindeer	30	16.9	11.5	2.8	–
Goat	19	4.5	2.9	4.1	0.8
Sheep	10	7.4	5.5	4.8	1.0
Rat	6	15.0	12.0	3.0	2.0

From Hambraeus L: Proprietary milk versus human breast milk in infant feeding: a critical appraisal from the nutritional point of view, *Pediatr Clin North Am* 24:17, 1977.

Several are listed in Table 4-1. Miscellaneous data are available on the milk of 150 more species, but almost no data are available for another 4000 species. Jenness and Sloan have compiled a summary of 140 species from which a sampling has been extracted (Table 4-2). The constituents of milk can be divided into the following groups, according to their specificity:

1. Constituents specific to both organ and species (e.g., most proteins and lipids)
2. Constituents specific to organ but not to species (e.g., lactose)
3. Constituents specific to species but not to organ (e.g., albumin, some immunoglobulins)

Normal Variations in Human Milk

In defining the constituents of human milk, it is important to recognize that the composition varies with the stage of lactation, the time of day, the sampling time during a given feeding, maternal nutrition, and individual variation. Many early interpretations of the content of human milk were based on spot samples or even pooled samples from multiple donors at different times and stages of lactation. Samples obtained by pumping may vary from those obtained by the suckling infant because some variation exists in content among the various methods of pumping. Banked donor milk differs from freshly

TABLE 4-2	Constituents of Milk (g/100 g) of Specific Mammals						
Mammalian Species (in Taxonomic Position)	Total Solids	Fat	Casein	Whey Protein	Total Protein	Lactose	Ash
Human	12.4	3.8	0.4	0.6	–	7.0	0.2
Baboon	14.4	5.0	–	–	1.6	7.3	0.3
Orangutan	11.5	3.5	1.1	0.4	–	6.0	0.2
Black bear	44.5	24.5	8.8	5.7	–	0.4	1.8
California sea lion	52.7	36.5	–	–	13.8	0.0	0.6
Black rhinoceros	8.1	0.0	1.1	0.3	–	6.1	0.3
Spotted dolphin	31.0	18.0	–	–	9.4	0.6	–
Domestic dog	23.5	12.9	5.8	2.1	–	3.1	1.2
Norway rat	21.0	10.3	6.4	2.0	–	2.6	1.3
Whitetail jackrabbit	40.8	13.9	19.7	4.0	–	1.7	1.5

Modified from Jenness R, Sloan RE: Composition of milk. In Larson BL, Smith VR, editors: *Lactation, vol. 3, Nutrition and biochemistry of milk/maintenance*, New York, 1974, Academic Press.

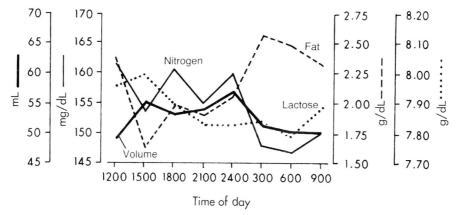

Figure 4-2. Mean concentrations of nitrogen, lactose, and fat in human milk by time of day. (Modified from Brown KH, Black RE, Robertson AD, et al: Clinical and field studies of human lactation: methodological considerations, *Am J Clin Nutr* 35:745, 1982.)

expressed, mature milk in nutrient content and energy value.[151]

Daytime consumption of milk in a given infant varies between 46% and 58% of the total 24-hour consumption, so that reliance on less than a 24-hour sampling may be misleading. Data from samples taken every 3 hours showed a variation in milk concentration of nitrogen, lactose, and fat, and in the volume of milk, by time of day (Figure 4-2). Furthermore, statistically significant diurnal changes occurred in the concentration of lactose and in the volume within individual subjects, but the times of those changes were not consistent for each individual. Some individuals varied as much as two-fold in volume production from day to day. A significant difference in the concentrations of both fat and lactose and the volume of milk produced by each breast was also found. At the extreme, the less productive breast yielded only 65% of the volume of the other breast.

The variation in the fat content has received some attention. Fat content changes during a given feeding, increasing as the feeding progresses. Fat content rises from early morning to midday; as reported in early studies, when feedings were controlled the volume increased from two to five times. Multiple studies in different countries and different decades, summarized by Jackson et al., reveal that some of the variation is related to other factors. Demand feeding (mothers in 1988 in Thailand) has a different circadian variation than scheduled feeding (mothers in 1932 in the United States) (Figure 4-3). In the later part of the first year of lactation, fat content diminishes. Work done by Atkinson et al.[11] that was confirmed by other investigators showed that the nitrogen content of the milk of mothers who deliver prematurely is higher than that of those whose pregnancies reach full term. For a given volume of milk, the premature infant would receive 20% more nitrogen than the full-term infant if each were fed his or her own mother's milk. Other constituents of milk produced by mothers who deliver prematurely have also been studied. Some milk banks now provide donor milk from mothers who have delivered prematurely.

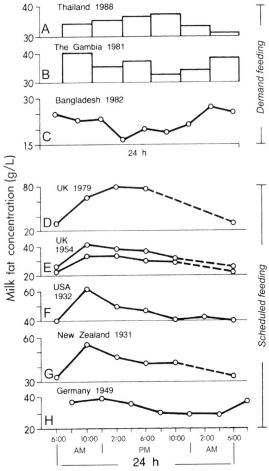

Figure 4-3. Circadian variation in fat concentration of breast milk from published studies. **A,** Thailand: Prefeed/postfeed expressed samples, 19 mothers studied for 24 hours each, infants aged 1 to 9 months. **B,** The Gambia: Demand feeding, pre/post expressed samples, 16 mothers studied for 24 hours each, infants aged 1 to 18 months. **C,** Bangladesh (Brown et al.): Samples collected at scheduled intervals by total breast extraction (breast pump), seven mothers studied for 24 hours each, infants aged 1 to 9 months. **D,** United Kingdom[79]: Prefeed/postfeed expressed samples, one mother studied for 72 hours. **E,** United Kingdom (Hytten): Samples collected by total breast extraction (breast pump). *Lower curve,* 29 mothers studied for 24 hours each, infants aged 3 to 8 days. *Upper curve,* 20 mothers studied for 24 hours each, infants aged 21 days to 4 months. **F,** United States (Nims et al.): Samples collected by total breast extraction (manual), three mothers studied, but values given only for one mother, for 24 hours on six occasions and 72 hours on one occasion, infant aged 6 to 60 weeks. **G,** New Zealand (Deem): Samples collected by total breast extraction (manual), 28 mothers studied for 24 hours each, infants aged 1 to 8 months. **H,** Germany (Gunther and Stainier): Collection of samples by total breast extraction (manual), two mothers studied for 24 hours each, six mothers studied for 52 hours each, infants aged 8 to 11 days. (Modified from Jackson DA, Imong SM, Silprasert A, et al: Circadian variation in fat concentration of breast milk in a rural northern Thai population, *Br J Nutr* 59:349, 1988; see article for complete bibliography.)

An additional consideration in reviewing information available on the levels of various constituents of milk is the technique used to derive the data. In 1975, Hambraeus reported less protein in human milk than originally calculated (see Table 4-1). The present techniques of immunoassay measure the absolute amounts; earlier figures were derived from calculations based on measurements of the nitrogen content. Of the nitrogen in human milk, 25% is nonprotein nitrogen (NPN). Cow milk has only 5% NPN.

A major concern about variation in content of human milk is related to the mother's diet. Maternal diet is of particular concern when the mother is malnourished or eats an unusually restrictive diet. Malnourished mothers have approximately the same proportions of protein, fat, and carbohydrate as well-nourished mothers, but they produce less milk. Levels of water-soluble vitamins, such as ascorbic acid, thiamin, and vitamin B_{12}, are quickly affected by deficient diets. "From a nutritional perspective, infancy is a critical and vulnerable period. At no other stage in life is a single food adequate as a sole source of nutrition," writes Picciano.[127] This results from the immaturity of the tissues and organs involved in the metabolism of nutrients, which limits the ability to respond to nutrition excesses and deficiencies. The system is species-specific and depends on the presence of the self-contained enzymes and ligands to facilitate digestion at the proper stage while preserving function (such as secretory immunoglobulin A [sIgA]). The system continues to facilitate absorption and utilization.

Mother's milk is recommended for all infants under ordinary circumstances, even if the mother's diet is not perfect, according to the Committee on Nutrition During Pregnancy and Lactation of the Institute of Medicine.[109]

The Cycles of Lactation

Two distinct phases occur during pregnancy, which have been identified as mammogenesis and lactogenesis I. Mammogenesis is the developmental differentiation that begins in early pregnancy. It includes the proliferation of the ductal tree, which results in the sprouting of multiple alveoli.

Mammogenesis results in the enlargement of the breast during pregnancy due to the proliferation of the ductoalveolar structure. Careful study of this development has been documented utilizing computerized breast measurement, first reported by Cox et al.[30] in 1999. Computerized breast measurement is an accurate noninvasive technology that is being used to determine changes in the size of human breasts (see Chapter 8, p. 261).

A longitudinal study using computerized breast measurement from before conception through pregnancy and lactation showed that growth began at week 10 of pregnancy. It was found that seven of eight women studied had an increase in breast size of about 170 mL with considerable individual variation on rate of change. Most women continued this growth immediately postpartum; at 1 month postpartum they had an average 211 mL of growth. The authors correlated this growth through pregnancy with an increase in placental lactogen.[30]

Stage I lactogenesis is the onset of milk secretion and begins with the early changes in the mammary gland during pregnancy and continues until full lactation has occurred after delivery. Stage I begins when small quantities of milk components such as casein and lactose are secreted. This amount is held in check by high levels of circulating progesterone. The first milk obtained by the newborn at birth is called colostrum, and the milk produced in the first 10 days is called transitional milk. Full volume is obtained in the next stage, lactogenesis II. The terms will be used in this text for clinical purposes (Figure 4-4). Neville et al.[111] state that the terms "colostrum" and "transitional milk" do not describe the mammary secretion product during the first 4 days or from days 4 to 10 postpartum. It has always been recognized that the content changes rapidly in the first 4 days and then more slowly in the next 6 days or so as a continuum. They suggest the abandonment of these terms. Colostrum and transitional milk are convenient clinical terms that are useful descriptive terms.

Prepartum Milk

Prepartum milk is the first stage of lactogenesis and is especially conspicuous in other species, such as the goat.[5] It provides evidence that the junctions between alveolar cells are "leaky" during pregnancy, allowing fluid and solutes to flow between the milk space and the interstitial fluid of the mammary gland.[112] Figure 4-5 illustrates the composition of this milk in humans. The lactose concentration is directly correlated with that of potassium, but sodium and chloride are inversely related to lactose (Tables 4-3 through 4-7).

Colostrum

The stages in the continuum of human milk in traditional nomenclature are colostrum, transitional milk, and mature milk, and their relative contents are significant for newborns and their physiologic adaption to extrauterine life.

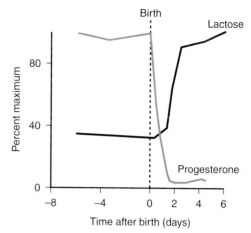

Figure 4-4. Progesterone withdrawal initiates lactogenesis II in women. The increase in lactose concentrations associated with increased synthesis of milk components coincides with a rapid decrease in progesterone concentration when the placenta is removed at parturition. (Modified from Kulski JK, Harman PE, Martin JD, et al: Effects of bromocriptine mesylate on the composition of the mammary secretion in non-breastfeeding women, *Obset Gynecol* 52:38, 1978; Czank C, Henderson JJ, Kent JC, et al: Hormonal control of lactation cycle. In Hale TW, Hartmann PE, editors: *Textbook of lactation*, Amarillo, Texas, 2007, Hale Publishing.)

The mammary secretion during the first few days consists of a yellowish, thick fluid: colostrum. The residual mixture of materials present in the mammary glands and ducts at delivery and immediately after is progressively mixed with newly secreted milk, forming colostrum. Human colostrum is known to differ from mature milk in composition, both in the nature of its components and in the relative proportions of these components. The first changes are in sodium and chloride concentrations and an increase in lactose, probably as a result of the closure of the tight junctions. The specific gravity of colostrum is 1.040 to 1.060. The mean energy value is 67 kcal/dL compared with 75 kcal/dL of mature milk. The volume varies between 2 and 20 mL per feeding in the first 3 days. The total volume per day also depends on the number of feedings and is reported to average 100 mL in the first 24 hours (which is different from the first day, depending on the time of delivery) (see Table 4-4). Tables 4-5 and 4-6 list the yield and composition of colostrum (1 to 5 days) and mature milk (14 days and beyond). The increased production of citrate is paralleled by the increase in volume (Figures 4-6 and 4-7). The result is a decrease in sodium and chloride and an increase in lactose concentration due to water dilution.[112,105]

The antepartum milk glucose level is 0.35 ± 0.16 mmol/L (see Table 4-3). Glucose levels vary among individuals. Glucose decreases during a feed as aqueous phase decreases and lipid increases.

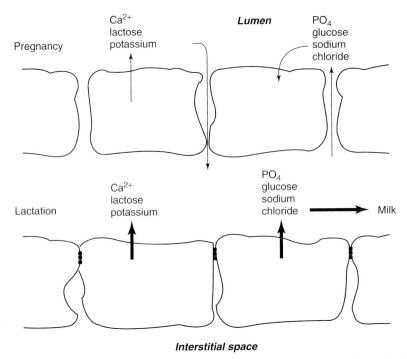

Figure 4-5. Model for directions of major fluxes of several macronutrients during pregnancy and lactation in women. (From Neville MC: Determinants of milk volume and composition. In Jensen RG, editor: *Handbook of milk composition*, San Diego, 1995, Academic Press.)

In early colostrum, glucose passes into the milk via the paracellular pathway and parallels lactose. When lactation is fully established, glucose levels are unrelated to lactose levels.[108] In mature milk, the level is 1.5 ± 0.4 mmol/L.

Dewey et al.[36] clearly demonstrate that in a well-established milk supply, volume depends on infant demand, and the residual milk available at each feeding is comparable in both low-intake and average-intake dyads. Infant birth weight, weight at 3 months, and total time nursing were positively associated with intake. The volume also varies with the mother's parity. Women who had other pregnancies, particularly those who previously nursed infants, have colostrum more readily available at delivery, and the volume increases more rapidly.

The yellow color of colostrum results from β-carotene. The ash content is high, and the concentrations of sodium, potassium, and chloride are greater than those of mature milk. Protein, fat-soluble vitamins, and minerals are present in greater percentages than in transitional or mature milk. sIgA and lactoferrin increase in concentration. The complex sugars, oligosaccharides, also

TABLE 4-3	Composition of Prepartum Human Milk*					
Milk Component	**Units**	**Mean ± SD (n)**	**Milk Component**	**Units**	**Mean ± SD (n)**
Mean days prepartum		20.21 ± 12.18 (11)	Calcium	mg/dL	25.35 ± 8.48 (10)
Lipid	%	2.07 ± 0.98 (11)	Magnesium	mg/dL	5.64 ± 1.44 (10)
Lactose	mM	79.78 ± 21.68 (9)	Citrate	mM	0.40 ± 0.17 (8)
Protein	g/dL	5.44 ± 1.71 (8)	Phosphate	mg/dL	2.32 ± 0.70 (9)
Glucose	mM	0.35 ± 0.16 (8)	Ionized calcium	mM	3.25 ± 0.84 (6)
Sodium	mM	61.26 ± 25.82 (10)	pH		6.83 ± 0.18 (6)
Potassium	mM	18.30 ± 5.67 (10)	Urea	mg/dL	14.87 ± 2.40 (9)
Chloride	mM	62.21 ± 17.44 (10)	Creatinine	mg/dL	1.47 ± 0.35 (9)

*Small samples of mammary secretion were obtained three times in prepartum period from each of 11 women. In some cases, volumes were insufficient for all analyses.

From Allen JC, Keller RP, Archer P, et al: Studies in human lactation: milk composition and daily secretion rates of macronutrients in the first year of lactation, *Am J Clin Nutr* 54:69, 80, 1991. SD = standard deviation.

TABLE 4-4 Average Milk Volume Outputs (mL/24 h) of Well-Nourished Mothers Who Exclusively Breastfed Their Infants

Country	No. Days Measured	Sex	Month of Lactation											
			<1		1-2		2-3		3-4		4-5		5-6	
			n	mL/24 h	n	mL/24 h	n	mL/24 h	n	mL/24 h	n	mL/24 h	n	mL/24 h
U.S.	2	M, F	–	–	3	691	5	655	3	750	–	–	–	–
U.S.	1-2	M, F	46	681	–	–	–	–	–	–	–	–	–	–
Canada	?	M, F	–	–	–	–	–	–	33	793	31	856	28	925
Sweden	?	M, F	15	558	11	724	12	752	–	–	–	–	–	–
U.S.	3	M, F	–	–	11	600	–	–	2	833	–	–	3	682
U.S.	3	M, F	–	–	26	606	26	601	20	626	–	–	–	–
U.K.	4	M	–	–	27	791	23	820	18	829	5	790	1	922
		F	–	–	20	677	17	742	14	775	6	814	4	838
U.S.	1	M, F	16	673±192 SD	19	756±170	16	782±172	13	810±142	11	805±117	11	896±122

Country	No. Days Measured	Sex	Month of Lactation					
			7	8	9	10	11	12
U.S.	1	M, F	875±142 SD	834±99	774±180	691±233	516±215	759±28

Modified from Ferris AM, Jensen RG: Lipids in human milk: a review, *J Pediatr Gastroenterol Nutr* 3:108, 1984.

TABLE 4-5 Yield and Composition of Human Colostrum and Milk from Days 1 to 28

Component	Day Postpartum						
	1	2	3	4	5	14	28
Yield (g/24 h)	50	190	400	625	700	1100	1250
Lactose (g/L)	20	25	31	32	33	35	35
Fat (g/L)	12	15	20	25	24	23	29
Protein (g/L)	32	17	12	11	11	8	9

Modified from Saint L, Smith M, Hartmann PE: The yield and nutrient content of colostrum and milk of women giving birth to 1 month postpartum, *Br J Nutr* 52:87, 1984.

TABLE 4-6 Composition of Human Milk from Days 1 through 36 Postpartum (Mean ± SD), British and German Donors

Day	Component (g/dL)		
	Total Protein	Lactose	Triacylglycerols
1	2.95 ± 0.86	4.07 ± 0.98	2.14 ± 0.86
3	1.99 ± 0.22	4.98 ± 0.76	3.01 ± 0.77
5	1.82 ± 0.21	5.13 ± 0.54	3.06 ± 0.45
8	1.73 ± 0.27	5.38 ± 0.97	3.73 ± 0.70
15	1.56 ± 0.42	5.42 ± 0.76	3.59 ± 0.86
22	1.51 ± 0.27	5.34 ± 0.96	3.87 ± 0.68
29	1.5 ± 0.27	4.01 ± 1.13	4.01 ± 1.13
36	1.4 ± 0.26	5.34 ± 1.31	4.01 ± 1.20

Modified from Hibberd CM, Brooke DG, Carter ND, et al: Variation in the composition of breast milk during the first five weeks of lactation, *Arch Dis Child* 57:658, 1982.

increase, adding to the infection protection properties at this stage. It has been suggested that the mammary gland is actually evolved in part as an inflammatory response to tissue damage and infection and that the nutritional function then followed the protective function.

The higher protein, lower fat, and lactose solution is rich in immunoglobulins, especially sIgA. The number of immunologically competent mononuclear cells is at its highest level. Fat, contained mainly in the core of the fat globules, increases from 2% in colostrum to 2.9% in transitional milk

and to 3.6% in mature milk. The concentration of fat in the prepartum secretion is only 1 g/dL, and the distribution among classes of lipids differs. Prepartum milk is 93% triglycerides, increasing to 97% in colostrum, with diglycerides, monoglycerides, and free fatty acids all increasing from prepartum to postpartum secretions. Phospholipid levels decline during the same period. Prepartum secretions contain higher amounts of membrane components such as phospholipids, cholesterol, and cholesteryl esters, which decline from colostrum to mature milk.

Cholesterol appears to be synthesized in the mammary gland. Beyond its use in brain tissue development, the myelinization of nerves, and as the base of many enzymes, the role of cholesterol in colostrum remains elusive. Little research has been done on cholesterol in colostrum.

Colostrum facilitates the establishment of *Lactobacillus bifidus* flora in the digestive tract. Colostrum also facilitates the passage of meconium. Meconium contains an essential growth factor for *L. bifidus* and is the first culture medium in the sterile intestinal lumen of the newborn infant. Human colostrum is rich in antibodies, which may provide protection against the bacteria and viruses that are present in the birth canal and associated with other human contact. Colostrum also contains antioxidants, which may function as traps for neutrophil-generated reactive oxygen metabolites.[18]

The progressive changes in mammary secretion in both breastfeeding and nonbreastfeeding women between 28 and 110 days before delivery and up to

TABLE 4-7 Fat Distribution in Milk

Measurement	Prepartum		Postpartum		
	Early	Late	Colostrum	Transitional	Mature
Fat (%)	–	2	2	2.9	3.6
Fat (g)	–	–	2.9	3.6	3.8
Lipid (g/dL)	1.15	1.28	3.16	3.49	4.14
Phospholipid (mg/dL)	37	40	35	31	27
Percentage of total lipid	3.2	3.1	1.1	0.9	0.6
Cholesterol (mg/dL)	–	–	29	20	13.5

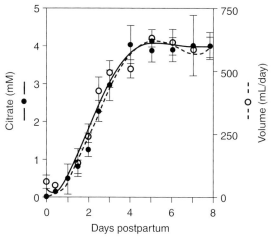

Figure 4-6. Changes in concentration of citrate in human milk in early postpartum period compared with increase in milk volume. (Data replotted from Neville et al., 1991.[116] Neville MC: Determinants of milk volume and composition. In Jensen RG, editor: *Handbook of milk composition*, San Diego, 1995, Academic Press.)

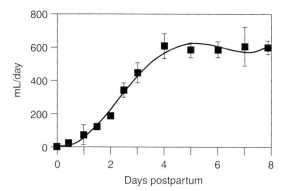

Figure 4-7. Milk volumes during first week postpartum. Mean values from 12 multiparous white women who testweighed their infants before and after every feeding for first 7 days postpartum. From Neville MC, Keller R, Seacat J, et al: Studies in human lactation: Milk volumes in lactating women during the onset of lactation and full lactation, *Am J Clin Nutr* 48:1375, 1988.

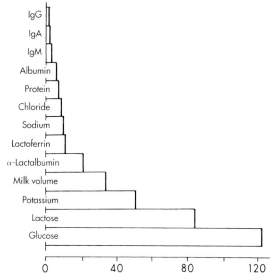

Figure 4-8. Relative increase in yield of milk components from day 1 to day 7 postpartum. Values presented are for day 7 expressed as percentage increase over day 1. (Modified from Kulski JK, Hartmann PE: Changes in human milk composition during the initiation of lactation, *Aust J Exp Biol Med Sci* 59:101, 1981.)

5 months after delivery were followed by Kulski and Hartmann to study the initiation of lactation. During late pregnancy the secretion contained higher concentrations of proteins and lower concentrations of lactose, glucose, and urea than those contained in milk secreted when lactation was well established. The concentrations of sodium, chloride, and magnesium were higher and those of potassium and calcium lower in colostrum than in milk. The osmolarity was relatively constant throughout the study. The authors described a two-phase development of lactation, with an initial phase of limited secretion in late pregnancy and a true induction of lactation in the second phase, 32 to 40 hours postpartum. Comparison with the

nonlactating women revealed similar secretion during the first 3 days postpartum. This, however, was abruptly reversed during the next 6 days as mammary involution progressed. Obtaining samples in these women, however, may have served to prolong the period of production. The authors point out that although breastfeeding was not necessary for the initiation of lactation in this study, it was essential for the continuation of lactation.

The yield of milk has been calculated from absolute values to demonstrate the increase in output of milk constituents during lactogenesis (Figure 4-8). Dramatic increases occurred in the production of all the milk constituents. The components synthesized by the mammary epithelium (lactose, lactalbumin, and lactoferrin) increased at a rate greater than those for IgA or proteins derived from the serum IgG and IgM. The greatest difference in yield between day 1 and day 7 postpartum was for glucose.[115]

A survey of the fatty acid components shows the lauric acid and myristic acid contents to be low in concentration the first few days. When the lauric and myristic acids increased, C_{18} acids decreased. Palmitoleic acid increased at the same rate as the myristic acid. From this, it was concluded that the early fatty acids are derived from extramammary sources, but the breast quickly begins to synthesize fatty acids for the production of transitional and mature milk (see Table 4-7). The total fat content may have a predictive value. It was shown that 90% of the women whose milk contained 20 g or more of fat per feeding on the seventh day were successfully breastfeeding 3 months later. Women who had only 5 to 10 g of fat on the seventh day had an 80% dropout rate by 3 months.

Colostrum's high protein and low fat are in keeping with the needs and reserves of the newborn at birth. Although the content of total nitrogen or any amino acid in breast milk in 24 hours is grossly related to the volume produced, the concentration in milligrams per deciliter (mg/dL) is not so related.[77] The relative distribution of the individual amino acids in each deciliter (100 mL) of milk differs in each mother. The colostrum may actually reflect a transitional maternal blood picture, which is associated with nitrogen metabolism of the postpartum period. The postpartum period is one of involution of body tissue and catabolism of protein in the mother (Figure 4-9).

Colostrum contains at least two separate antioxidants, an ascorbate-like substance and uric acid.[18] These antioxidants may function in the colostrum as traps for neutrophil-generated, reactive oxygen metabolites. The aqueous human colostrum interferes with the oxygen metabolic and enzymatic activities of the polymorphonuclear leukocytes that are important in the reaction to acute inflammation.[18] This supports the belief that human milk is antiinflammatory.

The mineral and vitamin reserves of the newborn infant are related to the maternal diet. A fetal supply of vitamin C, iron, and amino acids is adequate because infant blood levels exceed those of the mother. Colostrum is rich in fat-soluble vitamin A, carotenoids, and vitamin E. The average vitamin A level on the third day can be three times that of mature milk. Similarly, carotenoids in colostrum may be 10 times the level in mature milk, and vitamin E may be two to three times greater than in mature milk.

Studies that looked at multiparas versus primiparas showed that the volume of milk was significantly greater on day 5 with earlier appearance of the casein band in multiparas (Figure 4-10).[24]

SODIUM AS A PREDICTOR OF SUCCESSFUL LACTOGENESIS

Early in lactogenesis, the sodium levels are high but quickly drop from 60 to 20 mmol by day 3 in women who have been fully feeding their infant. Observations by Morton[104] have shown that high breast milk sodium concentrations on day 3 are suggestive of impending lactation failure. Even women who remove only a small amount of milk daily for research purposes have the physiologic drop in sodium.

Lactogenesis Stage II

Even though best practices recommend breastfeeding shortly after birth and frequently thereafter, Kulski et al. showed that milk removal is not needed for the programmed physiologic changes in mammary epithelium to trigger lactogenesis II. Studies by Woolridge confirmed this when no effect of breastfeeding in the first 24 hours was observed on later milk transfer to the infants. However, time of first breastfeeding and frequency of breastfeeding on day 2 are correlated with milk volume by day 5.[24] No relationship between concentration of prolactin in the plasma and the rate of milk synthesis in either the short or long term was found by Cox et al.[31]

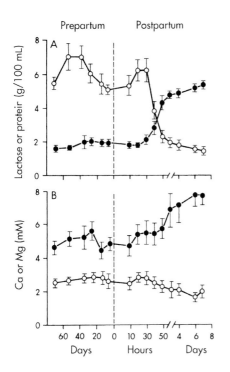

Key: calcium ○   magnesium ●   lactose ●   protein ○

Figure 4-9. The levels of milk constituents prepartum and postpartum change to reflect the maturation from colostrum to fully mature milk. Volume is driven by lactose production. (Modified from Dumas BR: Modifications of early milk composition during early states of lactation in nutritional adaptations of the gastrointestinal tract of the newborn. In Kretchmer N, Minkowski A, editors: *Nutritional adaptation of gastrointestinal tract of the newborn*, vol. 3, New York, 1983, Nestlé Vevey/Raven.)

TRANSITIONAL MILK

The milk produced between the colostrum and mature milk stages is transitional milk; its content gradually changes. The transitional phase is approximately from 7 to 10 days postpartum to 2 weeks postpartum. The concentration of immunoglobulins and total protein decreases, whereas the lactose, fat, and total caloric content increases. The water-soluble vitamins increase, and the fat-soluble vitamins decrease to the levels of mature milk.

In a study of transitional milks, breast milk samples were obtained from healthy mothers of term

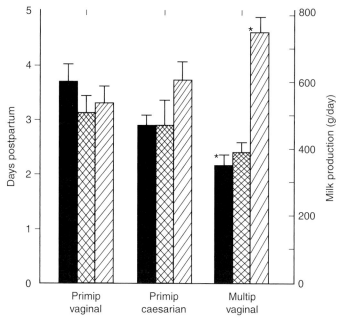

Figure 4-10. Effect of parity on measures of lactogenesis. Data show the mean time at which fullness of the breast was observed *(solid bar)*, the day on which the casein band first appeared *(crosshatched bar)* in an electrophoretic analysis of daily milk samples, and the volume of milk produced on day 5 *(hatched bar)* by primiparous (primip) women delivered vaginally (n=19), primiparous women delivered by cesarean section (n=5), and multiparous (multip) women delivered vaginally (n=16). * Significant difference (p<0.05) between multiparous and primiparous women delivered vaginally. The distance between the error bars represents two standard error of the mean (SEM). (Data from Chen DC, Nommsen-Rivers L, Dewey KG, et al: Stress during labor and delivery and early lactation performance, *Am J Clin Nutr* 68:335, 1998; Neville MC, Morton J, Umemura S: Breastfeeding 2001: the evidence for breastfeeding, *Pediatr Clin North Am* 48:35, 2001.)

infants on the 1st, 3rd, 5th, 8th, 15th, 22nd, 29th, and 36th days of lactation by Hibberd et al., who defined the first day of lactation to be the 3rd day postpartum. The researchers pooled 24-hour samples for analysis, and the remainder was fed to the baby. The authors found a high degree of variability, not only among mothers but also within samples from the same mother. The maximum value in almost every case was more than twice the minimum. They were able to show, however, that the changes in composition were rapid before day 8, and then progressively less change took place until the composition was relatively stable before day 36 (see Tables 4-5 and 4-6).

MATURE MILK

Water

In almost all mammalian milks, water is the constituent in the largest quantity, with the exception of the milk of some arctic and aquatic species, who produce milks with high-fat content (e.g., the northern fur seal produces milk with 54% fat and 65% total solids) (see Table 4-2). All other constituents are dissolved, dispersed, or suspended in water. Water contributes to the temperature-regulating mechanism of the newborn because 25% of heat loss is from evaporation of water from the lungs and skin. The lactating woman has a greatly increased

obligatory water intake. If water intake is restricted during lactation, other water losses through urine and insensible loss are decreased before water for lactation is diminished. Because lactose is the regulating factor in the amount of milk produced, the secretion of water into milk is partially regulated by lactose synthesis. Investigations by Almroth show that the water requirement of infants in a hot, humid climate can be provided entirely by the water in human milk.

Human milk is a complex fluid that scientists have studied by separating the several phases by physical forces.[76] These forces include settling; short-term, low-speed centrifugation; high-speed centrifugation; and precipitation by micelle-destroying treatments, such as using the enzyme rennin (chymosin) or reducing the pH. On settling, the cream floats to the top, forming a layer of fat (about 4% by volume in human milk) (Table 4-8).[71] Lipid-soluble components such as cholesterol and phospholipid remain with the fat. With a slow-speed spin, cellular components form a pellet. The high-speed spin brings the casein micelles into a separate phase or forms a pellet. On top of the protein pellet is a loose pellet referred to as the "fluff," composed of membranes.[112,114] Casein precipitation (0.2% by weight) is caused by acid destruction of the micelles. The aqueous phase is whey, which also contains milk sugar, milk proteins, IgA, and the monovalent ions.

TABLE 4-8 Estimates of the Concentrations of Nutrients in Mature Human Milk

Nutrient	Amount in Human Milk* (g/L ± SD)	Nutrient	Amount in Human Milk* (mcg ± SD)
Lactose	72.0 ± 2.5	Calcium	280 ± 26
Protein	10.5 ± 2.0	Phosphorus	140 ± 22
Fat	39.0 ± 4.0	Magnesium	35 ± 2
		Sodium	180 ± 40
		Potassium	525 ± 35
		Chloride	420 ± 60
		Iron	0.3 ± 0.1
		Zinc	1.2 ± 0.2
		Copper	0.25 ± 0.03
		Vitamin E	2.3 ± 1.0
		Vitamin C	40 ± 10
		Thiamin	0.210 ± 0.035
		Riboflavin	0.350 ± 0.025
		Niacin	1.500 ± 0.200
		Vitamin B_6	93 ± 8[¶]
		Pantothenic acid	1.800 ± 0.200
		Vitamin A, RE	670 ± 200 (2230 IU)
		Vitamin D	0.55 ± 0.10
		Vitamin K	2.1 ± 0.1
		Folate	85 ± 37[†]
		Vitamin B_{12}	0.97[‡,§]
		Biotin	4 ± 1
		Iodine	110 ± 40
		Selenium	20 ± 5
		Manganese	6 ± 2
		Fluoride	16 ± 5
		Chromium	50 ± 5
		Molybdenum	NR

IUs, International units; *NR,* not reported; *RE,* retinol equivalents; *SD,* standard deviation.

*Data from *Pediatric nutrition handbook,* ed 2, Elk Grove Village, Ill., 1985, AAP, p 363, unless otherwise indicated. Values are representative of amounts of nutrients present in human milk; some may differ slightly from those reported by investigators cited in text.

[†]From Brown CM, Smith CM, Picciano MF: Forms of human milk folacin and variation patterns, *J Pediatr Gastroenterol Nutr* 5:278, 1986.

[‡]From Sandberg DP, Begley JA, Hall CA: The content, binding, and forms of vitamin B_{12} in milk, *Am J Clin Nutr* 34:1717, 1981.

[§]Standard deviation not reported; range 0.33 to 3.20.

[¶]From Styslinger L, Kirksey A: Effects of different levels of vitamin B_6 supplementation on vitamin B_6 concentrations in human milk and vitamin B_6 intakes of breastfed infants, *Am J Clin Nutr* 41:21, 1985.

From Report of *Subcommittee, Institute of Medicine: nutrition during lactation,* Washington, D.C., 1991, National Academy Press.

Lipids

Intense interest in the lipids in human milk has been sparked by the reports from long-range studies of breastfed infants that show more advanced development at 1 year,[100] 8 to 10 years,[99] and now 18 years of age[70] compared with formula-fed infants. This attention has resulted from the interest in supplementing formula with various missing factors, such as cholesterol and docosahexaenoic acid (DHA).[125] These compounds function in a milieu of arachidonic acid, lipases, and other enzymes, and no evidence indicates that they are effective in isolation or that more is better. The value of

supplementing the mother's diet in pregnancy and lactation is an equally important question, because dietary DHA levels have declined in the last half century as women have reduced eggs and animal organs in their diet (see Chapter 9).

Lipids are a chemically heterogeneous group of substances that are insoluble in water and soluble in nonpolar solvents. Lipids are separated into many classes and thousands of subclasses. The main constituents of human milk are triacylglycerols, phospholipids, and their component fatty acids, the sterols. Jensen, a renowned milk lipidologist, and

TABLE 4-9   Compartments and Their Constituents in Mature Human Milk*

Compartment		Major Constituents	
Description	Content (%)	Name	Content (%)
Aqueous phase	87.0	Compounds of Ca, Mg, PO_4, Na, K, Cl, CO_2, citrate, casein	0.2 as ash
True solution (1 nm)			
Whey proteins (3-9 nm)		Whey proteins: α-lactalbumin, lactoferrin, IgA, lysozyme, serum albumin	0.6
		Lactose and oligosaccharides; 7.0% and 1.0%	8.0
		Nonprotein nitrogen compounds: glucosamine, urea, amino acids; 20% of total N	35-50 mg N
		Miscellaneous: B vitamins, ascorbic acid	
Colloidal dispersion (11-55 nm, 10^{16} mL^{-1})	0.3	Caseins: beta and kappa, Ca, PO_4	0.2-0.3
Emulsion			
Fat globules (4 μm, 1.1^{10} mL^{-1})	4.0	Fat globules: triacylglycerols, sterol esters	4.0
Fat-globule membrane interfacial layer	2.0	Milk-fat-globule membrane: proteins, phospholipids, cholesterol, enzymes, trace minerals, fat-soluble vitamins	2% of total lipid
Cells (8-40 μm, 10^4-10^5 mL^{-1})		Macrophages, neutrophils, lymphocytes, epithelial cells	

*All figures are approximate.
 From Jensen RG: *The lipids of human milk*, Boca Raton, Fla., 1989, CRC.

his coauthors[77] remind readers, in a comprehensive review of the lipids in human milk, of the nomenclature, such as palmitic acid (16:0), oleic acid (18:1), and linoleic acid (18:2). The figure to the left of the colon is the number of carbons and to the right is the number of double bonds. Polyunsaturated fatty acids (PUFAs) have a designation for the location of the double bond; in human milk, the designation is *cis* (*c*), which identifies the geometric isomer. Because milk is an exceptionally complex fluid, Jensen[79,80] and other scientists have found it helpful to classify components according to their size and concentration, with solubility in milk, or lack thereof, as additional categories (Table 4-9). The lipids fulfill a host of essential functions in growth and development,[15] provide a well-tolerated energy source, serve as carriers of messages to the infant, and provide physiologic interactions, including the following:

1. Allow maximum intestinal absorption of fatty acids
2. Contribute about 50% of calories
3. Provide essential fatty acids (EFAs) and PUFAs
4. Provide cholesterol

By percentage of concentration, the second greatest constituent in milk is the lipid fraction. Milk lipids provide the major fraction of kilocalories in human milk.[77] Lipids average 3% to 5% of human milk and occur as globules emulsified in the aqueous phase. The core or nonpolar lipids, such as triacylglycerols and cholesterol esters, are coated with bipolar materials, phospholipids, proteins, cholesterol, and enzymes. This loose layer is called the milk-lipid-globule membrane, which keeps the globules from coalescing and thus acts as an emulsion stabilizer.[77] Globules are 1 to 10 mm in diameter, with 1-mm globules predominating.[78]

Fats are also the most variable constituents in human milk, varying in concentration over a feeding, from breast to breast, over a day's time, overtime itself, and among individuals (Table 4-10). This information is significant when testing milk samples for energy intake, fat-soluble constituents, and physiologic variation and when clinically managing lactation problems.[63] Much of the early work was based on lactation in women who "nursed by the clock" rather than tuned into infant needs. When circadian variation in fat content was studied in a rural Thai population who had practiced demand feeding for centuries, Jackson et al. found fat concentrations in feeds in the afternoon and evening (1600 to 2000 hours) were higher than those during the night (400 to 800 hours). When Kent et al.[84] reexamined volume, frequency of breastfeedings, and the fat content of the milk throughout the day in 71 mother-infant dyads, they found similar trends. They found, however, that fat content was 41.1 ± 7.8 g/L and ranged from 22.3 to 61.6 g/L. It was not related to time after birth or number of breastfeedings during the day. No effect on the average milk fat content was related to the sex of the infant, clustered breastfeedings, or whether the infant fed at night. Fat content was

TABLE 4-10 Factors That Influence Human Milk Fat Content and Composition

Factor	Influence
Duration of gestation	Shortened gestation increases the long-chain polyunsaturated fatty acids secreted
Stage of lactation ($\uparrow$)	Phospholipid and cholesterol contents are highest in early lactation
Parity ($\downarrow$)	High parity is associated with reduced endogenous fatty acid synthesis
Volume ($\downarrow$)	High volume is associated with low milk fat content
Feeding ($\uparrow$)	Human milk fat content progressively increases during a single nursing
Maternal diet	A diet low in fat increases endogenous synthesis of medium-chain fatty acids (C6 to C10)
Maternal energy status ($\uparrow$)	A high weight gain in pregnancy is associated with increased milk fat

($\uparrow$) Increase; ($\downarrow$) decrease.
Modified from Picciano MF: Nutrient composition of human milk. Breastfeeding 2001, Part I: the evidence for breastfeeding, *Pediatr Clin North Am* 48:53, 2001.

higher during the day and evening compared with night and early morning. They recommended that infants be fed on demand day and night and not by schedule.

When milk of the mothers of preterm infants was measured ($6.6\% \pm 2.8\%$), the fat content was significantly higher in the evening ($7.9\% \pm 2.9\%$) than in the morning ($D < 0.001$).[97]

It is speculated that the altered posture at night, horizontal and relatively inactive, may redistribute fat. The larger the milk consumption at a feed, the greater is the increase in fat from beginning to end of the feed. Less fat change occurs during "sleep" feeds than in the daytime. Unless 24-hour samples are collected by standardized sampling techniques, results will vary. During the course of a feeding, the fluid phase within the gland is mixed with fat droplets in increasing concentration. The fat droplets are released when the smooth muscle contracts in response to the let-down reflex.

The lipid fraction of the milk is extractable by suitable solvents and may require more than one technique to extract all the lipids.[79,80] Complete extraction in human milk is difficult because the lipids are bound to protein. From 30% to 55% of the kilocalories are derived from fats; this represents a concentration of 3.5 to 4.5 g/dL. Milk fat is dispersed in the form of droplets or globules maintained in solution by an absorbed layer or membrane. The protective membrane of the fat globules is made up of phospholipid complexes.[71] The rest of the phospholipids found in human milk are dispersed in the skim milk fraction. Vitamin A esters, vitamin D, vitamin K, alkyl glyceryl ethers, and glyceryl ether diesters are also in the lipid fraction but do not fall into the classes listed.

Renewed interest in defining the constituents of human milk lipid has developed as investigators look for the causes of obesity, atherosclerosis, and other degenerative diseases and their relationship to infant nutrition. A number of reports of historic value have technical problems of sampling. Because the fat content of a feeding varies with time, spot samples give spurious results. Ferris and

Jensen have reviewed the literature exhaustively and describe the fractionated lipid constituents in detail.

Most studies on fat content of milk have been based on a geographically limited population. Milk fat changes with diet and maternal adipose stores; Yuhas et al.[153] studied milk samples from nine countries (Australia, Canada, Chile, China, Japan, Mexico, Philippines, the United Kingdom, and the United States). Saturated fatty acids were constant across countries, and monounsaturated fatty acids varied minimally. Arachidonic acid (C20: 4n-6) was also similar. DHA (22: 6n-3), however, was variable everywhere, but was dramatically different with milk from Japan having the highest values and the United States and Canada having the lowest values. Of note is the fact that the timing of collections was comparable in all countries. All samples were collected by electric pump, except in Japan where they were hand expressed.[153]

The average fat content of pooled 24-hour samples has been reported from multiple sources to vary in mature milk from 2.10% to 5.0% (Table 4-11). Maternal diet affects the constituents of the lipids but not the total amount of fat. A minimal increase in total lipid content was observed when an extra 1000 kcal of corn oil was fed to lactating mothers. A diet rich in polyunsaturated fats will cause an increased percentage of polyunsaturated fats in the milk without altering the total fat content. When the mother is calorie deficient, depot fats are mobilized, and milk resembles depot fat. When excessive nonfat kilocalories are fed, levels of saturated fatty acids increase as lipids are synthesized from tissue stores.

When fish oil supplementation is given during pregnancy it significantly alters the early postpartum breast milk fatty acid composition (omega-3 PUFA). Levels of omega-3 fatty acids are increased as are IgA and many other immunomodulatory factors (CD14).[40]

A 2-week crossover study of three nursing women was done by Harzer et al., alternating high fat/low carbohydrate and the reverse. The first diet

TABLE 4-11	Lipid Class Composition of Human Milk During Lactation					
	Percentage of Total Lipids at Lactation Day					
Lipid Class	**3**	**7**	**21**	**42**	**84**	**Immediate Extraction**
Total lipid, % in milk*	2.04 ± 1.32	2.89 ± 0.31	3.45 ± 0.37	3.19 ± 0.43	4.87 ± 0.62	
Phospholipid	1.1	0.8	0.8	0.6	0.6	0.81
Monoacylglycerol	–	–	–	–	–	ND
Free fatty acids	–	–	–	–	–	0.08
Cholesterol (mg/dL)[†]	1.3 (34.5)	0.7 (20.2)	0.5 (17.3)	0.5 (17.3)	0.4 (19.5)	0.34
1,2-Diacylglycerol	–	–	–	–	–	0.01
1,3-Diacylglycerol	–	–	–	–	–	ND
Triacylglycerol	97.6	98.5	98.7	98.9	99.0	98.76
Cholesterol esters (mg)[‡]						
Number of women	39	41	25	18	8	6

ND, Not done.
*Mean ± SEM.
[†]Total cholesterol content ranges from 10 to 20 mg/dL after 21 days in most milks.
[‡]Not reported, but in Bitman et al. (Bitman J, Wood DL, Mehta NR, et al: Comparison of the cholesteryl ester composition of human milk from preterm and term mothers, *J Pediatr Gastroenterol Nutr* 5:780, 1986), it was 5 mg/dL at 3 days and 1 mg/dL at 21 days and thereafter.
From Jensen RG, Bitman J, Carlson SE: Milk lipids. In: Jensen RG, editor: *Handbook of milk composition*, San Diego, 1995, Academic Press.

TABLE 4-12	Effects of Dietary Cholesterol, Phytosterol, and Polyunsaturate (P)/Saturate (S) Ratio on Human Milk Sterols		
Milk Component	**Maternal Ad Lib Diet (P/S 0.53) (mg/100 g fat)**	**Low-Cholesterol/High-Phytosterol Diet (P/S 1.8) (mg/100 g fat)**	**High-Cholesterol/Low-Phytosterol Diet (P/S 0.12) (mg/100 g fat)**
Cholesterol	240 ± 40	250 ± 10	250 ± 20
Phytosterol	17 ± 3	220 ± 30	70 ± 10
Dietary cholesterol	450 ± 30	130 ± 5	460 ± 90
Dietary phytosterol	23 ± 8	790 ± 17	80 ± 1
Total fat (%)	3.58 ± 0.56	2.69 ± 0.17	2.66 ± 0.16

From Lammi-Keefe CJ, Jensen RG: Lipids in human milk: a review, *J Pediatr Gastroenterol Nutr* 3:172, 1984.

was 50% fat, 15% protein, and 35% carbohydrate for a total of 2500 calories, which resulted in a reduction of triglycerides (4.1% to 2.6%) and an increase in lactose (5.2% to 6.4%) (Table 4-12).

The U.S. Department of Agriculture (USDA) has reported that the average American diet now includes 156 g of fat per day, up from 141 g in 1947. The significant change is from animal to vegetable fat, which is now 39% of total dietary fats, especially resulting from the switch from butter and lard. A change in fatty acid content to more long-chain fatty acids and a two-fold to three-fold increase in linoleic acid have occurred. Except for 18:2 content in mature milk, the fatty acid composition is remarkably uniform unless the maternal diet is unusually bizarre.

Polyunsaturated fats include C18:2 and C18:3, or linoleic and linolenic acid. The bovine ratio of polyunsaturated to saturated fats (P/S ratio) is 4. The P/S ratio has shifted as a result of recent dietary changes to 1.3 from 1.35 in human milk. The P/S ratio is significant in facilitating calcium and fat absorption. Calcium absorption is depressed by a 4:5 P/S ratio. The breast can dehydrogenate saturated and monounsaturated fatty acids in milk synthesis.

At least 167 fatty acids have been identified in human milk; possibly others are present in trace amounts. Bovine milk has 437 identified fatty acids. Major dietary changes would greatly change fatty acid composition.

Milk from vegetarians (lacto-ovo) contained a lower proportion of fatty acids derived from animal fat and a higher proportion of PUFAs derived from dietary vegetable fat. Women who consumed 35 g or more of animal fat per day had higher C10:0, C12:0, and C18:3 but lower levels of C16:0 and C18:0. Finley et al.[49] suggest that a maximum amount of C16:0 and C18:0 can be taken up from

TABLE 4-13 Effects of Maternal Vegetarian Diets on Saturated and Unsaturated Fatty Acids (wt%) in Human Milk Lipids (Mean ± SEM)

Lipid (%)/Fatty Acid	Vegetarian*	Control*	Vegan´	Vegetarian[†]	Omnivore[†]
Number	12	7	19	5	21
Saturates					
6:0	–	–	–	–	–
8:0	0.16 ± 0.03	0.22 ± 0.01	–	–	–
10:0	1.56 ± 0.13	1.57 ± 0.09	1.8 ± 0.40	1.3 ± 0.51	0.4 ± 0.23
12:0	7.07 ± 0.78	5.47 ± 0.66	6.6 ± 0.54	3.2 ± 0.49	1.7 ± 0.35
14:0	8.16 ± 1.00	6.54 ± 0.73	6.9 ± 0.58	5.2 ± 0.50	4.5 ± 0.35
16:0	15.31 ± 0.73	20.48 ± 0.64	18.1 ± 1.34	21.2 ± 1.07	25.1 ± 0.78
18:0	4.48 ± 0.37	8.14 ± 0.55	4.9 ± 0.36	7.4 ± 0.35	9.7 ± 0.68
20:0	0.54 ± 0.02	0.57 ± 0.03	–	–	–
Total	37.28	42.99			
Monounsaturates					
16:1	1.66 ± 0.14	3.35 ± 0.28	4.9 ± 0.24	2.9 ± 0.37	3.4 ± 0.35
18:1	26.89 ± 1.47	34.7 ± 0.86	32.2 ± 1.06	35.3 ± 1.94	38.7 ± 1.27
Total	28.55	38.06	37.10	38.2	42.1
Polyunsaturates					
n-6 Series					
18:2	28.82 ± 1.39	14.47 ± 1.98	23.8 ± 1.40	19.5 ± 3.62	10.9 ± 0.96
20:2	0.72 ± 0.03	0.50 ± 0.03	–	–	–
20:3	0.62 ± 0.03	0.56 ± 0.03	0.44 ± 0.03	0.42 ± 0.07	0.40 ± 0.08
20:4	0.68 ± 0.03	0.68 ± 0.03	0.32 ± 0.02	0.38 ± 0.05	0.35 ± 0.03
Total	30.84	16.21	31.4	27.5	18.4
n-3 Series					
18:3	2.76 ± 0.16	1.85 ± 0.16	1.36 ± 0.18	1.25 ± 0.22	0.49 ± 0.06
22:6	0.22 ± 0.08	0.27 ± 0.08	0.14 ± 0.06	0.30 ± 0.05	0.36 ± 0.07
Total	3.05	2.12	1.50	1.55	0.86

Dietary information

Vegetarian (col. 2): whole cereal grains, 50-60%; soup, 5%; vegetables, 20-25%; beans and sea vegetables, 5-10%; macrobiotic diet for a mean of 81 months; no meat or dairy products; occasional seafood, nuts, and fruit

Control: typical diet in the United States

Vegan´: No foods of animal origin

Vegetarian (col. 5): Exclude meat and fish

Omnivore: typical Western diet

*Modified from Specker BL, Wey HE, Miller D: Differences in fatty acid composition of human milk in vegetarian and nonvegetarian women: long-term effect of diet, *J Pediatr Gastroenterol Nutr* 6:764, 1987. New England donors: vegetarians, 3 to 13 months postpartum; control subjects, 1 to 5 months; capillary gas-liquid chromatography columns.

[†]Modified from Sanders TA, Reddy S: The influence of a vegetarian diet on the fatty acid composition of human milk and the essential fatty acid status of the infant, *J Pediatr* 120:S71, 1992. British donors: 6 weeks postpartum; packed GLC columns.

From Jensen RG, Bitman J, Carlson SE: Milk lipids. In Jensen RG, editor: *Handbook of milk composition*, San Diego, 1995, Academic Press.

the blood and subsequently secreted into milk (Table 4-13).

The milk of strict vegetarians has extremely high levels of linoleic acid, four times that of cow milk (see Table 4-13). Some researchers include other long-chain fatty acids (e.g., C20:2, C20:3, C24:4, C22:3) as essential nutrients because they are structural lipids in the brain and nervous tissue. The effects of diet are also discussed in Chapter 9.

One important outcome of linoleic and linolenic acids is the conversion of these compounds into longer-chain polyunsaturates. These metabolites have been shown to be important for fluidity of membrane lipids and prostaglandin synthesis. They are present in the brain and retinal cells. Long-chain polyunsaturates are needed for development of the infant brain and nervous system.[49] When Gibson and Kneebore studied fatty acid composition of colostrum and mature milk at 3 to 5 days and later at 6 weeks postpartum, they reported that mature milk had a higher percentage of saturated fatty acids, including medium-chain acids, lower monounsaturated fatty acids, and higher linoleic and linolenic acids and their long-chain polyunsaturated derivatives.

Infant intake of fatty acids from human milk over the first year of lactation (solids were started at 4 to 6 months) was studied by Mitoulas et al.[103] among mothers and infants in Australia. They determined the volume, fat content, and fatty acid composition of milk from each breast at each feed over 24 hours at 1, 2, 4, 6, 9, and 12 months. Volume of production was greater in the right breast (414 to 449 versus 336 to 360). Fat content also varied between breasts. Amounts of fat per 24 hours did not differ in the first year and only arachidonic acid and DHA differed between mothers. Changes in proportions of individual fatty acids may not result in commensurate changes in 24-hour infant intakes. The authors[84,103] note their findings were similar to Jensen's work in 1995 in the United States.

When this same group of investigators in Australia (Kent et al.[84] and Mitoulas et al.[103]) measured volume of milk, frequency of feedings, and fat content at 1 to 6 months of age in a normal group of mothers using demand feeding, they concluded infants should be fed on demand, day and night. They observed no relationship between total number of feeds and total volume. Furthermore fat content was 41.1 ± 7.8 g/L (range 22.3 to 61.6 g/L). Total fat was independent of frequency of feeding.

Prolonged lactation has long been suspected of providing reduced nutrition. It has been established that infection protection continues, but now there is evidence that high nutrition persists as well; 34 mother-baby dyads and 27 control dyads were studied by Mandel et al.[102] The mothers who were breastfeeding beyond 1 year (12 to 39 months) were older (34.4 ± 5.1, years), lighter ($59.8 \div 8.7$ kg), and with lower BMI (22.1 ± 3.0) than controls (breastfeeding 2 to 6 months; age 30.7 ± 2.9 years, weight 66.3 ± 11.8 kg, and BMI 24.5 ± 3.9). Feeding frequency per day was 5.9 ± 3.3 versus 7.36 ± 2.65 (controls). The milk of mothers who were breastfeeding beyond a year had significantly increased fat and increased energy content compared with controls.[102]

Factors affecting fatty acid composition include the stage of lactation, especially in specific fatty acids probably due to the recruiting of body fat stores. Milk from mothers of premature infants differs from that of mothers of full-term infants in fat content with higher levels of medium-chain fatty acids in premature milk. The significance of circadian rhythm on fatty acid composition is contradictory in the literature; therefore, studies of fat content should consider this in sample collection.[33]

Diet, on the other hand, has an extensive impact on fat content of milk with up to 85% derived from diet in the form of chylomicrons. This has led to dietary supplementation, especially utilizing the omega-3 fatty acids.[139]

Brain Development. To address the issue of nutrition during brain development, it is important to consider the different periods of brain development that have been described biochemically. First, cell division occurs, with the formation of neurons and glial cells, and second, myelination. In the rat brain, 50% of polyenoic acids of the gray matter lipids were laid down by the fifteenth day of life. The fatty acids characteristic of myelin lipids appeared later. Gray matter is largely composed of unmyelinated neurons, whereas white matter contains a very high proportion of myelinated conducting nerve fibers. Normal brain function depends on both. The synthesis and composition of myelin can be influenced by diet in the developing rat brain.

Myelin-specific messenger ribonucleic acid (mRNA) levels are developmentally regulated and influenced by dietary fat. The neonatal response to dietary fat is tissue specific at the mRNA level.[37]

The fatty acids characteristic of gray matter (C20:4 and C22:6) accumulate before the appearance of fatty acids characteristic of myelin (C20:1 and C24:1) in the developing brain. Arachidonic acid (C20:4) and DHA (C22:6) are synthesized from linoleic and linolenic acids, respectively, but the latter two must be obtained in the diet.

During the first year of life, the human brain more than doubles in size, increasing from 350 to 1100 g in weight. Of this growth, 85% is cerebrum; 50% to 60% of this solid matter is lipid. Cortical total phospholipid fatty acid composition in both term and preterm infants is greatly influenced by dietary fat intake. Phospholipids make up about one quarter of the solid matter and are integral to the vascular system on which the brain depends.[47] Brain growth is associated with an increase in the incorporation of long-chain PUFAs into the phospholipid in the cerebral cortex.[76] The transition from colostrum to mature milk leads to an increase in sphingomyelin and a decrease in phosphatidylcholine in the milk of mothers who deliver prematurely, along with a decrease in phospholipid content. Phospholipids are essential to brain growth, especially in a premature infant. Sphingomyelin and phosphatidylcholine are a source of choline, a major constituent of membranes in the brain and nervous tissue. Extreme dietary alterations in animal experiments have demonstrated an altered PUFA composition of the developing brain.

Such studies cannot be done in humans. Farquharson et al.[47] therefore examined the necropsy specimens of cerebrocortical gray matter obtained from 20 term and 2 premature infants, all of whom died within 43 weeks of birth. All were victims of sudden death and were genetically normal. The infants had either received exclusively breast milk or exclusively formula. The latter group was divided by formula type into three groups: mixture of formulas, SMA, or CGOST (cow milk or Osterfeed). (SMA and CGOST are formulas or mixtures of formulas sold in the United Kingdom.) Breastfed infants had greater concentrations of DHA in their cerebrocortical phospholipids than formula-fed infants in all groups. A compensatory increase in *n*-6 series fatty acids (arachidonic, docosatetraenoic, and docosapentaenoic) occurred in the SMA group. No significant differences were seen between saturated and monounsaturated fatty acids. The two premature infants had the lowest levels of DHA.

Cerebrocortical neuronal membrane glycerophospholipids are composed predominantly (95%) of phosphatidylcholine, phosphatidylethanolamine, and phosphatidylserine.[76] After birth, neuronal membranes and retinal photoreceptor cells derive most of their phospholipid DHA from diet and liver synthesis and not from fat reserves. Neither the liver nor the retinal and neuronal cells can synthesize DHA without reserves or a dietary supply. α-Linolenic acid, an EFA, is the precursor. If the enzymes are not activated or are inactivated by an excess of *n*-6 fatty acids, synthesis does not take place. Human milk provides the DHA and arachidonic acid.[61]

Dietary supplementation with fish oil in the latter part of pregnancy resulted in increased DHA status at birth when measured in the umbilical blood.[101] When postpartum women were supplemented with DHA by capsule in a blind study, breast milk levels of DHA ranged from 0.2% to 1.7% of total fatty acids, increasing with dose. Arachidonic acid levels and antioxidant status of plasma arachidonic acid and levels were unaffected.

Although DHA is essential to retinal development, levels peak in the retina at 36 to 38 weeks' gestation, suggesting that the most rapid rate of retinal accumulation occurs before term.[65] This further suggests that the premature infant is especially vulnerable to dietary deficiencies of DHA.

Dietary omega-3 (ω-3) fatty acids may not be essential to life, reproduction, or growth, but they are important for normal biochemical and functional development.[132] Long-chain ω-3 fatty acids, DHA in particular, form a major structural component of biologic membranes. When the ratio of omega-6 (ω-6) is high compared to ω-3, fatty acids aggravate the deficiency. Studies in monkeys have shown that DHA deficiency affects water intake and urine excretion, as well as ω-3 fatty acid levels in red blood cells.[132] Much remains to be learned about the effects of ω-3 fatty acids and DHA deficiency on developing human infants.

The EFAs, linoleic and linolenic acids, may have greater significance in the quality of the myelin laid down. Dick, observing the geographic distribution of multiple sclerosis worldwide, noted that the disease is rare in countries where breastfeeding is common. He postulated that the development of myelin in infancy is critical to preventing degradation later. Dick investigated the difference between human milk and cow milk in relation to myelin production in multiple sclerosis.

Experimental allergic encephalitis is a demyelinating condition and can be produced by shocking animals that have been sensitized to central nervous system (CNS) antigens. Newborn rats deficient in EFAs are more susceptible to this disease, which has been described as resembling multiple sclerosis pathologically.

Other Influences on Fat Content. Infections will alter milk composition. Mastitis does not alter fat content but does lower volume and lactose and increase sodium and chloride.

Parity has been cited as a major influence on fat content, with primiparous women having more fat than multiparous women. Prentice et al. found a significant relationship between fat content and triceps skinfold thickness. The authors found seasonal changes in The Gambia, where volume and fat were lowest following the rainy season, when nutrient resources are scarce.

Hyperlipoproteinemia

Milk from women with type I hyperlipoproteinemia has been investigated.[78] Because the primary deficiency is serum-stimulated lipoprotein lipase in the plasma, resulting in reduced transfer of dietary long-chain fatty acids from blood to milk, levels of fat as fatty acids were abnormally low (1.5%) and the amounts of 10:0 and 14:0 higher than normal (see Chapter 16).

Cholesterol

Cholesterol is an essential component of all membranes and is required for growth, replication, and maintenance. Infants fed human milk have higher plasma cholesterol levels than formula-fed infants. Animal studies suggest that early postnatal ingestion of a diet high in cholesterol protects against high-cholesterol challenges later.

The cholesterol content of milk is remarkably stable at 240 mg/100 g of fat when calculated by volume of fat. The range, depending on sampling techniques, is 9 to 41 mg/dL. The amount of cholesterol changed slightly over time, decreasing 1.7-fold over the first 36 days, as reported by Harzer et al., and stabilizing at approximately day 15 postpartum at 20 mg/dL. This resulted in a change in the cholesterol/triglyceride ratio. The authors found no uniform pattern of circadian variations between mothers.

Neonatal plasma cholesterol levels range between 50 and 100 mg/dL at birth, with equal distribution of low-density lipoprotein (LDL) and high-density lipoprotein (HDL). Plasma cholesterol increases rapidly over the first few days of life, with LDL predominating regardless of mode of feeding.[75] In breastfed infants, however, plasma cholesterol progressively increases compared with that in infants fed low to no cholesterol and high-PUFA formulas. This may have a lasting effect on the individual's ability to metabolize cholesterol, a point yet to be confirmed.[74] Low-birth-weight (LBW) premature infants are at risk for stimulation of endogenous cholesterol biosynthesis, resulting in marked elevations in plasma cholesterol as a result of intravenous nutrition.

The effect of breastfeeding on plasma cholesterol, body weight, and body length was studied longitudinally in 512 infants by Jooste et al.[81] Breastfed infants had higher plasma cholesterol than the formula-fed infants, created by a direct mechanism that persisted for as long as the infants were breastfed. Body length was similar in breastfed and formula-fed infants, but formula-fed infants weighed more.

Cholesterol has been a factor of great concern because of the apparent association with risk factors for atherosclerosis and coronary heart disease. At present, commercial formulas have high P/S ratios and little or no cholesterol compared with those of human milk. Dietary manipulation does not change the cholesterol level in the breast milk. When the dietary cholesterol level is controlled, however, a fall in the infant's plasma cholesterol level is associated with an increase in the amount of linoleic acid present in the milk.

Kallio et al.[83] followed 193 infants from birth, measuring concentrations of cholesterol, very-low-density lipoprotein (VLDL), LDL, HDL2, and, on a limited group of 36 infants, HDL3 and apoprotein B. The largest differences between exclusively breastfed and weaned infants were at 2 months (0.8 mmol/L), 4 months (0.6 mmol/L), and 6 months (0.5 mmol/L). The LDL and apoprotein B concentrations were lower in weaned infants. VLDL and HDL3 were independent of diet. The authors concluded that the low intake of cholesterol and high intake of unsaturated fatty acids greatly modify the blood lipid pattern in the first year of life.[83]

In a retrospective epidemiologic study of 5718 men in England born in the 1920s, 474 died of ischemic heart disease.[46] The infant-feeding groups were divided into those breastfed but weaned before 1 year, breastfed more than a year, and bottle fed. The first group had the lowest death rate from ischemic heart disease and had lower total cholesterol, LDL cholesterol, and apolipoprotein B than those who were weaned after a year and especially those who were bottle fed. In all feeding groups, serum apolipoprotein B concentrations were lower in men with higher birth weights and weights at 1 year.[107]

No long-range effect of serum cholesterol level has been identified, although Osborn described the pathologic changes in 1500 young people (newborns to age 20). He observed the spectrum of pathologic changes from mucopolysaccharide accumulations to fully developed atherosclerotic plaques. Lesions were more frequent and severe in children who had been bottle fed. Lesions were uncommon or mild in the breastfed children.

Animal investigations indicated that rats given high levels of cholesterol early in life were better able to cope with cholesterol in later life and maintained a lower cholesterol level.[37]

In a study of six breastfed and 12 formula-fed infants, ages 4 to 5 months, Wong et al. measured the fractional synthesis rate. The breastfed infants had higher cholesterol intakes (18.4 ± 4.0 mg/kg/day) than formula-fed infants (only 3.4 ± 1.8 mg/kg/day). Plasma cholesterol levels were 183 ± 47 versus 112 ± 22 mg/dL; LDL cholesterol levels were 83 ± 26 versus 48 ± 16 mg/dL. An inverse relationship existed between the fractional synthesis rate of cholesterol and dietary intake of cholesterol. The authors concluded that the greater cholesterol intake of breastfed infants is associated with elevated plasma LDL cholesterol concentrations. In addition, cholesterol synthesis in human infants may be efficiently regulated by coenzyme A (CoA) reductase when infants are challenged with dietary cholesterol.

A carefully designed, well-controlled longitudinal study is needed to determine the long-range impact of cholesterol because it is a consistent constituent of human milk throughout lactation. The brain contains cholesterol especially in early development.

n-3 Fatty Acids

The n-3 fatty acids are important components of animal and plant cell membranes and are selectively distributed among the lipid classes. The role of DHA (22: n-3) in infantile nerve and brain tissue and retinal development has been discussed. It is also found in high levels in testis and sperm. Human milk contains DHA, and studies to evaluate the effects of "fish oil" supplements to the diet suggest an elevation of the dose-dependent levels.

Eicosapentaenoic acid (20: 5n-3) is part of another group of n-3 fatty acids, the eicosanoids, which comprise two families: the prostanoids (prostaglandins, prostacyclins, and thromboxanes) and the leukotrienes.[78] The prostanoids are mediators of inflammatory processes. Leukotrienes are key mediators of inflammation and delayed hypersensitivity. The eicosanoids are highly active lipid mediators in both physiologic and pathologic processes.[136] Eicosanoids provide cytoprotection and vasoactivity in the modulation of inflammatory and proliferative reactions. Their precursors, long-chain PUFAs, can affect the generation of eicosanoids. The role of eicosanoids in physiologic and pathophysiologic processes is beginning to be identified. It clearly goes beyond adding a little DHA to the brew. Sellmayer and Koletzko[136] reviewed this work.

In other species, restriction of n-3 fatty acids results in abnormal electroretinograms, impaired visual activity, and decreased learning ability. The influence of dietary n-3 fatty acids on visual activity development in very-low-birth-weight (VLBW) infants was evaluated by Birch et al.,[14] using visual-evoked response and forced-choice preferential-looking procedures at 36 and 57 weeks postconception. Feeding groups were randomized to one of three diets: corn oil (only linoleic), soy oil (linoleic and linolenic), and soy/marine oil (added n-3 fatty acids). The marine oil group matched the "gold standards" of VLBW infants fed human milk. Visual activity parameters in the other infants who did not receive n-3 oils were considerably lower.

The n-3 fatty acids appear to function in the membranes of photoreceptor cells and synapses. Jensen and Jensen[80] suggest a daily intake of 18:3n-3 (0.5% of calories) with the inclusion of n-3 long-chain PUFA, which is available in human milk. Many studies affirm the value of n-3 fatty acids in the diet and as protection against heart disease, chronic inflammatory disease, and possibly cancer.[140] When synthetic DHA and arachidonic acid are added to infant formula, the measurements of visual acuity do not match those of human milk. The tolerance for these formulas is still undocumented and long-range outcomes unreported.

Carnitine

Carnitine is γ-trimethylamino-β-hydroxybutyrate and is essential for the catabolism of long-chain fatty acids. Only two conditions in life have been described when carnitine is indispensable: total parenteral nutrition lasting more than 3 weeks and early postnatal life. In older individuals it is synthesized in the liver and kidney from the essential amino acids lysine and methionine. Carnitine serves as an essential carrier of acyl groups across the mitochondrial membrane to sites of oxidation and,

therefore, has a central role in the mitochondrial oxidation of fatty acids in humans.[124]

Newborns undergo major metabolic changes during transition from fetal to extrauterine life, including the rapid development of the capacity to oxidize fatty acids and ketone bodies as fuel alternatives to glucose. The fatty acids derived from high-fat milk and endogenous fat stores become the preferred fuel of the heart, brain, and tissues with high-energy demands. In addition, a dramatic increase occurs in serum fatty acids in the first hours of life. After the interruption of the fetoplacental circulation and in the absence of an exogenous supply of carnitine, neonatal plasma levels of free carnitines and acylcarnitines decrease very rapidly. Carnitine administration seems to act by increasing ketogenesis and lipolysis. When serum carnitine and ketone body concentrations were measured in breastfed and formula-fed newborn infants, lower carnitine levels were found in infants fed formulas than in those fed breast milk.

The levels of carnitine range from 70 to 95 nmol/mL in breast milk (up to 115 nmol/mL in colostrum) and from 40 to 80 nmol/mL in commercial formula (Enfamil). The bioavailability of carnitine in human milk may be a significant factor in the higher carnitine and ketone body concentrations in breastfed babies. In omnivorous mothers, carnitine levels do not vary considerably over time.[15] Levels in the milk of lacto-ovovegetarian mothers were always consistently lower than those of omnivores. The lower serum level of lysine in these women is a possible cause of lower carnitine.

The carnitine levels in human milk were followed for 50 days postpartum and the mean level was found to be 62.9 nmol/mL (56.0 to 69.8 nmol/mL range) during the first 21 days and 35.2 ± 1.26 nmol/mL until days 40 to 50. Levels were not related to volume of milk secreted.

PROTEINS

All varieties of milks have been evaluated for their protein contents, which vary from species to species. Proteins constitute 0.9% of the contents in human milk and range up to 20% in some rabbit species. Proteins of milk include casein, serum albumin, α-lactalbumin, β-lactoglobulins, immunoglobulins, and other glycoproteins. Eight of 20 amino acids present in milk are essential and are derived from plasma. The mammary alveolar epithelium synthesizes some nonessential amino acids. Human milk amino acids occur in proteins and peptides, as well as a small percentage in the form of free amino acids and glucosamine[3] (Table 4-14; Figure 4-11).

Tikanoja et al. reported that postprandial changes in plasma amino acids in breastfed infants were proportional to dietary intake and were

TABLE 4-14	Free Amino Acid Concentrations in Human Milk		
Amino Acid	**Colostral Milk (μmol/dL)**	**Transitional Milk (μmol/dL)**	**Mature Milk (μmol/dL)**
Glutamic acid	36-68	88-127	101-180
Glutamine	2-9	9-20	13-58
Taurine	41-45	34-50	27-67
Alanine	9-11	13-20	17-26
Threonine	5-12	7-8	6-13
Serine	12	6-11	6-14
Glycine	5-8	5-10	3-13
Aspartic acid	5-6	3-4	3-5
Leucine	3-5	2-6	2-4
Cystine	1-3	2-5	3-6
Valine	3-4	3-6	4-6
Lysine	5	1-11	2-5
Histidine	2	2-3	0.4-3
Phenylalanine	1-2	1	0.6-2
Tyrosine	2	1-2	1-2
Arginine	3-7	1-5	1-2
Isoleucine	2	1-2	1
Ornithine	1-4	1	0.5-0.9
Methionine	0.8	0.3-3	0.3-0.8
Phosphoserine	8	5	4
Phosphoethanolamine	4	8	10
α-Aminobutyrate	1	0.4-1.4	0.4-1
Tryptophan	5	1	1
Proline	–	6	2-3

From Carlson SE: Human milk nonprotein nitrogen: occurrence and possible function, *Adv Pediatr* 32:43, 1985.

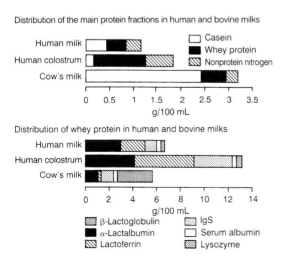

Figure 4-11. Distribution of main protein fractions *(top)* and whey protein *(bottom)* in human and bovine milk. (Modified from Dumas BR: Modifications of early human milk composition during early states of lactation in nutritional adaptation of the gastrointestinal tract of the newborn. In Kretchmer N, Minkowski A, editors: *Nutritional adaptation of gastrointestinal tract of the newborn*, vol. 3, New York, 1983, Nestlé Vevey/Raven.)

highest for the branched-chain amino acids. This was also found to be true for most semiessential and nonessential amino acids. The blood urea levels also reflect dietary intake, with values in breastfed infants being substantially lower than levels in bottle-fed infants. The sum of plasma free amino acids rose and the glycine/valine ratio fell after a feed. When breastfed and formula-fed infants were compared by Järvenpää, concentrations of citrulline, threonine, phenylalanine, and tyrosine were higher in formula-fed than in breastfed infants. Concentrations of taurine were lower in the formula-fed infants. The peak time was different for formula-fed and breastfed infants, which points out the need to standardize sampling times.

The DARLING (Davis Area Research on Lactation, Infant Nutrition, and Growth) Study was the first longitudinal study to follow a large group of mother-infant dyads to 12 months.[36] The investigators report protein intake to be positively associated with milk lipid concentrations after 16 weeks. Milk protein concentration was negatively related to milk volume at 6 and 9 months and positively related to feeding frequency at these times. Milk composition is more sensitive to maternal factors such as body composition, diet, and parity during later lactation than during the first few months.[119]

Casein

Milk consists of casein, or curds, and whey proteins, or lactalbumins. The term *casein* includes a group of milk-specific proteins characterized by ester-bound phosphate, high-proline content, and low solubility at a pH of 4.0 to 5.0.[79,93] Caseins form complex particles or micelles, which are usually complexes of calcium caseinate and calcium phosphate. When milk clots or curdles as a result of heat, pH changes, or enzymes, the casein is transformed into an insoluble caseinate-calcium phosphate complex. Physiochemical differences exist between human and cow caseins.[93] Casein has a species-specific amino acid composition.

When Lönnerdal and Forsum[93] originally measured the casein content of human milk by three different methods—isoelectric precipitation, sedimentation by ultracentrifuge, and indirect analysis—they consistently had three separate results.

Utilizing two newer techniques, Kunz and Lönnerdal[92] report confirming results revealing that casein synthesis is low or absent in early lactation, then increases rapidly, and then decreases. The concentration of whey proteins decreases from early lactation. The whey protein/casein ratios change accordingly from 90:10 in early milk to 60:40 in mature milk and 50:50 in late lactation. The authors suggest whey and casein are regulated by different mechanisms.[92]

Methionine/Cysteine Ratio

The cysteine content is high in human milk, whereas it is very low in cow milk. Because the methionine content is high in bovine milk, the methionine/cysteine ratio is two to three times greater in cow milk than in the milk of most mammals and seven times that in human milk. Human milk is the only animal protein in which the methionine/cysteine ratio is close to 1. Otherwise, this ratio is seen only in plant proteins.

Two significant characteristics of amino acid composition of human milk are the ratio between the sulfur-containing amino acids methionine and cysteine and the low content of the aromatic amino acids phenylalanine and tyrosine. Newborns and especially premature infants are poorly prepared to handle phenylalanine and tyrosine because of their low levels of the specific enzymes required to metabolize them.

Taurine

Taurine, 2-aminoethanesulfonic acid (so named because it was first isolated from the bile of the ox), is a third sulfur-containing amino acid that has been found in high concentrations in human milk and is virtually absent in cow milk. It is now being added to some prepared formulas. Free taurine and glutamic acid have been measured in breast milk in high concentrations. Taurine has been associated in the body at all ages with bile acid conjugation; in newborns, bile acids are almost exclusively conjugated with taurine.

Sturman et al. suggest that taurine may also be a neurotransmitter or neuromodulator in the brain and retina. Taurine in the nutrition of human infants was reviewed by Neville,[116] who reports that evidence is accumulating that taurine has a more general biologic role in development and membrane stability.

Taurine is found in very high concentrations in the milk of cats.[131] Kittens deprived of taurine by feeding with purified taurine-free casein diets after weaning develop retinal degeneration and blindness. The process can be reversed by feeding taurine, but not by feeding methionine, cysteine, or inorganic sulfate. The structural integrity of the retina of the cat has been shown to be taurine dependent. The taurine levels were more severely depleted in the brain tissue, but the significance of this finding has not yet been determined.[147] Both humans and cats are unable to synthesize taurine to any degree as newborns and young infants and are, therefore, wholly dependent on a dietary supply. The process requires cystathionase and cysteine-sulfinic acid decarboxylase, which are enzymes that convert methionine, cysteine, or cystine to taurine.

In studies of amino acid levels, only the concentrations of taurine in plasma and urine of breastfed term infants were higher than those of preterm infants fed formula. Levels in term infants were higher than those of preterm infants fed pooled human milk at a fixed volume. The effects of feeding taurine-deficient formula to human infants, which occurred before the addition of taurine to infant formula, are not as severe as seen in the kitten. The presence of taurine in human milk and predominance of taurine conjugates in the gut at birth suggest that bile acid conjugate status may be a controlling factor. When bile acid metabolism was measured in infants fed human milk, the infants consistently had higher intraluminal bile acid concentrations at all ages (1 to 5 weeks) than did formula-fed infants with and without additional taurine. Human milk also facilitated intestinal lipid absorption.[149]

Human infants conjugate bile acids predominantly with taurine at birth but quickly develop the capacity to conjugate with glycine. Those infants fed human milk continue to conjugate with taurine, whereas those fed formulas soon conjugate with glycine predominantly. The cat, in contrast, uses only taurine throughout life.[149] In humans the various pools of taurine in the body cannot be predicted by measurement of plasma taurine alone.

Since 1968, when scientists' attention was drawn to taurine, more than a thousand reports, including reviews, have been published. The physiologic actions of taurine have been reviewed exhaustively by Huxtable.[72] Nonmetabolic actions such as osmoregulation, calcium modulation, and interactions with phospholipid protein and zinc are reported. Taurine is also observed to be a product of metabolic action and a precursor of many other metabolic actions. All these actions demonstrate the careful balance in nature of a number of interdependent constituents. Taurine does not function in isolation. Because of the growing evidence for the role of taurine during development, the requirement for taurine for the neonate remains under investigation.

Whey Proteins

When clotted milk stands, the clot contracts, leaving a clear fluid called whey, which contains water, electrolytes, and proteins. The ratio of whey proteins to casein is 1.5 for breast milk and 0.25 for cow milk; that is, 40% of human milk protein is casein and 60% lactalbumin, and cow milk is 80% casein and 20% lactalbumin.[93]

Human milk forms a flocculent suspension with zero curd tension. The curds are easily digested. The total amount of protein has been recently measured to be 0.9%, which is lower than the previously reported 1.2%. The discrepancy is caused by recalculation of the data, in which the total amount of protein was determined by measuring the nitrogen content and multiplying by 6.25. Of the nitrogen content, 25% is NPN, whereas in bovine milk, 5% of the nitrogen is from NPN. Hambraeus has reported the composition of the nonprotein fraction to be urea, creatine, creatinine, uric acid, small peptides, and free amino acids (Table 4-15).

Closer examination of the whey proteins shows α-lactalbumin and lactoferrin to be the chief fractions, with no measurable β-lactoglobulin, which is the chief constituent of cow milk. The term *lactalbumin* includes a mixture of whey proteins found in bovine milk and should not be confused with α-lactalbumin, which is a specific protein that is part of the enzyme lactose synthetase. The α-lactalbumin content parallels lactose levels in

TABLE 4-15	Composition of Protein Nitrogen and Nonprotein Nitrogen in Human Milk and Cow Milk*			
	Human Milk		**Cow Milk**	
Protein nitrogen	1.43	(8.9)	5.3	(31.4)
Casein nitrogen	0.40	(2.5)	4.37	(27.3)
Whey protein nitrogen	1.03	(6.4)	0.93	(5.8)
β-Lactalbumin	0.42	(2.6)	0.17	(1.1)
Lactoferrin	0.27	(1.7)	Traces	
β-Lactoglobulin	–		0.57	(3.6)
Lysozyme	0.08	(0.5)	Traces	
Serum albumin	0.08	(0.5)	0.07	(0.4)
IgA	0.16	(1.0)	0.005	(0.03)
IgG	0.005	(0.03)	0.096	(0.06)
IgM	0.003	(0.02)	0.005	(0.03)
Nonprotein nitrogen	0.50		0.28	
Urea nitrogen	0.25		0.13	
Creatine nitrogen	0.037		0.009	
Creatinine nitrogen	0.035		0.003	
Uric acid nitrogen	0.005		0.008	
Glucosamine	0.047		?	
α-Amino nitrogen	0.13		0.048	
Ammonia nitrogen	0.002		0.006	
Nitrogen from other components	?		0.074	
Total nitrogen	1.93		5.31	

*Values refer to grams of nitrogen per liter; values within parentheses refer to grams of protein per liter.
From Forsum E, Lönnerdal B: Protein evaluation of breast milk and breast milk substitutes with special reference to the nonprotein nitrogen: effect of protein intake on protein and nitrogen composition of breast milk, *Am J Clin Nutr* 33:1809, 1980.

different species. Human milk is high in both lactose and α-lactalbumin. Many investigators, however, have continued to measure nitrogen compounds in human milk (see Table 4-15).

Lactoferrin

Lactoferrin is an iron-binding protein that is part of the whey fraction of proteins in human milk. Structurally, lactoferrin is a 78 to 80 kDa single peptide consisting of two lobes, each of which binds a molecule of iron.[143] It appears in very low amounts in bovine milk. Lactoferrin has been observed to inhibit the growth of certain iron-dependent bacteria in the gastrointestinal (GI) tract. It has been suggested that lactoferrin protects against certain GI infections in breastfed infants. Giving iron to newborn infants appears to inactivate the lactoferrin by saturating it with iron and promoting the growth of *Escherichia coli* in particular. It has other functions including cell growth regulation, deoxyribonucleic acid (DNA) binding, transcriptional activation of specific DNA sequences, natural killer cell activation, and antitumor activity. Lactoferrin also has enzyme activity. Those identified are protease, deoxyribonuclease, ribonuclease, adenosine triphosphatase (ATPase), phosphatase, and oligosaccharide hydrolysis. The role of these enzymes in lactoferrin's antimicrobial functions is under study.[33]

When lactoferrin is digested in the stomach by pepsin, the polypeptides produced also have biological functions including antimicrobial, antiviral, antitumor, and immunological functions. These proteins are under continued study because of their active infection protection. Regarding the impact of storage on lactoferrin, it was noted that 5 days of refrigeration does not change levels but 3 or more months of freezing significantly lowers the lactoferrin levels.

IMMUNOGLOBULINS

The immunoglobulins in breast milk are distinct from those of the serum, but are the key mechanism by which a mother passes immunity to the infant.[48] The main immunoglobulin in serum is IgG, which is present in the amount of 1210 mg/dL. IgA is found in the serum at 250 mg/dL, one fifth the level of IgG. The reverse is true of human colostrum and milk. Colostrum IgA is 1740 mg/dL, and milk IgA level is 100 mg/dL. Colostrum has 43 mg/dL of IgG, and milk has 4 mg/dL. The IgA and IgG in human milk are derived from serum and from synthesis in the mammary gland.

Lactation is associated with the appearance of catalytically active antibodies or abzymes (Abzs) with DNAse, RNAse, ATPase, amylolytic, protein

kinase, and lipid kinase activities in breast milk. Odintsova et al.[122] have demonstrated that the immune system of clinically healthy mothers can generate IgAs with β-casein-specific serine protease-like activity.

sIgA is the principal immunoglobulin in colostrum and milk and all human secretions. sIgA contains an antigenic determinant associated with a secretory component. It is synthesized in the gland from two molecules of serum IgA linked by disulfide bonds. sIgA levels are very high in colostrum the first few days and then decline rapidly, disappearing almost completely by the fourteenth day. sIgA is stable at low pH and resistant to proteolytic enzymes. It is present in the intestine of breastfed infants and provides a protective defense against infection by keeping viruses and bacteria from invading the mucosa. The protective qualities are further described in Chapter 5.

Nonimmunoglobulins

Human milk contains numerous nonimmunoglobulins that are being identified and their actions isolated and quantified.[152] Mucins and sialic acid-containing glycoproteins have been isolated and demonstrated to inhibit rotavirus replication and prevent experimental gastroenteritis. The rotavirus has been observed to bind to the milk mucin complex, inhibiting its replication both in vitro and in vivo. (See later discussion of oligosaccharides and glycoconjugates.)

Lysozyme

Lysozyme is a specific protein and basic polypeptide with lytic properties[64] found in high concentration in egg whites and human milk but in low concentration in bovine milk. It has been identified as a nonspecific antimicrobial factor. This enzyme is bacteriolytic against Enterobacteriaceae and gram-positive bacteria. It has been found in concentrations up to 0.2 mg/mL. Lysozyme is stable at 100°C (212°F) and at an acid pH. Lysozyme contributes to the development and maintenance of specific intestinal flora of the breastfed infant. (See later discussion of enzymes and Chapter 5 "Host Resistance Factors.")

Polyamines

Polyamines are ubiquitous intracellular cationic amines recognized as participants in cell proliferation and differentiation in many tissues, especially those of intestinal tract development, absorption, and biologic activity, in both sucklings and adults of the species.[129] The synthesis of polyamines is an active process in the mammary gland throughout lactation.[12]

Putrescine, spermidine, and spermine have been identified and quantitated in human milk by Pollack et al.[129] They reported mean values per liter of 0 to 615 nmol putrescine, 73 to 3512 nmol spermidine, and 722 to 4458 nmol spermine. In contrast, levels in formula are low and dependent on the protein source. Levels of spermine and spermidine increase greatly during the first few days of lactation, plateauing at levels 12 and 8 times, respectively, the levels immediately postpartum.[11] These findings have been confirmed by Romain et al.,[133] who noted that levels in human milk remained stable throughout lactation. They demonstrated the effects of spermine or spermidine on maturation and "gut closure" and suggest a protective effect of spermine against alimentary allergies.

NONPROTEIN NITROGEN

NPN accounts for 18% to 30% of the total nitrogen in human milk, compared with only 3% to 5% in cow milk. The NPN fraction of human milk is traditionally identified as the acid-soluble nitrogen remaining in the supernatant after protein precipitation or as the dialyzable nitrogen after dialysis of whole milk.[12] Because large-molecular-weight glycoproteins are also soluble in the acid, the fraction should be called acid-soluble nitrogen.[106]

Although there are large interindividual variations, acid-soluble nitrogen ranges from 350 to 530 mg/L. The total nitrogen ranges from 1700 to 3700 mg/L, depending on length of gestation, duration of lactation, and maternal diet. Some of the nitrogen contributes to the pool available for synthesis of nonessential amino acids in the neonate. Those compounds having more specialized roles are peptide hormone/growth factors, epidermal growth factor (EGF), amino sugars of oligosaccharides, free amino acids, amino alcohols of phospholipids, nucleic acids, nucleotides, and carnitine. Their importance is not based on percentage of concentration because they may serve roles as catalysts. Many protein factors in human milk serve roles other than growth, such as the host resistance factors (lactoferrin, sIgA, and lysozyme).

Table 4-16 presents the significance of these compounds and their relative concentrations. The wide variety of nitrogenous compounds within

TABLE 4-16	Levels and Significance of Nonprotein Nitrogen (NPN) Constituents of Human Milk		
	Concentration in Milk		
NPN	**Less Than 30 Days**	**More Than 30 Days**	**Significance**
Amino sugars			
N-Acetylglucosamine	230 mg N/L	150 mg N/L	Low oral osmotic load; controls gut colonization; constituent of gangliosides for brain development
N-Acetylneuraminic acid	63 mg N/L	3-27 mg N/L	Substrate for gut epithelium
Peptides	–	60 mg N/L	
Epidermal growth factor	88 ng/mL	–	Regulates intestinal mucosal development
Somatomedin-C/ insulin-like growth factor	18 ng/mL	6-8 ng/mL	Stimulates DNA synthesis and cell division in gut
Delta sleep-inducing peptide	30 ng/mL	5 ng/mL	Diurnal pattern highest at 2 PM and 8 PM; ? influences sleep/awake patterns
Insulin	21 ng/mL	2 ng/mL	? Regulates development of gut
Free amino acids			
Taurine	41-45 μmol/dL	27-67 μmol/dL	See under "Taurine" in paragraph below
Glutamic acid/ glutamine	2-9 μmol/dL	13-58 μmol/dL	Improves zinc absorption; precursor to brain glutamate
Carnitine	1.0 mg N/L	0.7 mg N/L	Brain lipid synthesis
Choline and ethanolamine	7-20 mg N/L	10-20 mg N/L	Possible growth requirement
Nucleic acid	–	19 mg N/L	Pool of DNA and RNA
Nucleotides	3 mg N/L	3 mg N/L	Growth and immune advantage
Polyamines	0.1 mg N/L	0.2 mg N/L	Increase rate of transcription, translation, and amino acid activation

DNA, Deoxyribonucleic acid; *N/L,* nitrogen per liter; *RNA,* ribonucleic acid.

the fraction of human milk is only beginning to be investigated and understood. This information clearly widens the chemical gap between human milk and proprietary formulas. Increasing evidence suggests that the premature infant reaps even more benefit than the term infant from mother's milk, based on the investigations of NPN alone.

While glutamic acid and taurine are the most abundant free amino acids in colostrum, taurine remains constant throughout lactation, but glutamic acid and glutamine increased from 2.5 to 20 times in the first 3 months in studies in 16 healthy lactating women.[3] The total content of free amino acids remains stable during that period so that over 50% of the total is glutamine and glutamic acid at 3 months. These components have been associated with growth and development, protecting intestinal mucosa and potentiating immune responses.

Maternal milk production and the protein nitrogen (but not NPN) fraction of human milk are well preserved when lactating women are subjected to marginal dietary protein intakes in the short term.[106] In nitrogen balance studies on poor Mexican women who were lactating, equilibrium was attained at 178.9 ± 25.8 mg nitrogen (1.1 g protein/kg body weight/day), which is close to current dietary standards.[34]

Interest in urea levels has been stimulated because women with various stages of renal failure were concerned about the effect of high serum levels of urea on their milk urea levels. Urea is 30% to 50% of the NPN in milk. Levels decrease from colostrum to mature milk (3.2 g/dL nitrogen in colostrum to 1.7 g/dL in milk). If the original milk urea was provided solely by passive diffusion from the maternal blood, a constant level of urea nitrogen would be anticipated at all stages of lactation instead of increasing from colostrum to mature milk.[12]

NUCLEOTIDES

Increased attention has been paid to the presence and role of nucleotides in human milk, as their relative absence in bovine milk has led to experimental supplementation of some infant formulas. Nucleotides have been identified as playing key roles in biochemical processes within the cell, acting as metabolic regulators and altering enzyme activities. A dietary requirement has not been established because they can be synthesized de novo in the adult. Human milk provides 20% of NPN as nucleotides; furthermore, human milk provides a larger percentage (30%) of nitrogen as NPN, three times more than other species. The daily intake from human milk is 1.4 to 2.1 mg of nucleotide nitrogen.[130] Cytidine, adenine, and uridine compose the majority of soluble nucleotides.

Nucleotides are compounds derived from nucleic acid by hydrolysis and consist of phosphoric acid combined with a sugar and a purine or pyrimidine derivative. The level and components of acid-soluble nucleotides of several species, including humans, have been studied extensively. Work has shown a characteristic nucleotide composition in the milk that differs from that of the mammary gland. The large numbers of purine and pyrimidine nucleotides present in various tissues have a number of functions in the cell. They are part of nucleic acid synthesis and metabolism and are also part of milk synthesis. It is well known that ATP supplies usable energy for biosynthetic reactions.

Free nucleotides in human milk have been recorded at 6.1 to 9.0 mmol/dL.[130] The levels in colostrum and mature milk are similar. The conspicuous difference in quality and quantity of nucleotides between the mammary gland and its secretion would indicate that nucleotides are secreted from the epithelial cells of the gland into the milk. Distinct species differences exist in composition and content of nucleotides as well. Cytidine monophosphate and uracil are the nucleotides in the highest concentration in human milk, which also contains uridine diphosphate-N-acetyllactosamine and other oligosaccharides. Human milk contains only a trace of orotic acid and no guanosine diphosphate fucose. Orotic acid is the chief nucleotide of bovine milk. Nucleotide levels fall rapidly in bovine milk to minimal levels in mature bovine milk. Synthetic nucleotides produced for formula have a very different profile.

When the nitrogen fraction of human milk was further identified overtime at 2, 4, 8, and 12 weeks, a variance was noted in the pattern of nucleotides (Table 4-17).[130] Levels of cytidine-5′-monophosphate and adenosine-5′-monophosphate

TABLE 4-17	Nucleotide Content of Human Milk
Nucleotide	**Mean* (mg/dL)**
Cytidine monophosphate	461 (17.9)
Uridine monophosphate	179 (19.8)
Adenosine monophosphate	175 (12.8)
Inosine monophosphate	228 (14.5)
Guanosine monophosphate	138 (8.5)
Uridine diphosphate	174 (12.8)
Cytidine diphosphate	474 (41.5)
Adenosine diphosphate	69 (17.9)
Guanosine diphosphate	96 (8.9)

*Mean nucleotide content of human milk at weeks 2, 4, 8, and 12 of lactation.

From Hendricks K: Nucleotide content human milk, *Semin Pediatr Gastroenterol Nutr* 2:14, 1991; Modified from Janas LM, Picciano MF: The nucleotide profile of human milk, *Pediatr Res* 16:659, 1982.

declined from 594 to 321 mg/dL and from 244 to 143 mg/dL, respectively, whereas levels of inosine-5′-monophosphate increased from 158 to 290 mg/dL. The total nucleotide nitrogen remained constant, accounting for 0.10% to 0.15% of the total NPN. The average intake per day of a normal breastfed infant would be 1.4 to 2.1 mg of nucleotide nitrogen. Measurement of adenosine-5′-monophosphate and cyclic guanosine monophosphate showed variation in concentration within 15 minutes, which fluctuated throughout 24 hours.[130] Milk concentration differed widely from maternal plasma levels collected at the same time.

The biologic effects of dietary nucleotides involve the immune system, the intestinal microenvironment, and the absorption and metabolism of certain other nutrients (see Table 4-17) so they are considered "semiessential" for newborns.[56] Whether inosine-5′-monophosphate contributes to the superior iron absorption is still unanswered.

Metabolic disturbances in nucleotide metabolism can result in abnormal accumulation of specific intermediates in cells and tissues, causing a variety of diseases. An example is Lesch-Nyhan syndrome, a genetic disease characterized by mental retardation, self-mutilation, and gout, which is caused by the absence of the purine salvage enzyme. On the other hand, disturbances from lack of nucleotides in the diet have not been identified.

Nucleotides are formed by de novo synthesis by capturing or scavenging partially degraded nucleotides or are obtained completely from the diet. Dietary nucleotides are absorbed by action of the microvillus membrane as nucleosides. The developing neonate has a reduced capacity to synthesize or salvage nucleotides. Exogenous nucleotides are potential stimuli, modulating not only the gene control of their own metabolism but also that of a number of functions in the cardiovascular, neurologic, and immune systems.[25] Nucleotides are important as coenzymes for the processes involved in the metabolism of lipids, carbohydrates, and proteins. Nucleotides are recognized as an integral part of the immune system, acting as the host defense against bacteria, viruses, and parasites, as well as various malignancies. Nucleotides are important in the process of protein synthesis, which is enhanced in the newborn infant by a dietary supply of nucleotides. A high protein diet (20%) does produce significant growth increase when nucleotides are added. This result may explain the satisfactory growth pattern of breastfed infants on relatively low protein intake and the more efficient protein utilization of breastfed infants.

Study of the exact role of nucleotides continues in vivo, although some effort to supplement formula with synthetic nucleotides has already begun.

Carbohydrates

The predominant carbohydrate of milk is lactose, or milk sugar. It is present in high concentration (6.8 g/dL in human milk and 4.9 g/dL in bovine milk). Lactose is a disaccharide compound of two monosaccharides, galactose and glucose. Lactose is synthesized by the mammary gland, described as a dynamic process.

A number of other carbohydrates are present in milk. They are classified as monosaccharides, neutral and acid oligosaccharides, and peptide-bound and protein-bound carbohydrates. Small amounts of glucose (1.4 g/dL) and galactose (1.2 g/dL) also are present in breast milk. Other complex carbohydrates are present in free form or bound to amino acids or protein, such as N-acetylglucosamine. The concentration of oligosaccharides in human milk is about 10 times greater than in cow milk. These carbohydrates and glycoproteins possess bifidus factor activity. Fucose, which is not present in bovine milk, may be important to the early establishment of L. bifidus as gut flora. The nitrogen-containing carbohydrates are 0.7% of milk solids.

In a study of carbohydrate content over the first 4 months of lactation, Coppa et al.[26] observed that lactose concentrations increased from 56 ± 6 g/L on day 4 to 68.9 ± 8 g/L on day 120.

Lactose is hydrolyzed selectively by a brush border enzyme called lactase located predominantly in the tip of the intestinal villi. Digestion of lactose is the rate-limiting step in its absorption. Although lactase activity develops later in fetal life than that of other disaccharidases, it is present by 24 weeks of fetal life. Lactase concentration is greatest in the proximal jejunum. Levels continue to increase throughout the last trimester, reaching concentrations at term of two to four times those levels at 2 to 11 months of age. Premature infants rapidly increase their lactase levels given a lactose challenge. A well-fed breastfed infant ingesting 150 mL of milk/kg/day receives 10 g of lactose/kg/day, which ensures the normal unstressed infant at least 4 mg/kg/min of glucose, which is considered the optimal rate.

Lactose does appear to be specific, however, for newborn growth. It has been shown to enhance calcium absorption and has been suggested as being critical to the prevention of rickets, in view of the relatively low calcium levels in human milk. Lactose is a readily available source of galactose, which is essential to the production of the galactolipids, including cerebroside. These galactolipids are essential to CNS development.

Interesting correlations have been made between the amount of lactose in the milk of a species and the relative size of the brain (Figure 4-12).[90] Because lactose is found only in milk and not in other animal and

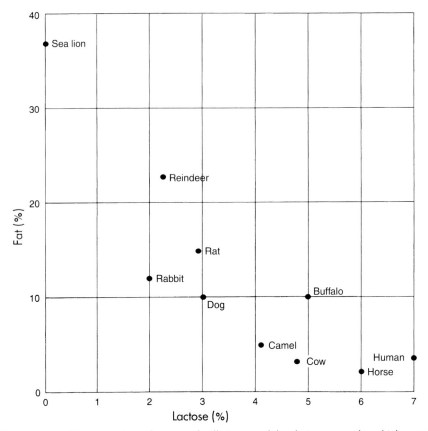

Figure 4-12. Concentration of lactose varies with source of milk. In general, less lactose, more fat, which can also be used by newborn animals as an energy source. (From Kretchmer N: Lactose and lactase, *Sci Am* 227:73, 1972. Copyright © 1972 by Scientific American, Inc. All rights reserved.)

plant sources, its high level in human milk is even more significant. Lactose levels are relatively constant throughout the day in a given mother's milk. Even in poorly nourished mothers, the levels of lactose do not vary. Because lactose is influential in controlling volume, the total output for the day may be diminished, but the concentration of lactose in human milk will be 6.2 to 7.2 g/dL.[115] An adequate source of carbohydrate is important for optimal lactation, which suggests that excessive amounts of sugar substitutes may have an effect on volume.[87]

OLIGOSACCHARIDES AND GLYCOCONJUGATES

Oligosaccharides have become an area of intense investigation and study in human milk science. Oligosaccharides are the third largest solid component in milk after lactose and triglyceride. They reach up to 20 g/L in early milk.[67] Most of the milk oligosaccharides contain lactose at the reducing end of the structure and may also contain fucose or sialic acid at the nonreducing end. More than 200 neutral and acidic oligosaccharides have been identified.[117] One liter of milk contains 5 to 10 g

of unbound oligosaccharides. The high amount and structural diversity are unique to humans.[16] The structural complexity of milk oligosaccharides hampers the assignment of specific functions to single carbohydrates. The interactions of milk oligosaccharides with intestinal microbiota and the mucosal immune system provide proof that breast milk provides much more than just nutrition.[67] The human milk metabolome reveals diverse oligosaccharide profiles. The variability in certain milk metabolites suggests possible roles in infant gut microbial development. Biochemically, oligosaccharides result from the sequential addition of monosaccharides to the lactose molecule in the mammary gland by glycosyl transferases. The presence and quantity of different types of oligosaccharides in human milk are genetically determined.[27] Of the 21 oligosaccharides studied in depth, the highest amount is present by day 4 with gradual decreasing by 20% by day 30. The physiologic role of human milk and oligosaccharides had been limited to the enhancement of the growth of *L. bifidus* flora and indirectly to the protection against GI infections. It is now known they act as soluble decoys preventing the adhesion of viruses, bacteria, and their toxins to their carbohydrate mucosal receptors.[67] Real efficacy has been demonstrated in core oligosaccharides against *Streptococcus pneumoniae*, *Helicobacter pylori*, *E. coli*, and influenza viruses.

The association between maternal milk levels of two-linked fucosylated oligosaccharide and the prevention of diarrhea as a result of campylobacter, caliciviruses, and all causes in breastfed infants was studied by Morrow et al.[143] Evidence was found that human milk oligosaccharides may offer clinically relevant protection against diarrhea.

Glycoproteins, glycosylated major milk proteins, include lactoferrin, immunoglobulins, and mucins. Their protective characteristics have been described as acting as receptor homologs, inhibiting the binding of enteropathogens to their host receptors. Research continues to link specific carbohydrate structures with protection against specific pathogens. These nonimmunoglobulin agents are also active against whole classes of pathogens.[113] The protective glyconjugates and oligosaccharides are unique to human milk and to date have not been replicated synthetically. They are synthesized exclusively in the mammary gland and only during lactation. Human oligosaccharides are distinct from other species with respect to quantity, quality, and diversity.[16] Human milk oligosaccharides, a major family of complex glycans are relevant to clinical illness in neonates and term infants. The newly emerging technologies for the biologic testing of these molecules open new opportunities to identify prophylactic and therapeutic agents that inhibit a variety of pathogens.

Minerals

Minerals represent a special category of constituents. Their pathways into milk vary from simple diffusion to both positive and negative pump mechanisms.[2] Table 4-18 records the measurements of the constituents in human milk compared with maternal serum. By examining this relationship, it can be estimated how the particular constituent reaches the milk, that is, by passive diffusion or positive or negative pump.

The total ash content of milk is species-specific and parallels the growth rate and body structure of the offspring. A number of metallic elements and organic and inorganic acids are present in milk as ions, unionized salts, and weakly ionized salts. Some are bound to other constituents. Sodium, potassium, calcium, and magnesium are the major cations. Phosphate, chloride, and citrate are the major anions.[28]

The monovalent ions are sodium, potassium, and chloride. The divalent ions are calcium, magnesium, citrate, phosphate, and sulfate.[11] The monovalent ions are among the most prevalent and contribute 30 mosmol, or one tenth of the total osmolarity of human milk.[8] The sum of the concentrations of the monovalent ions is inversely proportional to the lactose content across species. Monovalent ion concentration is regulated chiefly by the secretion mechanism in the alveolar cell, with humans having the highest lactose and lowest ion content.[153] This maintains osmolality close to that of serum.

Daily intakes of calcium, phosphorus, zinc, potassium, sodium, iron, and copper from breast milk were found to decrease significantly over the first 4 months of life, with only magnesium increasing. Despite seemingly low mineral intakes, growth during this time was found to be satisfactory by Casey et al.[22] High mineral content is associated with a rapid growth rate of specific species.

POTASSIUM AND SODIUM

Potassium levels are much higher than those of sodium, which are similar to the proportions in intracellular fluids (Table 4-19). Although sodium, potassium, and chloride are present as free ions, the other constituents appear as complexes and compounds. Ions can pass through the secretory cell membrane in both directions and in and out of the lumen. Intracellular sodium, chloride, and potassium are in equilibrium with the ions of the plasma and alveolar milk. An apical pumping mechanism has been calculated for chloride release, whereas sodium, potassium, and intracellular chloride pass into milk because of their electrochemical gradients. The cellular pumping mechanism maintains the ionic concentrations in the extracellular fluid and alveolar milk.

The Committee on Nutrition of the American Academy of Pediatrics[7] has stated that the daily requirement of sodium for growth is 0.5 mEq/kg/day between birth and 3 months of age, decreasing to 0.1 mEq/kg/day after 6 months of age (Table 4-20). To cover dermal losses, an additional 0.4 to 0.7 mEq/kg/day is needed, with a little for urine and stool losses. Infants fed human milk receive enough sodium to meet their needs for growth, dermal losses, and urinary losses. Studies by Keenan et al. have demonstrated an apparent regulation in the levels of milk sodium and potassium concentrations by adrenocorticosteroids as well as a circadian rhythm.

Sodium levels in cow milk are 3.6 times those in human milk (human: 7 mEq/L or 16 mg/dL; bovine: 22 mEq/L or 50 mg/dL). Hypernatremic dehydration has been associated with cow milk feedings. Experiments with newborn rats on high salt intakes have shown that hypertension can develop.

The diurnal variation in milk electrolytes was found to vary between 22% and 80%. These

TABLE 4-18 Difference in Composition of Human Milk and Blood Plasma

	Specific Gravity	Osmolarity	pH	Calories (kcal/dL)	Water (g%)	Sulfur (mg%)	Carbohydrates	Fat	Protein		Iron	Na$^+$ (mg%)	K$^+$ (mg%)
									Albumin (g%)	Globulin (g%)			
Human mature milk	1031	295	7.3	65	87.5	14	7.0 g% (lactose)	3.7 g%	0.3	0.2	0.15 mg%	15	57
Blood plasma	1033	285	7.4	35	92	2	80 mg% (glucose)	200 mg%	4.5	2.5	125 μg%	320	18

	Ca^{2+} (mg%)	Mg^{2+} (mg%)	Cl$^-$ (mg%)	Phosphorus (mg%)	Vitamins					
					A*	B$_1$ (μg%)	B$_2$ (μg%)	Niacin (μg%)	C (mg%)	D (IU/dL)
Human mature milk	35	4	43	15	280 IU/dL	20	50	172	5	5
Blood plasma	10	2.5	365	4	50 μg%	10	0.5	500	1	188

*1 μg of vitamin A corresponds to the activity of 3 IU of vitamin A.
Modified from Vorheer H: *The breasts: morphology, physiology, and lactation*, New York, 1974, Academic Press.

TABLE 4-19   Minerals in Human Milk and Cow Milk (per Deciliter)

Minerals	Colostrum	Transitional	Mature	Cow Milk
Calcium (mg)	39	46	35	130
Chlorine (mg)	85	46	40	108
Copper (μg)	40	50	40	14
Iron (μg)	70	70	100	70
Magnesium (mg)	4	4	4	12
Phosphorus (mg)	14	20	15	120
Potassium (mg)	74	64	57	145
Sodium (mg)	48	29	15	58
Sulfur (mg)	22	20	14	30
Total ash (mg)	–	–	200	700

From Food and Nutrition Board, National Research Council, National Academy of Sciences: *Recommended dietary allowances*, ed 10, Washington, D.C., 1989, U.S. Government Printing Office.

TABLE 4-20   Recommended Dietary Intake of Electrolytes for Infants

Age	Sodium (mg)	Potassium (mg)	Chloride (mg)
To 6 mo	115-350 (11.5 mg/kg)	350-925	275-700
6 mo-1 yr	250-750 (23 mg/kg)	425-1500	400-1200

From Food and Nutrition Board, National Research Council, National Academy of Sciences: *Recommended dietary allowances*, ed 10, Washington, D.C., 1989, U.S. Government Printing Office.

changes varied as the lactation period progressed but were independent of mother's diet. Sodium restriction did not influence milk levels. In a longitudinal study, sodium levels fell from 20 to 15 mEq/L in the first week. On day 8, levels were 8 mEq/L, and by the fifth week they were stabilized at 6 mEq/L.[107] Time-dependent changes in milk composition are also reported by Alaejos et al.[4] as a 25% or greater decrease in sodium, potassium, and citrate from 1 to 6 months. Calcium and glucose increase by 10% or more over this time. The authors suggest milk composition is always in transition.[5]

At a constant sodium intake, decreasing the sodium/potassium (Na/K) ratio in the diet by increasing potassium lowers blood pressure. The dietary Na/K ratio has an important role in determining the severity, if not the development, of salt-induced hypertension. The mechanism of potassium's antihypertensive effect is unclear, but the higher potassium and lower sodium levels of breast milk appear to be physiologically beneficial.

CHLORIDE

Little attention has been paid to the adequacy of chloride in the diet, and it has always been assumed to be sufficient until recent events focused attention on this cation.

Chloride deficiency in infants has become associated with a syndrome of failure to thrive with hypochloremia and hypokalemic metabolic alkalosis. This was first described in infants fed formula that was deficient in chloride but has also been described in a breastfed infant whose mother's milk contained less than 2 mEq/L chloride (normal is greater than 8 mEq/L).[9] This is a rare phenomenon caused by unexplained maternal production. This mother had previously successfully nourished five other infants.

TOTAL ASH

Cow milk has three times the total salt content of human milk (Table 4-21). All the minerals that appear in cow milk also appear in human milk. The phosphorus level is six times greater in cow milk; the calcium level is four times higher (Table 4-21).

The renal solute load of cow milk is considerably higher than that of breast milk. This is magnified by the metabolic breakdown products of the high protein content, which are in increased amounts as well. This is shown in the high urea levels in formula-fed infants (Table 4-23). Although the mean urea levels in breast milk are 37 mg/dL and only 15 mg/dL in cow milk, the blood urea levels

TABLE 4-21 Principal Salt Constituents in Bovine and Human Milks

Constituent	Bovine (mg/dL)	Human (mg/dL)
Calcium	125	33
Magnesium	12	4
Sodium	58	15
Potassium	138	55
Chloride	103	43
Phosphorus	96	15
Citric acid	175	20-80
Sulfur (total)	30	14 ± 2.6 (4.5 mmol/L)
Carbon dioxide	20	–

From Jenness R, Sloan RE: Composition of milk. In Larson BL, Smith VR, editors: *Lactation, vol. 3, Nutrition and biochemistry of milk/maintenance*, New York, 1974, Academic Press.

TABLE 4-22 Recommended Dietary Intake of Minerals for Infants*

Age	Calcium (mg)	Phosphorus (mg)	Magnesium (mg)	Iron (mg)	Zinc (mg)	Iodine (mg)
To 6 mo	400	300	40	6	5	40
6 mo-1 yr	600	500	60	10	5	50

*Because little information is available on which to base allowances, these amounts are provided in the form of ranges of recommended intakes.

From Food and Nutrition Board, National Research Council, National Academy of Sciences: *Recommended dietary allowances*, ed 10, Washington, D.C., 1989, U.S. Government Printing Office.

TABLE 4-23 Statistical Analysis by Student's T-test of Blood Urea Levels in 61 Healthy Infants Age 1 to 3 M

Infant Group	Number	Blood Urea, Mean ± SE (mg/dL)	Individual Values >40 mg/dL Number	Individual Values >40 mg/dL Total Observations (%)
A: breastfed	12	22.7 ± 1.6*	0	0[†]
B: artificial milk alone	16	47.4 ± 2.0[‡]	12	75[§]
C: artificial milk + solid foods	33	51.9 ± 1.8	29	88

*When compared with group B and group C: $p < 0.001$ ($t = 9.7$) and $p < 0.001$ ($t = 11.5$), respectively.
[†]When compared with group B and group C: $p < 0.001$ ($t = 6.9$) and $p < 0.001$ ($t = 15.5$), respectively.
[‡]When compared with group C: $p > 0.05$ ($t = 1.6$).
[§]When compared with group C: $p > 0.05$ ($t = 1.1$).
From Davies DP, Saunders R: Blood urea: normal values in early infancy related to feeding practices, *Arch Dis Child* 48:563, 1973.

in breastfed infants are about 22 mg/dL, whereas those of infants fed formula are 47 mg/dL and those of infants fed formula plus solids are 52 mg/dL (see Table 4-23). The plasma osmolarity of infants fed breast milk is lower and approximates the physiologic level of plasma.

CALCIUM/PHOSPHORUS RATIO

The calcium/phosphorus (Ca/P) ratio is considerably lower in cow milk (1:4) than in human milk (2:2). Many investigators have studied calcium and phosphorus values in human milk and found some variation from mother to mother and from study to study. The Ca/P ratio varied from 1.8 to 2.4, with the absolute values for calcium varying from 20 to 34 mg/dL and those for phosphorus varying from 14 to 18 mg/dL. Fetal and newborn plasma concentrations for calcium decline sharply from 10.4 mg/dL at birth to 8.5 mg/dL by day 4. Unlike calcium, phosphorus concentrations rise in the postnatal period. The drop in serum calcium levels in the bottle-fed infants was more marked than in the breastfed infants. Infant serum phosphorus concentrations rise during the postnatal period. When gestation is prolonged or the mother has preeclampsia, the concentrations are even higher at birth.

Longitudinal studies by Greer et al., measuring calcium and phosphorus in human milk and maternal and infant sera, have shown progressive increases in infant serum calcium in association with decreasing phosphorus content of breast milk and infant serum. Maternal serum calcium also increased, although the mother's dietary intake was below recommended levels for lactating women. Calcium uptake in the maternal duodenum is enhanced during lactation.

Although the Ca/P ratio has been stressed in the past, recent investigations have not found a statistical correlation between the calcium and phosphorus contents of plasma and corresponding breast milk Ca/P ratio. This finding suggests that Ca/P ratio is not critical in the low mineral loads present in breast milk. Calcium and phosphorus decrease over time during lactation.[7]

Lactating women contribute 210 mg of calcium per day in breast milk. A study of intestinal calcium absorption of women during lactation and after weaning revealed that serum calcium and phosphorus concentrations were greater in lactating compared with nonlactating postpartum women, but levels were the same after weaning.[82] Calcitriol, however, was greater in women after weaning compared with postpartum control subjects. Lactating women lost significantly more bone throughout the body and in the lumbar spine than nonlactating postpartum women in the first 6 months. After weaning, the lactating women regained significantly more bone in the lumbar spine than nonlactating women. Early resumption of menses was associated with a smaller loss and greater increase after weaning.[32] Parathyroid hormone concentrations are reported to be higher only after weaning.

Calcium supplementation does not prevent bone loss during lactation and only slightly enhances the gain in bone density after weaning.[82] Supplementation did not affect levels in the milk. Krebs et al.[89] reported that excesses of protein have a negative effect on calcium absorption in lactating women. The calcium/protein ratio appears to be critical to efficient utilization. Estradiol stimulated the osteoblastic proliferation and enhanced the collagen gene expression. Calcium was shown to be well absorbed in 5- to 7-month-old breastfed infants who had begun to receive beikost (solids and semisolids).

MAGNESIUM AND OTHER SALTS

Magnesium is present as a free ion and in complexes with casein and phosphate in caseinate micelles or citrate complexes. Cow milk has three times as much magnesium as human milk (12 mg/dL compared with 4 mg/dL) (see Table 4-21). Magnesium was measured

in human milk by Fransson and Lönnerdal,[54] who found 41.4 ± 15.4 mg/mL in whole milk samples, with most of the magnesium in the skim milk fraction but significant amounts in the fat fraction and less than 4% in the casein. The bound fraction was associated with low-molecular-weight proteins, thus enhancing bioavailability.

Longitudinal magnesium concentrations were measured by Greer et al. in milk and maternal sera and in the infants over a 6-month period. Progressive increases in serum magnesium level were seen in the breastfed infants in association with decreasing phosphorus content of the milk. Citrate is found in the milks of many species and is three to four times higher in cow milk than in human milk (see Table 4-21). The distribution of ions and salts differs among various milks and depends on the relative concentrations of casein and citrate.

Citrate is made in the mitochondria from pyruvate and transported into the cytoplasm, where it is available for lipid synthesis and for transport into the Golgi complex.[10] Citrate levels are not often measured in human milk, although citrate may be a marker of milk production potential (see Figure 4-5). Levels are high the first few days and rise as calcium levels rise.

Most of the sulfur in milk is in the sulfur-containing amino acids, with only about 10% present as sulfate ion. Some organic acids are present, and they appear as anions in milk.

Trace Elements

Tables 4-21 and 4-22 list the recommended daily intake of trace elements for infants.[50]

IRON

Because of the great emphasis on iron in the modern diet, and especially in the diet of the infant in the first year of life, the iron in human milk has been closely scrutinized. It has been determined that normal infants need 1500 mg of exogenous elemental iron in the first year of life, which can be translated into 8 to 10 mg/day (see Table 4-22). Prepared infant formulas currently supply 10 to 12 mg/day. Human milk has 100 mg/dL, which does not meet the requirements just given. Historically, however, breastfed infants have not been anemic (see Table 4-19).

In 350 samples of breast milk, there was a variation between less than 0.1 and 1.6 mg of iron/mL. Age, parity, and lactation history influenced the levels in some studies. The distribution of iron in various fractions of human milk of Swedish women was determined using multiple methods

limits, however, should not be considered deficient, especially in breastfed infants.

Selenium concentrations in human milk are consistent in samples collected from many parts of the world, according to work by Hadjimarkos and Shearer. The mean value was 0.020 ppm, which was similar to the value from many parts of the United States, where the range was 0.007 to 0.033 ppm.

Increased selenium requirements have been observed in pregnant and lactating women. Supplementation with different compounds, such as selenium-enriched yeast and selenomethionine, significantly influenced selected indices of selenium status, including milk concentrations.[4]

Selenium is considered an essential nutrient in humans. It is an integral component of glutathione peroxidase, an enzyme known to metabolize lipid peroxides, and deficiency states have been described. Questions have been raised about the detrimental effects of high selenium intake on dentition. Smith et al. assessed selenium status in infants exclusively fed human milk or infant formula for 3 months. Foremilk samples had a mean concentration of 15.7 ng/mL, hindmilk mean concentration was 16.3 ng/mL, and mean formula concentration was 8.6 ng/mL. Breastfed infants have greater intakes and higher serum levels of selenium than formula-fed infants in the first 3 months (see Table 4-24).

The concentration of chromium is highest in the organs of the newborn and declines rapidly during the first years of life. A longitudinal study of chromium in human milk was undertaken by Kumpulainen and Vuori.[91] Mothers collected samples at 8 to 18 days, 47 to 54 days, and 128 to 159 days postpartum, representing every feed during a 24-hour period with equal portions of foremilk and hindmilk. The mean concentration was 0.39 (SD = 0.15) ng/mL and the intake 0.27 mg/day (SD = 0.11). The values did not change overtime. These values are the same as those in human serum and urine. The mothers' dietary intake averaged about 30 mg/day, which is lower than the 50 to 200 mg recommended daily allowance.

When chromium metabolism was studied in 17 lactating postpartum subjects, breast milk chromium content was independent of dietary chromium intake and serum and urinary values.[7] Chromium intake did not correlate with serum or urinary chromium.

HDL cholesterol levels can be increased with chromium supplementation. Chromium also is reported to have a favorable effect on serum lipid profiles. Deficiency of chromium in infancy may be an issue with LBW infants or those with inadequate fetal stores. Chromium is present in all tissues of the body and is in high levels in nucleic acids.

Inordinately high levels of manganese have been found in infant formula, but little is known about its role in infant nutrition. Manganese is a component of comparatively few metalloenzymes, including pyruvate carboxylase and mitochondrial superoxide dismutase. It does, however, activate others. Deficiencies cause impaired growth and skeletal abnormalities in all species studied. In human milk, the major fraction of manganese is the 71% found in the whey, with 11% in the casein and 18% in the lipid. Levels in human milk in the first month of lactation decreased from a mean of 5.4 ± 1.6 μg/dL on day 1 to 2.7 ± 1.6 ng/mL from day 5 through day 28. The average intake of the breastfed infant in the first month was 2.0 μg/day. Elevated manganese levels have been associated with ADHD, hyperactive behaviors, and low verbal and visual memory.[146]

The main biochemical role of molybdenum in mammals is as a cofactor for several enzymes.[20] Deficiencies are rare, usually occurring in those receiving total parenteral nutrition. Molybdenum levels in human milk were measured from day 1 through day 38. Levels began at 15.0 ± 6.1 μg/dL and leveled off at 1 to 2 μg/dL at 1 month.[22]

Nickel is generally accepted as an essential trace element for animals, but its role in humans is undefined. Levels in human milk are stable over time at 1.2 μg/dl. The average daily intake of nickel at 1 month was 0.8 μg.

FLUORINE

Fluorine has been widely accepted as a significant dietary factor in decreasing dental caries (see Table 4-24). The effect has been associated with the conversion of the enamel hydroxyapatite to fluorapatite with a reduction in acid solubility. The presence of fluorine during the formation of hydroxyapatite may create less soluble, more resistant crystals.

Conflicting reports of the fluorine levels in human milk have led to the belief that breastfed infants needed supplementation.[94] More accurate studies in communities where fluoride has been in the public drinking water supply show 7 mg of fluorine per liter (range 4 to 14 mg/L).[44] The American Academy of Pediatrics no longer recommends routinely supplementing breastfed infants with fluorine[7] (see Chapter 9).

The significant development of deciduous and permanent teeth occurs after birth and depends on fetal stores of fluorine as well as on fluorine available in the diet. Studies comparing breastfed and bottle-fed infants show a distinct difference, with fewer dental caries and better dental health in breastfed infants. The role of fluorine and other factors, such as selenium, that predispose the breastfed infant to healthier teeth has yet to be defined completely. Nursing-bottle caries add to the total dental caries of the bottle-fed infant.

IODIDE

Many individuals are iodide deficient, especially women of reproductive age. Cause is unknown but the lack of use of iodized salt, the use of processed foods, and geographic location are considerations. This is of serious concern because iodine deficiency during pregnancy and lactation is associated with brain development in the offspring. The risk is greater with the increase in environmental pollutants such as nitrate, thiocyanate, and perchlorate. Pregnant and lactating women should take a supplement containing adequate iodide. Not all supplements contain enough. The American Thyroid Association and the National Academy of Sciences recommend that lactating women have a total intake of 290 μg of iodide per day, which usually requires a supplement with 150 μg of iodide. An intake of 150 μg of potassium iodide is equivalent to only 120 μg or less of iodide.[29] Environmental chemicals such as thiocyanate, nitrate, and perchlorate compete for transport by the sodium-iodide symporter (NIS). The NIS is an integral plasma membrane glycoprotein found in the thyroid gland and the breast, which mediates the iodide transport into thyroid cells, the first step in thyroid hormone synthesis. In the mammary gland, NIS mediates the transport of iodide into milk. Thiocyanate is found in cruciferous vegetables and tobacco smoke. Nitrate is found in some drinking water and root vegetables. Perchlorate is used in industry as an oxidizer and is found naturally in arid regions such as the southwestern United States. It has been detected in many foods, drinking water, and cow milk. The EPA developed regulations for perchlorate in drinking water in 2011. Worldwide agencies have taken similar steps.

Mothers should take at least 150 μg of iodide daily and use iodized table salt, according to the Council on Environmental Health of the AAP.[29] They should also avoid nitrates, especially from well water, which should be checked annually. Tobacco smoke and second hand smoke contain thiocyanates, which should also be avoided. The World Health Organization has also adopted similar guidelines for adults and children.

Spot urine tests of iodine in mcg/L

Mean UI Concentration (g/L)	Corresponding Intake (μg/dL)	Iodine Status
<20	<30	Severe deficiency
20-49	30-74	Moderate deficiency
50-99	75-149	Mild deficiency
100-199	150-299	Optimal
200-299	300-449	More than adequate
>299	>449	Possible excess

Assessment of iodine intake is most commonly done by random urinary spot iodine assessments. The World Health Organization has adopted these guidelines for adults and children.

PH AND OSMOLARITY

The pH range in human milk is 6.7 to 7.4, with a mean of 7.1. The mean pH of cow milk is 6.8. The caloric content of both human and cow milk is 65 kcal/dL or 20 kcal/oz. The specific gravities are 1.031 and 1.032, respectively.

The osmolarity of human milk approximates that of human serum, or 286 mosmol/kg of water, whereas that for cow milk is higher at 350 mosmol. The renal solute load of human milk is considerably lower than that of cow milk. Renal solute load is roughly calculated by totaling the solutes that must be excreted by the kidney. It consists primarily of nonmetabolizable dietary components, especially electrolytes, ingested in excess of body needs, and metabolic end products, mainly from the metabolism of protein. Renal solute load can be estimated by adding the dietary intake of nitrogen and three minerals—sodium, potassium, and chloride. Each gram of protein is considered to yield 4 mosmols (as urea), and each milliequivalent of sodium, potassium, and chloride is 1 milkeosmol. The renal solute load of cow milk is 221 milleosmol, compared with 79 milleosmols for human milk.

Dearlove and Dearlove investigated osmoregulation in human lactation in an effort to determine whether fluid loading was a valid clinical maneuver. It is known that an oral hypotonic fluid load results in suppression of prolactin in adults. After an intravenous hypotonic saline infusion, a significant correlation was seen between serum osmolarity and prolactin. No changes in serum prolactin, milk yield, serum, or breast milk osmolarity were noted, however, when normal lactating women were given a hypotonic fluid load in a controlled study.

CAROTENOIDS: LUTEIN

Lutein is the dominant carotenoid in the infant brain and the major carotenoid found in the retina of the eye. Its levels vary in breast milk reflecting the mother's dietary intake. Supplementation was studied in 89 lactating women[137] who were 4 to 6 weeks postpartum. They were randomly given a placebo of 0 mg/day of lutein, or 6 mg/day (low dose), or 12 mg/day (high dose). The dose was taken for 6 weeks along with their normal diet. Breast milk levels of plasma carotenoids were measured weekly by high performance liquid chromatography (HPLC) and at the end of the study. Infant plasma levels were measured at the end of the study and maternal plasma levels were assessed both at the beginning and the end of the study. No significant differences were found between dietary lutein plus zeaxanthin intake, and levels found of carotenoid in the milk, the infant plasma, or body mass index were higher by 170% and 250% in the treated groups compared to the placebo group. Other carotenoids were not affected.

VITAMINS

Vitamin A

Vitamin A content is 75 mg/dL or 280 international units (IUs) in mature human milk and only 41 mg/dL or 180 IU in cow milk (Table 4-25). Thus the supply of vitamin A and its precursors, carotenoids (e.g., β-carotene), is considered adequate to meet the estimated daily requirement, which varies from 500 to 1500 IU/day if the infant consumes at least 200 mL of breast milk per day (Table 4-26). Twice as much vitamin A is present in colostrum as in mature milk. During the first 6 months, the retinol equivalent (RE) content of term milk in developing countries is only 330 mg RE/L compared to 660 mg in developed countries.[118] Retinol content of milk of mothers who deliver prematurely is even higher. A single 60-mg supplement of β-carotene sustained elevated β-carotene concentrations in serum and milk longer than 1 week in normal mothers but did not affect concentrations of other major carotenoids, retinol, or tocopherol.[18] Vitamin A intake and serum vitamin A concentrations during pregnancy influence the composition of breast milk. Human milk is a vital source of vitamin A in developing countries, even beyond the first year of life.[123,126]

Vitamin A supplementation has been a major project of WHO. Technology used to test samples of milk for vitamin A before and after treatment have been studied.[45] HPLC gave higher values than iCheck. When checks are being done to measure change with treatment, the same method must be used throughout.

Vitamin D

Vitamin D has always been included in the fat-soluble vitamin group because that is the form in which it had been identified in nature. The levels in human milk were 0.05 mg/dL, previously reported in the fat fraction. Human milk was shown to have vitamin D in both the fat and the aqueous fractions. Investigators measured the water-soluble

TABLE 4-25	Vitamins and Other Constituents of Human Milk and Cow Milk (per Deciliter)			
Milk Elements	**Colostrum**	**Transitional**	**Mature**	**Cow Milk**
Vitamin A (μg)	151.0	88.0	75.0	41.0
Vitamin B$_1$ (μg)	1.9	5.9	14.0	43.0
Vitamin B$_2$ (μg)	30.0	37.0	40.0	145.0
Nicotinic acid (μg)	75.0	175.0	160.0	82.0
Vitamin B$_6$ (μg)	–	–	12.0-15.0	64.0
Pantothenic acid (μg)	183.0	288.0	246.0	340.0
Biotin (μg)	0.06	0.35	0.6	2.8
Folic acid (μg)	0.05	0.02	0.14	0.13
Vitamin B$_{12}$ (μg)	0.05	0.04	0.1	0.6
Vitamin C (mg)	5.9	7.1	5.0	1.1
Vitamin D (μg)	–	–	0.04	0.02
Vitamin E (mg)	1.5	0.9	0.25	0.07
Vitamin K (μg)	–	–	1.5	6.0
Ash (g)	0.3	0.3	0.2	0.7
Calories (kcal)	57.0	63.0	65.0	65.0
Specific gravity	1050.0	1035.0	1031.0	1032.0
Milk (pH)	–	–	7.0	6.8

From Food and Nutrition Board, National Research Council, National Academy of Sciences: *Recommended dietary allowances*, ed 10, Washington, D.C., 1989, U.S. Government Printing Office.

Age	Weight (kg)	Weight (lb)	Height (cm)	Height (in)	Protein (g)	Vitamin A (µg RE)[†]	Vitamin D (µg)[‡]	Vitamin E (mg α-TE)[§]
To 6 mo	6	13	60	24	kg × 2.2	395	7.5	3
6 mo-1 yr	9	20	71	28	kg × 1.6	375	10	4

TABLE 4-26 Recommended Daily Dietary Allowances of Fat-Soluble Vitamins for Infants*

*The allowances are intended to provide for individual variations among most normal persons as they live in the United States under usual environmental stresses. Diets should be based on a variety of common foods in order to provide other nutrients for which human requirements have been less well defined.

[†]RE = Retinol equivalents. 1 RE = 1 µg retinol or 6 µg carotene.

[‡]As cholecalciferol, 10 µg cholecalciferol = 400 IU vitamin D.

[§]α-Tocopherol equivalents. 1 mg d-α-tocopherol = 1 α-TE.

From Food and Nutrition Board, National Research Council, National Academy of Sciences: *Recommended dietary allowances*, ed 10, Washington, D.C., 1989, U.S. Government Printing Office.

sulfate conjugate of vitamin D and evaluated the biologic activity of the water-soluble metabolites. The water-soluble fraction is considered to be inactive metabolites. When activity is calculated by an assay that measures stimulation of intestinal calcium transport, human milk is found to contain 40 to 50 IU/L of vitamin D activity. The metabolite 25-hydroxyvitamin D_3 accounts for 75% of the activity; vitamins D_2 and D_3 account for 15%. Vitamin D sulfate, or any other as yet unidentified water-soluble metabolite of vitamin D, has not been proven to have significant biologic activity.

The impact of the maternal diet content of vitamin D was measured in a double-blind study of white mothers in a temperate climate in the winter. A direct relationship was seen between maternal and infant levels of 25-OH-vitamin D_3 and maternal diet.[150] An additional group of infants, whose mothers' diets were unsupplemented, received 400 IU of vitamin D per day and had even higher serum concentrations of 25-OH-vitamin D_3. When mothers have been given large doses of vitamin D, the content of vitamin D and D_3 in their milk increases as it does with exposure to sunshine. The level of 25-OH-vitamin D does not change. The majority of the activity in human milk is in the form of 25-OH-vitamin D. This may be an advantage for the breastfed infant, who utilizes this form most readily. Clearly, the levels vary and may be inadequate in human milk in some situations, especially in cold climates in the winter with little sunshine and for dark-skinned individuals.

In a review of vitamin D in adults, especially pregnant women, Hollis[69] clearly demonstrated that traditional levels of vitamin D of 400 IU/day or less are grossly inadequate today when few women get adequate sun exposure and many wear sunscreen or clothing that obstructs the exposure. Most recommendations were done before it was possible to measure circulating 25-(OH)-vitamin D, the true indicator of nutritional vitamin D status. The dose of 10 mg or 400 IU daily had little effect on adult 25-(OH)-vitamin D levels. When

submariners were given 600 IU/day for several months, they failed to maintain adequate 25-(OH)-vitamin D levels.[68] The dose that is adequate during pregnancy is a minimum of 1000 IU daily. Doses of 10,000 IU daily in adults did not elevate circulating 25-(OH)-vitamin D above the normal range, and doses of 1000 IU may not maintain normal levels. The resurgence of rickets in infants may well begin with inadequate levels in pregnancy.[150]

Cases of vitamin D-deficiency hypocalcemia and rickets in nonwhite infants have been reported in increasing numbers in exclusively breastfed infants.[23] The epidemic is aggravated by the use of sunscreen, ethnic traditions of covering the body, and lack of sunshine.[145] Serum 1,25-dihydroxyvitamin D concentrations are significantly higher in lactating compared with nonlactating women and among vegetarian compared with nonvegetarian women, report Specker et al.[142] All lactating women in a study by Chang had elevated serum parathyroid hormone levels (see Table 4-26). Levels of vitamin D are higher in colostrum than in mature milk.[95] Studies by Wagoner et al. provided high levels of vitamin D (4000 IU/day) to mothers to increase their milk levels.[149] A study of exclusively breastfed infants was conducted placing the infants at 1 month of age in one of four doses of vitamin D categories (200, 400, 600, 800 IU/day). At 1 month most of the infants had levels below normal. Seventy-two percent had levels below 88.2 + 23.0 nmol/L 25(OH) D concentrations. During the study, low levels were noted occasionally in all categories. Ziegler et al.[154] concluded that 400 IU/day should be standard for infants and that supplementation should start at birth.

It has been recommended by the AAP that all breastfed infants receive 400 IU of vitamin D beginning at birth. Until pregnant and lactating women who are at risk for inadequate intake receive adequate supplements, it will be necessary to supplement normal breastfeeding infants.[126,57]

The concern for toxicity of excessive vitamin D was based on the reported relationship with cardiac disease and supravalvular aortic stenosis syndrome and William syndrome, which has been proved to be genetic. Hypervitaminosis from high levels of vitamin D has resulted from therapeutic misadventures resulting in hypercalcium when the circulating 25-(OH)-vitamin D concentrations were over 100 ng/mL (normal levels of 25-(OH)-vitamin D are over 15 ng/mL serum). No case of hypervitaminosis D has been reported from sun exposure even though a half hour in the summer sun between 10 AM and 2 PM in a bathing suit (approximately 3 minimal erythemal dose exposures) will release about 50,000 IU or 1.25 mg/day of vitamin D within 24 hours in most white persons.[69]

Vitamin E

Vitamin E has been a subject of much interest. Levels in colostrum are 1.5 mg/dL, whereas transitional milk has 0.9 mg/dL and mature milk has 0.25 mg/dL. The difference at different stages has been found to be caused by α-tocopherol, because the contents of β- and γ-tocopherol are similar. Total tocopherol in mature milk correlates with total lipid and linoleic acid contents. Significantly higher tocopherol/linoleic acid ratios are found in both colostrum and transitional milk than in mature milk.

Cow milk has 0.07 mg/dL of vitamin E (see Table 4-25). Correspondingly, serum levels in breastfed infants rise quickly at birth and maintain a normal level, whereas cow milk-fed infants have depressed levels. Vitamin E includes a group of fat-soluble compounds (α, β, γ-, and δ-tocopherol) and their unsaturated derivatives (α-, β-, γ-, and δ-tocotrienol). An IU of vitamin E is equal to 1 mg of synthetic α-tocopherol or 0.74 mg of natural α-tocopherol acetate.

Vitamin E is required for muscle integrity, resistance of erythrocytes to hemolysis, and other biochemical and physiologic functions. The requirement for vitamin E is related to the PUFA content of the cellular structures and of the diet (see Table 4-26). Satisfactory plasma levels are 1 mg/dL, and these levels can be maintained by feedings with a vitamin E/PUFA ratio of 0.4 mg/g. The requirement for infants to age 6 months is 3 mg/day and after 6 months 4 mg/day. The requirement during lactation is 14 mg during the first 6 months and 17 mg/day after 6 months postpartum.

An estimate of the tocopherol/linoleic acid ratio in mature milk is 0.79 mg α-tocopherol equivalents per gram, which is comparable to a daily requirement of 0.5 mg for term infants but may be low for premature infants, especially those receiving iron supplements. Ordinarily, this would be supplied by 4 IU of vitamin E per day. Because human milk contains 1.8 mg/L or 40 mg of vitamin E per gram of lipid, it supplies more than adequate levels of vitamin E.[88]

Vitamin K

Vitamin K is essential for the synthesis of blood-clotting factors, which are normal in the serum at birth. The previous levels of vitamin K reported in human milk (15 mg/dL) have been replaced with those calculated by more accurate techniques and are lower: 2.1 mg/L for mature milk and 2.3 mg/L for colostrum,[21] which are less than the recommended daily intake of 12 mg/day (Table 4-27).

The measurements of the homologs of vitamin K have been equivocal. When mothers are given a single dose of 20 mg of phylloquinone (K_1), the milk level increases from 1 to 140 mg/L in 12 hours, dropping to 5 mg/L in 48 hours.

When infants are given 1 mg vitamin K_1 at birth, as is the practice in many countries, the concentration of K_1 in both breastfed and formula-fed infants in the first week of life remains elevated. When no neonatal prophylaxis is given, Büller et al.[17] reported no difference in coagulating factors among a sample of 113 breastfed, formula-fed, or combination-fed infants. They reported a case of low vitamin K levels in the milk of a mother whose infant died at 6 weeks from intracranial bleeding without neonatal prophylaxis.

Vitamin K is produced by the intestinal flora but takes several days in the previously sterile neonatal gut to be effective. Vitamin K-dependent clotting factors in normal breastfed infants were normal. The prothrombin time and partial thromboplastin time were similar in breastfed and bottle-fed infants. The Normotest and Thrombotest coagulation tests were significantly prolonged in the breastfed group. The authors concluded that 5% of breastfed children have possible vitamin K deficiency. In several case reports, 179 infants exclusively breastfed with no vitamin K given at birth developed late-onset hemorrhagic disease that responded to vitamin K administration. O'Connor et al.[120] note the association of vitamin K

TABLE 4-27	Recommended Daily Dietary Allowances of Vitamins for Infants*		
Age	Vitamin K (μg)	Biotin (μg)	Pantothenic Acid (mg)
To 6 mo	5 (1 μg/kg)	10	2
6 mo-1 yr	10	15	3

*The allowances are intended to provide for individual variations among most normal persons as they live in the United States under usual environmental stresses. Diets should be based on a variety of common foods in order to provide other nutrients for which human requirements have been less well defined.

From Food and Nutrition Board, National Research Council, National Academy of Sciences: *Recommended dietary allowances*, ed 10, Washington, D.C., 1989, U.S. Government Printing Office.

deficiency with home birth and suggest that the physician give vitamin K immediately as recommended by the American Academy of Pediatrics if it has been omitted.[7]

At 3 months of age, 165 breastfed infants who had received 1 mg vitamin K_1 at birth had reduced serum levels of vitamin K_1. Their clotting factors were unchanged. For complete protection, Cornelissen et al.[28] recommend a second oral dose of vitamin K_1 at 3 months. In a similar study, Greer et al. found that despite low plasma phylloquinone concentrations in the breastfed infant (less than 0.25 ng/mL) for the first 6 months, continued vitamin K_1 supplementation was not recommended. Canfield et al.[21] confirm the low levels of vitamin K_1 in breastfed infants compared with those in infants fed formula containing many times the recommended daily dose (0.5 ng/day). No requirements have been set for breastfed infants. No data are available regarding the potential toxicity of excessive vitamin K.

It is recommended that all infants receive vitamin K at birth, regardless of feeding plans, to prevent hemorrhagic disease of the newborn caused by vitamin K deficiency in the first few days of life.[7]

The vitamin content of common foods has been recalculated downward so that diets of average women are probably deficient in vitamin K. Furthermore, vitamin K levels in the serum of lactating women are not good markers of deficiency. Carboxylated prothrombin (des-γ-carboxyprothrombin) is produced in the absence of vitamin K and is a marker of vitamin K deficiency. Greer et al.[58] followed breastfed infants and found normal des-γ-carboxyprothrombin levels at birth and 4 weeks but elevations by 8 weeks. The authors recommend maternal supplementation during lactation.

Vitamin C

Vitamin C is part of several enzyme and hormone systems, as well as of intracellular chemical reactions. It is essential to collagen synthesis (Tables 4-28 and 4-29).

Human milk is an outstanding source of water-soluble vitamins and reflects maternal dietary intake (see Table 4-26). Increased vitamin C has been measured in the milk within 30 minutes of a bolus of vitamin C being given to the mother. Human milk contains 43 mg/dL (fresh cow milk contains up to 21 mg). Levels obtained in normal lactating women 6 months postpartum were 35 mg/L in those on normal diets and 38 mg/L in those supplemented with multivitamins containing 90 mg vitamin C.[138] Levels obtained in 16 lactating women of low-socioeconomic level were 53 mg/L for unsupplemented and 65 mg/L for supplemented mothers at 1 week postpartum and 61 and 72 mg/L, respectively, at 6 weeks postpartum. Several subjects in the unsupplemented low-socioeconomic group had levels too low to provide 35 mg vitamin C per day to their infants.

When lactating women were given 250, 500, or 1000 mg/day vitamin C for 2 days, milk levels remained within the range of 44 to 158 mg/L and did not differ significantly between dosages, even at 10 times the recommended dietary allowance (RDA). Total intake of the infant through the milk ranged from 49 to 86 mg/day. These findings suggest a regulatory mechanism for vitamin C levels in milk. When women received high doses of vitamin C, levels of the vitamin excreted in the urine also increased proportionately.[127]

VITAMIN B COMPLEX

Vitamin B_1

Vitamin B_1, or thiamin, levels increase with the duration of lactation but are lower in human milk (160 mg/dL) than in cow milk (440 mg/dL) (see Tables 4-28 and 4-29). In a study by Nail et al., levels obtained by normal lactating women showed significant increases between 1 and 6 weeks postpartum, but no difference in levels between supplemented (1.7 mg daily) and unsupplemented women

TABLE 4-28	Recommended Daily Dietary Allowances of Water-Soluble Vitamins for Infants*						
Age	Vitamin C (mg)	Thiamin (mg)	Riboflavin (mg)	Niacin (mg NE)[†]	Vitamin B_6 (mg)	Folacin[‡] (μg)	Vitamin B_{12} (μg)
To 6 mo	30	0.3	0.4	5	0.3	25	0.3
6 mo-1 yr	35	0.4	0.5	6	0.6	35	0.5

*The allowances are intended to provide for individual variations among most normal persons as they live in the United States under usual environmental stresses. Diets should be based on a variety of common foods in order to provide other nutrients for which human requirements have been less well defined.

[†]1 NE (niacin equivalent) is equal to 1 mg of niacin or 60 mg of dietary tryptophan.

[‡]The folacin allowances refer to dietary sources as determined by *Lactobacillus casei* assay after treatment with enzymes (conjugases) to make polyglutamyl forms of the vitamin.

From Food and Nutrition Board, National Research Council, National Academy of Sciences: *Recommended dietary allowances*, ed 10, Washington, D.C., 1989, U.S. Government Printing Office.

TABLE 4-29 Estimated Secretion of Nutrients in Mature Human Milk Compared with Increments in Recommended Dietary Allowances (RDA) for Lactating Women

A. Energy, protein, and fat-soluble vitamins

Measure	Energy (kcal)	Protein (g)	Vitamin A (μg RE)	Vitamin D (μg)	Vitamin E (mg of α-TE)	Vitamin K (μg)
Estimated secretion in milk*	420-700	6.3-10.5	400-670	0.3-0.6	1.4-2.3	1.3-2.1
Increment in RDAs†,‡ for following lactation periods						
0-6 mo	500	15	500	5	4	0
6-12 mo	500	12	400	5	3	0
Comments	Estimated 80% efficiency in conversion to milk energy	Estimated 70% efficiency in conversion to milk protein	None	Increment advised in part to maintain calcium balance	Estimated 75% absorption	No increment listed because intakes usually exceed RDA

B. Water-soluble vitamins

Measure	Vitamin C (mg)	Thiamin (mg)	Riboflavin (mg)	Niacin (mg of NE)	Vitamin B$_6$ (mg)	Folate (μg)	Vitamin B$_{12}$ (μg)
Estimated secretion in milk*	24-40	0.13-0.21	0.21-0.35	0.9-1.5	0.06-0.09	50-83	0.6-1.0
Increment in RDAs†,‡ for following lactation periods							
0-6 mo	35	0.5	0.5	5	0.5	100	0.6
6-12 mo	30	0.5	0.4	5	0.5	80	0.6
Comments	Estimated 85% absorption	Increment higher than secretion because of increased energy needs	Estimated 70% utilization for milk production	Increment higher than secretion because of increased energy needs	Milk concentration used is for unsupplemented women	Estimated 50% absorption; RDA based on 50 rather than 83 μg/L	RDA based on 0.6 rather than 1.0 μg/L

C. Minerals

Measure	Calcium (mg)	Phosphorus (mg)	Magnesium (mg)	Iron (mg)	Zinc (mg)	Iodine (µg)	Selenium (µg)
Estimated secretion in milk*	168-280	84-140	21-35	0.18-0.30	0.9-1.5§ 0.3-0.5¶	66-110	12-20
Increment in RDAs†,‡ for following lactation periods							
0-6 mo	400	400	75	0	7	50	20
6-12 mo	400	400	60	0	4	50	20
Comments	None	Based on desired 1:1 ratio for calcium/phosphorus intake	Estimated 50% absorption	Secretion during lactation is less than menstrual loss	Estimated 20% absorption	Based on need of infant, not maternal loss in milk	Estimated 80% absorption

α-TE, α-tocopherol equivalents; NE, niacin equivalents; RE, retinol equivalents.
*At volumes of 600-1000 mL/day, based on milk composition shown in Table 4-13.
†From National Research Council, Washington, D.C., 1989.
‡Women aged 25 to 50.
§0 to 6 months.
¶6 to 12 months.
From Report of Nutrition During Lactation Subcommittee, Institute of Medicine: Nutrition during lactation, Washington, D.C., 1991, National Academy Press.

was seen. Cases of beriberi in infants have been associated with a deficiency in the mother.

Because urinary excretion of thiamin is significantly higher in supplemented than in unsupplemented women, the amount of vitamin transferred into milk appears to be limited.[127] Malnourished women, however, do show significant increases in their milk when supplemented.[94] Thiamin is essential for the use of carbohydrates in the pyruvate metabolism (cofactor in pyruvic acid decarboxylation) and for fat synthesis. Insufficient thiamin produces insufficient carbohydrate oxidation with accumulation of intermediary metabolites such as lactic acid.

Vitamin B_2

Vitamin B_2, or riboflavin, is significant for the newborn in whom intestinal tract bacterial synthesis is minimal (see Tables 4-28 and 4-29). Riboflavin is involved in oxidative intracellular systems and is essential for protoplasmic growth. Levels are 36 mg/dL in human milk and 175 mg/dL in cow milk.

Levels obtained in normal lactating women showed significantly lower levels of riboflavin in the milk of the unsupplemented women (36.7 mg/dL) at 1 week compared with the milk of the supplemented women, who received 2 mg/day in a multivitamin (80.0 mg/dL). No significant difference was seen between 1 and 6 weeks in either group.

Niacin

Niacin (nicotinamide) is an essential part of the pyridine nucleotide coenzymes and is part of the intracellular respiratory mechanisms. Human milk has 147 mg/dL and cow milk has 94 mg/dL (see Tables 4-28 and 4-29). Levels respond to dietary supplementation.

Vitamin B_6

Vitamin B_6 (pyridoxine) forms the enzyme group of certain decarboxylases and transaminases involved in metabolism of nerve tissue. The supply of vitamin B_6 is vital to DNA synthesis, which is needed to form the cerebrosides in the myelination of the CNS. Human milk has 12 to 15 mg/dL of vitamin B_6 and cow milk has 64 mg/dL (see Tables 4-28 and 4-29). The principal form of vitamin B_6 in human milk is pyridoxal, but pyridoxine is the principal form of vitamin B_6 fortification in infant formulas. Levels of vitamin B_6 in the milk of mothers consuming more than 2.5 mg of the vitamin daily (RDA for lactating women is

2.5 mg/day) were significantly higher in the first week than were levels in the unsupplemented mothers' milk. Average maternal diets in several studies were consistently below the recommended levels of vitamin B_6.

The accumulated stores of vitamin B_6 during pregnancy are significant for the maintenance of adequate vitamin B_6 status of infants during the early months of breastfeeding. For some infants, human milk alone without supplementary foods may be insufficient to meet vitamin B_6 needs after 6 months of age.[66] The recommended daily intake for infants under 6 months of age is 0.30 mg. Vitamin B_6 deficiency has been associated with CNS disorders in three breastfed infants.

Long-term use of oral contraceptives has been shown to result in low levels of vitamin B_6 in maternal serum in pregnancy and at delivery and low levels in the milk of these mothers.[144] The relationship of vitamin B_6 supplements to suppression of prolactin and the treatment of galactorrhea is discussed under lactation failure (see Chapter 16). The doses used to suppress lactation (600 mg/day) far exceed the levels in multiple vitamins (1 to 10 mg) (see Table 4-29).

Pantothenic Acid

Pantothenic acid is part of CoA, a catalyst of acetylation reactions. The reaction of CoA with acetic acid to form acetyl-CoA is prime to intermediary metabolism. The levels of pantothenic acid in human milk were restudied by Johnston et al. because of the range of values in the literature. They found the mean to be 670 mg/dL in foremilk and hindmilk samples. No change occurred in concentrations from 1 to 6 months postpartum. They did find a positive correlation with dietary intake.

Folacin

Folacin (folic acid) is part of the conversion of glycine to serine. It is also involved in the methylation of nicotinamide and homocysteine to methionine. It is essential for erythropoiesis (see Table 4-28).

The folate (anionic form of folic acid) content of human milk produced by well-nourished women averages 80 to 130 mg/L (see Table 4-29).[120] These values are substantially greater than those reported in the literature previously because of difficulty in the analysis. Folate in human milk is quantitatively bound to folate-binding proteins and presents in multiple labile forms. Folate values typically increase as lactation progresses and are even maintained as maternal stores begin to be depleted.

Supplementation with folic acid in deficient mothers caused prompt increase in levels in the milk. When mothers and their infants were evaluated, folate levels were two to three times higher in the breastfed infants than in their mothers, and a correlation was seen between levels in the milk and in the infants' plasma. Folic acid has also been identified as a critical element in deficiency states during pregnancy, being associated with abruptio placentae, toxemia, and intrauterine growth failure as well as megaloblastic anemia.

Vitamin B_{12}

Early studies reported that vitamin B_{12} is found in human milk in a low concentration of 0.3 mg/L, whereas cow milk has 4.0 mg/mL. Well-nourished mothers on balanced diets appear to have adequate amounts for their infants.[144] Microbiologic assay has demonstrated that high concentrations of vitamin B_{12} appear in early colostrum but level off in a few days to those of serum. Samples of colostrum reported by Samson and McClelland have a mean binding capacity of 72 ng/mL; in mature milk the capacity is one third of this value. Vitamin B_{12} levels were compared by Sandberg et al.[134] in supplemented and unsupplemented mothers and were not significantly different. Levels were 33 to 320 ng/dL, with a mean of 97 ng/dL. When nutritionally deficient, low-socioeconomic lactating women were studied by Sneed et al., supplementation with a multivitamin did result in elevated vitamin B_{12} levels. This was true for folate as well.

Although cow milk has five to 10 times more vitamin B_{12} than mature human milk, cow milk has little vitamin B_{12}-binding capacity, which is substantial in human milk. Vitamin B_{12} functions in transmethylations such as synthesis of choline from methionine, serine from glycine, and methionine from homocysteine. It is involved in pyrimidine and purine metabolism. Vitamin B_{12} also affects the metabolism of folic acid. Megaloblastic anemia is a common symptom of vitamin B_{12} deficiency. Vitamin B_{12} occurs exclusively in animal tissue, is bound to protein, and is minimal or absent in vegetable protein.[126]

The recommendation for the minimum daily requirement of B_{12} for infants is 0.3 mg/day in the first year of life, when growth is rapid (see Table 4-28). Based on their data on omnivorous and vegetarian women, Specker et al.[141] conclude that the current RDA for infants provides little margin for safety (see Table 4-29).

ENZYMES

Considerable data have been collected on the enzymatic activities of many milks. Jenness and Sloan report 44 enzymes detected in bovine, human, and other milks. Xanthine oxidase, lactoperoxidase, uridine diphosphogalactose, galactosyl transferase, ribonuclease, lipase, alkaline phosphatase, acid phosphatase, and lysozyme have been isolated in crystalline form.

The role and significance of enzymes in human milk were reviewed by Hamosh,[62] who confirmed that more than 20 active human milk enzymes exist (Table 4-30). They can be categorized into three general groups by their activity: mammary gland function, which reflects physiologic changes occurring in the mammary gland itself during lactation; compensatory digestive enzymes in human milk, which have digestive functions in the neonate; and milk enzymes, important in stimulating neonatal development.[62] Some enzyme levels are significantly higher in colostrum than in mature milk. Most are whey proteins and contribute minimally to milk proteins. Some enzymes, like other proteins in milk, are probably produced elsewhere and transported to the breast via the bloodstream. The evidence to support the concept of local synthesis includes the demonstration of secretory tissue in the mammary gland. Amylase levels are twice as high in milk as in serum.[96] Casein proteins have been synthesized in vitro in cell-free mammary-derived mRNA-enriched systems. Mammary explants from mice, monkeys, and humans have accumulated lactose synthetase B. The enzymes of possible importance in infant digestion are those with pancreatic analogs: amylase, lipases, protease(s), and ribonuclease.

Amylase

Amylase, the chief polysaccharide-digesting enzyme, is not developed at birth even in full-term infants, who have only 0.2% to 0.5% of adult values. Mammary amylase is present, however, throughout lactation, with levels higher in colostrum than in mature milk. Human milk levels are 0.5 to 1.0 g/dL oligosaccharides of varying chain length. Milk levels of preterm mothers are comparable to term milk levels.

Milk levels are twice those of serum in the first 90 days and remain higher than serum over 6 months. When exposed to a pH of 5.3, this salivary-type amylase remains active; at a pH of 3.5, one half the original activity is present at 2 hours and one third at 6 hours. Amylase is stable at $-20°C$ to $-70°C$ ($-4°F$ to $-94°F$) for storage and at least for 24 hours at $15°C$ to $38°C$ ($59°F$ to $100°F$). Much milk amylase activity remains in the duodenum after a meal of human milk. This is significant for the digestion of starch because pancreatic amylase is still low in infants. Mammary amylase may be an alternate pathway of digestion of glucose polymers and of starch (Table 4-31).

Milk amylase is part of the isozyme group as salivary amylase and is thought to inhibit the growth of certain microorganisms.

Lipases

Milk fat is almost completely digestible. The emulsion of fat in breast milk is greater than in cow milk, resulting in smaller globules. Milk lipases play an active role in creating the emulsion, which yields a finer curd and facilitates the digestion of triacylglycerols. The newborn easily digests and completely uses the well-emulsified small fat globules of human milk. Free fatty acids are important sources of energy for the infant.

Lipase in human milk was first described in 1901. At least two different lipases (glycerol ester hydrolases) were described then. The lipases in human milk make the free fatty acids available in a large proportion even before the digestive phase of the intestine. The lipolytic milk-enzyme activity is similar to the activity of pancreatic lipase,

TABLE 4-30 Component Functions in Human Milk

Function	Component	Process
Biosynthesis of milk components in mammary gland	Phosphoglucomutase	Synthesis of lactose
	Lactose synthetase	Synthesis of lactose
	Fatty acid synthetase	Synthesis of medium-chain fatty acids
	Thioesterase	Uptake of circulating triglyceride fatty acids
	Lipoprotein lipase	Uptake of circulating triglyceride fatty acids
Digestive function in infant	Amylase	Hydrolysis of polysaccharides
	Lipase (bile salt-dependent)	Hydrolysis of triglycerides
	Proteases	Proteolysis (not verified)
	Xanthine oxidase	Carrier of iron, molybdenum
	Glutathione peroxidase	Carrier of selenium
	Alkaline phosphatase	Carrier of zinc, magnesium
Preservation of milk components	Antiprotease	Protection of bioactive proteins (i.e., enzymes and immunoglobulins)
	Sulfhydryl oxidase	Maintenance of structure and function of proteins containing disulfide bonds
Antiinfective agents	Lysozyme	Bactericidal
	Peroxidase	Bactericidal
	Lipases (lipoprotein lipase, bile salt-dependent lipase)	Release of free fatty acids that have antibacterial, antiviral, and antiprotozoan actions
Antiinflammatory agents	Vitamins A, C, and E	Scavenge oxygen radicals
	Catalase	Degrades hydrogen peroxide
	Glutathione peroxidase	Prevents lipid peroxidation
	Platelet-activating factor acetylhydrolase	Degrades platelet-activating factor
	α1-Antitrypsin	Inhibits inflammatory proteases
	α1-Antichymotrypsin	Inhibits inflammatory proteases
	Prostaglandin 1	Cytoprotective
	Prostaglandin 2	Cytoprotective
	Epidermal growth factor	Promotes gut growth and function
	Transforming growth factor-α	Promotes epithelial cell growth
	Transforming growth factor-β	Suppresses lymphocyte function
	Interleukin 10	Suppresses function of macrophages and natural killer and T cells
	Transforming growth factor-α receptors I and II	Binds to and inhibits transforming growth factor-α

From Hamosh M: Enzymes in human milk: their role in nutrient digestion, gastrointestinal function and nutrient delivery to the newborn infant. In Lebenthal E, editor: *Textbook of gastroenterology and nutrition in infancy*, ed 2, New York, 1989, Raven; Hamosh M: Bioactive factors in human milk. Breastfeeding 2001, Part I: the evidence for breastfeeding, *Pediatr Clin North Am* 48:69, 2001.

TABLE 4-31	Characteristics of Milk Enzymes Active in Infant Digestion	
Characteristic	**Amylase**	**BSSL**
High parity (≥10)	Low activity	?
Malnutrition	?	Decrease in activity
Diurnal and within feed activity	Constant	Constant
Prepartum	?	Present
Presence in preterm (PT) and term (T) milk	Equal activity PT and T	Equal activity PT and T
Pattern through lactation	Colostrum greater than milk	Colostrum lower than milk
Weaning	?	Activity constant independent of milk volume
Distribution in milk	Skim milk	Skim milk
Effect of milk storage −20°C to −70°C, 15°C to 38°C	Stable years Stable (≤24 h)	Stable years Stable (≤24 h)
Stability to low pH (passage through stomach)	pH >3.0	pH >3.0
Optimum pH	6.5-7.5	7.4-8.5
Enzyme characteristics	Salivary amylase isozyme	Identical with pancreatic carboxyl ester hydrolase
Evidence of activity in infant's intestine	Yes	Yes
Presence in milk of other species	?	Primates, carnivores, and rodents

BSSL, Bile salt-stimulated lipase.

From Hamosh M: Enzymes in human milk. In Jensen RG, editor: *Handbook of milk composition*, San Diego, 1995, Academic Press; Hamosh M: Bioactive factors in human milk. Breastfeeding 2001, Part I: the evidence for breastfeeding. *Pediatr Clin North Am* 48:69, 2001.

breaking down triglycerides to free fatty acids and glycerol. One enzyme is present in the fat fraction and is inhibited by bile salts.[62]

Milk from undernourished mothers may lose some of its ability to hydrolyze milk-lipid esters over the course of lactation; this ability remains constant in well-nourished mothers.[41] This would have an effect on the utilization of the esters of lipid-soluble vitamins A, D, and E.

It appears that the function of this enzyme, inhibited by bile salts, is to facilitate the uptake by the mammary gland of fatty acids from circulating triglycerides for incorporation with milk lipids, because lipase in vivo depends on added serum for

activity. Its presence in milk probably represents "leakage" from the mammary gland, and it is unlikely to play a major physiologic role in the lipolysis of milk triglycerides.

Additional lipases in the skim milk fraction are stimulated by bile salts. Bile salt-stimulated lipase (BSSL) has greater activity and splits all three ester bonds of the triglyceride. This lipase is also stable in the duodenum and contributes to the hydrolysis of the triacylglycerols in the presence of the bile salts. BSSL is identical to carboxyl ester hydrolase (carboxylesterase), a pancreatic enzyme. BSSL activity is lower in colostrum than in mature milk. No correlation appears to exist between the volume of milk at various stages and the volume of enzyme secreted.[51] BSSL is present in early prepartum secretions less than 2 months before delivery and in the milk expressed during weaning. For a given well-nourished woman, levels remain stable even after prolonged lactation. BSSL activity is protective against infection by virtue of the production of free fatty acids and monoglycerides, products of fat digestion that have antiinfective properties (see Table 4-31).[51]

The enzyme activity of BSSL is remarkably stable during prolonged storage up to 2 years at either −20°C or −70°C (−4°F or −94°F). It has also been noted to be stable at 15°, 25°, and 38°C (59°, 77°, and 100°F).[63]

Contrary to earlier suggestions, no association exists between jaundice and increased levels of free fatty acids produced as a result of high activity of milk lipase.[51]

Investigators have continued to study the action of these lipases in the presence of bile salts. The BSSL remains active during passage through the stomach because it is stable with a pH greater than 3.5 and only slowly inactivated by pepsin. The optimal bile salt concentration for activity is about 2 mmol/L, which is within the physiologic range in the newborn. Bile salts protect the enzyme from tryptic activity.

Glucose-6-Phosphate Dehydrogenase

Glucose-6-phosphate dehydrogenase is rich in the milk of mothers with normal red blood cell dehydrogenase and absent in mothers with glucose-6-phosphate dehydrogenase deficiency. Its levels depend on the increased rate of carbohydrate metabolism in the mammary gland.

Lactic and Malic Acid Dehydrogenases

Lactic and malic acid dehydrogenase levels are high in colostrum, are lower in mature milk, and are increased at the end of a feeding. The levels are higher in species with small body size; thus mice and humans have more than cows. Because no correlation exists with serum levels, these enzymes are thought to be synthesized in the mammary gland. A change occurs in these enzymes during lactation.

Lactose Synthetase

Lactose synthetase catalyzes the synthesis of lactose from UDP-galactose and glucose. This enzyme has two components: A-protein, a glycoprotein, and B-protein, an α-lactalbumin. The control mechanism for lactose biosynthesis by the A-protein and α-lactalbumin ensures that lactose is synthesized in the mammary gland only in response to specific hormones.[90]

Lysozyme

Lysozyme is a thermostable, nonspecific antimicrobial factor that catalyzes the hydrolysis of β-linkage between N-acetylglucosamine and N-acetylmuramic acid in the bacterial cell wall. It is bacteriolytic toward Enterobacteriaceae and gram-positive bacteria and is considered to play a role in the antibacterial activity of milk as well as a significant role in the development of intestinal flora. It also hydrolyzes mucopolysaccharides. Human lysozyme is antigenically and serologically different from the bovine enzyme. The content in human milk is 3000 times that in bovine milk and the activity 100 times that of bovine milk. Lysozyme is considered to be a spillover product from breast epithelial cells.

Phosphatases

Acid phosphatase is similar in human and bovine milk, but alkaline phosphatase is much less active in human milk by a factor of 40. Its level increases with the increase in fat concentration and increases as the feeding progresses. In 199 samples from 20 donors, no relationship to age, nationality, or other characteristics of the donor was found. Alkaline phosphatase concentrations appeared to be related to the fat concentration in human milk. Levels increased as lactation progressed.[2] Alkaline phosphatase is a metal-carrying enzyme with four zinc molecules and two magnesium atoms. It differs from the placental alkaline phosphatase.

Serum alkaline phosphatase is increased in pregnancy. The placenta produces alkaline phosphatase, which may contribute to this increase. The liver does not enlarge. The histologic appearance is normal. The spider angiomata and palmar erythema that are observed are attributed to the increase in estrogen.[55]

Proteases and Antiproteases

Several enzymes have caseinolytic activity and elastase-like activity. Beta casein and V-casein and galactothermin are probably the by-products of endogenous human milk proteolytic activity.[60] Also small peptides of only three to eight amino acids are derived from a casein group called β-casomorphins with specific physiologic activity. These peptides may be associated with the sleeping patterns of neonates and even have relevance to postpartum psychosis.

Proteases catalyze the hydrolysis of proteins. High levels of protease are found in human milk, suggesting that enzymes may provide the breastfed infant with significant digestive assistance immediately after birth.

Antiproteases' physiologic role is not entirely clear. The main protease inhibitors in human milk are α_1-antichymotrypsin and α_1-antitrypsin.[62] Trace amounts of others have been identified. One function may be to protect the mammary gland from local proteolytic activity by leukocytic and lysosomal proteases during different stages of lactogenesis. They may prevent the breakdown of proteins in stored milk.[60] The protection of immunoglobulins that are transferred intact to the neonate and the protection of growth hormones are probably other roles of the antiproteases. The presence of such inhibitors may restrain the invading bacterial enzymes in the host tissue (breast) or secretion (milk). Thus the presence of these inhibitors may protect the mammary gland and the recipient infant from infection.

Xanthine Oxidase

Xanthine oxidase catalyzes the oxidation of purines, pyrimidines, and aldehydes. Although bovine milk contains high levels, it was only after much effort that investigators were able to identify it in human milk. The activity in human milk peaks on the third day after birth and decreases with the progression of lactation. It differs from that in bovine milk in that it is not of bacterial origin and its activity is correlated with protein concentration.

Many enzymes are being studied in humans and other species. See Table 4-30 for a summary of the most significant enzymes. For an extensive discussion, see Hamosh.[62]

Hormones

Protein hormones, especially prolactin, and steroid hormones, such as gestagens, estrogens, corticoids, androgens, and opiate-like peptides, can be detected in human milk and in the milk of other mammals.[135]

Animal studies have shown that at least some of these hormones retain physiologic activity when ingested but not when pasteurized. Although their presence was recognized in the 1930s, advances in hormone assay techniques have brought more information to light.[86] Hormones with simple structures, such as steroids and thyroxine (T_4), can pass easily by diffusion into the milk from circulating blood. Peptide hormones such as hypothalamic-releasing hormones, because of their small size, also would be expected to appear in milk. Of the larger-molecular-weight pituitary hormones, only prolactin has been found so far. The hormones identified in human milk include gonadotropin-releasing hormone, thyroid-releasing hormone, thyroid-stimulating hormone (TSH; thyrotropin), prolactin, gonadotropins, ovarian hormones, corticosteroids, erythropoietin (EPO), cyclic adenosine monophosphate, and cyclic guanosine monophosphate (Tables 4-32 and 4-33).

The concentration of hormones changes during lactation, with prolactin decreasing over time and triiodothyronine (T_3) and T_4 increasing. Evidence indicates that the GI tract of suckling mammals possesses the ability to absorb various proteins with substantial preservation of their immunologic properties. The absorption of large-molecular-weight hormones has been demonstrated in suckling rats and mice, with measurable amounts appearing in serum and other tissues.

The thyroid hormones have received considerable attention because of the apparent protection of hypothyroid infants who are breastfed. TSH content was investigated by both direct I-TSH radioimmunoassay and indirect radioimmunoassay.

TSH was present in human milk in low concentrations comparable to those normally found in the serum of euthyroid adults. Experimentally, thyroidectomy of the lactating rat led to the disappearance of measurable T_4 and an increase in the level of TSH in the milk. In contrast, administration of T_3 decreased the TSH in the rat model.

Prolactin has been identified as a normal constituent of human milk. Levels are high in the first few days postpartum but subsequently decline rapidly. "Prolactin-like" biologic activity is measurable in human colostrum, with the highest levels on day 1. Concentrations in the milk tend to parallel concentrations in the blood plasma among different species. Three stages of neuroendocrine development are theorized: placental, milk, and autonomous, in which the milk phase is the adaptation to extrauterine life.[62]

The exact mechanism by which prolactin enters the milk is unclear. Prolactin-binding sites have been identified within the alveolar cells. The functional significance of prolactin also remains unclear. In rodents, milk prolactin influences fluid

TABLE 4-32	Nonpeptide Hormones in Human Milk
Hormone	**Concentration (ng/mL)**
Thyroid	
Thyroxine (T_4)	1-40.3-2.012.01.16-2.40.8-2.3
Triiodothyronine (T_3)	0.02-0.400.05-0.10
Reverse T_3	0.008-0.15
Adrenal gland: Cortisol	0.2-32.0 (5:10)*3.7
Sexual	
Progesterone	10-40
Pregnanediol	0-450
Estrogens	15-840 (15:60)*
Contraceptives	Biologically significant quantities

*Ratio of values in colostrum/values in mature milk.

Modified from Koldovsky O, Strbak V: Hormones and growth factors in human milk. In Jensen RG, editor: *Handbook of milk composition*, San Diego, 1995, Academic Press.

TABLE 4-33	Hormonally Active Peptides in Human Milk	
Peptide	**Concentration**	**Ratio (Colostrum/ Mature Milk)**
Erythropoietin	Bioassay	?
Growth factors		
Epidermal growth factor	3-107 ng/mL	2:10
Insulin	0-80 μU/mL	3:10
Insulin-like growth factor 1	1.3-7 ng/mL	2:3
Nerve growth factor	Present	
Transforming growth factor alpha (TGF-α)	0-8.4 ng/mL	1
Other growth factors	Present	?
Gastrointestinal regulatory peptides		
Gastrin	10-30 pg/mL	2:3
Gastric inhibitory peptide	33-59 ng/mL	1
Gastric regulatory peptide	31-55 pg/mL; 60-430 pg/mL	2:3
Neurotensin	7-15 pg/mL	2:3
Peptide histidine methionine	3-32 pg/mL	5:10
Peptide YY	15-30 pg/mL	2:3

Modified from Koldovsky O, Strbak V: Hormones and growth factors in human milk. In Jensen RG, editor: *Handbook of milk composition*, San Diego, 1995, Academic Press.

and ion absorption from the jejunum. It also may influence gonadal and adrenal function, as demonstrated in other species.

Endocrine responses in the neonate differ between breastfed and formula-fed infants. In a study of 34 healthy, 6-day-old full-term infants who were formula fed, plasma concentrations of insulin, motilin, enteroglucagon, neurotensin, and pancreatic polypeptide changed significantly after a feeding. Similar levels were measured in 43 normal breastfed infants, and little or no change was noted. Further, the basal levels of gastric inhibitory polypeptide, motilin, neurotensin, and vasoactive intestinal peptide were also higher in the bottle-fed than in the breastfed infants. Whether pancreatic and gut hormone-release changes affect postnatal development is yet to be determined.

EPO is synthesized in the maternal kidney and targets bone marrow where it stimulates erythropoiesis. The bioavailability of erythropoietin enterally is thought to be insufficient; however, when present in human milk, it may be different for newborns. In the rat model it has been shown to stimulate erythropoiesis in the suckling rat. It may have a physiologic effect on human breastfed newborns.[13]

PROSTAGLANDINS

In the investigation of the factors in human milk that may modify or supplement physiologic functions in the neonate, the role of prostaglandins comes under review. Prostaglandins include any of a class of physiologically active substances present in many tissues and originally described in genital fluid and accessory glands. Among the many effects are those of vasodepression, stimulation of intestinal smooth muscle, uterine stimulation, aggregation of blood platelets, and antagonism to hormones influencing lipid metabolism. Prostaglandins are a group of prostanoic acids often abbreviated PGE, PGF, PGA, and PGB with numeric subscripts according to structure.

The synthesis of prostaglandins occurs when dietary linoleic acid is converted in the body by a series of steps involving chain lengthening and dehydration to arachidonic acid, the principal (but not the only) precursor of prostaglandins. Although the prostaglandins are similar in structure, the biologic effects of various prostaglandins produced from a single unsaturated fatty acid can be profoundly different and, in some cases, antagonistic.

Because of the possible beneficial effects of prostaglandins on the GI tract of infants, several investigators[6,98] have measured levels in human milk. The measurements were made in colostrum, transitional milk, and mature milk with collections of both foremilk and hindmilk. PGE and PGF have

been shown to be present in breast milk in more than 100 times the concentration in adult plasma (Figure 4-13). The ratio of the principal metabolite of PGFM to PGF itself suggests a relatively long half-life. Although prostaglandins occur in cow milk, none was measurable in cow milk-based formulas. Two inactive metabolites were found in milk in levels similar to those in the control adult plasma.

It is thought that prostaglandins play a role in GI motility, possibly assisting peristalsis physiologically. Infantile diarrhea may occasionally be caused by excessive prostaglandin secretion into the mother's milk during menstruation, when maternal plasma levels of PGF may be raised. The difference in stool patterns between infants who are breastfed versus formula fed may be partially attributable to the presence of prostaglandins in human milk and not in formulas. The role of prostaglandins in the pathogenesis of food intolerance is also under study, because prostaglandins have a cytoprotective effect on the upper bowel and reportedly are increased in patients with abnormal peristalsis and irritable bowel syndrome.

Prostaglandins E_1, E_2, and $F_2\alpha$ (PGE_1, PGE_2, $PGF_2\alpha$) were determined in milk and plasma from mothers of term and preterm infants by Shimizu et al.[138] They found the concentration of PGE_1 in milk to be similar to that in plasma and the concentrations of PGE_2 and $PGF_2\alpha$ to be about 1.2 to 2 times higher in milk than in plasma. Foremilk and hindmilk levels, however, were similar, as were

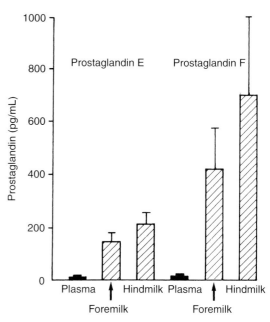

Figure 4-13. Prostaglandins E and F (PGE, PGF) (pg/mL ± SEM) in human milk and adult plasma. (From Lucas A, Mitchell MD: Prostaglandins in human milk, *Arch Dis Child* 55:950, 1980.)

term and preterm levels. Levels appeared to be constant throughout lactation. PGE_1 is credited with a variety of physiologic effects on the GI tract, including cytoprotection and a diarrhea-producing action. Other actions are expected and yet to be identified because of prostaglandins' stability throughout lactation and lack of degradation in milk and in the lumen of the gut.

In addition, human infants may require PGE_2 for maintenance of gastric mucosal integrity, as do adults. Therefore, it is not surprising that the use of prostaglandin synthesis inhibitors, such as indomethacin for closure of a patent ductus, is associated with necrotizing enterocolitis. PGE_2 in human milk may also promote the accumulation of phospholipids in the neonatal stomach, enhancing the gastric mucosal barrier.

Relaxin

Relaxin is a hormone with a polypeptide structure similar to that of insulin. It is produced by the corpus luteum during pregnancy as well as by the decidua and the placenta. Relaxin induces cervical softening, loosens the pelvic girdle, and decreases myometrial activity during pregnancy in many species.[43] Its role in humans remains under study.

It has been postulated that human mammary tissue is a target and a source of relaxin synthesis. Relaxin was measured by specific human relaxin radioimmunoassay in milk and sera of women delivering at term, prematurely at 3 days, and at 6 weeks postpartum.[43] Sera and milk levels were similar in term and preterm mothers; however, at 6 weeks, relaxin concentrations in milk were higher in the preterm group. The presence in milk at 6 weeks suggests a nonluteal site of synthesis. The authors suggest that before lactation, relaxin may aid the growth and differentiation of mammary tissue, and then in the neonate, it may act directly on the GI tract.

BILE SALTS

Another limiting factor in digestion in the newborn is the decreased bile salt pool and the low concentration of bile salts in the duodenum. The presence of some biologically active substances in human milk contributes to digestion in the newborn. For this reason, the role of bile salts was investigated, and cholate and chenodeoxycholate were found in all samples of milk obtained from 28 lactating women in the first postpartum week.[52] In both colostrum and milk, cholate predominated. Samples were randomly collected, and the range of concentration was wide. The ratio of maternal serum to milk levels was 1:1 for cholate and 4:1 for chenodeoxycholate. The significance of these findings is under study.

EPIDERMAL GROWTH FACTOR

EGF is a small polypeptide mitogen that has been identified in many species and isolated and characterized in human milk. Of the growth factors that have been purified to date, EGF is one of the most biologically potent and best characterized as to its physical, chemical, and biologic properties. EGF has been associated with neonatal maturation, mechanisms of milk collection, and various protective effects. It is well established that EGF stimulates the proliferation of epidermal and epithelial tissues and has significant biologic effects in the intact mammal, particularly in the fetus and the newborn. Effects verified in humans also include increased growth and maturation of the fetal pulmonary epithelium, stimulation of ornithine decarboxylase activity and DNA synthesis in the digestive tract, and acceleration of the healing of wounds of the corneal epithelium. Unrelated is the observation that EGF inhibits histamine- or pentagastrin-induced secretion of gastric acid. It has a maturational effect on duodenal mucosal cells and increased lactase activity and net calcium transport in suckling rats. EGF has been identified in plasma, saliva, urine, amniotic fluid, and milk. Human milk is known to be mitogenic for cultured cells. EGF is active when administered orally, stable in acid, and resistant to trypsin digestion.

Newborn puppies fed their mother's milk were found to have hyperplasia of the enteric mucosa as compared with formula-fed littermates. Furthermore, the intestinal weight, length, and DNA and RNA content were greater in the puppies fed their mother's milk.

Previous studies specified the presence of EGF in the aqueous portion of human milk only; however, Gullett et al.[59] have established that EGF and its receptor are found in all human milk compartments: aqueous, liposomal, and membranes (milk fat globule membranes [MFGMs]).

Studies of EGF in human milk first reported that human milk stimulates DNA synthesis in cell cultures in which growth had been arrested. The mitogenic activity of the milk was neutralized by the addition of an antibody to human EGF. These findings support the concept that EGF is a major growth-promoting agent in breast milk. Actual measurements of EGF in the milk of 11 mothers who delivered at term and 20 who delivered prematurely were also done. EGF concentrations were 68 ± 19 ng/mL (mean $\pm$ SEM) in those who delivered at term and 70 ± 5 ng/mL (mean $\pm$ SEM) in the milk of those who delivered prematurely. No significant change throughout 7 weeks and no diurnal variation were observed. The total EGF content was closely correlated with the volume of milk expressed, suggesting to the authors that EGF has a passive transport from the circulation as a function of plasma concentration.

Given that EGF has significant healing effects on injured GI tract mucosa and decreasing gestational age of neonates is associated with higher risk of developing GI disorders, the amount of EGF in milk is significant. Concentrations of EGF in human milk from extremely preterm (23 to 27 weeks) mothers were significantly higher than values obtained from preterm and full term mothers throughout the first month postpartum according to studies done by Dvorak et al.[42] They also noted that transforming growth factor (TGF-α) was also elevated in this group of mothers with extremely premature infants.

Using various techniques for assay, Iacopetta et al.[73] found 30 to 40 ng/mL EGF in human milk, less than 2 ng/mL in bovine milk, and none in several bovine milk-based formulas. Little change occurred with refrigeration or freezing. The role of EGF in promoting normal growth and functional maturation of the intestinal tract continues to be under study.

REFERENCES

1. Abrams SA, Wen J, Stuff JE: Absorption of calcium, zinc and iron from breast milk by five- to seven-month-old infants, Pediatr Res 41:384, 1996.
2. Adcock EW, Brewer ED, Caprioli RM, et al: Macronutrients, electrolytes and minerals in human milk: differences over time and between population groups. In Howell RR, Morriss FH, Pickering LK, editors: Human milk in infant nutrition and health, Springfield, Ill., 1986, Charles C. Thomas.
3. Agostonic C, Carratu B, Boniglia C, et al: Free glutamine and glutamic acid increase in human milk through a three-month lactation period, J Pediatr Gastroenterol Nutr 31(5):508–512, 2000.
4. Alaejos MS, Romero CD: Selenium in human lactation, Nutr Rev 53:159, 1995.
5. Allen JC, Keller RP, Archer P, et al: Studies in human lactation: milk composition and daily secretion rates of macronutrients in the first year of lactation, Am J Clin Nutr 54:69, 1991.
6. Alzina V, Puig M, de Echániz L, et al: Prostaglandins in human milk, Biol Neonate 50:200, 1986.
7. American Academy of Pediatrics: Section on breastfeeding: breastfeeding and the use of human milk, Pediatrics 129:e827–e841, 2012.
8. Ando K, Goto Y, Matsumoto Y, et al: Acquired zinc deficiency in a breast-fed mature infant: a possible cause of acquired maternal decreased zinc uptake by the mammary gland, J Am Acad Dermatol 29:111, 1993.
9. Asnes RS, Wisotsky DH, Migel PF, et al: The dietary chloride deficiency syndrome occurring in a breast-fed infant, J Pediatr 100:923, 1982.
10. Atkinson S, Alston-Mills B, Lönnerdal B, et al: Major minerals and ionic constituents of human and bovine milks. In Jensen RG, editor: Handbook of milk composition, San Diego, 1995, Academic Press.
11. Atkinson SA, Bryan MH, Anderson GH: Human milk: differences in nitrogen concentration in milk from mothers of term and premature infants, J Pediatr 93:67, 1978.
12. Atkinson SA, Lönnerdal B: Nonprotein nitrogen fractions of human milk. In Jensen RG, editor: Handbook of milk composition, San Diego, 1995, Academic Press.
13. Bernt KM, Walker WA: Human milk as a carrier of biochemical messages, Acta Paediatr 430(Suppl):27, 1999.
14. Birch EE, Birch DG, Hoffman DR, et al: Dietary essential fatty acid supply and visual activity development, Invest Ophthalmol Vis Sci 33:3242, 1992.
15. Bitman J, Wood DL, Neville MC, et al: Lipid composition of prepartum, preterm and term milk. In Hamosh M, Goldman AS, editors: Human lactation, maternal and environmental factors, vol. 2.
16. Bode L: Recent advances on structure, metabolism and function of human milk oligosaccharides, J Nutr 136: 2127–2130, 2006.
17. Büller H, Peters M, Burger B, et al: Vitamin K status beyond the neonatal period, Eur J Pediatr 145:496, 1986.
18. Buescher ES, McIlheran SM: Colostral antioxidants: separation and characterization of two activities in human colostrum, J Pediatr Gastroenterol Nutr 14:47, 1992.
19. Calvo EB, Galindo AC, Aspres ND: Iron status in exclusively breastfed infants, Pediatrics 90:375, 1992.
20. Canfield LM, Giuliano AR, Neilson EM, et al: Beta carotene in breast milk and serum is increased after a single beta carotene dose, Am J Clin Nutr 66:52, 1997.
21. Canfield LM, Hopkinson JM, Lima AF, et al: Vitamin K in colostrum and mature human milk over the lactational period: a cross-sectional study, Am J Clin Nutr 53:730, 1991.
22. Casey CE, Smith A, Zhang PC: Microminerals in human and animal milks. In Jensen RG, editor: Handbook of milk composition, San Diego, 1995, Academic Press.
23. Chang YT, Germain-Lee EL, Doran TF, et al: Hypocalcemia in non-white breastfed infants, Clin Pediatr 31:695, 1992.
24. Chen DC, Nommsen-Rivers L, Dewey KG, et al: Stress during labor and delivery and early lactation performance, Am J Clin Nutr 68:335, 1998.
25. Chu SW: Nucleotides: biochemistry and metabolism, Sem Pediatr Gastrol Nutr 2:11, 1991.
26. Coppa GV, Gabrielli O, Pierani P, et al: Changes in carbohydrate composition in human milk over 4 months of lactation, Pediatrics 91:637, 1993.
27. Coppa GV, Pierani P, Zampini L, et al: Oligosaccharides in human milk during different phases of lactation, Acta Paediatr 430(Suppl):91, 1999.
28. Cornelissen EAM, Kollee LAA, DeAbreu RA, et al: Effects of oral and intramuscular vitamin K prophylaxis on vitamin K1, PIVKA-II and clotting factors in breastfed infants, Arch Dis Child 67:1250, 1992.
29. Council on Environmental Health: Policy statement. Iodine deficiency, pollutant chemicals, and the thyroid: new information on an old problem, Pediatrics 133 (6):1163–1166, 2014.
30. Cox DB, Kent JC, Casey TM, et al: Breast growth and the urinary excretion of lactose during human pregnancy and early lactation: endocrine relationships, Exp Physiol 84 (2):421–434, 1999.
31. Cox DB, Owens RA, Hartmann PE: Blood and milk prolactin and the rate of milk synthesis in women, Exp Physiol 81:1007–1020, 1996.
32. Cross NA, Hillman LS, Allen SH, et al: Calcium homeostasis and bone metabolism during pregnancy, lactation, and post weaning: a longitudinal study, Am J Clin Nutr 61:514, 1995.
33. Czank C, Mitoulas LR, Hartman PE: Human milk composition: fat. In Hale TW, Hartmann PE, editors: Textbook of human lactation, Amarillo, Tex., 2007, Hale Publishing Inc.
34. DeSantiago S, Villalpando S, Ortiz N, et al: Protein requirements of marginally nourished lactating women, Am J Clin Nutr 62:364, 1995.
35. Dewey KG, Cohen RJ, Landa RI, et al: Effects of age of introduction of complementary foods on iron status of breastfed infants in Honduras, Am J Clin Nutr 67:878, 1998.
36. Dewey KG, Heinig MJ, Nommsen LA, et al: Maternal versus infant factors related to breast milk intake and residual milk volume: the DARLING Study, Pediatrics 87:829, 1991.

37. DeWille JW, Farmer SJ: Postnatal dietary fat influences mRNAs involved in myelination, *Dev Neurosci* 14:61, 1992.
38. Dorea JG: Is zinc a first limiting nutrient in human milk? *Nutr Res* 13:659, 1993.
39. Duncan B, Schifman RB, Corrigan JJ, et al: Iron and the exclusively breastfed infant from birth to six months, *J Pediatr Gastroenterol Nutr* 4:421, 1985.
40. Dunstan JA, Roper J, Mitoulas L, et al: The effect of supplementation with fish oil during pregnancy on breast milk immunoglobulin A, soluble CD 14, cytokine levels and fatty acid composition, *Clin Exp Allergy* 34:1237–1242, 2004.
41. Dupuy P, Sauniere JF, Vis HL, et al: Change in bile salt dependent lipase in human breast milk during extended lactation, *Lipids* 26:134, 1991.
42. Dvorak B, Fituch CC, Williams CS, et al: Increased epidermal growth factor levels in human milk of mothers with extremely premature infants, *Pediatr Res* 54(1):15–19, 2003.
43. Eddie LW, Sutton B, Fitzgerald S, et al: Relaxin in paired samples of serum and milk from women after term and pre-term delivery, *Am J Obstet Gynecol* 161:970, 1989.
44. Ekstrand J, Spak CJ, Falch J, et al: Distribution of fluoride to human breast milk following intake of high doses of fluoride, *Caries Res* 18:93, 1984.
45. Engle-Stove R, Haskell MJ, LaFrano MR, et al: Comparison of breast milk vitamin A concentration measured in fresh milk by a rapid field assay (the iCheck FLUORO) with standard measurement of stored milk by HPLC, *Eur J Clin Nutr* 68(8):938–940, 2014.
46. Fall CHD, Barker DJP, Osmond C, et al: Relation of infant feeding to adult serum cholesterol concentration and death from ischaemic heart disease, *Br Med J* 304:801, 1992.
47. Farquharson J, Cockburn F, Patrick WA, et al: Infant cerebral cortex phospholipid fatty-acid composition and diet, *Lancet* 340:810, 1992.
48. Filteau SM: Milk components with immunomodulatory potential. In Woodward B, Draper HH, editors: Advances in nutritional research, vol. 10, New York, 2001, Kluwer Academics/Plenum Publishers, p 327.
49. Finley DA, Lönnerdal B, Dewey KG, et al: Breast milk composition: fat content and fatty acid composition in vegetarians and non-vegetarians, *Am J Clin Nutr* 41:787, 1985.
50. Food and Nutrition Board, National Research Council, National Academy of Sciences: Recommended dietary allowances, ed 10, Washington, D.C., 1989, U.S. Government Printing Office.
51. Forsyth JS, Donnet L, Ross PE: A study of the relationship between bile salts, bile salt stimulated lipase, and free fatty acids in breast milk: normal infants and those with breast milk jaundice, *J Pediatr Gastroenterol Nutr* 11:205, 1990.
52. Forsyth JS, Ross PE, Bouchier IAD: Bile salts in breast milk, *Eur J Pediatr* 140:126, 1983.
53. Fransson GB, Lönnerdal B: Iron in human milk, *J Pediatr* 96:380, 1980.
54. Fransson GB, Lönnerdal B: Zinc, copper, calcium and magnesium in human milk, *J Pediatr* 101:504, 1982.
55. Gabbe SG, Niebyl JR, Simpson JL, et al: Obstetrics: normal and problem pregnancies, ed 4, Philadelphia, 2002, Churchill Livingstone, pp 92–93.
56. Gil A, Uauy R: Nucleotides and related compounds in human and bovine milk. In Jensen RG, editor: Handbook of milk composition, San Diego, 1995, Academic Press.
57. Greer F, Gartner L: Prevention of rickets and vitamin D deficiency: new guidelines for vitamin D intake, *Pediatrics* 111:908, 2003.
58. Greer FR, Marshal SP, Foley AL, et al: Improving vitamin K status of breastfeeding infants with maternal vitamin K supplements, *Pediatrics* 99:88, 1997.
59. Gullett SL, Baatz JE, Forsythe DW, et al: Establishing the presence of epidermal growth factor (EGF) and the EGFR in human milk's compartments, *ABM News Views* 9(4):26, 2003.
60. Hamosh M, Hong MH, Hamosh P: b-Casomorphins: milk b-casein derived opioid peptides. In Lebenthal E, editor: Textbook of gastroenterology and nutrition in infancy, 2 ed, New York, 1989, Raven.
61. Hamosh M: Breast milk jaundice, *J Pediatr Gastroenterol Nutr* 11:145, 1990.
62. Hamosh M: Enzymes in human milk. In Howell RR, Morriss FH, Pickering LK, editors: Human milk in infant nutrition and health, Springfield, Ill., 1986, Charles C Thomas.
63. Hamosh M: Lipid metabolism in pediatric nutrition, *Pediatr Clin North Am* 42:839, 1995.
64. Heine W, Braun OH, Mohr C, et al: Enhancement of lysozyme trypsin-mediated decay of intestinal bifidobacteria and lactobacilli, *J Pediatr Gastroenterol Nutr* 21:54, 1995.
65. Heird WC, Prager TC, Anderson RE: Docosahexaenoic acid and development and function of the infant retina, *Curr Opin Lipidol* 8:12, 1997.
66. Heiskanen K, Siimes MA, Perheentupa J, et al: Risk of low vitamin B_6 status in infants breast-fed exclusively beyond six months, *J Pediatr Gastroenterol Nutr* 23:38, 1996.
67. Hennet T, Weiss A, Borsig L: Decoding breast milk oligosaccharides, *Swiss Med Wkly* 144:w13927, 2014, http://dx.doi.org/10.444/smw.2014.13927.
68. Holick MF: Evolution, functions, and RDA. In Holick MF, editor: Vitamin D: physiology, molecular biology, and clinical applications, Totowa, N.J., 1999, Humana Press, p 1.
69. Hollis BW: Daily reference intake and lowest observed adverse effect level for vitamin D in the adult human subject with special emphasis on the pregnant women: a comparison of new and past data, *Am J Clin Nutr* 79:17, 2004.
70. Horwood LJ, Fergusson DM: Breastfeeding and later cognitive and academic outcomes, *Pediatrics* 101:e9, 1998.
71. Huston GE, Patton S: Membrane distribution in human milks throughout lactation as revealed by phospholipid and cholesterol analyses, *J Pediatr Gastroenterol Nutr* 5:602, 1986.
72. Huxtable RJ: Physiological actions of taurine, *Physiol Rev* 72:101, 1992.
73. Iacopetta BJ, Grieu F, Horlsberger M, et al: Epidermal growth factor in human and bovine milk, *Acta Paediatr* 81:287, 1992.
74. Innis SM, Hamilton JJ: Effects of developmental changes and early nutrition on cholesterol metabolism in infancy: a review, *J Am Coll Nutr* 11:635, 1992.
75. Innis SM: Human milk and formula fatty acids, *J Pediatr* 120(Suppl):556, 1992.
76. Jamieson EC, Abbasi KA, Cockburn F, et al: Effect of diet on term infant cerebral cortex fatty acid composition. In Galli C, Simopoulis AP, Tremoli E, editors: Fatty acids and lipids: biological aspects, *World Rev Nutr Diet* 75:139, 1994.
77. Jensen RG, Bitman J, Carlson SE: Milk lipids. A. Human milk lipids. In Jensen RG, editor: Handbook of milk composition, San Diego, 1995, Academic Press.
78. Jensen RG, Ferris AM, Lammi-Keefe CJ: Lipids in human milk and infant formulas, *Ann Rev Nutr* 12:417, 1992.
79. Jensen RG: Introduction. In Jensen RG, editor: Handbook of milk composition, San Diego, 1995, Academic Press.
80. Jensen RG: Lipids in human milk: a review, *Lipids* 34:243, 1999.
81. Jooste PL, Roosouw LJ, Steenkamp HJ, et al: Effect of breastfeeding on the plasma cholesterol and growth of infants, *J Pediatr Gastroenterol Nutr* 13:139, 1991.
82. Kalkwarf HJ, Specker BL, Bianchi DC, et al: The effect of calcium supplementation on bone density during lactation and after weaning, *N Engl J Med* 337:523, 1997.
83. Kallio MJT, Salmenperä L, Siimes MA, et al: Exclusive breastfeeding and weaning: effect on serum cholesterol

and lipoprotein concentrations in infants during the first year of life, *Pediatrics* 89:663, 1992.

84. Kent JC, Mitoulas LR, Cregan MD, et al: Volume and frequency of breastfeedings and fat content of breast milk throughout the day, *Pediatrics* 117:e387–e395, 2006.

85. Khoshoo V, Kjarsgaar DJ, Krafchick B, et al: Zinc deficiency in a full term breastfed infant: unusual presentation, *Pediatrics* 89:1094, 1992.

86. Koldovsky O, Strbak V: Hormones and growth factors in human milk. In Jensen RG, editor: *Handbook of milk composition*, San Diego, 1995, Academic Press.

87. Koski KG, Hill FW, Lönnerdal B: Altered lactational performance in rats fed low carbohydrate diets and its effect on growth of neonatal rat pups, *J Nutr* 120:1028, 1990.

88. Krebs NF, Hambidge KM: Zinc requirements and zinc intakes in breastfed infants, *Am J Clin Nutr* 43:288, 1986.

89. Krebs NF, Reidinger CJ, Robertson AD, et al: Bone mineral density changes during lactation: maternal, dietary, and biochemical correlates, *Am J Clin Nutr* 65:1738, 1997.

90. Kretchmer N: Lactose and lactase, *Sci Am* 227:73, 1972.

91. Kumpulainen J, Vuori E: Longitudinal study of chromium in human milk, *Am J Clin Nutr* 33:2299, 1980.

92. Kunz C, Lönnerdal B: Re-evaluation of whey protein/casein ratio of human milk, *Acta Paediatr* 81:107, 1992.

93. Lönnerdal B, Forsum E: Casein content of human milk, *Am J Clin Nutr* 41:113, 1985.

94. Lönnerdal B: Effects of maternal dietary intake on human milk composition, *J Nutr* 116:499, 1986.

95. Lammi-Keefe CJ: Vitamin D and E in human milk. In Jensen RG, editor: *Handbook of milk composition*, San Diego, 1995, Academic Press.

96. Lindberg T, Skude G: Amylase in human milk, *Pediatrics* 70:235, 1982.

97. Lubetsky R, Littner Y, Mimouni FB, et al: Circadian variations in fat content of expressed breast milk from mothers of preterm infants, *J Am Coll Nutr* 25:151–154, 2006.

98. Lucas A, Mitchell MD: Prostaglandins in human milk, *Arch Dis Child* 55:950, 1980.

99. Lucas A, Morley R, Cole TJ, et al: A randomised multicentre study of human milk versus formula and later development in preterm infants, *Arch Dis Child* 70:F141, 1994.

100. Lucas A, Morley R, Cole TJ, et al: Breast milk and subsequent intelligence quotient in children born preterm, *Lancet* 339:261, 1992.

101. Makrides M, Neumann MA, Gibson RA: Effect of maternal docosahexaenoic acid (DHA) supplementation on breast milk composition, *Eur J Clin Nutr* 50:352, 1996.

102. Mandel D, Lubetzky R, Dollberg S, et al: Fat and energy contents of expressed human breast milk in prolonged lactation, *Pediatrics* 116:e432–e435, 2005.

103. Mitoulas LR, Gurrin LC, Doherty DA, et al: Infant intake of fatty acids from human milk over the first year of lactation, *Br J Nutr* 90:979–986, 2003.

103a. Morrow AL, Ruiz-Palacios GM, Altahye M, et al: Human milk oligosaccharides are associated with protection against diarrhea in breast-fed infants, *J Pediatr* 145:297–303, 2004a.

104. Morton JA: The clinical usefulness of breast milk sodium in the assessment of lactogenesis, *Pediatrics* 93:802, 1994.

105. Moser PB, Reynolds RD: Dietary zinc intake and zinc concentrations of plasma, erythrocytes, and breast milk in antepartum and postpartum lactating and nonlactating women: a longitudinal study, *Am J Clin Nutr* 38:101, 1983.

106. Motil KJ, Thotathuchery M, Bahar A, et al: Marginal dietary protein restriction, reduced nonprotein nitrogen, but not protein nitrogen, components of human milk, *J Am Coll Nutr* 14:184, 1995.

107. Mott GE, Lewis DS, McGill HC Jr: Programming of cholesterol metabolism by breast or formula feeding. The childhood environment and adult disease, *Ciba Found Symp* 156:56, 1991.

108. National Academy of Science: *Nutrition during lactation. Institute of Medicine*, Washington, D.C., 1991, National Academy Press.

109. National Academy of Sciences: *Report of the subcommittee on nutrition during lactation. The Institute of Medicine*, Washington, D.C., 1991, National Academy Press.

110. Neville MC, Casey C, Hay WW: Endocrine regulation of nutrient flux in the lactating woman. In Allen L, King J, Lonnerdal B, editors: *Nutrient regulation during pregnancy, lactation, and infant growth*, New York, 1994, Plenum Press, p 85.

111. Neville MC, Morton J, Umenura S: Lactogenesis: the transition from pregnancy to lactogenesis, *Pediatr Clin North Am* 48:35, 2001.

112. Neville MC: Determinants of milk volume and composition. In Jensen RG, editor: *Handbook of milk composition*, San Diego, 1995, Academic Press.

113. Neville MC: Mammary gland biology and lactation: a short course. Presented at biannual meeting of the international society for research on human milk and lactation, Mass., October 1997, Plymouth.

114. Neville MC: Sampling and storage of human milk. In Jensen RG, editor: *Handbook of milk composition*, San Diego, 1995, Academic Press.

115. Neville MC: Volume and caloric density of human milk. In Jensen RG, editor: *Handbook of milk composition*, San Diego, 1995, Academic Press.

116. Neville MC, Zhang P, Allen JC: Minerals, ions, and trace elements in milk. A. Ionic interactions in milk. In Jensen RG, editor: *Handbook of milk composition*, San Diego, 1995, Academic Press.

117. Newburg DS: Oligosaccharides and glycoconjugates in human milk: their role in host defense, *J Mammary Gland Biol Neoplasia* 1:271, 1996.

118. Newman V: *Vitamin A, and breastfeeding: a comparison of data from developed and developing countries*, San Diego, 1993, Wellstart International.

119. Nommsen LA, Lovelady CA, Heinig MJ, et al: Determinants of energy, protein, lipid, and lactose concentrations in human milk during the first 12 months of lactation: the DARLING study, *Am J Clin Nutr* 53:457, 1991.

120. O'Connor DL, Tamura T, Picciano MF: Pteroylpolyglutamates in human milk, *Am J Clin Nutr* 53:930, 1991.

121. Obladen M: Milk demystified by chemistry, *J Perinat Med* 42(5):641–647, 2014. http://dx.doi.org/10.1515/jpm-2013-0288.

122. Odintsova ES, Buneva VN, Nevinsky GA: Casein-hydrolyzing activity of sIgA antibodies from human milk, *J Mol Recognit* 18:413, 2005.

123. Ortega RM, Andres P, Martinez RM, et al: Vitamin status during the third trimester of pregnancy in Spanish women: influence on concentrations of vitamin A in breast milk, *Am J Clin Nutr* 66:564, 1997.

124. Orzali A, Donzelli F, Enzi G, et al: Effect of carnitine on lipid metabolism in the newborn, *Biol Neonate* 43:186, 1983.

125. Oski FA: What we eat may determine who we can be, *Nutrition* 13:220, 1997.

126. Otten J, Pitze Hellwig J, Meyers L: *Dietary reference intake: the essential guide to nutrient requirements*, Washington, D.C., 2006, Institute of Medicine National Academy Press.

127. Picciano MF: Vitamins in milk. A. Water-soluble vitamins in human milk composition. In Jensen RG, editor: *Handbook of milk composition*, San Diego, 1995, Academic Press.

128. Pisacane A, DeVizia B, Valiante A, et al: Iron status in breast-fed infants, *J Pediatr* 127:429, 1995.

129. Pollack PF, Koldovsky O, Nishioka K: Polyamines in human and rat milk and in infant formulas, *Am J Clin Nutr* 56:371, 1992.

130. Quan R, Uauy R: Nucleotides and gastrointestinal development, *Sem Pediatr Gastrol Nutr* 2:3, 1991.

131. Rassin DK, Sturman JA, Gaull GE: Taurine in milk: species variation, *Pediatr Res* 11:449, 1977.
132. Reisbick S, Neuringer M, Connor WE, et al: Postnatal deficiency of omega-3 fatty acids in monkeys: fluid intake and urine concentration, *Physiol Behav* 51:473, 1992.
133. Romain N, Dandrifosse G, Jeusette F, et al: Polyamine concentration in rat milk and food, human milk and infant formulas, *Pediatr Res* 32:58, 1992.
134. Sandberg DP, Begley JA, Hall CA: The content, binding, and forms of vitamin B12 in milk, *Am J Clin Nutr* 34:1717, 1981.
135. Schams D, Karg H: Hormones in milk, *Ann N Y Acad Sci* 464:75, 1986.
136. Sellmayer A, Koletzko B: Long chain polyunsaturated fatty acids and eicosanoids in infants: physiological and pathophysiological aspects and open questions, *Lipids* 34:199, 1999.
137. Sherry CL, Oliver JS, Renzi LM, et al: Lutein supplementation increases breast milk and plasma lutein concentrations in lactating women and infant plasma concentrations but does not affect other carotenoids, *J Nutr* 144(8):1256–1263, 2014.
138. Shimizu T, Yamashiro Y, Yabuta K: Prostaglandin E1, E2, and F2a in human milk and plasma, *Biol Neonate* 61:222, 1992.
139. Shoji H, Shimizu T, Kaneko N, et al: Comparison of philosophical classes in human milk in Japanese mothers of term and preterm infants, *Acta Paediatr* 95:996–1000, 2006.
140. Simopoulas AP: Omega-3 fatty acids in health and disease in growth and development, *Am J Clin Nutr* 54:438, 1991.
141. Specker BL, Black A, Allen L, et al: Vitamin B12: low milk concentrations are reported to correspond to low serum concentrations in vegetarian women and to methylmalonic aciduria in their infants, *Am J Clin Nutr* 52:1073, 1990.
142. Specker BL, Tsang RC, Ho ML, et al: Effect of vegetarian diet on serum 1,25-dihydroxyvitamin D concentrations during lactation, *Obstet Gynecol* 70:870, 1987.
143. Suzuki YA, Shin K, Lönnerdal B: Molecular cloning and functional expression of a human intestinal lactoferrin receptor, *Biochemistry* 40:15771–15779, 2001.
144. Thomas MR, Sneed SM, Wei C, et al: The effects of vitamin C, vitamin B6, and vitamin B12, folic acid, riboflavin, and thiamin on the breast milk and maternal status of well-nourished women at 6 months postpartum, *Am J Clin Nutr* 33:2151, 1980.
145. Tomashek K, Nesby-O'Dell S, Scanlon KS, et al: Nutritional rickets in Georgia, *Pediatrics* 107:E45, 2001.
146. Tran TT, Chowanadisai W, Crinella FM, et al: Effects of neonatal dietary manganese exposure on brain dopamine levels and neurocognitive functions, *Neurotoxicology* 23 (4-5):645–651, 2002.
147. Vorbach C, Capecchi MR, Penninger JM: Evolution of the mammary gland from the innate immune system, *Bioessays* 28:606–616, 2006.
148. Vorherr H: *The breast: morphology, physiology, and lactation*, New York, 1974, Academic Press.
149. Wagner CL, Howard C, Lawrence RA, et al: Maternal vitamin D supplementation during lactation: a viable alternative to infant supplementation, *Pediatr Res* 53:255A, 2003.
150. Welch T, Bergstrom W, Tsang R: Vitamin D-deficient rickets: the reemergence of a once-conquered disease, *J Pediatr* 137:143, 2000.
151. Wojcik KY, Rechtman DJ, Lee ML, et al: Mactonutrient analysis of a nationwide sample of donor breast milk, *J Am Diet Assoc* 109:137–140, 2009.
152. Yolken RH, Peterson JA, Vonderfecht SL, et al: Human milk mucin inhibits rotavirus replication and prevents experimental gastroenteritis, *J Clin Invest* 90:1984, 1992.
153. Yuhas R, Pramuk K, Lien EL: Human milk fatty acid composition from nine countries varies most in DHA, *Lipids* 41:851–857, 2006.
154. Ziegler EE, Nelson SE, Jeter JM: Vitamin D supplementation of breastfed Infants. A randomized close-response trial, *Pediatr Res* 76(2):177–183, 2014.

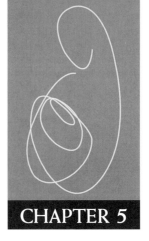

Host-Resistance Factors and Immunologic Significance of Human Milk

Some of the most dramatic and far-reaching advances in the understanding of the immunologic benefits of human milk have been made using newer techniques to demonstrate the specific contribution of the numerous "bioactive factors" contained in human milk (Table 5-1). The multifunctional capabilities of the individual factors, the interactive coordinated functioning of these factors, and the longitudinal changes in the relative concentrations of them for the duration of lactation make human milk unique. The immunologically active components of breast milk make up an important aspect of the host defenses of the mammary gland in the mother; at the same time, they complement, supplement, and stimulate the ongoing development of the infant's immune system.[130–132]

The explosion of research on all the immunologic properties and actions of breast milk in the last 10 years makes it impossible to summarize all the important aspects of what we now know about the immunologic benefits of breast milk. The recently developed technologies of genomic studies using microarrays and proteomics promise to continue this rapid expansion of knowledge on the biology of the mammary gland, human milk, and the infant's developing immune system.

The common comment about the immunologic benefits of breast milk, "It has antibodies," is a huge understatement. Antibodies in human milk play a relatively small role in the immune protection for the infant produced by breastfeeding. The intestinal microbiome, mucosal immunity, nucleotides, probiotics and prebiotics, oligosaccharides, and

glycans related to the ingestion of human milk are much more important components of the infant's immune protection.* The developing immunity of infants is a dynamic process. It is made all the more complex by the contextual nature of the interactions of various components in human milk with the developing gastrointestinal (GI) tract. This directly affects both local and systemic immunity over time. This chapter emphasizes the important concepts of these immunologic benefits and refers the interested reader to the most recent literature for more extensive information on the many specific components.

Overview

The immunologic benefits of human milk can be analyzed from a variety of perspectives:

1. Reviewing the published information on the protection of infants from specific infections that compares breastfed and formula-fed infants.
2. Comparing documented deficiencies in infants' developing immune systems and the actions of bioactive factors provided in breast milk.
3. Examining the proposed function of the active components contained in human milk: antimicrobial, antiinflammatory, and immunomodulating.
4. Considering the nature of the different factors: soluble, cellular, and hormone-like.
5. Examining the contribution of breast milk to immune protection of the mammary gland.

*21,87,158,236,237,254,328

TABLE 5-1 Immunologically and Pharmacologically Active Components and Hormones Observed in Human Colostrum and Milk

Soluble	Cellular	Hormones and Hormone-Like Substances
Immunologically specific	Immunologically specific	Epidermal growth factor
Immunoglobulin	T-lymphocytes	Prostaglandins
sIgA (11S), 7S IgA, IgG, IgM IgE, IgD, secretory component	B-lymphocytes	Relaxin
		Neurotensin
	Accessory cells	Somatostatin
	Neutrophils	Bombesin
T cell products	Macrophages	Gonadotropins
Histocompatibility antigens	Epithelial cells	Ovarian steroids
		Thyroid-releasing hormone
	Additional cells	Thyroid-stimulating hormone
Nonspecific factors	Stem cells	Thyroxine and triiodothyronine
Complement		Adrenocorticotropin
Chemotactic factors		Corticosteroids
Properdin (factor P)		Prolactin
Interferon		Erythropoietin
α-Fetoprotein		Insulin
Bifidus factor		Cytokines
Antistaphylococcal factor(s)		Interleukins
Antiadherence substances		
Epidermal growth factor		
Folate uptake enhancer		
Antiviral factor(s)		
Migration inhibition factor		
Gangliosides		
Nucleotides		
Antisecretory factor		
Spermine		
Soluble CD14		
Carrier proteins		
Lactoferrin		
Transferrin		
Vitamin B_{12}-binding protein		
Corticoid-binding protein		
Enzymes		
Lysozyme		
Lipoprotein lipase		
Leukocyte enzymes		

Modified from Ogra PL, Fishaut M: Human breast milk. In Remington JS, Klein JO, editors: *Infectious diseases of the fetus and newborn infant,* ed 4, Philadelphia, 1995, Saunders.

6. Determining the site of the postulated action of the specific factors (e.g., in the breast or in the infant) at the mucosal level (respiratory tract or GI tract) or at the systemic level.

7. Classifying the factors relative to their contribution to the constitutive defenses (innate immunity) versus the inducible defenses (adaptive immunity) of the infant's immune system.

8. Clarifying the mechanism of action of the proposed immunologic benefit (e.g., the mucosal-associated lymphoid tissue [MALT] forms bioactive factors at the level of the mucosa, which migrate to the breast and breast milk, activating cells at those sites).

9. Considering the contribution of human milk to the development of an infant's immune system relative to potential long-term immunologic benefits,

such as protection against allergy, asthma, autoimmune disease, or inflammatory bowel disease.

Protective Effect of Breast Milk

The protective effect of breast milk against infection was documented as early as 1892 in the medical literature. Data proved that milk from various species, including humans, was protective for offspring, containing antibodies against a vast number of antigens.[329]

Veterinarians have long known the urgency of offspring receiving the early milk of the mother. Death rates among human newborns not suckled at the breast in the Third World are at least five times higher than among those who receive colostrum and the mother's milk. The evidence that a lack of breastfeeding and poor environmental sanitation have a pernicious synergistic effect on infant mortality rate has been presented by Habicht et al.,[123] after studying 1262 women in Malaysia.

The evidence that breastfeeding protects against infections in the digestive and respiratory tracts has been reported for several decades.[326] However, many of the older studies were criticized for flawed methodology, and because they were performed in "developing countries," where the risk for infection due to poor sanitation was expected to be higher.[15,123,143] Various researchers have proposed specific criteria for assessing the methodology of studies reporting on the protective effects of breast milk, clearly identifying measurable outcomes and the definition of breastfeeding, with other methods to limit bias and to control for confounding variables.[15,59,180,182] More recent studies, which have incorporated many of the proposed methodologic criteria, continue to document that breastfeeding protects infants against diarrhea, respiratory infections,

and otitis media.* Individual papers report protection against urinary tract infections and neonatal sepsis.[7,132,266,333] Several papers document the decreased risk for dying in infancy associated with exclusive or predominant breastfeeding in Pakistan, Peru, Ghana, India, Nepal, and Bangladesh.[5,7,10,80,218] A systematic review by the Bellagio Child Survival Study Group predicted that exclusive breastfeeding for 90% of all infants through 6 months of age could prevent 13% of the childhood deaths occurring younger than 5 years of age.[165] Recent reviews on human breast milk document the evidence for protection against infectious diseases from breastfeeding, for resource-rich and resource-poor countries.[77,155,187]

Dose-Response Relationship

One of the important considerations relative to measuring the immunologic benefits of breast milk is the exclusivity and duration of breastfeeding. The basic concept is identifying a dose-response relationship between the amount of breast milk received by an infant during the period of observation and the immunologic benefit gained. This is equatable to the dose-response relationship for a medication and a specific measurable effect of that medication. In the case of breast milk, the "dose" or volume of breast milk consumed by the infant will be increased by the greater exclusivity and the longer duration of breastfeeding. Dr. Labbok and Krasovec[182] have carefully defined breastfeeding in terms of the patterns of breastfeeding relative to the amount of supplementation with formula or other fluids or foods (full/nearly full, medium or equal, low partial, or token) to standardize the use of equatable terms in different studies. Box 5-1 outlines these definitions

---

*3,8,18,54,64,70,150,202,243,252,269,273,292,338

BOX 5-1. Breastfeeding Definitions

Any breastfeeding	Full breastfeeding	Exclusive human breast milk only	Infant ingests no other nutrients, supplements, or liquids
		Almost exclusive	No milk other than human milk; only minimal amounts of other substances such as water, juice, tea, or vitamins
	Partial breastfeeding	High partial	Nearly all feeds are human milk (at least 80%)
		Medium partial	A moderate amount of feeds are breast milk, in combination with other nutrient foods and nonhuman milk (20%-80% of nutritional intake is human breast milk)
		Low partial	Almost no feeds are breast milk (less than 20% of intake is breast milk)
	Token		Breastfeeding primarily for comfort; nonnutritive, for short periods of time, or infrequent
Never breastfed	Infant never ingested any human milk		

of the "amount" of breastfeeding.[187] Raisler et al.[274] referred to a dose-response relationship when they studied the effect of "dose" of breast milk on preventing illness in more than 7000 infants. "Full breastfeeding" was associated with the lowest rates of illness (diarrhea, cough, or wheeze), and even children with "most" or "equal" breastfeeding had evidence of lower odds ratios of ear infections and certain other illnesses. A number of other long-term studies demonstrated greater protection from infection with increased exclusivity of breastfeeding and durations of at least 3 months. A couple of papers demonstrated a "dose" effect relative to decreased occurrence of late onset sepsis in very-low-birth-weight (VLBW) infants[95] and premature infants[294] associated with the infants' receiving at least 50 mL/kg per day of the mother's milk, compared with receiving other nutrition. The current recommendations from the American Academy of Pediatrics reinforce the importance of the dose-response relationship between breastfeeding and the benefits of breastfeeding. The AAP recommends exclusive breastfeeding for the first 6 months of life and at least partial breastfeeding after the introduction of solid foods for an additional 12 months or longer.* Another important consideration, relative to exclusive breastfeeding, is the potential effect of other foods and fluids in an infant's diet that could negatively influence immunologic benefits and infection-protective effects at the level of the GI mucosa.

Developmental Deficiencies in Infants' Immune Systems

The human immune system begins forming and developing in the fetus. Newborn infants' immune systems are immature and inadequate at birth. Immune systems rapidly adapt in the postnatal period. These are related to the natural maturation of the skin and mucosal barriers and in response to the exposure of infants to inhaled and ingested antigens and microbial agents in the extrauterine environment. Infants' immune systems develop throughout at least the first 2 years of life. Overall, infants have limited abilities to respond effectively and quickly to infectious challenges, which explains infants' ongoing susceptibility to infections.** Box 5-2 lists most of the better understood deficiencies in infants' immune systems. An extensive discussion of these developmental immune deficiencies affecting infants is presented by Lawrence and Pane.[187] The B-lymphocytes and immunoglobulin production are deficient in the amount and

---

*3,17,64,70,75,78,150,202,252,269,292,338
**56,106,107,109,148,339

BOX 5-2. Developmental Defects in Newborns

Phagocytes (function matures over the first 6 months of life):

Limited reserve production of phagocytes in response to infection

Poor adhesion molecule function for migration

Abnormal transendothelial migration

Inadequate chemotactic response

Qualitative deficits in hydroxyl radical production

Decreased numbers of phagocytes reaching the site of infection

Cell-mediated immunity:

Limited numbers of mature functioning (memory) T cells (gradual acquisition of memory T cells throughout childhood)

Decreased cytokine production: IFN-α, IL-2, IL-4, IL-10

Diminished NK cell cytolytic activity (matures by 6 months of age)

Limited antibody-dependent cytotoxic cell activity

Poor stimulation of B-cells (subsequent antibody production, isotype switching)

B-lymphocytes and immunoglobulins:

Limited amounts and repertoire of active antibody production

Poor isotype switching (primarily IgM and IgG1 produced in neonates)

IgG1 and IgG3 production is limited (matures at 1 to 2 years of age)

IgG2 and IgG4 production is delayed (matures at 3 to 7 years of age)

Serum IgA levels are low (less than adult levels through 6 to 8 years of age)

Deficient opsonization by immunoglobulins

Poor response to T cell independent antigens (polysaccharides) (matures at 2 to 3 years of age)

Complement cascade:

Decreased function in both the classical and the alternative pathways

Insufficient amounts of C5a

---

specificity of antibodies produced. There is limited isotype switching and slow maturation of the antibody response to specific antigens (polysaccharides).[140,216] The systemic cell-mediated immune response, including effector and memory T cells, is functionally limited in its response in infants.[304,331,341] Neutrophil activity in infants is also developmentally delayed, which directly contributes to infants' susceptibility to invasive bacterial infections during the first months of life.[192,209,300,309,342] The complement system in infants is characterized by low levels of complement components, and both the "classical" and alternative pathways have limitations for complement activation.[2,81,302,335] Numerous immune components are produced in limited amounts in infancy, including complement, interferon-γ, secretory immunoglobulin

A(sIgA), interleukins (IL-3, IL-6, IL-10), tumor necrosis factor (TNF)-α, lactoferrin, and lysozyme.[56,109]

Relative to these various immune deficits in infants, one can find various bioactive and immunomodulating factors in breast milk that are potentially capable of complementing and enhancing the development of infants' mucosal and systemic immune systems.[109,133] This concept of bioactive and immunomodulating factors in breast milk is an important area of evolving research that has been extensively reviewed in the literature.[109,110,133,176] The most intense focus of this research centers on the effects of human milk on infants' GI tract.[107,245]

Bioactive Factors

The bioactive factors being studied are as diverse as proteins (lactoferrin, lysozyme, etc.), hormones (erythropoietin, prolactin, insulin, etc.), growth factors (epithelial growth factor, insulin-like growth factor, etc.), neuropeptides (neurotensin, somatostatin, etc.), cytokines (TNF-α, IL-6, etc.), antiinflammatory agents (enzymes, antioxidants, etc.), and nucleotides (see Table 5-1). In the past, it was adequate to point to the lists of factors (especially immunoglobulins) to "explain" the immunologic benefit of breast milk. Today, it is necessary to understand not only the "actions" of the specific factors but to understand how they interact with and affect the action of multiple other factors acting on the same process or system. For example, it is important to understand how secretory IgA (sIgA) interacts with or affects the actions of other bioactive factors (lactoferrin, complement and mucins) at the level of the intestinal mucosa. The specific effects of the dynamic interactions of the numerous bioactive factors on mucosal immunity, the development of the infant's immune system, and local inflammation are only beginning to be understood.

From an evolutionary perspective, maternal antibodies are transmitted to the fetus by different pathways in different species.[109,193,313] An association has been recognized between the number of placental membranes and the relative importance of the placenta and the colostrum as sources of antibodies. By this analysis, horses, with six placental membranes, pass little or no antibodies transplacentally and rely totally on colostrum for protection of foals. Humans and monkeys, having three placental membranes, receive more of the antibodies via the placenta and less from the colostrum. The transfer of IgG in humans is accomplished by the active transport mechanism of the immunoglobulin across the placenta. Secretory IgA (sIgA) immunoglobulins are found in human milk and provide local protection to the mucous membranes of the GI tract. Other investigations have established that the

mammary glands and their secretion of milk are important in protecting the infant not only through the colostrum, but also through mature milk from birth through the early months of life.

Although the predominance of IgA in human colostrum and milk had long been described, the importance of this phenomenon was not fully appreciated until the discovery that IgA is a predominant immunoglobulin. It is present in mucosal secretions of other glands, in addition to the breast.

Mucosal Immunity

Mucosal immunity has become the subject of extensive research.[28,29,148,245] It is clear that considerable traffic of cells occurs between mucosal, epithelial, and secretory, or lymphoid, tissue sites.[263] The data support the concept of a general system of MALT, which includes the gut, lung, mammary gland, salivary and lacrimal glands, and the genital tract (Figure 5-2). Through the immune response of MALT, a reaction to an immunogen at a mucosal site may be an effective means of producing immunity at distant sites. Antibodies against specific antigens found in milk have also been found in the saliva, which is evidence for transfer of protection to two different distant sites simultaneously. Evidence suggests that the mammary glands may act as extensions of the gut-associated lymphoid tissue (GALT) and possibly the bronchiole-associated lymphoid tissue. The ability of epithelial surfaces exposed to the external environment to defend against infectious agents has been well documented for the GI, genitourinary, and respiratory tracts.[174] The sIgA and secretory IgM (sIgM) produced through the adaptive response of the mucosal-lymphoid immune system act by blocking colonization with pathogens and limiting the passage of harmful antigens across the mucosal barrier. Activated B-cells and cytokines pass to the mammary gland, where they contribute to the production of sIgA in breast milk. Direct contact between the antigen and the lymphoid cells of the breast is unlikely.[246] Peyer's patches, tonsils, and other MALT structures appear to be well developed at birth.[39] Even with the Peyer's patches, tonsils, and lymphoid tissue at the mucosal level being well developed at birth, there is inadequate production of sIgA and serum IgA in infancy. A breastfeeding infant, as part of the maternal-infant dyad exposed to the same antigens via their mucosal services, can receive protective sIgA and sIgM in the mother's breast milk, produced by the mother's MALT (Figure 5-2).

The protective properties of human milk can be divided into cellular factors and humoral factors for facility of discussion, although they are closely related in vivo. A wide variety of soluble and cellular components and hormone-like agents have been

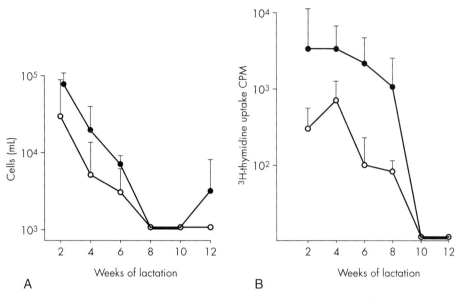

Figure 5-1. A, Longitudinal study of numbers of leukocytes. **B,** Longitudinal study of uptake of ^{3}H-thymidine in lymphocytes. Same subjects were examined during second through twelfth week of lactation. Data are presented as mean ± SD of macrophages-neutrophils (•) and lymphocytes (○) in A and of stimulated (•) and unstimulated (○) lymphocytes in B. (From Goldman AS, Garza C, Nichols BL, et al: Immunologic factors in human milk during the first year of lactation, *J Pediatr* 100:563, 1982.)

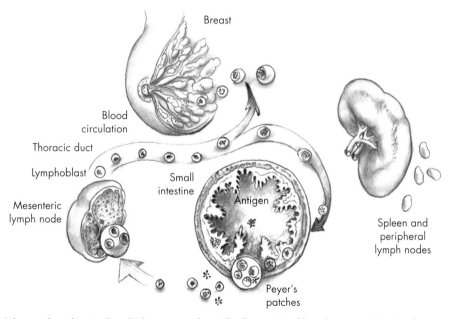

Figure 5-2. Schema of mechanism by which progeny of specifically sensitized lymphocytes originating from gut-associated lymphoid tissue may migrate to and infiltrate mammary gland and its secretions, supplying breast with immune cells. (Modified from Head JR, Beer AE: The immunologic role of viable leukocytic cells in mammary exosecretions. In Larson BL, editor: *Lactation, vol 4, mammary gland/human lactation/milk synthesis*, New York, 1978, Academic Press.)

identified in human milk and colostrum (see Table 5-1). Although the following discussion separates these elements, it is important to emphasize that the constituents of human milk are multifunctional and their functioning in vivo is interactive and probably coordinated and complementary.

Cellular Components of Human Colostrum and Milk

Cells are an important postpartum component of maternal immunologic endowment. More than

100 years ago, cell bodies were described in the colostrum of animals. As with much lactation research, further study of colostral corpuscles was undertaken by the dairy industry for commercial reasons in the early 1900s. This research afforded an opportunity to make major progress in the understanding of cells in milk. Initially, it was thought that these cells represented a reaction to infection in the mammary gland and were even described as "pus cells."

It has become clear that the cells of milk are normal constituents of colostrum in all species. Cells include macrophages, lymphocytes, neutrophils, and epithelial cells, and they total approximately 4000/mm[3]. Cell fragments and epithelial cells were examined by electron microscope in fresh samples from 30 women by Brooker.[35] He found that the membrane-bound cytoplasmic fragments in the sedimentation pellet outnumbered intact cells. The fragments were mostly from secretory cells that contained numerous cisternae of rough endoplasmic reticulum, lipid droplets, and Golgi vesicles containing casein micelles. Secretory epithelial cells were found in all samples and, after the second month postpartum, began to outnumber macrophages. Ductal epithelial cells were about 1% of the population of cells for the first week or so and then disappeared. All samples contained squamous epithelial cells, originating from galactophores and the skin of the nipple.

LEUKOCYTES

Living leukocytes are normally present in human milk.[174] The overall concentration of these leukocytes is of the same order of magnitude as that seen in peripheral blood, although the predominant cell in milk is the macrophage rather than the neutrophil. Macrophages compose about 90% of the leukocytes, and 2000 to 3000/mm[3] are present. Lymphocytes make up about 5% to 10% of the cells (200 to 300/mm[3]), which is a much lower concentration than in human blood.[113] The number of cells found in human milk increases with mastitis. Both large and small lymphocytes are present. By indirect immunofluorescence with anti-T cell antibody to identify thymus-derived lymphocytes, it has been shown that 50% of human colostral lymphocytes are T cells, and up to 80% of the lymphocytes in human milk are T cells.[334] Immunofluorescence procedures to detect surface immunoglobulins characteristic of B-lymphocytes identified 34% as B-lymphocytes.

The number of leukocytes and the degree of mitogenic stimulation of lymphocytes sharply decline during the first 2 or 3 months of lactation to essentially undetectable levels, according to Goldman et al. (Figure 5-1).[247] Enumeration of

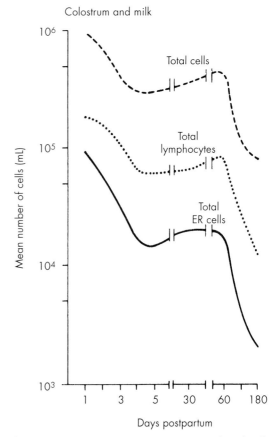

Figure 5-3. Geometric mean concentration of total cells, lymphocytes, and erythrocyte rosette-forming cells (ER) in colostrum and milk of 200 lactating women. (Modified from Ogra SS, Ogra PL: Immunologic aspects of human colostrum and milk. I. Distribution characteristics and concentrations of immunoglobulins at different times after the onset of lactation, *J Pediatr* 92:546, 1978.)

the total cell numbers in milk has been difficult, but when various techniques are compared (Coulter electronic particle counter, visual cell counting with special stains, filter trapping with fluorescent detection, and automated fluorescent cell counting), stains for deoxyribonucleic acid (DNA) were superior to the other techniques.

MACROPHAGES

Macrophages are large-complex phagocytes that contain lysosomes, mitochondria, pinosomes, ribosomes, and a Golgi apparatus. The monocytic phagocytes are lipid laden and were previously called the colostral bodies of Donne. They have the same functional and morphologic features as phagocytes from other human tissue sources. These features include ameboid movement, phagocytosis of microorganisms (fungi and bacteria), killing of bacteria, and production of complement components C3 and C4, lysosome, and lactoferrin. Other milk macrophage activities include the following:[265]

Phagocytosis of latex, adherence to glass
Secretion of lysozyme, complement components
C3b-mediated erythrocyte adherence
IgG-mediated erythrocyte adherence and phagocytosis
Bacterial killing
Inhibition of lymphocyte mitogenic response
Release of intracellular IgA in tissue culture
Giant cell formation
Interaction with lymphocytes

Data suggest these macrophages also amplify T cell reactivity by direct cellular cooperation or by antigen processing. The colostral macrophage has been suggested as a potential vehicle for the storage and transport of immunoglobulin. A significant increase in IgA and IgG synthesis by colostral lymphocytes, when incubated with supernatants of cultured macrophages, has been reported.[267]

The macrophage may also participate in the biosynthesis and excretion of lactoperoxidase and cellular growth factors that enhance growth of intestinal epithelium and maturation of intestinal brush-border enzymes.

The mobility of macrophages is inhibited by the lymphokine migration inhibitor factor, which is produced by antigen-stimulated sensitized lymphocytes. The activities of macrophages have been demonstrated in both fresh colostrum and colostral cell culture. Certain functions are altered compared with their counterpart in human peripheral blood.

POLYMORPHONUCLEAR LEUKOCYTES

The highest concentration of cells occurs in the first few days of lactation and reaches more than a million per milliliter of milk.

Colostrum (1 to 4 days postpartum) contains 10^5 to 5×10^6 leukocytes/mL, and 40% to 60% are polymorphonuclear cells (PMNs). Mature milk (i.e., after 4 days) has fewer cells (see Figure 5-3), approximately 10^5/mL with 20% to 30% PMNs. After 6 weeks, few PMNs are present. The functions of the PMNs normally include microbial killing, phagocytosis, chemotactic responsiveness, stimulated hexose monophosphate shunt activity, stimulated nitroblue tetrazolium dye reduction, and stimulated oxygen consumption.[41] When milk PMNs are compared with those in the serum, their activity is often less than that of serum PMN cells. Whether milk PMNs actually perform a role in the protection of the infant has been studied by many investigators using many techniques. Briefly, animal studies have shown that (1) the mammary gland is susceptible to infection in early lactation,

(2) a dramatic increase in PMNs occurs with mammary inflammation, and (3) in the presence of peripheral neutropenia during chronic mastitis, severe infection of the gland occurs. This implies, according to Buescher and Pickering,[41] that the primary function of milk PMNs is to defend the mammary tissue, per se, and not to impart immunocompetence to the newborn. This may explain the presence of large numbers of PMNs that are relatively hypofunctional early and then disappear over time. Evidence shows that neutrophils found in human milk demonstrate signs of activation, including increased expression of CD11b (an adherence glycoprotein), decreased expression of L-selectin, spontaneous production of granulocyte-macrophage colony-stimulating factor (GM-CSF), and the ability to transform into CD1$^+$ dendritic cells (DCs).[154] Human milk macrophages have the morphology and motility of activated cells. The movement of these cells in a three-dimensional system is greater than that of monocytes, their counterparts in peripheral blood. Such activated neutrophils may play a role in phagocytosis at the level of the mucosa of the GI tract, supplementing infants' poor ability to recruit phagocytes to that site.[169]

LYMPHOCYTES

Both T and B lymphocytes are present in human milk and colostrum and are part of the immunologic system in human milk. T cells are 80% of the lymphocytes in breast milk. Human milk lymphocytes respond to mitogens by proliferation, with increased macrophage-lymphocyte interaction and the release of soluble mediators, including migration inhibitor factor. Cells destined to become lymphopoietic cells are derived from two separate influences, the thymus (T) and the bursa (B) or bursal equivalent tissues. The population of the B cells makes up the smaller part of the total. They synthesize IgA antibody. The term B cell is derived from its origination in a different anatomic site from the thymus; in birds, it has been identified as the bursa of Fabricius. The B cells can be identified by the presence of surface immunoglobulin markers. The B cells in human milk include cells with IgA, IgM, and IgG surface immunoglobulins. B cells transform into plasma cells and remain sessile in the tissues of the mammary gland.

T CELL SYSTEM

More rapid mitotic activity occurs in the thymus gland than in any other lymphatic organ, yet 70% of the cells die within the cell substance. The thymus is the location for much of the T cell differentiation and selection and plays a major role in the development of infants' immune systems. Thymosin has been identified as a hormone produced by thymic epithelial cells to expand the peripheral lymphocyte population. After emergence from the thymus gland, T cells acquire new surface antigen markers. The T cells circulate through the lymphatic and vascular systems as long-lived lymphocytes, which are called the "recirculating pool." They then populate restricted regions of lymph nodes, forming thymic-dependent areas.[334] It is interesting to note that exclusively breastfed infants have a significantly larger thymus than formula-fed infants at 4 and 10 months.[134] The significance of the lymphocytes in human milk in affording immunologic benefits to breastfed infants continues to be investigated. It is suggested that lymphocytes can sensitize, induce immunologic tolerance, or incite graft-versus-host reactions. According to Head and Beer,[142] lymphocytes may be incorporated into sucklings' tissues, achieving short-term adoptive immunization of the neonate.

Studies of the activities of lymphocytes have been carried out by a number of investigators who collected samples of milk from lactating women at various times postpartum, examined the number of cell types present, and then studied the activities of these cells in vitro.[170,174] Ogra and Ogra[247] collected samples from 200 women and measured the cell content from 1 through 180 days (see Figure 5-3). They then compared the response of T lymphocytes in colostrum and milk with that of the T cells in the peripheral blood. T cell subpopulations have also been shown by surface epitopes to be similar to those in the peripheral blood.

The greatest number of cells appeared on the first day, with the counts ranging from 10,000 to 100,000/mm³ for total cells. By the fifth day, the count had dropped to 20% of the first day's count. In addition, the number of erythrocyte rosette-forming cells was determined by using sheep erythrocyte-rosetting technique. The erythrocyte rosette formation lymphocytes constituted a mean 100/mm³ on the first day and one tenth of that by the fifth day.

At 180 days, total cells were 100,000/mm³, lymphocytes were 10,000/mm³, and erythrocyte rosette formation lymphocytes were 2000/mm³. The investigators compared the values with those in the peripheral blood of each mother; the levels remained essentially constant.[246] In a similar study, Bhaskaram and Reddy[24] sampled milk over time from 74 women and found comparable cell concentrations. They examined the bactericidal activity of the milk leukocytes and found it to be comparable with that of the circulating leukocytes in the blood, irrespective of the stage of lactation or state of nutrition of the mother.

Ogra and Ogra[247] also studied the lymphocyte proliferation responses of colostrum and milk to antigens. Their data show response to stimulation from the viral antigens of rubella, cytomegalovirus (CMV), and mumps. Analysis of cell-mediated immunity to microbial antigens shows milk lymphocytes are limited in their potential for recognizing or responding to certain infectious agents compared with cells from the peripheral circulation. This is thought to be an intercellular action and not caused by lack of external factors. In contrast, the T cells and B cells have been shown to have unique reactivities not seen in peripheral blood.

Colostral lymphocytes are derived from mature rather than immature T cell subsets. The distribution of T cell subsets in colostrum includes both CD4+ and CD8+ cells.[278] The distribution of CD4 cells in colostrum and human milk is lower than in the serum, and fewer CD4 cells exist than CD8 cells.[334] The percentage of CD4 cells is higher than in the serum of either postpartum donors or normal control subjects. No correlation exists with length of gestation and number of cells (normal blood usually contains twice as many CD4+ as CD8+ lymphocytes).[166]

Parmely et al.[256] partially purified and propagated milk lymphocytes in vitro to study their immunologic function. Milk lymphocytes responded in a unique manner to stimuli known to activate T lymphocytes from the serum. The authors found milk lymphocytes to be hyporesponsive to nonspecific mitogens and histocompatibility antigens on allogenic cells in their laboratory. They found them unresponsive to *Candida albicans*. Significant proliferation of lymphocytes occurred in response to the K_1 capsular antigen of *Escherichia coli*.[146] Lymphocytes from blood failed to respond to the same antigen. This supports the concept of local mammary tissue immunity at the T lymphocyte level.

More recent experiments in rodents have provided evidence that T lymphocytes that are reactive to transplantation alloantigens can adoptively immunize a suckling newborn. Foster nursing experiments performed in rodents have shown that newborn rats exposed to allogenic milk manifested alterations in their reactivity to skin allografts of the foster mother's strain. In animals, mothers may give their suckling newborn immunoreactive lymphocytes. The influence of maternal milk cells on the development of neonatal immunocompetence has been demonstrated in several different immunologic contexts. Congenitally, athymic nude mice nursed by their phenotypically normal mothers or normal foster mothers had increased survival. The mothers contributed their T-cell-helper activity to the suckling newborn.

Colostral lymphocytes proliferate in response to various mitogens, alloantigens, and conventional antigens. Colostral cells survive in the neonatal stomach and in the gut of experimental animals, some remaining viable in the upper GI tract for a week. No evidence, however, indicates that trans-epithelial migration takes place when neonatal mice are foster-nursed by newly delivered animals whose colostral cells were tagged with ^{3}H-thymidine.[41]

Cells in human milk have been studied using the same markers employed with cells in the peripheral blood; 80% of the lymphocytes are T cells that are equally distributed between CD4$^+$ and CD8$^+$ subpopulations, and their T cell receptors are principally of the α/β type. CD4$^+$ cells are common leukocyte cells of the helper and suppressor-inducer subsets, and CD8$^+$ cells are leukocytes of the cytotoxic and noncytotoxic subsets. T cells in human milk are presumed activated because they display increased phenotypic markers of activation, including HLA-DR and CD25 (IL-2 receptor). The majority of T cells in human milk are CD45RO$^+$, consistent with effector and memory T cells.[284,334] These cells are effective producers of interferon-γ, which is consistent with their phenotypic features. Here again, human milk may supplement the infant with a functioning immune cell to compensate for an identified deficiency in the infant, a paucity of memory T cells.

B CELL SYSTEM

Juto[166] studied the effect of human milk on B-cell function. Cell-free, defatted, filtered colostrum, as well as mature breast milk, showed an enhancing effect on B-cell proliferation and generation of antibody secretion. This was not seen with formula. Juto suggested that this could represent an important immunologic mechanism. Goldblum et al.[104] were able to show a B-cell response in human colostrum to E. coli given to the mother orally, which was not accompanied by a systemic response in the mother. This suggests that the breast and breast milk reflect sites of local, humoral, or cell-mediated immunity, which were initially induced at a distant site such as the gut and transferred via reactive lymphoid cells migrating to the breast. Head and Beer[142] provided a scheme to describe this mechanism (see Figure 5-2). The diagram depicts the progeny of specifically sensitized lymphocytes that originated in GALT, specifically Peyer's patches, as they migrate to the mammary gland. As they infiltrate the mammary gland and its secretion, they supply the breast with immune cells capable of selected immune responses. Ogra and Ogra[246,247] suggest that the cells may selectively accumulate in the breast during pregnancy. The responses of milk cells and their antibodies are not representative of an individual's total immunity.[256] Most of these immunocompetent cells, initially stimulated in GALT, recirculate to the external mucosal surface and populate the lamina propria as antibody-producing plasma cells. A substantial number of these antigen-sensitized cells selectively home-in to the stroma of the mammary glands and initiate local IgA antibody synthesis against the antigens initially encountered in the respiratory or intestinal mucosa.[24] More recent work on human milk-derived B-cells demonstrates that breast milk contains activated memory B-cells, different than those in the blood. These cells express mucosal adhesion molecules ($\alpha_4\beta_7^{-/+}$, $\alpha_4\beta_1^+$, CD44$^+$, CD62L$^-$), suggesting an origin in the mammary gland, but similar to GALT-associated B-cells.[320] The mucosae-associated epithelial cytokine CCL28 may contribute to migration of and retention of these cells in the mammary gland.[332] This information supports the concept of the mammary gland as an effector site of the mucosal immune system.

The accumulated epidemiologic research supports the concept that colostrum and milk provide human infants with immunologic benefits. Both T- and B-lymphocytes found in breast milk are reactive against organisms invading the intestinal tract. However, the proof of specific viral or bacterial protection, secondary to the action of immunologically active B-cells, has not been demonstrated.

Survival of Maternal Milk Cells

Although it is clear that cells are provided in the colostrum and milk, the effectiveness and impact of these cells on the neonate depend on their ability to survive in the GI tract. It has been demonstrated in several species, including humans, that the pH of the stomach can be as low as 0.5, but the output of hydrochloric acid is minimal for the first few months, as is the peptic activity. Immediately after a feeding begins, the pH rises to 6.0 and returns to normal in 3 hours. The cells from milk tolerate this. Studies in rats have also shown that intact nucleated lymphoid cells are found in the stomach and intestines.[19] These cells, when removed from rat stomachs, are capable of phagocytosis. Lymphoid cells in milk have been shown to traverse the mucosal wall.

When human milk is stored, however, the cellular components do not tolerate heating to 63°C (145.4°F), cooling to −23°C (−9.4°F), or lyophilization. Although a few cells may be identified in processed milk, they are not viable.[105]

STEM CELLS

Interest in mammary stem cells (MaSCs) has blossomed since Cregan et al.[62] reported the presence of MaSCs in human breast milk. Their research was based on the demonstration of the cytokeratin 5 MaSC marker on cells isolated from human breast milk. Additional analysis showed cells from human milk with both the multipotent stem cell marker, nestin, and the cytokeratin 5 marker. There are several areas of interest relative to these MaSCs in humans: the potential ready availability of multipotent mesenchymal stem cells for autologous stem cell therapies; the identified cell markers and signaling pathways on these cells, which could lead to more targeted breast cancer therapies; the role of stem cells in the dynamic states of the breast, especially lactation; the potential correlation between MaSCs and transplantation tolerance; and the state of microchimerism of MaSCs in the infant and the potential effects on the infant.*

The mammary gland is an attractive target in the search for stem cells, in that it is a dynamic, metabolically active tissue. It has the capacity to proliferate and hypertrophy through adolescent development, pregnancy, lactation, and the subsequent involution phase of the breast. Embryonic stem cells have a tremendous differentiation potential, in that they can develop into every cell type in the body. Adult stem cells constitute a small portion of organ cells that can mature into multiple specific cell types. Adult stem cells can also produce new stem cells to maintain the population of these cells in the organ. They are said to remain quiescent within "stem cell niches" within an organ.[336] DeOme et al. noted the existence of adult stem cells in mammary tissue in 1959. Other investigators investigated the renewal capacity of these cells and considered them to be a multipotent stem cell.[69] The search for such pluripotent stem cells continued, using a variety of markers (Sca 1) and characteristics (Hoechst dye efflux), which led to the identification of mammary gland stem cell progenitors (MG-SP). These are able to differentiate into both the K18+ luminal and K14+ myoepithelial cell lineages.[58] Dontu et al. demonstrated that MaSCs grown in "mammospheres" (under anchorage independent conditions) expressed the surface cell markers CD49f, K5, and CD10. Some additional markers, characteristic of luminal and myoepithelial cells, were expressed. Some of these same cells were treated with prolactin and developed into functional alveolar cells, secreting beta-casein. Other investigators demonstrated that these progenitor cells, raised in mammospheres, were capable of differentiating in three types of cells (luminal, myoepithelial, and alveolar). They were clonally derived and could retain multipotent capacity after propagation through several passages.[72] Others have employed label-retention studies to characterize MaSCs as label-retention cells (LRCs) and been able to demonstrate asymmetric division in their nonquiescent

states.[301] Subsequent research has identified signaling pathways related to stem cell propagation including Wnt/beta-catenin, Notch, Hedgehog (Hh) transforming growth factor (TGF)-beta, phosphatase and tensin homologue, and Bmi.[336] Stem cells have many of the features of tumor cells, including self-renewal and the ability to replicate indefinitely.[337] The question is what might distinguish normal progenitor cells from tumorigenic progenitor cells. Other investigators searching for such tumorigenic mammary gland stem cells identified MaSCs with the surface markers Lin⁻ CD29hiCD24+, which were capable of generating a functional mammary gland in the mouse.[299]

The exact mechanism of acquired tolerance to noninherited maternal antigens (NIMA) is unknown. It has been suggested that exposure of the fetus during pregnancy and exposure during breastfeeding to NIMA may be the explanation for transplantation tolerance in breastfed persons.[4,214] Breast milk contains a variety of major histocompatibility complex antigens from the mother. Molitor et al. demonstrated high levels of NIMA HLA proteins in both the cord blood and breast milk, emphasizing the potential role of human breast milk in exposing the infant to NIMAs. The existence of mammary derived stem cells in the infant suggests a degree of microchimerism in infants directly from maternal breast cells in breast milk. Dutta and Burlingham propose that stem cell microchimerism in infants is related to tolerance to NIMAs.[79]

Human milk contains a heterogeneous cell population. Early lactation milk and colostrum contain larger numbers of leukocytic origin cells, and mature breast milk contains more cells of epithelial origin. There also exists variability in the breast milk cell content and composition between breastfeeding women and within an individual woman over the time period of lactation.[136] Hassiotou et al. have proposed a broad degree of differentiation of breast milk stem cells (hBSCs) found in human milk. The proposed lineage includes differentiation in breast cells (myoepithelial, ductal, alveolar, and secretory), stromal type cells (osteoblast, chondrocytes, and adipocytes), neural progenitor type cells, and endodermal cell types (hepatocytes and pancreatic cells).[135,137] There remains much more to be understood about the existence of human breast stem cells in human milk and their possible role in health in the infant and later in life.

Humoral Factors

IMMUNOGLOBULINS

All classes of immunoglobulins are found in human milk. The study of immunoglobulins has been

*16,85,135,136,203,257,290,299,318,336

enhanced through the techniques of electrophoresis, chromatographics, and radioimmunoassay. More than 30 components have been identified; of these, 18 are associated with proteins in the maternal serum, and the others are found exclusively in milk. The concentrations are highest in the colostrum of all species, and the concentrations change as lactation proceeds.[210] IgA, principally sIgA, is highest in colostrum. Although postpartum levels fall throughout the next 4 weeks, substantial levels are maintained throughout the first year, during gradual weaning between 6 and 9 months, and even during partial breastfeeding (when the infant receives solid foods) in the second year of life (Figure 5-4 and Table 5-2). Specific sIgA antibodies to *E. coli* persist through lactation and may even increase (see Figure 5-4).

The main immunoglobulin in human serum is IgG; IgA content is only one fifth the level of IgG. In milk, however, the reverse is true. IgA is the most important immunoglobulin in milk, not only in concentration but also in biologic activity. sIgA is likely synthesized in the mammary alveolar cells[307] or by lymphocytes that have migrated from Peyer's patches in the GI tract or from lymphoid tissue in the respiratory tract via the lymphatics to the breast. Cytokines cause isotype switching of local IgM+ B-cells to become IgA+ B-lymphocytes.[107,297,330] These isotype switched cells travel to the breast, where they are transformed into plasma cells producing secretory, dimeric IgA. It is through this "enteromammary" pathway that the mother provides increased amounts of sIgA to the infant against the microorganisms present in the mother's and infant's environment.[313]

Brandtzaeg[29] has proposed a model for the transport of IgA (polymeric) and IgM (pentameric), produced by plasma cells, across the secretory epithelium. The model involves the formation of sIgA and IgM, through binding, with the secretory component attached to the epithelial membrane. This occurs in the membrane of mammary epithelial cells during lactation.[30,115]

Quantitative determinations of immunoglobulins in human milk were made from milk collected at birth to as long as 27 months postpartum by Peitersen et al.[259] and by Goldman et al.[114] The IgA content was high immediately after birth, dropping in 2 to 3 weeks, and then remaining constant. Similar observations were made on IgG levels and IgM levels. Ogra and Ogra[246,247] have compared serum and milk levels at various times postpartum. Samples obtained separately from the left and right breasts showed similar values. The levels remained constant during a given feeding and throughout a 24 hour period. In all quantitative determinations, IgA is the predominant immunoglobulin in breast milk, constituting 90% of all the immunoglobulins in colostrum and milk.

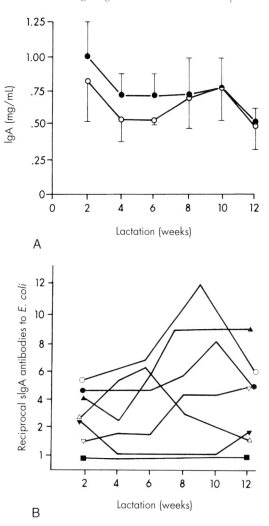

Figure 5-4. Same subjects in Figure 5-3 were examined during second through twelfth week of lactation. **A,** Longitudinal study of total IgA and sIgA. Total (•) and secretory IgA (○). **B,** Longitudinal study of reciprocal of sIgA antibody titers to *E. coli* somatic antigens in human milk. The sIgA antibody titers to *E. coli* somatic antigens from each subject are represented by a different symbol (open and closed circles, diamonds, and squares). (From Goldman AS, Garza C, Nichols BL, et al: Immunologic factors in human milk during the first year of lactation, *J Pediatr* 100:563, 1982.)

Ogra and Ogra[246–248] studied the serum of postpartum lactating mothers and nonpregnant matched control subjects. They noted that the individual and mean concentrations of all Ig classes were lower in the postpartum subjects. The levels were statistically significant for IgG; they were 50 to 70 mg higher in the nonpregnant women.

Immunoglobulin levels, particularly IgA and IgM, are very high in colostrum and drop precipitously in the first 4 to 6 days, but IgG does not show this decline. The volume of mammary secretion, however, increases dramatically in this same period; thus the absolute amounts of immunoglobulins

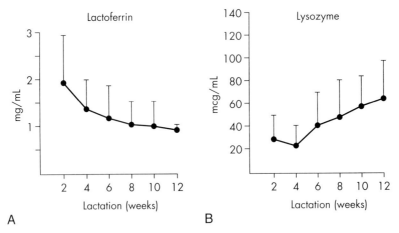

Figure 5-5. Same subjects in Figure 5-3 were examined during second through twelfth week of lactation. Data in longitudinal studies are presented as mean ± SD. **A,** Concentration of lactoferrin progressively decreased through first 8 weeks ($r = 0.69$) (2 vs. 8 weeks; $p < 0.02$), but not thereafter. **B,** In contrast, lysozyme levels steadily increased from fourth through twelfth week ($r = 0.76$) (4 vs. 12 weeks; $p < 0.01$). (From Goldman AS, Garza C, Nichols BL, et al: Immunologic factors in human milk during the first year of lactation, *J Pediatr* 100:563, 1982.)

TABLE 5-2	Concentrations of Immunologic Components in Human Milk Collected During Second Year of Lactation		
	Duration of Lactation (mo)		
Component	**12**	**13-15**	**16-24**
IgA (mg/mL)			
Total	0.8±0.3	1.1±0.4	1.1±0.3
Secretory (sIgA)	0.8±0.3	1.1±0.3	1.1±0.2
Lactoferrin (mg/mL)	1.0±0.2	1.1±0.1	1.2±0.1
Lysozyme (mcg/mL)	196±41	244±34	187±33
sIgA antibodies (reciprocal titers to *E. coli* somatic antigens)	5±6	9±10	6±3

Data are presented as the mean ± SD.

From Goldman AS, Goldblum RM, Graza C: Immunologic components in human milk during the second year of lactation, *Acta Paediatr Scand* 72:461, 1983.

remain more nearly constant than it would first appear. Local production and concentration of IgA, and probably IgM, may take place in the mammary gland at delivery.

IgE and IgD have also been measured in colostrum and milk. Using radioimmunoassay techniques, colostrum was found to contain concentrations of 0.5 to 0.6 IU/mL IgE in 41% of samples and less in the remainder.[11] IgD was found in all samples in concentrations of 2 to 2000 mg/dL. Plasma levels were poorly correlated. The findings suggest possible local mammary production rather than positive transfer. The question of whether IgE or IgD antibodies in breast milk have similar specificities for antigens as the IgA antibodies in milk remains unanswered.[208] Keller et al.[171] examined the question of local mammary IgD production, and its possible participation in a mucosal immune system, by comparing colostrum and plasma levels of total IgD with specific IgD antibodies. From their work comparing colostrum/plasma ratios for IgG, IgD, and albumin and measuring IgD against specific antigens, the authors reported evidence for IgD participation in the response of the mucosal immune system, with increases in total IgD and IgD against specific antigens found in colostrum.

Butte et al.[45] addressed the question of total quantities of immunologic components secreted into human milk per day and available to an infant. They did so by measuring the amounts of sIgA, sIgA antibodies to *E. coli*, lactoferrin, and lysozyme ingested per day and per kilogram per day in the first 4 months of life (Figures 5-6 through 5-10). Lactoferrin, sIgA, and sIgA antibodies gradually declined in amount ingested per day and per kilogram per day. Lysozyme, in contrast, rose during the same period in total amount available and amount per kilogram per day. The authors[45] suggest that production and secretion of these immunologic factors by the mammary gland may be linked to the catabolism of the components at an infant's mucosal tissues. When the concentrations of sIgA, IgG, IgM, α_1-antitrypsin, lactoferrin, lysozyme, and globulins C3 and C4 were compared in relationship to parity and age of the mother, no consistent trend was observed. When maturity of the pregnancy was considered, however, mean concentrations of all these proteins were higher, except for IgA, when the delivery was premature. Because

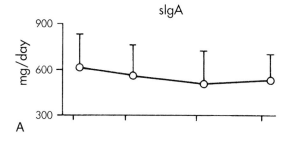

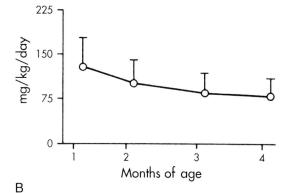

Figure 5-6. Amounts of sIgA and sIgA antibodies to *E. coli* somatic antigens in human milk ingested per day (**A**). Per kilogram per day (**B**). Data are presented as mean ± SD. (From Butte NF, Goldblum RM, Fehl LM, et al: Daily ingestion of immunologic components in human milk during the first four months of life, *Acta Paediatr Scand* 73:296, 1984.)

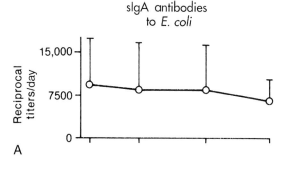

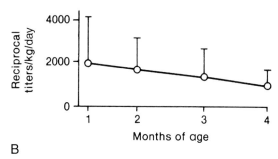

Figure 5-7. Amounts of sIgA antibodies to *E. coli* somatic antigens in human milk ingested as reciprocal titers per day (**A**). Per kilogram per day (**B**). Data are presented as mean ± SD. (From Butte NF, Goldblum RM, Fehl LM, et al: Daily ingestion of immunologic components in human milk during the first four months of life, *Acta Paediatr Scand* 73:296, 1984.)

several proteins in human milk have physiologic functions in infants, Davidson and Lönnerdal[66] examined the survival of human milk proteins through the GI tract. Crossed immunoelectrophoresis showed that three human milk proteins transversed the entire intestine and were present in the feces: lactoferrin, sIgA, and α_1-antitrypsin.

Miranda et al.[213] reported on the effect of maternal nutritional status on immunologic substances in human colostrum and milk. Maternal malnutrition was characterized as lower weight-to-height ratio, creatine/height index, total serum proteins, and IgG and IgA. In malnourished mothers, the colostrum contained one third the normal concentration of IgG, less than half the normal level of albumin, and lower IgA and complement C4. Lysozyme, complement C3, and IgM levels were normal. Levels improved with development of mature milk and improvement in maternal nutrition. According to one report in 2003, moderate exercise during lactation does not affect the levels of IgA, lactoferrin, or lysozyme in breast milk.[199] Immunologic components contained in human milk during the second year of lactation become a significant point as more infants are nursed longer. For a longitudinal study of lactation into the second year by Goldman

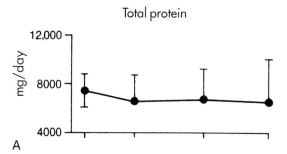

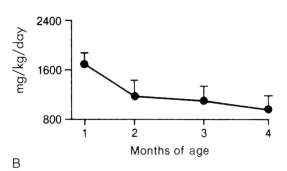

Figure 5-8. Amount of total protein in human milk ingested per day (**A**). Per kilogram per day (**B**). Data are presented as mean ± SD. (From Butte NF, Goldblum RM, Fehl LM, et al: Daily ingestion of immunologic components in human milk during the first four months of life, *Acta Paediatr Scand* 73:296, 1984.)

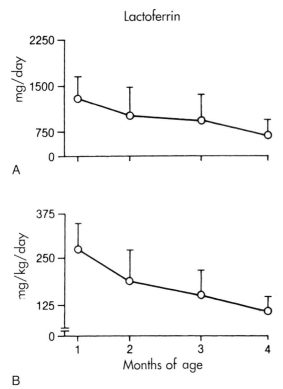

Figure 5-9. Amount of lactoferrin in human milk ingested per day (**A**). Per kilogram per day (**B**). Data are presented as mean±SD. (From Butte NF, Goldblum RM, Fehl LM, et al: Daily ingestion of immunologic components in human milk during the first four months of life, *Acta Paediatr Scand* 73:296, 1984.)

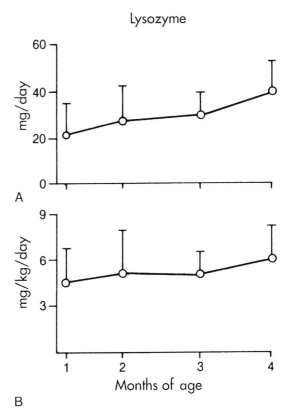

Figure 5-10. Amount of lysozyme in human milk ingested per day (**A**). Per kilogram per day (**B**). Data are presented as mean±SD. (From Butte NF, Goldblum RM, Fehl LM, et al: Daily ingestion of immunologic components in human milk during the first 4 months of life, *Acta Paediatr Scand* 73:296, 1984.)

et al.,[111] women were included who had fully breastfed their infants for 6 months to a year and were continuing to partially breastfeed. Samples were collected by fully emptying the breast by electric pump. Table 5-2 summarizes the concentrations of the measured factors. No leukocytes were detected. Concentrations of total IgA and sIgA, lactoferrin, and lysozyme were similar to those 7 to 12 months postpartum and during gradual weaning. sIgA antibodies to *E. coli* were produced in the second year, demonstrating significant immunologic benefit to the infant with continued breastfeeding.[111] IgA, IgM, and IgG were measured in nursing women from the beginning of lactation and simultaneously in the feces of their children by Jatsyk et al.[161] at the Academy of Medicine in Moscow. They reported IgA to be very high in the milk and rapidly increasing in the feces. IgG and IgM levels, however, were low in both milk and feces. In normal full-term bottle-fed infants, IgA appeared in the feces at 3 to 4 weeks of age, but at much lower levels than in breastfed infants. Koutras and Vigorita[179] reported that in the first 8 weeks of life increased amounts of sIgA were found in the stools

of breastfed infants compared with formula-fed infants. The authors ascribed this phenomenon to the presence of sIgA in human milk and a stimulation of the local GI production of immunoglobulin.

Savilahti et al.[291] measured serum levels of IgG, IgA, and IgM in 198 infants at 2, 4, 6, 9, and 12 months of age. By 9 months, the exclusively breastfed infants had IgG and IgM levels significantly lower than those who had been weaned early (before 3.5 months) to formula. Six infants were still exclusively breastfed at 12 months, and their IgA levels had also lowered to levels found at 2 months with bottle feeders. Infection rates were similar. Two months after the children were weaned to formula, the IgG and IgM levels were comparable. Iron and zinc levels were the same in all children.

SPECIFICITY OF IMMUNOGLOBULINS

sIgA antibodies have been identified in human milk that recognize a large variety of microorganisms. The sIgA antibodies that recognize bacteria, viruses, parasites, and fungi are listed in Table 5-3. Some sIgA antibodies recognize various bacteria, including

TABLE 5-3	Antibodies in Human Milk		
Factor	Shown, In Vitro, to Be Active Against:	Assay	Effect of Heat
Secretory IgA	Enteroviruses		
	Poliovirus types 1, 2, 3	ELISA, NA, Precipitin	Stable at 56°C for 30 min; some loss (0%-30%)
	Coxsackievirus types A₉, B₃, B₅	NA	Stable at 62.5°C for 30 min; destroyed by boiling
	Echovirus types 6 and 9	NA	
	Herpesvirus		
	CMV	ELISA, IFA, NA	
	Herpes simplex virus	NA	
	HIV		
	Semliki Forest virus	IFA	
	Respiratory syncytial virus	IFA	
	Rubella	IFA, HAI	
	Reovirus type 3	ELISA, NA	
	Rotavirus		
	Measles		
	Norovirus		
	Escherichia coli (EIEC, EAEC, EPEC)		
	Shigella		
	Salmonella		
	Campylobacter		
	Vibrio cholerae		
	Haemophilus influenzae type b		
	Streptococcus pneumoniae		
	Clostridium difficile		
	Clostridium botulinum (toxin B16S)		
	Clostridium perfringens enterotoxin A		
	Klebsiella pneumoniae		
	Streptococcus group B, type III		
	Listeria monocytogenes		
	Staphylococcus aureus		
	Staphylococcal toxic shock syndrome toxin-1		
	Staphylococcal enterotoxin C		
	Helicobacter pylori		
	Entamoeba histolytica		
	Strongyloides		
	Giardia		
	Candida albicans		
IgM, IgG	CMV		Stable at 56°C for 30 min; IgG decreased by a third at 62.5°C for 30 min
	Respiratory syncytial virus		
	Rotavirus		
	Rubella		
IgE	Parvovirus B19	ELISA	

CMV, Cytomegalovirus; *EAEC,* enteroadherent *E. coli; EIEC,* enteroinvasive *E. coli; ELISA,* enzyme-linked immunosorbent assay; *EPEC,* enteropathogenic *E. coli; HAI,* hemagglutination inhibition; *HIV,* human immunodeficiency virus; *IFA,* immunofluorescent assay; *NA,* neutralizing assay.

E. coli, Shigella, Salmonella, Campylobacter pylori, Vibrio cholerae, Haemophilus influenzae, Streptococcus pneumoniae, Group B *Streptococcus* type III, *Staphylococcus aureus, Clostridium difficile, Clostridium botulinum, Klebsiella pneumonia,* and *Listeria monocytogenes.* Some sIgA antibodies recognize *Entamoeba histolytica, Giardia, Strongyloides stercoralis,* and *C. albicans.*[107,240] The list of viruses for which sIgA antibodies exist in human milk is equally long, including enteroviruses (poliovirus, coxsackie, and echovirus), CMV, herpes simplex virus, human immunodeficiency virus (HIV), Semliki Forest virus, respiratory syncytial virus (RSV), rubella, reovirus type 3, rotavirus, measles, Norovirus, and porcine coronavirus. IgG and IgM antibodies also exist in human milk against CMV, RSV, and rubella, as well as IgE antibodies against parvovirus B19. Noguera-Obenza and Cleary[240] reviewed the role of breast milk sIgA in providing protection for infants against various agents specifically causing bacterial enteritis.

STABILITY OF IMMUNOGLOBULINS

Preservation of human milk at −20°C for up to 3 months does not decrease significantly the levels of IgA, IgG, IgM, C3, C4, lactoferrin, or lysozyme.[84,91,194,249] The preservation of sIgA, IL-6, and TNF-α with freezing at −4°C or −20°C was recently confirmed by Hines et al.[145]

A variety of different heat treatments have been applied to milk to protect against bacterial contamination or to protect against infection with specific infectious agents (especially HIV and CMV). Heat treatments include low-temperature, short-time at 56°C for 15 minutes; Holder pasteurization at 62.5°C for 30 minutes; high-temperature, short-time at 70 to 73°C for 15 seconds; boiling at 100°C for greater than 1 minute; sterilization, variable time periods, Pretoria pasteurization at 56 to 62.5°C for approximately 15 minutes[162]; flash heating at 56°C for approximately 6 minutes with a peak temperature at 72°C[156,157]; and microwave heating, with milk temperatures of 20 to 77°C for 30 seconds.[272] Boiling or sterilization essentially destroys 100% of immunologic activity. sIgA and lysozyme activities drop by 20% with Holder pasteurization and by 50% at 65°C. Neither low-temperature, short-time nor high-temperature, short-time reduces the sIgA or lysozyme content markedly. IgG and IgM are greatly reduced by Holder pasteurization.

sIgA differs antigenically from serum IgA. IgA can be synthesized in the nonlactating, as well as in the lactating, breast. It is a compact molecule and resistant to proteolytic enzymes of the intestinal tract and the low pH of the stomach. The sIgA present in human milk is primarily manufactured by plasma cells in the mammary gland, modified in its translocation across the mammary epithelia, and only minimally produced by the cellular

lymphocytes in milk. Levels in milk are 10 to 100 times higher than in serum. Levels in cow milk are very low, that is, a tenth of the level in mature human milk (0.03 mg/dL). Later in life, the human intestinal tract's subepithelial plasma cells secrete IgA. The intestinal secretion of sIgA does not occur in the neonatal period but increases between 4 and 12 months of life.

Discussion continues as to whether any antibodies are absorbed from the intestinal tract, although probably 10% are absorbed. Almost 75% of ingested IgA from milk survives passage through the intestinal tract and is excreted in the feces. All immunoglobulin classes have been identified in the feces.[277] A large body of evidence demonstrates the activity of the immunoglobulins, especially IgA, at the mucosal level of the GI and respiratory tracts. These antibodies provide local intestinal protection against microorganisms, which may infect the mucosa or enter the body through the gut or respiratory tract.

Other Bioactive Factors

BIFIDUS FACTOR

It is well established that the predominant bacteria found in breastfed infants are bifid bacteria. Bifid bacteria are gram-positive, nonmotile, anaerobic bacilli. Many observers have shown the striking difference between the flora of the guts of breastfed and bottle-fed infants. Gyorgy[122] demonstrated the presence of a specific factor in colostrum and milk that supported the growth of *Lactobacillus bifidus.* Bifidus factor has been characterized as a dialyzable, nitrogen-containing carbohydrate that contains no amino acid.

In vitro studies by Beerens et al.[20] showed the presence of a specific growth factor for *Bifidobacterium bifidum* in human milk, which they called BB. Other milks, including cow milk, sheep milk, pig milk, and infant formulas, did not promote the growth of this species but did show some activity supporting *B. infantis* and *B. longum.* This growth factor was found to be stable when the milk was frozen, heated, freeze-dried, and stored for 3 months. Growth-promoting factors were present for the six strains studied, which varied in their resistance to physical change. Because all these factors were active in vitro, they did not require the presence of intestinal enzymes for activation. It has not been possible to show the presence of this growth factor in other mammalian milks; thus it may contribute to the implantation and persistence of *B. bifidum* in a breastfed infant's intestine.

Lactobacillus has been described as one of a number of probiotic bacteria, which provide an immune protective benefit to their host. *Lactobacillus* reportedly stimulates antibody production and improves phagocytosis by blood leukocytes.[167,261] The use of probiotic bacteria has reportedly produced benefits in a variety of situations associated with infections. The addition of such bacteria to formula is another example of trying to make formula better by making it more like breast milk. Hatakka et al.[138] examined the possible effect of adding probiotic bacteria to formula on the occurrence of infection in children attending daycare. They reported modest reductions in the number of children with complicated respiratory infections or lower respiratory tract infections, as well as the number of children receiving antibiotics for a respiratory infection, in the group of children receiving formula supplemented with *Lactobacillus rhamnosus* GG compared with children receiving unsupplemented formula.

RESISTANCE FACTOR

It was well known in the preantibiotic era that human milk protects human infants throughout lactation against staphylococcal infection. Gyorgy[122] identified the presence of an "antistaphylococcal factor" in experiments with young mice that had been stressed with staphylococci. This factor, with no demonstrable direct antibiotic properties, was termed resistance factor and described as nondialyzable, thermostable, and part of the free-fatty acid part of the phosphide fraction, probably C18:2, but distinct from linoleic acid.

LYSOZYME

Human milk contains a nonspecific antimicrobial factor, lysozyme, which is a thermostable, acid-stable enzyme. This enzyme is a 130-amino-acid-containing glycoprotein that can hydrolyze the 1 to 4 linkage between *N*-acetylglucosamine and *N*-acetylmuramic acid in bacterial cell walls. It is found in large concentrations in the stools of breastfed infants and not in stools of formula-fed infants; thus it is thought to influence the flora of the intestinal tract.

Goldman et al.[114] describe an initial fall in lysozyme levels from 85 to 90 mg/mL to 25 mg/mL at 2 to 4 weeks and then an increase during 6 months to 250 mg/mL (see Figure 5-5). Lysozyme levels show an increase over time during lactation; this finding is more apparent in Indian women than in those of the Western world. Reddy et al.[276] studied the levels of lysozyme in well-nourished and poorly nourished women in India and found no difference between them (Table 5-4). As shown in this study, lysozyme levels increase during lactation. Levels in human milk are 300 times the level in cow milk. Lysozyme is bacteriostatic against Enterobacteriaceae and gram-positive bacteria.[265] It is secreted by neutrophils and some macrophages and is present in many body secretions in the adult.

In a study of immunologic components in human milk in the second year of lactation, Goldman et al.[97] reported that concentrations of lysozyme, lactoferrin, and total IgA and sIgA were similar to those in uninterrupted lactation and in gradual weaning at 6 to 9 months. sIgA antibodies to *E. coli* were also produced during the second year. The authors state that "this supports the idea that the enteromammary lymphocyte traffic pathway, which leads to the development of lymphoid cells in the mammary gland that produce IgA antibodies to enteric organisms, operates throughout lactation."[111] When cow milk formula is added to human milk, it reduces the effect of lysozyme; however, powdered human milk fortifier (Enfamil) did not inhibit the antiinfective properties.[173]

TABLE 5-4	Antibacterial Factors in Colostrum and Mature Milk in Well-Nourished and Undernourished Indian Women						
Group	Hemoglobin (g/dL)	Serum Albumin (g/dL)	Immunoglobulins (mg/dL)			Lysozyme (mg/dL)	Lactoferrin (mg/dL)
			IgA	IgG	IgM		
Colostrum (1-5 days)							
Well-nourished women	11.5±0.37	2.49± 0.065	335.9±37.39 (17)*	5.9±1.58 (17)	17.1±4.29 (17)	14.2±2.11 (15)	420±49.0 (28)
Undernourished women	11.3±0.60	2.10± 0.081	374.3±42.13 (10)	5.3±2.30 (10)	15.3±2.50 (10)	16.4±2.39 (21)	520±69.0 (19)
Mature milk (1-6 months)							
Well-nourished women	12.8±0.43	3.39± 0.120	119.6±7.85 (12)	2.9±0.92 (12)	2.9±0.92 (12)	24.8±3.41 (10)	250±65.0 (17)
Undernourished women	12.6±0.56	3.47± 0.130	118.1±16.2 (10)	5.8±3.41 (10)	5.8±3.41 (10)	23.3±3.53 (23)	270±92.0 (13)

*Figures in parentheses indicate number of samples analyzed.

From Reddy V, Bhaskaram C, Raghuramula N, et al: Antimicrobial factors in human milk, *Acta Paediatr Scand* 66:229, 1977.

LACTOFERRIN

Lactoferrin is an iron-binding protein closely related to the serum iron transport protein, transferrin, and is part of the larger transferrin protein family. Lactoferrin is found in mucosal secretions (tears, saliva, vaginal fluids, urine, nasal and bronchial secretions, bile, GI fluids) and, notably, in milk and colostrum. A bacteriostatic effect of lactoferrin is well established for a wide range of microorganisms, including gram-positive and gram-negative aerobes, anaerobes, viruses, parasites, and fungi. The original proposed mechanism of action for its bacteriostatic effect was depriving the microorganism of iron. A second antibacterial action, involving direct action with bacterial surfaces, binds negatively charged molecules (lipoteichoic acid) on the surface of gram-positive bacteria. This neutralizes the surface charge, allowing the action of other antibacterial factors (like lysozyme or binding lipid A) on gram-negative bacteria, which releases the lipid, producing damage to the cell membrane. Another antibacterial action is binding bacterial adhesions blocking host cell interaction.[116] Lactoferrin can kill *C. albicans* and *C. krusei* by changing the permeability of the fungal cell surface. Lactoferrin now is considered a multifunctional, immunoregulatory protein.

The biologic role of lactoferrin has been reviewed in several studies.[197,198,242,289] They point out that lactoferrin reversibly binds two ferric ions and that its affinity for iron is 300 times greater than that of transferrin, retaining iron down to a pH of 3. Human lactoferrin is strongly basic. Lactoferrin is normally unsaturated with iron,[44] and it is usually less than 10% saturated with iron in human milk.[93,289] Oral iron therapy for an infant can interfere with the bacteriostatic action of lactoferrin, which depends on its unsaturated state for some portion of its bacteriostatic function. Reddy et al.[276] showed that giving iron to the mother did not interfere with the saturation of lactoferrin in the milk or, thus, its potential bacteriostatic effect. Protein energy malnutrition, rather than iron supplies, influences lactoferrin synthesis in the mammary gland. Malnourished but nonirondeficient mothers are lactoferrin deficient.

The concentration of lactoferrin is high in colostrum—600 mg/dL—then progressively declines over the next 5 months of lactation, leveling at about 180 mg/dL. Breast milk also contains small amounts of transferrin (10 to 15 mg/mL). Lactoferrin is 10% to 15% of the total protein content of human milk.[197] Lactoferrin is resistant to proteolysis, especially in its iron-saturated form. Intact lactoferrin is detectable in the stool of infants, with higher proportions of lactoferrin measurable in the stool of premature infants.[71] Both intact lactoferrin

and fragments have been detected in the urine of premature infants, although absorption is less likely in full-term infants.[130] The absorption of iron from breast milk is directly enhanced by lactoferrin.[198]

Many bacteria require iron for normal growth, and one bacteriostatic effect of lactoferrin has been ascribed to its iron-binding action. In neutrophils, lactoferrin within neutrophilic granules tightly binds iron, but neutrophils with excessive iron are inefficient at destroying bacteria. Lactoferrin does not limit the growth of all microorganisms; *Helicobacter pylori* and Neisseria, Treponema, and Shigella species all have receptors for lactoferrin, directly binding iron and allowing adequate growth.

Some evidence supports various other proposed mechanisms of action for lactoferrin's antimicrobial effect. Lactoferrin has been shown to limit the formation of biofilms by specific organisms, inhibit adhesion to host cells by other organisms, and directly bind to viral particles of herpes simplex virus, HIV, and adenovirus. A proteolytic action of lactoferrin appears to inactivate virulence factors of some organisms. Separately, lactoferrin binds directly to glycosamino glycans (GAGs) and integrins interrupting the binding of various viruses (herpes simplex virus, HIV, adenovirus, CMV, hepatitis B virus [HBV]) to host cells. Pepsin hydrolysate products of lactoferrin (B or H) may exert a direct bactericidal effect by binding to lipopolysaccharide of gram-negative organisms and disrupting bacterial membranes.[317] Lactoferrin may cause an increased release of cytokines by cells including antiinflammatory cytokines such as IL-10.[63,191] Others have shown that lactoferrin suppresses the release of IL-1, IL-2, IL-6, IL-8, and TNF-α, all proinflammatory cytokines, which would be more of an immune-modulating effect.[191] Other investigators using a recombinant human lactoferrin (talactoferrin) demonstrated evidence of lactoferrin causing increased maturation of DCs[303] and talactoferrin causing the recruitment and activation of neutrophils and macrophages[281] as other examples of how lactoferrin affects the innate immune protection of the growing infant. Several other effects have been proposed for lactoferrin, including inhibition of hydroxyl radical formation, decreasing local cell damage; lipopolysaccharide binding, also leading to a diminished inflammatory response; and DNA binding, affecting transcription and possibly regulation of the production of cell products.[242] Activation of natural killer (NK) cells, modulation of complement activity, and blocking of adhesion of enterotoxigenic *E. coli* and *Shigella flexneri*[103] are other proposed actions of lactoferrin.

A specific region of lactoferrin, near the N-terminus of the molecule, is strongly basic and is reported to mediate some of lactoferrin's antimicrobial activity. "Lactoferricins," small peptides containing this basic region and produced by proteolytic cleavage, reportedly bind to lipopolysaccharide, leading to disruption of the bacterial cell wall and cytoplasmic membrane.[317]

In another area of immune protection, lactoferrin may limit cancer development.[191] The proposed mechanisms of its anticancer effects include increasing NK cell cytotoxicity, increased production of IL-18 and inhibition of angiogenesis, augmented apoptosis of cancer cells, and initiation of cell cycle arrest in growing tumor cells.[191]

The multiple roles and proposed mechanisms of action of lactoferrin in breastfed infants continue to be more specifically elucidated.

INTERFERON

Colostral cells in culture have been shown to be stimulated to secrete an interferon-like substance with strong antiviral activity up to 150 National Institutes of Health units/mL.[265] This property has not yet been identified in the supernatant of colostrum or milk. Interferon-γ has been produced by T cells from human milk when stimulated in vitro.[265] The T cells isolated from human milk were the CD45RO phenotype and have been identified as a source of interferon. Srivastava et al.[305] have measured low levels of interferon-γ in not only colostrum, but also transitional and mature milk. They postulated that the low level of interferon-γ (0.7 to 2 pg/mL) might be adequate to protect against infection without hyperactivation of T cells. Interferon is produced by NK cells and by T cells, phenotypically Thy0 and Thy1. It can cause increased expression of major histocompatibility complex molecules, increase macrophage function, inhibit IgE and IL-10 production, and produce antitumor and antiviral activity. The exact role of interferon-γ in breast milk has not been delineated.

COMPLEMENT

The C3 and C4 components of complement, known for their ability to fuse bacteria bound to a specific antibody, are present in colostrum in low concentrations compared with their levels in serum. IgG and IgM activate complement. C3 proactivator has been described, and IgA and IgE have been identified as stimulating the system. Activated C3 has opsonic, anaphylactic, and chemotactic properties and is important for the lysis of bacteria bound to a specific antibody. No functional role for complement in breast milk has been identified.

VITAMIN B$_{12}$-BINDING PROTEIN

Unsaturated vitamin B$_{12}$-binding protein of high molecular weight has been found in very high levels in human milk, and in the meconium and stools of breastfed infants, compared with its levels in infant formulas and infants who are formula fed. The protein binding renders the vitamin B$_{12}$ unavailable for bacterial growth of *E. coli* and *Bacteroides*.[121]

GLYCANS AND OLIGOSACCHARIDES

Glycans are complex carbohydrate structures attached to various other structures (a lactose moiety, a lipid component, peptides, proteins, or aminoglycans) that are present in large amounts in human milk.[233] They include glycoproteins, glycolipids (gangliosides), glycosaminoglycans, mucins, and oligosaccharides. Oligosaccharides are composed of a basic core structure derived from glucose, galactose, or *N*-acetylglucosamine. They are linked to a variety of terminal fucose linkages or sialic acid linkages to create numerous different compounds. Oligosaccharides compose the major portion of glycoconjugates in milk and are present in the milk-fat globule membrane and in skim milk.[229,233,235] Gangliosides are glycolipids found in the plasma membrane of cells, especially in cells in the gray matter of the brain. More specifically, gangliosides are glycosphingolipids that contain sialic acid, hexoses, or hexose amines as the carbohydrate component and ceramide as the lipid component of the molecule. Human milk oligosaccharides (HMO) are poorly absorbed and poorly digested and remain in the gut. Their probable functions are antipathogenic, immunomodulatory, antiinflammatory, and prebiotic.[236]

The predominant gangliosides in human milk are GM1, GM2, GM3, and GD3, as reported by Newburg.[231] A diverse abundance of these complex carbohydrates are synthesized by the many glycosyltransferases contained in the mammary gland. Mucin and lactadherin are two glycoproteins included in this group that have antimicrobial effects.[286] Some of these carbohydrate molecules are structurally similar to glycans on the surface of small intestine epithelial cells that act as receptors for microorganisms. One proposed mechanism for the antimicrobial effect of these soluble substances is direct binding with the potential pathogenic organisms.[230,231] After studying the adhesion of S-fimbriated *E. coli* to buccal epithelial cells, Schroten et al.[296] proposed that mucins contained in the human milk-fat globule membrane can block bacterial adhesion throughout the intestine.

Gangliosides appear to be responsible for blocking the activity of heat-labile enterotoxin from *E. coli* and the toxin from *V. cholerae* in rat intestinal loop preparations.[251] Another toxin from *Campylobacter jejuni*, with similar binding specificity, also seems to be inhibited by GM1.[184,283] Globotriaosylceramide, another glycolipid in human milk, is the natural cell surface receptor for the toxin from *Shigella dysenteriae* and verotoxin released by entero-hemorrhagic *E. coli*.[232] The proposed mechanism of action of these glycolipids is that, by binding to the toxin, they form a stable complex that prevents the toxin from binding to the appropriate receptors on intestinal cells. However, Crane et al.[61] proposed, from their studies, that the oligosaccharide binds to the toxin receptor to block the action of the heat-stable enterotoxin of *E. coli*. Human milk gangliosides may be important in protecting infants against toxin-induced diarrhea, but this has not been specifically demonstrated in vivo in controlled trials.[232,251] Evidence exists that human milk glycans inhibit a broad range of pathogens (Table 5-5).[229-234] Newberg et al.[232] document the constitutive expression of various fucosylated glycans in human milk and secretions and present "typical" concentrations of these active agents in human milk from the literature. Their secretion is related to the "secretor" and Lewis genes, which control the individual differences in expression of Lewis blood group types.

Chaturvedi et al.[55] have recently examined the survival of oligosaccharides from human milk in infants' intestines. They demonstrated that the concentrations of oligosaccharides were higher in the infants' feces than in mothers' milk and higher in feces than urine. The profile of oligosaccharides found in the infants was similar to that found in their mothers' milk. The formula-fed infants had lower concentrations of oligosaccharides, and the profiles of the oligosaccharides were different from those found in the breastfed infants. The oligosaccharides remained intact passing through the intestine. A small percentage are absorbed and excreted intact in the urine. The oligosaccharides were available at these sites to block intestinal and urinary pathogens. Two other groups of researchers have documented variation of the composition of glycans in human milk over the first 4 months of lactation[60] and variations in the composition of glycans in diverse populations.[83] Others have analyzed the oligosaccharide composition of donor human milk (Holder pasteurized) and compared that to samples of human milk obtained directly from the mothers.[204] The total amount of HMO was lower in donor human milk. The concentrations of specific oligosaccharides (lacto-*N*-tetraose, lacto-*N*-neotetraose, lacto-*N*-fucopentaose I, and disialyllacto-*N*-tetraose) were significantly lower in donor milk. The concentrations of 3'-sialyllactose and 3-fucosyllactose were higher in human milk obtained directly from the mothers.[204] Therefore, a diverse repertoire of glycans are present in large amounts in human milk, which persist intact in the intestine and reach the urine, and have demonstrated inhibitory effects on a variety of pathogens.

TABLE 5-5	Nonimmunoglobulin Antipathogen Factors in Human Milk
Antipathogen	**Pathogen**
Ganglioside GM$_1$	Cholera toxin
	Labile toxin of *Escherichia coli*
	Toxin of *Campylobacter jejuni*
Globotriaosylceramide	*Shigella* toxin I
	Shigella-like toxin of *E. coli*
GM3	Enteropathogenic *E. coli*
Fatty acids	Enveloped viruses
	Giardia lamblia
Chondroitin sulfate	HIV
Sulfatide	HIV
Glycoprotein (mucin)	Inhibition: rotavirus in vitro and in vivo
Glycoprotein (mucin, glycosaminoglycan)	HIV
Lactadherin	Rotavirus
Mucin	Adherence: S-fimbriated *E. coli*
MUC 1	Poxviruses, HIV
Glycoprotein (mannosylated)	*E. coli* intestinal adherence
Large macromolecule	Respiratory syncytial virus
Macromolecule-associated glycans	Norovirus, *Pseudomonas aeruginosa*
Oligosaccharides	Adherence: *Streptococcus pneumoniae* and *Haemophilus influenzae*, enteropathogenic *E. coli*
	Listeria monocytogenes
Fucosylated oligosaccharide	Adherence, invasion, *C. jejuni*, stable toxin of *E. coli* stable toxin in vivo, *Vibrio cholera*
Sialyllactose	Cholera toxin, *E. coli*, *Pseudomonas aeruginosa*, Influenza virus
	Aspergillus fumigates, Polyomavirus, *Helicobacter pylori*

GM, Granulocyte-macrophage; *HIV*, human immunodeficiency virus.

Modified from Newburg DS, Ruiz-Palacios GM, Morrow AL: Milk glycans protect infants against enteric pathogens, *Ann Rev Nutr* 25:37-58, 2005.

These components constitute a major contribution of human milk to innate immunity at the level of an infant's gut. There is variability in the amounts of specific HMO in the milk of different mothers, at different times through each mother's period of lactation and in human donor milk. The importance of the "match" of the mother-infant dyad based on HMO composition and quantity and the benefits to the infant still need to be elucidated.

Other authors propose that the gangliosides GD3 and GM3 may play an immunomodulatory role early in lactation by affecting DCs, decreasing the production of ILs (IL-10 and IL-12), and suppressing the expression of various cluster designation (CD) markers and major histocompatability complex class II on DCs.[34]

INTERLEUKINS

ILs are considered a "subgroup" of cytokines.[195] Originally, when cytokines were first hypothesized, it was thought that they were primarily produced by leukocytes and acted on other leukocytes, and therefore they could be called ILs. Although much of their effect is on lymphocyte activation and differentiation, it is now known that ILs act on and are produced by a variety of cells.[113]

Goldman et al.[113] identified IL-1β, IL-6, IL-8, and IL-10 in breast milk (Table 5-6). Srivastava et al.[305] reported measuring moderate amounts of IL-6, IL-8, and IL-10 in the different stages of breast milk. Very low amounts of IL-1β were detected, especially in comparison with the amount of IL-1 receptor antagonist (RA), which presumably could block the activity of the small amount of IL-1.

TABLE 5-6	Bioactivity and Concentrations of Cytokines in Human Milk	
Agents	**Bioactivity in Milk**	**Concentrations***
IL-1β	±	1130±478
IL-6	+	151±89
IL-7	?	79-100±19†
IL-8	?	3684±2910
IL-10	+	3400±3800
TNF-α	+	620±183
G-CSF	?	~358
M-CSF	+	17,120
Interferon-γ	?	?
EGF	+	~200,000
TGF-α	+	~2200-7200
TGF-β2	+	130±108

CSF, Colony-stimulating factor; *EGF*, epidermal growth factor; *G*, granulocyte; *IL*, interleukin; *M*, macrophage; *TGF*, transforming growth factor; *TNF*, tumor necrosis factor.
*The concentrations of these agents were determined by enzyme-linked immunosorbent assay (ELISA) except for IL-1β and EGF by radioimmunoassay. Concentrations are expressed as pg/mL except for M-CSF (U/mL).
†From Ngom PT, Collinson AC, Pido-Lopez J, et al: Improved thymic function in exclusively breastfed infants is associated with higher interleukin 7 concentrations in their mothers' breastmilk, *Am J Clin Nutr* 80:722-728, 2004.
From Goldman AS, Chheda S, Garofalo R, Schmalstieg FC: Cytokines in human milk properties and potential effects upon the mammary gland and the neonate, *J Mammary Gland Biol Neoplasia* 1:251, 1996.

Hawkes et al.[139] reported on the amount of cytokines in breast milk over the first 12 weeks of lactation. The proposed "proinflammatory" cytokines, IL-1β, IL-6, and TNF-α, were present in only 7 of 36 mothers who donated samples at each point throughout the study. A broad range of concentrations of each of these cytokines was seen during the course of the study. The "antiinflammatory" cytokines, TGF-α1 and TGF-β2, were present in significant amounts in all samples. IL-2 has also been reported in breast milk in 81% of the mothers tested, with milk (aqueous) levels correlating with plasma IL-2 levels. IL-2 was constitutively produced from 57% of milk cell samples, and IL-2 production was markedly increased by stimulation of the cells with Con A.[37]

IL-6 has been identified in breast milk by other investigators, especially in the first 2 days of life.[253,282] The authors suggest that IL-6 in human milk may augment the newborn's immune functions before the body can begin full production of cytokines. Specifically, this is accomplished by increasing antibody production, especially IgA; enhancing phagocytosis; activating T cells; and increasing α1-antitrypsin production by mononuclear phagocytes. IL-7 is a chemokine known to improve thymic output in animals and appears related to the proliferation and survival of T cells in all stages of development.[238] Ngom et al.[238] have described improved thymic function in exclusively breastfed infants associated with higher IL-7 concentrations in the mother's breast milk. The breast milk of Gambian mothers contained variable levels of IL-7, but the geometric mean levels were higher in the first 8 weeks postpartum in mothers whose infants were born in the "harvest-season" (January to June) compared with those mothers whose infants were born in the "hungry-season." The authors postulate that IL-7 in breast milk enhances T cell proliferation and survival and overall thymic development in the infant, leading to long-term benefits in protection from infection.

IL-8 is a chemokine capable of attracting and activating neutrophils and attracting CD45RA+ T cells. IL-8 is produced by mammary epithelial cells.[253] Srivastava et al.[305] also detected messenger ribonucleic acid (mRNA) for IL-8, suggesting that cells in breast milk were capable of producing IL-8. The exact function of IL-8 in breast milk remains to be elucidated.

IL-10 is thought to have antiinflammatory effects, including decreasing the production of interferon-γ, IL-12, and other proinflammatory cytokines. It has been reported to enhance IgA, IgG, and IgM synthesis.

IL-18 has been identified in colostrum, early milk, and mature milk, with the highest levels occurring in colostrum and in association with preterm deliveries and complications of pregnancy in the mothers.[312] The levels of IL-18 were correlated with soluble Fas ligand in colostrum. IL-18 was detected by immunohistochemical staining in actively secreting epithelial cells in a lactating breast. IL-18 has been shown to be produced by intestinal epithelial cells and activated macrophages. It leads to the production of other chemokines (GM-CSF, IL-2, TNF-α). It induces the expression of Fas ligand on lymphocytes. The authors suggested that IL-18, present in colostrum, may play a role in stimulating a systemic T_H1 response and causing NK cell and macrophage activation in neonates.

The interaction and the direct effect of these ILs in breast milk must be clarified. The amount of T cells bearing markers of recent activation is increased in human milk compared with the results in peripheral blood of adults. Wirt et al.[334] have described a marked shift from virginal to antigen-primed (memory) T cells in human milk, which suggests certain functional capacities for these cells. The phenotypic pattern of T cells may result from T-cell-activating substances or selective homing of T cells to the breast. These activated T cell populations are transferred to the infant through breast milk, along with a variety of ILs at a time when infants are capable of only limited production of ILs. A complex interaction of ILs and cells in human milk and at the mucosal level may provide antimicrobial and antiinflammatory benefits to the infant.

CYTOKINES

Of the many bioactive substances that have been identified in human milk, cytokines are some of the most recently identified and investigated agents. Their existence has long been suspected in attempts to explain certain immunologic and protective effects of breast milk on infants. More than 40 cytokines have been described,[200] and more than 10 of these have been identified in human milk.[113,305] Cytokines are small proteins or glycoproteins that, through binding to receptors on immune and nonimmune cells, produce a broad range of effects (many still unidentified) through autocrine, paracrine, and endocrine actions. Cytokines are produced predominantly by immune cells and function in complex associations with other cytokines to stimulate and control the development and normal functioning of the immune system. The nomenclature and abbreviations used are complicated and confusing. Newer systems of classification have been established according to which cells produce them or what their general functions are[195] or based on the relative position of their cysteine residues or their receptor types (CCR, CXCR,

BOX 5-3. Nomenclature and Abbreviations for Various Cytokines	
Interferon Alpha, Beta, Gamma	**IFN-α, -β, -γ**
Granulocyte colony-stimulating factor	G-CSF
Macrophage colony-stimulating factor	M-CSF
Stem cell factor	SCF
Interleukins 1, 2, 4, 6, 8, 10	IL-1, -2, -4, -6, -8, -10
Interleukin 1 beta	IL-1β
Interleukin 1 receptor antagonist	IL-1RA
Soluble interleukin 2 receptor	sIL-2R
Transforming growth factor beta$_2$	TGF-β_2
Tumor necrosis factor alpha	TNF-α
Transforming growth factor alpha	TGF-α
Macrophage inflammatory protein	MIP
Regulated on activation, normal T cell expressed and secreted	RANTES
Epidermal growth factor	EGF
Growth-regulated oncogene	GRO
Monocyte chemoattractant protein 1	MCP-1
Leukocyte inhibitory factor	LIF

and CX3CR).[200] Box 5-3 provides a simplified list with abbreviations.

Little evidence demonstrates specific in vivo activity of the different cytokines. Based on general information on the function and interaction of the particular cytokines, as well as consideration of as yet unexplained effects of breast milk, proposed functions of the cytokines include initiation of development of host defense; stimulation of host defenses; prevention of autoimmunity, antiinflammatory effects in the upper respiratory tract and GI tract; and stimulation of the development of the digestive system, especially the mucosal immune system of the alimentary tract and the proximal respiratory tract. The maternal breast may respond to feedback stimulation or suppression by secreted cytokines, influencing the growth, differentiation, and secretory function of the breast. As shown in other situations, cytokines may enhance receptor expression on cells in the respiratory and GI tracts for major histocompatibility complex molecules or immunoglobulins. Various cell types in the mucosal immune system may be activated or attracted to specific sites in the GI tract by the action of cytokines.

Beyond these proposed beneficial effects of cytokines, newer studies are identifying specific immunologic and protective roles for different cytokines in developing infants. For example, extensive work has been done on epidermal growth factor (EGF), and other growth factors (HB-EGF,

G-CSF, EPO, and EPO-like growth factors) have been studied relative to their role in preventing necrotizing enterocolitis (NEC) and gut homeostasis.[223] A number of potential roles for EGF in gut homeostasis have been proposed and studied, including intestinal development, proliferation and adaptive response to damage, repair, and regeneration and diminishing inflammatory responses to various stimuli. TGF-β has been studied for its role in initiating and stimulating IgA production early on in infancy.[244]

The actual measurement of cytokines in breast milk has been complicated by a number of factors, including different assays used (bioassays, enzyme-linked immunosorbent assay [ELISA], radioimmunoassay), binding to proteins, their existence in monomeric or polymeric forms, the presence of antagonists, and their varying presence in colostrum, early milk, or mature milk.[9] Goldman et al.[113] reported on the bioactivity and concentration of cytokines in breast milk from their own work and that of others (see Table 5-6). Srivastava et al.[305] obtained some conflicting results using different assays in colostrum, early milk, and mature milk. They confirmed the presence of M-CSF throughout lactation, as well as TGF-β_1 and -β_2, IL-1RA, GRO-α, MCP-1, RANTES, and IL-8, but reported insignificant amounts of GM-CSF, stem cell factor, LIF, MIP-1α, IL-2, IL-4, IL-11, IL-12, IL-13, IL-15, sIL-2R, and IFN-α (see Box 5-3 for nomenclature). Srivastava et al.[305] also used reverse transcriptase (RT) polymerase chain reaction (PCR) to measure the production of cytokine mRNA by cells in breast milk. They reported the presence of mRNA for MCP-1, IL-8, TGF-β_1, TGF-β_2, M-CSF, IL-6, and IL-1β, which may be another source of these cytokines in breast milk. Hawkes et al.[139] demonstrated that human milk cells from lactating women at 5 weeks postpartum are capable of active cytokine production in vitro (IL-1β, IL-6, and TNF-α), with and without exposure to lipopolysaccharide. Continued cytokine production by human milk cells is another explanation for the variable amounts of cytokines identified in breast milk and is further evidence that the cells are capable of responding to an infectious stimulus.

In their investigations of the possible antiinflammatory effects of breast milk, Buescher and Malinowska[40] examined milk for the presence of soluble receptors and cytokine antagonists. They demonstrated soluble intercellular adhesion molecule 1, soluble vascular cell adhesion molecule 1, and soluble E-selectin in colostrum and at lower levels in mature milk, as well as high levels of soluble TNF-α receptor I (sTNF-αRI), sTNF-αRII, and IL-1RA. Also, they identified that most TNF-α did not exist "free" in breast milk, but was associated with TNF receptors. The in vivo significance of these findings remains to be assessed.

Given the complex interaction and regulation of cytokine production and cytokines' relation to coordinated inflammatory and antiinflammatory responses in tissues, one should assume that the interaction of cytokines in breast milk and the effect of cytokines, cytokine receptors (soluble and expressed on various cell types), and cytokine antagonists on the infant will be equally complex. A new methodology, antibody-based protein arrays, has been applied to identify cytokines in human milk.[181] Kverka et al.[181] analyzed colostrums and milk samples from the first 4 days postpartum, using two different arrays capable of detecting 42 and 79 cytokines. Three cytokines (EGF, IL-8/CXCL8, and GRO/CXCL1-3) were detected in all of the tested samples. Nineteen cytokines were present in more than 50% of the samples. An additional 32 cytokines were identified in human milk for the first time. The concentration of cytokines varied in the different women and varied over time. Continued investigation with this and other assays will be essential to understanding the significance and specific effects of these substances in breast milk.

Nucleotides

Nucleotides, nucleosides, nucleic acids, and related metabolic products are essential to many biologic processes. Although they are not essential nutrients, because they can be synthesized endogenously and recovered from in vivo "salvage" sources, their presence in the diet may carry significant benefits under various conditions (i.e., "conditionally essential").[53,224,322,344] In situations of disease, stress, rapid growth, or limited dietary intake, supplementation of the diet with nucleotides may decrease energy expenditure to synthesize or salvage nucleotides, which optimizes the host response to these adverse situations.[344]

Nucleotides exist in relatively large amounts in human milk (15% to 20% of the nonprotein nitrogen), suggesting that they have some nutritional significance, although no clinical syndromes have been associated with nucleotide deficiency to date. Nucleotides are present in the natural milk of different species in varying amounts and composition. The nucleotide content and composition of bovine milk are particularly less and different from human milk. Infant formulas supplemented with nucleotides contain roughly the same amounts of nucleotides as human milk, from 20 to 70 mg/L.[50,51,188] Unsupplemented formulas contain lesser amounts of nucleotides.

Mammalian cells contain a large variety of nucleotides and related products, which have many metabolic functions, including the following[51–53]:

1. Energy metabolism: adenosine triphosphate is a major form of available cellular energy.
2. Nucleic acid precursors: the monomeric units for RNA and DNA are present.
3. Physiologic mediators: cyclic adenosine monophosphate and cyclic guanosine monophosphate serve as "messengers" for cellular processes; adenosine diphosphate is necessary for platelet aggregation; and adenosine has been shown to affect vasodilatation.
4. Related products function as coenzymes in metabolic pathways: nicotinamide-adenine dinucleotide, flavin adenine dinucleotide, and coenzyme A.
5. Related products function as intermediate carrying molecules in synthetic reactions: uridine diphosphate glucose in glycogen synthesis and guanosine diphosphate mannose, guanosine diphosphate-fucose, uridine diphosphate-galactose, and cytidine monophosphate sialic acid in glycoprotein synthesis.
6. Allosteric effectors: the intracellular concentrations of nucleotides influence the progression of certain steps of metabolic pathways.
7. Cellular agonists: extracellular nucleotides influence intracellular signal transduction (e.g., cyclic adenosine monophosphate and inositol-calcium pathway).

Nucleotide concentrations in cells and tissues are maintained by de novo synthesis and salvage from intermediary metabolism and diet (Figure 5-11).[271] Nucleosides are the predominant product absorbed in the small intestine. Nucleosides are probably transported by passive diffusion and a carrier-mediated process; purines and pyrimidines are transported by passive diffusion at high concentrations and by a sodium-dependent active mechanism at low concentrations (Figure 5-12).[271] The digestion and absorption of nucleotides, nucleosides, and pyrimidines and purines also involve polymeric and monomeric nucleotides and other adducts (nucleosides in a biologically active moiety).

In early reports on the nucleotide and nucleoside content of milk, various methods of measurement were used, and the amounts were described as either the monomeric fraction of nucleotides or the total RNA. Leach et al.,[188] recognizing the complex nature of digestion and absorption of nucleotides and related products, attempted to measure the total potentially available nucleosides (TPANs) in human milk. They used solid-phase extraction, high-performance liquid chromatography analysis, and enzymatic hydrolysis of the various fractions. They analyzed breast milk samples at various stages throughout lactation (colostrum, transitional, early, and late mature milk) from 100 European women and 11 American women. They used an aqueous TPAN-fortified solution containing ribonucleosides, 5'-mononucleotides, polymeric RNA, and nucleoside-containing adducts to estimate the accuracy of their process.

The mean ranges of TPAN values were similar for European women from different countries and American women, although broad ranges were seen and the composition of individual nucleotides varied.[188] The mean TPAN value was lowest in colostrum but did not show a consistent upward or downward trend in transitional, early, or late mature milk. The mean ranges of TPAN values were 82 to 164 mmol/L for colostrum, 144 to 210 mmol/L for transitional milk, 172 to 402 mmol/L for early

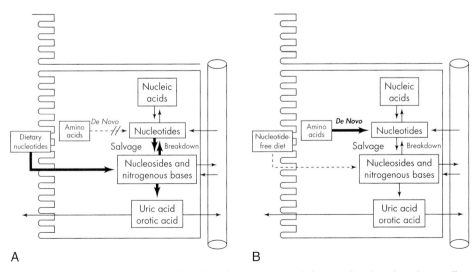

Figure 5-11. Metabolic regulation of cellular nucleotide pools in presence and absence of nucleotide in diet. **A,** Effect of dietary nucleotide activating salvage pathway. **B,** De novo nucleotide synthesis is enhanced with nucleotide-free diet. (From Quan R, Barness LA: Do infants need nucleotide supplemented formula for optimal nutrition? *J Pediatr Gastroenterol Nutr* 11:429, 1990.)

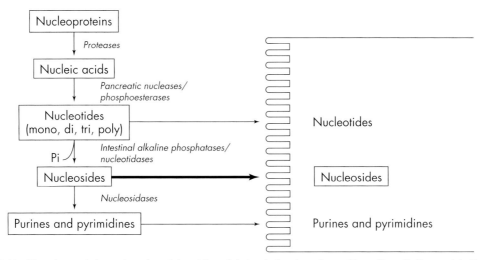

Figure 5-12. Digestion and absorption of nucleic acids and their relational products. (From Quan R, Barness LA: Do infants need nucleotide supplemented formula for optimal nutrition? *Pediatr Gastroenterol Nutr* 11(4):429, 1990.)

mature milk, and 156 to 259 mmol/L for late mature milk (Table 5-7). Monomeric and polymeric nucleotides were the predominant forms of TPAN in pooled samples. Cytidine, guanosine, and adenosine were found mainly in these fractions, whereas uridine was found primarily as free nucleotide and adduct (Table 5-8). The methods used recovered 90% to 95% of the true TPAN values compared with the TPAN-fortified solution, although the uridine and guanosine content was underestimated. Tressler et al.[319] measured the TPAN in pooled breast milk samples from Asian women demonstrating average levels in colostrum, transitional milk, and mature milk and found it to be similar to the levels in European and American women.

Leach et al.[188] concluded that their process of estimating TPANs, including sequential enzymatic hydrolyses, and measuring the entire nucleotide fraction provides a reasonable estimate of the in vivo process and the nucleotides available to the infant from human milk.

Proposed effects of dietary nucleotides include effects on the immune system, iron absorption, intestinal flora, plasma lipoproteins, and growth of intestinal and hepatic cells. Effects on the immune system, related to nucleotide supplementation to the diet, have mainly been reported from animal studies. They include increased mortality rate from graft-versus-host disease; improved delayed-type cutaneous hypersensitivity and alloantigen-induced lymphoproliferation; reversal of malnutrition and starvation-induced immunosuppression; increased resistance to challenge with *S. aureus* and *C. albicans*; and enhanced T cell maturation and function.[264] Spleen cells of mice fed a nucleotide-free diet produce lower levels of IL-2, express lower levels of IL-2 receptors, and have

decreased NK cell activity and macrophage activity.[51,52] Presumably, these nucleotide-associated changes are related to T-helper/inducer cells and the initial phases of antigen processing and lymphocyte proliferation.[52,53,322]

In vitro and in vivo experiments documented that ingested nucleotides increased iron absorption, perhaps affecting xanthine oxidase.[271] Although in vitro studies showed that added nucleotides enhanced the growth of bifidobacteria, conflicting results have been obtained on the influence of dietary nucleotides on the fecal flora of infants receiving breast milk or nucleotide-supplemented formula.[12,271] Clinical studies in infants receiving nucleotide-supplemented formula demonstrated increased high-density lipoprotein cholesterol, lower very-low-density lipoprotein cholesterol, increased long-chain polyunsaturated fatty acids (PUFA), and changes in red blood cell membrane phospholipid composition.[12] Supplementation studies in animals have shown enhanced GI tract growth and maturation, improved intestinal repair after diarrhea, stimulation of hepatic growth, and augmented recovery from hepatectomy.[264]

A recent review discusses the effects of dietary nucleotides on the immune system and protection against infection reported in studies in the literature.[293] Carver et al.[52] compared infants receiving breast milk to those receiving commercially available infant formula and formula supplemented with nucleotides at a level of 32 mg/L. At 2 and 4 months, NK cell activity and IL-2 production were higher in the breastfed and nucleotide-supplemented groups compared with those receiving formula without nucleotide supplements. Infections occurred infrequently in all groups, but slightly less in the breastfed group. No differences were noted in

TABLE 5-7 Nucleotide and Total Potentially Available Nucleoside (TPAN) in Pooled Human Milk by Stage of Lactation (μmol/L)*

	Uridine	Cytidine	Guanosine	Adenosine	TPAN
Colostrum					
Site 1	27	84	22	20	153
Site 2	21	33	15	13	82
Site 3	30	82	26	26	164
Site 4	24	84	20	22	150
Mean	26	71	21	21	137
Transitional milk					
Site 1	23	82	22	19	146
Site 2	33	76	19	17	144
Site 3	37	84	43	42	206
Site 4	36	100	36	38	210
Mean	32	86	30	29	177
Early mature milk					
Site 1	30	86	28	28	172
Site 2	50	79	23	21	173
Site 3	44	96	36	37	214
Site 4	67	146	91	97	402
Mean	48	102	45	46	240
Late mature milk					
Site 1	36	73	22	25	156
Site 2	58	106	29	27	219
Site 3	49	81	20	24	173
Site 4	45	124	40	49	259
Mean	47	96	28	31	202
Grand mean	38	88	31	32	189
SD	13	24	18	20	70
Range	21-67	33-146	19-92	13-97	84-402
American pool†	37	70	30	24	161

*Data from 100 individual samples collected at four sites and combined into 16 pooled samples (5-7 individual samples per site per stage of lactation). *Site 1*, Rouen and Mount Saint Aignau, France; *Site 2*, Mainz, Germany; *Site 3*, Bolzano, Italy; *Site 4*, Treviso, Italy.
†Pooled sample of milk collected from 11 American women between 2 and 4 months postpartum.
From Leach JL, Baxter JH, Molitor BE, et al: Total potentially available nucleosides of human milk by stage of lactation, *Am J Clin Nutr* 61:1224, 1995.

TABLE 5-8 Percentage of Total Potentially Available Nucleoside (TPAN) in Pooled Human Milk as Adducts, Polymeric Nucleotides, Monomeric Nucleotides, and Nucleosides*

	Uridine	Cytidine	Guanosine	Adenosine	TPAN
Polymeric nucleotides	19±7	57±12	59±21	47±11	48±8
Monomeric nucleotides	36±12	37±13	34±14	35±10	36±10
Nucleosides	18±14	5±5	1±2	5±4	8±6
Adducts†	27±12	1±1	7±15	13±9	9±4

*x±SD. Based on the mean of entire pool of human milk collected from 100 individuals at four stages of lactation at four sites.
†Adducts are of the form nucleoside-phosphate-phosphate-X, where X is a biologically relevant moiety (e.g., uridine diphosphate-galactose or nicotinamide-adenine dinucleotide).
From Leach JL, Baxter JH, Molitor BE, et al: Total potentially available nucleosides of human milk by stage of lactation, *Am J Clin Nutr* 61:1224, 1995.

hematologic profiles and plasma chemistry values, and no toxicity or intolerance was associated with nucleotide supplementation. The sample size was small, marked variability was seen in the IL-2 measurements, and the differences noted at 4 months were less than at 2 months. Therefore, the authors concluded that dietary nucleotides may contribute to improved immunity in breastfed infants.

Brunser et al.[36] examined the effect of a nucleotide-supplemented formula on the incidence of diarrhea in 392 infants in Chile, studied through 6 months of age. Although the infants receiving the supplemented formula (20 mg/L) experienced less diarrhea, the difference in the duration of diarrhea was small. The numbers were too small to comment on the causative agents of diarrhea, although no apparent protection against any one agent was seen. The beneficial effect of nucleotides against diarrhea was proposed to be secondary to enhanced immune response to intestinal pathogens or improved intestinal integrity or a combination of both. In a larger study of 3243 infants younger than 6 months of age, the severity of the diarrhea (duration and number of bowel movements), as well as the incidence of diarrhea, was lower in the nucleotide-supplemented group.[185]

Two groups of premature infants fed either nucleotide supplemented (20 mg/L) or unsupplemented formula were followed, and the concentration of plasma immunoglobulins throughout the first 3 months of life was measured.[224] IgG plasma concentrations were not different in the two groups during the study period. IgM plasma levels were higher in the nucleotide-supplemented group at 20 to 30 days and 3 months of life, while IgA plasma levels were significantly higher at 3 months of age in the supplemented group.

Pickering et al.[264] published a 12-month, controlled, randomized study of 311 infants to examine the effect of added nucleotides at levels comparable to human milk on infants' immune responses to various vaccine antigens; 103 nonrandomized infants received breast milk for at least 2 months and then either human milk or a standard infant formula. Another 208 infants were randomized to receive either a standard infant formula or one supplemented with nucleotides. The amount and actual nucleotide content added were based on TPANs, as measured by Leach et al.,[188] equaling 72 mg/L. Overall growth and nutrition tolerance were similar in each group. The nucleotide group had significantly higher geometric mean titers of *H. influenzae* type b antibody and diphtheria antibody than the control group or the breastfed infants. No significant difference was seen between the nucleotide and control groups for the IgG response to oral poliovirus vaccine or tetanus. Infants who were breastfed for longer than 6 months had significantly higher antibody responses to oral poliovirus

vaccine than children breastfed for less than 6 months, or either of the two formula-fed groups. No significant differences were found between the different groups with respect to total IgG, IgA, or IgE. Differences were seen in the number of children who experienced at least one episode of diarrhea: the nucleotide group (4/27, 15%), versus the control group (13 of 32, 41%, $p < 0.05$), and the breastfed group (6 of 27, 22%). Notably, the breastfed group was heterogeneous, relative to the amount of breast milk received and the duration of feeding, whereas the nucleotide group received supplementation for the entire 12 months.

Questions that remain concerning nucleotides and their proposed beneficial effects in an infant's diet include the following:

- What are the proven mechanisms of action of these proposed benefits?
- What form and concentration of nucleotides are necessary to affect these benefits?
- Is adequate information available to justify using nucleotides in infant formula in higher amounts and different compositions than are currently used?

Debate and research to answer these and other questions concerning nucleotides will continue.

Mucosal Immune System

A primary function of each of the body's different mucosal surfaces is immunologic. Each distinct mucosal surface has multiple other physiologic functions including gas exchange (in the lungs), nutrient absorption (in the gut), sensory detection (in the eyes, nose, and mouth), and reproduction (in the uterus and vagina). The thin, permeable nature of these barrier mucosal surfaces, their large surface area, and the constant exposure to microorganisms, foreign proteins, and chemicals predispose the mucosal membranes to damage and infection. During the first year(s) of life, when the infant's immune system is developing and maturing, it is doing so on a systemic and a mucosal basis, as well as involving both innate and adaptive immune mechanisms. That development must include the ability to respond to and protect against invasive pathogens, and at the same time "tolerate" or "ignore" the multitude of commensal organisms that reside at these surfaces. During this early development, breast milk contains numerous bioactive factors that supplement the immune protection at the mucosal level, while limiting inflammation. Additionally, these factors contribute to the immune modulation and growth stimulation of infants' mucosal and systemic immune defenses.*

*106,107,108,109,110,133

The mucosal immune system involves both innate mechanisms and adaptive immune mechanisms functioning in concert. The development of the mucosal immune system occurs in the prenatal period and continues in the postnatal period. The functional mucosal barrier includes the action of enzymes, chemicals, acidity or pH, mucus, immune globulins, and indigenous flora. In as early as 8 weeks of gestational age, researchers have identified changes in the intestinal barrier with the development of enterocytes, goblet cells, and enterochromaffin cells, along with evidence of development of tight junctions between the epithelial cells.[255,268] Mucus production, which can block adherence of pathogens to epithelial cells, demonstrates both pre- and postnatal development, beginning with evidence of expression of the *muc2* gene as early as 12 weeks' gestational age.[43] This is approximately the same time that Paneth cells appear in intestinal crypts. These cells secrete various products, including α-defensin, lysozyme, secretory phospholipase A_2, and TNF α, which contribute to protection from pathogens, enhance stem cell protection within the epithelial layer, and influence the selection and number of commensal organisms.[219,288] Secretory immune globulins sIgA and IgM act at the epithelial surface, largely without inflammation, by limiting adherence and transmigration and facilitating phagocytosis of potential pathogens.

Mucosal-Associated Lymphoid Tissue

The well-recognized MALT is present in localized areas beneath the mucosal surfaces: tonsils and adenoids in the nasopharynx, and Peyer patches and isolated lymphoid follicles in the intestine. Overlying the isolated lymphoid follicles of the gut are specialized epithelial cells called M-cells. M-cells (membrane, microfold, or multifenestrated cells) come in direct contact with microorganisms and antigens due to a lack of a surface glycocalyx covering. These remarkable cells endocytose, phagocytose, and transcytose molecules and antigens, from their luminal surface to their basal surface. Antigen-presenting cells and lymphocytes process the trancytosed molecules, presenting them to submucosal aggregates of lymphocytes. The activated lymphocytes that have responded to the specifically presented antigens migrate via the lymphatics to the thoracic duct and into the blood. These lymphocytes circulate in the blood, until they return to mucosal tissues, predominantly the same ones they originated from, where they now function as effector lymphocytes in the lamina propria. This process of "directed migration" to specific sites occurs due to the influence of cytokines and adhesion molecules, such as chemokine CCL28 (mucosal epithelia chemokine), expressed in the colon

and salivary glands, and CCL25 (thymus-expressed chemokine), which effects the site-specific migration.[263] The immune response of lymphocytes in the submucosa, and the subsequent directed migration to the same and other mucosal sites, produces a focused response to a selected repertoire of antigens at those sites. The lactating mammary gland is an essential component of MALT. A mother makes a mature effective immune response to microorganisms in her and her infant's environment through antigenic stimulation of MALT in the mother's gut and respiratory mucosa. The maternal immune response produces activated lymphocytes, cytokines, immunoglobulins, and other factors against the specific microorganism. There is a subsequent "directed migration" of these activated lymphocytes, immunoglobulins, cytokines, and bioactive factors to the breast and into the breast milk. These specific factors in the breast milk add to the protective effect of breast milk against specific microorganisms in the mother's and infant's environment. This is a well-recognized example of how breast milk can provide additional immune protection to the infant. It is also one of the reasons to continue breastfeeding when a mother or the infant has a possible infection.

The mucosal immune system undergoes significant postnatal development, in part due to the dramatic exposure of the mucosa to large numbers of microorganisms in early postnatal life. Peyer patches are rudimentary, and few immunoglobulin-producing intestinal plasma cells are present until several weeks after birth.[31] After several weeks, germinal centers within the lymphoid follicles develop, and the number of IgM- and IgA-producing cells in the intestine increase. Immunoglobulin-producing intestinal plasma cells (primarily IgA-producing cells) in the lamina propria increase in number from 1 to 12 months of age.[308] With normal maturation of the mucosal immune system, large numbers of immunoglobulin-producing cells locate in the intestinal lamina propria. The monomeric IgA produced by these plasma cells is transported through epithelial cells to the mucosal lumen. Attachment of an epithelial glycoprotein, the membrane secretory component to two IgA molecules, leads to the formation of a dimeric molecule. The sIgA molecule is "secreted" at the mucosal surface. IgM, in the form of a pentamer, contains a polypeptide J-chain and is transported by the same mechanism.[32] A portion of the secretory component remains attached to the sIgA and IgM, which protects these molecules against proteolysis and contributes to their stability. Large amounts of sIgA and IgM are produced, in a similar fashion, by the mammary glands and delivered to the infant via breast milk. The sIgA and IgM remain stable in saliva and feces[128] and provide specific protection by blocking adherence and entry. They also facilite inactivation, neutralization, and agglutination of a wide variety of microorganisms.

Distinct from the action of immunoglobulins, a large number of bioactive factors in breast milk act at the mucosal level to supplement the innate defenses.[126] These include lactoferrin, lysozyme, casein, oligosaccharides, glycoconjugates, and lipids. Mucin-1, lactadherin, and a glycosaminoglycan are antimicrobial components, which are part of the milk-fat globule. Free-fatty acids and monoglycerides, digested components of the milk-fat globule, can cause lysis of enveloped viruses, bacteria, fungi, and protozoa. Lauric and linoleic acids, which constitute a large percentage of the FFE in human milk, are two such acids produced by lipolysis in the stomach.[127]

Additional factors contained in breast milk with demonstrated activity at the level of the mucosa include cytokines, hormones, and growth factors. IL-10 and IFN-γ act by influencing the epithelial barrier.[96] Other factors that are considered to contribute to mucosal growth and development are TGF-α, EGF, and hormones (insulin and insulin-like growth factor).[71] Many other factors contained in breast milk have the potential for activity at the level of the mucosa, including nutrients, vitamins, nucleotides, enzymes, and soluble molecules with receptor-like structures (soluble CD14, soluble toll-like receptor (TLR) 2).[183,189,324]

Toll-Like Receptors

TLRs and the complex interaction between indigenous bacterial flora and the intestine are important aspects of research into the development of the mucosal immune system. Forchielli and Walker[90] have reviewed many of these immune mechanisms acting at the mucosal level. TLRs are transmembrane receptors (pattern recognition receptors) that are capable of detecting and discriminating among various groups of potential pathogens and initiate different immune responses to them. TLRs "recognize" pathogen-associated molecular patterns, or conserved features in the pattern of molecules expressed by pathogens and commensal organisms. Specific TLRs recognize a particular repertoire of patterns: TLR2 identifies bacterial lipoproteins and peptidoglycan molecules; TLR3 recognizes double-stranded DNA; and TLR4 identifies lipopolysaccharide. Ten TLRs are recognized in humans to date; some have identified legends (pathogen-associated molecular patterns from viruses, bacteria, and protozoa) to which they bind. TLRs are present on some epithelial cells, but are predominantly expressed on macrophages and DCs.[275] Intestinal epithelial cells are influenced by gut flora and local immune response to express specific TLRs. The recognition of specific antigen patterns by epithelial cells, macrophages, and dendritic cells within the gut via the different toll-like receptors on these cells leads to the different T-lymphocyte immune responses. It has been postulated that the ongoing immune stimulation elicited by the microbial flora in the gut "programs" the host to predominately express different T-helper cell responses: T_H1-like, T_H2-like, and T_H3-like. This is referred to as "cross-talk" between the indigenous intestinal flora and the body's immune system. The T_H1-like response is described as delayed-type hypersensitivity or cellular immunity. It is characterized by the predominant release of IL-2, IL-12, and interferon-γ. The T_H2-like response is primarily involved with humoral immunity and antibody production (especially IgE) associated with ILs: IL-4, IL-5, and IL-6. The T_H3-like response is related to oral tolerance and antiinflammatory effects in association with the release of IL-10 and TGF-10. A theoretical "ideal" for this system is the ability of the host to respond to various stimuli with balanced protection against the microbial invasion, without excessive inflammation or damage to the host. An imbalanced (or poorly regulated) response of this system could result in an allergic reaction against food proteins (T_H2 excess) or an autoimmune inflammatory response against self-antigens (T_H1 excess).[90]

Ongoing research continues to explore these molecular mechanisms, and their potential contribution to allergy, autoimmune disease, and normal immune function development within a fetus, infant, and young child. The role of breast milk in the development of the systemic and mucosal immune systems takes on new significance when considering these concepts and mechanisms. This is especially true when examining the role of breast milk in adding to the innate and adaptive immune response at the level of the mucosa. The postulated effects of breast milk on the intestinal microbiota and the inflammatory state within the intestine must also be considered when considering the issues of allergy, autoimmune disorders, and normal immune function development. Vorbach et al.[327] postulated that the mammary gland evolved from a protective immune gland as part of the innate immune system. They present a list of various protective molecules that are part of both mucosal secretions and human milk. They discuss how specific nutritional factors in human milk have dual functions: nutritional and protective. This highlights the dual role of the breast as a nutritional and immune organ and should stimulate further research into the breast's role in innate immunity, as a component of the mucosal immune system.

Microbiota, Probiotics, and Prebiotics

Investigation into the microbial colonization of the intestinal tract has exploded. Much of this investigation has been driven by new molecular techniques involving the analysis of ribosomal RNA sequences of microbes that might not have been identified by traditional culture techniques. The diversity of the microbiota (all the microbes which colonize the GI tract) can be viewed from different perspectives, based on the technical methods used.[306] Culture independent methods for identifying breast milk microbiota and the human infant intestinal microbiome are expanding our understanding of the complex nature of human microbiota and their role in the developing infant. Probiotics have been broadly defined as microorganisms that can exist within a host while affording benefits for the organisms and the host. Prebiotics are substances that (through different mechanisms) increase the growth and survival of probiotic bacteria within the host. Commonly recognized probiotic bacteria are *L. rhamnosus GG, B. infantis, Streptococcus thermophilus, Bacillus subtilis, Saccharomyces boulardii,* and *Bifidobacteria bifidus.* Many more organisms are considered to be probiotic, some of which are commercially available.[68,217] Prebiotics are predominantly nondigestible oligosaccharides that ferment within the colon, changing the ambient pH and producing small-chain fatty acids. Breast milk, with its significant composition of oligosaccharides, functions as a prebiotic source for an infant, facilitating the growth of bifidobacteria and lactobacilli.[65,298]

Ongoing research is exploring the potentially mutually beneficial relationship between the microbes and the host. Researchers are paying particular attention to nutrition (the availability of nutrients, energy sources, and synthesis of vitamins as influenced by the microbes);[22] the developing GI tract (including angiogenesis and mucosal barrier repair);[97,147,226,254] the maturation of mucosal immunity,[172,262] both the innate system[147] and adaptive system;[147,314] and the bioavailability and metabolism of drugs and chemicals in the GI tract.[73,149] Specific proposed mechanisms of how probiotic bacteria and prebiotic substances[220] contribute to an infant's developing immune system include competition with pathogenic bacteria for colonization; strengthening the tight junctions to enhance the mucosal barrier; producing antimicrobial bacteriocidins; stimulating mucus production; stimulating peristalsis; influencing the secretion of sIgA; stimulating the crosstalk interaction between intestinal cells; colonizing bacteria to affect the mucosal immune development; and increasing the production of certain cytokines (IL-10 and interferon-γ).[97,172,260,262]

The complex role of the infant's intestinal microbiota in immunity, inflammation, and intestinal homeostasis continues to be explored. Various authors have summarized the current concepts surrounding the microbiota and immunity and intestinal homeostasis.[21,108,110,158,328] The relationship between the bacteria that constitute the microbiota within the infant host can be commensal,

mutualistic, and parasitic. This depends on the timing, location, and situation, in addition to the nutritional status of the infant, co-infection with other specific organisms, and the genetic make-up of the infant. The homeostatic balance (eubiosis) is associated with the normal development of the infant's immunity and intestinal maturity. Imbalances of the homeostasis (dysbiosis) seem to contribute to pathologic conditions such as allergy, autoimmunity, and inflammatory conditions. Jain and Walker have eloquently described the maturation of the intestinal mucosal barrier and mucosal immune system as related to the effect of human milk on the microbiota and nutritional balance of the infant.[158] They discuss the influence of human milk on the interactions between nutrition, intestinal microbiota, and developing mucosal and systemic immunity. They consider the effects of microbiota on epithelial cell proliferation and how the development of the intestinal mucosa villi and crypts affect the mucosal barrier. Jain and Walker discuss probable mechanisms of these effects being the modulation of occludin and caludin proteins, as well as the epithelial cell signaling to enhance mucosal integrity. The microbiota is also essential to the development of the intestinal lymphoid tissue, in particular, the isolated lymphoid tissue and cryptopatches in the lamina propria. The next line of lymphoid defense, Peyer's patches and mesenteric lymph nodes, is also affected. DCs, lymphoid cells, and effector cytokines and chemokines are influenced by the complex interactions of intestinal microbiota. This leads to combating infection, dampening inflammation, and aiding in tissue repair of the barrier function more effectively. Breast milk's direct effect on the microbiota and the nutritional milieu is both conditioning and developmental. This is mediated through the effect on the intestinal cell expression and activity of toll-like and C-type lectin receptors. These affect the detection of microbe associated molecular patterns (MAMPS), leading to further development of isolated lymphoid follicles and Peyer's patches, which are essential to the maturation of B-cell response and sIgA production. Specific actions of bacteria have been identified with specific effects on the immune system. *Bacteroides fragilis* produces polysaccharide A (PSA), which induces and expands Treg cells, which produce IL-10. Other intestinal bacteria produce quantities of short-chain fatty acids (SCFA) as a fermentation product, which includes butyrate as a well-known SCFA. Butyrate contributes to the induction of and function of the Treg cell network and its activity in the gut.[21] Some commensal bacteria contribute to "colonization resistance,"[42] which is the direct competition with pathogenic organisms for the same nutrients. Thus colonization by pathogenic organisms is limited. Other commensals produce specific antimicrobial peptides that can limit the growth or survival of particular pathogens.[125] In addition to the intestinal microbiota affecting local immune responses, there are data suggesting that alterations in intestinal commensal organism spectrum and amount can diminish systemic T and B cell response to influenza. Alternatively, this may improve neutrophil killing of *S. pneumoniae* and *S. aureus*.[22,57] Separately, there are data suggesting that any alteration of the microbiota or alteration of the local inflammatory environment can lead to bacterial translocation and systemic infection. Conversely, an intestinal infection or inflammatory state can lead to disruption of the local microbiota (dysbiosis).[33,215] There is a large amount of research on the role of intestinal microbiota in combination with genetics and the host immune system contributing to the development of inflammatory bowel disease.[201] Cystic fibrosis is another chronic illness that has been ascribed to a genetic defect leading to dysbiosis and ongoing activation of the immune system leading to chronic inflammation and infections.[26] Intestinal cancer is associated with inflammation of the GI tract and microbiota activated inflammation.[82] There is ample and growing evidence that eubiosis is associated with the normal development of the infant's immunity and intestinal maturity and that dysbiosis plays a role in chronic inflammatory diseases.

Gastrointestinal Commensal Organisms

The microbial colonization of an infant's intestinal tract begins at birth; organisms from the maternal flora are the first colonizers. Numerous additional factors directly influence the composition of the intestinal microbiota in early infancy, including gestational age, ingestion of breast milk or formula, initiation of solid foods, mode of delivery, the route of delivery of food, the time of onset of feeding, exposure to other microbes through contact (with family, animals, persons from other environments), antibiotics, and intercurrent or chronic illness.[86,121,149,261]

Breast milk is known to transmit bacteria, fungi, parasites and viruses to the infant. Human milk has been analyzed by both culture and molecular techniques to identify its microbiota, which predominately includes organisms associated with the skin or the intestine.[46,87,153,163,262] Next-generation sequencing is the newest method and involves direct extraction of bacterial DNA from the milk and pyrosequencing to identify particular

---

BOX 5-4. Bacteria Commonly Found in Breast Milk

Phyla	Genera
Firmicutes	***Staphylococcus, Streptococcus, Leuconostoc, Lactococcus,*** *Enterococcus, Clostridia, Veillonella, Gemella, Bifidobacterium, Lactobacillus*
Actinobacteria	***Corynebacterium***, *Propionibacterium, Actinomyces*
Proteobacteria	***Pseudomonas, Serratia, Sphingomonas, Ralstonia***, *Escherichia, Enterobacter, Acinetobacter, Bradyrhizobium*
Bacteroidetes	*Prevotella*

Bolded bacteria are most prevalent populations detected.
Derived from Cabrera-Rubio et al. (2012), Fernandez et al. (2012), and Hunt et al. (2011).

---

species. Despite the broad diversity of bacteria in human milk[87] there are four dominant phyla in the human intestine: Actinobacteria, Bacteroides, Firmucutes, and Proteobacteria.[47] (See Box 5-4. Bacteria Commonly Found in Breast Milk.) The microbiota of human milk changes from being very diverse in colostrum to becoming less diverse, with organisms similar to the oral and skin flora of infants over the period of lactation.[46,153] There has been discussion of the potential mechanisms of entry of bacteria into human milk: from the mother's skin (nipple and surrounding areola); retrograde passage from the infant's mouth into the breast; migration of leukocytes and/or DCs; with intracellular bacteria, which move from the mother's intestine to the mammary gland and into the milk; and from the maternal breast tissue/cells into the milk (Fernandez L: Pharm Res 2013,[87] LaTuga MS: Semin Reprod Medicine 2014[186]). There has even been a distinct microbiota of human breast tissue identified with Proteobacteria and Firmicutes, also in high abundance in the breast as noted for human milk.[321,340]

The predominant flora of breastfed infants are *L. bifidus* and *Bifidobacterium* spp., which constitute up to 95% of the culturable organisms. The remaining minority of bacteria include *Streptococcus, Bacteroides, Clostridium, Micrococcus, Enterococcus, E. coli,* and other uncommon organisms in small numbers.[217,226,343] *L. bifidus* metabolizes milk saccharides, producing large amounts of acetic acid, lactic acid, and some formic and succinic acids, which create the low pH of the stool of breastfed infants. *L. bifidus* also produces SCFA in the course of colonization. Large numbers of bifidobacteria can lower the pH of the intestine, which limits the growth of some pathogens such as *E. coli, Bacteroides,* and staphylococci. The flora of bifid bacteria is inhibitory to certain pathogenic bacteria. Substantial clinical evidence is available to demonstrate protection against intestinal infections from *S. aureus*, *Shigella*, *Salmonella*, *V. cholerae*, *E. coli*, rotavirus, *Campylobacter*, and protozoa.[103] Two facilitory actions of breast milk are apparent. The first encourages the growth of *L. bifidus* and thus crowds out the growth of other bacteria. In the second, the number of pathogens is also kept low by the direct action of lysozyme and lactoferrin. When the number of pathogenic bacteria is kept low, multiple other factors can contribute to keeping the growth of potentially pathogenic bacteria under control and limit the invasion of bacteria through the gut wall into the bloodstream. These other potentially beneficial factors and mechanisms include intestinal motility, gastric acid secretion, intestinal mucin, oligosaccharides, intestinal integrity as a permeability barrier, subepithelial cells in lymphoid follicles (phagocytic and non-phagocytic [DCs]), cytokines, chemokines, and, potentially, immunomodulatory nutrients (glutamine, arginine, nucleotides, and PUFA).[227]

The intestinal flora of formula-fed infants is made up of predominantly gram-negative bacteria, especially coliform organisms, *Bacteroides*, and *Clostridium*, *Enterobacter*, and *Enterococcus*.[343]

Studies have demonstrated that potentially four distinctly different "microhabitats" for microflora exist; within the GI lumen, within the mucus layer, separately within crypt mucus, and directly on the surface of the intestinal epithelium. The significance of these microhabitats and the effect of specific microorganisms have yet to be determined.[97] At weaning, the facultative anaerobes decline in number, and obligate anaerobes (*Bacteroides*) become the predominant organisms in the intestine. Preterm infants are colonized with different types and numbers of bacteria than are full-term infants. The environment of neonatal intensive care units (NICUs) influences the microbial colonization. Factors of the NICU environment include incubators, widespread use of antibiotics and parenteral nutrition, and illness. The short- and long-term effects of the different and changing GI microbiota are a concern.[227,250] This is particularly true when one considers the contributing factors or causes for sepsis, NEC, chronic lung disease, or poor neurologic outcome in NICUs.

The question of a causal role of intestinal microflora and the development of NEC in premature and VLBW infants has been proposed.[151,211] Gewolb et al.[101] suggested that a low percentage of *Bifidobacterium* and *Lactobacillus* in the stool of VLBW infants within the first month of life is a risk factor for infection. Some studies on the use of probiotics and the occurrence of NEC have demonstrated a lower incidence of NEC in infants receiving probiotics.[25,152,196] Here again, the use of the mothers' breast milk for premature infants

and VLBW infants decreases the risk to the infant of sepsis, NEC, and infection-related events.[73,245] In a controlled prospective study of high-risk, low-birth-weight infants in India using donor human milk, significantly fewer infections and no major infections were found in the group receiving human milk. The control infants experienced diarrhea, pneumonia, septicemia, and meningitis.[225] There is evidence that probiotics or a human milk diet can prevent NEC in preterm infants.[144,258,280,311]

It is clear that the intestinal microbiota is essential to the maturation of the GI tract and the developing immune system. Human breast milk is an important determining factor in the make-up of the microbiota. The microbiota, in combination with many of the bioactive factors in breast milk, is crucial to maintaining a eubiotic state in the intestinal tract and programming both the local GI immune milieu and a normal systemic immune response.*

Genetics and Epigenetics

As research pushes to identify all the benefits of human breast milk for the developing infant and corroborate the etiologic effect of factors in breast milk that lead to specific outcomes in neonates, the how and why of these effects become more important. The high level of variability in breast milk composition, and the potential link between breast milk variation and neonatal outcomes, suggests genetic or epigenetic effects or both. Baumgartel and Conley presented a systematic review of publications of genetic studies that utilized RNA and DNA found in human breast milk and the potential effects on BM compositional variability and neonatal outcomes.[16] They identified 13 articles which focused on gene expression and three articles on epigenetics. A number of methods for the analyses of genes were utilized in these studies: Northern blot, RT-PCR, spectrophotometry, microarrays, and Western blots. Bisulfite conversion, PCR amplification, and pyrosequencing were used for epigenetic analysis. In addition to "cataloging" these studies, the authors outlined the limitations of these studies. They made recommendations for the methodology of future studies on breast milk, concerning gene expression and epigenetic effects. The related gene products examined in these studies included important proteins contained in breast milk (β-casein, α-lactalbumin, M-ficolin, and parathyroid hormone-related protein), transporter proteins, cytokines, and ILs. The epigenetic studies examined methylation of specific genes, for

---

*14,21,141,158,159,314,328

example: kallikrein-related peptidase 6 (KLK6), retinol binding protein (RBP1), and glutathione S-transferase (GSTP1), among others. This small collection of studies only emphasizes how much work there is to do to understand the genetics and epigenetics of breast milk and breastfeeding.

The complexity of the breast, its various stages of development, the stages of lactation, and the variable composition of human breast milk suggest a complex interplay between genetic, epigenetic, environmental, and lifestyle factors. These all affect milk production and influence the benefits of lactation for the mother and infant. Epigenetics may play a pivotal role in our understanding of the benefits of breastfeeding. The word "epigenetics" means "atop" or "surrounding" genetics. Various definitions of epigenetics enhance our understanding of its essential features: (a) "changes in gene function which do not alter the underlying structure of DNA but result in genes being switched on or off in a reversible way"[270] and (b) "stable heritable phenotype resulting from changes in a chromosome without alterations in the DNA sequence."[23] Broadly, this implies any mitotically or meiotically heritable change that leads to different gene expression without actually changing the DNA sequence. The true implication is that each individual "adapts" to their environment through some of these epigenetic mechanisms, leading to potentially different health outcomes for the individual.

Berger et al. discuss three "categories of signals" leading to the epigenetic change, which becomes a stably heritable state: epigenator, epigenetic initiator, and epigenetic maintainer. The epigenator is an external or environmental signal, which affects the cell, leading to the activation of the initiator. The intracellular epigenetic initiator "selects" the location of chromosomal/chromatin change, which leads to a change in gene expression. The epigenetic maintainer preserves the new epigenetic chromatin state. The major epigenetic mechanisms for changing gene expression and maintaining it are DNA methylation, histone modification, chromatin remodeling, and noncoding RNAs (ncRNA) [microRNA (miRNA) is one of the ncRNAs]. DNA methylation and histone modification can influence the transcription of specific genes. ncRNAs can affect either transcription (production of an RNA copy of specific genes) or interference with translation (the production of an amino acid sequence from messenger RNA [mRNA]). DNA methylation often results in the "silencing" of the affected gene. Methylation in humans happens at a cytosine next to a guanine nucleotide (CpG site). The critical periods for the occurrence of DNA methylation are early in gestation and early in infancy. "Genomic imprinting" is a specific example of DNA methylation. Imprinting is the inactivation of one of the two copies of a gene inherited from one's parents, leading to the expression of the other copy of the gene. Imprinting has been described in a percentage of children with Beckwith-Wiedemann syndrome (BWS); a change in DNA methylation leads to genomic imprinting and, subsequently, the disorder. As noted in adults and children, there are genes involved in DNA methylation regulation that are mutated in acute myeloid leukemia.[270] Histone modification changes how the DNA and proteins are "packaged" to form chromatin. Either the chromatin is formed in the "inactive form," leading to transcriptional repression, or in the "active form," leading to active transcription and gene expression.

Verduci et al. summarized a number of possible epigenetic effects of human breast milk components on specified health outcomes.[323] They describe in vitro animal studies correlating specific breast milk components with variable gene expression and potential health outcomes. These include lactoferrin reducing NF-κB expression and leading to less NEC; prostaglandin J decreasing the expression of cholesterol biosynthesis enzymes and prevention of nonalcoholic fatty liver disease (NAFLD); and long-chain PUFA $n-3$ (LCPUFA $n-3$) causing diminished expression of hepatic hydroxymethyl glutaryl coenzyme A (HMGCoA) reductase, limiting the development of high total blood cholesterol in adult mice. They also note several epigenetic effects hypothesized in humans: prostaglandin J, which leads to increased perioxisome proliferator-activated receptor γ (PPARγ) and less obesity in adolescents; and undigestible oligosaccharides, which promote the growth of various commensal bacteria and lead to diminished inflammation through the inhibition of nuclear factor kappa-light-chain (NF-κB) activation of B-cells. Each of these is an example of the types of epigenetic changes that could occur in humans due to exposure to specific factors in human breast milk. Verduci et al. refer to dietary factors leading to changes in gene expression as "nutritional epigenetics."[323]

Kosaka et al. have described the existence of microRNA in breast milk and its potential as an immune regulatory agent through transfer from mother to infant (Kosaka N et al. Silence 2010[178]). After the extraction of RNA from human breast milk, they performed a miRNA microarray analysis. They identified specific miRNAs as abundant in human milk. These were related to T and B cell maturation and regulation, neutrophil proliferation, and activation and regulation of TLRs. They also demonstrated that extracted human milk miRNA was resistant to degradation by low pH (pH 1), freezing and thawing, and RNase digestion. As a result, it is highly likely that infants ingest a good amount of miRNA. Thus this miRNA in

263. Picker LJ, Treet JR Jr, Ferguson-Darnell B, et al: Control of lymphocyte recirculation in man. II. Differential regulation of the cutaneous lymphocyte-associated antigen, a tissue-selective homing receptor for skin-homing T cells, *J Immunol* 150(3):1122–1136, 1993.

264. Pickering LK, Granoff DM, Erickson JR, et al: Modulation of the immune system by human milk and infant formula containing nucleotides, *Pediatrics* 101(2):242, 1998.

265. Pickering LK, Kohl S: Human milk humoral immunity and infant defense mechanisms. In Howell RR, Morriss RH, Pickering LK, editors: *Human milk in infant nutrition and health*, Springfield, Ill., 1986, Charles C Thomas.

266. Pisacane A, Graziano L, Mazzarella G, et al: Breast-feeding and urinary tract infection, *J Pediatr* 120(1):87, 1992.

267. Pitt J: The milk mononuclear phagocyte, *Pediatrics* 64(5 Pt 2 Suppl):745, 1979.

268. Polak-Charcon S, Shoham J, Ben-Shaul Y: Tight junctions in epithelial cells of human fetal hindgut, normal colon, and colon adenocarcinoma, *J Natl Cancer Inst* 65 (1):53–62, 1980.

269. Popkin BM, Adair L, Akin JS, et al: Breast-feeding and diarrheal morbidity, *Pediatrics* 86(6):874, 1990.

270. Puumala SE, Hoyme HE: Epigenetics in pediatrics, *Pediatr Rev* 36(1):14–21, 2015. http://dx.doi.org/10.1542/pir.36-1-14.

271. Quan R, Barness LA: Do infants need nucleotide supplemented formula for optimal nutrition? *J Pediatr Gastroenterol Nutr* 11(4):429, 1990.

272. Quan R, Yang C, Rubenstein S, et al: Effects of microwave radiation on anti-infective factors in human milk, *Pediatrics* 89(4):667–669, 1992.

273. Quigley MA, Kelly YJ, Secker A: Breastfeeding and hospitilization for diarrheal and respiratory infection in the United Kingdom Millenium Cohort Study, *Pediatrics* 119(4): e837, 2007.

274. Raisler J, Alexander C, O'Campo P: Breast-feeding and infant illness: a dose-response relationship? *Am J Public Health* 89:25, 1999.

275. Rasmussen SB, Reinert LS, Palludan SR: Innate recognition of intracellular pathogens. detection and activation of the first line of defense, *APMIS* 117:323–337, 2009.

276. Reddy V, Bhaskaram C, Raghuramulu N, et al: Antimicrobial factors in human milk, *Acta Paediatr Scand* 66(2):229, 1977.

277. Remington JS, Klein JO: Current concepts of infections of the fetus and newborn infant. In Remington JS, Klein JO, editors: *Infectious diseases of the fetus and newborn infant*, ed 5, Philadelphia, 2001, WB Saunders, pp 1–69.

278. Richie ER: Lymphocyte subsets in colostrum. In Howell RR, Morriss RH, Pickering LK, editors: *Human milk in infant nutrition and health*, Springfield, Ill., 1986, Charles C Thomas.

279. Rigas A, Rigas B, Glassman M, et al: Breast-feeding and maternal smoking in the etiology of Crohn's disease and ulcerative colitis in childhood, *Ann Epidemiol* 3 (4):387, 1993.

280. Robinson J: Cochrane in context: probiotics for prevention of necrotizing enterocolitis in preterm infants, *Evid Based Child Health* 9(3):672–674, 2014. http://dx.doi.org/10.1002/ebch.1977.

281. de la Rosa G, Yang D, Tewary P, et al: Lactoferrin acts as an alarmin to promote the recruitment and activation of APCs and antigen-specific immune responses, *J Immunol* 180 (10):6868–6876, 2008.

282. Rudloff HE, Schmalstieg FC Jr, Palkowetz KH, et al: Interleukin-6 in human milk, *J Reprod Immunol* 23(1):13, 1993.

283. Ruiz-Palacios G, Torres J, Torres NI, et al: Cholera-like enterotoxin produced by *Campylobacter jejuni, Infect Immun* 43:314, 1984.

284. Sabbaj S, Ghosh MK, Edwards BH, et al: Breastmilk-derived antigen-specific CD8+ T cells: an extralymphoid effector memory cell population in humans, *J Immunol* 174:2956–2961, 2005.

285. Sadeharju K, Knip M, Virtanen M, et al: Maternal antibodies in breast milk protect the child from enterovirus infections, *Pediatrics* 119:941–946, 2007.

286. Saeland E, Jong Nabatob AA, Kalay H, et al: MUC1 In human milk blocks transmission of human immunodeficiency virus from dendritic cells to T cells, *Mol Immunol* 46(11-12):2309–2316, 2009.

287. Saito S, Yoshida M, Ichijo M, et al: Transforming growth factor-beta (TGF-beta) in human milk, *Clin Exp Immunol* 94 (1):220, 1993.

288. Salzman NH, Underwood MA, Bevins CL: Paneth cells, defensins, and the commensal microbiota: a hypothesis on intimate interplay at the intestinal mucosa, *Semin Immunol* 19(2):70–83, 2007.

289. Sanchez L, Calvo M, Brock JH: Biological role of lactoferrin, *Arch Dis Child* 67(5):657, 1992.

290. Sani M, Hosseini SM, Salmannejad M, et al: Origins of the breast milk-derived cells; an endeavor to find the cell sources, *Cell Biol Int* 39(5):611–618, 2015. http:// dx.doi.org/10.1002/cbin.10432 (Epub ahead of print) PMID: 25572907.

291. Savilahti E, Salmenpera L, Taino VM, et al: Prolonged exclusive breast-feeding results in low serum concentrations of immunoglobulin G, A and M, *Acta Paediatr Scand* 76(1):1, 1987.

292. Scariati PD, Grummer-Strawn LM, Fein SB: A longitudinal analysis of infant morbidity and the extent of breastfeeding in the United States, *Pediatrics* 99(6):E5, 1997.

293. Schaller JP, Buck RH, Rueda R: Ribonucleotides: conditionally essential nutrients shown to enhance immune function and reduce diarrheal disease in infants, *Semin Fetal Neonatal Med* 12(1):35–44, 2007.

294. Schanler RJ, Lau C, Hurst NM, et al: Randomized trial of donor human milk vs. preterm formula as substitutes for mothers' own milk in the feeding of extremely premature infants, *Pediatrics* 116:400–406, 2005.

295. Schlesinger JJ, Covelli HD: Evidence for transmission of lymphocyte responses to tuberculin by breast-feeding, *Lancet* 2(8037):529, 1977.

296. Schroten H, Hanisch FG, Plogmann R, et al: Inhibition of adhesion of S-fimbriated *Escherichia coli* to buccal epithelial cells by human milk fat globule membrane components: a novel aspect of the protective function of mucins in the nonimmunoglobulin fraction, *Infect Immun* 60:2893, 1992.

297. Schultz CL, Coffman RL: Control of isotype switching by T cells and cytokines, *Curr Opin Immunol* 3:350, 1991.

298. Sghir A, Chow JM, Mackie RI: Continuous culture selection of bifidobacteria and lactobacilli from human faecal samples using fructooligosacchirade as selective substrate, *J Appl Microbiol* 85(4):769–777, 1998.

299. Shackleton M, Vaillant F, Simpson KJ, et al: Generation of a functional mammary gland from a single stem cell, *Nature* 439(7072):84–88, 2006.

300. Shigeoka AO, Santos JI, Hill HR: Functional analysis of neutrophil granulocytes from healthy, infected, and stressed neonates, *J Pediatr* 95(3):454–460, 1979.

301. Smith GH: Label-retaining epithelial cells in mouse mammary gland divide asymmetrically and retain their template DNA strands, *Development* 132:681–687, 2005.

302. Sonntag J, Brandenburg U, Polzehl D: Complement system in healthy term newborns: reference values in umbilical cord blood, *Pediatr Dev Pathol* 1(2):131–135, 1998.

303. Spadaro M, Caorsi C, Ceruti P, et al: Lactoferrin, a major defense protein of innate immunity, is a novel maturation factor for human dendritic cells, *FASEB J* 22:2747–2757, 2008.

304. Splawski JB, Jelinek DF, Lipsky PE: Delineation of the functional capacity of human neonatal lymphocytes, *J Clin Invest* 87(2):545–553, 1991.

305. Srivastava MD, Srivastava A, Brouhard B, et al: Cytokines in human milk, *Res Commun Mol Pathol Pharmacol* 93(3):263, 1996.

306. Rajilic-Stojanovicć M, Smidt H, de Vos WM: Diversity of the human gastrointestinal tract microbiota revisited, *Environ Microbiol* 9(9):2125, 2007.

307. Stoliar OA, Pelley RP, Kaniecki-Green E, et al: Secretory IgA against enterotoxins in breast-milk, *Lancet* 1 (7972):1258, 1976.

308. Stoll BJ, Lee FK, Hale E, et al: Immunoglobulin secretion by the normal and the infected newborn infant, *J Pediatr* 122(5Pt 1):780–786, 1993.

309. Strauss RG, Snyder EL: Activation and activity of the superoxide-generating system of neutrophils from human infants, *Pediatr Res* 17(8):662–664, 1983.

310. Strober W, Kelsall B, Fuss I, et al: Reciprocal IFN-gamma and TGF-beta responses regulate the occurrence of mucosal inflammation, *Immunol Today* 18:61, 1997.

311. Sullivan S, Schanler RJ, Kim JH, et al: An exclusively human milk-based diet is associated with a lower rate of necrotizing enterocolitis than a diet of human milk and bovine milk-based products, *J Pediatr* 156(4):562–567, 2010. http://dx.doi.org/10.1016/j.jpeds.2009.10.040. Epub 2009 Dec 29.

312. Takahata Y, Takada H, Nomura A, et al: Interleukin-18 in human milk, *Pediatr Res* 50(2):268, 2001.

313. Telemo E, Hanson LA: Antibodies in milk, *J Mammary Gland Biol Neoplasia* 1(3):243, 1996.

314. Thaiss CA, Levy M, Suez J, et al: The interplay between the innate immune system and the microbiota, *Curr Opin Immunol* 26:41–48, 2014. http://dx.doi.org/10.1016/j.coi.2013.10.016. Epub 2013 Nov 22.

315. Thorpe LW, Rudloff HE, Powell LC, et al: Decreased response of human milk leukocytes to chemoattractant peptides, *Pediatr Res* 20(4):373, 1986.

316. Tiede B, Kang Y. From milk to malignancy: the role of mammary stem cells in development, pregnancy and breast cancer. Cell Res. 2011 Feb;21(2):245-57. doi: 10.1038/cr.2011.11. Epub 2011 Jan 18. Review. PMID: 21243011.

317. Tomita M, Takase M, Wakabayshi H, et al: Antimicrobial peptides of lactoferrin, *Adv Exp Med Biol* 357:107, 1995.

318. Tow J: Heal the mother, heal the baby: epigenetics, breast-feeding and the human microbiome, *Breastfeed Rev* 22 (1):7–9, 2014 Mar.

319. Tressler RL, Ramstack MB, White NR, et al: Determination of total potentially available nucleosides in human milk from Asian women, *Nutrition* 19(1):16, 2003.

320. Tuaillon E, Valea D, Becquart P, et al: Human milk-derived B cells: a highly activated switched memory cell population primed to secrete antibodies, *J Immunol* 182(11):7155–7162, 2009.

321. Urbaniak C, Cummins J, Brackstone M, et al: Microbiota of human breast tissue, *Appl Environ Microbiol* 80 (10):3007–3014, 2014. http://dx.doi.org/10.1128/AEM .00242-14. Epub 2014 Mar 7.

322. Van Buren CT, Kulkarni AD, Fanslow WC, et al: Dietary nucleotides, a requirement for helper/inducer T lymphocytes, *Transplantation* 40(6):694, 1985.

323. Verduci E, Banderali G, Barberi S, et al: Epigenetic effects of human breast milk, *Nutrients* 6(4):1711–1724, 2014. http://dx.doi.org/10.3390/nu6041711.

324. Vidal K, Donnet-Hughes A: CD14: a soluble pattern recognition receptor in milk, *Adv Exp Med Biol* 606:195–216, 2008.

325. Viirtanen SM, Rasanen L, Aro A, et al: Infant feeding in Finnish children less than 7 yr of age with newly diagnosed IDDM, Childhood Diabetes in Finland Study Group, *Diabetes Care* 14(5):415, 1991.

326. Villalpando S, Hamosh M: Early and late effects of breast-feeding: does breast-feeding really matter? *Biol Neonate* 74 (2):177, 1998.

327. Vorbach C, Capecchi MR, Penninger JM, et al: Evolution of the mammary gland from the innate immune system? *Bioessays* 28:606–616, 2006.

328. Walker WA: Initial intestinal colonization in the human infant and immune homeostasis, *Ann Nutr Metab* 63(Suppl 2):8–15, 2013. http://dx.doi.org/10.1159/000354907. Epub 2013 Nov 8.

329. Wheeler TT, Hodgkinson AJ, Prosser CG, et al: Immune components of colostrum and milk: a historical perspective, *J Mammary Gland Biol Neoplasia* 12:237–247, 2007.

330. Whitmore AC, Prowse DM, Haughton G, et al: Ig isotype switching in B lymphocytes. The effect of T cell-derived interleukins, cytokines, cholera toxin, and antigen on isotype switch frequency of a cloned B cell lymphoma, *Int Immunol* 3:95, 1991.

331. Wilson CB, Lewis DB: Basis and implications of selectively diminished cytokine production in neonatal susceptibility to infection, *Rev Infect Dis* 12:410–420, 1990.

332. Wilson E, Butcher EC: CCL28 Controls immunologlobulin (Ig)A plasma cell accumulation in the lactating mammary gland and IgA antibody transfer to the neonate, *J Exp Med* 200:805–809, 2004.

333. Winberg J, Wessner G: Does breast milk protect against septicaemia in the newborn? *Lancet* 1:1091, 1971.

334. Wirt DP, Adkins LT, Palkowetz KH, et al: Activated and memory T lymphocytes in human milk, *Cytometry* 13:282, 1992.

335. Wolach B, Dolfin T, Regev R, et al: The development of the complement system after 28 weeks' gestation, *Acta Paediatr* 86:523–527, 1997.

336. Woodward WA, Chen MS, Behbod F, et al: On mammary stem cells, *J Cell Sci* 118(Pt 16):3585–3594, 2005.

337. Woodward WA. Breast cancer stem cell targets, Oncology (Williston Park) 25(1):34, 2011. 36.

338. Wright AL, Holberg CJ, Martinez FD, et al: Breast feeding and lower respiratory tract illness in the first year of life, Group Health Medical Associates., *BMJ* 299(6705): 946, 1989.

339. Xanthou M: The development of the immune system. In Xanthou M, Bracci R, Prindull G, editors: *Neonatal haematology and immunology. II*, Amsterdam, 1993, Elsevier, pp 113–122.

340. Xuan C, Shamonki JM, Chung A, et al: Microbial dysbiosis is associated with humanbreast cancer, *PLoSONE*9(1): e83744, 2014. http://dx.doi.org/10.1371/journal.pone. 0083744.

341. Yabuhara A, Kawai H, Komiyama A: Development of natural killer cytotoxicity during childhood: marked increases in number of natural killer cells with adequate cytotoxic abilities during infancy to early childhood, *Pediatr Res* 28:316–322, 1990.

342. Yasui K, Masuda M, Tsuno T, et al: An increase in polymorphonuclear leukocyte chemotaxis accompanied by a change in the membrane fluidity with age during childhood, *Clin Exp Immunol* 81:156–159, 1990.

343. Yoshioka H, Iseki K, Fujita K: Development and differences of intestinal flora in the neonatal period in breast-fed and bottle-fed infants, *Pediatrics* 72:317, 1983.

344. Yu VY: Scientific rationale and benefits of nucleotide supplementation of infant formula, *J Paediatr Child Health* 38:543, 2002.

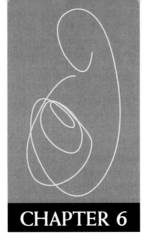

CHAPTER 6

Psychological Impact of Breastfeeding

The mental health of the mother will have a significant impact on her postpartum recovery and a dramatic influence on the infant's well-being. Breastfeeding has a significant impact on the outcome for both mother and infant especially during the first year postpartum.

Although the previous chapters provide more than adequate information to support the preference for breastfeeding in almost every case, the critical impact in the return to breastfeeding in modern cultures rests with the issue of a mother's role and her perception of breastfeeding as a biologic act. The maternal influences include psychophysiologic reactions during nursing, long-term psychophysiologic effects, maternal behavior, sexual behavior, and attitudes toward men. All professionals providing support care in the perinatal period need to have a clear view, not only of the biologic benefits of breastfeeding, but also of their own psychological attitudes about the breast itself.

"For men, breasts are sexual ornaments—the crown jewels of femininity."[60] This is not true worldwide, however, and other body parts (e.g., small feet, nape of neck, buttocks) are sexually charged, with much of the fascination resulting from full or partial concealment. Until the fourteenth century, the nursing Madonna was the prevailing image, but in truth, the availability of a mother's milk meant life or death for every newborn.

The breast has assumed many roles throughout history, moving from sacred to domestic to political to erotic. The definition of the breast has been provided by moralists, historians, poets, pornographers, lovers, and women themselves. Much of the rhetoric today is about the breast in crisis: "The breast is torn between nurturance, eroticism,

and the fear of cancer."[60] In the eyes of the beholder, babies see food, men see sex, physicians see disease, business sees dollar signs, and religion sees spiritual symbols. Psychoanalysis places breasts in the center of the unconscious. The breast has a privileged place in human thought. Perhaps the love affair with science has turned women from being comfortable with their breasts as a source of infant nurturance to being uncomfortable and ashamed of breastfeeding and yet has them searching through science and medicine for the perfect size or shape.[60]

The breast has been regarded as a sex object in the Western world for more than a century, and its biologic benefits have been downplayed. This is clearly demonstrated by the conflicting mores that permit pornographic pictures in newspapers, movies, and nude theaters but insist on the arrest of a mother for indecent exposure who is discreetly nursing her baby in public.

Proponents of breastfeeding have generally accepted, even before the upsurge of interest and research in attachment, that the major reason to breastfeed is to provide the special relationship and closeness that accompany nursing. Conversely, the major contraindication to breastfeeding was lack of desire to do so. This was evidenced by it being considered more appropriate to present breastfeeding as a matter of personal choice with no compelling reasons to urge a mother to consider nursing. The concern about creating guilt in the mother who chooses not to nurse has been significant, and it often resulted in a passive attitude on the part of the clinician so that the mother received no prenatal counseling about infant feeding.[31] As efforts to educate the public in general and women in particular about the benefits of breastfeeding have been increased, guilt is being used as a defense for doing nothing. Far more disturbing have been the aggressive attacks on breastfeeding promotion justified by the fear of producing guilt in the mother who chooses not to breastfeed.[47] Other public health campaigns have not been muted or halted for fear of producing guilt in those who are obese, smoke, or abuse drugs.

Bonding and the Impact of Breastfeeding

The studies performed to understand bonding have largely been done without reference to breastfeeding. A supposedly comprehensive book, *Attachment and loss* by Bowlby,[7] which reviews early mother-infant interactions extensively, never mentions breastfeeding. In addition, suckling is given extensive treatment without making a distinction between bottle and breast or implying that an alternative to the bottle exists. The emphasis in the 1940s was on the effects of disrupting already-formed attachments. Separation in the neonatal period was ignored, and infant socialization was studied from 6 months of age.

Work by Spitz[52] and others has identified the devastating effects on infants deprived of long-term maternal contact. These investigators demonstrated major deficits in both mental and motor development, as well as general failure to thrive. The impact on the mother had not yet been described. Klaus and Kennell[29] provided those data in their many writings on mother-infant interactions, which are summarized in their book *Parent-infant bonding*. Evidence indicates that the maternal-infant bond is the strongest human bond when two major facts are considered: an infant's early growth is within the mother's body and survival after birth depends on her care. Although the process had not been meticulously described yet, Budin[9] noted in 1907 that when a mother was separated from her infant and was unable to provide the early care of her sick child, she lost interest and even abandoned the infant.

The immediate emotional reactions of mothers to their newborns were studied by Robson and Kumar in 193 women (two groups of primiparas, $n = 112$ and $n = 41$, and one group of multiparas, $n = 40$); 40% of the primiparas and 25% of the multiparas recalled that their predominant emotional reaction when holding their babies for the first time was indifference. Maternal affection was more likely to be lacking if the mother had an amniotomy or painful labor or had received more than one dose of meperidine (pethidine) unrelated to cesarean or forceps delivery. The authors found no difference between mothers who breastfed or bottle fed. The feelings of indifference persisted for a week or longer. This study points out that normal women may be initially indifferent toward their babies, whereas others experience great elation.

The development of positive feelings in primiparous women toward their normal newborns occurred before delivery in a third of women, immediately at birth or on the first day for 42%, and by the second or third day for 19% in a study by Pascoe and French.[45] Mothers who breastfed were more likely to express positive feelings. Labors of less than 9 hours were associated with positive feelings, but no association with social class, infant sex, type of delivery, or duration of initial mother-infant contact was found.

Klaus and Kennell[29] noted that mothers in the United States showed different attachment behavior when permitted early contact with their premature infants compared with mothers who had first contact at 3 weeks of age. Mothers of full-term infants who were allowed contact within the first 2 hours and subsequent extra contact behaved differently at 1 month and 1 year with their babies compared with control subjects. Jackson et al.[25] made similar observations in the Yale Rooming-In Unit from 1945 to 1955 but failed to provide control observations.

In part because of the thought-provoking work of Klaus and Kennell[29] in the 1970s, remarkable changes have taken place in labor, delivery, and postpartum services in hospitals in the United States and around the world. Mothers have been "allowed" to have their infants to hold and cuddle as soon as possible after delivery, and fathers have been "allowed" to participate in the birth experience. The take-charge attitude of health care professionals has relaxed, and gradually hospital perinatal care has been humanized. In the meantime, a number of investigators have challenged the power of bonding. In a critical review of early and extended maternal-infant contact research, Siegel suggests that, although many longitudinal experiences affect parenting behavior in complex ways, reasonable judgment supports early and extended contact whenever possible.

When a normal, healthy infant born to an unmedicated mother is placed on the mother's abdomen immediately after the cord is cut, the infant crawls to the breast, finds the nipple, and latches on, beginning to suckle.[50] This event takes place unassisted by the mother or an attendant. The warmth of the mother maintains the infant's body temperature. This is described as a series of events beginning with the infant resting and occasionally looking at the mother, then moving toward the breast with some lip smacking and mouthing.

Approaching the breast, the infant turns from one to the other breast before finally moving toward one nipple, bobbing over it, and grasping the areola and suckling (Figure 6-1). Experiments that involve washing one breast demonstrate that the infant chooses the unwashed breast. When the mother has been medicated during labor, the "medicated" infant struggles to find the breast and often fails. Infants who are left with their mothers seldom cry during this awake, alert period.[50] If unimpeded, this process takes 40 to 45 minutes, which suggests the original baby-friendly mandate of initiating breastfeeding within a half hour may have been hasty. Physiologically, the stimulus to the mother's nipple and the stimulus to the infant's mouth trigger the release of vital hormones in both mother and infant, beginning the maturation of the intestinal mucosa and enhancing nutrient absorption for both mother and infant.

This awake, alert period immediately after delivery provides an opportunity for receiving the first measure of colostrum, which is not only nourishing but also protective from an immunologic and infectious standpoint.

When a newborn is separated from the mother in the first hours postpartum, crying occurs and stops on reunion.[27] The cry has been studied by sound spectrographic analysis in a group of infants in contact with their mothers for the first 90 minutes compared with those kept in a crib. The separated infants cried 10 times more than the contact infants. On analysis, the cry was characterized as a discomfort cry compared with patterns seen in cries of hunger or pain.

The impact of early mother-infant interaction and breastfeeding on the duration of breastfeeding has been reported; no data appear to be available as to whether mothering is different between mothers who breastfeed and bottle feed in this early period. Sosa et al.[51] reported the effect of early mother-infant contact on breastfeeding, infection, and

growth. Breastfeeding mothers who were permitted early contact but not early breastfeeding were compared with mothers without early contact who also breastfed. The mothers with early contact were observed to nurse 50% longer than the control subjects. The early-contact infants were heavier and had fewer infections. Sosa et al.[51] conducted a similar study in Brazil, in which each mother nursed immediately on delivery and the infant was kept beside the mother's bed until they went home. At home, they had a special nurse make regular visits to help in the breastfeeding. The control subjects had traditional therapy, that is, contact at feeding times after an early glimpse. Infants were housed in a separate nursery. At 2 months, 77% of the early-contact mothers and only 27% of the control mothers were successfully nursing. The early and continued contact may have been accompanied by increased support and assistance from the nursery staff. This added support could facilitate breastfeeding and thus be the cause of the improved outcome.

An additional study of early contact by deChâteau et al. in Sweden investigated a group of 21 mothers with early contact and 19 control mothers, all of whom were breastfeeding in the hospital.[10a] The only difference in management was the first 30 minutes of early contact because 24-hour rooming-in was provided for all mothers after 2 hours postpartum. The length of breastfeeding differed: for the early-contact group, 175 days, and for the control subjects, 105 days. Follow-up observations at 3 months showed different mothering behavior. The study group displayed more attachment behavior, fondling, caressing, and kissing than the control group.

Unless heavy medication or difficult delivery intervenes, an infant experiences a period when the eyes are wide open and the infant can see, has visual preferences, turns to the spoken word, and responds to the environment. Similar periods in the state of consciousness of the infant

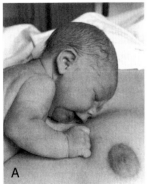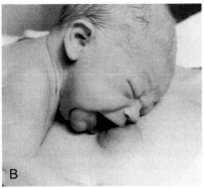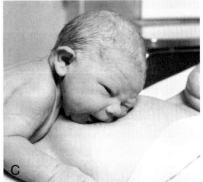

Figure 6-1. Infant crawling to breast (**A**), making mouthing and sucking movements (**B**), then taking breast (**C**). (From Righard L, Alade MO: Effect of delivery room routines on success of first breast-feed, *Lancet* 336:1105, 1990.)

may last only a few seconds or minutes during the next 1 to 2 days.

Although some mothers begin the attachment process when the decision to have an infant is made, after conception the physiologic changes in the maternal body strengthen the developing bond. During pregnancy, listening to the fetal heart and watching echocardiographic images of fetal movements are confirming factors created by modern medicine. The first picture in an infant's scrapbook may be of the infant as a 12-week fetus. The moment of delivery, the first glimpse, and the first hours are intense opportunities for further "bonding" to occur. For some, however, the process will take a day or a week before the mother feels true love for the infant. Unfortunately, studies investigating this timeline do not distinguish women who breastfeed from those who bottle feed.

As in every area of medicine, new ideas and new theories invite criticism. The best type is neither partisan nor polemical and serves to dispassionately repeat the studies and confirm or disprove.[17] Many investigators have affirmed the "bonding" theory. Other critics,[1] however, have been hostile yet unable to disprove that biologic factors might play a significant role in a mother's response to her infant. A new group has called the theories "a bogus notion," reflecting medicine's need to control women and to enhance market demands and the status of medicine itself.[14] Further, it is argued that bonding is demeaning to women because it rests on the idea of instinct. These critics agree that increased contact between mother and infant in the first few days increases maternal emotional response, that early contact enhances breastfeeding, and that early extended contact decreases the incidence of child abuse, with effects solely on the parents, not the child.

Further study is needed, although randomly assigning a mother to a restricted contact control group would be difficult, if not unethical, today. Skin-to-skin versus clothed contact and hormonal components in relationship to behaviors remain to be explored. The father's and siblings' roles also deserve additional attention. Despite his criticism of bonding research, Lamb[30] has been supportive of the trend toward humanizing childbirth to provide a rich emotional experience for parents.

Sensitive periods in biologic phenomena are times when events alter later behavior. The existence of a sensitive period in human behavior is disputed, although it has been shown to exist in other species. Human bonding occurs in a longer period of time.[30] The power of attachment enables mother and father to make many sacrifices necessary

for their infant.[28] More than 50 years of investigation have confirmed the observations that the human maternal-infant bond can be facilitated, supported, and encouraged by more caring sensitive processes beginning with labor and throughout the perinatal period.

Human relationships are complex. A newborn brings joy, fear, anxiety, frustration, and triumph, reminds Righard. Adaptability and compensation in the developmental processes are part of human existence. The concept of bonding has drawn attention to this period of life and began the process of understanding the mother-infant relationship.

Body Contact and Cultural Tradition

If we look at other mammals, lactation behavior, including the duration and frequency of feedings, is species specific and predictable because it is a genetically controlled behavioral characteristic of the species. Only those animals kept in zoos or laboratories reject their young. Among higher primates, learning plays a significant role; monkeys reared without role models have to be taught how to groom and feed their young. In humans, breastfeeding behavior is highly variable from one culture to the next. Different cultures of the world have different sets of "rules" about lactation as they do about many other aspects of life and death. Cultural tradition dictates the initiation, frequency, and termination of breastfeeding. Learning plays a key role in the lactation process, but the learning is focused on the beliefs, attitudes, and values of the culture.

The degree of body contact permitted by the culture is a fundamental difference.[42] Simpson-Herbert describes the degree of mother-infant body contact as the physical and social distance that mothers keep from their babies. The physical distance is viewed as a reflection of the social distance sanctioned by the culture.

Cultures prescribe how often infants will be held or carried and how they will be carried (e.g., in the arms, a pouch, or a sling, or on a cradleboard). How infants are clothed, where they are placed when not held, and where they spend the night are culturally determined and affect breastfeeding. The cultural constraints that control maternal behavior include those on the kinds and amounts of maternal clothing, acceptability of breast exposure, and beliefs on frequency and length of feedings.[3]

The effect of increased carrying of infants was studied by Hunziker and Barr[24] in a group of primiparous breastfeeding women in Montreal.

---

[1]References 4,14–19.

The crying pattern of normal infants in industrialized societies has been reported to increase until 6 weeks of age, followed by a decline to 4 months, with most crying occurring in the evening. The investigators had the study families increase carrying the infants either in the arms or in a carrier to a minimum of 3 hours per day, whereas control infants were placed in a crib or a seat with a mobile in view. At 6 weeks, significantly less (43%) crying was observed in the "carried" infants, especially in the evening. Similar but smaller differences were noted at 4, 8, and 12 weeks.

When Cunningham et al. randomly provided either soft baby carriers or plastic infant seats to a group of low-income women in a clinic in New York City, they found the infants carried in a soft carrier were more securely attached than those placed in a seat when tested with the Ainsworth Strange-Situation Study. The study and control infant groups had an equal number of mothers who breastfed, and thus the authors found no effect of breastfeeding on study results. They concluded that in low-income groups, mother-infant relationships benefited from early use of soft carriers and "contact comfort."

Although the mean length of breastfeeding was similar in both groups, the breastfeeding was not defined, that is, as exclusive, partial, or minimal. Also, time spent holding to breastfeed versus time spent holding to bottle feed was not noted. There were 21 women who breastfed and 28 women who bottle fed. Although it is helpful to use carriers with bottle-fed infants, it should not be done to the abandonment of breastfeeding support programs.

Anthropologic studies of 60 societies by Whiting[59] considered mother-infant body contact. He classified these cultures as high or low in contact as shown in Figure 6-2.

Other factors influence the development of cultural mores, including climate and means of food gathering. Simpson-Herbert points out that when infants are heavily clothed and swaddled, as in cold climates, they are neat packages that can be put down easily. Inuit people are an exception, however, traditionally keeping infants inside mothers' parkas for warmth and frequent feedings. Breastfeeding is almost axiomatic in warm climates where clothing is loose or absent; frequent holding and carrying are common, and the breast is readily accessible.

The diet of hunter-gatherer societies is not conducive to early weaning because meat, roots, nuts, and berries are difficult for infants to chew and digest, whereas the softer foods of the agricultural societies can be prepared for early infant feeding.

Study of specific world societies reveals that North American and European women are concerned with the beliefs that it is indecent to expose

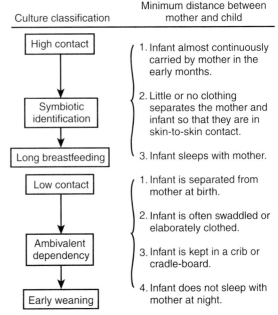

Figure 6-2. Anthropologic studies of mother-infant body contact in 60 societies. (From Whiting JWM: Causes and consequences of the amount of body contact between mother and infant. In Munroe RL, Munroe RD, Whiting BB, editors: *Handbook of cross-culture human development,* New York, 1980, Garland.)

the breast, it is possible to spoil an infant with too much handling, and early weaning is a sign of infant development. Western mothers keep their distance from their babies. Mothers in high-body contact societies spend at least 75% of the time in contact with their babies, whereas low-contact societies spend less than 25%.

Since the 1990s, infant care in Western societies has included carrying infants in carriers close to the parent's body. Co-sleeping with the infant for easy access to the breast through the night and the concept of the family bed has emerged as more conducive to good parent-infant attachment. Breastfeeding increases sleep duration for new parents according to a study by Doan et al.[13] They demonstrated that supplementing with formula at night resulted in more sleep loss similar to that of bottle-feeding parents. Exclusive breastfeeding resulted in 40 to 45 minutes more of sleep.

The practice of co-sleeping and bed sharing, although customary in many cultures, is rare in industrialized societies. Careful scientific study of co-sleeping has revealed a number of benefits, but present custom is based on the bottle-feeding philosophy that embraces separation of parent and child. Where the infant sleeps is not just a family issue but a medical one according to McKenna,[40] who has performed the seminal studies on co-sleeping and pointed out the benefits of bed

BOX 6-1. Safe Sleeping Environments for Infants

Families should be given all the information that is known about safe sleeping environments for their infants, including the following:

- Place babies in a supine position for sleep.
- Use a firm, flat surface and avoid waterbeds, couches, sofas, pillows, soft materials, and loose bedding.
- Use only a thin blanket to cover the infant. Assure the head will not be covered. In a cold room the infant could be kept in an infant sleeper to maintain warmth.
- Avoid the use of quilts, duvets, comforters, pillows, and stuffed animals in the infant's sleep environment.
- Never put an infant down to sleep on a pillow or adjacent to a pillow.
- Never leave an infant alone on an adult bed.
- Inform families that adult beds have potential risks and are not designed to meet federal safety standards for infants.
- Ensure that there are no spaces between the mattress and headboard, walls, and other surfaces that may entrap the infant and lead to suffocation.

sharing. As a result of extensive study on the subject, the Academy of Breastfeeding Medicine has developed "A Guideline on Co-Sleeping and Breastfeeding" (Box 6-1).[1]

Breastfeeding is often enhanced by bed sharing, and providing that precautions are taken, bed sharing is safe and healthy. Bed sharing has been singled out by the AAP Committee on SIDS as a major cause of SIDS. This is not true when associated with breastfeeding. It is true when associated with drugs, smoking, and alcohol. The alternative to bed sharing while breastfeeding is the very hazardous sofa, lounge chair, or rocker.

Psychological Difference Between Breastfeeding and Bottle-Feeding

Professionals have spent decades reassuring mothers that they can capture the same emotional and behavioral experience by feeding an infant from a bottle as they can feeding with the breast, with the same warmth and love. Technically speaking, the same warmth is not present because lactating breasts have been shown to be warmer than nonlactating breasts. This warmth can be demonstrated by infrared pictures and thermograms. Responses to stress appear to be muted in lactating women. Using graded treadmill exercises, lactating women had significantly decreased plasma levels of adrenocorticotropic hormones, or corticotrophin, cortisol, and epinephrine compared with match-control nonlactating women. Plasma glucose did not rise as it did in nonlactating women.[16]

At 1 to 12 months postpartum Mezzacappa and Katkin examined subjective stress as well as individual differences in both mothers who breastfed and those who bottle fed. They administered the Perceived Stress Scale and the trait component of the State-Trait Personality Inventory. The 10-item Perceived Stress Scale is widely used to index subjective stress, and the State-Trait Personality Inventory is a 30-item questionnaire assessing anxiety, anger, and curiosity. Mothers who breastfed had significantly less perceived stress in the month preceding the test than did the those who bottle fed. No significant differences were seen among groups in anxiety, anger, or curiosity. Maternal age, time postpartum, parity, and work status were controlled for. In a second experiment, the authors examined the acute psychological effects of breastfeeding and bottle-feeding. Positive and negative mood were assessed in the same mother before and after a feeding. They recruited mothers who were both breastfeeding and bottle-feeding, studying them in two sessions a week apart, randomly sequenced. The mothers completed the Positive and Negative Affect Scale, rested 10 minutes, fed the infant, rested 10 minutes, and retook the test. The mood was significantly less positive after bottle-feeding than after breastfeeding. Mood became significantly less negative after breastfeeding than after bottle-feeding. A possible explanation is the surge of oxytocin during let-down.[56] Uvnäs-Moberg[53a,56] has reported mood effects of breastfeeding mediated by oxytocin. She describes oxytocin levels as inversely related to negative moods and emotions. The higher the levels of oxytocin, the more calm the mother (Figure 6-3).

Mezzacappa and Katkin conclude that the results confirm that breastfeeding buffers mood. They attributed this to psychological effects of breastfeeding itself and not to the differences between women who breastfeed and those who bottle feed because the participants did both and were their own controls.

Newton and Newton[43] suggest that special caution should be used in evaluating statistical associative studies that purport to investigate the hypothesis that breastfeeding and bottle-feeding are psychological equivalents. "Because breastfeeding involves a large measure of personal choice and because it is related to attitudinal and personality factors, no groups of breastfeeders and bottle feeders are likely to be equal in other respects. Therefore the relation of breastfeeding to any particular psychosocial measure may not be cause and effect, but simply the differences due to other uncontrolled covariables."[43] A human mother's care

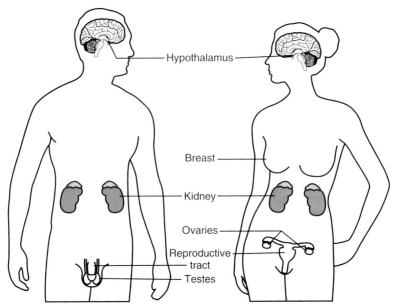

Figure 6-3. Sites of oxytocin action in humans. Oxytocin acts on multiple organ systems in men and women to regulate various physiological processes. In women, these include the milk let-down response by the smooth muscle of the breast, and uterine contractions; in men, they include contractions of the smooth muscles of the reproductive tract. Oxytocin is also involved in regulation of water balance by the kidneys and is released by central neurons to influence behavior. (Redrawn from McCarthy MM, Altemus M: Central nervous system actions of oxytocin and modulation of behavior in humans, *Mol Med Today* 3:269, 1997 (Figure 1).)

of her infant is derived from a complex mixture of her genetic endowment, the response of the infant, a long history of interpersonal relationships, her family constellation, this and previous pregnancies, and the community and culture.

The method chosen to feed a baby is but one item in a whole style of maternal-child interaction. It is unlikely that this style is determined by the method of feeding; according to Righard. Breastfeeding is a different activity when it is carried out by a small minority compared with breastfeeding that is commonplace in the community. After many years of promoting artificial feedings, breastfeeding has become the norm as it had been historically for centuries.

In a study of patterns of variation in breastfeeding behaviors, Quandt[48] offers three explanations: cultural, biologic, and bicultural. Predictions of exclusive breastfeeding duration were most accurate for women with a breastfeeding style of infrequent feedings and therefore early weaning, whereas predictions for women with a style of frequent feeding were confounded by cultural factors that independently affected supplementation.

Before reviewing specific psychological attributes relating to breastfeeding, the distinction between styles of nursing in Western societies should be considered. The Interagency Group for Action on Breastfeeding developed a schema for breastfeeding definitions. Newton and Newton,[43] however, have described two distinct styles—unrestricted breastfeeding and token breastfeeding—that are important to understanding maternal choices.

Unrestricted Breastfeeding

Unrestricted breastfeeding means the infant is put to the breast whenever he or she cries or fusses. Feeding is ad lib and not by the clock, usually leading to 10 or more feedings per day. The infant receives no bottles, and solids are not introduced until the second half of the first year. Breast milk continues to be a major source of nourishment beyond the first year of life. It is interesting that this was routine practice in the United States in the beginning of the twentieth century, as attested by writings on the subject of child rearing. The present recommendation of WHO and major professional organizations (i.e. American Academy of Pediatrics [AAP], American College of Obstetrics/Gynecology [AGOG], American Academy of Family Practice [AAFP]) is unrestricted exclusive breastfeeding for 6 months.

Token Breastfeeding

Token breastfeeding means feeding characterized by rules and regulations. Both frequency and duration of feeding are determined by the clock. It is deemed unnecessary to permit unlimited suckling.

Weaning usually occurs by the third month, if not before. Supplementary bottles and solids are not uncommon. As a result, the let-down reflex is never well established. Engorgement may occur. An infant is frequently too frantic from crying or too sleepy to feed well at the appointed times.

New definitions of breastfeeding (i.e., exclusive, partial) have been published to standardize statistical comparisons (see Chapter 1) but do not reflect the psychosocial differences between unrestricted and token breastfeeding. The American Academy of Pediatrics Section on Breastfeeding recommends exclusive breastfeeding for 6 months and the gradual inclusion of solids (never before 4 months), preferably at 6 months or later.

A University of Rochester study[32] of urban physicians revealed that those pediatricians who prescribed solids by 3 months or earlier also suggested supplementary bottles and had been in practice 20 years or longer. Most of the physicians in the family medicine program in the same community, however, provided no supplements and no solids until 6 months and had been in practice less than 20 years. More than 50% of mothers in that community who planned to breastfeed had made contact with some childbirth or breastfeeding program and chose their physician according to practice style.

Definition of breastfeeding in the United States has been undertaken by the Breastfeeding Promotion Consortium convened by the U.S. Department of Agriculture semiannually since 1990.[19] The report points out that many definitions (legal, programmatic [for WIC food allotments], surveillance, and monitoring) were used for policies and guidelines and for research. Descriptively, it includes initiation, duration, and intensity. The Breastfeeding Promotion Consortium is concerned about monitoring for surveillance purposes. The clinician needs to know frequency per day, length of a feeding, and the provision of any other liquids or foods.[31] The CDC has assumed the responsibility of monitoring breastfeeding trends annually.

Imprinting, Pacifiers, and Dummies

Scores of infants are being introduced to pacifiers or dummies shortly after birth, all too often by an impatient perinatal staff member who knows a breastfed infant should not be bottle fed. Free pacifiers are being provided as gifts by some formula companies eager to beat the competition. The UNICEF/WHO's 10 steps to becoming a baby-friendly hospital (see Chapter 1) include the exclusion of pacifiers from the hospital's provisions. Do pacifiers have a long-range impact on infants? For bottle-fed infants, probably not, if possible dental problems are excluded; a pacifier will provide the sucking a bottle-fed infant may not receive during a feeding. For a breastfed infant, the answer may be different.

Human imprinting is little discussed in pediatric textbooks and rarely noted when discussing infant feeding, yet human infants, like any other mammalian newborns, recognize the mother by the oral, tactile, and olfactory modes. "The most sensitive organ and the one over which a newborn mammal has the most control, its mouth, is the organ central to mammalian and human imprinting," states Mobbs. It is thought that the imprinting process, or "stamping" as it was initially termed, takes place for a brief period early in postnatal development when an animal seeks a particular class of stimuli (i.e., objects of a particular shape). Having found such an object or one resembling it, the animal responds with an unlearned pattern of attachment behavior. The process is innate. Comfort sucking and formation of nipple preference are genetically determined behaviors for imprinting to the mother's nipple. The recognition of the mother is at first through the distinctive features of the nipple. Although imprinting is multisensory and varies from species to species, it is oral/tactile for humans and other higher mammals.

Mistakes and mishaps can occur in the process when a newborn fixes on a rubber nipple (bottle), thumb, or pacifier (Table 6-1). In birds,

TABLE 6-1	Instinctive Fixation on Sucking Objects in the Process of Oral, Tactile, Mother Recognition			
	Objects of Fixation			
	Human Breast	Filled Nursing Bottle	Thumb/Finger/Knuckles	Empty Bottle/Pacifier (Dummy)/Cloth
Nutritive	Yes	Yes	No	No
Animate	Yes	No	Yes	No
Nonself	Yes	Yes	No	Yes
Infant control	No	No	Yes	No

From Mobbs EJG: Human imprinting and breastfeeding: are the textbooks deficient? In Llewellyn-Jones D, Abraham S, editors: *Proceedings: 16th annual congress,* Pokolbin, South Wales, March 1989, Australian Society for Psychosomatic Aspects of Reproductive Medicine.

innate responses are preferentially selective to supernormal-size stimuli. Nonnutritive sucking on thumbs or pacifiers is displacement activity that would normally be directed at imprinting to mother's nipple and reflects a tendency toward supernormal size. In other species with multiple births or litters, the offspring imprints to one teat throughout the lactation period. The one nipple preference sometimes reflects emotional attachment to the object rather than a preoccupation with a need for sucking. According to Passman and Halonen,[46] who found 42% of the interaction with the dummy to be nonsucking attachment, the preference for one nipple was maintained.

Mothers of thumb-sucking infants are less likely to breastfeed successfully, as was demonstrated in a study of 93 mother-infant pairs. Those who used a dummy or pacifier breastfed a shorter period (mean of 5.5 months compared with 7.5 months). Nonnutritive sucking on objects was added to the list of causes of lactation failure by Lilburne et al. after this study. Margaret Mead stated that in those societies where access to the breast is unlimited and frequent suckling is accepted, no thumb sucking occurs.[49]

A randomized prospective study of 750 mother-infant pairs was performed by Howard et al.[23] The pairs were randomly assigned to early pacifier at 2 weeks or no pacifier. A significant negative impact on duration of breastfeeding was seen in the group given a pacifier early.

Although the term "nipple confusion" has been questioned in the medical literature, strong psychosomatic evidence does show that human imprinting can be altered by introducing a foreign object during the process of imprinting.

Personality Differences Between Mothers Who Breastfeed and Mothers Who Bottle Feed

Clear differences exist between mothers who practice unrestricted breastfeeding and those who bottle feed. Even some distinctions between women who do token breastfeeding and those who bottle feed have been noted. It has been said that maternal personality is more important than either breastfeeding or bottle-feeding per se to the development of the infant's personality.

Experimenters looking at these factors have provided a wealth of somewhat conflicting information. Chamberlain studied the differences between mothers who bottle fed and those who practiced unrestricted breastfeeding with their second child. The groups were similar in age, education, parity, intelligence, and socioeconomic status. The

mothers who breastfed were less defensive about their method of feeding, were more oriented toward home life, and had higher radicalism scores. The mothers who bottle fed confirmed the hypothesis that they had problems with trying to breastfeed their first child because of inadequate lactation, possibly a psychosomatic reaction. They also had a greater incidence of sexual performance problems, as indicated by a higher surgency score. A higher surgency score indicates increased gaiety, enthusiasm, effervescence, and impulsiveness and an increase in conversion reaction symptoms (hysteria) and sexual anomalies. The mothers who breastfed wanted their children to do things typical of children; the mothers who bottle fed preferred their children to be conservative and other-person oriented and urged them to be more adult. A study of stress and mood measured the differences between exclusive breast-feeders and formula feeders.[18] Breastfeeders have more positive moods and perceived less stress. Serum prolactin levels were inversely related to stress and mood. Higher serum cortisol, lower stress, and lower anxiety were seen in breastfeeders compared to formula feeders and controls (undergraduate and graduate nursing students). Breastfeeding appeared to be somewhat protective of negative moods and stress. Breastfeeding was associated with higher prolactin levels (Groer).

Call studied the emotional factors favoring successful breastfeeding and noted that of 104 consecutive mothers delivering at an Air Force hospital, 42.6% of the multiparas and 50% of the primiparas chose bottle-feeding. Of the mothers who breastfed, 48% of the multiparas and 40% of the primiparas were successful beyond 3 weeks. Failure was associated with engorgement, lack of let-down reflex, and psychological conflict. The two conflicts seen in those who did not nurse and those who failed were as follows:

1. They had a conflict in accepting the biologic maternal role in relation to the infant versus other roles society holds for women. The maternal role is considered a general class attitude in middle-class American society.
2. They had a conflict regarding the functioning of the breast itself, that is, as an organ for nourishment of the young versus a sexual organ, affording the breast the same psychological value as the penis in the male. Nursing thus became a "castration" threat.

Psychophysiologic Reactions During Nursing

Newton and Newton[43] have equated psychophysiologic reactions during nursing to the degree of successful lactation. During unrestricted suckling, the gentle stroking of the nipple by undulating motion of the infant tongue occurs 3000 to 4000 times in a single feeding. This should result in an increase in temperature of the mammary skin and rhythmic contraction of the uterus. Failure to experience these signs in early lactation is associated with failure to produce adequate milk.

Let-Down Reflex

When an unrestricted breastfed infant cries, the mother has the urge to suckle the infant because the cry has triggered her let-down reflex. The breast is turgescent and ready for the infant. Unrestricted crying is rarely seen in these infants. With token breastfeeding, such a response does not occur on schedule, and from feeding to feeding the milk supply may be little or, conversely, gushing. The infant is unable to cope with the unpredictability. Insufficient milk is rarely a problem when infants are carried and fed frequently.

The role of various hormones in inducing maternal behaviors in animals has been extensively studied. Rosenblatt showed that both male and female rats, including virgin females, manifest maternal behavior after 5 to 7 days of contact with foster pups. Manipulation of estrogen, progesterone, and prolactin has demonstrated that estrogen is the most potent inducer of maternal behavior, progesterone usually is inhibitory, and prolactin strangely ineffective.

More recently, evidence indicates that prolactin does have a role in stimulating maternal behaviors in rats, but only when it is primed by placental lactogens that affect the maternal brain (medial preoptic area) regarding maternal responses at birth. The brain of the maternally behaving rat is altered as a result of the dam's behavior toward her pups. Morphologic changes are seen in the supraoptic nucleus, which contains oxytocinergic neurons important for lactation. The supraoptic nuclei of lactating animals have a higher incidence of dendritic bundling compared with those of nonmaternal virgin rats.[59] These experiments support the concept that maternal behavior in lactating animals can have a profound effect on the morphology and physiologic functioning of oxytocinergic neurons in the hypothalamus (Figure 6-4).

When oxytocin was administered intranasally to humans, it played a key role in social attachment thus increasing the benefits from social interactions. It specifically affects a person's willingness to accept social risks and causes a substantial increase in trust among humans. The mother-infant bond depends upon human trust. Studies using animals have confirmed the effects of oxytocin on the regulation of behavior. In pregnancy and postpartum, oxytocin affects bonding and parenting behaviors. The actions of oxytocin on the brain are regulated by gonadal steroid hormones, particularly estrogen. Studies comparing lactating and nonlactating postpartum women's behavior have assumed there were higher oxytocin levels in the lactating women. Results suggest[39] that breastfeeding within 1 hour of birth, when oxytocin levels are high, causes long lasting enhancement of bonding and interactive behavior between mother and infant.

Other studies have also found this when the oxytocin levels were not sampled during breastfeeding; oxytocin levels were thought to be related to bonding behaviors such as gaze, vocalizations, and affectionate touch.[15]

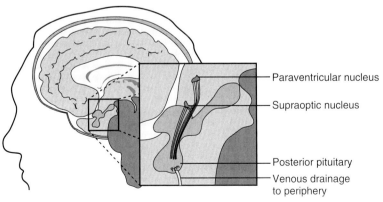

Figure 6-4. The source of oxytocin. Oxytocin is supplied to the posterior pituitary from neurons located in the paraventricular and supraoptic nuclei of the hypothalamus. It is then released from the pituitary into the circulation in response to appropriate stimuli. These same neurons, in addition to accessory oxytocinergic neurons located elsewhere in the brain, project broadly throughout the central nervous system. Receptors for oxytocin are discretely distributed in the brain and, in most mammalian species, are found in the hypothalamus and components of the limbic system. (Redrawn from McCarthy MM, Altemus M: Central nervous system actions of oxytocin and modulation of behavior in humans, *Mol Med Today* 3:269, 1997 (Figure 2).)

When levels were measured in 22 puerperal women, the suckling-induced oxytocin during nursing was pulsatile, with discrete, short pulses. When the women were subjected to the stress of loud noise (70 dB) by earphones or to the stress of performing mathematical problems, the frequency of pulsatile release of oxytocin was significantly lower. No difference was seen in prolactin levels or milk yield. These data suggest that psychological relaxation is necessary for a successful let-down response, confirming what Newton and Newton[43] had observed more than 50 years ago.

The induction of maternal behavior after administration of oxytocin experimentally in rats by Pedersen and Prange demonstrated that estrogen priming is necessary for the effect, but oxytocin may be the triggering hormone for maternal behaviors. A strong relationship between the peptide hormones native to the central nervous system and the reproductive hormones results not only in endocrine effects but also in behavioral effects.[22]

Unrestricted Nursing

The long-term psychophysiologic response to unrestricted nursing is a more even mood cycle than the mood swings associated with ovulation and menstruation. Unrestricted nursing is associated with secondary amenorrhea for as long as 16 months. In relating the rate of success in breastfeeding to experiences at birth, Jackson et al.[25] reported that the more difficult the labor, the less successful the breastfeeding. A direct correlation has also been made with the amount of medication and anesthetic given during labor and delivery and subsequently the sleepiness of the infant and, ultimately, the inadequacy of the suckling. Newton and Newton[43] observed that mothers who talked to their babies on the second day nursed their babies longer, that is, beyond the second month.

Modahl and Newton[41] measured mood state differences between mothers who breastfed and those who bottle fed when feeding and not feeding. They used the Curran and Cattel questionnaire, which measures transient mood states rather than personality traits. Bottle feeders showed significantly more anxiety, stress, depression, regression, fatigue, and guilt than breastfeeders. Mothers measured while bottle-feeding reported higher levels of these states and more extroversion than the control group of those who bottle fed tested in a nonfeeding situation. Members of another control group who were lactating but also gave bottles were measured while not feeding and showed less anxiety, stress, depression, regression, fatigue, and guilt than the average population. Measurements were taken at home with no examiner present.

The psychophysiologic responses of mothers who breastfeed and those who bottle feed to their infants' signals were measured by Wiesenfeld et al., using physiologic monitoring, while mothers observed previously prepared videotapes of their own infants while they smiled, were quiescent, and cried. Strikingly different response patterns characterized mothers who breastfed and those who bottle fed across all response measures. Mothers who breastfed were physiologically more relaxed but were more apt to want to interact with their child and expressed greater satisfaction with the feeding experience. The authors interpreted these patterns as suggesting a physiologic influence of breastfeeding rather than maternal personality factors influencing the choice of feeding mode.

When 60 primiparous mothers' maternal role adjustments were analyzed by measuring mother-infant mutuality and maternal anxiety scores, the infant-feeding method (breast, bottle, or both) was found to account for considerable variation by Virden. Women who breastfed had scores indicating less anxiety and more mutuality, a central factor in maternal adjustment, than women who bottle fed. The Maternal Attitude Scale was used. The findings are compatible with other studies showing breastfeeding to be emotionally gratifying and that breastfeeding stimulates a sense of emotional union between mother and infant.[49]

Oxytocin, known to be an important activator in the let-down reflex, has been shown to be important throughout the life cycle in both sexes. Oxytocin has been shown to enhance human trust (Kosfeld). Oxytocin has modulatory effects on neural functioning that are important in the regulation of behavior including parenting. The action of oxytocin in the brain is regulated by gonadal steroid hormones particularly estrogen.[39] Oxytocin has an essential role in prosocial approach behavior as well as other social behaviors. Oxytocin may well be essential in the difference between women who breastfed and those that do not.

Impact of Society, Medical Profession, and Family

SOCIETY

Newton[44] has pointed out that a woman's joy in, and acceptance of, the female biologic role in life may be an important factor in her psychosexual behavior, which includes lactation. She found that women who wished to bottle feed also often believed that the male role was the more satisfying role. Nulliparous women who planned to breastfeed their children more often stated their satisfaction with the female role, according to Adams.[2]

Breastfeeding behavior has been related to a woman's role in life as influenced by her cultural locale, education, social class, and work. Breastfeeding rates and weaning times vary in the United States by geographic area. The smaller the community, the longer is the duration of breastfeeding. Cross-cultural studies in large cities show variation in rates of nursing. These rates are influenced by education, and in the current generation, the higher the education, the higher the incidence of breastfeeding.

MEDICAL PROFESSION

An enthusiastic physician in the practice can influence the number of mothers who breastfeed; this has been demonstrated. If the physician provides knowledgeable medical and psychological support, the success rate of the patients who intended to breastfeed will increase. Some patients who had not formed an opinion or given it any thought in their preparation for motherhood will be persuaded to try. In addition, this physician will attract patients to the practice who are already successfully breastfeeding but find their own physician unable or unwilling to support their efforts.

A study was done at the University of Rochester in a small community where more than 50 pediatricians practiced.[33] The pediatricians described their own practices according to the number of mothers who breastfeed (high, 75%; moderate, 50%; low, 25%). They were also asked when the mothers started solid foods, general practice "regulations," and finally, how their own children were fed. The physicians with a high incidence of breastfeeding in their practices recommended starting solids after 4 months and had few rules and regulations about the practice, and usually their own children had been breastfed. Physicians with a high number of women who bottle fed recommended starting solids by 6 weeks and had many rules and regulations about the practice, and their own children had been bottle fed. When asked about using lay groups to help their patients breastfeed, female physicians were more apt than male physicians to discredit what these lay mothers could do to help other mothers.

A national survey conducted among a representative sample of obstetricians, pediatricians, and family physicians by mailed questionnaire reinforced the observation that a physician's attitude and personal beliefs about breastfeeding influence the advice given.[46] It further confirmed that not all physicians were informed about current knowledge on human lactation, not all physicians discussed lactation with their pregnant patients, and not all believed it was worth counseling time when problems arose. Despite national efforts to increase

physicians' knowledge base regarding breastfeeding,[47] there remains a residual cluster of physicians who do not support breastfeeding. The correlation to the feeding mode of their own children is clear. When trained in a program that supports breastfeeding, this trend is muted.

THE FAMILY

Impact on Infants

For infants, differences exist between breastfeeding and bottle-feeding in the alleviation of hunger, the mother-infant interaction, oral gratification, activity, development, personality, and adaptation to the environment. Often mother and baby are alone together during breastfeeding, and the mother gives her full attention to the baby with stroking and fondling. Social interaction with the baby is less frequent during bottle-feeding, and the mother is often in a distracting social situation or someone else feeds the infant. The breastfed infant has control of what is happening, or at least shares control, whereas the mother controls the bottle and the bouts of sucking.

In a study of newborns at 6 to 7 days of age, the effects of breastfeeding, giving breast milk by bottle, and just holding the infant were measured.[37] Results suggest that the total mother-infant interaction during breastfeeding has a positive influence on neonatal behavior. It induces a more stable state for an infant compared with that generated by giving the same human milk in a bottle and increases some sucking and holding times.

The attitudes of the husband, close family, and friends influence a mother's attitude toward breastfeeding. More important, these attitudes influence the rate of success and the age at weaning more negatively than positively. One study showed that a grandmother's interest did not influence the mother's decision to nurse as frequently as did a friend's (peer's) decision to bottle feed. A woman whose husband is not supportive of breastfeeding weans early or does not start at all.[26]

DEVELOPMENT

Early assessment of newborns in the first and second weeks of life shows more body activity with breastfed than bottle-fed infants. They are more alert and have stronger arousal reaction. Statistics reported by Douglas on age of learning to walk in Great Britain showed a distinct difference, with breastfed infants starting 2 months earlier than bottle-fed infants. The longer the infant was nursed, the more striking the differences. Thus prolonged breastfeeding does not impede development as has been implied by advocates of early weaning. A study in Illinois compared children exclusively breastfed for 4 months, 9 months, and more than a year with bottle-fed infants.[21] The children who were exclusively breastfed for 4 and 9 months scored significantly higher on achievement tests, but the difference was reversed beyond a year. Exclusive breastfeeding beyond a year increased morbidity as well, which is in keeping with the concept that solids should be added in the second half of the first year as promoted by WHO, the AAP, and others.

A cross-cultural study of 50 3-year-old children in Hawaii, reflecting the cultural diversity of the islands, provided periodic behavioral assessments as part of the heptachlor toxicity exposure study. The study, which used the McCarthy scales, showed that the duration of breastfeeding was correlated with general cognition, verbal and quantitative scores, and memory, regardless of socioeconomic status, sex, or pesticide exposure. No associations to motor skills at 3 years of age were seen in this study.[4]

An extensive study by Morrow-Tlucak et al. investigated differences between breastfed and bottle-fed infants. Batteries of infant assessment measures and maternal interviews were conducted by trained examiners blind to the risk factors during home visits when the infant was 6, 12, and 24 months of age. The 350 children were born to women at the Cleveland Metropolitan General Hospital who were part of a study of child development and psychosocial risk factors. The Bayley scales and the Home Observation Measurement of Environment were done. A significant difference among bottle-fed children, children breastfed 4 months or less, and those breastfed 4 months or more was found at all points, with extended breastfeeding showing a positive effect.

Animal research has also shown a relationship of weaning time to learning skills. Because it has become evident that species-specific proteins and amino acids exist, it is possible that the brain develops more physiologically with the precise basic nutrients. Comparisons with animal species show that the more intelligent and skillful groups within a species are nursed longer.

PERSONALITY

The personality and adjustment of infants as related to their early feeding experiences has been the subject of much discussion. The personality of the mother and the temperament of the child need to be considered. Some conflicting information is reported in studies retrospectively analyzing the effects of breastfeeding on outcome in terms of security and behavior. The emphasis has been on the duration of the breastfeeding rather than on the quality of the relationship.

In a prospective study of a birth cohort of New Zealand children followed to the age of 8 years, both maternal and teacher assessments of conduct disorder showed a statistically significant tendency for conduct disorder scores to decline with increasing duration of breastfeeding.[16] Overall, however, the authors suggest that no real evidence indicates that breastfeeding is protective against conduct disorders.

When abrupt weaning takes place, it may be psychologically traumatic for infant and mother. In animals, when the mother is stressed while lactating, the nursling's plasma cortisone levels are elevated. The psychologically depressed mother may not experience postpartum depression until the infant is weaned from the breast. It has been accepted that early experience, including feeding experience, does influence later behavior in the long run. The performance in young college women on an anxiety scale questionnaire Institute for Personality and Ability Testing (IPAT) and a personality inventory Eysenck Personality Inventory (EPI) showed that women who had been bottle fed had higher anxiety scores and greater neuroticism than women who had been breastfed, irrespective of duration of breastfeeding. Study continues to be done measuring the impact of nursing at the breast and the complexity of life's events.

Impact on the Father

Since the birthing process moved into the hospital setting, fathers have been moved farther from the nucleus of the new family. In recent years, this trend has been reversed. Research on interaction with infants focused on the mother until Parke et al. observed all three together. In the triadic situation, a father tends to hold the baby twice as much and touches the baby slightly more but smiles significantly less than the mother. The father plays the more active role when both are present. The study was conducted with middle-class participants who had been to childbirth classes, but the same results were obtained among low-income families without preparation or the presence of the father in the labor and delivery room. The infant had to be relatively active and responsive to capture the father's attention. The investigators believed that fathers were far more involved in, and responsive toward, their infants than our culture had acknowledged. Other studies have shown that when fathers were asked to undress their babies and establish eye contact with them in the first few days of life, they showed more caregiving behavior 3 months later than did control subjects.

Newton and Newton[43] describe the early attachments of the new family as follows:

Father interacts with baby: Engrossment
Mother interacts with baby: Bonding
Baby interacts with mother: Attachment

Fathers have been brought back into the childbirth scene as coaches. The coach role has been described as the father's role in shared childbirth. The idea of coaching can have negative connotations because a coach is one who presses the players to work and try harder but always to win. Ideally, the father should be a partner and supporter in labor, delivery, and breastfeeding. Raphael[49] has suggested that the father may well play the role of a doula. A doula is one who provides psychological encouragement and physical assistance to the newly delivered mother. Raphael further indicates that the lack of a doula to support the mother predisposes her to failure with breastfeeding.[49]

The stress placed on sharing responsibilities of parenthood implies an across-the-board division of labor. This implies that parenting is equal for women and men. Fathers and mothers have complementary activities. Parents are not equally able to do all things. Nurturing an infant is more than just feeding. Therefore, the father should play a significant role with the infant. For instance, when an infant is fussy and does not need to be fed, comforting is often best done by the father; nonnutritive cuddling is best done by a father. "Nonnutritive Cuddler" is an important role for the father and equally as important in the balance of parenting roles.

According to Waletzky,[58] a father's most common negative reaction to breastfeeding is jealousy of the physical and emotional closeness of the nursing mother and child. The degree of jealousy may reflect how much and how happily the mother breastfeeds. Actually, fathers may express distress because they have no similar way to bring food and contentment to their baby. Male envy of female sex characteristics and reproductive capacity has been identified by Lerner[34] as "a widespread and conspicuously ignored dynamic." Improving the birth experience for fathers is a significant means of helping them feel closer to their babies and better about themselves as fathers, according to Waletzky.[58]

Fathers who object to their wives' breastfeeding may do so because they do not want to share this part of their lover with an infant. Some fathers express concern that the breast will leak and destroy any sexual mystique. On the other hand, many men take great pride in the knowledge that their infants will be breastfed and support their wives in this effort. The decision to breastfeed should be made with full involvement of the father.

Impact on Siblings

Although some information is available about siblings and breastfeeding with regard to behavior patterns, no known studies compare siblings of bottle-fed and breastfed infants. Just as siblings frequently want to try the infant's bottle, they may want to nurse at the breast. The child will reflect the mother's attitude toward breasts and nursing. If the mother nurses secretly or in private and isolates herself from the family, it may cause concern in the sibling and produce feelings of shame or guilt toward breasts.

Breastfeeding and Feminism

"Breastfeeding empowers women and contributes to gender equality [and therefore] is an important feminist, human rights and women's issue," states Van Esterik.[57] Despite Eyer's statement that the results of mother-infant research "will be shaped to address social and political agendas ... and women inspired by feminism helped to precipitate a reform movement that actively embraces bonding,"[14] Van Esterik points out that writers on feminist theory almost always ignore the breasts and motherhood as well. Breastfeeding advocates have been criticized as wanting to tie women down.

Policy makers have consulted with women's groups before breastfeeding legislation was drafted, and new legislation has improved the work environment for nursing women and public opinion about the breastfeeding dyad. Progress has been made to make breastfeeding the medical and social norm. Breastfeeding is an emotional issue for many women, and strategies should be developed for framing the issue in nonjudgmental ways.

Possible negative effects, such as employers threatening to fire women rather than provide maternity entitlements, have been anticipated and dealt with. Breastfeeding campaigns have stressed the welfare of both mother and child.

Intimacy and Breastfeeding

Breastfeeding is an intimate activity for some women, but most health professionals tend to present it in the context of the biopsychosocial model.[12] The closeness of the mother-infant dyad is a feminine image.

According to McAdams,[38] the definition of intimacy includes 10 characteristics in the exchange between people: joy and mutual delight, reciprocal dialog, openness, contact, union, receptivity, perceived harmony, concern for the other's well-being, surrender of manipulative control and the desire to master, and being in an encounter.

The theoretical definition for intimacy, states Timmerman,[55] is "a quality of a relationship in which the individuals must have reciprocal feelings of trust and emotional closeness toward each other and are able to openly communicate thoughts and feelings with each other. The conditions that must be met for intimacy to occur include reciprocity of trust, emotional closeness and self-disclosure."

Breastfeeding provides body contact with another and is the source of comfort, security, warmth, and nourishment for the infant and reciprocity for the mother. A mother's perception of breastfeeding as intimate describes her concept of the mother-infant relationship. The spouse's perception, however, may have the greatest effect on the success and duration of breastfeeding. Jordan and Wall[26] suggest that "supporting the father during breastfeeding may help improve the mother's satisfaction with breastfeeding, the duration of breastfeeding and adaptation of both parents to parenting."

Abuse and Neglect

A 15-year prospective cohort study of 7223 Australian mother-infant dyads (full term) examined the incidence of child maltreatment including neglect, physical abuse, and emotional abuse. As substantiated by child protective reports, potential confounders included socioeconomic status, pregnancy "wantedness," substance abuse, employment, and anxiety and depression; 512 children (4.3%) had been maltreated (i.e., maternal abuse or neglect). As breastfeeding decreased, the risk for abuse increased. Nonbreastfed children were 4.8 times more likely to be abused, and, when adjusted for confounding factors, the risk was still 2.6 times higher. Infants who were breastfed were nonneglected.[54]

When a woman has been abused, this may affect her ability to breastfeed and her fear of further abuse. Studies of women in Brazilian ghettos have correlated low rates of breastfeeding with experiences with abuse, especially spousal abuse.[10] Chin[10] also reported on a community-based participatory research project that emphasizes the life experiences and perspectives of its low-income population with respect to the cultural logic that forms infant-feeding choices.

Psychosocial Risk Factors and Early Weaning

Support from clinicians and maternal depressive symptoms have been associated with breastfeeding duration.[54] In a prospective cohort study of low-risk mothers enrolled at a health maintenance organization (HMO), the dyads were randomized to home visits or not. Of the original group of 1163, 1007 (87%) were breastfeeding at birth, 872 (75%) were breastfeeding at 2 weeks postpartum, and 646 (55%) were breastfeeding at the 12-week interview. Mothers who were breastfeeding at 12 weeks had received encouragement from their clinician. Breastfeeding discontinuation was associated with clinical depression and, for some, returning to work. The authors associated stress with depression and the discontinuance of breastfeeding.

Psychosocial well-being was also investigated by Li et al.[35] in relation to breastfeeding duration. Experience of stressful life events during pregnancy increased the odds for early cessation of breastfeeding independent of maternal sociodemographic parameters. They reported that separation, divorce, financial problems, and residential moves were important predictors for shorter duration of breastfeeding. Posttraumatic stress syndrome symptoms have been described by mothers in the national survey "New Mothers Speak Out." Using a 17-point scale to measure posttraumatic stress disorder, the survey identified 18% of mothers with some symptoms, and 9% appeared to meet all the criteria for the diagnosis. Black non-Hispanic mothers had the highest score (26%), compared with non-Hispanic whites (17%) and Hispanic mothers (14%) ($p < 0.01$). The higher scores were associated with unplanned pregnancy, low education, and low income, but not traumatic birth.[11]

In this same survey mothers were also asked to answer the seven-question short version of the Postpartum Depression Screening Scale. The questions involved feelings in the 2 weeks before the survey. A score of 14 or higher was found in 63% of the women (i.e., two out of three) (Table 6-2); 5% of mothers reported suicidal thoughts, a troubling proportion. Among mothers who had cesarean delivery, 8 of 10 had pain in the first two months. Among women with a vaginal birth, almost half (48%) had perineal pain, with 15% complaining that it was a major problem, which usually involved an episiotomy. Pain associated with an episiotomy was more likely to interfere with activity.[22]

When this group of mothers who took the survey were asked to report words that came to mind about the first 2 months postpartum, *tired, messy, unsure,* and *isolated* were mentioned frequently. Only 19% of first-time mothers were confident (and only 23% of multiparas). Breastfeeding intentions were high before birth (61% planned to exclusively breastfeed and only 20% to feed formula). After birth 23% dropped breastfeeding if they had cesarean delivery, and 7% of mothers who delivered vaginally discontinued. All mothers commented

TABLE 6-2   Mothers' Experience of Dimensions of Depression in 2 Weeks Before Survey*

Base: All Mothers n = 1573	Strongly Disagree (%)	Disagree (%)	Neither Agree nor Disagree (%)	Agree (%)	Strongly Agree (%)
Had shifting emotions	26	15	10	27	21
Experienced sleep disturbance	32	19	6	25	17
Felt anxious about baby	29	23	15	21	11
Experienced loss of sense of self	40	21	11	16	11
Had mental confusion	43	19	12	17	9
Felt guilty about mothering behavior	44	24	11	12	8
Had suicidal thoughts	78	11	5	3	2

*Results of short version of Postpartum Depression Screening Scale (PDSS), which was licensed and used in survey; contact Western Psychological Services for exact language of this proprietary screening tool.

From Declercq ER, Sakala C, Corry MP, et al: New mothers speak out: national survey results highlight women's postpartum experiences, N.Y., 2008, Childbirth Connections. Available at www.childbirthconnection.org/newmothersspeakout (Accessed 01.08.09.); LTMI = Listening to Mothers I.

on the hospital environment where free formula and pacifiers were distributed regardless of mother's wishes. They also noted a lack of support for breastfeeding and that it was too difficult to get breastfeeding established; 14% tried breastfeeding and did not like it. Success at breastfeeding and at breastfeeding for as long as a mother had planned appeared to be clearly related to having a partner and education and somewhat to income.[22]

The most poignant commentaries were those volunteered by mothers indicating that childbirth can be scary, disruptive, and exhausting. Other thoughts included that the mothers felt they were not in control even when they had carefully planned ahead.[11]

When Borra et al.[6] examined whether breastfeeding influenced the risks of postnatal depression, they found the beneficial effects were strongest at 8 weeks postpartum and weaker after 8 months. For mothers who had no symptoms before birth, the risk of postpartum depression was greatest among women who had not intended to breastfeed. The effect of breastfeeding on maternal depression was highly heterogeneous and very dependent upon intentions during pregnancy. Mothers not depressed during pregnancy that planned to breastfeed and did had the lowest risk of depression. Those that planned to breastfeed but were unable to for various reasons were at an increased risk. They also found that providing specialized support to new mothers who were unable to breastfeed was essential to diminishing the risk of depression postpartum.[6]

Why Some Women Do Not Breastfeed

Before the trend toward bottle-feeding can be permanently reversed, one has to understand why some women do not breastfeed. It cannot be blamed on society or the medical profession when a woman cannot accept this as part of the biologic role of a mother. A physician who does not understand the complexities of rejecting breastfeeding cannot hope to assist a mother to succeed in breastfeeding.

Exploring the question of whether body satisfaction and maternal attachment affect breastfeeding, 38 women at approximately 35 weeks' gestation were given the maternal-fetal attachment scale, the eating disorders examination, and the body satisfaction scale; 30 women who intended to breastfeed were more satisfied with their gravid shape and had higher levels of maternal-fetal attachment. The mother's age and body mass index did not differ between those who breastfed and those who bottle fed. Mothers with high-body dissatisfaction did not breastfeed. Not surprisingly, five mothers with a history of bulimia had difficulty breastfeeding, and three thought it was distasteful and adversely affected their appearance.[52] In a report of six women with bulimia nervosa who had bilateral reduction mammaplasty, the surgeons report that postoperatively the women were relieved of their physical symptoms and had improvement in their psychological well-being.[53] Previously, women with eating disorders had been disqualified for plastic surgery. Macromastia can cause a distortion of the body image and in such cases can be the root cause of the bulimia.[36]

Our society has assumed that no valid intellectual stimulation can occur in the company of young children. Mothers are made to feel intellectually stagnant and uncreative while breastfeeding. Indeed, they are also made to feel asexual at the peak of their sexual cycle. In response, new mothers struggle in panic to maintain their social and professional ties. They feel they must produce tangible works to be productive. Bloom poignantly points out that one of the greatest intellectual voyages of our time was undertaken when Jean Piaget sat at his son's crib and observed the child's successive attempts to grasp a rattle. A nursing mother learns about her child through many internal, subjective, and kinesthetic modes that were not open to Piaget. When a mother wrote of her observations in this setting, her writing was ignored as unscientific and trivial.

Bentovim[5] has taken a systems approach to successful breastfeeding, pointing out that a range of physical, psychological, and sociologic factors are involved. "Breastfeeding is a systemic product of many interacting factors rather than a product of individual behavior only,"[5] according to Bentovim. A good experience with breastfeeding can ensure an intense interaction and synchronous response of giving and taking. According to Brazelton,[8] this is the essence of the infant's beginning to create a secure world for the self.

Beliefs and attitudes toward breastfeeding influence the choice and the success of breastfeeding. Bentovim[5] points out that it may be possible to restore breastfeeding as the natural choice. Society has begun to accept breasts not only as good for the infant and development, but also as the object of less ambivalent and secret pleasure. The role of the health professional in this area is important. Hendrickse[20] states that the biggest block in the minds of women relates to feelings of shame associated with breastfeeding. More than half the women in the Newcastle survey were prevented from choosing breastfeeding because of a sense of shame. The shame is a result of relating the breast to concepts of sexuality.

Failure at Breastfeeding: Grief, Shame, Guilt, or Anger

When a mother who had planned to breastfeed is unable because of illness in herself or her baby, or when a mother begins to breastfeed and must stop, a grief reaction often occurs. A mother experiences a great loss. Prolonged mourning and depression may occur. Some women report feeling more distant from this child than from her other children if the others had been successfully breastfed. The stronger the commitment had been to breastfeed, the stronger is the grief reaction. Few mothers found help, according to Righard in this study, from either professionals or lay support groups. Professionals failed to understand the feeling of failure or loss. The support groups tended to magnify the guilt and sense of failure.

The emotions are complex surrounding this intimate activity. Physicians who must recommend discontinuing breastfeeding for medical reasons should be aware of the impact and provide for

appropriate support for mothers. A woman's choice of feeding method does not make her a good or bad mother, and her inability to produce adequate milk for her infant does not make her a bad mother. Lactation failure is often a reflection on the system and the culture rather than the person.

A random sampling of educated middle-class women in a university neighborhood revealed that a number of women had difficulty breastfeeding. The study did not describe methodology or how it was randomized, but the report reflected much shame, guilt, and finally anger. Failure of breastfeeding by a woman or her friends can be a powerful influence against deciding to breastfeed a future child.

Fear, shame, and guilt were regarded by Freud as different forms of anxiety. Objective anxiety is fear (fear of failure) and arises from external dangers; social anxiety is shame resulting from the criticisms of others; and conscience anxiety is guilt. Real external dangers produce normal anxiety, but when one overreacts, this is neurotic anxiety. Defenses against guilt feelings include repression, rationalization, and projection. Any guilt can be borne more easily if someone else has had a similar experience. Thus knowing other women have failed to breastfeed successfully relieves guilt.

Lasting anger after lactation failure has become more visible. The woman who writes an angry tirade against breastfeeding in a letter-to-the-editor after a news story supporting breastfeeding deserves understanding and support. She is likely a victim of poor medical management and inadequate social support to breastfeed. Letter writing can be therapeutic, but it is never a cure for the underlying hurt.

In our clinical experience, well-educated women who have difficulty producing enough milk or who have an infant who fails to thrive are driven to find out why. The Lactation Study Center has received many calls from women who may even have had trouble feeding one or more other infants and wants to be "tested" to find the cause. Testing resources are limited and reveal little more than can be identified with a good history of breast response in pregnancy and postpartum. The mother's need usually involves a desire to know that the situation is out of her control. The best management beyond ruling out simple remediable causes (positioning, timing, or reduction of fatigue) may be the therapy of a good listener and the reassurance that one is still a good mother.[54] Confirming that the prolactin levels are low can be a great source of comfort for the mother that it was not her fault (Table 6-3).

Avoiding Guilt as a Reason Not to Promote Breastfeeding

In many interactions physicians, especially obstetricians, are encouraged to provide enough information about breastfeeding to a woman prenatally to allow

TABLE 6-3	Reasons for Breastfeeding Discontinuation Vary by Weeks				
	Week of Breastfeeding Discontinuation				
Main Reason for Discontinuation	**0-1 (n = 105) (%)**	**2-3 (n = 74)* (%)**	**4-6 (n = 112) (%)**	**7-9 (n = 53) (%)**	**10-12 (n = 19) (%)†**
Infant still hungry/not enough milk	27	18	38	28	11
Problems sucking/latching on	23	12	1	1	5
Breast pain/soreness	14	14	4	0	0
Mother returned to work or school	4	14	29	34	58
Mother sick or on medication	2	12	6	11	11
Bottle-feeding easier or more convenient	8	9	7	13	0
Lack of energy/desire to discontinue	4	8	7	2	4
Other‡	18	13	8	11	11

*Mothers were asked, during the 2- and 12-week interviews, to report when they discontinued and the reason for breastfeeding discontinuation. Of the 135 women who discontinued breastfeeding at 2 weeks, 132 (98%) women responded to this question.
†Of the 321 additional women who discontinued breastfeeding after 2 weeks, 231 (72%) responded to this question.
‡Other reported reasons for discontinuation included infant not gaining weight or sick, breast milk intolerance, and infant spitting up.
From Taveras EM, Capra AM, Braveman PA, et al: Clinical support and psychosocial risk factors associated with breastfeeding discontinuation, *Pediatrics* 112:108–115, 2003.

her to make an informed choice. The response often is, "No, I don't want to make a mother feel guilty, so I say nothing."

No studies in the literature support this position. In the dozens of reports on efforts to increase breastfeeding among many cultures, no report on producing guilt feelings is available. Women interviewed with open-ended questionnaires have not mentioned guilt feelings in response to the questioning. The only individuals who ever mention guilt are those in the older generation whose daughters are now choosing breastfeeding. The grandmother feels guilty because no one ever told her; no one ever encouraged her to breastfeed; "If only she had known ... if only her doctor had told her... ." In the interest of good health, physicians counsel their patients about good nutrition, weight gain, smoking, drinking, and a number of detrimental personal behaviors without any concern for the guilt they might produce because of the importance of the issue. The feeding choice has an equally important impact for both mother and infant.

In a study at the University of Rochester prenatal clinic, women were randomly assigned to the group attending the Best Start program to encourage breastfeeding or to the control group spending the same time in "counseling" about pregnancy and delivery but nothing about breastfeeding.[33] After delivery, interviewed mothers in both groups were comfortable about their own infant-feeding decision. Those who received breastfeeding encouragement and chose to bottle feed said it was right for them and denied any guilt feelings.

Summary

Decades of research have shown that the breast plays an important role in the growth, development, identity, and psychological well-being of women. Not all women have the same level of comfort with their breasts or see them in the same way with respect to their primary purpose, nourishment of the newborn offspring. The infant, on the other hand, when given the opportunity, will find the breast, seek out and latch on, and suckle. Infants at birth are programmed to breastfeed. Their innate reflexes of rooting and suckling are designed for breastfeeding. Infants also can be taught other mechanisms for feeding. The intricacies of how women choose infant-feeding methods remain to be identified. This choice is influenced by culture, community, personal experiences, education, and the opinions of those close to the mother. The greatest external influence is the primary health care provider, the obstetrician or midwife.

Physicians can make a difference. Women indicate that they rely heavily on the messages they hear from their physicians. The issue of guilt is no more important in choosing to breastfeed than it is in choosing to smoke, drink, abuse drugs, or give in to problems of overeating. The physician's role in the latter situations has always been clear: take a firm stand and provide guidelines for the patient. In addition to providing information and support regarding infant-feeding choices, the physician is in a critical position to facilitate breastfeeding in its early hours and to be supportive and constructive in ensuring its success with appropriate monitoring of progress, not only in the hospital but in the first weeks and months of the infant's life. Midwives do this intuitively.

The impact of breastfeeding on the mother herself is more difficult to identify. Mothers who breastfeed are not different at the onset but do change in their relationship with their infant. Breastfeeding does have an impact psychologically on both mother and infant.

REFERENCES

1. Academy of Breastfeeding Medicine: A guideline on co-sleeping and breastfeeding clinical guideline no. 6. Revision; March, 2008, *Breastfeed Med* 3(38), 2008.
2. Adams AB: Choice of infant feeding technique as a function of maternal personality, *J Consult Clin Psychol* 23:143, 1959.
3. Barr RG: Nursing interval and maternal responsivity: effect of early infant crying, *Pediatrics* 81:529, 1988.
4. Bauer G, Ewald S, Hoffman J, et al: Breastfeeding and cognitive development of three year old children, *Psychol Rep* 68:1218, 1991.
5. Bentovim A: Shame and other anxieties associated with breast feeding: a systems theory and psychodynamic approach. In *Ciba foundation symposium, no. 45, breast feeding and the mother*, Amsterdam, 1976, Elsevier Scientific.
6. Borra C, Lacovour M, Sevilla A: New evidence on breast-feeding and postpartum depression: the importance of understanding women's intentions, *Matern Child Health J*, 2015. http://dx.doi.org/10.1007/s10995-014-1591-z.
7. Bowlby J: *Attachment and loss*, London, 1969, Hogarth.
8. Brazelton TB: The early mother-infant adjustment, *Pediatrics* 32:931, 1963.
9. Budin P: *The nursling*, London, 1907, Caxton.
10. Chin N: Cultural differences in breastfeeding. Presented at the first annual summit on breastfeeding: first food—the essential role of breastfeeding, Washington, D.C., June 2009, *Breastfeed Med* 4(Suppl 1):541, 2009.
10a. deChâteau P, Homberg H, Jakobsson K, et al: A study of factors promoting and inhibiting lactation, *Dev Med Child Neurol* 19:575, 1977.
11. Declercq ER, Sakala C, Corry MP, et al: *New mothers speak out: national survey results highlight women's postpartum experiences*, New York, 2008, Childbirth Connections, Available at www.childbirthconnection.org/newmothersspeakout (Accessed 01.08.09.).
12. Dignam DM: Understanding intimacy as experienced by breastfeeding women, *Health Care Women Int* 16:477, 1995.
13. Doan T, Gardiner A, Gay CL, et al: Breastfeeding increases sleep duration of new parents, *J Perinat Neonatal Nurs* 21(3):200–216, 2007.
14. Eyer D: *Mother-infant bonding: a scientific fiction*, New Haven, 1992, Yale University Press.
15. Feldman R, Weller A, Zagoory-Sharon O, et al: Evidence for a neuroendocrinological foundation of human affiliation, *Psychol Sci* 18:965–970, 2007.
16. Fergusson DM, Horwood LJ, Shannon FT: Breastfeeding and subsequent social adjustment in six- to eight-year-old children, *J Child Psychol Psychiatry* 28:378, 1987.
17. Foster SF, Slade P, Wilson K: Body image, maternal fetal attachment and breast feeding, *J Psychosom Res* 41:181, 1996.
18. Groer MW: Differences between exclusive breastfeeders, formula-feeders, and controls in study of stress, mood, and endocrine variables, *Biol Res Nurs* 7(2):106–117, 2005.
19. Grummer-Strawn LM, Li R, Perrine CG, et al: Infant feeding and long-term outcomes: results from the year 6 follow-up of children in the infant feeding practices study II, *Pediatrics* 134(Suppl 1):S1–S3, 2014. http://dx.doi.org/10.1542/peds.2014.0646B.
20. Hendrickse RG: *Discussion from Ciba foundation symposium, no. 45, breast feeding and the mother*, Amsterdam, 1976, Elsevier Scientific.
21. Hoefer C, Hardy MC: Later development of breast fed and artificially fed infants, *JAMA* 92:615, 1929.
22. Hollander E, Liebowitz MR, Cohen B, et al: Prolactin and sodium lactate-induced panic, *J Psychiatr Res* 28:181, 1989.
23. Howard CR, Howard FM, Lanphear B, et al: A randomized clinical trial of pacifier use and bottle or cup feeding and their effect on breastfeeding, *Pediatrics* 111:511, 2003.
24. Hunziker UA, Barr RG: Increased carrying reduces infant crying: a randomized controlled trial, *Pediatrics* 77:64, 1986.
25. Jackson EB, Wilkin LC, Auerbach H: Statistical report on incidence and duration of breast feeding in relation to personal-social and hospital maternity factors, *Pediatrics* 17:700, 1956.
26. Jordan PL, Wall VR: Supporting the father when an infant is breastfed, *J Hum Lact* 9:31, 1993.
27. Kennell JH, Klaus MH: Bonding: recent observations that alter perinatal care, *Pediatr Rev* 19:4, 1998.
28. Kennell JH, Trause MA, Klaus MH: Evidence for a sensitive period in the human mother. In *Ciba symposium, no. 33, parent-infant interaction*, Princeton, N.J., 1975, Excerpta Medica, Associated Scientific Publishers.
29. Klaus M, Kennell J: *Parent-infant bonding*, St Louis, 1982, Mosby.
30. Lamb M: Early contact and maternal-infant bonding: one decade later, *Pediatrics* 70:763, 1982.
31. Lawrence RA: *Review of the surgeon general's workshop in breastfeeding and human lactation for the American public health association meetings*, San Diego, C.A., November 1984.
32. Lawrence RA: Practices and attitudes toward breast-feeding among medical professionals, *Pediatrics* 70:912, 1982.
33. Lawrence RA: Unpublished data, 1996.
34. Lerner H: Early origins of envy and devaluation of women: implications for sex role stereotypes, *Bull Menninger Clin* 38:538, 1974.
35. Li J, Kendall GE, Henderson S, et al: Maternal psychosocial well-being in pregnancy and breastfeeding duration, *Acta Paediatr* 97:221–225, 2008.
36. Losee JE, Serletti JM, Kreipe RE, et al: Reduction mammaplasty in patients with bulimia nervosa, *Ann Plast Surg* 39(5):443, 1997.
37. Maekawa K, Nara T, Hoash E: Influence of breastfeeding on neonatal behavior, *Acta Paediatr Jpn* 27:608, 1985.
38. McAdams D: *Power, intimacy, and the life story: personological inquiries into identity*, New York, 1988, Guilford.
39. McCarthy MM, Altemus M: Central nervous system actions of oxytocin and modulation of behavior in humans, *Mol Med Today*(June):269–275, 1997.
40. McKenna JJ, Thoman EB, Anders TF, et al: Infant-parent co-sleeping in an evolutionary perspective: implications for understanding infant sleep development and the sudden infant death syndrome, *Sleep* 16:263, 1993.
41. Modahl C, Newton N: Mood state differences between breast and bottle feeding mothers. In Carenza L, Zinchella L, editors: Emotion and reproduction, *Proc Serano Symp* 20B:819, 1979.
42. Montague A: *Touching*, New York, 1986, Harper & Row.
43. Newton N, Newton M: Psychological aspects of lactation, *N Engl J Med* 277:1179, 1967.
44. Newton N: Psychologic differences between breast and bottle feeding. In Jelliffe DB, Jelliffe EFR, editors: Symposium: the uniqueness of human milk., *Am J Clin Nutr* 24:993, 1971.

45. Pascoe JM, French J: The development of positive feelings in primiparous mothers toward their normal newborns: a descriptive study, *Am J Dis Child* 142:382, 1988 (abstract).

46. Passman RH, Halonen JS: A developmental survey of young children's attachments to inanimate objects, *J Genet Psychol* 134:165, 1979.

47. Petersen M: Breastfeeding ads delayed by a dispute over content, *N Y Times* (December 4), 2003, C1, C4.

48. Quandt SA: Patterns of variation in breastfeeding behaviors, *Soc Sci Med* 23:445, 1986.

49. Raphael D: *The tender gift: breastfeeding*, New York, 1976, Schocken.

50. Righard L, Alade MO: Effect of delivery room routines on success of first breast-feed, *Lancet* 336:1105, 1990.

51. Sosa R, Kennell JH, Klaus M: The effect of early mother-infant contact on breast feeding: infection and growth. In *Ciba foundation symposium, no. 45, breast feeding and the mother*, Amsterdam, 1976, Elsevier Scientific.

52. Spitz RA: An inquiry into the psychiatric conditions in early childhood, *Psychoanal Study Child* 1:53, 1945.

53. Stein A, Fairburn C: Children of mothers with bulimia nervosa, *Br Med J* 299:777, 1989.

53a. Strathearnl L, Mamun AA, Najim JM, et al: Does breastfeeding protect against substantiated child abuse and neglect? A 15-year Cohort Study, *Pediatrics* 123:483–493, 2009.

54. Taveras EM, Capra AM, Braveman PA, et al: Clinical support and psychosocial risk factors associated with breastfeeding discontinuation, *Pediatrics* 112:108–115, 2003.

55. Timmerman G: A concept analysis of intimacy, *Issues Ment Health Nurs* 12:19, 1991.

56. Uvnäs-Moberg K, Widstrom AM, Nissen E, et al: Personality traits in women 4 days postpartum and their correlation with plasma levels of oxytocin and prolactin, *J Psychosom Obstet Gynaecol* 11:261, 1990.

57. Van Esterik P: Breastfeeding and feminism, *Int J Gynaecol Obstet* 47(Suppl):S41, 1994.

58. Waletzky LR: Husband's problems with breast feeding, *Am J Orthopsychiatry* 49:349, 1979.

59. Whiting JWM: Causes and consequences of the amount of body contact between mother and infant. In Munroe RL, Munroe RD, Whiting BB, editors: *Handbook of cross-culture human development*, New York, 1980, Garland.

60. Yalom M: *A history of the breast*, New York, 1997, Knopf.

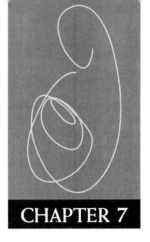

CHAPTER 7

Benefits of Breastfeeding for Infants/Making an Informed Decision

Breastfeeding is not a matter of choice, it is a public health matter, strongly stated the section on Breast-feeding of the American Academy of Pediatrics in its policy statement in 2012. The American College of Obstetrics and Gynecology (ACOG) has also signed on to this statement as has the American Academy of Family Practice (AAFP). "The discussion is over, human milk is for human infants" proclaimed Myers at the twenty-fifth Surgeon General's Workshop in 2009. The evidence is overwhelming. The Old Testament states firmly that women should breastfeed their children. The Koran also indisputably commanded mothers to breastfeed their infants until they were 2 years old. Christians had been conspicuously silent until 1995 when Pope John Paul II spoke out and proclaimed that the women of the world should breast-feed their children.

So why are we still discussing it? The evidence of the value of breastfeeding for both mother and child continues to mount. Along with the dozens of studies confirming what we already knew, there have been published challenging papers where the evidence is carefully culled to present a different picture. Studies analyzing the benefits have compared the "ever breastfed" to the formula-fed child. Ever breastfed includes any infant who went to breast only once. The most challenging problem is setting up a controlled study randomly assigning women to breastfeed or including controls that were not to breastfeed; such a study is neither ethical nor possible. Formula feeding has been called the largest experiment in life with no science to prove it is safe or efficacious. Formula is a necessary commodity only because not all women can or will breastfeed.

The evidence of the benefits of breastfeeding presented here is selected from the best of medical research. There has never been a study done that proves formula is better nor, in fact, even equal. Formula is adequate when human milk is not available.

Compelling Reasons to Breastfeed

SPECIES SPECIFICITY

Species specificity encompasses all the benefits of being breastfed for human infants because breast milk is more than just good nutrition. Human breast milk is specific for the needs of human infants, just as the milk of thousands of other mammalian species is specifically designed for their offspring. For optimal growth of brain and body, as well as protection against infection and development of immunity, human milk is specifically designed for all the needs of human infants.

NUTRITIONAL BENEFITS

Many benefits of breastfeeding are related to how children eat rather than what they eat as they get older. Breastfeeding eating is different from bottle-feeding, which depends on the maternal feeding style and her control of the process. The more frequently the infant bottle feeds (regardless of bottle

214

content) the more likely the mother focuses on giving the infant enough. Mother encourages finishing every drop. This continues with later feeding habits to clean the plate and take more. This behavior is often the basic problem with obesity. In breastfeeding, the infant takes what he wants, no more. Feeding at the breast is a satisfying experience so that additional suckling is rarely needed.

The unique composition of breast milk provides the ideal nutrients for human brain growth, especially in the first year of life. Cholesterol, docosahexaenoic acid (DHA), and taurine are particularly important. Cholesterol is part of the fat globule membrane and is present in approximately equal amounts in both cow milk and breast milk. Maternal dietary intake of cholesterol has no impact on breast milk's cholesterol content. Formula naturally lacks human DHA and taurine. The cholesterol in cow milk, however, has been removed in infant formulas, which are cholesterol-free. These elements—cholesterol, DHA, and taurine—are readily available from breast milk and are essential nutrients for human infants, especially for growth of the brain. Regardless of what additives are manufactured and added to bovine formula, they all have their origin from some other species and have been chemically extracted and subjected to extensive heat.

The maximum bioavailability of essential nutrients, including micro minerals, means that digestion and absorption are highly efficient. Comparison of the biochemical percentages of constituents of breast milk and infant formula fails to reflect the highly efficient bioavailability and utilization of constituents in breast milk compared with modified cow milk, from which only a small fraction of some nutrients is absorbed.

Nourishment with breast milk is a combination event, in which nutrient-to-nutrient interaction is significant. The process of mixing isolated single nutrients in formula does not guarantee the nutrient or nonnutrient benefits that result from breastfeeding. The composition of human milk is a delicate balance of macronutrients and micronutrients, each in the proper proportion to enhance absorption. Ligands bind to some micronutrients to enhance their absorption. Enzymes also contribute to the digestion and absorption of all nutrients. All enzymes and hormones have been destroyed by processing in infant formulas.

An excellent example of balance is the action of lactoferrin, which binds iron to make it unavailable for *Escherichia coli*, which depends on iron for growth. When the iron is bound, *E. coli* cannot flourish and the normal flora of the newborn gut, *Lactobacillus bifidus (Bifidobacterium bifidum)*, can thrive. In addition, the small amount of iron in human milk is almost totally absorbed, whereas only about 10%

of the iron in formula is absorbed by the infant. Nutrients such as proteins are examples of constituents in human milk with multiple functions, which include preventing infection and inflammation, promoting growth, transporting micro minerals, catalyzing reactions, and synthesizing nutrients.[93]

IMPACT ON CARDIOVASCULAR HEALTH

A study asking the question of whether perinatal supplementation of long-chain polyunsaturated fatty acids prevents hypertension in later life concluded that long-chain polyunsaturated fatty acids depended upon other nutrients as well. Thus it was concluded that breastfeeding the infant can protect against insulin resistance and hypertension in later life.[18] A meta-analysis by Martin et al.[58] involving 15 studies and 17,503 subjects revealed that a small reduction in diastolic blood pressure was associated with breastfeeding, which confers long-term benefits on cardiovascular health. Another study by Martin et al.[59] reported a reduced risk for atherosclerosis by breastfeeding as recorded in the 65-year follow-up of the Boyd Orr Cohort. The Boyd Orr Cohort is an historical cohort based on the Carnegie Survey diet and health in prewar Britain 1937 to 1939. This cohort involves 4999 participants of 1343 families in 16 centers in England and Scotland who participated in a 1-week diet survey when 0 to 19 years old between 1937 and 1939. The trace rate was 88 when they were sent follow-up surveys. In 2002, 2563 of the original cohort were alive and living in Britain. Controlling for numerous variables, socioeconomic status, smoking, and alcohol made little difference.[57] A prospective cohort study of 2512 men between 45 and 59 years of age were studied according to their infant feeding history. There was a positive association between breastfeeding and coronary heart disease mortality and incidence. There was no evidence of a duration-response effect. Breastfeeding was not associated with stature, blood pressure, insulin resistance, total cholesterol (TC), or fibrinogen. These data, however, only compared ever breastfed and bottle fed. Small studies of exclusively breastfed infants have shown breastfeeding impacts blood pressure. Large studies use all subjects if ever breastfed and the significance is muted. Studies of TC and low-density lipoprotein (LDL) cholesterol showed that levels were higher in infants while consuming breast milk which contains cholesterol. (Formula contains no cholesterol.) Levels in adult life are lower in breastfed infants suggesting that breastfeeding has long-term benefits for cardiovascular health.[74] Adult glucose tolerance tests showed lower 120 minute glucose levels in -individuals who had been breastfed.[79]

In this same Boyd Orr Cohort, Martin et al.[59] studied the impact of breastfeeding and social mobility after 60 years. Prevalence of breastfeeding varied from 45% to 86% by district but not with household income, number of siblings, birth order, or social class in childhood. Breastfeeding was associated with upward social mobility; the longer the duration, the greater the probability, an effect that was not explained by other factors. Childhood obesity and infant feeding has also been evaluated by systematic review of published studies on Medline since 1966.[74,35,36] In 28 studies involving 298,900 subjects providing odds ratios, breastfeeding was associated with a reduced risk for obesity compared to formula-fed infants. Even in six studies adjusted for parental obesity, maternal smoking, and social class the effect was reduced but present.

For decades, growth in infancy had been measured according to data collected on infants who were exclusively formula fed, until the publication of data in the 1990s on the growth curves of infants who were exclusively breastfed.[25] The physiologic growth curves of breastfed infants show a pattern similar to that of formula-fed infants at the 50th percentile, with significantly fewer breastfed infants in the 90th percentile. This is most evident in the examination of the Z-scores, which indicate that formula-fed infants are heavier compared with breastfed infants, meaning that more are obese.[25,24] The World Health Organization (WHO) constructed an international study involving seven countries, rich and poor, to record how children should grow.[101] All participants were exclusively breastfed and had good health. The growth curves from these observations are available worldwide and should replace old curves that demonstrate how children grow, the tall and the short, the fat and the thin, the sick and well. These old curves which included all children are mathematical averages of the good and bad. These growth issues are discussed more completely in Chapter 11.

A study of adolescents, assessing body composition including height, weight, skinfolds, and waist circumferences, showed an effect of being breastfed if "never breastfed" was compared to breastfed over 4 months in a European multicentered study. Breastfeeding for at least 1 year or more had a profound effect on the development of obesity in Hispanic toddlers. Breastfeeding in this group was associated with a reduced intake of sugar-sweetened beverages.[20,83]

INFECTION PROTECTION

Leukocytes, specific antibodies, and other antimicrobial factors protect breastfed infants against many common infections. Protection against gastrointestinal infections is well documented.[36] Protection against infections of the upper and lower respiratory system and the urinary tract is less recognized but equally well documented. These infections lead to more emergency room visits, hospitalizations, treatments with antibiotics, and health care costs for the infant who is not breastfed.[2]

The incidence of acute lower respiratory infections in infants has been evaluated in a number of studies examining the relationship between respiratory infections and breastfeeding or formula feeding in these infants.[77] These studies confirm that breastfed infants are less likely to be hospitalized for respiratory infection and, if hospitalized, are less seriously ill.[11] In a study of infant deaths from infectious disease in Brazil, the risk for death from diarrhea was 14 times more frequent in formula-fed infants, and the risk for death from respiratory illness was 4 times more frequent.

According to the report from the Agency for Health Research Quality (AHRQ) in 2007,[36] breastfeeding for 4 or more months is associated with a reduction in the risk for hospitalization secondary to lower respiratory tract disease.

The association of wheezing and allergy with infant feeding patterns has also shown a significant advantage to breastfeeding. In a report from a 7-year prospective study in South Wales, the advantage of breastfeeding persisted to age 7 years in nonatopic infants, and in at-risk infants who were breastfed the risk for wheezing was 50% lower (after accounting for employment status, passive smoking, and overcrowding).[10] Breastfeeding is thought to confer long-term protection against respiratory infection as well.

Upper and lower respiratory tract infections have been evaluated in case-control studies, cohort-based studies, and mortality studies in both clinic attended and hospitalized children in many countries of the developed world.[20,15,52] The results show clearly that breastfeeding has a protective effect, especially in the first 6 months of life. Acute respiratory infections (ARIs) were studied by Vereen et al. because they are a major cause of infant morbidity. Ever breastfed were compared with never breastfed in a cross-sectional analysis of viral severity in 629 mother-infant dyads. When the infant had ARI, breastfeeding was associated with a decreased risk of having lower versus upper respiratory tract infection. A randomized, controlled trial indicated that withholding cow milk and giving soy milk provided no such protective effect.[12] The incidence of acute otitis media in formula-fed infants is dramatically higher than in breastfed infants,[1,3] not only because of the protective constituents of human milk but also because of the process of suckling at the breast, which protects the inner ear. When an infant feeds by bottle, the eustachian tube does not close, and formula and secretions are regurgitated in the tubes. Child care exposure increases the risk for otitis media, and bottle-feeding amplifies this risk.[15,52] The longer the breastfeeding, the more prolonged the protection.[36]

IMMUNOLOGIC PROTECTION

In addition to the protection provided by breastfeeding against acute infections, epidemiologic studies have revealed a reduced incidence of childhood lymphoma,[21] both acute lymphocytic and acute myelogenous leukemia,[36,5,48] and type 1 insulin-dependent diabetes,[96] as well as type 2 diabetes and Crohn disease,[45] in infants who have been exclusively breastfed for at least 4 months, compared with formula-fed infants. In a systematic review and meta-analysis of breastfeeding and childhood cancer published in 49 references between 1966 and 2004, the authors report lower risks such as decreased incidence of acute lymphoblastic leukemia, Hodgkin's disease, and neuroblastoma. These findings were based on "ever breastfed," not inclusive breastfeeding for 6 months.[60] Within this cohort, a meta-analysis by Kwan et al.[49] strongly supported the impact of breastfeeding on limiting the risk of childhood leukemia. It demonstrated that longer breastfeeding reduced the risk.

ALLERGY PROPHYLAXIS

Breastfed infants at high risk for developing allergic symptoms such as eczema and asthma by 2 years of age show a reduced incidence and severity of symptoms in early life.[10] Some studies suggest the protective effect continues through childhood.[9,43] A significant reduction in risk for childhood asthma at age 6 years was reported by Oddy et al.[72] if exclusive breastfeeding is continued for at least 4 months. Available evidence regarding full-term infants in developed countries suggests that exclusive breastfeeding for at least 3 months is associated with a reduced risk for atopic dermatitis in children with a family history of atopy.[30]

Prolonged breastfeeding may improve subsequent lung function at 10 years old. Forced vital capacity, forced expiratory volume, and peak expiratory flow were measured in 1456 children who were part of the Isle of Wight Study; 196 were not breastfed, 243 were breastfed less than 2 months, 142 were breastfed more than 2 months but less than 4 months, and 374 were breastfed at least 4 months. Lung volume was enhanced in the breastfed children. The authors[4] speculate that the effect on airflow was mediated by lung volume changes, which could be the result of prolonged suckling at the breast, providing a mechanical stimulus to improve the mechanics of ventilation.[4]

PSYCHOLOGICAL AND COGNITIVE BENEFITS

The prevailing impression from large epidemiological studies is that being breastfed results in higher cognitive function and higher performance intellectually. Does breastfeeding alter early brain development? Morphometric brain imaging has supported this premise.[23] Increased white matter and subcortical gray matter volume and parietal lobe cortical thickness have been observed. When quiet magnetic resonance imaging (MRI) scans were used to compare measurements of white matter microstructure in 133 healthy children aged 10 months through 4 years who were exclusively breastfed a minimum of 3 months with those formula fed or fed a mixture, the breastfed children had increased white matter in frontal and associated brain regions. Other regions were anatomically consistent with improvements in cognitive and behavior performance measures. The developmental advantages associated with breastfeeding are supported by the hypothesis that breastfeeding promotes healthy neural growth and white matter development, according to investigators.[23]

Nielsen and O'Hara[71] noted that children who had been breastfed were more mature, secure, and assertive, and they progressed farther on the developmental scale than nonbreastfed children. More recently, studies by Lucas et al.[56] and other investigators[38] found that premature infants who received breast milk provided by tube feeding were more advanced developmentally at 18 months and at 7 to 8 years of age than those of comparable gestational age and birth weight children who had received formula by tube. Such observations suggest that breast milk has a significant impact on the growth of the central nervous system. This suggestion is further supported by studies of visual activity in premature infants who were fed breast milk compared with those who were fed infant formula. When similar studies were performed in full-term infants, visual acuity developed more rapidly in the breastfed infants.[40] Even when DHA was added to formula, the performance by breastfed infants was still better.[39]

An 18-year longitudinal study reported by Horwood and Fergusson[33] demonstrates a small but detectable increase in childhood cognitive and educational achievement in infants who were breastfed. The effects were confirmed in a range of measures, including standardized tests, teacher ratings, and academic outcomes in high school and young adulthood. More than 1000 children in New Zealand participated. Children who were breastfed for 8 months or longer had a mean test score at age 18 that was 0.11 to 0.30 standard deviation units higher than those not breastfed.

To examine the association between duration of infant breastfeeding and intelligence in young adult life, Mortensen et al.[68] conducted a prospective longitudinal cohort study of more than 3000 individuals in Denmark born between 1959 and 1961. They concluded that, independent of a wide range of possible confounding factors, a significant positive association between duration of breastfeeding and intelligence test results existed, using two separate intelligence tests.

In an effort to examine the minimum duration of exclusive breastfeeding for optimal neurologic outcome, Bouwstra et al.[6] assessed the quality of general movements at 3 months of 147 breastfeeding, healthy term infants. General movement quality is considered a sensitive marker of neurologic status according to the authors. They demonstrated a positive effect between breastfeeding duration and general movement quality with a saturation effect at about 6 weeks. They concluded that exclusive breastfeeding for at least 6 weeks might improve neurologic outcome.

Evidence-Based Systematic Reviews

In 2007, two careful, comprehensive assessments of the value of human milk and breastfeeding were published: one from the AHRQ,[36] the other from the Department of Child and Adolescent Health and Development of WHO. The AHRQ reviewed the evidence on the effects of short- and long-term breastfeeding on infants and maternal health outcomes in developed countries. More than 9000 abstracts were screened and 400 individual studies reviewed. The data supported a long list of advantages (Tables 7-1 and 7-2) but did not support the increase in cognitive performance. The relationship between breastfeeding and cardiovascular disease was unclear. Maternal risk reduction is noted in Table 7-3, and only weight loss and osteoporosis reduction was unclear from the studies. The authors did comment that breastfeeding did not mean exclusive breastfeeding.[36] The Irish Nursing Homes Organization (INHO) analysis also reflected a lack of clarity in terms of impact on intellectual performance, cardiovascular disease, and obesity.[61] When the analysis was complete, however, they were able to confirm that long-term subjects who were breastfeeding experienced lower mean blood pressure and TC and higher performance on intelligence tests. The prevalence of overweight and obesity and type 2 diabetes was lower among breastfeeding infants. Although all

TABLE 7-1	Advantages of Breastfeeding as Determined by AHRQ
Full-Term Infant Outcomes	**Reduction in Relative Risk**
Acute otitis media	50% reduction
Atopic dermatitis	Equivocal
Gastrointestinal infections	64% reduction
Lower respiratory tract disease	72% reduction
Asthma	27% reduction
Cognitive development	Equivocal because of confounding factors
Obesity	24%, 7%, 4% for each month of breastfeeding
Risk for cardiovascular disease	Blood pressure: up to 1.5 monthly reduction; LDL cholesterol: 7.0–7.7 mg/dL reduction; all-cause CV mortality: needs further investigation
Type 2 diabetes	39% reduction (confounders not well controlled)
Childhood leukemias	19% reduction (all); 15% (AML)
SIDS	36% reduction

AHRQ, Agency for Health Research Quality; *AML*, acute myelogenous leukemia *CV*, cardiovascular; *LDL*, low-density lipoprotein; *SIDS*, sudden infant death syndrome.
  Summarized from AHRQ report no. 153[35,36].

TABLE 7-2	Maternal Advantages of Breastfeeding as Determined by AHRQ
Mother Outcomes	**Reduction in Relative Risk**
Return to prepregnancy weight	Unclear
Maternal type 2 diabetes	2%-12%
Osteoporosis	Unclear
Postpartum depression	Too few studies
Breast cancer	28% for 12 or more months (4.3% for each year of breastfeeding)
Ovarian cancer	21%

Intensity and duration of breastfeeding were not defined in most studies, thus diluting the magnitude of the effects.[44]
  AHRQ, Agency for Health Research Quality.

were statistically significant some differences were modest. The definition of breastfeeding, exclusive or partial, and length of breastfeeding remain significant factors in measuring outcome.

Since these two meta-analyses were performed, several new studies have been published that further support advancement in intellectual skills.[51]

TABLE 7-3	Reduction of Risk for Disease	
Infant	Risk for acute otitis media	No evidence
	Nonspecific gastroenteritis	Cognitive performance
	Severe lower respiratory tract infection	Cardiovascular disease
	Atopic dermatitis	Infant mortality is developed
	Asthma	
	Obesity	
	Type 1 and 2 diabetes	
	Childhood leukemia	
	SIDS	
	Necrotizing enterocolitis	
Maternal	Risk for type 2 diabetes	No relationship
	Breast cancer	Osteoporosis
	Ovarian cancer	Return to prepregnancy weight
	Postpartum depression	Weight loss?

Breastfeeding for 3 months or longer was found to enhance language skills and motor skills in a cross-sectional study of 22,399 children with concerns about language decreasing the longer they were breastfeeding.[22]

Evidence from a large randomized trial examining breastfeeding and cognitive development in 17,046 healthy breastfeeding infants, 81.5% of whom were followed for 6.5 years, showed exclusive breastfeeding at 3 months of 43.3% in the experimental group and only 6.4% in the control group and a higher rate of breastfeeding at all ages through 12 months. This was part of the Promotion of Breastfeeding Intervention Trial (PROBIT) study group in Belarus.[46] The experimental group had higher mean scores in the Wechsler Abbreviated Scales of Intelligence, which measures both verbal and performance intelligence quotient (IQ). Teachers' academic ratings were significantly higher.

The authors considered it strong evidence that prolonged and exclusive breastfeeding improves children's cognitive development.[46]

Using the data from the National Longitudinal Study of Adolescent Health (26,000 schools in the United States) on sibling pairs, it was estimated that the effect of having been breastfed on high school graduation, high school GPA, and college attendance was significant. Cognitive ability and adolescent health seemed interrelated to breastfeeding.[82] A novel approach utilized in 2011 to improve the causal inference in observational studies compared high, middle, and low income cohorts. Breastfeeding was thought by these authors to have a causal relationship to intelligence. The causal effects of breastfeeding on IQ were determined in a systematic review that looked at the role of confounders. Walfisch concluded that the apparent effect on intelligence was due to confounding. Confounding was based on failure to control for parental IQ.

Although data on cognitive ability was impressive, it did not meet AHRQ scrutiny. Nevertheless, evidence continues to mount. The original studies[56,31] actually were done on premature infants, measuring visual activity and auditory acuity, both of which are electroencephalographic responses to standard stimuli. The reactions are unrelated to demographics such as intellectual scores or socioeconomic status of the parents. The value of receiving human milk was clearly demonstrated. A more accurate assumption is that breastfeeding allows a child to reach his/her full potential. It is clear that no study has ever suggested that artificial feedings contribute to good brain growth.

Does Breastfeeding Reduce the Risk for Sudden Infant Death Syndrome?

The policy statement for the American Academy of Pediatrics on Sudden Infant Death Syndrome (SIDS) released in 2011 again affirmed the value of supine sleeping for infants and recommends a pacifier for sleep time along with the list of cautions against soft surfaces, soft covers, and toys.[94] It is stated that co-sleeping is a major cause of SIDS. Concern has arisen about co-sleeping deaths occurring in hospitals in the first few days of life. Fifteen deaths and three near deaths were reported occurring between 1999 and 2013 as reported by members of the National Association of Medical Examiners. The problem is believed to be underreported. Associated circumstances were falling asleep while breastfeeding in eight cases, obesity, and swaddling, but all were bed sharing.[95] The committee states that breastfeeding infants are more easily aroused than formula-fed infants, a safety factor. They also state that some epidemiological studies have proven a relationship between breastfeeding and reduction of SIDS, but others have not. The committee acknowledged[16] the value of breastfeeding but did not recommend breastfeeding as a strategy to reduce SIDS.

The recommendation for pacifier use included a delay in beginning a pacifier in a breastfeeding infant until 1 month of age. It is also stated that if the pacifier falls out of the mouth during sleep that it not be reinserted. There is an increased incidence of plagiocephaly from positioning, and the increase in malocclusion and otitis media from pacifier use was acknowledged. A paper published in 2009 by Vennemann et al.[96] reported that the population-based, case-control study of 333 cases of SIDS and 998 matched controls from Germany showed breastfeeding reduced the risk for SIDS by 50% at all ages; 73% of infants died before 6 months of age.

In a letter to the editor in 2014, the Taskforce[94] states that the Taskforce supports the value of breastfeeding in preventing SIDS.

Benefits of Breastfeeding for Mother

Breastfeeding may provide a mother with a number of benefits, which should be included during discussions about making an informed decision regarding how to feed one's infant.

EMPOWERMENT

In addition to clinically proven medical benefits, breastfeeding empowers a woman to do something special for her infant. The relationship of a mother with her suckling infant is considered the strongest of human bonds. Holding an infant to the mother's breast to provide total nutrition and nurturing creates an even more profound and psychological experience than carrying the fetus in utero. These observations have been tested in animal experiments in which oxytocin and prolactin have triggered parenting behavior with nonpregnant subjects.

In studies of young women enrolled in the Women, Infants, and Children (WIC) program in Kentucky who were randomly assigned to breastfeed or not to breastfeed and who were provided with a counselor/support person throughout the first year postpartum, the women who breastfed changed their behavior.[32] They developed self-esteem and assertiveness, became more outgoing, and interacted more maturely with their infants than did the women assigned to artificial feeding. The women who breastfed turned their lives around by completing school, obtaining employment, and providing for their infants.

POSTPARTUM RECOVERY

Women who breastfeed return to a prepregnancy state more promptly than women who do not, and they have a lower incidence of obesity in later life (Box 7-1).[93,87] The presence of oxytocin stimulates the uterus to contract and involute with each feeding so that the uterus returns to the prepregnant state within 6 weeks. The extra pregnancy tissue storage is utilized in the production of milk, and the return to prepregnancy weight is thus facilitated.

> **BOX 7-1. Benefits of Breastfeeding**
>
> INFANT
> - Species specificity
> - Nutritional advantages
> - Infection protection
> - Immunologic protection
> - Allergy prophylaxis
> - Psychological benefits
>
> MOTHER
> - Postpartum recovery
> - Psychological benefits, empowerment
> - Improved health risks

DECREASED RISK FOR OSTEOPOROSIS

The risk for osteoporosis in later life is greatest for women who have never borne an infant, somewhat less for those who have borne infants, and measurably less for those who have borne and breastfed infants.[41–89] The bone mineral loss experienced during pregnancy and lactation is temporary. Bone mineral density returns to normal after pregnancy and even after extended lactation when mineral density may exceed the original baseline. Serum calcium and phosphorus concentrations are greater in lactating than in nonlactating women. Lactation stimulates the greatest increases in fractional calcium absorption and serum calcitriol after weaning.[42] Postweaning concentrations of parathyroid hormone are significantly higher than in other stages, and urinary calcium loss is significantly lower.[17] Studies reporting the history of fractures in postmenopausal women do not address exclusivity or duration of breastfeeding nor do they account for body mass index (BMI) or hormone replacement therapy.[36]

MATERNAL RISK FOR CARDIOVASCULAR DISEASE, HYPERLIPIDEMIA, AND DIABETES

The occurrence of cardiovascular disease in women has become an urgent consideration since heart attack and stroke have become more common in women. The correlation with breastfeeding and reduction of risk for cardiovascular disease has been reported for more than two decades.[86] The influence of initial infant feeding on cardiorespiratory risk factors in adults in 9377 persons born during 1 week in 1958 in England has been reported by Rudnicka et al.[85] Breastfeeding was described as never breastfeeding, partially or wholly for less than a month, or breastfeeding more than a month. Little impact was found except for reduced waist circumference, waist/hip ratio, and lower odds of obesity.[81] One month of some breastfeeding would hardly be expected to have a long-range impact.

On the other hand, a study from the Women's Health Initiative of over 139,000 women more than 63 years of age with at least one live birth concluded that increased duration of lactation was associated with a lower prevalence of hypertension, diabetes, hyperlipidemia, and cardiovascular disease in women who reported 12[44,91] or more months of lactation in their lifetime. In a study of 1262 women, it was demonstrated that for every 6 months of breastfeeding the risk of developing type II diabetes, was reduced further. It has been suggested that the role of body weight may reduce the effect.

PROTECTION AGAINST OVARIAN CANCER

A woman's increasing number of pregnancies, increasing length of oral contraceptive use, and increasing duration of lactation are generally agreed to be protective against ovarian cancer.[99] When the relationship between lactation and epithelial ovarian cancer was studied from a multinational database, short-term lactation was as effective as long-term lactation in decreasing the incidence of ovarian cancer in developed countries where ovulation suppression may be less prolonged in relation to lactation.[83] In a study of black women, who are known to have a lower incidence of ovarian cancer, breastfeeding for 6 months or longer, as well as four or more pregnancies and oral contraceptive use, further reduced the incidence of ovarian cancer.[37]

Siskind et al.[88] studied the modifying effect of menopausal status on the association between lactation and risk for ovarian cancer in 824 cancer patients and 855 community control subjects. No association was noted in women whose cancer occurred postmenopausally; however, breastfeeding was somewhat protective against ovarian cancer before menopause in this study. Breastfeeding of more than 12 months cumulative duration was associated with a reduction of the risk for ovarian cancer compared with never breastfeeding. Ovarian cancer was reported in the subgroups of pre- and postmenopausal women but had less robust evidence according to the AHRQ report.[36]

REDUCED INCIDENCE OF BREAST CANCER

A mother with a new diagnosis of breast cancer should not nurse her infant in the interest of having definitive treatment immediately because prolactin levels remain high during lactation, and the role of prolactin in the advancement of mammary cancer is still in dispute. Although endogenous prolactin by itself may not be a risk factor, it could, along with

sex steroids, contribute to the acceleration of malignant growth.[92] All lumps in the lactating breast are not cancer and are not even benign tumors. The lactating breast is lumpy, and the "lumps" shift day by day. If a mass is located and the physician thinks it should be biopsied, this can be done under local anesthesia without weaning the infant.

Surgeons have performed many such procedures after referrals in the past 40 years without postoperative complications. The diagnosis of a benign mass was made in most cases. Immediate surgery relieved tremendous anxiety without unnecessarily sacrificing breastfeeding. With noninvasive mammary imaging techniques such as ultrasound, computed tomography (CT) scanning, and MRI, careful diagnosis can be made without interfering with lactation and without delaying diagnosis.

Relationship to Breastfeeding

Is cancer more or less common in women who breastfeed? The answer is not easy to find, but in countries where breastfeeding is common, breast cancer is uncommon. In the United States, the incidence of breast cancer has steadily risen while the frequency of breastfeeding has declined. It has been suggested that nursing protects a woman against breast cancer. This concept has been investigated in many international studies.[26] Breastfeeding does not predispose a woman to cancer and may protect her.[29] How breastfeeding-induced mammary differentiation confers protective effects against breast cancer is not understood. Accessing the normal cellular hierarchy of the fully differentiated gland has been compared to the cellular hierarchy of breast cancer subtypes. Shared transcription factors of normal breast stem cells and certain aggressive breast tumors suggest that it is an imbalance of certain gene regulatory networks that causes this disease.

A case-controlled study of 453 white women with breast cancer and 1365 white women without breast cancer from upstate New York showed an inverse relationship between length of breastfeeding and incidence of breast cancer in premenopausal women that has not been seen in postmenopausal women.[10] The authors found this apparent protective effect persisted throughout the childbearing years, with statistical control for age, parity, age at first pregnancy, age of menarche, and education. The women with cancer had had a higher incidence of lactation failure caused by "insufficient milk." The authors[10] suggest that the significance of this study may be that women who are unsuccessful at lactation are at increased risk for cancer rather than that breastfeeding is protective.

The combination of low parity and late age at first birth was associated with a sevenfold increase in risk for breast cancer at ages 66 to 80 in a study by Lubin et al.[55] of more than 1400 women in Canada. At all ages, the authors found an increased cancer risk associated with relative infertility, benign breast disease, and not breastfeeding.

Marriage has been established as a negative risk factor for breast cancer. Mortality rates for most causes of death are higher among single women than among ever-married women.

The statistics associating pregnancy and breast cancer influence the picture. In an epidemiologic study, the risk for breast cancer had a linear relationship to the time interval between puberty and childbirth.[67,70] The risk was reduced by one third for women who bore their first child before 18 years of age compared with those women who had their first infant when they were older. The risk for breast cancer for women who become pregnant before 20 years old was about half that of those who first become pregnant after 25 years of age. Births after the first full-term pregnancy did not influence the statistics. Women whose first pregnancy appeared after 30 to 35 years of age had a risk for breast cancer four times that of nulliparous women in the same age group.[68,70]

The incidence of breast cancer is low among groups who nursed their infants, including lower economic groups, foreign-born groups, and those in sparsely populated areas.[68,70] The frequency of breast cancer in mothers and sisters of a woman with breast cancer is two to three times that expected by chance. This influence could be genetic or environmental. Since the isolation of the "breast cancer gene," women who are at risk are being identified. Cancer actually is equally common on both sides of the family of an affected woman. If breast milk were the cause, it should be transmitted from mother to daughter.[103] When mother-daughter incidence of cancer was studied, no relationship was found to breastfeeding. The association between breastfeeding and the incidence of breast cancer among 89,887 women in the U.S. Nurses Healthy Study was sought through an additional questionnaire. The authors[65] suggest that no important association exists between breastfeeding and the occurrence of breast cancer. Data gathered since 1996 have changed the conclusions about breastfeeding being protective.[36]

Unilateral breastfeeding (limited to the right breast) is a custom of Tanka women of the fishing villages of Hong Kong. Ing et al.[34] investigated the question, "Does the unsuckled breast have an altered risk for cancer?" They studied breast cancer data from 1958 to 1975. Breast cancer occurred equally in the left and the right breasts. Comparison of patients who had nursed unilaterally with nulliparous patients and patients who had borne children but had not breastfed indicated a highly significant increase in risk for cancer in the unsuckled breast. The authors conclude that in postmenopausal women who have breastfed unilaterally, the risk for cancer is significantly higher in the unsuckled breast.[63] They think that breastfeeding may help protect the suckled breast against cancer.[34]

Other authors[47] have suggested that Tanka women are ethnically a separate people and that it is possible that left-sided breast cancer is related to their genetic pool and not to their breastfeeding habits. No mention has been made of other possible influences; for instance, the impact of their role as "fishermen" or any inherent trauma to the left breast.[34]

As early as 1926, Lane-Claypon[50] stated that breasts that never lactated were more liable to become cancerous. Nulliparity and absence of breastfeeding had been considered important risk factors for breast cancer.

In a collective review of the etiologic factors in cancer of the breast in humans, Papaioannou concludes, "Genetic factors, viruses, hormones, psychogenic stress, diet and other possible factors, probably in that order of importance, contribute to some extent to the development of cancer of the breast."

Gradually, studies have appeared challenging the dogma. Brinton et al.,[8] McTiernan and Thomas,[64] and Layde et al.[54] showed the clearly protective effects of breastfeeding. Another example is a study conducted to clarify whether lactation has a protective role against breast cancer in Asian people, regardless of confounding effects of age at first pregnancy, parity, and closely related factors.[102] Similar results were reported by Zheng et al.[104] in a study in Shandong Province, China, in both pre- and postmenopausal women who had a reduced risk for breast cancer. The more months of breastfeeding, the lower the risk. In a hospital-based, case-control study of 521 women with breast cancer and 521 women without breast cancer, statistical adjustment for potential confounders and a likelihood ratio test for linear trend were done by unconditional logistic regression. Total months of lactation, regardless of parity, was the discriminator. Regardless of age at first pregnancy and parity, lactation had an independent protective effect against breast cancer in Japanese women.[102] Breastfeeding over 6 months, regardless of a family history of breast cancer, was protective in a large group of Spanish women whose records were reviewed retrospectively. The authors suggested that the recent increase in breast cancer paralleled the absence of breastfeeding. Although breast cancer incidence is influenced by genetics, stress, hormones, and pregnancy, in most reports, clearly breastfeeding has a protective effect.[69] A systematic review and meta-analysis do not support the theory that $BRCA_1$ and $BRCA_2$ mutation carriers are protected from cancer by breastfeeding.

Two large prospective studies[65,47] did not report a protective effect of breastfeeding. Populations of 50,274 and 89,887 identified 2130 and 459 patients with breast cancer. The odds ratios indicate 1.01 (0.98 to 1.05) and 0.95 (0.86 to 1.06), respectively. As with most studies of this nature, the cancers are well defined but not the breastfeeding. No attempt was made to note exclusivity and associated amenorrhea. The studies obtained breastfeeding histories when the women were older than 45 years old and included all those who ever breastfed. Insufficient milk supply has not been associated with increased risk of breast cancer when a large number of reports were reviewed by Cohen et al.[14]

The concern for exposure to estrogen early in life has been part of breast cancer assessment.[73] In utero exposure to estrogen is greater in twin pregnancies and when the mother is older. Estrogen levels in smokers, however, are lower. Weiss et al.[98] analyzed cancer risk in a population-based, case-control study in the United States (2202 with breast cancer and 2009 control subjects under 55 years of age). Twins were at greater risk than singletons, but no association with maternal age at delivery was found. A reduced breast cancer risk was seen among women who had themselves been breastfed as infants. Following Cochrane guidelines in performing a Medline search of papers from 1990 to 2002, a reduction of women's relative risk for breast cancer and a protective effect against ovarian cancer in women who breastfed their children was demonstrated. Results from meta-analyses in the AHRQ report concluded that there was a reduction in the risk for breast cancer in women who breastfeed their infants.[36] A lifetime breastfeeding history of more than 12 months was especially protective.

In an effort to understand the relationship between breastfeeding and breast cancer, Newton[70] points out that over the past two centuries, women have changed from being pregnant or lactating 60% of the time between menarche and menopause to fewer pregnancies and shorter lactation periods. Thus the amount of time a woman lives with unopposed estrogen (the proliferative phase of the menstrual cycle) was 15% in 1800 and 45% in 1996. Case-control epidemiologic studies consistently show a protective effect (Table 7-4). The most important predictors may be duration of the amenorrheal/hypoestrogenic state and the exposure to breast milk as an infant, according to Newton.[70] Breast cancer mortality is disproportionally high in black women of all ages. African-American women who do not breastfeed are at higher risk for aggressive breast cancer according to Palmer.[75] Women with children who never breastfed were more likely to develop estrogen receptor-negative breast tumors compared to those who never had children. Data from 3700 black breast cancer patients revealed the risk of not breastfeeding. A black mother who had four or more children but never breastfed was more likely to develop estrogen receptor-negative breast cancer compared to a woman with only one child whom she breastfed. According to Palmer,[75] breastfeeding represents a modifiable factor that could reduce the number of cases of estrogen-receptor negative breast cancer and reduce the number of African-American women dying from this disease.

Radiation Therapy to Breast

Ionizing radiation is carcinogenic to female mammary tissue. Women in Hiroshima and Nagasaki and those subjected to therapeutic radiation for mastitis were followed for many years.[87] The risk for cancer is 3.2 times greater in irradiated breasts, increasing with time after the irradiation. A linear relationship to radiation dose also exists.

TABLE 7-4	Breast Cancer and Lactation		
Study	**Population**	**Odds Ratio**	**95% Confidence Interval**
Likelihood of Breast Cancer			
Pillay et al.[76]	All	0.93	0.83-1.03
	BF >2 yr	1.11	0.90-1.38
Lawrence[53]	Premenopausal, BF >2 yr	0.53	0.23-1.41
Thach[95]	All	0.39	0.25-0.62
Byers et al.[10]	BF >2 wk	0.87	0.7-1.0
Yang et al.	Premenopausal, failed to BF	3.0	1.6-5.4
Yoo et al.[102]	All	0.62	0.37-1.04
	Premenopausal, BF >7 mo	0.39	0.15-0.97

BF, Breastfed.

From Newton ER Jr: Does breastfeeding protect women from breast cancer? *ABM News Views* 2:1, 1996.

In the late 1940s and early 1950s, radiation of the breast was performed as a treatment for mastitis. Although this approach seems irrational today, no antibiotics were readily available at that time, and women were hospitalized for mastitis. Sulfa drugs were not identified until the 1940s and penicillin shortly thereafter. The compounds were used only for life-threatening diseases. The effect of radiation on the infected breast was to clear the mastitis dramatically, stop lactation overnight, and seemingly solve the problem. The mother would continue to nurse on the other breast. The long-term follow-up of these women reveals a high incidence of cancer in the radiated breast.[87]

Radiation usually causes destruction to lobules, condensation of the cytoplasm in cells lining the ducts, and fibrosis. Successful lactation after radiation for carcinoma, however, has been reported in a 36-year-old woman with one previous pregnancy and lactation experience 6 years earlier.[19]

PROTECTIVE EFFECT OF BEING BREASTFED

Davis[20] first reported the reduction of childhood-onset cancers in children who have been exclusively breastfed for at least 4 months. The fear of cancer in the breastfed female offspring of a woman with breast cancer does not justify avoiding breastfeeding. Breastfed women have the same breast cancer experience as nonbreastfed women, and no increase occurs in benign tumors.[62] Daughters of women with breast cancer have an increased risk for developing benign and malignant tumors by merit of their heredity, not their breastfeeding history.[68,66] This is confirmed with the identification of a breast cancer gene.

The critical question remains: does being breastfed increase any child's risk for developing breast cancer, especially female offspring? This haunting question, first posed by an experimental scientist, created tremendous publicity and genuine concern among physicians queried by patients. The available data need to be explored.

No documented evidence indicates that women with breast cancer have ribonucleic acid (RNA) of a tumor virus in their milk. No correlation between cancer and RNA-directed deoxyribonucleic acid (DNA) polymerase activity has been found in women with a family history of breast cancer. RNA-directed DNA polymerase activity, a reverse transcriptase, is a normal feature of the lactating breast.[13–84]

PROTECTION AGAINST CHILD ABUSE AND NEGLECT

Many professionals in the field have commented that they had never seen a child who had been abused or neglected that had been breastfed by the mother. There were no studies and no evidence.

A cohort of 7223 Australian mother-infant pairs have been monitored prospectively for more than 15 years by Strathearn et al.[90] They analyzed the duration of breastfeeding with respect to child neglect, physical abuse, and emotional abuse in 6621 cases (91.7%) based on substantiated child protection agency records. The odds ratio for maternal maltreatment increased as breastfeeding duration decreased. The odds of maternal maltreatment in bottle-fed infants were 4.8 times greater than for children breastfeeding for 4 months or longer. With adjustment for possible confounding, the odds were still 2.6 times greater in mothers who bottle fed. Maternal neglect was especially common among nonbreastfeeding women. Biologically, considering the impact of oxytocin on the brain, the authors found the results understandable.

Contraindications to Breastfeeding

In reviewing the contraindications to breastfeeding, it is important to look at the entities that put the mother or infant at significant risk and are not remediable. Contraindications are medical; the disadvantages tend to be social. The physician needs to have a clear understanding of the benefits of breastfeeding to measure the risks for a particular mother-infant dyad. The risk/benefit ratio can be determined only by the clinician in a position to weigh all the data, usually the pediatrician for the infant or the obstetrician for the mother or the family physician.

INFECTIOUS DISEASES

In general, acute infectious diseases in the mother are not a contraindication to breastfeeding, if such diseases can be readily controlled and treated.[15] In most cases the mother develops the infection during breastfeeding. By the time the diagnosis has been made, the infant has already been exposed, and the best management is to continue breastfeeding so that the infant will receive the mother's antibodies and other host resistance factors in breast milk.[53] This is true for respiratory infections such as the common cold. Infections of the urinary tract or other specific closed systems, such as the reproductive tract or gastrointestinal tract, do not pose a risk for excreting the virus or bacteria in the breast milk unless generalized septicemia occurs. In certain situations, given the relative virulence and infectivity of the organism, such as with β-hemolytic streptococcus group A, both mother and infant should be treated, but breastfeeding is not contraindicated (Table 7-5).[15,52] When the offending organism is especially virulent

TABLE 7-5 Possible Medical Contraindications to Breastfeeding*

Problem	Breastfeeding acceptable	Conditions
Infectious diseases		
Acute infectious disease	Yes	Respiratory, reproductive, gastrointestinal infections
HIV	No	HIV positive in developed countries
Active tuberculosis	Yes	After mother has received 2 or more weeks of treatment
Hepatitis		
A	Yes	As soon as mother receives gamma globulin
B	Yes	After infant receives HBIG, first dose of hepatitis B vaccine should be given before hospital discharge
C	Yes	If no coinfections (e.g., HIV)
Venereal warts	Yes	
Herpesviruses		
Cytomegalovirus	Yes	
Herpes simplex	Yes	Except if lesion on breast
Varicella-zoster (chickenpox)	Yes	As soon as mother becomes noninfectious
Epstein-Barr	Yes	
Toxoplasmosis	Yes	
Mastitis	Yes	
Lyme disease	Yes	As soon as mother initiates treatment
HTLV-I	No	
Over-the-counter/prescription drugs and street drugs (see Chapter 12)		
Antimetabolites	Variable	Temporarily pump and discard
Radiopharmaceuticals		
Diagnostic dose	Yes	After radioactive compound has cleared mother's plasma
Therapeutic dose	No	
Drugs of abuse	No	Exceptions: cigarettes, alcohol
Other medications	Yes	Drug-by-drug assessment
Environmental contaminants		
Herbicides	Usually	Exposure unlikely (except workers heavily exposed to dioxins)
Pesticides		
DDT, DDE	Usually	Exposure unlikely
PCBs, PBBs	Usually	Levels in milk very low
Cyclodiene pesticides	Usually	Exposure unlikely
Heavy metals		
Lead	Yes	Unless maternal level ≥40 mcg/dL
Mercury	Yes	Unless mother symptomatic and levels measurable in breast milk
Cadmium	Usually	Exposure unlikely
Radionuclides	Yes	Risk greater to bottle-fed infants

DDE, Dichlorodiphenyldichloroethane; *DDT*, dichlorodiphenyltrichloroethane; *HBIG*, hepatitis B immune globulin; *HIV*, human immunodeficiency virus; *HTLV-1*, human T-cell leukemia virus type 1; *PBBs*, polybrominated biphenyls; *PCBs*, polychlorinated biphenyls.
*This table provides a brief summary. Each situation must be decided individually. Contraindications are rare.
Modified from Lawrence RA: A review of the medical benefits and contraindications to breastfeeding in the United States. In *Maternal and child health technical information bulletin*, Arlington, Va., 1997, National Center for Education in Maternal and Child Health.

or infection occurs through direct contact or respiratory droplets, separation of the infant and mother is indicated regardless of the mode of feeding (formula or breast milk). Examples of such infections include smallpox and tuberculosis. In these situations, giving the infant expressed breast milk without maternal contact is appropriate. A mother who bottle feeds also exposes her child by contact but provides no protective properties because they are not present in formula. See Chapter 13 for discussion of management of infectious diseases during lactation.

Many agents in breast milk protect against infection, and their presence is not affected by nutritional status. Protection against infection is important in the United States, especially among infants exposed to multiple caregivers, child care outside the home, compromised environments, and less attention to the spread of organisms.[32] One of the most important and thoroughly studied agents in breast milk is secretory immunoglobulin (sIg, specifically, sIgA), which is present in high concentrations in colostrum and early breast milk and in lower concentrations throughout lactation, when the volume of milk is increased.[32] sIgA antibodies may neutralize viruses, bacteria, or their toxins and are capable of activating the alternate complement pathway.[15] The normal flora of the intestinal tract of the breastfed infant, as well as the offspring of all other mammalian species studied until weaning, is bifidobacteria or lactobacilli.[32] These bacteria further inhibit the growth of bacterial pathogens by producing organic acids. This is in striking contrast to formula-fed infants, who have comparatively few bifidobacteria and many coliform bacteria and enterococci. In addition, although the attack rates of certain infections are similar in breastfed and formula-fed infants in the same community, the manifestations of the infections are much less evident in the infants who are breastfed. This appears to result from antiinflammatory agents in breast milk.[52]

For a few specific infectious diseases, the possible infectious risk for breastfeeding outweighs the benefits.[15,53,80] See the following section and refer to Chapter 13.

LIFE-THREATENING ILLNESSES

Life-threatening or debilitating illness in the mother may necessitate avoiding lactation. This clinical judgment should be made with the mother and father with all facts presented. Although one woman may be able to overcome all obstacles and prove she can nurse her baby, it does not necessarily mean that another patient with the same diagnosis can.[8,7] If a mother wants some lay reading on the subject, the clinician should be familiar with available material so any apparent inconsistencies of opinion can be discussed. (See management of specific maternal illnesses in Chapter 16.)

OVER-THE-COUNTER/PRESCRIPTION DRUGS AND STREET DRUGS

Medications

Much concern and anxiety have been expressed regarding the question of medications taken by lactating women and the risk to the suckling infant. In reality, very few drugs are contraindicated during breastfeeding.[53] Each situation should be evaluated on a case-by-case basis by the physician. The important factors include the pharmacokinetics of the drug in the maternal system and the absorption, metabolism, distribution, storage, and excretion in the recipient infant. Variables to consider in the decision include gestational age, chronologic age, body weight, breastfeeding pattern, and other dietary practices. Ultimately, the decision is made by assessing the risk/benefit ratio (i.e., the risk for a small amount of the drug compared with the tremendous benefit of being breastfed).

See Chapter 12 for a full discussion of drugs, medications, and environmental toxins. The contraindications are few but include radioactive medications, antimetabolites, and street drugs (see Table 7-5).

Drug Abuse

Breastfeeding is contraindicated in women who are IV drug abusers.[93] The possibility of the infant receiving substantial amounts of drug through the milk is real; deaths have been reported in the recipient neonate. IV drug abusers have high incidences of hepatitis, HTLV-I/II, or HIV, which may be transmitted to the breastfed infant from the infected mother (see Chapter 12).

Disadvantages of Breastfeeding

Because no known disadvantages exist for normal infants, the disadvantages of breastfeeding are those factors perceived by the mother as an inconvenience to her. (In the rare circumstance of galactosemia in the neonate, which involves an inability to tolerate lactose, breastfeeding is contraindicated; see Chapter 14.) In cultures in which nursing in public is commonplace, nursing is not considered inconvenient because the infant and the feeding are always available.

The mother's commitment to the infant for 6 to 12 feedings per day for months may be overwhelming to a woman who has been free and independent. Motherhood itself changes a woman's lifestyle.[12]

Guilt from failure, shame, and other anxieties are of considerable concern. Surveys evaluating the decline of breastfeeding have revealed that mothers describe feelings of shame, immodesty, embarrassment, and distaste. These feelings are more common in lower economic groups. Research on wider sociologic and psychological factors regarding the feelings and attitudes toward breastfeeding can have considerable influence on the choice to breastfeed and will be helpful in dealing with these issues.

Professionals and lay persons, under the banner of "supporting breastfeeding," occasionally get caught up in a rush to "convert" all mothers and parents to breastfeeding. Sometimes the push is to change many hospital routines and regulations to facilitate without assessing the full impact of those changes on all mothers and infants. A sense of balance should be maintained. It is important to appreciate that some normal women cannot or will not nurse their babies. Their babies will survive and grow normally. Each woman, infant, and family should be supported in their choice of infant feeding; it is their choice to make. The education and support should be specific for the particular needs of each mother-infant dyad.

The sharp letter by Fisher[28] brings this to focus when she describes the frustrations and disappointments of others and dispels what she calls the myths about breastfeeding. She expresses anger over her failure to successfully breastfeed her child. Her anger is an outward sign of inner guilt about this perceived failure.

The popular press has drawn attention to parenting trends that divide responsibility for the infant equally between mother and father after the birth. This, of course, necessitates some bottle feeding. The justification is division of labor and equal opportunity for both parents to serve the needs of the baby. This is probably another way of expressing breast envy and jealousy. Some husbands are jealous because they have no similar way to provide food and contentment to their infants, according to Waletzky.[97] "A certain manliness was required to foster breastfeeding in one's family when society as a whole was hostile to it," according to Pittenger and Pittenger.[78] They point out that the perinatal period is a breeding ground for marital and parental maladjustment. Shared responsibility does not mean that the father must feed his baby half the time. The father can take primary responsibility for another of the numerous needs, such as bathing or dressing the infant or nourishing the mother while she breastfeeds. Fathers can become "nonnutritive cuddlers" for infants, a very important role.

Many writers, however, have described participation in childbirth as a potentially beneficial experience for men. The father's feelings are useful during labor and delivery. These experiences contribute to heightened self-concepts and better adjustments to roles as husband and father. The quality of the birth experience has been cited as the major determinant of paternal attachment. Paternal attachment has led to greater pride in breastfeeding and a more secure, self-confident support person for the mother who is breastfeeding.

Perinatal counseling of prospective new parents may anticipate these reactions, and the professional will have an opportunity to facilitate the best experience possible.[12]

REFERENCES

1. Alho OP, Koivu M, Sorri M, et al: Risk factors for recurrent acute otitis media and respiratory infection in infancy, Int J Pediatr Otorhinolaryngol 19:151, 1990.
2. Ando Y, Matsumoto Y, Nakano S, et al: Long-term follow-up study of HTLV-I infection in bottle-fed children born to seropositive mothers, J Infect 46:9, 2003.
3. Aniansson G, Alm B, Andersson B, et al: A prospective cohort study on breastfeeding and otitis media in Swedish infants, Pediatr Infect Dis J 13:183, 1994.
4. Barclay L, Vega C, Scudder L, et al: Prolonged breastfeeding may improve subsequent lung function thorax 1, on line 10 November 2008 (first issue).
5. Bener A, Denic S, Galadari S: Longer breast-feeding and protection against childhood leukaemia and lymphomas, Eur J Cancer 37:234, 2001.
6. Bouwstra H, Boersma ER, Boehm G, et al: Exclusive breastfeeding of healthy term infants for at least 6 weeks improves neurological condition. Nutritional Neuro-sciences Research Communication, J Nutr 133:4243, 2003.
7. Brewster DP: You can breastfeed your baby, even in special situations, Emmaus, Pa., 1979, Rodale Press.
8. Brinton LA, Potischman NA, Swanson CA, et al: Breastfeeding and breast cancer risk, Cancer Causes Control 6:199, 1995.
9. Burr ML, Limb ES, Maguire MJ, et al: Infant feeding, wheezing, and allergy: a prospective study, Arch Dis Child 68:724, 1993.
10. Byers T, Graham S, Rzepka T, et al: Lactation and breast cancer, Am J Epidemiol 121:664, 1985.
11. Chantry CJ, Howard CR, Auinger P: Breastfeeding fully for 6 months vs. 4 months decreases risk of respiratory tract infection, ABM News Views 9:29, 2003.
12. Chaudron LH, Klein MH, Remington P, et al: Predictors prodromes and incidence of postpartum depression, J Psychosom Obstet Gynaecol 22(2):103–112, 2001.
13. Chopra H, Ebert P, Woodside N, et al: Electron microscopic detection of simian-type virus particles in human milk, Nat New Biol 243:159, 1973.
14. Cohen JM, Hutcheon JA, Julien SG, et al: Insufficient milk supply and breast cancer risk: a systematic review, PLoS ONE 4(12):e8237, 2009.
15. Committee on Infectious Diseases: American Academy of Pediatrics: report of the committee on infectious diseases, ed 6, Elk Grove Village, Ill., 2003, American Academy of Pediatrics.
16. Common sudden infant death. American Academy of Pediatrics: policy statement sudden infant death, Pediatrics 116, 2005.
17. Cross NA, Hillman LS, Allen SH, et al: Calcium homeostasis and bone postweaning: a longitudinal study, Am J Clin Nutr 61:514, 1995.
18. Das UN: Can perinatal supplementation of long-chain polyunsaturated fatty acids prevent hypertension in adult life? Hypertension 38:e6–e8, 2001.
19. David FC: Lactation following primary radiation therapy for carcinoma of the breast, Int J Radiat Oncol Biol Phys 11:1425, 1985.
20. Davis MK: Review of the evidence for an association between infant feeding and childhood cancer, International Union Against Cancer (UICC, WHO) workshop: nutritional morbidity in children with cancer—mechanisms, measures and management, Int J Cancer 11 (Suppl):29, 1998.
21. De Martino M, Tovo PA, Tozzi AE, et al: HIV-1 transmission through breast-milk: appraisal of risk according to duration of feeding, AIDS 6:991, 1992.
22. Dee DL, Li R, Lee L-C, et al: Associations between breastfeeding practices and young children's language and motor development, Pediatrics 119:S92–S98, 2007.
23. Deoni SCL, Dean DC III, Piryatinsky I, et al: Breastfeeding and early white matter development: a cross-sectional study, Neuroimage 82:77–86, 2013.

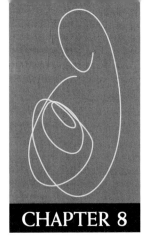

CHAPTER 8

Practical Management of the Mother-Infant Nursing Couple

Management of lactation begins with understanding the physiologic process of suckling and the physiologic process involved in latching on to the breast. For thousands of years, women fed their young by breastfeeding. They learned the art from senior women in the family. It was not a medical issue. The social structure of the family has changed, and the natural learning pathways are gone. The physician now has a critical role in the management of human lactation.

Successful nursing depends on the successful interaction of mother and infant, with appropriate support from the father, the family, and available health care resources. Because mothers and infants vary, no simple set of rules in hospitals can be outlined to guarantee success. In fact, one of the difficulties has been that rigid systems were established for initiating lactation in hospitals that did not fit all mother-infant couples. Many physicians have not received formal education about breastfeeding; thus they resort to gaining information from a variety of sources, including personal experiences, and may assume that this is the correct way to approach the situation.

Nowhere in medicine do one's personal interests or prejudices become more evident than in the area of counseling about childbirth and breastfeeding. Having a child does not make one an expert on the subject. Conversely, not having a child does not preclude the development of exceptional knowledge. Some of the world's most revered experts in human lactation have neither had a child nor nursed an infant, but they have brought to the situation the eye of a skilled observer and the experience of a broadly trained clinician, unencumbered by emotional bias and personal prejudices.

Historically, rigid dogmas have directed management of lactation. In the effort to replace these with what was perceived as more rational management, new dogmas have arisen. Once there was a paucity of literature; now there is a deluge from all sources, some valid, others questionable. The careful art and science of breastfeeding are being lost in the rage of righteousness. No rules exist for breastfeeding. As in all other areas of medicine, a clinician adapts the recommendations to individual patients and their circumstances.[151]

It is not ordinarily a physician's role to teach a mother how to breastfeed. Instead, nursing staff who interact in the perinatal period, including obstetric office nursing, labor/delivery, nursery, postpartum, birth center, pediatric office personnel, and midwives, have job descriptions that include hands-on assistance for a mother in the process of breastfeeding. A physician does, however, need to understand the anatomy and physiology and the basics of breastfeeding to recognize problems and determine their solutions (Table 8-1). This chapter addresses the basic breastfeeding process. It is not a "how-to" manual for mothers, but the physician should be familiar with one or two good sources of information to suggest for patients, such as K. Huggins' *The Nursing Mother's Companion*, now in its 6th edition after 25 years of inspiring mothers to breastfeed. *The Womanly Art of Breastfeeding* from La Leche League International is also available.

The references for this chapter are not an exhaustive list of all material written on the topic; rather, they are intended to assist a reader in locating research that supports the evidence-based concepts described here.[108,126]

TABLE 8-1	Common Breastfeeding Conditions and Symptoms and Their Connection with Breast Anatomy	
Clinical Condition	**Symptoms**	**Anatomic Relationship**
Glandular anomaly		
Hypoplasia	Low milk production	Possible deficiency of glandular tissue
Hyperplasia	Excessive breast growth, lymphedema, possible necrosis	Excess glandular tissue
Breast surgery		
Reduction mammoplasty	Low milk production	Large volume of glandular tissue removed, severing milk ducts (fewer in number than previously thought); possible nerve damage inhibiting milk ejection reflex
Breast augmentation	Low milk production	Possible compression of milk ducts by implant; possible deficiency in volume of glandular tissue
Palpable mass		
Blocked duct	Mass (small or large) with or without pain; possible reduction in milk production	Compression of ducts: possible cause of blocked duct; if large lobe affected a significant reduction in milk production may occur; identification of the level of duct obstruction by ultrasound ensures treatment of entire affected area
Galactocele	Mass (generally small)	Possible ductal abnormality
Benign mass (cyst, fibroadenoma)	Mass	Possible compression of ducts causing blocked duct; possible obstruction of milk flow in the area of attachment of the infant to the breast
Malignant mass	Palpable nonresolving mass	Irregularly shaped mass that may be mistaken for a blocked duct or galactocele; ultrasound with or without mammography needed for diagnosis
Infant sucking mechanism	Ineffective suck	Lack of milk sinuses and evidence that vacuum plays a major role in milk removal may alter intervention
Milk expression	Differences in efficiency of pumping	Theorized that women with large milk ducts or duct dilations at milk ejection express milk quickly
	Differences in effectiveness of pumping	Poor shield fit may result in compression of superficial ducts and inhibit milk flow
Milk ejection	Time of increased milk availability	Small ducts lacking lactiferous sinuses do not store a large amount of milk; optimization of milk removal during milk ejection will improve milk removal from the breast

From Geddes DT: Inside the lactating breast: the latest anatomy research, *J Midwifery Women's Health* 52(6), November/December 2007.

Infant feeding and care practices were assessed by the Department of Health and Human Services and published as a supplement to *Pediatrics* in 2008. It documents various aspects of infant feeding, as reported by more than 2000 women nationally for 1 year postpartum in 2004 and compares results with a similar study in 1993. This report serves as a reality check for many routines held dear.[36]

The home access to e-technologies was evaluated by Laborde et al.[69] in France. They noted that women with available technologies were more apt to be employed, did not use pacifiers, and did not smoke. Duration of breastfeeding was not different overall, suggesting that technology has not replaced good health resources and support systems yet.[28]

The key to the management of the mother-infant nursing couple is establishing a sense of confidence in the mother and supporting her with simple answers to her questions when they arise. Good counseling also depends on understanding the science of lactation. Then, when a problem arises, a mechanism already is in place for a mother to receive help from her physician's office before the problem creates a serious medical complication.

Peripartum Breastfeeding Management

All pregnant women should receive education about the benefits and management of breastfeeding to provide an opportunity to make an informed decision. The obstetrician with prenatal consultation should make an assessment of the potential for successful breastfeeding if a problem is identified. Labor and delivery with the presence of a doula has been shown to enhance breastfeeding. Mode of delivery and use of anesthesia and medications also impact breastfeeding. Provision for breastfeeding within the first hour of life and the availability of rooming-in are also essential. The Academy of Breastfeeding Medicine (ABM) provides a helpful protocol for successful peripartum management.

A model of breastfeeding policy is also provided by the ABM, which is designed so that hospitals can incorporate it into their own policies.[101] It meets requirements for the Baby Friendly Hospital Initiative.

The Science of Suckling

The ability to lactate is characteristic of all mammals, from the most primitive to the most advanced. The divergence of suckling patterns, however, makes it urgent that human patterns be studied specifically. Some aquatic mammals, such as whales, nurse under water; others, such as the seal and sea lion, nurse on land. A variety of erect or recumbent postures are assumed by different terrestrial mammals.[24] Nursing may be continuous, as in the joey attached to a marsupial teat, or at widely different intervals characteristic of the species and parallel to the nutrient concentrations of the milk. The intervals may be a half hour for dolphins, an hour for pigs, a day for rabbits, 2 days for tree shrews, or a week for northern fur seals.

New anatomy research gathered for the first time in 160 years since the brilliant work of Sir Ashley Cooper has been generated in the laboratory of Peter Hartmann in Australia and his eclectic team of scientists. They have had access to the latest digital technology. They have shown that the milk ducts of the breast are small (Figure 8-1), compressible, superficial, and closely intertwined.[40] There are no "dilated sinuses" that store large amounts of milk. The amount of adipose tissue in the breast is very variable and not a measure of the amount of glandular tissue; there is twice as much glandular tissue as fat.[32] Magnetic resonance imaging has identified some central ducts in the breasts of lactating women. The anatomy of the lactating breast was redefined with ultrasound imaging in Hartmann's laboratory.[103] Ducts were found to number four to eight, and branches drain glandular tissue directly beneath the nipple and merge into a collecting duct very close to the nipple. They do increase in diameter during milk ejection. Milk production is not dependent on neural stimulation but is hormonal. Milk ejection is critical to successful lactation. Failure to remove milk results in

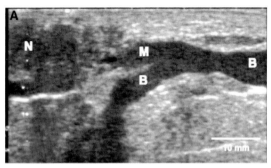

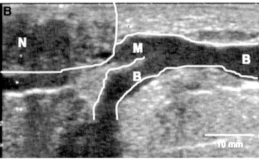

Figure 8-1A and **B.** Ultrasound image of a main milk duct (Toshiba, Aplio). The nipple is the round hypoechoic *(dark)* structure in the left of the image (N). The main duct (M) branches into two ducts (B) approximately 5 mm from the nipple. Note the small diameter of the ducts (approximately 3 mm). (From Geddes DT: Inside the lactating breast: the latest anatomy research. *J Midwifery Women's Health* 52(6), November/December 2007, Figure 3.)

decreased milk production. Multiple milk ejections occur during breastfeeding, even though a women usually only senses the first milk ejection.

Although many anatomic distinctions exist as well, the principal mechanism of milk removal common to all mammals is the contractile response of the mammary myoepithelium under the hormonal influence of oxytocin released from the neurohypophysis.[145]

The key function in all species is effective control of milk delivery to the young in the right amount and at the appropriate intervals, which requires a production system, exit channels, a prehensile appendage, an expulsion mechanism, and a retention mechanism. The primary, secondary, and tertiary ducts form an uninterrupted channel for the passage of milk from the milk-producing alveoli to the prehensile appendage. A process of erection of the areolar region facilitates prehension by the young during suckling. The principal object of the suction produced by the facial musculature of the young is to draw the nipple into the mouth and retain it there. Positive pressure is used to expel milk from the gland by the contractile changes in the mammary gland provided by the myoepithelial cells (see Figure 3-15). The sympathetic nervous stimuli can oppose milk ejection by increasing vasoconstrictor tone, thereby reducing access of circulating oxytocin to the mammary myoepithelium. Sympathetic activity also can occur during conditions of apprehension or muscular exertion. The milk-ejection reflex can be blocked by emotional disturbance or reflex excitation of the neurohypophysis. The central nervous system control of milk ejection indeed suggests that restraining mechanisms exist to ensure that milk ejection can only occur under circumstances wholly conducive to the effective removal of milk by the suckling young.

In all species that have been studied, a rise in intramammary pressure and flow of milk occurs as a reflex event in suckling. The excitation of the neurohypophysis results in the release of oxytocin, which is conveyed via the bloodstream to mammary capillaries, where it evokes contraction of the myoepithelium. The successive ejection pressure peaks, demonstrated in lactating women, can be duplicated more accurately by a series of separate oxytocin injections than by the same total dose as a single injection or by a continuous infusion of the hormone. This strongly suggests that oxytocin is released from the neurohypophysis in spurts. The study of suckling patterns in all species shows a high degree of ritualization, which in turn suggests a close neural connection between cognitive or behavioral and hormonal responses.

Attention has focused on the mechanisms that control suckling behavior, on its incidence, on events that precipitate and terminate it, on the effects of stress, and on how development modifies it. Suckling is characteristic of each species and is vital for survival. *Suckling* means to take nourishment at the breast and specifically refers to "breastfeeding" in all species. *Sucking*, however, means to draw into the mouth by means of a partial vacuum, which is the process employed when bottle feeding. *Sucking* also means to consume by licking.

Although suckling has been studied in young and mothers in other species, a large portion of human data have been collected using a rubber nipple and bottle. Other mammals suckle only in the nutritive mode, whether receiving milk from the nipple or not. Human infants were noted to have two distinct patterns with rubber nipples: a nutritive mode and a nonnutritive mode.[145,146] When this work was repeated using the breastfeeding model, no difference between nutritive and nonnutritive suckling rates, but rather a continuous variation of suckling rate in response to milk-flow rate, has been seen.[15] Suckling rates in other species correlate with milk composition and species-specific feeding schedules (one suck per second in great apes and four to five sucks per second in sheep and goats).

In further experiments, an inverse linear relationship was found between milk flow and suckling rate. Thus the higher the milk flow, the lower the suckling rate. In human infants younger than 12 weeks of age, suckling will terminate with sleep and be reinstated on awakening, a pattern that is well described in other species. In infants older than 12 weeks, suckling is not always terminated by sleep. At 12 to 24 weeks, infants will play with the nipple, explore the mother, and not always elicit nipple attachment. Continuous measurement of milk intake during a given feeding from one breast showed a progressive reduction in intake volume per suck and an increase in the proportion of time spent pausing between bursts of sucking.

Using the miniature Doppler[147] ultrasound flow transducer, Woolridge and Baum[148] studied 32 normal mother-baby pairs from 5 to 9 days postpartum. Intakes during trials averaged 34.2 g (± 3.7 g) on the first breast and 26.2 g (± 3.5 g) on the second breast. At the start of feeds, the average suck volume was about 0.14 mL/suck, which decreased to about 0.10 mL/suck or less. The mean latency for release of milk was 2.2 minutes after the infant began to suckle. The researchers also noted that on the first breast the flow increased and stabilized after 2 minutes, with concomitant slowing and stabilizing of sucking pattern during the remainder of the feed. On the second breast the suck volume fell off dramatically toward the end of the feed (50% reduction from peak to end of feed) (Figure 8-2).

These observations support the theory that infants become satiated at the breast, and milk remains unconsumed in the breast. During the first month of life, infants consume a given amount of fluid with decreasing investment of time.[148] The amount of fluid per suck increases over time. The control of intake appears to come under intrinsic control of the infant during the first month of life.[98]

A cineradiographic study of breastfeeding was done by Ardran et al.[7] in 1957 and compared with a similar study of bottle feeding.[8] The nipples and areolae of 41 breastfeeding mothers were coated with a paste of barium sulfate in lanolin, and cineradiographic films were taken with the infant at breast. These were then reviewed meticulously. Box 8-1 lists the authors' conclusions in their original description. These observations are of historic interest, but newer techniques in imagery have more accurately described the understanding of human suckling.

The development of real-time ultrasound improved the definition of images. Several studies have been published using this noninvasive technique to observe the action of the infant's tongue and buccal mucosa and the maternal nipple areola. Using a video recorder in the 1980s that allowed frame-by-frame analysis and recorded simultaneous respiration, the pattern of suck, swallow, and

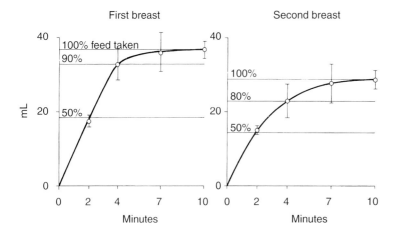

Figure 8-2. Mother-infant pattern of milk flow. (From Lucas A, Lucas PJ, Baum JD: Pattern of milk flow in breast-fed infants, *Lancet* 2:57, 1979.)

breathing was documented during a period of active suckling at the breast. A suck was defined by Weber et al.[137] as the beginning of one indentation of the nipple by the tongue to the beginning of the next. Weber et al. had examined six breastfed and six bottle-fed infants between 1 and 6 days of life. Not all sucks were associated with a swallow. Box 8-2 summarizes the process.

Observations of suckling using improved techniques from 2 to 26 weeks showed that suckling starts with a series of fast sucking movements and then stabilizes. In a 2-week-old breastfeeding infant, sucking and breathing pattern proportions alternated smoothly at about two sucks to one breath, with swallowing occurring with every suck. Bottle feeding patterns were variable and sometimes asynchronous with sucking and breathing.

BOX 8-1. Radiographic Interpretation of Suckling at Breasts

1. The nipple is sucked to the back of the baby's mouth, and a teat is formed from the nipple and the adjacent areola and underlying tissues.
2. When the jaw is raised, this teat is compressed between the upper gum and the tip of the tongue resting on the lower gum. The tongue is applied to the lower surface of the teat from the front backward, pressing it against the hard palate; the teat is reduced to approximately half its former width. As the tongue moves toward the posterior edge of the hard palate, the teat shortens and becomes thicker.
3. When the jaw is lowered, the teat is again sucked to the back of the mouth and restored to its previous size.
4. Each cycle of jaw and tongue movement takes place in approximately 1.5 seconds. The pharyngeal cavity becomes airless and the larynx closes every time the upward movement of the tongue against the teat and hard palate is completed.

BOX 8-2. Ultrasound Interpretation of Suckling at Breasts

1. The lateral margins of the tongue cup around the nipple, creating a central trough.
2. The suck is initiated by the tip of the tongue against the nipple followed by pressure from the lower gum.
3. There is peristaltic action of the tongue toward the back of the mouth.
4. The tongue elevation continues to move the bolus of milk into the pharynx.

The process of suckling has been described as a pulsating process similar to peristalsis along the rest of the gastrointestinal (GI) tract. This undulating motion, as described by cineradiography, did not involve stroking or friction, as was clearly pointed out by Woolridge.[147] The nipple should not move in and out of the infant's mouth if the breast is positioned correctly. The tip of the tongue does not move along the nipple. The positive pressure of the tongue against the teat (areola and nipple), coupled with ejection of the milk from increased intraductal pressure, evacuates the milk, not suction. The negative pressure created in the mouth holds the nipple and breast in place and reduces the "work" to refill the ducts. Visual observations and videotapes made in our laboratory to study suckling show the undulating motion of the external buccal surfaces even in newborns. Ultrasound confirms the molding of buccal mucosa and tongue around the teat, leaving no space.

In breastfeeding the tongue action is a "rolling," or peristaltic, action from the tip of the tongue to the base, not side to side. In bottle feeding the tongue action is more piston like or squeezing. When the infant rests between sucks, the human nipple is indented by the tongue, and the latex teat is expanded in bottle feeding (Figures 8-3 and 8-4).

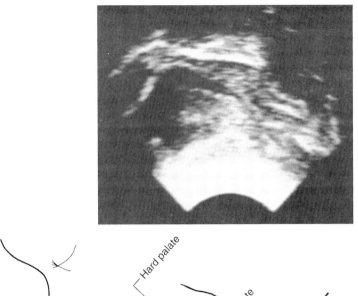

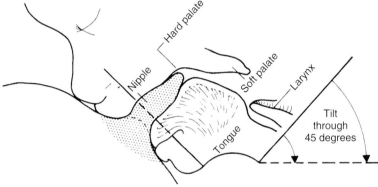

Figure 8-3. Ultrasound of infant at breast. Still picture of ultrasound scan frame from video recording. Scanner head is at bottom, with a sector view of 90 degrees. Below is an artist's impression of image showing key features. Image is seen best when tilted through 45 degrees so that the infant's head is vertical. Picture corresponds to point in sucking cycle when maximum point of compression of nipple by tongue has almost reached tip of nipple. Once nipple has become fully expanded, fresh cycle of compression will be initiated at base of nipple and will then move back. (From Weber F, Woolridge MW, Baum JD: An ultrasonographic study of the organization of sucking and swallowing by newborn infants, *Dev Med Child Neurol* 28:19, 1986.)

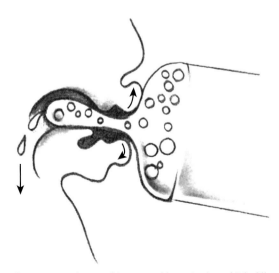

Figure 8-4. Infant sucking on rubber nipple, which fills mouth and thus prevents tongue action and provides flow without tongue movement. Flow occurs even if lips are not tight around rubber hub.

The change in nipple dimensions during suckling is detailed by Smith et al.,[123] who also used ultrasound and examined 16 term infants ages 60 to 120 days and their mothers. They demonstrated that human nipples are highly elastic and elongate during active feeding, including approximately 2 cm of areola, to form a teat approximately twice its resting length. They also showed that infants' cheeks (buccal membranes), with their thick layer of fatty tissue, known as sucking fat pads, act to make a passive seal to create a vacuum (as opposed to the concept that the cheeks are sucked in by the negative pressure). Milk ejection was noted to occur after maximal compression of the nipple.

COORDINATION OF SUCK AND SWALLOW

The ability to swallow is developed in utero during the second trimester and has been well demonstrated by fetal ultrasound. Fetal swallowing of amniotic fluid is an important part of the complex regulation of amniotic fluid. The suck is actually part of the oral phase of the swallow. Little was done to examine the role of swallowing on the suckling rate until Burke[17] studied the role of swallowing in the organization of suckling behavior, although with a bottle and solutions of 5% and 10% sucrose solution. The author reported two major observations: "First, the frequency of swallowing in newborns increased significantly as a function of increasing concentration and amount of sucrose solution given per criterion suck. Second, there was a significant difference in the duration of the sucking interresponse times that immediately followed the onset of swallowing and the duration of interresponse times not associated with swallowing." These observations explain those of previous investigators regarding nutritive and nonnutritive sucking.

The coordination of sucking and swallowing was observed by ultrasound by Weber et al.[137] as a movement of the larynx. By 4 days of age, both breastfed and bottle-fed infants were swallowing with every suck. Later in the feeding the ratio of sucks to swallows changed to 2:1 or more until sucking stopped. Swallowing occurred in the end-expiratory pause between expiration and inspiration (see Figure 8-3). The change in suck/swallow ratio seemed to be a function of the availability of milk.

FACTORS THAT INFLUENCE SUCKLING

As one manages infants with difficulty feeding, a number of rituals are often initiated to enhance infant behavior. Only a few of these have been evaluated for their effect.[95] The effect of the infant's position, that is, supine or supported upright to a 90-degree angle, was found to have no influence on the sucking pattern or pressure. The effect of temperature, however, was found to be significant. Sucking pressure decreased as environmental temperature increased from 80°F to 90°F (26.6°C to 32.2°C), which may have application in encouraging an infant to nurse. This effect was shown to increase from the third to the fifth day of life. Higher sucking pressures have been recorded in the morning than in the afternoon.

When the size of latex nipples was studied, the large nipple elicited fewer sucks and a slower sucking rate than smaller nipples, although the volume of milk delivered was the same, in this study, with all nipple sizes. Although human nipple size cannot be altered, this knowledge may help in assessing the response of a newborn in specific situations. Increasing nipple size and decreasing sucking rate may be significant in considering using an adult finger for finger feeding.

The volume of each swallow was calculated during breastfeeding in 1905 by Süsswein,[127] who counted swallows and made test weighings. His observations were later confirmed with elaborate electronic equipment.[148] The average swallow of a newborn is 0.6 mL, which is also the exact amount drawn from a bottle equipped with an electromagnetic flowmeter transducer and a valve that responds to negative pressure at each suck in modern studies, even though the sucking mechanism between breast and bottle is different.[118] The size of the hole in the nipple influences the volume of the suck only in the valved bottle. When breastfed infants were compared with a group fed by cup from birth and a group fed by bottle, the breastfed infants had a stronger suck than either of the other two groups, who did not differ from each other in sucking skill.[24,26]

Patterns of milk intake using electronic weighings in interrupted feeds were studied. Fifty percent of a feed from each breast was consumed in 2 minutes and 80% to 90% by 4 minutes, with minimal feeding from each breast in the last 5 minutes. Bottle-fed infants, evaluated with the same technique of test weighings, took 84% of the feeding in the first 4 minutes. Bottle feeding patterns were linear, whereas the breastfed infant had a biphasic pattern when nursed on both breasts. The total intake of the two types of feeds was similar in volume in the same 25 minutes of total time.

FAT CONTENT AND SUCKLING

The high concentration of fat in breast milk toward the end of a feed was hypothesized as a satiety signal to terminate the feeding. When this was studied using high- and low-fat formulas, it was found that high-fat milk did not act to cue babies to slow or stop feeding.[92] In fact, babies appeared to feed more actively on high-fat milk, sucking in longer bursts with less resting. When human milk of low- and high-fat content was fed from bottles, switching the baby from low-fat breast milk to high-fat breast milk, the babies did not alter either milk intake rate or sucking patterns.

To test the hypothesis fully, a study carefully observed infants switching from the first to the second breast and back to the first breast. Infants were 2 months old and well established at exclusive breastfeeding. No significant difference was seen in the time taken to attach to the new breast and the time taken to reattach to the previously suckled breast. Mean milk intake from the first breast was 91.7 g (range 58 to 208 g), higher than that from the second breast (mean 52.5 g, range 8 to 75 g). The mean fat contents before and after nursing on the first breast were 23 and 52 g/L, whereas on the second breast they were 24 and 48 g/L. This shows that infants will nurse when fat content is higher, contrary to the theory that increasing fat causes satiation.[92]

Studies of 3-day-old bottle-fed infants fed sucrose and glucose solutions show that they manifest tongue movements of greater amplitude when fed stronger concentrations of carbohydrate, even though they do not respond to fat content in formula. Sensory apparatus responsible for assessing sweetness is apparently competent in the newborn.

BREATHING AND SUCKING DURING FEEDING

Breathing and sucking during feeding were studied in normal full-term infants from 1 to 10 days of age, measuring breathing, sucking, and flow of fluid from a feeding bottle with a flow meter. No infant aspirated water, but 8 of 18 infants inhaled saline. Even from a bottle, breast milk was associated with more regular breathing than was formula feeding. It has been demonstrated in other species that newborns will become apneic when fed milk from species other than their own. The coordination of breathing and swallowing improves with an increase in milk availability and with the maturity of the infant.[137]

SUCKLING PATTERNS AS INDICATORS OF PROBLEMS OR PATHOLOGY

The behavior of an infant at birth is the first opportunity to observe the infant's adeptness at suckling. In a careful analysis of videotapes of newborns in the first 90 minutes of life, Widström and Thingström-Paulsson[141] observed a consistent pattern. Licking movements preceded and followed the rooting reflex in alert infants. The tongue was placed in the bottom of the mouth cavity during distinct rooting. The authors suggest that forcing the infant to the breast might disturb reflex action and tongue position. They further observed that a healthy infant should be given the opportunity to show hunger and optimal reflexes and attach to the mother's nipple by itself.[141]

Righard and Alade[110] observed that an infant placed on the mother's abdomen will self-attach to the breast and suckle correctly in less than 50 minutes. They further reported that when the infants were separated from their mothers for delivery room procedures, the initial suckling attempts were disturbed, and many infants were too drowsy to suckle at all.[110]

Righard and Alade[111] also investigated the prognostic value of suckling technique (faulty vs. correct) during the first week after birth in relation

to the long-term success of breastfeeding. For assessment of breastfeeding technique, 82 healthy mother-infant pairs were observed before discharge. The authors defined correct sucking as the infant's mouth being wide open, the tongue under the areola, and the milk expressed in slow, deep sucks. Incorrect sucking was defined as the infant positioned as if bottle feeding, using the nipple as a teat. The oral searching reflex was defined as the infant opening the mouth wide in response to proximity of the nipple to the lips and thrusting the tongue forward in preparation to taking the breast. This reflex is a part of the normal response to circumoral stimulus, resulting in rooting by the infant, who comes forward, opens the mouth wide, and extends the tongue when stimulated centrally on the lower lip and even the upper lip. Stimulus on the side of the mouth or cheeks elicits turning to that side.

It was first noted by Barnes et al.[12] that mothers with difficult labors and deliveries had more problems breastfeeding. The influence of mode of delivery on the initiation of breastfeeding has been reported. For infants delivered by vacuum extraction or cesarean delivery, suckling was delayed and they received more supplements, C-section patients also received postdelivery narcotics, which changed suckling patterns.[117] Parity increases chances of success in lactation, according to Dewey et al.[30] They confirmed the influence of mode of delivery, duration of labor, labor medications, and the use of artificial feedings and pacifiers as well.[2] When these factors are present, extra care should be made to support the mother's efforts to breastfeed (Figure 8-5),[30] particularly monitoring at day 3 and the day of discharge.

C-section rates have risen and fewer women who deliver by C-section breastfeed. Initiation rates require more support and monitoring for C-section patients.[67] At 6 months the long-term success, however, is the same for both vaginal and operative patients who breastfeed.

Medications During Labor and Epidural Anesthesia

Because of repeated concerns about the possible effect of intrapartum epidural anesthesia on a newborn infant's ability to suckle and the rising incidence of epidurals in some hospitals (more than 50% of vaginal deliveries), Rosen and Lawrence[114] investigated 83 mother-infant dyads who either exclusively breastfed or bottle-fed. An infant's ability to nurse at the breast or take a bottle was scored from multiple observations. Weight loss in the first few days was also evaluated. Epidural anesthesia

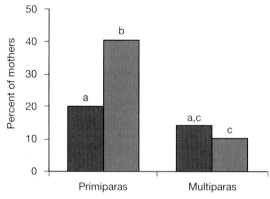

Figure 8-5. Percentage of mothers with delayed onset of milk production, by parity and infant birth weight, adjusted for mode of delivery, duration of stage II labor, maternal body mass index, and flat or inverted nipples (bars with different letters are significantly different, $p < 0.05$). Vertical bars, birth weight ≤ 3600 g; horizontal bars, birth weight > 3600 g. $N = 69$ primiparas with infants ≤ 3600 g, 61 primiparas with infants > 3600 g, 40 multiparas with infants ≤ 3600 g, and 71 multiparas with infants > 3600 g. (From Dewey KG, Nommsen-Rivers LA, Heinig MJ, Cohen RJ: Risk factors for suboptimal infant breastfeeding behavior, delayed onset lactation, and excess neonatal weight loss, *Pediatrics* 112:607, 2003.)

had no apparent effect (although analgesics showed a relationship) on ability to feed or initial weight loss. However, prolonged epidural use (beyond 4 hours or repeated dosing) may well have an effect because the drug has time to be absorbed into the systemic circulation.

The question of duration of epidural anesthesia was investigated by Bader et al.,[11] who found that maternal venous and umbilical venous levels of fentanyl and bupivacaine were relatively constant whether the epidural lasted 1 hour or up to 15 hours. Total doses varied between 27 and 200 mg for bupivacaine and 22 to 300 mg for fentanyl. Significantly, however, bupivacaine was measurable in the umbilical venous sample of the infants $(0.15 \pm 0.06$ mg/mL). The significance of fetal tissue uptake is unclear. Umbilical artery blood gases and neurobehavioral scores were normal. Neonatal urine in another study[16] had small, but measurable, bupivacaine metabolites 36 hours after delivery when spinal anesthesia was used for cesarean delivery. It is noteworthy that usually the infant is delivered within 15 minutes of medication administration for cesarean delivery, so fetal exposure is minimal when used for C-sections.

The effect on infants of different doses of meperidine given to mothers in labor has been clearly demonstrated. Most hospitals no longer use meperidine.

The sucking rhythms of infants with a normal perinatal course were compared with those of infants with perinatal distress. The analysis showed that rhythms of nonnutritive sucking were significantly different from rhythms of normal control subjects even when no gross neurologic signs were present.[63] Subtle difficulties with feeding are sometimes the only perinatal evidence of the impact of hypoxia, as noted by low Apgar scores.

Infants whose mothers received bupivacaine epidural anesthesia were described to be less alert and have less ability to orient over the first month of life. Bupivacaine and its metabolites are found in the circulation of infants for the first 3 days of life whose mothers had epidural anesthesia. More recent studies report use of lower doses of bupivacaine and either fentanyl or sufentanyl.[74] Less sufentanyl appeared in the cord blood. Only the Rosen and Lawrence study[114] reported the effects of epidural anesthesia on feeding ability of the neonates.

Cesarean Delivery

The effect of cesarean delivery on breastfeeding has long been thought to be significant. With the rise in rates of cesarean delivery, the question becomes imperative. A study of 97 women who had infants by cesarean delivery and 88 who delivered vaginally was designed to determine milk production rates at each feed in the first week of life.[33] The volume of milk transferred to the infants born by cesarean delivery was significantly less than that received by the infants born vaginally from days 2 to 5, but volumes were comparable by day 6. Birth weight was regained on day 6 by 40% of the vaginally delivered infants but only 20% of the infants born by cesarean delivery.

A comparison of early sucking dynamics during breastfeeding after C-section showed minor differences in suckling itself; duration and milk intake were similar in both section and vaginally delivered women. Successful initiation, however, required additional lactation support and monitoring in women who were delivered by C-section.[117]

Sucking Stimulus and Prolactin

When lactating postpartum women nurse their infants, the prolactin level increases from a high baseline level to levels several times over the mean baseline.[5] When nursing women played with but did not feed their infants, prolactin did not rise, despite the initiation of milk dripping. Substitution of a breast pump at regular intervals caused prolactin elevations similar in timing and magnitude to those induced by sucking. When normal, menstruating, nonlactating adult women were stimulated with a breast pump for 30 minutes, significant prolactin increases occurred in 7 of the 18 women. No response was obtained in normal men.

When the prolactin response was used as a measure of "success" in establishing lactation in the first week postpartum, no difference in prolactin levels was seen between women who had been considered good producers and those who were considered poor producers.[54] Mothers whose infants were in the special care unit, and who were using a breast pump to establish lactation, had minimal prolactin response to pumping but produced a mean of 86 g of milk per pumping. When prolactin levels were measured after use of the breast pump at uniform settings, all three groups were similar. This and the work of others[84] demonstrates that infant suckling plays a significant role in adequate milk production.

Knowledge about infant suckling has been accumulating rapidly, but only recently has it involved study of suckling at the breast. It has been established that the patterns are different mechanically. At the breast, nutritive and nonnutritive suckling varies only in rate, not in pattern. Infants can suckle immediately at birth and tolerate mother's milk (colostrum) best as the pattern of respirations remains physiologic. Inadequate suckling can influence maternal production, but inadequate suckling can be improved.

Management of breastfeeding is best discussed in terms of the three stages: (1) prenatal period, (2) immediate postpartum, or hospital, period, and (3) postnatal, or posthospital, period.

Prenatal Period

It is most effective to prepare for breastfeeding well in advance of delivery. Prospective parents should consider feeding plans for an infant during the prenatal period, after the pregnancy is well established. Once quickening (awareness of fetal movement) has occurred, an infant becomes more of a reality for the mother and she can relate to planning. Except in sophisticated cultures, the parents generally will not initiate this decision-making discussion, and it is appropriately introduced by the obstetrician, family physician, or midwife in the second trimester. Use of ultrasound and the presentation of an ultrasound picture of the fetus to the parents confirms the reality of a baby. Particularly with first children, it is appropriate to suggest to the parents that they select a pediatrician early. They should request a prenatal conference with the pediatrician to discuss not only feeding but also points of management and child rearing about which they might have questions. If the mother is receiving

prenatal care from a family practice physician, then this step is automatic.

Many mothers decide long before the pregnancy about feeding the infant, but those who choose bottle feeding admit they could have been persuaded, if only someone had cared enough to tell them how important breastfeeding is to the infant. All women know mother's milk is best. Clearly, health care providers have made breastfeeding too complicated and burdened mothers with so many rules and regulations that they cannot cope and default to bottle feeding. When health care workers try to persuade a woman to breastfeed, they perpetuate the image of a difficult chore by saying, "Why not give it a try? It's not that bad," or "You'll be surprised. It isn't that hard," instead of conveying opportunity and good experience with, "It is a marvelous opportunity for you and your baby," or "It will be a special joy." Employment is often cited as the cause of early weaning, but it is actually unemployed women who are at home bottle feeding (see Chapter 18). Any time spent breastfeeding is worthwhile for a working mother and her infant.

The medical profession has been hesitant to take anything but a neutral position in discussions of breastfeeding for fear of pressuring mothers. The evidence is stronger than ever that breastfeeding has distinct advantages for infants and mothers. Parents have the right to hear the data. They can make their own choices. Fear of instilling guilt is a poor reason to deprive a mother of an informed choice, especially because women generally do not feel guilty about their own informed decision. After interviews with hundreds of mothers, half of whom chose to bottle feed, not one felt guilty, but some were disappointed that their physician did not discuss infant feeding.[114]

The prenatal discussion should also include any questions the parents may have about the lactation process and a mother's ability to provide adequately for the infant. An examination of the breasts is part of good prenatal care and an excellent opportunity to discuss breastfeeding. If any anatomic abnormalities exist, then they should be discussed. The breast tissue should be checked for lumps and cysts that might need treatment. The amount of mammary tissue is not correlated with the ability to produce milk. The more generous gland usually results from a more generous fat pad. During pregnancy the fat is replaced by proliferating acini. A woman with small breasts should not be discouraged from nursing.

Breast texture should be assessed by palpation. An inelastic breast gives the impression it is firmly knit together, and the overlying skin is taut and firm so it cannot be picked up. The elastic breast is looser, the overlying skin is free, and the tissue is more easily picked up. Inelastic breasts are more prone to engorgement and seem improved by prepartum massaging and close attention to prevention of engorgement (Figure 8-6).

Examination of the areola and nipple is equally important to identify any anatomic problems that may need attention before delivery. Gross malformations and inversion of the nipple can be easily detected, but lesser problems may go unnoticed. One must test for freedom of protrusion. When the areola is compressed and the nipple retracts instead of protrudes, it indicates a "tied nipple," or inverted nipple, caused by the persistence of fibers from the original embryologic invagination of the mammary dimple (Figure 8-7).

Although a physician may provide literature on breastfeeding or suggest reading sources for the patient, one should avoid dismissing the parents' questions by merely suggesting appropriate readings, because their decision making will be enhanced by open discussion with a knowledgeable professional. Although parents may have access to childbirth preparation programs in the community, they should not be dismissed to get all their information from such sources. When parents have no opportunity to discuss with their care provider issues such as early infant contact, nursing the infant in the delivery room, and family-centered maternity care, they often experience tremendous disappointment and misunderstanding.

The concerns most frequently expressed by mothers considering breastfeeding are related to themselves, not the infant. Mothers who are more concerned about their own well-being have more trouble adjusting to motherhood and should be provided with more support in adapting to the role. They may be helped by selecting a doula to support them, because our modern culture tends to isolate young couples. Raphael describes a doula as one of "those individuals who surround, interact with, and aid the mother at any time within the perinatal period, which includes pregnancy, birth and lactation."[104] Doulas have been further studied by Klaus and Kennell,[64] who found a clear relationship between the presence of a doula in labor and the outcome of delivery, the

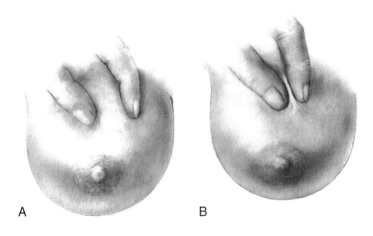

Figure 8-6. Texture of breast tissue can be assessed by picking up skin of breast. **A,** Inelastic breast tissue. **B,** Elastic breast tissue.

A   B

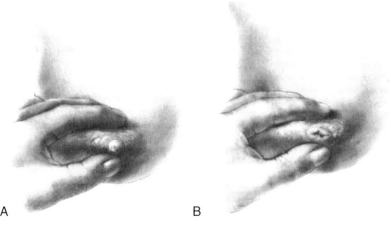

Figure 8-7. A, Normal nipple averts with gentle pressure. **B,** Inverted or tied nipple inverts with gentle pressure.

A   B

mother's personal experience, and her recovery period (including breastfeeding).

Concerns most frequently expressed prenatally by mothers include the following:

1. What is the effect on the mother's figure? Data indicate that breasts are affected by heredity, age, and pregnancy in that order and only minimally by lactation. Women who have never borne children may "lose their figures" long before a multipara who nurses her infants. Pregnancy enlarges breasts temporarily, as does early lactation, but the effect is temporary. Poor diet and lack of exercise will destroy a figure in both men and women long before any other influence.

2. What is the effect on the mother's freedom? Obviously, only a mother can breastfeed an infant; however, ample data support that it is possible to maintain a career, keep a job, or just get away from the house and still nurse in today's world. Mothers in primitive cultures have returned to the fields, or some form of productivity outside the home, out of sheer necessity for generations. Mothers concerned about this often are best reassured by their peers—that is, mothers who are nursing. In communities with nursing mother groups, it is a simple referral. Employment statistics have revealed that women do successfully return to the work force and continue breastfeeding. Employment is rarely a reason for not breastfeeding, but it may influence duration (Chapter 18).

3. Many women are concerned about exposing their breasts. Despite the constant barrage of publicity about breasts in the modern press, many women are embarrassed to consider baring their breasts. As pointed out in Chapter 6, shame and embarrassment are important considerations when helping a mother accept breastfeeding. Shame and anxieties arise from the influence of one's life history and previous events; thus intervention is necessary at many levels. Clothes that make discreet breastfeeding possible are readily available and fashionable. Considerable body exposure is not necessary for breastfeeding. In a public survey performed in the Midwest, few people, male or female, in any age group considered breastfeeding embarrassing, and 82% would want their child breastfed. Universal publicity about breastfeeding in public places has created a more accepting attitude in most people, so that a nursing mother no longer needs to hide to feed her infant.

Preparation of the Breasts

The prenatal period is a time for a couple to prepare for their new role as parents and to learn as much as possible about breastfeeding. Most mothers do no special preparation and are successful. Carefully controlled studies do not support the contention that fair-skinned women, especially redheads, are more prone to developing cracked, sore nipples than are others. Mothers who have had trouble with tender, cracked nipples when nursing a previous infant will need extra assistance in putting the infant to breast properly in the first few days, but elaborate rituals prenatally may actually cause problems. Nipple preparation has a negative effect on some women who are not ready to handle their breasts for these preparations during pregnancy and has not proved to make a difference. Proper positioning is highly important.

Bathing should be as usual, with minimal or no soap directly on the nipples and thorough rinsing. Some recommend patting the nipple dry with a soft towel, but this should not be done except after a shower or bath. Persistent removal of natural oils of the nipple and areola actually predisposes the skin to irritation. Montgomery glands in the areola secrete a sebaceous material for the cleansing and lubrication of the areola and nipple. This should not be removed by soaps or chemicals. Tincture of benzoin, alcohol, and other drying agents are contraindicated because they predispose the nipples to cracking during early lactation.[84] Wearing protective brassieres, modern women do not experience the friction to the nipples that looser clothing causes, which may be why cracked nipples are a common problem in modern society but almost unheard of in developing countries and among other mammals. In Scandinavia, it is suggested that pregnant women get as much air and sunshine as possible directly on the breasts before delivery. Wearing a nursing brassiere with the flaps down to expose the nipples under loose clothing serves the same purpose. However, aggressive and abrasive treatment of the nipples does not prevent nipple pain postpartum and may aggravate it. Gentle love making involving the breasts is usually safe and is the most effective preparation.

The use of lanolin, which is miscible with water and thus allows normal evaporation from the skin, does no apparent harm but in controlled studies also made no difference prenatally. Women allergic to wool will also be allergic to lanolin. The use of vitamin A and D ointment prophylactically also makes no difference, having an effect only in the treatment of fissures later. In climates with average to high humidity, ointments are not routinely recommended for breasts and may interfere with Montgomery gland secretion. In extremely dry climates, using ointments sparingly is often necessary.

Some believe gentle traction to the point of discomfort, but not pain, reduces perception of pain in the first week of lactation. A study, carefully controlled to eliminate subjective discrepancies of interpretation, revealed no significant difference in nipple sensitivity or trauma in those who practiced prenatal nipple rolling, application of breast cream, or expression of colostrum compared with those who had untreated breasts.[58] No increased pain or trauma was reported among fair-skinned participants in the study, treated or untreated. Because many women are not inclined to manipulate their breasts before delivery and might be discouraged from breastfeeding if it is implied that this must be done, physicians should prescribe treatment only when an indication exists.[146]

Preparation of the Nipples

Flat nipples or inverted nipples do not preclude breastfeeding. Flat nipples respond to the same passive treatment with a breast shell that works for inverted nipples. The shells can be worn during the last trimester by women who choose to do so (Figure 8-8). They should be recommended only after careful examination and discussion about advantages and disadvantages by the physician. Follow-up at subsequent prenatal visits is also appropriate.

Alexander et al.[3] estimated that 10% of pregnant women have inverted or nonprotractile nipples, which are thought to contribute to breastfeeding problems.[3] Breast shells (plastic disks with holes in the center and a domed cover) (see Figure 8-8) and Hoffman exercises[52] (stretching and pulling of the nipple and areola, vertically and horizontally) are the most common treatments suggested. Alexander et al.[3] compared use of shells with no treatment and found more sustained improvement in the untreated group. The difference in use of

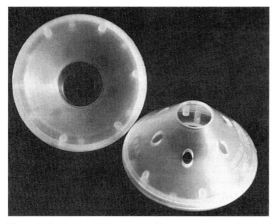

Figure 8-8. Breast shells: vented domes worn over ring that allows nipple to evert. Shell is slipped into cup of well-fitting brassiere. Available in several styles and designs.

shells/no shells was 52% and 60%, which is not significant. A large multicenter trial of shells, Hoffman exercises, and no prenatal treatment showed "no treatment" to be most effective.[107] Nipple stretching has had no significant impact and is contraindicated because of its tendency to initiate uterine contractions. The most significant finding was that more women who were instructed to wear shells or do nipple exercises than control subjects who had no prenatal preparation failed to initiate breastfeeding at delivery. More study women also discontinued breastfeeding by 6 weeks compared with control subjects. The women complained that shells caused discomfort, embarrassment, sweating, rash, or milk leakage or were conspicuous.

Such studies illustrate some of the risks of using untried methods to solve problems, although some women probably benefit by using shells. The question deserves further study. The process of assessing anatomic problems and initiating management should not be a deterrent to breastfeeding.

Inverted nipples (see Figure 8-7) can be diagnosed by pressing the areola between the thumb and the forefinger. A flat or normal nipple will protrude; a truly inverted nipple will retract. True inverted nipples are actually rare. Mildly retracting nipples can be improved with gentle stretching to evert them, preferably done before delivery.

One or both nipples may be pierced and may have jewelry inserted. The jewelry should be removed during pregnancy, or as soon as observed, to allow the nipple to recover and avoid any infection. Usually nursing proceeds without a problem. Sometimes milk will leak from the piercings. It can be absorbed by keeping a washcloth handy. The jewelry should not be worn while breastfeeding. The major risk to the mother is infection, which can be avoided by good hygiene and not wearing the jewelry. The risk of the infant swallowing the jewelry if left in place is monumental.

Nipple Stimulation to Induce Labor

The obstetric literature abounds with articles about the use of nipple stimulation in place of the traditional oxytocin challenge test to induce uterine contraction; only a few are cited here.[20,21,79] Using a breast pump or manual expression to produce colostrum is reported to induce labor or increase the strength of contractions in desultory labor.

Taylor and Green[128] reported a case of severe abruptio placentae after nipple stimulation. A series of patients induced labor with self-manipulation of the breasts with a 45% success rate. All patients in the series showed some ripening of the cervix with dilatation and effacement in 3 days of breast stimulation. Lipitz et al.,[73] Amatayakul et al.,[5] and Taylor and Green[128] reported a relatively high incidence (45.5%) of exaggerated uterine activity in response to a breast-stimulation stress test, usually within 7 minutes of initiation of stimulation. Although all the cases and series cannot be reported here, it is clear that nipple stimulation in the third trimester can initiate uterine contractions and, in some, labor. Under the direction of an obstetrician, breast stimulation can be effective therapeutically, but it should not be attempted without obstetric evaluation and guidance.

Suggesting stretching (Hoffman) exercises is not advised, especially in women with a tendency to early labor. No study since Hoffman's initial report of two cases[52] has shown the process to be effective in the nipples. Stretching the areola forcefully can damage the delicate Montgomery glands. Prepartum mastitis has also occurred with prenatal expression of colostrum. Whether manipulating the breast prenatally provides the mother with greater comfort in breastfeeding has not been demonstrated. Mothers who choose to bottle feed have told us that having to "exercise" their breasts is one of the "rules" that kept them from breastfeeding.

Pumping with a pulsatile electric pump with a soft Silastic flange has been shown to facilitate latch-on with flat or inverted nipples after delivery. The breast is gently pumped on low settings until the teat is drawn out, and then the infant is offered the breast. Similar pumping is done on the second breast, when that nipple is also inverted, before placing the infant on that breast. Usually the pumping can be discontinued after a few days, or a hand pump is adequate if preferred. Pumping needs to be continued at home to evert the nipples.

These approaches avoid the risk for never initiating breastfeeding. They also provide one-on-one support from the nursing staff, which is very different from sending the mother home to use a strange plastic device.

An infant breastfeeds. An infant does not nipple-feed. If the nipples are flat or inverted, extra care is needed to provide enough areolar tissue in the infant's mouth to allow latch-on. Experienced postpartum nurses can facilitate the breastfeeding experience by assisting with the initial latch to the breast.

Surgical Correction

Inverted nipples have been known to medicine for centuries. Treatment has included various exercises, use of older vigorous infants to suckle, and the use of adults who are hired for this purpose in difficult cases. The first surgical procedure was described in 1873. Other techniques have since been advanced.[46,105] A primary indication for surgical repair of the inverted nipple is the chronic occurrence of central pockets of inflammation of the nipple, leading to the spread of infection and infectious mastitis. A simple method for correction without division of the lactiferous ducts involves using a purse-string suture and traction of holding sutures. The procedure can be done in the office under local anesthesia, according to Hauben and Mahler.[46] A truly inverted nipple may have fewer ducts. The microscopic pathologic examination of severely inverted nipples indicates the ducts are abnormal.

Hand Expression Prenatally

Some breastfeeding instructions suggest hand expressing the breast to produce a few drops of colostrum every day for the last few weeks of pregnancy. Fortunately, the instructions usually suggest the patient consult her physician first. Manual or any kind of pumping of the breasts may stimulate the uterus to contract. Hand expression has no particular benefit and means that the early-sequestered cells are expressed away in the drops of colostrum before delivery and are lost to the infant. Occasionally, prepartum mastitis has developed from this treatment. The risks far outweigh any seeming benefit.

Summary

1. During the first trimester, make the initial breast examination. Initiate the discussion about how the infant is to be fed and the benefits of breastfeeding. If anatomic variations may interfere with lactation, mention them and discuss possible remedies.
2. At each prenatal visit, offer information about breastfeeding.
3. Investigate the mother's knowledge of breastfeeding, and document her information base to fill in the gaps and correct misinformation. Also inquire about any treatments or routines she has initiated on her own, so that the total management is appropriate.
4. Once quickening has been experienced, the parents are ready to plan more concretely about the baby. Suggest a visit with the pediatrician.
5. As delivery approaches, initiate discussion about feeding the infant immediately after birth, feeding protocols, and the mother's special needs or requests.
6. Be familiar with community resources so that patients can be wisely referred for peer support or assistance unavailable from one's office staff.

or tipped down slightly. The palmar grasp can be used when there is nipple pain, soreness, or trauma. It is also useful when the mother's hand is too small for a large breast. The mother should be encouraged to use the hand position that is most natural and comfortable.

DAYS IN THE HOSPITAL

A physician should see that patients are permitted to have their infants with them as much as they wish, within the guidelines of reasonable medical care. Only the few patients with difficult deliveries, cesarean delivery with medication, postpartum complications, or eclampsia need to be excluded. The mother's physician should make that judgment.

The influence of mode of delivery on initiation of breastfeeding was examined in 370 primiparas. Cesarean delivery and other surgical delivery procedures (e.g., vacuum extraction) were associated with a sleepy infant, late start to feeding after delivery, increased incidence of bottle supplementation, less frequent night feedings, and delayed milk production in the hospital.[133] Despite many interventions, breastfeeding can succeed with sufficient support. An experienced nursing staff is critical to the management of the nursing mother in the first few days postpartum. Advice should be reasonable and consistent, and nurses should be cautioned against interjecting their own personal opinion or experience. When too many individuals are involved in postpartum care, mothers are easily overwhelmed with information, especially if each person says something different. The hospital should provide at least one staff member who is also a board-certified licensed lactation consultant for every 15 postpartum patients.

Key points in management should include the following:[100]

1. Feed when the infant is showing signs of hunger (Box 8-3).
2. Help the mother find a comfortable position. No rules should exist about sitting up or lying down on her side or on her back.

BOX 8-3. Signs of Hunger in an Infant

1. Begins to stir.
2. Brings hand(s) to mouth.
3. Shows increasing efforts to root.
4. Increasing activity, arms and legs flexed, hands in fists.
5. If not picked up, progresses to frantic movements, whimpering.
6. Cries (a late sign of hunger).

---

3. Help the infant to the breast. The infant should be held so that the ventral surface of the infant faces the ventral surface of the mother.
4. Help the mother hold her breast for her baby, choosing the better grasp for the situation, and draw the baby to the breast by moving her arm toward her chest. Note: Never push the infant's head toward the breast because the infant will push back, often arching away from the breast. Holding or pushing the infant's head has been associated with persistent arching by the infant (arching reflex).
5. Help the mother reposition the infant on the second breast if the infant is still interested after releasing the first side. Moving may be difficult for the mother immediately postpartum.
6. If the infant falls asleep after the first breast, the mother should be shown how to break the suction with her finger. Nonnutritive suckling while asleep is especially irritating to the nipple in the first few days. The mother should wait a little, wake the baby, and then move the infant to the second side.
7. When waking an infant to initiate feeding, unwrapping the blanket and using gentle stimulus are appropriate. Jackknifing is never appropriate and may cause regurgitation, aspiration, or trauma to vital organs. Usually infants feed best when they are ready.
8. The infant will nurse on the first breast until satisfied. After gentle burping, if the infant is still awake, the second side can be offered. The next feeding should be initiated on the second side. This will balance the stimulus to the breasts in the critical early days when milk production is just beginning.
9. Signs of satiety: Sounds of swallowing dwindle and stop, nonnutritive suckling occurs in brief bursts, arms and legs relax, and the infant falls asleep and usually releases the nipple.

Stopwatch timing is not appropriate. It takes 2 to 3 minutes for the let-down reflex to produce milk in the early days, so the feeding must allow for the let-down. It is helpful for some mothers to have guidelines or estimates from which to work. Usually, infants nurse about 10 to 15 minutes per feeding in the first days. Nursing continually hour after hour may be counterproductive. Frequent small feedings will provide good stimulation to the breast without stressing the mother. The milk supply, however, is best stimulated by suckling.[98] The policy of the nursery should be to have all breastfed infants taken to their mothers when they awaken during the night,[71] if they are not already rooming-in.

In keeping with the Baby Friendly Hospital Initiative (see Chapter 1), infants should be nursed on demand around the clock and receive no other food or drink. A mother and infant should be housed together unless there is a medical contraindication. Modern hospitals are a hubbub of activity, though, and with liberal visiting hours, the mother has no time to rest unless naps are scheduled. In the early days of the Rooming-In Unit at the Yale–New Haven Hospital, Barnes et al.[12] insisted that all postpartum mothers have a nap after lunch. Every day the shades were drawn and traffic decreased on the unit for an hour. This is part of mothering the mother. In primitive cultures, mothers are groomed, fed, and protected after delivery, often for weeks. Furthermore, adequate rest is essential to successful lactation. In 1953, Jackson, with Barnes and other colleagues,[12] prepared a classic description of the management of breastfeeding that remains the single most valuable source of information on the subject.

Diagnosing Breastfeeding Problems

To solve the problem of unsuccessful nursing, someone should observe a mother feeding the infant. Often the problem is a simple one, such as a mother so uncomfortable and tense that the letdown reflex will not trigger or perhaps an infant with a poor suck or poor latch. In these cases and others the diagnosis can be made most easily by direct observation.

In addition to a mother's hand position, the manner in which the infant is held or placed to breastfeed is important. There is no one right position. Shortly after birth, lying down may be preferable for the mother. She lies on her side and the infant is placed on his or her side facing the breast, which the mother supports with her upper hand. She can use her lower hand to cradle the infant and bring him or her close. Pillows help sustain the mother's position with one against her back and one between her knees. The pillow between the knees is essential to keep her from rolling over should she drift asleep. She may also lie semiinclined. When a mother is sitting up, the cradle position, with the mother bringing the infant to the breast while cradling the infant in her bent elbow, is the most common and natural position, especially once a mother is home.

Head control can be a problem with the cradle position the first few days, as the infant requires more support to hold the head.

The cross-cradle or cross-over hold works best with mother sitting erect and one to two pillows in her lap so the baby is just at the level of the breast and not above the breast. Short women may only need one small pillow. The infant is held with the opposite arm so that the infant's head and

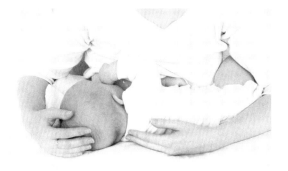

Figure 8-12. Cross-cradle position.

shoulders are held (Figure 8-12). The thumb is below one ear and the fingers are below the other ear. With the head tipped back slightly and the infant brought to the breast, the nipple can stroke the infant's lower lip. Visual demonstration of the latch is available online. "Fifteen-Minute Helper" is a physician-produced video for the physician audience created by Jane Morten, MD, from Stanford University. There is a link at www .nursingmotherscompanion.com/resources.

The football hold is a misnomer; the infant is not tucked under the arm like a football but rather forward so that mother supports the infant's head with her hand and the infant is supported by the mother's arm. The infant must be squarely facing the breast.

These traditional postures were called into question by Colson et al.,[22] who observed less effective breastfeeding and declining duration in spite of aggressive maternal training in their programs. They studied 40 mothers and infants in England and France doing feeding videotapes during the first month. They described and compared primitive neonatal reflexes, investigating whether certain feeding behaviors and positions, termed *biological nurturing*, are associated with the release of these reflexes that they thought were pivotal to establish successful breastfeeding. When mothers chose their own body positions, they selected semiinclined positions, making the infant an abdominal feeder displaying antigravity reflexes, which aid in latching. Gravity pulled the infant's chin and tongue forward, triggering mouth opening to achieve attachment. At the very least, it suggests that alternatives to side lying and sitting upright are viable positions to initiate lactation.[22]

Introducing all the possible positions is overwhelming at first and should be avoided. With a little practice, mothers will find what works best.

Understanding the mechanism of suckling in the neonate (Figure 8-13), however, is essential to recognizing ineffective sucking. As the breast is offered to the infant, the mouth opens wide and

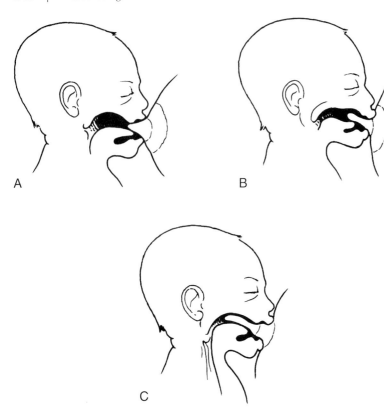

Figure 8-13. A, As infant grasps breast, tongue moves forward to draw in nipple. **B,** Nipple and areola move toward palate as glottis still permits breathing. **C,** Tongue moves along nipple, pressing it against hard palate and creating pressure. Ductules under areola are milked, and flow begins as a result of peristaltic movement of tongue. Glottis closes. Swallow follows.

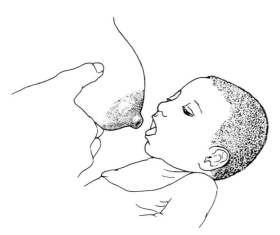

Figure 8-14. Latch-on response. In response to stimulating infant's lower lip with nipple, mouth opens wide. This response has been called oral searching reflex. It is part of the circumoral rooting reflex. (From Righard L, Alade MO: Sucking technique and its effect on success of breastfeeding, *Birth* 19:185, 1992.)

the tongue is extended as the nipple is drawn into the mouth (Figure 8-14). In a rhythmic motion, the tongue moves up against the hard palate, as it draws the nipple and areola into the mouth, creating an elongated teat. The cheeks fill the mouth because

of the sucking fat pads and provide further negative pressure because they do not collapse. The tongue undulates along the teat, while remaining in place, compressing the collecting ductules in the areola and "milking" them toward the nipple.

This undulation is peristalsis, which continues from tongue to pharynx and the entire gastrointestinal track. Milk flows from the nipple and is swallowed as the swallowing reflex is triggered, and the peristaltic wave continues to the posterior tongue and pharynx and down the esophagus.

If an infant has a fluttering tongue that is discoordinate, it may not be as productive in stimulating ejection. If the infant cannot coordinate suck and swallow, choking occurs. Sometimes, if letdown is strong, the first rush of milk will cause choking. Stopping and starting again should solve the problem. If the mother's milk flows abundantly with first let-down, she may need to express manually (and save) the first few milliliters to avoid choking the infant. Usually the flow moderates in the next few days. This problem is temporary or is limited to times when the infant has not been nursed for an unusually long interval. Positioning the infant over the breast with the mother on her back may diminish the flow due to gravity in these special cases.[22]

If an infant's jaw is slightly receding, the nipple may not stay in place. Gentle support from the mother's index finger at the angle of the jaw, bringing it forward, will help. She may always have to support the breast with her hand (see Chapter 14).

An infant who is given a bottle or rubber nipple to suck can become confused because the milking action is different (see Figure 8-4). The relatively inflexible rubber nipple may keep the tongue from its usual rhythmic action. In addition, the flow from the bottle may be so rapid, even without sucking, that the infant learns to put the tongue against holes in the rubber nipple to slow down the flow. Some infants who have been breastfed gag when the relatively large rubber nipple is put in their mouths. When infants use the same tongue action needed for a rubber nipple while at the breast, they may even push the human nipple out of the mouth. When infants cannot grasp an engorged areola properly, they will clamp down on the nipple with the jaws, causing pain in the nipple and disrupting the ejection reflex. Manual expression of a little milk will soften the areola, permitting compression by the mother's hand and an easier grasp by the infant.

A study of suck-swallow-breathe, oxygenation, and heart rate patterns had not been performed in breastfeeding infants. No measurements had been taken over the first 4 months of lactation in term infants. Fifteen infants were studied by Sakalidis et al.[117]

Simultaneous recordings of vacuum, tongue movement respiration, swallowing, oxygen saturation, and heart rate were measured at about 1 month and at 2 to 4 months.

Suck bursts became longer, pauses became shorter, vacuum levels decreased, oxygen saturation increased, and heart rate decreased as the infants matured. They consumed a similar amount of milk in a shorter time period (Figures 8-15 and 8-16).

When observing an infant being breastfed, take note of the following:
1. Position of mother, body language, and tension. Pillows may provide support for the arms or the infant.
2. Position of infant. The infant's ventral surface should be to the mother's ventral surface, with the lower arm, if not swaddled, around the mother's thorax. The infant cannot swallow if the head has to turn to the breast, and grasp of the areola will be poor. The infant's head should be in the crook of the mother's arm and moved toward the breast by the mother's arm movement if cradle hold is used.
3. Position of mother's hand on breast is not in the way of proper grasp by infant.
4. Position of infant's lips on areola about 1 to 1½ inches (2.5 to 3.7 cm) from the base of nipple, thus facilitating the formation of the teat.
5. Lips should be flanged and lower lip not folded in so that the infant does not suck it.
6. Actual events around presenting breast and assisting the infant to latch on.
7. Response of the infant to lower lip stimulus by opening mouth wide (see Figure 8-14).
8. Motion of masseter muscle during suckling and sounds of swallowing.
9. Ratio of sucks to swallows should move to 1:1 as feeding progresses.
10. Mother is comfortable with no breast pain.

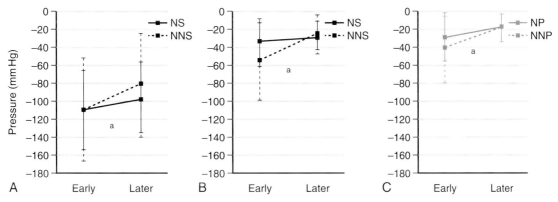

Figure 8-15. Significant relationships for vacuum between burst type and visit. Average vacuum levels for **(A)** peak, **(B)** baseline, and **(C)** pausing vacuums during early and later lactation. *NNP,* nonnutritive pausing; *NNS,* nonnutritive sucking; *NP,* nutritive pausing; *NS,* nutritive sucking. [a]*P<0.05* for interaction with burst type and visit. (From Sakalidis VS, Kent JC, Garbin CP, et al.: Longitudinal changes in suck-swallow-breathe, oxygen saturation, and heart rate patterns in term breastfeeding infants, *J Hum Lact* 29(2):236–245, 2013.)

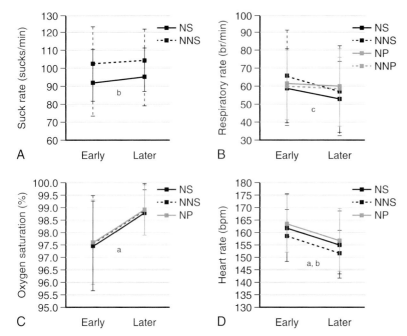

Figure 8-16. Significant relationships with burst type and visit **(A)** suck rate, **(B)** respiratory rate, **(C)** oxygen saturation, and **(D)** heart rate. *NNP,* nonnutritive pausing; *NNS,* nonnutritive sucking; *NP,* nutritive pausing; *NS,* nutritive sucking. [a]$P < 0.05$ for visit. [b]$P < 0.05$ for burst type. [c]$P < 0.05$ for interaction with burst type and visit. (From Sakalidis VS, Kent JC, Garbin CP, et al.: Longitudinal changes in suck-swallow-breathe, oxygen saturation, and heart rate patterns in term breastfeeding infants, *J Hum Lact* 29(2):236–245, 2013.)

ENGORGEMENT

The best management of engorgement is prevention. The degree of engorgement lessens for a woman with each infant, because the time during which the milk "comes in" seems to shorten in multiparas. The primipara suffers most from engorgement.

Breast engorgement was carefully documented by Humenick et al.[55] for 14 days postpartum in 114 breastfeeding women. Four distinct patterns emerged, varying from minimal engorgement to intense engorgement and including a bell-shaped and a multimodal pattern. Characteristics of mothers, infants, and feeding frequency were similar across all patterns. Engorgement in these women was increased in women breastfeeding for the second time, with women breastfeeding for the first time peaking at about 108 hours and second-time feeders at 100 hours. Engorgement cleared more quickly the second time. Clearly, mothers' experiences differ under seemingly similar circumstances. With early discharge, mothers are already home when it occurs.

A number of often conflicting theories and explanations regarding engorgement have been proposed in the professional and lay literature. The dictionary defines engorgement as "swollen with blood," and pathologists define it as "congestion." Engorgement of the breast involves three elements: (1) congestion and increased vascularity, which is the physiologic response that follows removal of the placenta and does not depend on suckling; (2) accumulation of milk, also a physiologic response to placental

removal; and (3) edema secondary to the swelling and obstruction of drainage of the lymphatic system by vascular increases and fullness of the alveoli. No parallel exists in nature because the underlying process is physiologic. Engorgement is not injury, hemorrhage, or trauma. When the physiologic process proceeds smoothly, no pain, discomfort, or excessive swelling occurs. When edema is identifiable, the surface of the breast pits with pressure. The process is then out of control, and intervention is necessary.[51] It is important to distinguish engorgement from mastitis and gigantomastia, which are discussed in Chapter 16.

Engorgement may involve only the areola, only the body of the breast (so-called peripheral engorgement), or both. A little bit of engorgement is normal. When the breast does not respond with engorgement and "fullness," this is abnormal and requires attention.

Areolar Engorgement

When the areola is engorged, it obliterates the nipple and makes properly grasping the areola impossible for the infant. If the infant sucks only the nipple, it is exquisitely painful, because this is the only area of the breast with pain fibers. In addition, the collecting ductules are not "milked" and therefore do not empty, and the infant is frustrated by lack of milk.

The treatment is directed toward reducing the engorgement so that the infant can nurse effectively, which will further reduce the overdistended

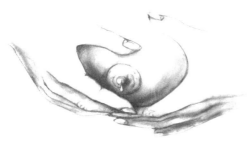

Figure 8-17. Position for manual expression of breast. Thumbs are brought toward areola, compressing areola between thumb and supporting fingers. With areola grasped, pressure is applied toward chest wall, and then pressure is released. This compression and pressure stimulate milking action.

ducts. Gentle manual expression by the mother usually produces a small amount of flow and softens the areola. The presence of milk on the nipple will further encourage the infant's sucking. Warm soaks just before a feeding may facilitate manual expression. Every mother should be taught how to express milk manually (Figure 8-17). When an infant is put to the breast, the mother should compress the areola between two fingers to make it easier for the infant to grasp. Offering the breast this way makes it easier for any infant to grasp, especially when the infant needs encouragement to nurse (Figure 8-18).

Peripheral Engorgement

Initially after delivery the breasts increase in vascularity and begin to swell. This usually starts in the second 24-hour period after delivery. Engorgement at this stage is vascular; thus pumping mechanically briefly to stimulate the breast, when the infant is not nursing adequately, is appropriate. Pumping "to relieve engorgement" will yield little milk and may traumatize the hypervascular breast.

The mother should be advised to wear a well-fitting but adjustable nursing brassiere that does not have thin straps or permanent plastic lining. She should wear it 24 h/day initially. With moderately severe engorgement, the breasts become full, hard, and tender. The swelling starts at the clavicle and goes to the lower rib cage and from the midaxillary line to the midsternum. The breasts may even become hard, tense, and warm. The mother typically complains of throbbing and aching pain and can find no comfortable position except to lie flat on her back and very still (Figure 8-19).

Management centers on making the mother comfortable so that she can continue to nurse and stimulate milk production, as well as nourish the infant. Proper support to elevate the breasts is important. The axillae are particularly painful, probably as a result of the tension on the Cooper ligament. Cold packs reduce vascularity. Warm packs aggravate the swelling. Having the mother stand in a warm shower, however, and manually express some milk at the same time may be the best preparation to feed the infant. Some find comfort in alternating hot and cold water. Other mothers find leaning over a large mixing bowl filled with warm water just before feeding facilitates let-down and milk flow and is less disruptive than taking a shower.

After a feeding, cold packs reduce the swelling, edema, warmth, and pain. Acetaminophen or ibuprofen may give the mother some relief and is safe for the nursing infant. A codeine preparation can be recommended if there is no response to the simple medications. Codeine is cleared well by the mother, peaking in her serum at 30 to 60 minutes.

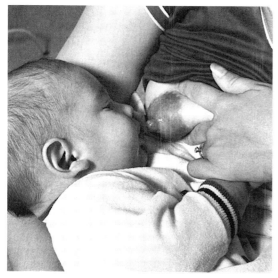

Figure 8-18. When breast is offered to infant, areola is gently compressed between two fingers and breast is supported to ensure that infant is able to grasp areola adequately.

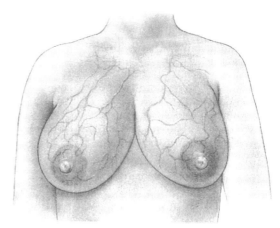

Figure 8-19. Marked mammary engorgement, predominantly vascular in nature.

Breastfeeding should be avoided for approximately 2 hours after dosing. The mother may need some sleep medication. Medications should be timed so that the least amount possible reaches the mother's milk and the baby. With ibuprofen, acetaminophen, codeine, or short-acting barbiturates, if the medication is taken immediately before nursing, the pain will be relieved, but the drug will not reach the milk for more than a half hour.

It is important to maintain drainage of the ducts during this period of engorgement to prevent back pressure in the ducts from developing and eventually depressing milk production. Intraductal pressure can lead eventually to atrophy of both the secreting and the myoepithelial cells and a diminishing milk supply. The best treatment is breastfeeding frequently around the clock, because suckling by the infant is the most effective mechanism for removal of milk. Relief is based on establishment of flow. The infant may have trouble grasping or may not be interested in nursing frequently in the first few days, so manual expression may also be necessary. Every mother should be taught manual expression by the perinatal nursing staff before discharge.[84]

MANUAL EXPRESSION

The mother should support the breast with her fingers and place her thumbs distally and massage gently toward the areola, rotating gradually around the breast to include all quadrants. Then, once the peripheral lobules have been softened, areolar expression should be used to encourage complete emptying of the collecting ducts in the areola. Placing the thumb and forefinger at the margins of the areola and pressing back in toward the chest and then bringing the fingers together, rhythmically simulating the action of the infant's jaw, will start the flow and soften the tense tissue. This is a procedure best done by the mother, but it takes a skilled and experienced nurse to teach this technique. In women with significant engorgement, it may be helpful to use an electric pump, set at low pressure and rate, which is effective because of its gentle milking action (see Chapter 21). The breast should be massaged distally before and during pumping.

Hand pumps can be used but exert only negative pressure on the areola. Unless accompanied by manual expression of the distal segments, they are only temporizing.

TREATMENT WITH CABBAGE LEAVES

A favorite treatment for severe engorgement is cabbage leaves. Cabbage leaves have been used in Europe for generations to relieve edema in other body parts, including the ankles. Chopped fresh leaves are applied to ankles overnight as a poultice and wrapped with a towel. When chilled whole cabbage leaves and chilled gel packs were compared as breast treatments for breast engorgement, no difference was found. Pain was relieved within 1 to 2 hours with both treatments in 68% of women. The mothers preferred the cabbage treatment.[113]

Severe engorgement occurs between the third and seventh day postpartum, and the breasts are described as full, red, hard, and warm. The literature on this therapy is sparse, but two reports have been published. An Australian study involved a series of cases in which the treatment was applied.[115] There were no failures, but in several women the treatment was interrupted by other staff who applied ice and medications for pain without success. When cabbage leaves were reapplied, symptoms were relieved in 2 to 24 hours. Relief was often within 2 hours. Clinicians treated 30 patients and reported on 9 in detail. Rosier[115] tried the treatment first with women who were engorged but were not nursing. No side effects have been reported.

A second randomized, controlled trial was undertaken in South Africa by Nikodem et al.,[89] who studied 120 breastfeeding women. At 72 hours postpartum, they were randomized to control or treatment group. Treatment was application of cool (from refrigerator) cabbage leaves to breasts, leaving just the nipple exposed. The leaves were applied after four feedings for 20 minutes or so until the leaves wilted. The cabbage used was *Brassica oleracea L var. capitata.* All mothers were also taught routine breast exercises, which consisted of bending the arms at the elbow, moving the arms across the chest, with hands facing the same shoulder, so elbows touched, and swiping across the breast a total of 10 times. This exercise, known by various names, including the Johannesburg salute, is used as a preventive treatment for engorgement. Although the experimental group reported less engorgement, it was not statistically significant. Exclusive breastfeeding at 6 weeks was 76% compared with 58% among controls ($p = 0.09$). Mean duration of breastfeeding was 36 versus 30 days in control subjects ($p = 0.04$). However, this study had more multiparas in the control group, and engorgement is rarely a serious problem in multiparas.

Whether cabbage leaves have prophylactic value may be challenged, but their value in the therapy of severe engorgement is worth noting. Whether it is the coolness of the leaves or an innate property of cabbage itself that is therapeutic has not been proved. In Duke's *Handbook of Medicinal Herbs,*[38] cabbage (*Brassica oleracea*) is referred to as a *galactogogue.* The most common variety of cabbage, *Brassica capitata* (*B. capitata*), is the one used in engorgement therapy. This handbook also lists cabbage with other angiosperms as capable of causing hypoglycemia. Cabbage is noted to contain sinigrin (allyl isothiocyanate) and rapine. Herbalists consider rapine to be an antifungal antibiotic. The text lists galactogogues and lactation suppressants found in other plants but does not mention any mammary effects of cabbage when applied to the breasts.

A product is available on the market called Cabbage Gel (Pure Necessities, 15036 Beltway, Addison, TX 75244). This pale green gel has a gentle odor of peppermint, is made of aloe vera, and contains peppermint oil and "herbal infusions," and apparently no cabbage. It is intended for use alone or with fresh cabbage leaves to help keep the leaves in place and cool the engorged breast. Care must be taken to remove the gel before feeding the infant, because aloe vera can be a powerful purgative.

As breastfeeding has become more common, more devices and preparations to solve every problem have become available. Most have not been subjected to any scientific review. Nursing pads and nipple ointments are an example. Lanolin has been modified so that it no longer causes an allergic response (Lasinoh®). Gel pads are also available, some made of glycerin, others of hydrogel, that are applied to the nipple and areola and worn between feedings. ABM Clinical Protocol 20 discusses the diagnosis and management of engorgement.

Going Home from the Hospital

Currently, uncomplicated maternity patients are going home from the hospital in 24 to 48 hours, driven by insurance coverage. This is certainly before lactation is well established and before engorgement is full blown. When maternity floors were run so rigidly that ad lib breastfeeding was an impossible feat, it was often suggested that a mother go home and get away from the negative hospital atmosphere to a place where she could relax and concentrate on feeding the infant and resting. This is the point at which the doula, so well described by Raphael,[104] could make the difference between success and failure. It may be appropriate for the obstetrician to order the mother to have some assistance at home, whether from her husband, her mother, or a friend. "The common denominator for success in breastfeeding is the assurance of some degree of help from some specific person for a definite period of time after childbirth."[104]

Raphael studied mothers in the cycle of anxiety, while she became the doula for them at about 6 to 10 days postpartum. The calm that can be experienced in the presence of a confident, caring

person will relax the mother. The infant senses the calm and confidence and sleeps. When feeding again, the infant nurses well. Breaking the cycle of panic that seizes a new mother when she finds herself home alone with a new infant who needs frequent feeding requires someone to instill confidence. This individual does not need to be a health professional but should be a calm, reassuring, nonthreatening person who is supportive of breastfeeding.

Although physicians are rarely the doula, they can be sure that a family understands the need and can suggest community resources if no personal ones are available. A lactation consultant should be available in the office or the community. Successful breastfeeding is not automatic, as demonstrated by the failure rate. Some problems have been generated by the disturbance of the synchronized interaction between mother and infant by rigid hospital protocol. A Baby Friendly certified hospital will avoid these problems, but does not protect against lack of local support services. The office practice should be available by telephone. Ideally, the office nurse practitioner makes a home visit in the first week. The AAP recommends that an office visit with the pediatrician be scheduled within a week of birth, or sooner if a problem exists, especially for a weight check or hyperbilirubinemia.

Most communities have an international board certified lactation consultant (IBCLC) available for new mothers or any mother with a problem. The physician should be familiar with the available lactation consultants if the practice does not have one on its staff.

The First Visit to the Baby's Physician

According to the ACOG and AAP,[6] the first postpartum visit to the infant's physician should take place at 3 to 5 days of age and certainly before the seventh day. When the caregiver has been specially trained in lactation, the breastfeeding outcome for mothers and infants shows more prolonged breastfeeding.[68] Studies have demonstrated the value of postresidency training in breastfeeding when practitioners did not receive such training in residency.

NIPPLES
Painful Nipples

Presumably, the nipples will adapt to the nursing experience naturally; however, discomforts often arise. The initial grasp of the nipple and first suckles typically cause discomfort in the first few days of lactation because it is a new experience for the mother. This is not cause for alarm but does require maternal reassurance. The sensation is created by the negative pressure on the ductules, which are not yet filled with milk. Later, when lactation is well established and the let-down reflex has matured, mothers describe a turgescence, which is the increased fluid pressure being relieved by suckling. If the pain persists throughout the feeding, the situation demands immediate attention. It should not hurt to breastfeed.[85]

Nipple pain was studied in 102 women in the first 96 hours postpartum.[71] Engorgement was most closely associated with nipple discomfort, which may be enhanced by the general discomfort of the breast. Prenatal breast preparation was unrelated to soreness. Length of time spent suckling was also unrelated. No record was kept on nonnutritive suckling, although others have found suckling without swallowing to be more traumatic early in lactation. How the breast is presented to the infant is the most critical factor (maternal hand position and infant squarely facing breast).[35,33] This is the time actually to observe the feeding, to check the latch, and to look for malpositioning or other abnormalities.

The most common cause of painful nipples in the first few days is positioning. This should be reviewed in detail, making sure that the areola is softened sufficiently to have the infant grasp adequately.[34,33] The infant's lower lip is checked to ensure it is flanged around the breast and not drawn into the mouth, which can abrade the nipple. The tongue should be under the teat and cupped around it.

Specific areas of pain may have specific causes. Soreness on the top of the nipple or on the tip usually results from poor latch-on or from tongue thrusting in an infant who is also bottle-fed. Soreness can also be caused by tipping the nipple upward so that it grazes the hard palate from overzealous use of the palmar grasp or C-hold. Pain on the underside of the nipple is caused by presenting the breast with the nipple tipped up, usually because of more pressure by the mother's thumb on top than the fingers below the breast, so the infant "strokes" the underside of the nipple. The tip of the nipple may also graze the hard palate. The nipple may be bruised, scabbed, or blistered, depending on how long the problem has continued (Figure 8-20). Normally, the peristaltic motion of the tongue below the nipple is not uncomfortable.

If no abnormality is found, the pain may be caused by a "barracuda baby" with a vigorous suck. Occasionally, an infant will have a discordant suck, clamping down on the nipple. This may have a

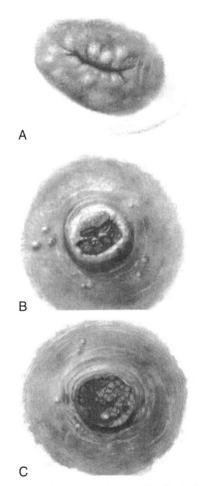

Figure 8-20. Various types of cracks in abraded lactating nipples. **A,** Crack across nipple. **B,** Multiple cracks (stellate). **C,** Crack at lower base.

neurological cause. Suck training may help.[1] The breast will gradually adapt, and this pain will not last indefinitely. Sometimes the maternal tissues are unusually tender and delicate. Brief dry heat may help between feedings in humid climates. The mother should remove the waterproofing from her brassiere and expose her breasts to air briefly after each feeding. Vitamin A and D ointment may help in dry climates.

Even more effective, especially in humid climates, is the use of an electric hair dryer set on warm and fanned across the breast about 6 to 8 inches (15 to 20 cm) away for 2 to 3 minutes only

[1]Suck training is a special technique developed to help an infant who cannot coordinate the undulating (peristaltic) movement of the tongue. It involves using the gloved finger of the lactation consultant and stimulating the infant's tongue with the finger pad to the tongue. The infant will gradually learn to suck. Using a feeding tube attached to a syringe of milk along the finger will provide the infant with milk when sucking is correct. This is called finger feeding.

to avoid overdrying. This brings remarkable comfort and can be done sitting, standing, or lying down. In dry climates, however, wetting the tissues is the preferred treatment. The breast will be moist with milk right after a feeding. This should not be wiped away but allowed to dry on the skin. Many primitive cultures treat irritations of the skin with human milk.[99] The surface-drying effect of the treatment helps counteract the increase in moisture experienced in the first days of lactation.[100]

Stabbing pain that radiates through the breast so the mother feels like the ducts are liquid fire may be associated with *Candida* infection of the breasts, often seen after antibiotic treatment. This deserves special attention by the physician.[31] Not all burning pain is due to *Candida* infection. Sore nipples that occur beyond the first weeks of breastfeeding may be caused by infections such as *Staphylococcus* or by vasospasm. These causes are discussed in Chapters 13 and 16.

Ointments

The appropriate treatment of sore nipples is based on removing the cause and facilitating healing. Positioning is the most common cause, but repositioning will not heal a seriously damaged nipple without some medical intervention. The most appropriate application depends not only on cause but also on environmental conditions. With high humidity, greasy moisture-sealing ointments aggravate the skin. If the atmosphere is dry (e.g., at high altitudes or in desert climates), creams may be appropriate.

All treatments are not appropriate to all lesions. Cool, wet tea bags, for instance, serve as an astringent because of the tannic acid, causing drying and cracking, and are not usually recommended.[70]

The routine application of ointments to the nipple, areola, or breast should be discouraged, however, except in cases of extremely dry skin where the tissue needs to be lubricated.

Lanolin is most hazardous to anyone with a wool allergy. Lansinoh is a purified, alcohol-free, and "allergen-free" ointment, however, and should be safe if an ointment is indicated. Some ointments and creams contain irritants. The sebaceous and Montgomery glands of the areola and nipple are easily plugged by repeated applications of oily substances during pregnancy and lactation. Preparations with vitamins A and D are innocuous, but those with vitamin E or hormones are unsafe unless prescribed for a specific problem by the physician.

Moist wound healing for sore or cracked nipples has been proposed by some dermatologists and is comparable to treatment for other areas of the body. Early soreness may be caused by insufficient moisture present in the skin, coupled with the friction of malpositioning.[107] Wetness on the surface caused by the milk and occlusive plastic-lined nursing pads does cause irritation. The moisture within the tissue, however, should be preserved by the application of a nonirritating ointment after a feeding when the nipple has been gently dried.[122] Local anesthetic creams should not be used because they can lead to allergic reactions. More important, they can interrupt the let-down reflex and dangerously affect the infant by numbing the infant's mouth and throat. The use of ice to numb the pain before feeding does not correct the cause and may interfere with the let-down reflex, which is easily intercepted by cold as well as by pain. If ice numbs the areola, it may numb the nervous response. Irritation or rash should first be treated by discontinuing any ointments or other self-medicating material. This is usually the first step in the treatment of any dermatologic problem. Chronic or intractably sore nipples require more aggressive intervention. It may be necessary to discontinue breastfeeding and resort to manual expression or gentle pumping with an electric pump. A Silastic flange is the least irritating kind of pump attachment. The milk must be removed from the breast frequently. When positioning has been ruled out as a cause as well as infection with *Staphylococcus* or *Candida albicans*, the clinician must determine a means of healing. Some clinicians use all-purpose nipple cream, which contains an antifungal, an antibiotic, a corticosteroid, and a local anesthetic. The contraindications for these constituents have been discussed. Dermatologists almost never use a cream with more than one active ingredient because the bad effects often outweigh the good. The cause of the nipple pain should be determined and the appropriate treatment used. Some clinicians recommend plastic wrap over the ointment to reduce the friction of clothing. The patient should be reminded to use a large piece and to remove it before pumping or feeding. Vaseline gauze can be used in severe cases much as it is used in burn therapy. If antiinflammatory treatment is indicated, preparations of halobetasol propionate (e.g., Ultravate) are best and much more effective than hydrocortisone cream. Usually 2 to 3 days of treatment is sufficient. A tiny amount is rubbed into the nipple after each feeding. It is absorbed promptly and does not need to be removed to feed the infant.

Nipple Shields

A nipple shield is a device made of rubber or synthetic materials that is worn over the nipple and areola while an infant is suckling. A makeshift shield of a nursing-bottle nipple should never be used. Shields differ from the shells designed to

Resters

Resters prefer to nurse a few minutes and then rest a few minutes. If left alone, they often nurse well, although the entire procedure will take much longer. They cannot be hurried.

WEIGHT LOSS

Newborns usually lose some weight, which tends to be a function of whether they are appropriate, large, or small for gestational age, as well as how many kilocalories they ingest in the first few days. Breastfeeding infants of multiparas often lose little weight because the milk "comes in" so quickly. Conversely, the normal primipara may not have a full supply for 72 to 96 hours. If the weight loss is more than 5% (150 g in a 3-kg infant), evaluate the process to identify any problems before they become serious. A 7% loss is maximum, and weight should plateau by 72 hours. A 10% weight loss is acceptable only if all else is going well, voiding 6 × daily and stooling 1 × daily, and the physical examination is negative. It should be justified in the record, and the infant should be seen shortly after discharge from the hospital to ensure resolution of the problem. An increasing number of mothers are receiving epidurals and having caesarian deliveries, which are usually accompanied by intravenous (IV) fluids. These added fluids will affect the fluid volume of the fetus and ultimately the birth weight of the newborn, who has to excrete the extra fluid. Increasingly, infants are dropping 10% of their birth weight in 72 hours as a result of the fluid load and not of failed breastfeeding. IV fluids during labor are an important part of the evaluation history of apparent excess weight loss after birth. If discharge home has taken place in 48 hours or less, it is imperative that the pediatrician's office keep in touch with the mother. Many offices have a nurse practitioner who makes the follow-up telephone calls or a home visit.

Newton[86] described a simple observation of breastfeeding mothers that was an accurate predictor of ultimate lactation success (Table 8-2). All the observations were related to the milk-ejection reflex (i.e., uterine pain, milk dripping on sight of baby, and relief of nipple discomfort on initiation of sucking). Successful breastfeeders had significantly more uterine pain during suckling on day 2 postpartum ("afterpains"), more dripping of the opposite breast, more dripping on sight of infant, and cessation of nipple discomfort.[106] In further evaluation, Newton[87] compared the amount of milk left in the breast after feeding that was available with a dose of synthetic oxytocin (Pitocin) and pumping. Successful breastfeeding women had only 27% left, and unsuccessful breastfeeding women had 47% left. This technologic measurement is no better measure of success than the simple observations of the let-down reflex (see Table 8-2). This observation parallels the observations by ultrasound of Hartmann on storage capacity of the breast, which varies from woman to woman.[45]

Provision of early formula supplementation in the hospital was also associated with less successful lactation.[143] A strong predictor of the need for supplementation was excessive time from delivery to first breastfeeding. When water and sugar water were routinely provided, there was greater weight loss in the infant and a lower lactation success rate.[66]

Early weight loss nomograms for exclusively breastfeeding newborns were developed by Flaherman et al.[38] at University of California San Francisco following 161,471 term newborns, of which 83,433 were delivered vaginally and 25,474 by C-section. Differential loss by delivery mode was evident in 6 hours and persisted over time. Only 5% of vaginally delivered infants and more than

TABLE 8-2	Percentage of Women Reporting Symptoms of Milk Ejection With Significant Difference Between Successful and Unsuccessful Breastfeeders			
Symptoms	Successful Breastfeeders (%)	Unsuccessful Breastfeeders (%)	Probability (p)
Uterine pain (cramps) during suckling: day 2	64	38	<0.05
Dripping from opposite breast during suckling: day 6	95	67	<0.01
Dripping before suckling (as oxytocin is triggered by sight or expectation of baby or other times): day 5	78	56	<0.05
Cessation of nipple pain (as milk flow counteracts negative pressure produced by suckling)			
Day 4	89	69	<0.05
Day 5	89	69	<0.01
Day 6	89	69	<0.05
All symptoms: all days	59	48	<0.01

From Newton N: The quantitative effect of oxytocin (Pitocin) on human milk yield, *Ann NY Acad Sci* 652:484, 1992.

10% of C-section–delivered infants had lost more than 10% of their birth weight in 48 hours. The nomograms from this study are seen in Figure 8-22 and can be used for early identification of neonates on a trajectory for greater weight loss and possible morbidities.

Breastfeeding duration and weight gain trajectory in infants who were followed with weight and length measurements ($n = 595$) were noted to have short breastfeeding periods. The authors developed an obesity risk index, which included maternal BMI, education, and smoking during

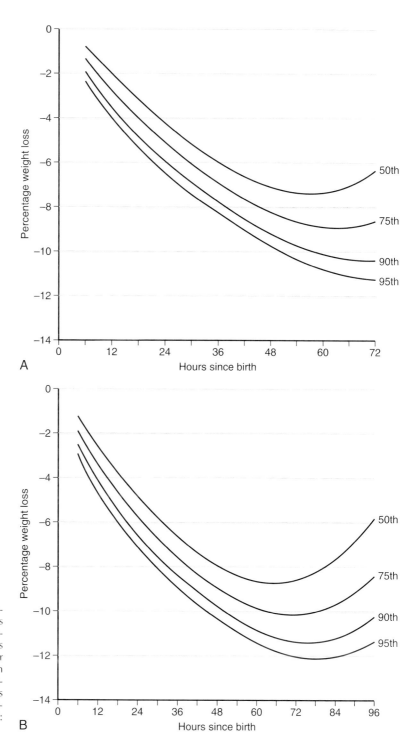

Figure 8-22. A, Estimated percentile curves of percent weight loss by time after birth for vaginal deliveries. **B,** Estimated percentile curves of percent weight loss by time after birth for cesarean deliveries. (From Flaherman VJ, Scharfer EW, Kuzniewicz MW, et al.: Early weight loss nomograms for exclusively breastfeeding newborns, *Pediatrics* 135(1): e16–e23, 2015, Figure 2.)

maternal behavior at the appropriate time and plays a significant role in sustaining maternal behavior during lactation.[96]

The milk-ejection reflex can be at least partially blocked by large amounts of alcohol, which seems to have a central effect preventing the release of oxytocin, because the mammary gland and uterine response to injected oxytocin are not changed by alcohol. Studies on mothers with diabetes insipidus suggest that the patient retains the ability to synthesize and release oxytocin despite being unable to produce antidiuretic hormone (ADH, vasopressin) in response to stimuli. Artificial cervical dilatation postpartum will also cause milk ejection. Vaginal stimulus also initiates let-down in all species.

Injection of oxytocin reproduces the effect of suckling. A rapid series of injections of 1 to 10 mU IV will simulate suckling. A continuous drip is less effective. Use of Pitocin as a snuff or nasal spray is the best method for home use of oxytocin to initiate let-down. The oxytocin concentration in the blood rises with suckling, which supports the hypothesis that suckling elicits the release of oxytocin.

The data on the question of ADH release during suckling are contradictory, but it would seem that release of oxytocin and of ADH are independent.

In the first weeks of lactation, the threshold dose of oxytocin to cause let-down is low, averaging 0.65 mU from the fifth day (see Figure 8-23). Thirty days after weaning, it is 100 mU. Vasopressin is not as effective and requires 100 times the dosage of oxytocin to produce the same effect during lactation. Deaminooxytocin is 1.5 times as potent as oxytocin on the third postpartum day, but the difference disappears over time, probably because of the rapid breakdown of natural oxytocin by oxytocinase early in the postpartum period.

An objective assessment of milk ejection can be obtained by using ultrasound as described by Hartmann and Prosser.[45] The diameter of the milk ducts just below the nipple area can be visualized. In mothers who carried to term, there is an acute increase in milk duct diameter in the free breast while the infant feeds from the other (Figure 8-25). The same is true if one breast is pumped. The visualization of the increase in diameter, Hartmann and Prosser indicate, is positive evidence of the effect and the let-down reflex.[45]

Prostaglandins (PGs) have been shown to have a number of physiologic effects, including an effect on mammary epithelium to increase mammary duct pressure. In a blinded crossover study, oxytocin, IV PG, and nasal PG were given and the intraductal pressures measured. The most effective IV PGs were 16-phenoxy-PGE2 and PGF2α, which were then tried nasally, but only PGF2α was effective nasally. The potential of nasal PGF2α treatment in engorgement and failure of let-down is possible but is as yet unexplored clinically.[16]

PRACTICAL ASPECTS OF MILK-EJECTION REFLEX

When the nipple is stimulated, the receptors in the nipple and areola are stimulated, and nervous impulses are transmitted to the hypothalamus via the somatic afferent nerves.[130] The hypothalamus stimulates the pituitary gland to secrete prolactin, which induces the alveoli in the breast to produce and secrete milk. The cell membranes release fat globules and protein into the lumen. This produces the hind milk, which has a higher protein and fat content. Part of the foremilk has been present since the previous nursing and is released first. It is a more dilute, less fatty solution. The ejection reflex induces the holocrine excretion of milk from the cells. The posterior pituitary gland secretes oxytocin, which stimulates the myoepithelial cells to contract and eject the milk from the ducts.[131]

Early in lactation, if engorgement is marked, the ejection reflex may be inhibited by the congested blood flow to the target organ, the myoepithelial cell. Therefore, when suckling is initiated and oxytocin is released into the bloodstream, the ejection

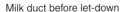

Milk duct before let-down   Milk duct after let-down

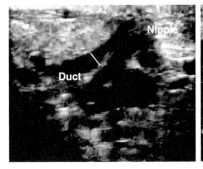
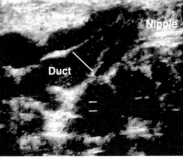

Figure 8-25. Ultrasonography of breast before *(left)* and during *(right)* let-down, demonstrating the filling of the duct system with milk. Before milk ejection the ducts near the nipple are 2 to 8 mm in basal diameter. (Courtesy Peter Hartmann, PhD, University of Western Australia, Perth, Australia.)

TABLE 8-3	Milk-Ejection Reflex*
Maternal Disturbance	**Mean Amount of Milk Obtained by Infant (g)**
No distractions (no injection)	168
Distraction (saline injection)	99
Distraction (oxytocin injection)	153

*Interrupted milk flow can be restarted with hormone injection.
Modified from Newton M, Newton N: The let-down reflex in human lactation, *J Pediatr* 91:1, 1977.

reflex message is delayed in reaching the myoepithelial cell with the message because of vascular congestion. Preparing the breast with warm soaks, gentle massage, and manual expression of a little milk may facilitate let-down.

Newton[87] studied the milk-ejection reflex and clearly showed the effect of distraction on the let-down reflex. In the clinical experiment, distractions included immersing feet in ice water (reported to be the worst); being asked mathematic questions in rapid series, which resulted in an electric shock if a wrong answer was given; or having painful traction on the big toe (Table 8-3). In practice, pain, stress, and mental anguish interfere with let-down in some mothers. When simple adjustments such as making the mother more comfortable, playing soft music or leaving the mother in a quiet room do not work, other techniques should be tried.

Gentle stroking of the breast may help to decrease anxiety and stimulate flow. Use of tactile warmth as opposed to cold may improve release. Ice should not be used to make the nipple erect because it interferes with let-down. Cold is known to interrupt the neuropathway and cause vasoconstriction.[88] Hyperactive let down can produce such a flood of milk that the infant is overwhelmed and often chokes and coughs. This overactivity occurs in the early days of lactation and gradually diminishes. The best approach is to have mother express and save the first 5 to 10 mL of milk before putting the infant to the breast. The expressed milk can be frozen for later use. If the second breast is exposed when the infant latches on, it too will let down and then will be defused when the infant attempts to latch on.

Excessive milk supply is more common in primiparas and is characterized by continued dripping between feedings, excessive amounts released during a feeding, and let-down at the slightest stimulus. Treatment is a firm, well-constructed brassiere. If necessary, a Velcro binder and cool packs can be applied between feedings. Dripping between feedings can be reduced by folding the nipple over before applying the breast pads. If it persists beyond 2 to 3 weeks, the mother should be evaluated for hyperprolactinemia or hyperthyroid or hypothyroid state (see Chapter 3).

A rapid computerized breast measurement system has been developed by Hartmann and his laboratory[45] for the determination of breast volume. Using patterns of 64 horizontal light stripes (moiré topography) projected onto the breast and chest wall allowed the calculation of volume by a digitalized camera image analysis (Figure 8-26). The technique was verified by before and after test weighing of both the infant and the mother. Using this technology, they have been able to measure the amount of milk present, the storage capacity, and the amount of milk removed.

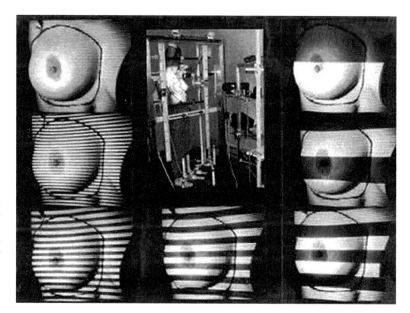

Figure 8-26. The computerized breast measurement system. Mother is positioned in the ultrasound machine. The breast images demonstrate the use of moiré patterning to measure change in breast volumes. (Courtesy Peter Hartmann, PhD, University of Western Australia, Perth, Australia.)

SOLID FOODS

Successful nursing mothers are rarely as impatient to start the baby on solid foods as mothers who bottle-fed frequently are. Milk, and especially human milk, supplies the appropriate nutrients. At approximately 6 months, a normal infant begins to deplete iron stores. This is probably an appropriate time to start solid foods, especially iron-containing ones. This permits the entire process of weaning to cup and solid foods to be gradual. An infant does not need teeth to eat baby food and, conversely, does not have to be weaned from the breast because teeth have erupted. By 6 months, the number of feedings usually decreases. The timing and volume begin to cycle to a schedule that resembles three meals per day and some snacks.

EXCLUSIVE BREASTFEEDING FOR 6 MONTHS

There is no objective evidence that solids are needed before 6 months, according to a WHO/UNICEF meta-analysis.[65] Solids do not solve any problems. A reduced morbidity rate due to GI infections was observed in infants breastfed exclusively for 6 months or more and no observable deficits in growth. No benefits of introducing solids between 4 and 6 months have been identified, except for iron needs in special infants, which are best treated by iron drops. A breastfed infant usually starts some solids by 6 months of age.[65]

CARRYING AND HOLDING

Carrying and holding young infants have been considered by some, in the era of peak bottle feeding, as predisposing to spoiling the infants. In many cultures around the world, infants are carried with the mother night and day.[77] In Western cultures, infants are tightly swaddled, that is, wrapped up like a package and put down. In a randomized controlled study of primiparous breastfeeding women, Hunziker and Barr[56] showed that increased carrying reduces infant crying and colicky behavior. Conversely, they showed that lack of carrying predisposes to crying and colic.

SLEEPING

Sleeping through the night has been assumed to be an important developmental milestone dependent on maturation. First-time parents ($n = 26$) of exclusively breastfed infants were randomly assigned to a treatment or control group.[97] The treatment group was instructed to offer a "focal feed" between 10 PM and midnight and then offer reswaddling, diapering, walking, and rocking to postpone the next feeding to 5 AM, minimizing light and sound. By 3 weeks, the treatment group was sleeping significantly longer. By 8 weeks, 100% of the treated group, compared with 23% of control infants, was sleeping at least from midnight to 5 AM. They fed more frequently during the day, especially early morning. Milk intakes for 24 hours between the two groups were not different. Pinilla and Birch[97] concluded that parents can teach their breastfed infants to lengthen nighttime sleep periods. Parents should be encouraged to develop management plans that they find most comfortable. Whether they share the family bed or keep the newborn in the same room or in the next room is their decision. Continuing night feeds is associated with longer duration of breastfeeding and more abundant milk supply.

Milk composition influences infant sleep latency. Tryptophan concentrations are higher in human milk than in formula. Tryptophan is known to increase sleep in adults. When breastfed and formula-fed infants were compared using formulas with different levels of tryptophan, they had shorter sleep latency with high levels of tryptophan.[125] In a survey of new mothers nationally, almost one in five mothers (18%) indicated that their infant always slept in bed with them in the first 6 months; 10% more reported the infant often did, and 16% said they sometimes did. Thirty-six percent of black non-Hispanic women reported always, but 30% of Hispanic mothers, and only 12% of white mothers, reported always sleeping with their baby. The AAP has spoken out against co-sleeping and has launched a vigorous campaign against co-sleeping. The ABM has developed a protocol regarding the issue.

In the report by Hauck et al.,[47] the main reasons for bed-sharing were to calm a fussy baby, facilitate breastfeeding, and help both mother and infant sleep better. The rates of bed sharing were 42% at 2 weeks, 34% at 3 months, and 27% at 12 months. Failure to comply with supine sleeping arrangements at night was 26% at 3 months, 29% at 6 months, and 36% at a year. Non-Hispanic black mothers were more likely to use nonsupine positions and to bed share. SIDS was not included in the report.

Colic and Crying

By definition, colic is spasmodic contractions of smooth muscle causing pain and discomfort. It can be experienced in many organs, such as the GI or genitourinary tract, and at all ages. When the term *colic* is used in reference to infants, it usually means a syndrome in which a young infant has unexplained paroxysms of irritability, fussing, and crying for a prolonged period, often at the same time of day, in the early months of life. The infant usually draws the legs up as if in pain. A myriad of remedies are directed at various possible causes, including allergy, hypertonicity, and hormone withdrawal. However, it may be a matter of parenting style and expectations that brings a parent to complain about colic. Colic does occur in premature infants but usually not until they reach 42 weeks' adjusted gestation.[49]

Infantile colic has been reported to occur equally among breastfed (20%), formula-fed (19%), and mixed breastfed and formula-fed (21%) infants in a study of almost 1000 infants.[1] Fecal α-antitrypsin and fecal hemoglobins were not different in colicky infants. The series had no evidence of dietary protein hypersensitivity.[129] Lactose as a cause of colic has also been ruled out in several studies.[72]

Characteristically, an infant will cry and scream as if in pain from 3 to 4 hours at a stretch, often between 6 and 10 PM. The infant will nurse frequently and then scream and pull away from the breast as if in pain, only to cry a few minutes later. Sometimes the infant can be comforted by another adult such as the father or grandmother. The infant will respond to gentle rocking when held against a warm shoulder. If the infant is put down, the screaming starts again. If the nursing mother holds the infant, the infant is frantic unless nursed and yet does not need to be fed. This may disturb a new mother, who wonders why she cannot console her infant (Is her milk weak? Does it disagree with her infant? Is she an inadequate mother?). None of these is true, but smelling the mother's milk makes the infant behave as if it needs to nurse. Anyone who is not nursing can quickly quiet the infant. Picking up the infant does not spoil the child, and rocking and cuddling are appropriate. Warm pressure is usually palliative; a warm hot water bottle or warm shoulder with some pressure or massage is comforting. The use of rhythmic incessant sounds or lights (e.g., vacuum cleaner, TV out of focus so it is a changing pattern) has variable success.

A carefully taken history and physical examination are always in order to rule out other pathologic conditions, such as otitis media, anal fissure, hair tourniquet, or hernia before a diagnosis of colic is made. Hunger should be ruled out. Sometimes an infant who was just fed needs to be fed again. True colic, however, is characterized by an inconsolable infant who continues to fret, fuss, and cry. If true colic is diagnosed because of the consistency of the screaming for several hours each day at the same time, treatment is in order.[61]

INFLUENCE OF COW MILK IN MATERNAL DIET

The literature is not straightforward on the issue of the effect of cow milk in the maternal diet and infantile colic. Information was first published on congenital sensitization to food, especially eggs and cow milk, in humans in the early twentieth century, which was manifested as clinical allergy in breastfed infants. Research techniques are far superior today, and information is accumulating. Gerrard and Shenassa[41] report sensitization caused by substances in breast milk thought to be due to two types of food allergies one is immunoglobulin E (IgE) mediated and triggered by trace amounts of antigen, and the other is not IgE mediated and is triggered by large amounts of antigen. GI transport of macromolecules in the pathogenesis of food allergy is under investigation, as is T-cell-mediated immunity in food allergy. However, the present state of scientific knowledge has not resolved the issue of colic and cow milk for clinicians.

Clinical studies have been done to test the association of dairy products in mothers who breastfed and their babies with colic. Jakobsson and Lindberg[58] described a cause-and-effect relationship in a group of 18 mothers, which was criticized because it was not a double-blind study. Evans et al.[34,35] then reported that they found no such relationship when they did a double-blind crossover study in which mothers received cow milk protein for 2 days and then a placebo for 2 days. Jakobsson and Lindberg[59] repeated their work using a double-blind crossover study design in the mother-baby pairs in which the infants had colic; 35% of the infants improved on maternal diets free of cow milk. A torrent of mail to the journals confirmed these conclusions in small clinical practice trials as well.

Jakobsson et al.[60] found bovine β-lactoglobulin in the milk of 18 of 38 mothers chosen at random. Three mothers had high amounts, and their infants had colic that was relieved by a maternal diet free of bovine milk products. Dietary modification with a low-allergen diet should be considered in the mothers of healthy breastfed infants with colic, according to Hill et al.,[50] who reported a community-based study. They also restricted the diet by eliminating artificial color, preservatives, and milk, eggs, wheat, and nuts.[50]

Colic has been investigated in breastfed and formula-fed infants by measuring breath hydrogen (H_2) production, a product of lactose metabolism.[82] H_2 levels were significantly higher at both 6 weeks and 3 months of age in infants who developed colic. The authors suggest that increased lactose malabsorption may be related to colic. Studies that used lactase to minimize the effect of

45. Hartmann PE, Prosser CG: Physiological basis of longitudinal changes in human milk yield and composition, *Fed Proc* 43:2450, 1984.

46. Hauben DJ, Mahler D: A simple method for the correction of the inverted nipple, *Plast Reconstr Surg* 71:556, 1983.

47. Hauck FR, Signore C, Fein SB, et al: Infant sleeping arrangements and practices during the first year of life, *Pediatrics* 122:S113–S120, 2008.

48. Heck LJ, Erenberg A: Serum glucose levels in term neonates during the first 48 hours of life, *J Pediatr* 110:119, 1987.

49. Hide DW, Guyer BM: Prevalence of infant colic, *Arch Dis Child* 57:559, 1982.

50. Hill DJ, Hudson IL, Sheffield LJ, et al: A low allergen diet is a significant intervention in infantile colic: results of a community-based study, *J Allergy Clin Immunol* 96:886, 1995.

51. Hill PD, Humenick SS: The occurrence of breast engorgement, *J Hum Lact* 10:79, 1994.

52. Hoffman JB: A suggested treatment for inverted nipples, *Am J Obstet Gynecol* 66:346, 1953.

53. Howard CR, Howard FM, Lanphear B, et al: A randomized clinical trial of pacifier use and bottle or cup feeding and their effect on breastfeeding, *Pediatrics* 111:511, 2003.

54. Howie PW, McNeilly AS, McArdle T, et al: The relationship between suckling-induced prolactin response and lactogenesis, *J Clin Endocrinol Metab* 50:670, 1980.

55. Humenick SS, Hill PD, Anderson MA: Breast engorgement: patterns and selected outcomes, *J Hum Lact* 10:87, 1994.

56. Hunziker UA, Barr RG: Increased carrying reduces infant crying: a randomized controlled trial, *Pediatrics* 77:641, 1986.

57. Jain E: Tongue-tie (ankyloglossia). Presented at first annual international meeting, Academy of Breastfeeding Medicine: physicians and breastfeeding—a new alliance, Rochester, NY, 1996.

58. Jakobsson I, Lindberg T: Cow's milk as a cause of infantile colic in breast-fed infants, *Lancet* 2:437, 1978.

59. Jakobsson I, Lindberg T: Cow's milk proteins cause infantile colic in breast-fed infants: a double-blind crossover study, *Pediatrics* 71:268, 1983.

60. Jakobsson I, Lindberg T, Benediksson B, et al: Dietary bovine β-lactoglobulin is transferred to human milk, *Acta Paediatr Scand* 74:342, 1985.

61. Karp H: *The happiest baby on the block: the new way to calm crying and help your newborn baby sleep longer*, New York, 2003, Bantam.

62. Kent JC, Mitoulas LR, Cregan MD, et al: Volume and frequency of breastfeeding and fat content of breast milk throughout the day, *Pediatrics* 117:e387–e395, 2006.

63. Klaus MH: The frequency of suckling, *Obstet Gynecol Clin North Am* 14:623, 1987.

64. Klaus MH, Kennell JH: The doula: an essential ingredient of childbirth rediscovered, *Acta Paediatr* 86:1034, 1997.

65. Kramer MS, Kakuma R: *The optimal duration of exclusive breastfeeding: a systematic review*, Geneva, 2002, World Health Organization, Department of Nutrition for Health and Development. www.NCBI.NLM.NIHI/gov/pubmed/22895934.

66. Kurinij N, Shiono PH: Early formula supplementation of breastfeeding, *Pediatrics* 88:745, 1991.

67. Kuyper E, Vitta B, Dewey K: Implications of cesarean delivery for breastfeeding outcomes and strategies to support breastfeeding, 52(6):556–563, 2007.

68. Labarere J, Gelbert-Baudino N, Ayral A-S, et al: Efficacy of breastfeeding support provided by trained clinicians during an early, routine, preventive visit: a prospective, randomized, open trial of 226 mother-infant pairs, *Pediatrics* 115(2):e139–e146, 2005.

69. Laborde L, Gelbert-Baudino N, Fulcher J, et al: Breastfeeding outcomes for mothers with and without home access to e-technologies, *Acta Paediatr* 96:1071–1075, 2007.

70. Lavergne NA: Does application of tea bags to sore nipples while breastfeeding provide effective relief, *J Obstet Gynecol Neonatal Nurs* 26:53, 1997.

71. L'Esperance CM: Pain or pleasure: the dilemma of early breastfeeding, *Birth Fam J* 7:21, 1980.

72. Liebman WM: Infantile Colic Association with lactose and milk intolerance, *JAMA* 245:732–733, 1981.

73. Lipitz S, Barkai G, Rabinovici J, et al: Breast stimulation test and oxytocin challenge test in fetal surveillance: a prospective randomized study, *Am J Obstet Gynecol* 157:1178, 1987.

74. Loftus JR, Hill H, Cohen SF: Placental transfer and neonatal effects of epidural sufentanil and fentanyl administered with bupivacaine during labor, *Anesthesiology* 83:300, 1995.

75. Lothe L, Ivarsson S-A, Ekman R, et al: Motilin and infantile colic, *Acta Paediatr Scand* 79:410, 1990.

76. Lust KD, Brown JE, Thomas W: Maternal intake of cruciferous vegetables and other foods and colic symptoms in exclusively breast-fed infants, *J Am Diet Assoc* 96:47, 1996.

77. Maekawa K, Nara T, Hoashi E: Influence of breastfeeding on neonatal behavior, *Acta Paediatr Jpn* 27:608, 1985.

78. Marshall WM, Cumming DC, Fitzsimmons GW: Hot flushes during breastfeeding? *Fertil Steril* 57:1349, 1992.

79. Mashini IS, Devoe LD, McKenzie JS, et al: Comparison of uterine activity induced by nipple stimulation and oxytocin, *Obstet Gynecol* 69:74, 1987.

80. Millard AV: The place of the clock in pediatric advice: rationales, cultural themes, and impediments to breastfeeding, *Soc Sci Med* 31:211, 1990.

81. Miller AR, Barr RG: Infantile colic: is it a gut issue? *Pediatr Clin North Am* 38:1407, 1991.

82. Moore DJ, Robb TA, Davidson GP: Breath hydrogen response to milk containing lactose in colicky and non-colicky infants, *J Pediatr* 113:979, 1988.

83. Neifert MR: Prevention of breastfeeding tragedies, *Pediatr Clin North Am* 48:273, 2001.

84. Neifert MR, Seacat JM: A guide to successful breastfeeding, *Contemp Pediatr* 3:16, 1986.

85. Newton N: Nipple pain and nipple damage: problems in the management of breast feeding, *J Pediatr* 41:411, 1952.

86. Newton N: The quantitative effect of oxytocin (Pitocin) on human milk yield, *Ann NY Acad Sci* 652:481, 1992.

87. Newton N: The relation of the milk-ejection reflex to the ability to breastfeed, *Ann NY Acad Sci* 652:484, 1992.

88. Newton M, Newton NR: The let-down reflex in human lactation, *J Pediatr* 33:698, 1948.

89. Nikodem VC, Danziger D, Gebka N, et al: Do cabbage leaves prevent breast engorgement? A randomized controlled study, *Birth* 20:61, 1993.

90. Nissen E, Lilja G, Widström A-M, et al: Elevation of oxytocin levels early postpartum in women, *Acta Obstet Gynecol Scand* 74:530, 1995.

91. Notestine GE: The importance of the identification of ankyloglossia (short lingual frenulum) as a cause of breastfeeding problems, *J Hum Lact* 6:113, 1990.

92. Nysenbaum AN, Smart JL: Sucking behavior and milk intake of neonates in relation to milk fat content, *Early Hum Dev* 6:205, 1982.

93. O'Connor NR, Tanabe KO, Siadaty MS, et al: Pacifiers and breastfeeding: a systematic review, *Arch Pediatr Adolesc Med* 163(4):378–382, 2009.

94. Parker SJ, Barrett DE: Maternal type A behavior during pregnancy, neonatal crying and early infant temperament: do type A women have type A babies? *Pediatrics* 89:474, 1992.

95. Paul K, Dittrichová J, Papousek H: Infant feeding behavior: development in pattern and motivation, *Dev Psychobiol* 29:563, 1996.

96. Pedersen CA: Oxytocin control of maternal behavior: regulation by sex steroids and offspring stimuli, *Ann NY Acad Sci* 807:126, 1997.

97. Pinilla T, Birch LL: Help me make it through the night: behavioral entrainment of breastfed infants' sleep patterns, *Pediatrics* 91:436, 1993.

98. Pollitt E, Consolazio B, Goodkin F: Changes in nutritive sucking during a feed in two-day and thirty-day-old infants, *Early Hum Dev* 5:201, 1981.

99. Prentice A, Addey CV, Wilde CJ: Evidence for local feedback control of human milk secretion, *Biochem Soc Trans* 17:489, 1989.

100. Protocol Committee Academy: Breastfeeding medicine protocol #5—peripartum breastfeeding management for the healthy mother and infant at term. *Breastfeeding Med* 3(2):129–132, 2008. Available www.abm.com.

101. Protocol Committee Academy Breastfeeding Medicine: Protocol #7 model breastfeeding policy, *Breastfeed Med* 1:50, 2007.

102. Ramsay DT, Kent JC, Owens RA: Ultrasound imaging of milk ejection in the breast of lactating women, *Pediatrics* 113:361, 2004.

103. Ramsey DT, Kent JC, Owens RA, et al: Ultrasound imaging of the lactating breast redefined with ultrasound imaging, *J Anatomy* 206:525–534, 2005.

104. Raphael D: *The tender gift: breast feeding*, New York, 1976, Schocken.

105. Rayner CR: The correction of permanently inverted nipples, *Br J Plast Surg* 33:413, 1980.

106. Reiff MI, Essock-Vitale SM: Hospital influences on early infant-feeding practices, *Pediatrics* 76:872, 1985.

107. Renfrew MJ, McCandish R: With women: new steps in research in midwifery. In Roberts H, editor: *Women's health matters*, London, 1992, Routledge.

108. National Center for Education in Maternal and Child Health: *Report of the second surgeon general's workshop on breastfeeding and human lactation*, Washington, D.C., 1991, National Center for Education in Maternal and Child Health.

109. Righard L: Are breastfeeding problems related to incorrect breastfeeding technique and the use of pacifiers and bottles? *Birth* 25:40, 1998.

110. Righard L, Alade MO: Effect of delivery room routine on success of first breastfeed, *Lancet* 336:1105, 1990.

111. Righard L, Alade MO: Sucking technique and its effect on success of breastfeeding, *Birth* 19:185, 1992.

112. Righard L, Flodmark C-E, Lothe L, et al: Breastfeeding patterns: single and two-breast principles vis à vis infant behavior, *Birth* 20:182, 1993.

113. Robert KL: A comparison of chilled cabbage leaves and chilled gelpaks in reducing breast engorgement, *J Hum Lact* 11:11, 1995.

114. Rosen AR, Lawrence RA: The effect of epidural anesthesia on infant feeding, *J Univ Roch Med Ctr* 6(1):3, 1994.

115. Rosier W: Cool cabbage compresses, *Breastfeed Rev* 12:28, 1988.

116. Saadeh R: Major findings and priority actions of the WHO scientific review and technical consultation on nutrition and HIV/AIDS in Africa. In *International Congress of Nutrition*, Durban, South Africa, August 2005.

117. Sakalidis VS, Williams TM, Hepworth AR, et al: A comparison of early sucking dynamics during breastfeeding after cesarean section and virginal birth, *Breastfeed Med* 8(1):79–85, 2013.

118. Salisbury DM: Bottle-feeding: influence of teat hole size on suck volume, *Lancet* 1:655, 1975.

119. Schubiger G, Schwarz U, Tönz O, et al: UNICEF/WHO baby friendly hospital initiative: does the use of bottles and pacifiers in the neonatal nursery prevent successful breastfeeding? *Eur J Pediatr* 156:874, 1997.

120. Schutzman DL, Hervada AR, Branca PA: Effect of water supplementation of full-term newborns on arrival of milk in the nursing mother, *Clin Pediatr* 25:78, 1986.

121. Section of Breastfeeding American Academy Pediatrics: Breastfeeding and the use of human milk, *Pediatrics* 115(2):496–506, 2005.

122. Sharp DA: Moist wound healing for sore or cracked nipples, *Breastfeed Abstr* 12(2):19, 1992.

123. Smith WL, Erenberg A, Nowak A: Imaging evaluation of the human nipple during breastfeeding, *Am J Dis Child* 142:76, 1988.

124. Ståhlberg M-R, Savilahti E: Infantile colic and feeding, *Arch Dis Child* 61:1232, 1986.

125. Steinberg LA, O'Connell NC, Hatch TF, et al: Tryptophan intake influences infants' sleep latency, *J Nutr* 122:1781, 1992.

126. St. James-Roberts I: Persistent infant crying, *Arch Dis Child* 66:653, 1991.

127. Süsswein J: Zur Physiologie des Trinkens beim Säugling, *Arch Kinderheilkd* 40:68, 1905.

128. Taylor RN, Green JR: Abruption placentae following nipple stimulation, *Am J Perinatol* 4:94, 1987.

129. Thomas DW, McGilligan K, Eisenberg LD, et al: Infantile colic and type of milk feeding, *Am J Dis Child* 141:451, 1987.

130. Uvnäs-Moberg KU: *The oxytocin factor*, Cambridge, Mass., 2003, DaCapo Press.

131. Uvnäs-Moberg K, Widström A-M, Werner S, et al: Oxytocin and prolactin levels in breastfeeding women, *Acta Obstet Gynecol Scand* 69:301, 1990.

132. van Gelderen WF, Goosen A: Mammographic features of unilateral breastfeeding, *Clin Radiol* 5:134, 1996.

133. Vestermark V, Hogdall CK, Birch M, et al: Influence of the mode of delivery on initiation of breastfeeding, *Eur J Obstet Gynecol Reprod Biol* 38:33, 1990.

134. Victora CG, Behague DP, Barros FC, et al: Pacifier use and short breastfeeding duration: cause, consequence or coincidence? *Pediatrics* 99:445, 1997.

135. Victora CG, Tomasi E, Olinto MTA, et al: Use of pacifiers and breastfeeding duration, *Lancet* 341:404, 1993.

136. Waldenstrom U, Sundelin C, Lindmark G: Early and late discharge after hospital birth: breastfeeding, *Acta Paediatr Scand* 76:727, 1987.

137. Weber F, Woolridge MW, Baum JD: An ultrasonographic study of the organization of sucking and swallowing by newborn infants, *Dev Med Child Neurol* 28:19, 1986.

138. Weitzmen RE, Leake RD, Rubin RT, et al: The effect of nursing on neurohypophyseal hormone and prolactin secretion in human subjects, *J Clin Endocrinol Metab* 51:836, 1980.

139. Weizman Z, Alkrinawi S, Goldfarb D, et al: Efficacy of herbal tea preparation in infantile colic, *J Pediatr* 122:650, 1993.

140. Whitfield MF, Kay R, Stevens S: Validity of routine clinical test weighing as a measure of the intake of breast-fed infants, *Arch Dis Child* 56:919, 1981.

141. Widström A-M, Thingström-Paulsson J: The position of the tongue during rooting reflexes elicited in newborn infants before the first suckles, *Acta Paediatr* 82:281, 1993.

142. Widström A-M, Wahlberg V, Matthiesen A-S, et al: Short-term effects of early suckling and touch of the nipple on maternal behavior, *Early Hum Dev* 21:153, 1990.

143. Wight NE: Management of common breastfeeding issues. Breastfeeding 2001. Part I: the evidence for breastfeeding, *Pediatr Clin North Am* 48(2001):321, 2001.

144. Win NN, Binns CW, Zhao Y, et al: Breastfeeding duration in mothers who express breast milk: a cohort study, *Int Breastfeed J* 1:28, 2006.

145. Wolff PH: The serial organization of sucking in the young infant, *Pediatrics* 42:943, 1968.

146. Woolridge MW: Aetiology of sore nipples, *Midwifery* 2:172, 1986.

147. Woolridge MW: The "anatomy" of infant sucking, *Midwifery* 2:164, 1986.

148. Woolridge MW, Baum JD: Recent advances in breastfeeding, *Acta Paediatr Jpn* 35:1, 1993.

149. Woolridge MW, Fisher C: Colic, "overfeeding," and symptoms of lactose malabsorption in the breast-fed baby: a possible artifact of feed management, *Lancet* 2:382, 1988.

150. Woolridge MW, Ingram JC, Baum JD: Do changes in pattern of breast usage alter the baby's nutrient intake? *Lancet* 336:395, 1990.

151. Work Group on Breastfeeding: American Academy of Pediatrics: breastfeeding and the use of human milk, *Pediatrics* 100:1035, 1997.

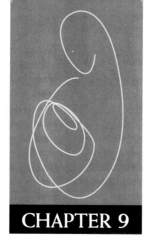

CHAPTER 9

Maternal Nutrition and Supplements for Mother and Infant

Lactation is the physiologic completion of the reproductive cycle. The maternal body prepares during pregnancy for lactation, not only by developing the breast to produce milk but also by storing additional nutrients and energy for milk production. The transition to fully sustaining an infant should not be complex or require major adjustments for a woman. After delivery, mothers usually note an increase in appetite and thirst and a change in some dietary preferences. In some cultures, anthropologists have noted that, traditionally, the birth of a baby means that members of the community take gifts of special foods—usually high in protein, nutrients, and calories—for the mother to ensure she will make good milk for the infant. This tradition may have affected some early studies in which relatively malnourished women were noted to produce milk comparable with that produced by well-nourished women in industrialized countries.

After an exhaustive study of the world's literature and current scientific evidence, the Subcommittee on Nutrition During Lactation of the Committee on Nutritional Status During Pregnancy and Lactation of the Food and Nutrition Board of the Institute of Medicine at the National Academy of Sciences[112] published its first report. The subcommittee stated that breastfeeding is recommended for all infants in the United States under ordinary circumstances. Women living in a wide variety of circumstances in the United States and elsewhere are capable of fully nourishing their infants by breastfeeding them. Furthermore, exclusive breastfeeding is preferred for the first 4 to 6 months. The report further stated that mothers with less than perfect diets could make good milk.

The overwhelming evidence indicates that women are able to "produce milk of sufficient quantity and quality to support growth and promote the health of infants—even when the mother's supply of nutrients is limited." Nonetheless, the depletion of the mother's nutrient stores is a risk if efforts to achieve adequate food intake are not made to replace maternal stores.

Most material for nursing mothers regarding maternal diet during lactation set up complicated "rules" about dietary intake that fail to consider the mother's dietary stores, normal dietary preferences, and cultural patterns. Thus, one barrier to breastfeeding for some women is the "diet rules" they see as being too hard to follow or too restrictive.[40] All over the world, women produce adequate and even abundant milk on inadequate diets. Women in cultures with modest but adequate diets produce milk without any obvious detriment to themselves and with none of the fatigue and loss of well-being that some well-fed Western mothers experience. Insufficient milk is a problem in Western cultures and rarely in developing countries.

Impact of Maternal Diet on Milk Production

Although much has been learned about dietary requirements for lactation by studying women from many cultures and various levels of poor nutrition, some of the information is conflicting, principally because of varying sampling techniques and the improvement over time in laboratory analysis. Extensive reviews of the current literature on various nutrients in human milk and the influence of maternal dietary intake have been referenced.* Those readers needing access to the original studies are referred to the bibliographies from these reviews, which include hundreds of items, a listing beyond the scope of this text.

MILK VOLUME

The volume of milk produced varies over the duration of lactation from the first few weeks to 6 months and beyond but is remarkably predictable except during extreme malnutrition or severe dehydration. In periods of acute water deprivation, manifested in a healthy mother by an acute bout of vomiting and diarrhea, the volume of milk will diminish only after the maternal urine output has been significantly compromised (10% dehydration).

Malnutrition, however, is complex, and single-nutrient deficiencies are rare. Malnutrition does seem to have an effect on the total volume of milk produced. In the extreme, when famine occurs, the milk supply dwindles and ceases, with ultimate starvation of the infant. The classic study is the report of Smith[105] on the effects of maternal undernutrition on the newborn infant in the Hunger Winter in Holland in 1944 to 1945. It was reported that the volume of milk was slightly diminished, but the duration of lactation was not affected. The latter is a testimony to courage rather than diet. Analysis of milk produced showed no significant deviations from normal chemical structure. Milk was produced at the expense of maternal tissue.

These data from the Dutch famine in the 1940s during World War II were reexamined by Stein et al.,[109] who pointed out that women who conceived during the famine did develop some maternal stores in anticipation of lactation that were not accounted for by the fetus, placenta, or amniotic fluid, even though the fetus was a pound lighter at birth. They reported fetal weight down by 10% but maternal weight down by only 4%. This demonstrates the maternal body's strong biologic commitment to preparing for lactation during pregnancy.

There is a wide range of volume of milk intake among healthy breastfed infants, averaging 750 to 800 g/day and ranging from 450 to 1200 g/day.[13] Any factor that influences the frequency, intensity, or duration of suckling by an infant influences the volume.[85] In a study of wet nurses in the 1920s, Macy et al.[75] reported human capacity at 3500 mL/day. Compared with the 800 mL from mothers with singletons, studies of mothers producing for multiples, done by Saint et al., confirmed production of 2 to 3 L/day for twins and triplets. At 3 months of age for all populations, the volume averages 770 g/day (range 500 to 1200 g/day).[61,88] The self-regulation of milk supply by the infant has been confirmed by a study by Dewey et al.[29] in which additional milk was pumped after each feeding for 2 weeks, thus increasing the milk supply. The infants, however, remained at baseline consumption during the pumping. The residual milk supply of healthy women (i.e., that which can be extracted after a full feeding) is about 100 g/day, even when an infant consumes comparatively low volumes of milk.[29,84,86]

Topographic computer imaging has been used to study breast production and storage capacities in the laboratory of Hartmann. Using moiré patterns projected onto the breast, it has been possible to calculate the volume of milk produced. As the breast expands with increasing milk, the moiré patterns change. By correlating the maternal weights before and after a feeding and the imagery patterns, data were converted to accurate milk volumes. This technique has remarkable potential for clinical use. Hartmann reports the normal range of milk production from 1 to 6 months postpartum to be between 440 and 1220 g/day for mothers who gave birth at full term.

Prentice and Prentice[99] described "energy sparing adaptations" that were associated with normal lactation when energy intake is limited. These were decreases in basal metabolic rate, thermogenesis, and physical activity.

When well-nourished mothers reduced their intake by 32% for 1 week, consuming no less than 1500 kcal/day, no reduction in milk volume occurred, although plasma prolactin levels increased. Mothers who consumed less than 1500 kcal/day for a week did experience decreased milk volumes compared with those of the control group and the group consuming more than 1500 kcal.

Exercise, manual labor, and losing weight do not usually alter an established milk volume. Milk production will increase with infant demand, but infant demand will only increase with growth, which depends on sufficient nourishment.[61] Having the mother take supplements could improve production and stimulate the infant's appetite.

*References 40, 80, 83, 87.

ENERGY SUPPLEMENTATION AND LACTATION PERFORMANCE

When women received supplements during the last trimester of pregnancy, no effect was noted in their milk production. This suggests that short-term supplementation may be ineffective. Other studies that provided supplementation of a maximum of 900 kcal/day for 2 weeks resulted in an increase in milk production (662 to 787 g/day).[114] No increase in infant weight compared with the control group's infants was seen in this period of 2 weeks.

The problem of insufficient milk supply for a baby is reported in well-nourished as well as poorly nourished populations, but in cross-cultural studies it appears to be unrelated to maternal nutrition status.[116] The effect of supplementation may be more psychologic than physiologic.

In countries where food supplies vary with the season, milk supplies drop 1 dL/day during periods of progressively greater food shortages. Studies continue on lactation performance of poorly nourished women around the world, including Burma, The Gambia, Papua New Guinea, and Ethiopia as well as among Navajo people. Results continue to reflect an impact on quantity, not quality, of milk.[13,23,65,105]

The interrelationship of milk volume, nutrient concentration, and total nutrient intake by the infant must be considered.[29] The reason for low protein content in a given sample may be lack of protein stores, lack of total energy content, or lack of vitamin B_6, a requirement of normal protein metabolism.

Of concern, however, is the report of dietary supplementation of Gambian nursing mothers in whom lactational performance was not affected by increased calories (700 kcal/day).[100] The supplement produced a slight initial improvement in maternal body weight and subcutaneous fat but not in milk output. Whether the mothers utilized the increased energy to work harder farming or whether the infants did not stimulate increased milk production is unresolved. Food supplementation of lactating women in areas where malnutrition is prevalent has generally had little, if any, impact on milk volume.[112] Such supplementation improves maternal health and is more likely to benefit the mother than the infant except where milk composition had been affected by specific deficiencies.

PROTEIN CONTENT

Since the work of Hambraeus reestablished the norms for protein in human milk to be 0.8 to 0.9 g/dL in well-nourished mothers, figures from previous studies have been recalculated to consider that all nitrogen in human milk is not protein; 25% of the nitrogen is nonprotein nitrogen (NPN) in human milk, and only 5% of the nitrogen is NPN in bovine milk. The protein content of milk from poorly nourished mothers is surprisingly high, and malnutrition has little effect on protein concentration. An increase in dietary protein increases volume but not overall protein content, given the normal variations seen in healthy, well-nourished women.

Observations made over a 20-month period of continued lactation showed that milk quality did not change, although the quantity decreased slightly, which has been attributed to the decreasing demand of a child who is receiving other nourishment. Therefore, the total protein available with the decreased volume of milk and increased weight of the child decreased from 2.2 g/kg of body weight to 0.45 g/kg. The need for additional protein sources from other foods for the child after 1 year of age becomes obvious.

The composition of human milk is maintained even with less-than-recommended dietary intake of macronutrients. The concentrations of major minerals, including calcium, phosphorus, magnesium, sodium, and potassium, are not affected by diet. Maternal dietary intakes of selenium and iodine, however, are positively affected: an increase in the diet increases the level in the milk. The proportion of different fatty acids in human milk varies with the maternal dietary intake.

In Zaire,[83] lactating mothers with protein malnutrition were given 500 kcal (2093 kilojoules [kJ]) and 18 g of protein as a cow milk supplement for 2 months, after which their nutritional status improved significantly.[31] The volume of milk did not change (607 versus 604 mL). Their breastfed infants, however, did show significant improvement in their mean serum albumin levels, and their growth matched that of healthy infants of the same age.

The effect of very-low-protein (8% of energy) and very-high-protein (20% of energy) diets on the protein and nitrogen composition of breast milk in three healthy Swedish women "in full lactation" was significant.[50] High-protein diets produced higher production and greater concentrations of total nitrogen, true protein, and NPN. The increased NPN was caused by increased urea levels and free amino acids. The 24-hour outputs of lactoferrin, lactalbumin, and serum albumin were not significantly higher.

When marginally nourished women were provided a mixed-protein diet predominantly from plant sources up to 1.2 g/kg/day, equilibrium was achieved at a protein intake of 1.1 g/kg. In a study of healthy women given marginal protein intakes, Motil et al.[82] reported that maternal milk production and the

TABLE 9-3	Lipid Concentrations of Mature Human Milk					
	Diet			**Lipid Concentration in Milk**		
Study	**Plan**	**Saturation of Fat***	**Cholesterol (mg/day)**	**Cholesterol (mg/dL)**	**Triglyceride (g/dL)**	**Phospholipid (mg P/dL)**
I ($n=7$)	A	S	580	$18.1 \pm 2.7^{\dagger}$	3.42 ± 0.61	4.04 ± 0.71
	B	P	110	19.3 ± 3.6	3.57 ± 0.82	4.18 ± 0.91
II ($n=3$)	C	S	380	23.3 ± 2.3	4.11 ± 0.42	
	D	P	345	21.3 ± 2.4	4.12 ± 0.56	

*S, rich in saturated fatty acids (P/S ratio ~0.07); P, rich in polyunsaturated fatty acids (P/S ~1.3).
†Mean ± SEM.
From Potter JM, Nestel PJ: The effects of dietary fatty acids and cholesterol on the milk lipids of lactating women and the plasma cholesterol of breast-fed infants, *Am J Clin Nutr* 29:54, 1976.

Thus, no evidence is available that concentrations of cholesterol and phospholipids can be changed by diet. Milk cholesterol is stable at 100 to 150 mg/L even in hypercholesterolemic women and increases only in severe cases of pathologic hypercholesterolemia, according to Jensen.[60] The fat globule membrane contains both cholesterol and phospholipids, and their secretion rates are related to the total quantity and are not influenced by diet. This supports the conclusion that cholesterol is essential to the diet of the infant.

Where maternal undernutrition is commonplace, the percentage of maternal body fat may influence the concentration of fat in the milk.[96] Milk fat concentrations in Gambian women were positively correlated with maternal skinfold thickness and decreased over the course of lactation. Women with parity of 10 and above appear to have a decreased capacity to synthesize milk fat and thus have lower milk fat concentrations in their milk.

The synthesis of fatty acids up to the carbon number of 16, as well as the direct desaturation of stearic acid into oleic acid, can take place in the mammary gland, whereas longer-chain fatty acids come directly from plasma triglycerides[55,61] (see Chapter 4). The intake of both carbohydrate and fat must be taken into account when evaluating maternal diet because high-carbohydrate diets increase lauric acid and myristic acid and moderate levels of carbohydrate influence linoleic acid.

When serum lipids are measured in African women accustomed to a low-fat intake, the levels are relatively low and the women are virtually free of coronary heart disease.[3,100] Among long-lactating (1 to 2 years minimum) African mothers, the amount of fat in their daily milk is of the same order as that ingested in their habitual diet.[120] Despite this, they are not significantly hypolipidemic when compared with nonlactators.

Human milk samples obtained from women living in five different regions of China showed the great diversity of milk fatty acids. The docosahexaenoic acid (DHA) concentrations in women from the marine region were twice as high as those from rural areas.[91] The milk concentrations of DHA varied greatly (0.44 ± 0.29 to 2.78 ± 1.20 g/100 g total fat), with pastoral regions being lowest and the marine region highest. Seafood consumption was high in the marine group. Similarly, AA, when stated as a ratio (AA/DHA, g/g), was 2.77 in pastoral areas and 0.42 in the marine region. AA has been associated with infant growth and DHA with brain and retinal growth. Similar findings are reported in Alaskan Inuit people who have a diet high in fish and fish oil. When women's diets were supplemented with fish and fish oils, the blood concentrations of DHA in the maternal plasma and red blood cells (RBCs) were increased.[23] Infants showed a 35% DHA increase in RBCs and 45% increase in plasma, which supports the concept that maternal diet can influence the DHA levels in newborns. The fatty acid patterns of human milk correlate with the current American diet, which has a high P/S ratio; there is a shift toward higher levels of C18:2 fatty acids, linoleic acid, and C18:3 linolenic acid.[61,69,70] Depot fat reflects dietary fatty acid patterns and thus the pool for mammary gland synthesis of milk fats. The mammary gland can dehydrogenate saturated and monosaturated fatty acids.[103]

Diet composition affects milk fat synthesis. When a woman is in energy balance, the fatty acids from the diet account for about 30% of the total fatty acids in her milk.

The habitual diet of healthy primiparas in Finland was associated with breast milk containing 3.8% fat.[118] Their diet was 16% protein, 39% fat, and 45% carbohydrate. Half the fatty acids of the diet and the milk were saturated, and one third were monoenoic. PUFAs were 15% of the diet and 13% of the breast milk, with a P/S ratio of 0.3 for both. The maternal diet had no effect on total fat content of the milk except for the low level of oleic acid, which is apparently peculiar to Finnish breast milk.

DHA, a long-chain fatty acid (22:6, omega-3), has attracted attention because deficiency has been associated with visual impairment in offspring of rhesus monkeys. Essential *n*-3 fatty acids in pregnant women have been linked to visual acuity and neural development in their term infants. Some pregnant women in the United States have been found to be deficient in DHA.[57] A descriptive meta-analysis of 106 studies worldwide was culled to 65 to include only those utilizing modern analysis methods to obtain fatty acid profiles. The highest DHA concentrations were found in coastal populations and associated with consumption of fish. DHA was 0.32% + 0.22% and 0.47% + 0.13% for AA, representing the mean concentrations worldwide. Omega-3 DHA is important to the fetus and to the offspring through breastfeeding, and emerging science suggests it may protect against preterm delivery, and postpartum depression as well.[12]

FISH CONSUMPTION DURING LACTATION

Maternal fish consumption during pregnancy has been correlated with cognitive and visual abilities in offspring. Maternal omega-3(*n*-3) LCPUFA supplementation during pregnancy was evaluated comparing early childhood cognitive and visual development in mother's with and without supplementation. A systematic review and meta-analysis of randomized controlled trials failed to prove or disprove that omega-3 LCPUFA supplementation in pregnancy improves cognitive and visual development of the children.[45]

Fish oil is an excellent dietary source of DHA, and women who consistently eat fish have higher levels in their milk. In a study, Finley et al.[34] found that vegetarians have higher DHA levels in their milk than omnivore control subjects. Many formulas have been supplemented with synthetically derived DHA in an effort to mimic human milk. They do not, however, contain cholesterol, and no data support the concept that synthetically derived DHA is as effective as natural DHA in human milk.

A strong association exists between the body fat of the mother and lipid in her milk. Lovelady et al.[73] found that the best predictor of milk lipids was overall "fatness" rather than the distribution of that fat. Dietary fat was not associated with milk fat in the "fat" women (27% or more body fat) but was positively correlated with diet in lean women (less than 27% body fat).

When healthy pregnant women are supplemented with fish oil capsules from the thirtieth week of gestation, the fatty acid compositions of the phospholipids isolated from umbilical plasma and umbilical vessel walls differ from those of unsupplemented mothers, with more *n*-3 and less *n*-6 fatty acids.[117] This suggests that DHA status can be altered at birth.

A group of lactating women were given supplements of different doses of fish oil concentrates rich in omega-3 fatty acids, including DHA.[53] Receiving 5 g/day for 28 days, 10 g/day for 14 days, and 47 g/day for 8 days, each experienced significant dose-dependent increases in DHA in their milk and plasma. Baseline levels in milk were 0.1% of total fatty acids, and levels rose from 0.8% to as high as 4.8% on the 47 g/day diet. This suggests that relatively small supplements of DHA can enhance levels in the milk. Preformed dietary DHA is known to be better synthesized into nervous tissue than that synthesized from linolenic acid, and other essential fatty acids can inhibit this transformation to DHA. The consumption of fish during pregnancy and lactation is an important dietary consideration in preference to fish oil capsules. The concern rests with possible mercury contamination. Fish, however, provides lean protein, and an abundance of vitamins B, zinc, iodine and selenium as well as naturally rich sources of long-chain omega-3 fatty acids and vitamin D. It has been recorded that women who do not eat fish during pregnancy put their infants at risk for suboptimal visual, cognitive, motor, and behavior skill outcomes.[57] International studies have shown the value of fish in pregnancy and lactation. The most thorough was a 15-year follow-up of infants breastfed on the Seychelles Islands by mothers with a high intake of fish, measurable mercury levels, and developmental growth scores that were higher with greater consumption of fish and greater levels of breastfeeding. The Food and Drug Administration (FDA) has stated that, while fish oil supplements are beneficial for those who cannot eat fish, fish has the full range of nutrients. The FDA recommends a minimum of two meals of fish per week (up to 12 ounces) during lactation.[89]

Studies of linoleic acid supplementation from 20 weeks' gestation in normal women showed that levels increased in those with low linoleic acid levels to match those with high levels.[1] The neonatal linoleic acid status did not change. Linoleic acid supplementation did result in slightly but significantly higher total amounts of *n*-6 long-chain polyenes in umbilical plasma. Linoleic acid (18:2, *n*-6) is essential to the maintenance of the epidermal water barrier and is the ultimate dietary precursor of eicosanoids, which include leukotrienes, prostaglandins, and thromboxanes. Linoleic acid is not synthesized by humans and must be supplied by diet.

TABLE 9-5 Dietary Reference Intakes: Recommended Intakes for Individuals, Macronutrients (Food and Nutrition Board, Institute of Medicine, National Academies)

Life Stage Group	Total Water[a] (L/day)	Carbohydrate (g/day)	Total Fiber (g/day)	Fat (g/day)	Linoleic Acid (g/day)	α-Linolenic Acid (g/day)	Protein[b] (g/day)
Females							
9-13 yr	2.1	130	26	ND	10	1.0	34
14-18 yr	2.3	130	26	ND	11	1.1	46
19-30 yr	2.7	130	25	ND	12	1.1	46
31-50 yr	2.7	130	25	ND	12	1.1	46
51-70 yr	2.7	130	21	ND	11	1.1	46
>70 yr	2.7	130	21	ND	11	1.1	46
Pregnancy							
14-18 yr	3.0	175	28	ND	13	1.4	71
19-30 yr	3.0	175	28	ND	13	1.4	71
31-50 yr	3.0	175	28	ND	13	1.4	71
Lactation							
14-18 yr	3.8	210	29	ND	13	1.3	71
19-30 yr	3.8	210	29	ND	13	1.3	71
31-50 yr	3.8	210	29	ND	13	1.3	71

apparent. Levels of water-soluble vitamins in milk are raised or lowered by changes in the maternal diet. The body's requirement for vitamin C increases under stress, including lactation. Furthermore, the vitamin C content of human organs at autopsy is much higher in the neonate than at any other time of life. This is true of all the major organs, including the brain.

The influence of maternal intake of vitamin C on the concentration of vitamin C in human milk and on the intake of vitamin C by the infant has been carefully measured in 25 well-nourished lactating women. Supplements ranged from 0 to 1000 mg vitamin C daily (more than 10 times the RDA). Concentrations in milk ranged from 44 to 158 mg/L and were not correlated significantly with maternal intakes, which ranged from 156 (0 mg supplement) to 1123 mg (1000 mg supplement). Dietary vitamin C had no effect on the volume of milk produced. Maternal excretion of vitamin C in urine was correlated with maternal intake. Regardless of the level of maternal intake of vitamin C, the mean vitamin C concentration in breast milk was twice that recommended for infant formula. Vitamin C levels in milk did not increase in response to increasing maternal intake despite tenfold increases, whereas urinary excretion did suggest that mammary tissue becomes saturated.

It is postulated that a regulatory mechanism prevents an elevation in concentration of vitamin C beyond a certain level in milk. Vitamin C levels were at the same or higher levels in exclusively breastfed infants at 6 and 9 months of age compared with levels of supplemented bottle-fed control infants. Levels were dependent on maternal nutrition and vitamin C levels in milk. Low levels of vitamin C are recorded in 6% of well-nourished healthy mothers. In malnourished women, tissue stores may take time to replenish, which explains why 35 mg/day supplementation failed to increase low plasma levels. Data from multiple studies suggest that there is a level above which further vitamin C supplementation will not affect milk vitamin C levels.

The level of B vitamins, also water soluble, reflects dietary intake. The levels are affected acutely by maternal diet. Infantile beriberi is not unheard of in seemingly normal infants nursed by apparently well-nourished mothers with thiamin-deficient diets. The influence of maternal diet has been pointed out dramatically in reported cases of megaloblastic anemia, methylmalonic aciduria, and homocystinuria in the breastfed infants of strict vegetarians. Vitamin B_{12} exists in all animal protein but not in vegetable protein. A strict vegetarian would require vitamin B_{12} supplements during pregnancy and lactation.[41,52] Vitamin B_{12} deficiency in infants has also been seen in New Delhi, where malnourished mothers produced vitamin B_{12}-deficient milk. These infants also had megaloblastic anemia.

Infants of vegetarians who have low vitamin B_{12} serum and milk levels have methylmalonic acid in their urine inversely proportional to their vitamin B_{12} levels, even though they are asymptomatic.[107] Other authors[41,52] have concluded that the current RDA for infants provides little margin of safety: 0.3 or 0.05 mg/kg body weight is close to the intake below which infant urinary methylmalonic acid measures are elevated.

TABLE 9-6   Dietary Reference Intakes: Tolerable Upper Intake Levels[a]—Elements (Food and Nutrition Board, Institute of Medicine, National Academies)

Life Stage Group	Arsenic[b]	Boron (mg/day)	Calcium (g/day)	Chromium	Copper (μg/day)	Fluoride (mg/day)	Iodine (μg/day)	Iron (mg/day)	Magnesium (mg/day)[c]	Manganese (mg/day)[c]	Molybdenum (μg/day)	Nickel (mg/day)	Phosphorus (g/day)	Potassium	Selenium (μg/day)	Silicon[d]	Sulfate	Vanadium (mg/day)[e]	Zinc (mg/day)	Sodium (g/day)	Chloride (g/day)
Pregnancy																					
14-18 yr	ND[f]	17	2.5	ND	8000	10	900	45	350	9	1700	1.0	3.5	ND	400	ND	ND	ND	34	2.3	3.6
19-50 yr	ND	20	2.5	ND	10,000	10	1100	45	350	11	2000	1.0	3.5	ND	400	ND	ND	ND	40	2.3	3.6
Lactation																					
14-18 yr	ND	17	2.5	ND	8000	10	900	45	350	9	1700	1.0	4	ND	400	ND	ND	ND	34	2.3	3.6
19-50 yr	ND	20	2.5	ND	10,000	10	1100	45	350	11	2000	1.0	4	ND	400	ND	ND	ND	40	2.3	3.6

[a]UL = The maximum level of daily nutrient intake that is likely to pose no risk of adverse effects. Unless otherwise specified, the UL represents total intake from food, water, and supplements. Due to lack of suitable data, ULs could not be established for arsenic, chromium, silicon, potassium, and sulfate. In the absence of ULs, extra caution may be warranted in consuming levels above recommended intakes.

[b]Although the UL was not determined for arsenic, there is no justification for adding arsenic to food or supplements.

[c]The ULs for magnesium represent intake from a pharmacologic agent only and do not include intake from food and water.

[d]Although silicon has not been shown to cause adverse effects in humans, there is no justification for adding silicon to supplements.

[e]Although vanadium in food has not been shown to cause adverse effects in laboratory animals and these data could be used to set a UL for adults but not children and adolescents. The UL is based on adverse effects in laboratory animals and these data could be used to set a UL for adults but not children and adolescents.

[f]ND = Not determinable due to lack of data of adverse effects in this age group and concern with regard to lack of ability to handle excess amounts. Source of intake should be from food only to prevent high levels of intake.

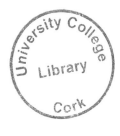

TABLE 9-7 Dietary Reference Intakes: Estimated Average Requirements for Groups (Food and Nutrition Board, Institute of Medicine, National Academies)

Life Stage Group	CHO (g/day)	Protein (g/day)	Vit A (µg/day)[a]	Vit C (mg/day)	Vit E (mg/day)[b]	Thiamin (mg/day)	Riboflavin (mg/day)	Niacin (mg/day)[c]	Vit B6 (mg/day)	Folate (µg/day)[d]	Vit B12 (µg/day)	Copper (µg/day)	Iodine (µg/day)	Iron (mg/day)	Magnesium (mg/day)	Molybdenum (µg/day)	Phosphorus (µg/day)	Selenium (µg/day)	Zinc (mg/day)
Females																			
9-13 yr	100	28	420	39	9	0.7	0.8	9	0.8	250	1.5	540	73	5.7	200	26	1055	35	7.0
14-16 yr	100	38	485	56	12	0.9	0.9	11	1.0	330	2.0	685	95	7.9	300	33	1055	45	7.3
19-30 yr	100	38	500	60	12	0.9	0.9	11	1.1	320	2.0	700	95	8.1	255	34	580	45	6.8
31-50 yr	100	38	500	60	12	0.9	0.9	11	1.1	320	2.0	700	95	8.1	265	34	580	45	6.8
51-70 yr	100	38	500	60	12	0.9	0.9	11	1.3	320	2.0	700	95	5	265	34	580	45	6.8
>70 yr	100	38	500	60	12	0.9	0.9	11	1.3	320	2.0	700	95	5	265	34	580	45	6.8
Pregnancy																			
14-18 yr	135	50	530	66	12	1.2	1.2	14	1.6			520	2.2	785	160	23	335	40	1055
19-30 yr	135	50	550	70	12	1.2	1.2	14	1.6			520	2.2	800	160	22	290	40	580
31-50 yr	135	50	550	70	12	1.2	1.2	14	1.6			520	2.2	800	160	22	300	40	580
Lactation																			
14-18 yr	160	60	885	96	16	1.2	1.3	13	1.7			450	2.4	985	209	7	300	35	1055
19-30 yr	160	60	900	100	16	1.2	1.3	13	1.7			450	2.4	1000	209	6.5	255	36	580
31-50 yr	160	60	900	100	16	1.2	1.3	13	1.7			450	2.4	1000	209	6.5	265	36	580

Note: This table presents estimated average requirement (EARs), which serve two purposes: for assessing adequacy of population intakes, and as the basis for calculating recommended dietary allowances (RDAs) for individuals for those nutrients. EARs have not been established for vitamin D, vitamin K, pantothenic acid, biotin, choline, calcium, chromium, fluoride, manganese, or other nutrients not yet evaluated via the DRI process.

[a] As retinol activity equivalents (RAEs). 1 RAE = 1 mg retinol, 12 mg b-carotene, 24 mg a-carotene, or 24 mg b-cryptoxanthin. The RAE for dietary provitamin A carotenoids is twofold greater than retinol equivalents (RE), whereas the RAE for preformed vitamin A is the same as RE.

[b] As α-tocopherol. α-Tocopherol includes RRR-α-tocopherol, the only form of -tocopherol that occurs naturally in foods, and the 2R-stereoisomeric forms of α-tocopherol (RRR-, RSR-, RRS-, and RSS-α-tocopherol) that occur in fortified foods and supplements. It does not include the 2S-stereoisomeric forms of α-tocopherol (SRR-, SSR-, SRS-, and SSS-α-tocopherol), also found in fortified foods and supplements.

[c] As niacin equivalents (NEs). 1 mg of niacin = 60 mg of tryptophan.

[d] As dietary folate equivalents (DFEs). 1 DFE = 1 mg food folate = 0.6 g of folic acid from fortified food or as a supplement consumed with food = 0.5 mg of a supplement taken on an empty stomach.

Sources: Dietary Reference Intakes for Calcium, Phosphorous, Magnesium, Vitamin D, and Fluoride (1997); Dietary Reference Intakes for Thiamin, Riboflavin, Niacin, Vitamin B6, Folate, Vitamin B12, Pantothenic Acid, Biotin, and Choline (1998); Dietary Reference Intakes for Vitamin C, Vitamin E, Selenium, and Carotenoids (2000); Dietary Reference Intakes for Vitamin A, Vitamin K, Arsenic, Boron, Chromium, Copper, Iodine, Iron, Manganese, Molybdenum, Nickel, Silicon, Vanadium, and Zinc (2001), and Dietary Reference Intakes for Energy, Carbohydrate, Fiber, Fat, Fatty Acids, Cholesterol, Protein, and Amino Acids (2002). These reports may be accessed via www.nap.edu. Copyright 2002 by the National Academy of Sciences. All rights reserved.

TABLE 9-8 Suggested Measures for Improving Nutrient Intake of Women with Restrictive Eating Patterns

Type of Restrictive Eating Pattern	Corrective Measures
Excessive restriction of food intake, i.e., ingestion of less than 1800 kcal/day, which ordinarily leads to unsatisfactory intake of nutrients compared with amounts needed by lactating women	Encourage increased intake of nutrient-rich foods to achieve energy intake of at least 1800 kcal/day; if mother insists on curbing food intake sharply, promote substitution of foods rich in vitamins, minerals, and protein for those lower in nutritive value; in individual cases, it may be advisable to recommend a balanced multivitamin-mineral supplement and discourage use of liquid weight-loss diets and appetite suppressants
Complete vegetarianism, i.e., avoidance of all animal foods, including meat, fish, dairy products, and eggs	Advise intake of regular source of vitamin B_{12}, such as special vitamin B_{12}-containing plant food products or a 2.5-μg vitamin B_{12} supplement daily
Avoidance of milk, cheese, or other calcium-rich dairy products	Encourage increased intake of other culturally appropriate dietary calcium sources, such as collard greens for blacks from southeastern United States; provide information on appropriate use of low-lactose dairy products if milk is being avoided because of lactose intolerance; if correction by diet cannot be achieved it may be advisable to recommend 600 mg of elemental calcium per day taken with meals
Avoidance of vitamin D-fortified foods, such as fortified milk or cereal, combined with limited exposure to ultraviolet light	Recommend 10 μg of supplemental vitamin D per day

From the Subcommittee on Nutrition During Lactation, Committee on Nutritional Status During Pregnancy and Lactation, Food and Nutrition Board, et al: *Nutrition During lactation,* Washington, D.C., 1991, National Academies Press.

Thiamine (vitamin B_1) has been studied infrequently, but maternal supplementation does not increase milk levels beyond a certain limit. Urinary excretion of thiamine is significantly higher in supplemented compared with unsupplemented women. In malnourished women, evidence indicates that supplementation does increase thiamine levels in milk. It is recommended that thiamine intake be at least 1.3 mg/day (the RDA for nonpregnant, nonlactating women of 1.1 mg/day plus an increment for milk secretion of 0.2 mg/day) when the calorie intake is less than 2200 kcal/day.

Riboflavin (vitamin B_2) requirements of lactating women in a controlled study in The Gambia showed the minimum to be 2.5 mg/day to maintain normal biochemical status in the mother and adequate levels of vitamin B_2 in her milk.[10] This level is higher than what is recommended in the United States and the United Kingdom.

Niacin (vitamin B_3) content of human milk has been reported to parallel dietary intake. In unsupplemented diets, low vitamin B_3 levels usually parallel low levels of other B vitamins and low protein intakes.

Pyridoxine (vitamin B_6) intake and milk levels were studied in healthy lactating women. There were marked diurnal variations of vitamin B_6 levels, with peaks occurring in those mothers taking supplements 3 to 5 hours after a dose. Those taking less than 2.5 mg/day had much lower milk levels. Vitamin B_6 concentrations in human milk change rapidly with maternal intake.[6] When supplemented, the level in the milk is a direct reflection of amount ingested. Plasma pyridoxal-5′-phosphate levels and birth weight are the strongest predictors of infant growth.[64]

When lactating mothers received supplements of vitamin B_6 ranging from 0 to 20 mg pyridoxine hydrochloride, the levels of vitamin B_6 measurable in the milk paralleled the intake, with levels peaking 5 hours after ingesting the supplement. When maternal intakes of vitamin B_6 approximated 2.0 mg/day, breastfed infants were unlikely to receive the current RDA of 0.3 mg vitamin B_6 per day. The AAP Committee on Nutrition[18] recommends a minimum of 0.35 mg vitamin B_6/100 kcal milk from birth to 12 months. The RDA for vitamin B_6 for lactating women is 0.5 mg daily. Vitamin B_6 is the vitamin in milk that is most likely to be deficient, because pyridoxine levels in milk are closely influenced by dietary intake.[6,64] Supplementing with an additional 2.5 mg/day results in levels twice as high as in unsupplemented women.[6] The increment in the RDA for vitamin B_6 in lactation is more than five times the estimated secretion of this vitamin in milk,[112] which varies between 0.01 and 0.02 mg/L early in lactation to 0.10 to 0.25 mg/L in mature milk. The recommendation is to advise diets rich in vitamin B_6, such as poultry, meat, fish, and some legumes, and reserve supplementation for special-risk cases.

Pantothenic acid levels in milk are strongly correlated with maternal intake for the preceding day, although some pantothenic acid is stored in the

on postprandial milk sodium or potassium concentrations.[33] Dietary potassium may influence milk potassium more significantly. RDI in lactation is 5.1 g/day. With increasing numbers of women with cardiac and renal disease choosing to lactate, potassium levels in the diet would be of significance, in addition to concerns about necessary medications that are known to deplete potassium levels.

Chlorine level in the breast milk is not thought to be affected by maternal diet. Chlorine deficiency reported in a breastfed infant was associated with normal maternal serum and dietary intake[8] but with deficit levels in the milk (less than 2 mEq/L). Normal is greater than 8 mEq/L. This deficit in the milk was assumed to be a defect of breast function. Daily requirement is 2.3.

The concentration of electrolytes (sodium, potassium, chloride) in milk is determined by an electrical potential gradient in the secretory cell rather than by maternal nutritional status.[112]

Iron

The iron content of milk is not readily affected by the iron content of the diet or the maternal serum iron level. Increases in dietary iron that increase serum levels do not increase iron in the milk. It is important, however, for the mother to replace her iron stores postpartum.[94] It has not been established that increases in tissue iron are advantageous. Iron that is added to human milk will bind to lactoferrin and may interfere with its function. Infants exclusively breastfed for 7 months or longer were not found to be anemic at 12 or 24 months.[94] Half the infants breastfed for a shorter period were anemic at 12 months because additional dietary iron from solids was not provided.

A large study, however, involving children from Sweden and Honduras examined whether iron supplements affect growth and morbidity.[28] Children were assigned to supplements or a placebo. If the hemoglobin was less than 110 g/L at onset, iron had a therapeutic effect. Growth measurements were significantly lower in length and head circumference in those who received iron. Those who had hemoglobin greater than 110 g/L and received iron had more diarrhea. The authors suggest that iron not be given unless it is needed. In another observational study involving more than 900 children at 8 and 12 months, it was noted that those who combined 6 or more breastfeedings or 600 mL or more cow milk per day had higher levels of anemia. The authors recommend more iron containing solids and less milk for this age group.[54]

The requirement for iron is 1.8 times higher for vegetarians due to the lower bioavailability of iron from vegetarian sources.[90]

Iron supplementation appeared safe according to Friel et al.,[37] who conducted a double-blind, randomized control trial of iron supplementation in early infancy in a total of 77 healthy term breastfed infants using 7.5 mg/day of elemental iron as ferrous sulfate or a placebo from 1 to 6 months of age. Iron supplementation produced higher hemoglobin and mean corpuscular volume at 6 months of age as well as higher visual acuity and psychomotor development index at 13 months of age.

Dietary iron for lactating women is set at 9 mg/day, which is offset by the suppression of menses during lactation.

Phosphorus, Magnesium, Zinc, and Copper

Phosphorus, magnesium, zinc, and copper levels in milk are not affected by dietary administration of these elements.[67] Again, however, it is important for the mother to replenish her stores.[94]

According to the RDA, many lactating women are receiving marginal amounts of magnesium.[77] The amount recommended for lactation is two to three times the amount estimated to be in the milk or 310 to 320 mg/day.

Zinc has a RDA during lactation of 4 to 13 times higher than the amount estimated to be in the milk on the basis that it is poorly absorbed (20%). Studies done with stable isotopes in lactating women show that absorption was 59% to 84% of intake. Zinc absorption during pregnancy increases dramatically and during lactation decreases slightly but is double the prepregnant rates, presumably in response to the demand by the breast for milk synthesis.[39] Milk levels are unaffected by supplementation and gradually decline over time from 2 mg/day.[68] Supplementation does result in increased maternal absorption and increased plasma levels.

Prolactin is a zinc-binding hormone that is associated with the initiation and maintenance of lactation. Zinc is also thought to be involved with synthesis, storage, and secretion of prolactin. Increasing zinc availability is thought to inhibit formation and secretion of prolactin from the pituitary. The relationships among plasma zinc, prolactin, milk transfer, and milk zinc were studied by O'Brien et al.[87] No differences in milk transfer or prolactin levels were found between those who were zinc supplemented and those who were not. Low zinc levels are seen in those with a history of long-term alcohol ingestion. Their daily requirement is doubled.

Although no major health risks have been associated with low zinc intakes, zinc is known to be important to immune function.[59] RDA for zinc is 12 to 13 mg/day during pregnancy and lactation.

Recommended intake for infants 0 to 6 months of age is 4 mg/day.

Iron supplementation has no significant effect on levels of copper, selenium, and zinc in mother's serum and breast milk.[7]

Selenium

A correlation exists between selenium in human milk and maternal dietary intake.[72] Maternal plasma levels vary with the form of selenium supplementation (selenomethionine or selenium-enriched yeast).[76] The original source of selenium is the soil, and levels vary geographically. It is transferred to plants and works up the food chain. Breastfed infants are known to have higher intake and utilization than infants fed formula or cow milk because of bioavailability.[2] Many selenoproteins have been identified, but glutathione peroxidase is involved with producing a variety of organic hydroperoxides or reactive oxygen radicals in the liver. Although selenium toxicity is possible, deficiency from low intake is a problem.[74] Two diseases showing selenium deficiency are Keshan disease and Kashin-Beck disease, which are associated with accumulation of lipid peroxides. Dietary studies have shown that intake can affect the mother's plasma and milk levels.[2] RDI is 70 μg daily during lactation, compared with 55 μg for nonlactators.

Chromium

Breast milk levels of chromium are reported to be 3.54 ± 40 nmol/L (0.18 ng/mL) and independent of dietary intake.[5] Total absorption for lactating women was 0.79 ± 0.08 mmol/dL, which was greater than that of nonlactators. Serum levels were correlated with urinary chromium excretion, a good indicator of serum levels. The estimated RDA for breastfed infants is 10 mg, which is much greater than the levels measured in the study by Anderson et al.[5] The RDA for adults is 45 mg during lactation and 25 mg for nonlactating women of the same age.[36]

Iodine

Iodine in milk does depend on dietary content. The breast is able to raise the concentration of iodine in the milk above that in the blood, and thus there is an increased danger in giving radioactive iodine to the lactating woman. With iodized salt, bread dough conditioners, and common use of iodine-containing cleansers, excessive iodine intake is a risk.

The question of possible iodine deficiency, however, has been raised in breastfed infants around the globe as well as in the United States. A study of women in Boston found a mean breast milk concentration of 155 μg/L with a mean urinary iodine level of 144 μg/L; 47% of the women had milk insufficient in iodine.[93] Smoking is also recognized to reduce iodine concentrations in breast milk to a mean level of 26 μg/L. The authors suggest that lactating women should take iodine supplements, such as an iodine-containing vitamin preparation with at least 150 μg per dose. The daily requirement is 290 μg; however, more than 450 μg daily is considered excessive.[92] Urinary iodine concentrations optimally are 100 to 199 μg/L with a corresponding intake of 150 to 299 μg/day. Infants need 110 μg/day.

Milk iodine concentrations are higher now than were reported in the 1930s. Mean breast milk iodide levels ranged from 29 to 490 mg/L, averaging 178 mg/L, above the RDA for infants. In a study of pregnant and lactating women in Bangkok, iodine levels were 70.6 and 138.0, respectively, following supplementation with 200 mg iodine daily. Cord blood TSH was reduced with supplementation and in the infants, this demonstrated that maternal supplementation did improve the milk and subsequently the thyroid function of the infants in iodine poor regions.

Fluorine

Human milk contains 16 ± 5 mg fluoride per liter and reflects, to some degree, the level in the water supply. The risk for excessive fluoride has been pointed out by Walton and Messer,[123] who report dental mottling and milk fluorosis in supplemented breastfed infants. The AAP Committee on Nutrition, therefore, has stated, "It may not be necessary to give fluoride supplements to breastfed infants who are living in an area where water is adequately fluoridated." If the water is not fluoridated or mother drinks fluoride-free bottled water, she should be supplemented.

Fluoride concentrations of infant foods and drinks have been found to vary widely, ranging from 0.01 to 0.72 mg/kg, so that no need exists for supplementation if the diet is well balanced when solid foods are initiated.[120]

Summary

Table 9-12 summarizes constituent levels in human milk and changes over time.

TABLE 9-12   Representative Values for Constituents of Human Milk*

Constituent (per Liter)*	Early Milk (<28 Days Postpartum)	Mature Milk (≥28 Days Postpartum)
Energy (kcal)		**650-700**
Carbohydrate		
Lactose (g)	20-30	67
Glucose (g)	0.2-1.0	0.2-0.3
Oligosaccharides (g)	22-24	12-14
Total nitrogen (g)	**3.0**	**1.9**
Nonprotein nitrogen (g)	0.5	0.45
Protein nitrogen (g)	2.5	1.45
Total protein (g)	**16**	**9-12.6**
Total casein (g)		
β-Casein (g)	3.8	5.7
κ-Casein (g)	2.6	4.4
Whey proteins		6.7
α-Lactalbumin (g)	3.62	3.26
Lactoferrin (g)	3.53	1.94
Serum albumin (g)	0.39	0.41
sIgA (g)	2.0	1.0
IgM (g)	0.12	0.2
IgG (g)	0.34	0.05
Amino acids (g)[†]		
Alanine	0.65-1.71	0.26-0.42
Arginine	1.16-1.42	0.25-0.40
Aspartic acid	1.18-3.52	0.54-0.92
Cystine	0.47-1.41	0.11-0.23
Glutamic acid+glutamine	2.03-4.75	1.26-1.97
Glycine	0.36-1.42	0.10-0.27
Histidine	0.41-0.67	0.15-0.25
Isoleucine	0.43-1.27	0.33-0.57
Leucine	1.48-2.80	0.82-0.94
Lysine	0.72-2.06	0.30-0.90
Methionine	0.16-0.45	0.09-0.19
Phenylalanine	0.50-1.52	0.26-0.36
Proline	0.93-2.51	0.57-1.05
Serine	1.27-2.59	0.42-0.62
Threonine	0.65-1.94	0.32-0.42
Tryptophan	0.25-0.42	0.09-0.17
Tyrosine	0.76-0.54	0.31-0.47
Valine	0.88-1.66	0.35-0.51
Total lipids (%)	**2**	**3.5**
Triglyceride (% total lipids)	97-98	97-98
Cholesterol[‡] (% total lipids)	0.7-1.3	0.4-0.5
Phospholipids (% total lipids)	1.1	0.6-0.8
Fatty acids (weight %)	**88**	**88**
Total % saturated fatty acids	43-44	44-45
C12:0		5
C14:0		6
C16:0		20
C18:0		8
Total % monounsaturated fatty acids		40
C18: 1ω-9	32	31

Continued

TABLE 9-12	Representative Values for Constituents of Human Milk—cont'd	
Constituent (per Liter)	Early Milk (<28 Days Postpartum)	Mature Milk (≥28 Days Postpartum)
Total % polyunsaturated fatty acids (PUFA)	13	14-15
Total ω-3	1.5	1.5
C18: 3ω-3	0.7	0.9
C20: 5ω-3	0.2	0.1
C22: 6ω-3	0.5	0.2
Total ω-6	11.6	13.06
C18: 2ω-6	8.9	11.3
C20: 4ω-6	0.7	0.5
C22: 4ω-6	0.2	0.1
Water-soluble vitamins		
Ascorbic acid (mg)		80-100
Thiamin (μg)	20	200
Riboflavin (μg)		400-600
Niacin (mg)	0.5	1.8-6.0
Vitamin B_6 (mg)		0.09-0.31
Folate (μg)		80-140
Vitamin B_{12} (μg)		0.5-1.0
Pantothenic acid (mg)		2.0-2.5
Biotin (μg)		5-9
Fat-soluble vitamins		
Retinol (mg)	2	0.3-0.6
Carotenoids (mg)	2	0.2-0.6
Vitamin K (μg)	2-5	2-3
Vitamin D (μg)		0.33
Vitamin E (mg)	8-12	3-8
Major minerals		
Calcium (mg)	250	200-250
Magnesium (mg)	30-35	30-35
Phosphorus (mg)	120-160	120-140
Sodium (mg)	300-400	120-250
Potassium (mg)	600-700	400-550
Chloride (mg)	600-800	400-450
Trace minerals		
Iron (mg)	0.5-1.0	0.3-0.9
Zinc (mg)	8-12	1-3
Copper (mg)	0.5-0.8	0.2-0.4
Manganese (mg)	5-6	3
Selenium (mg)	40	7-33
Iodine (mg)		150
Fluoride (mg)		4-15

The values are expressed per liter of milk as a percentage on the basis of milk volume or weight of total lipids. Values as mean values or ranges of means. ω-3, Omega-3; ω-6, omega-6.

*All nutrient values except for amino acids are modified from Picciano MF: Appendix: representative values for constituents of human milk, *Pediatr Clin North Am* 48:263, 2001.

†Modified from George DR, De Francesca BA: Human milk in comparison to cow milk. In Lebenthal E, editor: *Textbook of gastroenterology and nutrition in infancy and childhood,* ed 2, New York, 1989, Raven Press, pp 242–243.

‡The cholesterol content of human milk ranges from 100 to 200 mg/L in most samples of human milk after day 21 of lactation.

Maternal Nutrition: Immunologic Substances and Leukocyte Activity

Substances in colostrum and mature milk confer important infection protection on breastfed infants. Maternal malnutrition was associated with lower levels of immunoglobulins G and A (IgG, IgA) in a group of Colombian women studied by Miranda et al.[81] The colostrum contained only one third the normal levels of IgG and less than half the normal albumin. Significant reductions in IgA and complement C4 were observed in colostrum, but lysozyme, C3, and IgM were normal. Titers against respiratory syncytial virus were unaffected by nutritional status. The protective deficiencies improved in mature milk over time and with improvement of nutritional status. The total leukocyte concentrations as well as their bactericidal capacity were similar in well-nourished and undernourished women.[11]

Prentice et al. measured breast milk antimicrobial factors of rural Gambian mothers. The concentrations and daily secretions of all immunoproteins, except lysozyme, decreased during the first year and then remained steady. Compared with those in Western women, levels of IgG, IgM, C3, and C4 were higher in Gambian women; IgA and lactoferrin were similar; and lysozyme was lower. Dietary supplement in Gambian women did not raise the breast milk immunoproteins in this study.

The Subcommittee on Nutrition During Lactation has concluded that the effects of maternal nutritional status on the immunologic system in human milk are controversial.[112] Some studies suggest that malnutrition decreases the production and secretion of some components of the immunologic system, but further investigation clearly is necessary.

Recommendations for Nutritional Support During Lactation

The previous section noted that the quantity, protein content, and calcium content of milk are relatively independent of maternal nutritional status and diet. Amino acids lysine and methionine, certain fatty acids, and water-soluble vitamin contents vary with intake. It is important to point out that stores of calcium, minerals, and fat-soluble vitamins need to be replenished.[124] Much of the data collected have varied, depending on the method used in collection. The daily intakes thought necessary for infants were determined by feeding infants processed human milk in a bottle, which is not a physiologic standard.[24] It is known, for example, that putting the entire sample in one container removes the natural variation in fat from beginning to end of the feeding.

The Subcommittee on Nutrition During Lactation[39,115] has recommended a balanced diet comparable to one for the nonlactating postpartum mother, with a few additions. Although the calculated caloric cost of producing 1 L of milk is 940 kcal, during pregnancy most women store 2 to 4 kg of extra tissue in the physiologic preparation for lactation.[35] Thus, it is probably necessary to add only 500 kcal to the diet, except in women with known high metabolic rates.

Preparation for lactation begins in pregnancy, if not before. The major daily increases for pregnancy are 300 kcal; 20 g of protein; a 20% increase in all vitamins and minerals except folic acid, which is doubled; and a 33% increase in calcium, phosphorus, and magnesium. In comparing the RDAs for lactating women with those for nonlactating adult women, the increases suggested should provide ample nutrition and replace stores (Table 9-7).

When dietary supplements are suggested, concern arises about increased costs. Cost increases are modest for the standard diet and minimal for the low-budget diet, as demonstrated by Worthington-Roberts. Although one rarely chooses breastfeeding or bottle-feeding on the basis of cost, the price of a few extra maternal kilocalories versus the cost of formula feeding makes a reassuring comparison. Hypoallergenic formulas are even more costly, estimated to be more than $5 per day.

After the report of the Subcommittee on Nutrition During Lactation,[112] an additional report was prepared, *Nutrition during pregnancy and lactation: an implementation guide*.[113] Its purpose is to offer practical guidance to primary care providers by including a sample nutrition screening questionnaire, indications for supplementation, nutritional assessment guidelines, and how and when to refer patients to registered dietitians.

The subcommittee did not propose a food guide because it recognized that diverse ways are available to meet nutrient needs and that culturally appropriate foods are important, especially in the perinatal period. It did offer the following recommendations[113]:

- Avoid diets and medications that promise rapid weight loss.
- Eat a wide variety of breads and cereal grains, fruits, vegetables, milk products, and meats or meat alternatives each day.
- Consume three or more servings of milk products daily.
- Make a greater effort to eat vitamin A-rich vegetables or fruits often. Examples of foods high in vitamin A include carrots, spinach or other cooked greens, sweet potatoes, and cantaloupe.

- Be sure to drink when thirsty. Lactation requires more fluid than usual.
- If you drink coffee or other caffeinated beverages, such as cola, do so in moderation. Two servings daily are unlikely to harm the infant. Caffeine passes into the milk.

MALNUTRITION: SPECIAL SUPPLEMENTATION FOR THE LACTATING WOMAN

It has been suggested that supplementing the diet of malnourished mothers with a special formula would be the best way to achieve ideal nourishment for mother and child. Infants will then gain the additional advantages of human milk, such as protection against infection.[65] Such formulas have been devised. Sosa et al.[106] successfully tried this approach in Guatemala. When nutritional supplements are recommended, ideally they are given to the mother. Such studies have been repeated in many geographic areas. The results confirm that the provision of supplemental food improves milk production and the duration of exclusive breastfeeding among undernourished women.[25] In contrast, well-nourished women do not show any benefits from supplementation.[44,124]

With the ready availability of well-balanced nutrition supplements today in the form of stable powders in both supermarkets and drugstores, it should not be difficult to initiate a high-protein, vitamin-enriched diet supplementation that is also palatable for an occasional mother who is at nutritional risk. With the inclusion of breastfeeding as a goal in the Women, Infants, and Children (WIC) program, dietary counseling and supplementation are available for mothers at poverty level to encourage these mothers to breastfeed and to give them nutritional support while doing so. Infants in the WIC programs will receive the greatest benefit from being breastfed. Present WIC supplements focus on improved maternal diet and were improved and expanded in 2009.

Because studies have revealed a negative effect of malnutrition on infection protection properties as well as on galactopoietic hormones (corticosteroids are greatly increased and prolactin decreased), nourishing the mother is the most effective way of benefiting the infant rather than supplementing the infant to meet growth standards.

The impact of dietary supplementation on lactating women with restricted diets has been reported to be inconsistent with respect to lactational amenorrhea.[115] Most recently, a study in Sri Lankan women did not show an effect on menstruation or ovulation with supplementation.[113] However, the study did result in a longer duration of full breastfeeding in supplemented women, which may have had an effect in suppressing ovulation. No difference was seen between supplemented and unsupplemented women regarding lactational amenorrhea.[115]

ALLERGY

In families with a strong history of allergy, a hypoallergenic diet avoiding common allergens such as wheat and eggs should be recommended. Interest in the transfer of cow milk proteins to infants via breast milk has increased as case reports appear detailing breastfed infants' reaction to cow protein. β-Lactoglobulin has been identified in breast milk and appears to be related to long-term exposure to cow milk products.[38] Controlling intake has also been reported to reverse the presence of β-lactoglobulin in breast milk. Ovalbumin has been identified in human milk in only a fraction of mothers tested, although average intake was four eggs per week (see Chapter 17).

VEGETARIAN DIET

The growing interest in vegetarianism has necessitated a better understanding of the several types of diets and their potential for adequate nutrients and growth as well as the motivation for these diets (see Table 9-13). In general, serious vegetarians usually have a greater knowledge of and commitment to good nutrition.[16]

Reports of malnutrition among breastfed infants of vegetarians usually focus on the very strict groups, such as vegans and those on macrobiotic diets. The dietary risks involved are chiefly with the B vitamins because these vitamins are usually associated with protein, which is also proportionally lower from vegetable sources.[101] An additional concern is the availability of various amino acids in specific concentrations to utilize them for protein synthesis. The net protein utilization of a food may be considerably lower than total protein content; therefore, it is important when using vegetable sources of protein to use foods with "complementary protein" at the same meal. Vegetarian cookbooks emphasize this. Throughout history, culturally traditional meals have ensured complementary proteins. Concentrations of polychlorinated biphenyls are lower in the breast milk of vegetarians.

Vitamin B_{12} deficiency has been described in vegans because of the absence of animal protein. It is advisable in these cases to supplement the diets of pregnant or lactating women and of infants or growing children with up to 4 mg/day of vitamin B_{12}. It has been shown that fermented soybean foods do contain vitamin B_{12} as do the single-cell proteins such as yeast because even single-cell

TABLE 9-13 Vegetarianism and Associated Risks

Type of Vegetarian	Diet Includes	Diet Avoids	Risks
Semivegetarian	Vegetables, milk products, seafood, poultry	Red meat	Minerals*
Ovolactovegetarian	Vegetables, milk products, eggs	Flesh foods (meat, seafood, poultry)	Minerals,* esp. zinc
Lactovegetarian	Vegetables, milk products	Flesh foods, eggs	Minerals,* esp. zinc, protein[†]
Ovovegetarian	Vegetables, eggs	Flesh foods, milk products	Minerals,* esp. iron and zinc, protein,[†] riboflavin, vitamin D, vitamin B_{12}
Vegan	Only vegetables	Flesh foods, milk products, eggs	Minerals,* protein,[†] riboflavin, vitamin D, vitamin B_{12}
Macrobiotic	Gradual progression to a diet of only cereals		Advanced stage nutritionally inadequate

*Excessive dietary phytates and dietary fiber inhibit absorption of minerals such as iron, zinc, and calcium. *Phytates* are organic chemicals present in many vegetables and unleavened bread that bind with minerals.
[†]Diets not using complementary proteins may be deficient in net protein because the net protein utilization is low.

animal species contain small amounts of vitamin B_{12}. In a study of vegetarian mothers and their infants, a large proportion of the infants had elevated methylmalonic acid levels, indicative of vitamin B_{12} deficiency.[107] A significant number of vegetarian women, both lactators and nonlactators, had elevated methylmalonic acid levels and low vitamin B_{12} levels.

. As noted previously, vegetarians have lower levels of DHA.[103] Comparison of umbilical cord blood of infants born to South Asian vegetarian women showed less DHA in the plasma and cord artery phospholipids than in infants born to omnivores.[103] Early onset of labor, incidence of cesarean delivery, lower birth weight, head circumference, and length, after adjusting for maternal height, duration of gestation, parity, smoking, and sex of infant, were also related to DHA levels.

Reports of growth curves in vegetarian children in the first few years show them to be shorter and leaner than standard, with the greatest effect among those whose mothers were on the most restricted diets.[34] Studies of children from birth to 10 years in The Netherlands reared in a macrobiotic tradition showed the greatest growth retardation with fat and muscle wasting and slower psychomotor development between 6 and 18 months of age.[23] The breast milk of their mothers, who breastfed an average of 13.6 months, contained less vitamin B_{12}, calcium, and magnesium compared with matched omnivorous control subjects.[23,32] Breastfed vegetarian infants are usually on the norms for growth, with the exception of those receiving minimal vitamin D and calcium, as reported in dark-skinned mothers in cloudy climates. The mean serum 1,25-dihydroxyvitamin D concentrations were 37% higher in lactating vegetarian women than nonvegetarian women. The serum parathyroid hormone was elevated in all lactators

compared with nonlactators. It is postulated that the low calcium in the vegetarian diet stimulates the elevated 1,25-dihydroxyvitamin D level, and this in turn stimulates the increased absorption of calcium to meet the needs of milk production.[107]

A study of the milk from vegetarian mothers compared with that from nonvegetarian mothers looked at fat and fatty acid composition.[23] Those fats and fatty acids produced de novo by the breast were not different.[108] The precursors of arachnodonic acid (AA) were higher in vegetarians, yet the AA level in the milk was lower and continued to decrease the longer the vegetarian diet was maintained. Linoleic acid was greater among vegetarians. The amounts of DHA were not different. Among 34 breastfed infants at 7 months in the Tufts study, 3 were below the 10th percentile for height and weight, 1 had low weight for length, and 3 had high weight for length, whereas of the 51 who were not breastfed, 6 were below the 10th percentile, 2 had low weight for length, and 4 had high weight for length.

Four vegetarian children between 8 and 24 months of age were reported by Hellebostad et al.[51] to have vitamin D-deficient rickets (three with tetany and seizures) and vitamin B_{12} deficiency. All the infants were initially breastfed by mothers whose diets were low in vitamin D, high in fiber and phytate (which interferes with enterohepatic circulation of vitamin D), and low in calcium and phosphate.

Cereals are the primary source of dietary zinc in vegetarian diets. The bioavailability of zinc is affected by the presence of phytates, fiber, calcium, or other zinc absorption inhibitors, which results in poor absorption of zinc in vegetarian diets.[90] Vitamins B_6 and B_{12}, vitamin A, and calcium, because of a high content of oxalic acid, are poorly absorbed.

Selenium is dependent on the selenium content of the soil, as is zinc. Increased dietary sources or supplementation are required in vegetarians.

General recommendations for lactating vegetarian women are as follows:

1. Supplement with soy flour, molasses, and nuts.
2. Use complementary protein combinations.
3. Avoid excessive phytates and bran.
4. Watch protein and iron intake. Calcium should be supplemented if bone mineralization decreases because the milk levels will be adequate.
5. Supplement with 10 μg vitamin D plus adequate sunshine.
6. Know that vitamins B_{12} and B_2 (riboflavin) are low in vegetarian diets and should be supplemented.

If the mother does not supplement herself, the infant must be supplemented.

SUPPLEMENTATION OF BREASTFED INFANTS' DIETS

For newborn infants, human milk is the ideal food, containing all the necessary nutrients. In establishing dietary norms for infants fed cow milk, many nutrients identified as being needed in the diet were found to exist in greater amounts in cow milk than in human milk. This does not consider the probability that the nutrient may be in a more bioavailable form in human milk. The specific items in question are protein, sodium, iron, vitamin D, and fluorine.

When a breastfed infant must be supplemented with formula, however, it is preferable that a formula low in iron be used to avoid providing excessive iron that will bind with lactoferrin and interfere with its infection protective activity.

The AAP Committee on Nutrition[18] has noted that iron deficiency is rare in breastfed infants and attributes this to increased absorption and the absence of microscopic blood loss into the gastrointestinal tract, which is seen in bottle-fed infants. The Section on Breastfeeding of the AAP recommends a source of iron in solid foods (fortified infant cereal) at 6 months of age for breastfed infants.[4]

The AAP no longer recommends fluoride supplements in all breastfed infants. Many breastfed infants have done without fluorine supplementation and have had no adverse dental problems, but the decision should be based on individual determinants, including family dental history and level of fluoride in the water supply, which is ideally between 0.7 and 1.0 ppm. If the level is less than 0.3 ppm, 0.25 mg of daily fluoride should be given. Maternal supplementation may be the better choice in this case.

The AAP now recommends 400 IU vitamin D daily for all breastfed infants starting at birth unless they are also receiving 500 mL fortified formula daily.[18] Maternal supplementation is a preferred alternative. The Section on Breastfeeding of the AAP, however, tailors the recommendation to the dyad, using supplements of vitamin D to the infant as a last resort.

EXERCISE WHILE BREASTFEEDING

There are usually no contraindications to exercise in moderation during lactation. The most common obstacle is having sufficient time. The availability of home exercise equipment does offer an option for home programs. Exercise baby carriages, which have large wheels for greater speed and rough terrain, are another option. Because they tip somewhat easily, infants may need a helmet and a safety strap. A safety strap that attaches to the runner's wrist prevents the vehicle from getting away. These carriages are excellent for brisk walks as well.

The impact of programmed exercise on milk volume, milk composition, and ultimately milk acceptability has been studied.[26] Women who exercise excessively, especially those who jog, may have trouble maintaining their milk supply. This difficulty has been attributed to any activity that results in persistent motion of the breasts and excessive friction of clothing against the nipples. A firm athletic brassiere made of cotton will reduce this effect. No data are available on the impact of jogging with or without support on later breast sagging.

The production of lactic acid during exercise has been studied in relation to lactation by Wallace et al., who had mothers report whether their infants refused to nurse or fussed when breastfed after exercise. The study demonstrated that seven healthy lactating women who normally spent more than 30 minutes in aerobic activity (jogging, running, swimming, biking, and aerobics), as well as some who did calisthenics and racket sports, had an increase in their blood lactic acid levels after exercise. When a standardized treadmill exercise was used to maximal voluntary effort, blood lactic acid level increased at 10 minutes compared with that of the at rest sample, but the level at 30 minutes had returned almost to the at rest level. Milk samples at 10 and 30 minutes continued to have elevated lactic acid, although wide variation was seen among subjects.

In a larger sample, when 26 women between 2 and 6 months postpartum who normally exercised during pregnancy and postpartum were exercised on a standardized treadmill to maximal voluntary effort, the levels of lactic acid were correlated to infant acceptance of the milk. The breasts were wiped with a dry towel before milk collection. Milk samples collected before exercise and at 10 and 30 minutes after exercise revealed an increase in lactic acid levels over baseline at both 10 and 30 minutes. In a double-blind order of samples, the infants were offered milk by dropper and were less likely to accept samples with high lactic acid. The authors noted that the levels of lactic acid were high enough for adults to detect when offered water solutions at the same concentrations (1.6 mmol). Human milk is sweet, but lactic acid is known to be bitter/sour. Infants have been noted to make a puckering facial expression to a sour taste as early as a few hours of age.[110] Studies of sucking in newborns have shown more rapid rates with sweet than sour, with some change in heart rate, respiratory rate, and sucking patterns.[61] The lactic acid level can remain elevated in the milk for as long as 90 minutes, according to Wallace and Rabin.

When exercise studies were undertaken by Wallace et al.,[121,122] comparing the effects of a typical workout and a standard maximal exercise regimen, significant differences were noted. The milk lactate level before exercise was 0.61 ± 0.14 mM and after typical exercise was 1.06 ± 33 mM. After maximal exercise in the same women, the level was 2.88 ± 0.80 mM. Seventeen percent of the subjects had lactate levels above the reported adult taste threshold of 1.5 mM. Milk rejection probably is a function of lactate concentration in the milk and infants' sensitivity to taste. Women who exercised with full breasts developed a peak postexercise lactate concentration at 10 minutes, whereas women who exercised with empty breasts did not peak for 30 minutes.[121] Many of the studies reported may have not measured peak lactate when samples were collected only at 10 minutes.

Mothers have reported that their infants may reject their milk after exercising. Women reported to the Lactation Study Center that their infants were fussy and colicky for as long as 4 to 6 hours after the mother's strenuous exercise. Exercise generates sweat high in sodium and chloride, and lactic acid may change the pH. Although these studies are being expanded, the following precautions might be recommended when breastfeeding after strenuous exercise:

- Shower, or at least wash the breast of perspiration.
- Manually express 3 to 5 mL of milk from each breast and discard.
- If infant displays puckering facial expression, postpone feeding or replace feeding with previously pumped milk.

Levels of prolactin and adrenal activation have been studied in eumenorrheic and amenorrheic women who exercise regularly. Prolactin levels after exercise are elevated for 20 to 40 minutes.[27] The effect appears to be unrelated to anaerobiosis. The hypothalamic-pituitary-adrenal axis is known to be activated under the influence of various forms of stress, including exercise. How this activation might affect milk production or oxytocin-stimulated milk let-down after exercise has yet to be determined.

Serum prolactin and growth hormone increased severalfold during prolonged acute exercise in normal women and runners with and without menses, demonstrating that a threshold of exercise intensity must be reached for this reaction to occur.[17] There was no correlation to menstrual dysfunction.

When the lactation performances of eight physically fit, exercising women were compared with those of sedentary control subjects, no significant differences in milk volume or composition were observed despite wide variations in energy intake and expenditure.[73] Exercising women compensated by increasing energy intake; thus no net difference was seen between the groups. It has been reported that lactating women exercising on a regular basis expend an average of 2630 kcal/day exclusive of milk energy output, compared with the 1800 to 1900 kcal/day expenditures of women who did not exercise.[112]

Dewey et al.[30] studied the impact of regular exercise on the volume and composition of breast milk and further confirmed that breastfeeding women can safely exercise. Although previous studies were done on exercising fit women, this study randomly assigned sedentary women to exercise with supervised aerobic exercise to 60% to 70% of the heart rate reserve for 45 minutes per day, 5 days a week for 12 weeks. The control group remained breastfeeding but sedentary. Measurements of energy expended, dietary intake, body composition, and milk volume and composition were collected at 6 to 8 weeks, 12 to 14 weeks, and 18 to 20 weeks postpartum. Maximum oxygen uptake and plasma prolactin response in 2 hours after nursing were measured at the first and last assessment times. No significant differences were seen in maternal weight and fat losses, volume or composition of milk, infant weight gain, or plasma prolactin response between exercising and sedentary women. No women reported difficulty nursing after moderate exercise. The authors[31] did note that the 300 kcal/day mean extra energy expenditure of the exercise group at midpoint in the study decreased toward the end as they cut back on other activities to compensate. This suggests that high levels of energy expenditure[30] may be difficult to sustain while lactating because of fatigue and time limitations (Figures 9-4 and 9-5).

Lovelady et al.[73,74] further evaluated this same study group, randomly assigned to exercise or to remain sedentary. Exercise marginally increased

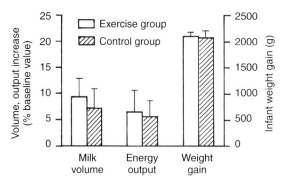

Figure 9-4. Percent increase in breast-milk volume and energy output and absolute increase in infants' weight in exercise and control groups during a 12-week study. Values shown are means±SE. To convert kilocalories to megajoules, multiply by 0.004186. None of the differences between the groups was significant. The 95% confidence intervals were as follows: for the percent change in milk volume, 2% to 17% for the exercise group and −1% to 16% for the control group ($p=0.66$); for the percent change in energy output in breast milk, −2% to 15% for the exercise group and −1% to 12% for the control group ($p=0.85$); and for infant weight gain, 1871 to 2279 g for the exercise group and 1733 to 2355 g for the control group ($p=0.86$). (Modified from Dewey KG, Lovelady CA, Nommsen-Rivers LA, et al: A randomized study of the effects of aerobic exercise by lactating women on breast-milk volume and composition, *N Engl J Med* 330:449, 1994.)

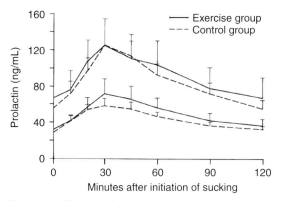

Figure 9-5. Plasma prolactin response to nursing in control and exercise groups at beginning and end of study. Values shown are mean±SE. Study began 6 to 8 weeks postpartum and ended 18 to 20 weeks postpartum. Change in the area under the curve from beginning to end of the study was not significantly different between the two groups ($p=0.38$). (Modified from Dewey KG, Lovelady CA, Nommsen-Rivers LA, et al: A randomized study of the effects of aerobic exercise by lactating women on breast-milk volume and composition, *N Engl J Med* 330:449, 1994.)

high-density lipoprotein cholesterol levels but did not affect other lipid concentrations. Further, at rest metabolic rate did not change overtime. Weight and body fat percentage declined similarly in both groups. No difference was found between exercising and sedentary groups regarding insulin, glucose, or thermal response. The authors concluded that

sedentary women can initiate moderate exercise programs during lactation but that exercise does not increase weight loss or fat loss without dietary control, that is, by avoiding compensatory increased intake. In a similar randomized study of 33 women, Potter et al.[95] and Prentice[97] reported that moderate exercise sufficient to improve cardiovascular fitness without marked changes in energy expenditure, dietary intake, and body weight and composition does not jeopardize lactation performance.

Maternal exercise did not alter the mineral content of the milk in a randomized crossover trial measuring phosphorus, calcium, magnesium, sodium, and potassium. Samples were drawn before and during rest periods after 10, 30, and 60 minutes of maximal graded exercise. Thus, with the exception of a temporary rise in milk lactate after prolonged heavy exercise, exercise has no apparent impact on milk composition.[71]

DIETING WHILE BREASTFEEDING

The Subcommittee on Nutrition During Lactation[112] stated in its report that the average rate of weight loss postpartum while maintaining adequate milk volume is 0.5 to 1.0 kg (1 to 2 lb) per month. In individuals who are significantly overweight, a weight loss of up to 1 to 2 kg (about 4 to 5 lb) per month should not affect milk volume, although weight gain and feeding pattern in the infant should be monitored. The subcommittee[112] considers rapid weight loss, that is, more than 2 kg per month after the first month, ill-advised. In addition, because no data exist about curtailing maternal energy intake during the first 2 to 3 weeks postpartum, dieting immediately postpartum is not recommended and could be associated with poor milk supply. Energy intake must be balanced with the level of physical activity. The subcommittee does not recommend intakes less than 1500 kcal/day; however, brief fasts, perhaps for religious reasons, of less than a day are unlikely to affect milk supply. Liquid diets or weight-loss medications are not recommended. In studies of food-deprived rats, a clear correlation exists between adequate milk production and adequate food intake. This finding was amplified if diet was also restricted during pregnancy.

Studies of weight loss during lactation are scarce. Many women in developed countries experience an appetite surge with lactation and may experience no weight loss in the first months beyond the weight lost in the first weeks. They may not return to prepregnancy weight for 6 months. Women who are prone to gaining weight may be more apt to gain on an unregulated diet. Maternal nutrition status in the United States, as measured by anthropometric indices prenatally and postpartum, is unrelated to milk volume, according to the studies of Butte et al.[13] and Dewey.[26] Total energy expenditure of sedentary women, including those housebound with a new baby, averages 1800 kcal/day, exclusive of the energy put into the milk produced.[76]

No consistent relationship was reported in a study of 411 postpartum women between mode (i.e., breast or bottle) of feeding and postpartum weight loss.[95] Despite the energy deficiency of breastfeeding women, the trend was to greater weight loss in nonlactators. Women who gained more during pregnancy lost more postpartum regardless of their pregnancy weight. No dietary intake was recorded because the data were collected retrospectively.

The Stockholm Pregnancy and Weight Development Study prospectively investigated trends in eating patterns, physical activity, and sociodemographic factors in relation to postpartum body weight development, following 1423 pregnant women.[88] Weight retention 1 year postpartum was greater in women who increased their energy intake during and after pregnancy. Weight retention also increased in those who not only increased their snacking to three or more times per day but also decreased their lunch frequency. Sedentary lifestyle was correlated with 5 kg or more weight gain over prepartum weight. The authors summarized their findings as being related most closely to a change in lifestyle after pregnancy.[88]

The tremendous variability in women's responses to the stress of reproduction and lactation suggests that there is very low stress per unit time. Thus, many different variables exist during the perinatal period to rebalance the energy equation, according to Prentice and Prentice.[99] Some women are energy sparing and some energy profligate. Although generally beneficial, the interaction between exercise and skeletal integrity is influenced by hormonal status and many exercise variables.

During lactation, many women do not need additional dietary supplements as often recommended according to work by Hartmann et al. They reported considerable variation among individual women for the energy output in milk and the energy actually mobilized from maternal stores for milk synthesis, and they recommend that energy should be calculated for each mother depending on her energy stores and milk demands. Even a low-fat diet could be appropriate to maximize the de novo synthesis of fatty acids for milk triacylglycerols, if one were sure there was AI of long-chain PUFAs and basic nutrients. Further, they demonstrated that perceived inability to make milk was usually a function of inappropriate suckling, scheduled feeds, and other

TABLE 9-14	Dietary Reference Intakes: Additional Macronutrient Recommendations
Macronutrient	**Recommendation**
Dietary cholesterol	As low as possible while consuming a nutritionally adequate diet
Trans fatty acids	As low as possible while consuming a nutritionally adequate diet
Saturated fatty acids	As low as possible while consuming a nutritionally adequate diet
Added sugars	Limit to no more than 25% of total energy

From Dietary Reference Intakes for Energy, Carbohydrate, Fiber, Fat, Fatty Acids, Cholesterol, Protein, and Amino Acids, Washington, D.C., 2002, Food and Nutrition Board, Institute of Medicine, National Academies.

lactation management issues, not lack of substrate (Table 9-14).

Weight loss during lactation is greatest between 3 and 6 months. Dietary advice for women who choose to diet while lactating should include the following[112]:

- Diet must include balanced, varied foods rich in calcium, zinc, magnesium, vitamin B_6, and folate.
- Minimum energy intake should be 1800 kcal.
- Calcium and multivitamin-mineral supplements may be necessary to replace stores if diet is marginal.

Foods to Avoid

The concern about foods causing gas in breastfed babies has no scientific basis. The normal intestinal flora produce gas from the action on fiber in the intestinal tract. Neither the fiber nor the gas is absorbed from the intestinal tract, and they do not enter the milk, even though they may cause the mother some discomfort. The acid content of the maternal diet also does not affect the milk because it does not change the pH of the maternal plasma. Essential oils are present in foods such as garlic and some spices that have characteristic odors and flavors. These oils may pass into the milk, and occasionally an infant objects to their presence.

Twenty-four-hour colic studies by Mennella and Beauchamp[78,80] show that the diet of the lactating woman alters the sensory qualities of her milk. They found that garlic ingestion significantly and consistently increased the intensity of the milk odor as perceived by blinded adult panelists. The odor was not apparent at 1 hour, peaked at 2 hours, and decreased thereafter. Similar observations have been made in other species. Garlic is one of the most potent of the volatile sulfur-containing foods (onions, broccoli, etc.). Garlic consumption by the mother increased the length of time spent suckling and the rate of suckling of the next feeding.[80] This behavior is usually associated with a tendency of the breast to make more milk. The authors suggest that the mouth movements made during sucking facilitated the retronasal perception of the garlic volatile oils in the milk. This study reports only the first 4 hours postingestion and makes no reference to the period between 4 and 24 hours after ingestion, a time occasionally associated with colic in breastfed infants after ingestion of certain foods by the mothers (often called 24-hour colic).

When these mothers and infants were tested over an 11-day period, those infants who had garlic previously showed no response to reexposure; that is, suckling pattern and volume ingested were unchanged.[79] Garlic odor of amniotic fluid has been noted when the mother consumed garlic before delivery or amniocentesis. These investigators also report that alcohol, mint, and cheese flavors are transmitted to milk. When mothers were fed carrot juice while lactating, the infant subsequently preferred cereal mixed with carrot juice rather than with plain formula or milk.[78]

Animal studies show that odors in utero and early in life are associated with a preference for them after birth. Breastfed infants experience a wide variety of odors and flavors during maternal lactation, which may enhance their weaning to solid foods. This suggests that infants fed standard formulas experience a constant set of flavors, thus missing significant sensory experiences. In experiments with rats, Mennella and Beauchamp[80] found a mother's milk contains gustatory cues reflecting the flavor of the mother's diet and that these cues are sufficient to influence dietary preferences at weaning.

Extensive clinical experience suggests, however, that some infants do not tolerate certain foods in the mother's diet, particularly specific vegetables and fruits. Garlic and onions may cause 24-hour colic in some infants. Cabbage, turnips, broccoli, or beans may bother others, making them colicky for 24 hours. The same has been said of rhubarb, apricots, and prunes. If a mother questions the effect of a food, she should avoid it or document its effect carefully by watching for colic in the 24 hours after ingestion. In the summer, a heavy diet of melon, peaches, and other fresh fruits may cause colic and diarrhea in the infant. Chocolate rarely lives up to its reputation and can be consumed in moderation without causing colic, diarrhea, or constipation in most infants.

Red pepper, which contains capsaicin and related compounds, has been reported to cause dermatitis in breastfed infants within an hour of milk ingestion.[20] The rash can last 12 to 48 hours and differs from the contact dermatitis known to occur from capsaicin applied directly. When hot peppers are prepared with bare hands, an intensely painful reaction can occur. In countries where red pepper dishes such as kimchi are common (Korea), a perianal rash has long been seen in breastfed infants whose mothers ingested these hot dishes.

FOOD ADDITIVES

Artificial sweeteners are the most common food additives. Saccharin and cyclamate are not known to be teratogenic, but the remote relationship to cancer in rats has led to the recommendation that they be used in moderation. The same pertains during lactation. Cyclamate is a cyclohexylamine, an indirectly acting sympathomimetic amine that has been banned from use.

Aspartame is a dipeptide sweetener, aspartyl-L-phenylalanine methyl ester, that metabolizes to phenylalanine and aspartic acid. Thus, it poses a risk to those with phenylketonuria. Normal individuals can consume 50 mg/kg/day without adverse effects. In large doses of 75 mg/kg/day, individuals increase their excretion of formate and methanol. When given aspartame, lactating women were noted to have phenylalanine levels four times the normal in their plasma.[108] Milk levels of phenylalanine and tyrosine were only slightly elevated. Aspartame in moderation during lactation is presumed safe unless the infant has phenylketonuria.

Color of Milk and Maternal Diet

The color of mature human milk is bluish white (foremilk), initially changing to creamy white (hindmilk). The color of colostrum is yellow to yellow-orange. Mothers occasionally report changes in the color of their milk. Most of these changes can be traced to pigments consumed in the diet, medications, or herbal remedies. The infant's urine may also turn color.

PINK OR PINK-ORANGE MILK

Pink-orange milk was traced to Sunkist orange soda, which contains red and yellow dyes. A case of a breastfed infant with pink to orange urine was reported by Roseman.[104] This combination of food dyes is also used in other brands of soda, fruit drinks, and gelatin desserts. Even fresh beets can change the urine of both mother and infant to a red-pink hue.

GREEN MILK

Several cases of green milk have been reported to our study center. A careful search of the diet for the offending substance was made in each case. The effect of ingestion of the identified culprit and its avoidance were then tested to confirm the association with the milk's color. Several items have been clearly identified. Gatorade (the green beverage), kelp and other forms of seaweed (especially in tablet form), and natural vitamins from health food sources have been associated with one or more cases of green milk and usually green urine.

BLACK MILK

Minocycline hydrochloride therapy was associated with black milk galactorrhea in a 24-year-old woman who received the compound for pustulocystic acne for 4 years.[9] Examination of the fluid revealed that the macrophages contained hemosiderin, thus causing the black color. This drug is known to cause black pigmentation of the skin. A second case was reported in a 29-year-old woman who had weaned but could express black milk 3 weeks after beginning oral minocycline therapy. Hunt et al.[56] found iron-staining pigment particles in the macrophages and suggested it was an iron chelate of minocycline.

SUMMARY

Supplements recommended during lactation for mothers are unnecessary unless the mother's diet is deficient. Finishing the prenatal vitamin supply postpartum is more than adequate. Having adequate vitamin D stores during pregnancy and lactation is important. Continued studies are being conducted to determine the efficacy of large doses of vitamin D for mothers so that supplementing infants can be avoided.

Supplements for breastfeeding infants are ordinarily unnecessary in exclusively breastfed infants unless a deficiency is identified. The AAP does recommend vitamin D 400 mg beginning at birth. Iron needs should be addressed with appropriate solid foods after 6 months of exclusive breastfeeding. Fluoride supplementation is unnecessary if the mother is adequately resourced; if not, the mother should take fluoride.

REFERENCES

1. Al MD, Houwelingen AC, Badart-Smook A, et al: Some aspects of neonatal essential fatty acid status are altered by linoleic acid supplementation of women during pregnancy, *J Nutr* 125:2822, 1995.
2. Alaejos MS, Romero CD: Selenium in human lactation, *Nutr Rev* 53:159, 1995.
3. Alexander RP, Walker BF, Bhamjee D: Serum lipids in long-lactating African mothers habituated to a low-fat intake, *Atherosclerosis* 44:175, 1982.
4. American Academy of Pediatrics: Section on breastfeeding: breastfeeding and the use of human milk, *Pediatrics* 129(3):e827–e841, 2012.
5. Anderson RA, Bryden NA, Patterson KY, et al: Breast milk chromium and its association with chromium intake, chromium excretion, and serum chromium, *Am J Clin Nutr* 57:519, 1993.
6. Andon MB, Reynolds RD, Moser-Veillon PB, et al: Dietary intake of total and glycosylated vitamin B6 and the vitamin B6 nutritional status of unsupplemented lactating women and their infants, *Am J Clin Nutr* 50:1050, 1989.
7. Arnaud J, Prual A, Preziosi P, et al: Effect of iron supplementation during pregnancy on trace element (Cu, Se, Zn) concentrations in serum and breast milk from Nigerian women, *Ann Nutr Metab* 37:262, 1993.
8. Asnes R, Wisotsky DH, Migel PF, et al: The dietary chloride deficiency syndrome occurring in a breastfed infant, *J Pediatr* 100:923, 1982.
9. Basler RS, Lynch PJ: Black galactorrhea as a consequence of minocycline and phenothiazine therapy, *Arch Dermatol* 121:417, 1985.
10. Bates CJ, Prentice AM, Watkinson M, et al: Riboflavin requirements of lactating Gambian women: a controlled supplementation trial, *Am J Clin Nutr* 135:701, 1982.
11. Bhaskaram P, Reddy V: Bactericidal activity of human milk leukocytes, *Acta Paediatr Scand* 70:87, 1981.
12. Brenna JT, Varamini B, Jensen RG, et al: Docosahexaenoic and arachidonic acid concentrations in human breast milk world wide, *Am J Clin Nutr* 85:1457–1464, 2007.
13. Butte NF, Garza C, Stuff JE, et al: Effect of maternal diet and body composition on lactational performance, *Am J Clin Nutr* 39:296, 1984.
14. Byrne J, Thomas MR, Chan GM: Calcium intake and bone density of lactating women in their late childbearing years, *J Am Diet Assoc* 87:883, 1987.
15. Chappell JE, Clandinin MT, Kearney-Volpe C: Trans fatty acids in human milk lipids: influence of maternal diet and weight loss, *Am J Clin Nutr* 42:49, 1985.
16. Christoffel K: A pediatric perspective on vegetarian nutrition, *Clin Pediatr* 20:632, 1981.
17. Chulei R, Xiaofang L, Hongsheng M, et al: Milk composition in women from five different regions of China: the great diversity of milk fatty acids, *J Nutr* 125:2998, 1995.
18. Committee on Nutrition, American Academy of Pediatrics: *Pediatric nutrition handbook*, ed 7, Elk Grove, Ill., 2014, American Academy of Pediatrics, pp 6, 71, 307, 793.
19. Connor WE, Lowensohn R, Hatcher L: Increased docosahexaenoic acid levels in human newborn infants by administration of sardines and fish oil during pregnancy, *Lipids* 31:5183, 1996.
20. Cooper RL, Cooper MN: Red pepper-induced dermatitis in breast-fed infants, *Dermatology* 193:61, 1996.
21. Crozier SR, Harvey NC, Inskip HM: Maternal vitamin D status in pregnancy is associated with adiposity in the offspring, *Am J Clin Nutr* 96(1):57–63, 2012.
22. Daaboul J, Sanderson S, Kristensen K, et al: Vitamin D deficiency in pregnant and breastfeeding women and their infants, *J Perinatol* 17:10, 1997.
23. Dagnelie PC, van Staveren WA: Macrobiotic nutrition and child health: results of a population-based, mixed-longitudinal cohort study in the Netherlands, *Am J Clin Nutr* 59(Suppl):1187S, 1994.
24. Dagnelie PC, van Staveren WA, Roos AH, et al: Nutrients and contaminants in human milk from mothers on macrobiotic and omnivorous diets, *Eur J Clin Nutr* 46:355, 1992.
25. DeSouza MJ, Maguire MS, Maresh CM, et al: Adrenal activation and the prolactin response to exercise in

eumenorrheic and amenorrheic runners, *J Appl Physiol* 70(6):2378, 1991.

26. Dewey KG: Does maternal supplementation shorten the duration of lactational amenorrhea? *Am J Clin Nutr* 64: 377, 1996.

27. Dewey KG, Domellof M, Cohen RJ, et al: Iron supplementation affects growth and morbidity of breast-fed infants: results of a randomized trial in Sweden and Honduras, *J Nutr* 132:3249–3255, 2002.

28. Dewey KG, Finley DA, Lönnerdal B: Breast milk volume and composition during late lactation (7-20 months), *J Pediatr Gastroenterol Nutr* 3:713, 1984.

29. Dewey KG, Heinig MJ, Nommsen LA, et al: Maternal vs infant factors related to breast milk intake and residual milk volume: the Darling study, *Pediatrics* 87:829, 1991.

30. Dewey KG, Lovelady CA, Nommsen-Rivers LA, et al: A randomized study of the effects of aerobic exercise by lactating women on breast-milk volume and composition, *N Engl J Med* 330:449, 1994.

31. Donnen P, Brasseur D, Dramaix M, et al: Effects of cow's milk supplementation on milk output of protein deficient lactating mothers and on their infants' energy and protein status, *Trop Med Int Health* 2:38, 1997.

32. Dwyer JT, Palombo R, Thorne H, et al: Preschoolers on alternate lifestyle diets, *J Am Diet Assoc* 72:264, 1978.

33. Ereman RR, Lönnerdal B, Dewey KG: Maternal sodium intake does not affect postprandial sodium concentrations in human milk, *J Nutr* 117:1154, 1987.

34. Finley DA, Lönnerdal B, Dewey KG, et al: Breast milk composition: fat content and fatty acid composition in vegetarians and non-vegetarians, *Am J Clin Nutr* 41:787, 1985.

35. Food and Drug Administration: Draft risk benefit assessment, report of quantitative risk and benefit assessment of consumption of commercial fish, Available from: www.cfsan.fda.gov/udms/mehgrb.html, 2009 (Accessed 19.03.09.).

36. Food and Nutrition Board, Institute of Medicine, National Academies: *Dietary reference intakes (DRIs): recommended intakes for individuals,* Washington, D.C., 2006, The National Academic Press.

37. Friel JK, Aziz K, Andrews WJ, et al: A double-masked randomized control trial of iron supplementation in early infancy in healthy term breast-fed infants, *J Pediatr* 143:582, 2003.

38. Fukushima Y, Kawata Y, Onda T, et al: Consumption of cow milk and egg by lactating women and the presence of b-lactoglobulin and ovalbumin in breast milk, *Am J Clin Nutr* 65:30, 1997.

39. Fung EB, Ritchie LD, Woodhouse LR, et al: Zinc absorption in women during pregnancy and lactation: a longitudinal study, *Am J Clin Nutr* 66:80, 1997.

40. Gabriel A, Gabriel KR, Lawrence RA: Cultural values and biomedical knowledge: choices in infant feeding—analysis of a survey, *Soc Sci Med* 23:501, 1986.

41. Gambon RC, Lentze MJ, Rossi E: Megaloblastic anaemia in one of monozygous twins breast fed by their vegetarian mother, *Eur J Pediatr* 145:570, 1986.

42. Gartner LM, Greer FR: Prevention of rickets and vitamin D deficiency: new guidelines for vitamin D intake, *Pediatrics* 111:908, 2003.

43. Gogia S, Sachelev HS: Maternal postpartum vitamin A supplementation for prevention of mortality and morbidity in infancy: a systematic review of randomized controlled trials, *Internet J Epidemiol* 39:1217–1226, 2010.

44. Gonzalez-Cossio T, Habicht JP, Rasmussen KM, et al: Impact of food supplementation during lactation on infant breast-milk intake and on the proportion of infants exclusively breast-fed, *J Nutr* 128:1692, 1998.

45. Gould JF, Smithers LG, McKrides M: The effect of maternal omega-3(*n*-3) LCPUFA supplementation during pregnancy on early childhood cognitive and visual development: a systematic review and meta-analysis of randomized controlled trials, *Am J Clin Nutr* 97:531–544, 2013.

46. Greer FR, Marshall SP, Severson RR, et al: A new mixed-micellar preparation for oral vitamin K prophylaxis: comparison with an intramuscular formulation in breast-fed infants, *Arch Dis Child* 79:300, 1998.

47. Greer FR, Marshall SP, Suttle JW: Improving the vitamin K status of breast-feeding infants with vitamin K supplements, *Pediatrics* 99:88, 1997.

48. Greer FR, Tsang RC, Levin RS, et al: Increasing serum calcium and magnesium concentrations in breast-fed infants: longitudinal studies of minerals in human milk and in sera of nursing mothers and their infants, *J Pediatr* 100:59, 1982.

49. Griffin IJ, Abrams SA: Iron and breastfeeding, *Pediatr Clin North Am* 48:401, 2001.

50. Gushurst CA, Mueller JA, Green JA, et al: Breast milk iodide: reassessment in the 1980s, *Pediatrics* 73:354, 1984.

51. Hellebostad M, Markestad T, Halvorsen KS: Vitamin D deficiency rickets and vitamin B12 deficiency in vegetarian children, *Acta Paediatr Scand* 74:191, 1985.

52. Higginbottom MC, Sweetman L, Nyhan WL: A syndrome of methylmalonic aciduria, homocystinuria, megaloblastic anemia and neurologic abnormalities in a vitamin B12 deficient breastfed infant of a strict vegetarian, *N Engl J Med* 299:317, 1978.

53. Hollis BW, Pittard WB III, Reinhardt TA: Relationships among vitamin D, 25-hydroxyvitamin D, and vitamin D-binding protein concentrations in the plasma and milk of human subjects, *J Clin Endocrinol Metab* 62:41, 1986.

54. Hopkins D, Emmwtt P, Steer C, et al: Infant feeding in the second 6 months of life related to iron. status: an observational study, *Arch Dis Child* 92:850–854, 2007.

55. Hopkinson J: Nutrition in lactation. In Hale TW, Hartmann PE, editors: *Textbook of human lactation,* Amarillo, Tex., 2007, Hale Publishing.

56. Hunt MJ, Salisbury ELC, Grace J, et al: Black breast milk due to minocycline therapy, *Br J Dermatol* 134:943, 1996.

57. Innes SM, Friesen RW: Essential *n*-3 fatty acids in pregnant women and early visual acuity maturation in term infants, *Am J Clin Nutr* 87(3):548–557, 2008.

58. Insull W, Hersch J, James T, et al: The fatty acids of human milk. II. Alterations produced by manipulation of caloric balance and exchange of dietary fats, *J Clin Invest* 38:443, 1959.

59. Jackson MJ, Giugliano R, Giugliano LG, et al: Stable isotope metabolic studies of zinc nutrition in slum dwelling lactating women in the Amazon valley, *Br J Nutr* 59:193, 1988.

60. Jensen RG: *The lipids of human milk,* Boca Raton, Fla., 1989, CRC.

61. Johnson P, Salisbury DM: Preliminary studies on feeding and breathing in the newborn. In Weiffenbach JM, editor: *Taste and development: the genesis of sweet preference,* Bethesda, Md., 1977, Public Health Service, National Institutes of Health, Department of Health, Education and Welfare Publication (NIH).

62. Johnston L, Vaughn L, Fox HM: Pantothenic acid content of human milk, *Am J Clin Nutr* 34:2205, 1981.

63. Kalkwarf HJ, Specker BL, Herbi JE, et al: Intestinal calcium absorption of women during lactation and after weaning, *Am J Clin Nutr* 63:526, 1996.

64. Kang-Yoon SA, Kirksey A, Giacoia G, et al: Vitamin B6 status of breastfed neonates: influence of pyridoxine supplementation on mothers and neonates, *Am J Clin Nutr* 56:548, 1992.

65. Kliewer RI, Rasmussen KM: Malnutrition during the reproductive cycle: effects on galactopoietic hormones and lactational performance in the rat, *Am J Clin Nutr* 46:926, 1987.

66. Kramer M, Szöke K, Lindner K, et al: The effect of different factors on the composition of human milk and its variations.

III. Effect of dietary fats on the lipid composition of human milk, *J Nutr Diet* 7:71, 1965.

67. Krebs NF, Hambidge KM, Jacobs MA, et al: The effects of a dietary zinc supplement during lactation on longitudinal changes in maternal zinc status and milk zinc concentrations, *Am J Clin Nutr* 41:560, 1985.

68. Krebs NF, Reidinger CJ, Hartley S, et al: Zinc supplementation during lactation: effects on maternal status and milk zinc concentrations, *Am J Clin Nutr* 61:1030, 1995.

69. Lammi-Keefe CJ, Jensen RG: Lipids in human milk: a review. II. Composition and fat-soluble vitamins, *J Pediatr Gastroenterol Nutr* 3:172, 1984.

70. Lammi-Keefe CJ, Jensen RG, Clark RM, et al: Alpha tocopherol total lipid and linoleic acid contents of human milk at 2, 6, 12, and 16 weeks. In Schaub J, editor: *Composition and physiological properties of human milk*, Amsterdam, 1985, Elsevier Science.

71. Larson-Meyer DE: Effect of postpartum exercise on mothers and their offspring: a review of the literature, *Obes Res* 10:841–853, 2002.

72. Levander OA, Moser PB, Morris VC: Dietary selenium intake and selenium concentrations of plasma, erythrocytes, and breast milk in pregnant and postpartum lactating and non-lactating women, *Am J Clin Nutr* 46:694, 1987.

73. Lovelady CA, Lönnerdal B, Dewey KG: Lactation performance of exercising women, *Am J Clin Nutr* 52:103, 1990.

74. Lovelady CA, Nommsen LA, McCrory MA, et al: Effects of exercise on plasma lipids and metabolism of lactating women, *Med Sci Sports Exerc* 27:22, 1995.

75. Macy IG, Huncher HA, Donelson E, et al: Human milk flow, *Am J Dis Child* 6:492, 1930.

76. McGuire MK, Burgent SL, Milner JA, et al: Selenium status of lactating women is affected by the form of selenium consumed, *Am J Clin Nutr* 58:649, 1993.

77. Mellies MJ, Ishikawa TT, Gartside P, et al: Effects of varying maternal dietary cholesterol and phytosterol in lactating women and their infants, *Am J Clin Nutr* 31:1347, 1978.

78. Mennella JA, Beauchamp GK: Maternal diet alters the sensory qualities of human milk and nursling's behavior, *Pediatrics* 88:737, 1991.

79. Mennella JA, Beauchamp GK: The effects of repeated exposure to garlic-flavored milk on the nursling's behavior, *Pediatr Res* 34:805, 1993.

80. Mennella JA, Beauchamp GK: The early development of human flavor preferences. In Capaldi ED, editor: *Why we eat what we eat: the psychology of eating*, Washington, D.C., 1996, American Psychological Association.

81. Miranda R, Saravia NG, Ackerman R, et al: Effect of maternal nutritional status on immunological substances in human colostrum and milk, *Am J Clin Nutr* 37:632, 1983.

82. Motil KJ, Thotathuckery M, Bahar A, et al: Marginal dietary protein restriction reduced nonprotein nitrogen, but not protein nitrogen components of human milk, *J Am Coll Nutr* 14:184, 1995.

83. National Academy of Sciences: Dietary reference intakes, 2000, 2001, 2002, 2003, 2004, 2005. Available from: www.nap.edu.

84. Nelson TR, Pretorius DH, Schiffer LM: Menstrual variation of normal breast NMR relaxation parameters, *J Comput Assist Tomogr* 9:875, 1985.

85. Neville MC: Volume and caloric density of human milk. In Jensen RD, editor: *Handbook of milk composition*, San Diego, 1995, Academic Press, p 99.

86. Neville MC: Anatomy and physiology of lactation, In Schanler RJ, editor: Breastfeeding 2001, Part I. The evidence for breastfeeding, *Pediatr Clin North Am* 48(1):13, 2001.

87. O'Brien CE, Krebs NF, Westcott JL, et al: Relationships among plasma zinc, plasma prolactin, milk transfer and milk zinc in lactating women, *J Hum Lact* 23(2):179–183, 2007.

88. O'Connor DL: Folate status during pregnancy and lactation, *Adv Exp Med Biol* 352:157, 1994.

89. Oken E, Radesky JS, Wright RO, et al: Maternal fish intake during pregnancy, blood mercury levels, and child cognition at age 3 years in a US cohort, *Am J Epidemiol* 167(10):1171–1181, 2008.

90. Otten JL, Heilwig UP, Meyers LD, editors: *Dietary reference intakes-the essential guide to nutrient requirements*, Washington, D.C., 2006, Institute of Medicine, The National Academies Press.

91. Parkinson AJ, Cruz AL, Heyward WL, et al: Elevated concentrations of plasma omega-3 polyunsaturated fatty acids among Alaskan Eskimos, *Am J Clin Nutr* 59:384, 1994.

92. Pearce EN: National trends in iodine nutrition: is everyone getting enough? *Thyroid* 17(9):823–827, 2007.

93. Pearce EN, Leung AM, Blount BC, et al: Breast milk iodine and perchlorate concentrations in lactating Boston-area women, *J Clin Endocrinol Metab* 92(5):106–1677, 2007.

94. Picciano MF: Nutrient composition of human milk, *Pediatr Clin North Am* 48:53, 2001.

95. Potter S, Hannum S, McFarlin B, et al: Does infant feeding method influence maternal postpartum weight loss? *J Am Diet Assoc* 91:441, 1991.

96. Prentice A: Maternal calcium requirements during pregnancy and lactation, *Am J Clin Nutr* 59(Suppl):477S, 1994.

97. Prentice A: Should lactating women exercise? *Nutr Rev* 52:358, 1994.

98. Prentice A, Jarjou LM, Cole TJ, et al: Calcium requirements of lactating Gambian mothers: effects of a calcium supplement on breast milk calcium concentration, maternal bone content, and urinary calcium excretion, *Am J Clin Nutr* 62:58, 1995.

99. Prentice AM, Prentice A: Energy costs of lactation, *Annu Rev Nutr* 8:63, 1988.

100. Prentice A, Prentice AM, Cole TJ, et al: Breast milk antimicrobial factors of rural Gambian mothers. I. Influence of stage of lactation and maternal plane of nutrition, *Acta Paediatr Scand* 73:796, 1984.

101. Rana SK, Sanders TAB: Taurine concentrations in diet, plasma, urine, and breast milk of vegans compared with omnivores, *Br J Nutr* 56:17, 1986.

102. Rassin DK, Sturman JA, Gaull GE: Taurine and other free amino acids in milk of man and other mammals, *Early Hum Dev* 2:1, 1978.

103. Reddy S, Sanders TAB, Obeid O: The influence of maternal vegetarian diet on essential fatty acid status of the newborn, *Eur J Clin Nutr* 48:358, 1994.

104. Roseman BD: Sunkissed urine, *Pediatrics* 67:443, 1981 (letter).

105. Smith CA: Effects of maternal undernutrition upon newborn infants in Holland (1944-1945), *J Pediatr* 30:229, 1947.

106. Sosa R, Klaus M, Urrutia JJ: Feed the nursing mother, thereby the infant, *J Pediatr* 88:668, 1976.

107. Specker BL, Black A, Allen L, et al: Vitamin B12: low milk concentrations are related to low serum concentrations in vegetarian women and to methylmalonic aciduria in their infants, *Am J Clin Nutr* 52:1073, 1990.

108. Specker BL, Wey HE, Miller D: Differences in fatty acid composition of human milk in vegetarian and nonvegetarian women: long-term effect of diet, *J Pediatr Gastroenterol Nutr* 6:764, 1987.

109. Stein ZA, Susser MW, Saenger G, et al: *Famine and human development: the Dutch Hunger Winter of 1944-45*, New York, 1975, Oxford University Press.

110. Steiner JE: Facial expressions of the neonate indicating the hedonics of food-related chemical stimuli. In Weifferbach JM, editor: *Taste and development: the genesis of sweet preference*, Bethesda, Md., 1977, Public Health Service, National Institutes of Health, Department of Health, Education and Welfare Publication (NIH).

111. Steingrimsdottir L, Brasel JA, Greenwood MRC: Diet, pregnancy, and lactation: effects on adipose tissue, lipoprotein lipase, and fat cell size, *Metabolism* 29:837, 1980.

112. Subcommittee on Nutrition During Lactation, Committee on Nutritional Status During Pregnancy and Lactation, Food and Nutrition Board, et al: *Nutrition during lactation,* Washington, D.C., 1991, National Academy Press.

113. Suitor CW, Olson C, Wilson J: Nutrition care during pregnancy and lactation: new guidelines from the IOM, *J Am Diet Assoc* 93:478, 1993.

114. Tennekoon KH, Karunanayake EH, Seneviratne HR: Effect of skim milk supplementation of the maternal diet on lactational amenorrhea, maternal prolactin and lactational behavior, *Am J Clin Nutr* 64:238, 1996.

115. Thomas DW, Greer FR: Probiotics and prebiotics in pediatrics clinical report, *Am Acad Pediatr* 126:2009.

116. Tully J, Dewey KG: Private fears, global loss: a cross-cultural study of insufficient milk syndrome, *Med Anthropol* 9:225, 1985.

117. Van Houwelingen AC, Sorensen JD, Hornstra G, et al: Essential fatty acid status in neonates after fish-oil supplementation during late pregnancy, *Br J Nutr* 74:723, 1995.

118. Vlachou A, Drummond BK, Curzon MEJ: Fluoride concentrations of infant foods and drinks in the United Kingdom, *Caries Res* 26:29, 1992.

119. Wagner CL, Greer F: Section on breastfeeding and committee on nutrition: prevention of rickets and vitamin D. Deficiency in infants, children and adolescents, *Pediatrics* 122(5):1142–1152, 2008.

120. Walker ARP, Walker BF, Bhamjee D, et al: Serum lipids in long-lactating African mothers habituated to a low fat intake, *Atherosclerosis* 44:175, 1982.

121. Wallace JP, Ernsthausen K, Inbar G: The influence of the fullness of milk in the breasts on the concentration of lactic acid in post exercise breast milk, *Int J Sports Med* 13:395, 1992.

122. Wallace JP, Inbar G, Ernsthausen K: Infant acceptance of post exercise breast milk, *Pediatrics* 89:1245, 1992.

123. Walton JL, Messer LB: Dental caries and fluorosis in breast-fed and bottle-fed children, *Caries Res* 15:124, 1981.

124. Winkvist A, Habicht JP, Rasmussen KM: Linking maternal and infant benefits of a nutritional supplement during pregnancy and lactation, *Am J Clin Nutr* 68:656, 1998.

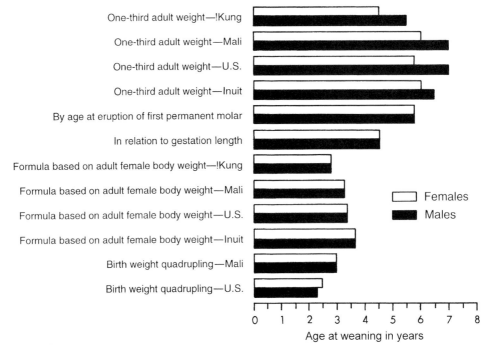

Figure 10-1. Natural age at weaning according to technique used. (Modified from Dettwyler KA: A time to wean. In Stuart-MacAdam P, Dettwyler KA, editors: *Breastfeeding: biocultural perspectives,* New York, 1995, Aldine de Gruyter.)

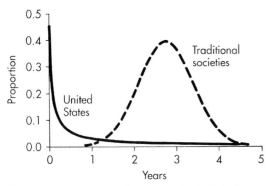

Figure 10-2. Comparison of age at weaning in United States and 64 traditional societies. (Modified from Dettwyler KA: A time to wean. In Stuart-MacAdam P, Dettwyler KA, editors: *Breastfeeding: biocultural perspectives,* New York, 1995, Aldine de Gruyter.)

additional source of protein becomes necessary toward the end of the first year of life because the grams of protein needed per kilogram of body weight can no longer be supplied by milk alone as the infant grows heavier. The content of protein in the milk begins to drop slightly after 9 months of lactation. A human infant also needs bulk, or roughage, in the diet. The exact time this need becomes apparent is not known, but it may well be by the end of the first year (Table 10-1).

Developmentally, an infant is ready to learn to chew solids instead of suckle liquids at about 6 months. It has been suggested that there is a "critical period of development" during which infants can and must learn to chew. Chewing is an entirely different motion of the tongue and mouth from sucking. The sucking fat pads in the cheeks begin to disappear at the end of the first year. The rooting reflex has been lost. Even though all the teeth are not in, the development of good dentition requires chewing exercise.

Role of Development in Initiation of Weaning

Although the developmental milestones of infant behavior are noted to influence the introduction of weaning foods, the development of the gastrointestinal tract plays an equal role. Even the taste buds, which can be identified at the seventh week of fetal life as collections of elongated cells on the dorsal surface of the tongue, are fully innervated over the next weeks. The fetus is known to suck and swallow in utero; sucking is discussed in Chapters 3 and 8.

When taste becomes a factor in feeding is not known, although a lack of discrimination has been noted in the first weeks of life: infants have consumed formula with high salt or absence of chloride with morbid results. As more women are pumping and storing their milk, a notable number of women have their infants reject the stored milk, which is

TABLE 10-1 Recommendations on Duration of Breastfeeding

WHO	Exclusive for 6 months	Continue 2 years and beyond
AAP	Exclusive for 6 months	Continue 1 year and as long as mother/infant wish
AAFP	About 6 months exclusive	Continue 1 year/mutually desired
ACOG	About 6 months exclusive	As long as possible
Healthy People 2010	75% at birth	25% at 6 months
Healthy People 2020	Exclusive for 6 months	Continue for 1 year

AAP, American Academy of Pediatrics; *AAFP,* American Academy of Family Practice; *ACOG,* American College of Obstetrics and Gynecology; *WHO,* World Health Organization.

Modified from Dettwyler KA: A time to wean: the hominid blueprint for the natural age of weaning in modern human populations. In Stuart-MacAdam P, Dettwyler KA, editors: *Breastfeeding: biocultural perspectives,* New York, 1995, Aldine de Gruyter.

noted to smell sour. See discussion of lipase and sour milk. Because of the variation in the composition of mother's milk over a feeding, over a day, and from time to time according to maternal dietary intake, a breastfed infant has a richer range of experience in tasting than a formula-fed infant. Breastfed infants are, therefore, more accustomed to new taste experiences. Similarly, feeding problems in infants are rare in breastfed infants.

Both sucking and chewing are complex movements, having reflexive as well as learned components. The development of the chew-swallow reflex is necessary for the successful introduction of solids. This skill develops sequentially with neuronal development and then is a learned behavior conditioned by oral stimulation. Before this point, when a spoon is introduced, the infant purses the lips and pushes the tongue against the spoon. By 4 to 6 months, the tongue is depressed in response to the spoon and the food accepted, and by 7 to 9 months, rhythmic biting movements occur regardless of the presence of teeth. Biting and masticatory strength and efficiency progress throughout infancy. If a stimulus is not applied when the neural development is taking place, the chewing reflex will not develop and the infant will always be a poor chewer. There is a relationship between prolonged sucking without solids and poor eating. The clinical model for this is a child sustained on

parenteral feedings or gastrostomy beyond a year who has tremendous difficulty accepting solids.

For a human infant, nursing also plays a role as a comfort and emotional support, a mechanism often referred to as "comfort nursing." Inadequate nipple contact may lead to thumb sucking or the substitute use of a pacifier. Young monkeys and apes in the wild do not suck their thumbs, but they do in captivity when bottle fed. Infants of the !Kung tribes in Africa do not suck their thumbs.[12] They are carried by the mother and breastfed in frequent short bursts.

In summary, an infant is ready to explore new feeding experiences at approximately 6 months. Feeding is an important social as well as nutritional encounter. Eating solids and learning to drink from a cup are important social achievements as well. This readiness does not mean the infant is taken from the breast, but that the diet is expanded and now includes solid foods, other liquids, and breast milk. Although a range of qualitative, quantitative, and temporal practices are known, the optimal approach matches the needs and requirements of a given child with the functions and capacities of the body.

Introduction of Solids

The World Health Organization (WHO), the Canadian Pediatric Society, the Paediatric Society of New Zealand, and similar groups in England and Scotland[55] emphasize that weaning is not the termination of breastfeeding but the addition of solids while continuing breastfeeding. The key recommendation on length of exclusive breastfeeding reads as follows:

> ...to strengthen activities and develop new approaches to protect, promote and support exclusive breastfeeding for six months as a global public health recommendation, taking into account the findings of the WHO expert consultation on optimal duration of exclusive breastfeeding, and to provide safe and appropriate complementary foods, with continued breastfeeding for up to two years of age or beyond, emphasizing channels of social dissemination of these concepts in order to lead communities to adhere to these practices.

The intake of supplementary foods may add nutrients in a less bioavailable form, and it decreases the bioavailability of nutrients in human milk and the intake of other important factors in human milk. Investigators have shown that when solid foods are introduced in the diet of breastfed infants, energy intake per kilogram of body weight does not increase.[43] Solid foods displaced energy intake from in lactation and the regression of the mammary gland occur slowly with gradual weaning.

When an infant is fully breastfeeding and solids are initiated, a feeding of solids is given during the day and breastfeeding continues on demand. As solids are increased and a three-meals-per-day schedule is reached, breastfeeding still continues on demand, although nursings may be fewer or briefer. No nursings need be intentionally omitted in this scheme, although it is important to give the scheduled solids before breastfeeding the infant.

The study of the composition of milk during abrupt weaning revealed that the secretory capability of the mammary gland of women changed dramatically after complete cessation of breastfeeding but that the involuting gland remained partially functional for 45 days. After termination that occurred in 1 day, sample collections were attempted for each breast by manual expression at the same time on days 1, 2, 4, 8, 16, 21, 31, 42, and 45. The concentrations of lactose and potassium decreased, while sodium, chloride, fat, and total protein increased progressively over 42 days. The milk becomes notably salty, but the infants continue to drink the salty fluid. The increase in protein was related to increases in the concentrations of lactoferrin, IgA, IgG, IgM, albumin, lactalbumin, and casein. Concentrations from each breast were similar throughout.

The involution in other species is rapid. For example, complete reabsorption occurs in 7 days in cows. The threshold dose of oxytocin required to elicit milk ejection increased progressively for at least 30 days after termination of breastfeeding. It is thought that a psychological nursing stimulus contributes to this effect in humans because they continue contact with their infants, whereas other species are separated. Experimental animals given oxytocin after weaning also show a delay in involution.

Weaning ages and techniques in a sample of American women who practiced extended breastfeeding were reported by Sugarman and Kendall-Tackett.[51] Women were recruited from La Leche League meetings in the area and nationally, utilizing survey forms (closed-end, self-administered, 96-item questionnaires). Based on 134 mothers and 211 children, the weaning age ranged from 1 month to 7 years 4 months. For those who weaned three children, as well as the entire sample, the tendency was to nurse the youngest the longest, perhaps because it was not supplanted by a sibling.

Reasons for weaning were predominantly child-led for about 60% of children, but weaning was the mother's decision in up to 15.8% in the youngest child (Tables 10-2 and 10-3). Those who were still nursing responded to the question, "Have you thought about weaning this child?" predominantly with a "no" (Table 10-4).[51]

A normal, well-adjusted mother may experience some depression and sadness at the reality of the last feeding.[48] It may be difficult to deal with this experience. It is important to recognize this as a physiologic phenomenon as well as an emotional one. If a mother is forced by circumstances beyond her control to wean early, she may need understanding and encouragement to cope with the disappointment. If she had pressure from friends or relatives to breastfeed, she may need to face what she considers failure and recognize that one can bottle feed and still mother very well.

TABLE 10-2	Reasons for Weaning and Types of Methods		
	Child A* (n=25)	Child B* (n=125)	Child C* (n=69)
Reasons for weaning (%)			
Lack of information	5.3	4.2	8.7
Lack of support or opposition	2.6	4.2	8.7
Next pregnancy affected taste or supply of milk	7.9	14.3	8.7
Next pregnancy affected mother's motivation	5.3	21.8	24.6
Illness or separation from child	5.3	5.9	11.6
Child-led, happened naturally	63.2	57.1	52.2
Mother's decision that child was ready	15.0	13.4	10.1
Mother's decision based on family circumstance	7.9	5.0	4.3
Other	0.0	5.9	1.4
How weaning was accomplished (mean %)			
Sudden	12.8	7.6	8.8
Gradual	56.4	60.2	45.6
Child-led	53.3	56.7	54.1
Mother deliberately weaned	2.6	11.0	13.2
Mother encouraged weaning by talking to child	23.1	31.4	20.6
Substituted thumb, pacifier	2.6	3.4	1.5
Other	1.7	1.8	1.7
Number of reasons (mean)	1.8	1.8	1.7

*A, B, and C represent three consecutive children, child A being the youngest.

From Sugarman M, Kendall-Tackett KA: Weaning ages in a sample of American women who practice extended breast feeding, *Clin Pediatr* 34:642, 1995.

TABLE 10-3 Percentage of Mothers Who Indicated That Specified Reasons Were Important in Their Decision to Stop Breastfeeding, According to Infants' Age at Weaning

Reasons Cited as Important	Infants' Age When Breastfeeding Was Completely Stopped (mo)					Average
	<1	1-2	3-5	6-8	≥9	
Lactational factor						
My baby had trouble sucking or latching on*	51.7	27.1	11.0	2.6	1.5	19.2
My nipples were sore, cracked, or bleeding*	36.8	23.2	7.2	5.7	4.2	15.4
My breasts were overfull or engorged*	23.9	12.3	4.8	1.6	1.2	8.8
My breasts were infected or abscessed*	8.1	5.7	3.1	3.1	3.1	4.6
My breasts leaked too much*	14.1	8.0	3.8	1.6	1.9	5.9
Breastfeeding was too painful*	29.3	15.8	3.4	3.7	4.2	11.3
Psychosocial factor						
Breastfeeding was too tiring*	19.8	17.2	11.0	7.8	5.3	12.2
Breastfeeding was too inconvenient*	20.4	22.4	18.6	12.5	4.2	15.6
I wanted to be able to leave my baby for several hours at a time*	11.2	24.1	18.2	15.6	7.3	15.3
I had too many household duties*	12.6	14.0	9.6	5.2	18	9.0
I wanted or needed someone else to feed my baby*	16.4	23.2	21.0	17.2	6.1	16.8
Someone else wanted to feed the baby*	13.5	15.5	120	5.7	3.4	10.0
I did not want to breastfeed in public*	14.9	18.6	15.1	4.7	4.6	11.6
Nutritional factor						
Breast milk alone did not satisfy my baby*	49.0	55.6	49.1	49.5	43.5	49.5
I thought that my baby was not gaining enough weight*	23.0	18.3	11.0	14.1	8.4	15.0
A health professional said my baby was not gaining enough weight*	19.8	15.2	8.6	9.9	5.0	11.7
I had trouble getting the milk flow to start*	41.4	23.2	19.6	14.6	5.7	20.9
I didn't have enough milk*	51.7	52.2	54.0	41.8	26.0	45.5
Lifestyle factor						
I did not like breastfeeding*	16.4	10.9	6.2	1.1	1.9	7.7
I wanted to go on a weight-loss diet*	6.6	7.2	10.3	10.9	6.5	8.3
I wanted to go back to my usual diet*	5.5	9.5	7.2	5.2	5.0	6.5
I wanted to smoke again or more than I did while breastfeeding	6.0	5.2	3.4	1.0	0.8	3.3
I wanted my body back to myself*	8.9	13.2	16.8	18.8	15.7	14.7
Medical factor						
My baby became sick and could not breastfeed*	9.5	7.4	5.5	6.3	19	6.1
I was sick or had to take medicine	14.4	16.3	14.8	12.5	8.0	11.2
I was not present to feed my baby for reasons other than work	3.2	6.9	5.2	5.2	2.7	4.6
I became pregnant or wanted to become pregnant again*	1.7	3.4	3.4	6.8	12.2	5.5
Milk-pumping factor						
I could not, or did not want to, pump or breastfeed at work*	11.2	22.4	21.3	13.5	4.6	14.6
Pumping milk no longer seemed worth the effort that it required*	16.7	21.2	23.1	17.7	11.5	18.2
Infant's self-weaning factor						
My baby began to bite*	5.2	5.7	13.4	38.5	31.7	18.9
My baby lost interest in nursing or began to wean himself or herself*	13.2	19.7	33.1	47.9	47.3	32.2
My baby was old enough that the difference between breast milk and formula no longer mattered*	5.2	11.4	16.5	26.6	28.2	17.6

*$p < 0.01$ for association between each reason and weaning age after adjustments for maternal age, marital status, parity, education, poverty, WIC participation, race, and region.

From Li J, Fein SB, Chen J, et al: Why mothers stop breastfeeding: mothers' self-reported reasons for stopping during the first year, *Pediatrics* 122:S69–S76, 2008.

TABLE 10-4 Reasons for Weaning or Not Weaning (Have You Thought about Weaning This Child?)

Response	Frequency (%)
No, weaning should be child-led	75.9
No, enjoy the nursing relationship	72.3
Yes, for a specific reason (pregnancy, returning to work)	4.8
Yes, child is ready/child is biting	7.8
Yes, due to social pressure	3.6
Yes, child is nursing too frequently for age	3.6

From Sugarman M, Kendall-Tackett KA: Weaning ages in a sample of American women who practice extended breastfeeding, *Clin Pediatr* 34:642, 1995.

TABLE 10-5 Main Reasons for Premature Weaning

Reason	N	%
Not enough, inadequate, or "weak" milk	307	30.9
Child refused breast	177	17.8
Illness of child	159	16.0
Mother needed to go to work	149	15.0
Correct age for bottle-feeding	139	14.0
Other reasons	64	6.3
Total	995	100.0

From Gunn TR: The incidence of breastfeeding and the reasons for weaning, *NZ Med J* 97:360, 1984.

Historically, weaning has varied from strict to permissive schedules depending upon cultural norms.[10] Rigid feeding schedules were associated with early weaning.[7] Weaning has varied from early strict denial to slow and gentle withdrawal. In the twentieth century, the time considered proper for weaning gradually shortened from 2 or 3 or 4 years to as soon as 6 to 8 months or less for some mothers and infants. Public opinion has overlooked an infant's needs in favor of what are considered the mother's rights. It is not necessary to have a specific plan for weaning in the early weeks of nursing unless constraints on the mother's time are an issue. Weaning should be done with an infant's needs as a guide. If an infant younger than 1 year of age rejects the breast, it is unusual but not abnormal and should not be considered by the mother as a personal rejection. Some bottle-fed infants throw down the bottle at 9 months as well.

Studies of weaning practices are few. In a study of primigravidas, the women introduced solids because their infants seemed hungry and less satisfied and woke more frequently. The average time to introduce nonmilk food in bottle-fed infants was 3 months and in breastfed infants, 5 months. Most observations are done on duration of feeding when the success rate is low.

The reasons given why women in Dunedin, New Zealand, elected to wean their infants early included concern about their milk supply and other maternal problems.[25] One of the most significant factors in lactation termination was mismanagement of breastfeeding by health professionals. A similar study in Sweden reported that 66% of the mothers weaned because they thought their milk was drying up.

Brazil had also experienced a decline in breastfeeding. The study was undertaken to understand the causes of early weaning to develop better means of encouraging longer breastfeeding and delaying weaning. The bottle was introduced at birth by 24% of women, at 2 months by 72.6%, and at 6 months by 88.0%.

Table 10-5 lists the main reasons given for weaning. A third of the mothers believed their milk was weak. In general, most studies of weaning practices indicated that most weaning is mother initiated, often because she thinks her milk is no longer adequate. The primary cause of failing milk supply reported by most investigators is inadequate help or instructions about milk production from medical personnel. In a study of 750 mother-baby dyads, Howard et al.[26] showed a clear relationship to early weaning, decreased exclusive breastfeeding, and the early introduction of a pacifier. In most studies, those who breastfeed longer tend to be older than 25 years, well-educated, middle class, self-educated about lactation, and enjoy breastfeeding.[21]

The problem of recall bias when reporting breastfeeding duration was investigated by Huttly et al.,[28] who compared responses given at 11, 23, and 47 months postpartum by the mothers of 1000 children; 24% misclassified weaning time at 23 months and 30% at 4 years. Those in the better-educated, higher socioeconomic group were more apt to report longer breastfeeding.

In worldwide epidemiologic studies, the interruption of breastfeeding because of pregnancy may play a significant role. The mean monthly bias introduced was to reduce breastfeeding by 2 months. In Third World countries, infant death also lowers the duration of breastfeeding inversely to the mother's education; that is, the less educated the mother, the greater the risk for infant death from infection and accident.

Why Women Wean

In 2001 using the National Survey of Family Growth to analyze breastfeeding behaviors of a national probability sample of 6733 first-time mothers in the United States from 15 to 44 years of age, Taylor et al. found 3267 women who breastfed.[52] Among these women, 46%, 68%, 78%, and 85% had weaned by 3, 6, 9, and 12 months, respectively. The reason 1091 women stopped was because their infant was "old enough to wean." This reason was claimed by 15%, 34%, and 78% at the same 3-month intervals. White and Hispanic women had similar weaning patterns. For black women who stopped because their child was "old enough to wean," greater numbers weaned sooner (22%, 46%, 68%, and 86% stopped at 3, 6, 9, and 12 months, respectively).[29]

Physical and medical problems were the next most common reasons (26.9%), followed with "job or schedule" (only 17.9%), and "preferred to bottle feed" (15.3%) (Table 10-6). Differences by race revealed black women stopped because they "preferred to bottle feed." Hispanic women had a few more infants who refused the breast (3.7%) compared to black women (0.5%) and white women (2.1%).

In 2006 to 2007, the Infant Feeding Practices Study II (IFPS II), a mail survey supported by the Division of Nutrition of the Centers for Disease Control and Prevention, was focused on why women stop breastfeeding, and the reasons were not significantly different.[36] In a forced answer questionnaire the statements were slightly different but the three top explanations were that infant was not satisfied, the child was old enough to wean, and concern about nutritional issues. In the first 2 months, mothers were concerned that the milk was inadequate; after 2 months, however, mothers were concerned that infants' activities were meant to self-wean, and later weaning took place for social reasons such as work or maternal freedom. When infants were approximately 1 year old, the misconception that it was the age to wean was a factor. Clearly, each of these issues could be addressed through adequate counseling. When data were extracted from the Pregnancy Risk Assessment Monitoring System (PRAMS) to examine breastfeeding behaviors, periods of vulnerability for breastfeeding cessation, predelivery intentions, and breastfeeding behaviors, it was clear that younger women with limited economic resources stopped early.[1] Those who planned to breastfeed were more likely to continue than those who did not plan ahead to breastfeed. Early postpartum cessation was due to physical discomforts of breastfeeding and the uncertainty about milk supply. Professional intervention early might well change these figures.

A longitudinal observational study involving appropriate controls and mothers who delivered healthy term infants at Yale-New Haven Hospital and planned to take them to the clinic showed that a mother's knowledge and problems with lactation were not associated with early stopping of breastfeeding.[16] Those who lacked confidence in their success and those who believed the baby preferred formula were most likely to stop in 2 weeks. The rates of discontinuation were 27%, 37%, 70%, and 89% by 1, 2, 8, and 16 weeks, respectively. In this population of minority women, 91% of whom were already enrolled in WIC, the authors[32] recommended that the focus needs to shift from increasing knowledge and problem management to enhancing a mother's confidence and correcting misconceptions about an infant's preferences. The probability of early weaning is increased by the occurrence of stressful life events during pregnancy such as separation, divorce, financial stresses, and residential moves. This was independent of hospital care and delivery issues.[37]

Reasons why mothers wean sooner than they had planned were analyzed from 1177 mothers over 18 years of age who responded to monthly surveys from the IFPS II conducted by the Food and Drug Administration (FDA) and the Centers for Disease Control (CDC).[44] Sixty percent of these mothers stopped sooner than they had planned. The major reasons given were (1) difficulties breastfeeding, (2) concern for infant nutrition and weight gain, (3) maternal illness or need to take medicine, and (4) the time and effort associated with pumping. Continued professional intervention is suggested as a possible solution (Table 10-7).

In a subsequent study from the IFPS II that included 1334 mothers who reported a 7-day food frequency questionnaire monthly, determination was made of the exact time mothers were introducing solids. Of those in the study, 24.3% of breastfed, 52.7% of formula-fed, and 50.2% of mixed-fed infants started before 4 months.[9] The mean age of introduction was 11.8 weeks, and 9.1% of mothers who were formula feeding started before 4 weeks. It was claimed that a doctor suggested it for 55.5% of mothers and 46.4% of mothers were told that solids would help the baby sleep. The odds of these behaviors were higher for formula-fed infants (Table 10-8). Breastfeeding mothers tend to feel more satisfied with the infant feeding experience.

Mother-infant dyads with unlimited access to lactation consultants had slower introduction of solid foods at the initial complementary feeding period, compared to dyads followed in the well-baby clinic at the University of Iceland.

Infant-Initiated Weaning

Infant-initiated weaning in the first year of life was investigated by Clarke and Harmon,[8] who studied

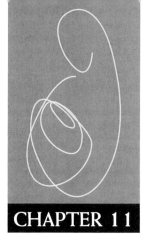

CHAPTER 11

Normal Growth, Failure to Thrive, and Obesity in Breastfed Infants

Normal Growth

The focus on growth evaluations in childhood have relied on averages: averages of the fat, the thin, the tall, the short, the sick, and the well. The real science is looking at ideal growth in ideally fed children anywhere in the world.

The growth of exclusively breastfed infants has become the focus of much interest among pediatricians, researchers, and nutritionists.[12] Historically, the Boyd-Orr cohort study in the 1920s and 1930s showed that breastfed children were taller in childhood and adulthood.[80] Stature was associated with health and life expectancy. Adult leg length is very sensitive to environment factors and diet in early childhood because this is the time of most rapid leg growth. After infancy, chest growth is rapid before puberty and is sensitive to stress and illness. Cross-sectional association between cardiovascular risk factors and components of stature (total height, leg length, and trunk length) was demonstrated. The risk of coronary heart disease was inversely related to leg length but not trunk length in the Caerphilly study in South Wales.[110]

A number of long-range follow-up studies have been initiated to address the issues of growth during the critical first year of life, when brain growth is greater than it ever will be again in postnatal life. An interest in height and weight increments and ratios is only part of the concern about obesity and the long-range issues of adiposity. Does breastfeeding protect against adult obesity? Does human

milk protect against cholesterol "intolerance" in adult life? The questions are clear, but the answers are not unless one assumes the teleological approach: human milk is ideal for human infants, with its low protein, controlled calories, and persistent unchangeable cholesterol.

The questions are actually, "Is it safe to overfeed an infant with formula?"; "Is it safe to deprive an infant of cholesterol during a period of critical brain growth when brain growth depends on cholesterol?"; and "When infants are deprived of cholesterol in early infancy, are they less able to tolerate it later?"

Antiquated data and anthropometric standards have led to the belief that the growth curves and tables of normal height and weight do not reflect the growth of most healthy, well-fed breastfeeding infants.[83] Reliability of weight gain as a measure of growth has developed because it is a measurement easily obtained.[83] Measurement of length, however, is considered a better standard.[93] Weight gain and linear growth are not always correlated. Furthermore, during infancy and childhood, the lower leg grows at a higher rate than the rest of the body. Knee-heel length can be expressed as a percentage of total length and increases with age: 25% at birth, 27% at 12 months, and 31% in adult life. During several decades of formula feeding, "normal" growth curves were developed based only on formula-fed infants. Furthermore, whole cow milk is fortunately almost totally abandoned, and the recommendations for introduction of solid food at 6 months and older have been universally adopted by nutrition-conscious physicians and parents. World Health Organization (WHO) and United Nations International Children Education Fund (UNICEF) have reconfirmed that breastfeeding should be exclusive for the first 6 months. Growth curves have been developed based on breastfed infants on delayed solids.

Bottle-fed infants gain more rapidly in weight and length during the first months of life than do breastfed infants.[26] Therefore, evaluating an infant's physical growth by standards set by bottle-fed infants predisposes one to the diagnosis of failure to thrive.

Forman et al.[35] reported a longitudinal study of breastfed and bottle-fed infants during the first few months of life that demonstrated the 10th and 90th percentile values for weight and length of the two groups were similar at birth, and the 10th percentile values of the two groups were similar at age 112 days. The significant difference was in the values for the 90th percentile. Bottle-fed infants were above this percentile in substantially greater numbers. These differences were attributed to caloric intake rather than the difference in composition of the diet. Fomon et al. showed that the bottle-fed infant not only gains more in weight and length, but also gains more weight for a unit of length. This gain reflects the overfeeding of the bottle-fed infants.[34]

Most studies of growth in breastfed infants have been plagued with the problem of variation in supplementation and the occurrence of partial weaning.

The effects on growth of specific protein and energy intake in 4- to 6-month-old infants who were either breastfed or formula fed with high and low protein were measured by Axelsson et al.[3] No significant differences were found in the growth rate of crown-heel length and head circumference or weight gain. The authors concluded that the differences in protein intake between breastfed and formula-fed infants without differences in growth indicate that the formulas may provide a protein intake in excess of the needs. When milk intake and growth in exclusively breastfed infants were carefully documented in the first 4 months by Butte et al.,[11] energy and protein intakes were substantially less than current nutrient allowances. Infant growth progressed satisfactorily when compared with National Center for Health Statistics (NCHS) standards, despite that energy dropped from 110 ± 24 kcal/kg/day at 1 month to 71 ± 17 kcal/kg/day at 4 months.[11] Similarly, protein intake decreased from 1.6 ± 0.3 g/kg/day at 1 month to 0.9 ± 0.2 g/kg/day at 4 months. Reevaluation of protein and energy requirements is essential.

Weight-for-length and weight gain were significantly correlated with total energy intake but not with activity level during the first 6 months of life in breastfed infants studied by Dewey et al.[24,22]

Energy intake was considerably lower than recommended—85 to 89 kcal/kg/day—when compared with the 115 kcal/kg/day recommended dietary allowances of the National Academy of Sciences in 1980.[17] Presently energy recommendations suggested by the Institute of Medicine (IOM) are expressed as: $(89 \times wt[kg] - 100) + 175$ kcal.

Those infants who consumed the most breast milk became the fattest. A 4-kg infant would require 105 kcal/kg/day.

When patterns of growth are examined in the infants of marginally nourished mothers, weight gain is comparable to a reference population but does not permit recovery of weight differential at birth, which was significantly small for gestational age (SGA).[7] The intakes of energy and protein by individual infants were reflected in their weight gain but were below internationally recommended norms.[30] Maternal milk alone, when produced in sufficient amounts, can maintain normal growth up to the sixth month of life. Exclusive breastfeeding in Chilean infants of low-middle and low socioeconomic families produced the highest weight gain and practically no illness or hospitalization.[59]

In the Copenhagen Cohort Study in 1994, exclusively breastfed term infants had a mean intake of 781 and 855 mL/24 hours at 2 and 4 months, respectively.[82] The median fat concentration of human milk was 39.2 g/L and was positively associated with maternal weight gain during pregnancy. This supports the concept that maternal fat stores laid down during pregnancy are easier to mobilize during lactation than other fat stores. This may limit milk fat when pregnancy fat stores are exhausted.

The effect of prolonged breastfeeding on growth has been an issue of concern, especially in developing countries.[35] In a review of 13 studies, Grummer-Strawn[42] pointed out in 1993 that eight reported a negative relationship, two had a positive relationship, and three had mixed results. Grummer-Strawn identified the flaws in study design and suggested that until better information is available, women should nurse as long as possible because the benefits to infant health exceed the risks in these geographic areas.

In addition to recognizing the importance of genetic, metabolic, and environmental influences in producing significant differences in growth patterns, Barness[5] suggests that recommendations for nutrition of healthy neonates may be too high for some and too low for others. However, the benchmark for nutritional requirements of the full-term infant remains milk from the infant's healthy, well-nourished mother.

Gain in physical growth is not as critical as gain in brain growth, but measurements of brain growth are only indirectly implied from growth of the head. In evaluating any infant's progress, head circumference hind milk. If the mother is interrupting the feeding to go to the other side, a period of feeding exclusively on one breast during each feeding may change the gaining pattern. If necessary, the level of fat in the milk can be checked by doing a "creamatocrit," comparing milk before and after the timing change (see Chapter 21). By weighing the infant before and after a feeding with a digital readout scale, an accurate measurement of breast milk intake can be recorded. A gainer will have good intake.

In a schema for classifying failure to thrive at the breast, the causes associated with infant behavior and problems are distinguished from those related to maternal problems (Figure 11-1). The causes in the infant can be further evaluated by looking at net intake, which may be associated with poor feeding, poor net intake from additional losses, or high energy needs. The maternal causes can be divided into poor production of milk and poor release of milk. When a poor let-down reflex continues long enough, it will eventually cause a decrease in milk production. Several factors may affect the outcome, and more than one management change may be indicated.

Evaluation of Infant

Examination of the infant should suggest any underlying physical problems, such as hypothyroidism, congenital heart disease, mechanical abnormalities of the mouth (e.g., cleft palate), or major neurologic disturbances.[6] An infant's ability to root, suck, and coordinate swallowing should be observed. Today, a greater risk for missing subtle structural problems exists because infants spend much of their hospital life out of the newborn nursery away from the eyes of experienced nurses and are discharged before problems become manifest.

The routine observation of a feeding by an infant's physician should be part of the discharge examination from the hospital. If this is not practical, such an examination should be incorporated into the first office or clinic visit within the first week of life. The mother should be asked to let you see how the baby feeds. The focus, however, should be to watch the positioning of the mother and the infant, placement of the mother's hands, and initiation of latch-on (see Chapter 8). A small number of infants will be identified with physical abnormalities that need medical attention (Box 11-2).

Lukefahr[76] identified 38 infants younger than 6 months of age in a suburban pediatric practice as having failure to thrive while breastfeeding. Only 2 of 28 infants (7.1%) who presented in the first 4 weeks had underlying illnesses (salt-losing adrenogenital syndrome and congenital hypotonia); 5 of the 10 presenting between 1 and 6 months had underlying disease (all of whom actually presented with a problem by 4 months). This report stresses the importance of ruling out underlying disease and the urgency of having a pediatrician evaluate a child when the symptom of poor weight gain is first suspected, thus avoiding the serious complications of dehydration and metabolic disorders that may result when "home remedies" for lactation problems are used.

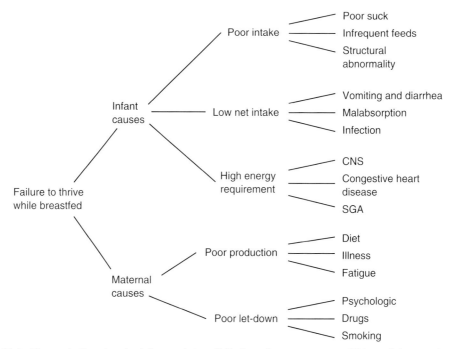

Figure 11-1. Diagnostic flowchart for failure to thrive. *CNS,* Central nervous system; *SGA,* small for gestational age.

BOX 11-2. Conditions Associated with or Causing Disorders of Sucking and Swallowing

Absent or Diminished Suck	Mechanical Factors Interfering with Sucking	Disorders of Swallowing Mechanism (Not Including Esophageal Abnormalities)
Maternal anesthesia or analgesia	Macroglossia	Choanal atresia
Anoxia or hypoxia	Cleft lip	Cleft palate
Prematurity	Fusion of gums	Micrognathia
Trisomy 21	Tumors of mouth or gums	Postintubation dysphagia
Trisomy 13-15	Temporomandibular	Palatal paralysis
Hypothyroidism	ankylosis or hypoplasia	Pharyngeal tumors
Neuromuscular abnormalities		Pharyngeal diverticula
Kernicterus		Familial dysautonomia
Werdnig-Hoffmann disease		
Neonatal myasthenia gravis		
Congenital muscular dystrophy		
Central nervous system infections		
Toxoplasmosis		
Cytomegalovirus infection		
Bacterial meningitis		

Oral Motor Problems: Feeding Skills Disorder. Growth failure secondary to feeding skills disorder is the terminology proposed by Ramsay et al.[97] to replace nonorganic failure to thrive. The authors describe a series of children who were referred for nonorganic failure to thrive who had displayed subtle problems since birth. The criteria include early abnormal feeding-related symptoms present shortly after birth, such as impaired oral function, suggesting the infants are minimally neurologically abnormal, sometimes associated with borderline low Apgar scores. Difficulties during earlier stages of feeding development not only may interfere with the development of more mature feeding skills, but also may contribute eventually to difficulties in mother-infant interaction. The common finding among all infants with failure to thrive was underlying feeding-related symptoms that were neurophysiologic but manifested in different degrees of oral sensorimotor (and pharyngeal) impairment. The neurologic impairment may vary from obvious cerebral palsy to symptoms that are not apparent on casual observation but lead to abnormal feeding-related symptoms in early life. When the mother copes and adapts, the disorder goes unnoticed until solid foods are added. Diagnosis requires oral sensorimotor assessments and a neurologic examination sensitive enough to measure minimal neurologic impairment in an apparently healthy child who is failing to gain. Early history is also critically important.

Small-for-Gestational-Age Infant. A SGA infant will be identified if gestational age and birth weight are scrutinized. This infant is small at birth despite full gestation time in utero. An SGA infant has a large nutritional deficit from intrauterine failure to grow. The cause of the intrauterine problem should be assessed: placental insufficiency, maternal disease, toxemia, heavy smoking, or intrauterine infection, such as toxoplasmosis.

SGA infants are difficult to feed initially by any method and often require tube feedings for a few days. Their caloric needs parallel the needs of an infant of appropriate weight for gestation rather than their actual low weight. SGA infants should be placed on frequent feedings, every 2 to 3 hours by day and every 4 hours at night. They should be awakened for feedings if they sleep long periods. If they have not been nursing well, the breast may not have been stimulated to produce to its full capability. The mother may need to express milk manually or mechanically pump milk to enhance her production. Her milk may then be given by a passive means such as a tube, a small cup, or the lactation supplementing device, which provides additional stimulus to the breast while providing the extra calories needed (see Chapter 19).

An infant who is sufficiently starved in utero may have a degree of inanition that prevents active suckling at first, predisposing to further starvation. The successful nursing of an SGA infant may require extended efforts by the mother to ensure adequate growth. Such efforts are well worth the trouble if one considers the impact of intrauterine growth failure on the central nervous system. It is to the infant's advantage to have the critical amino acids, such as taurine and the lipids of human milk, with which to "catch up" brain growth. As noted earlier, SGA infants are more likely to close the growth gap more rapidly if breastfed.[12]

Jaundice. An infant with an elevated bilirubin level from any cause may be neurologically depressed and lethargic and, therefore, may not nurse well. If the infant appears jaundiced, laboratory evaluation to determine the cause and its appropriate treatment should be undertaken. Visible jaundice under 24 hours of age requires a full evaluation and is not related to breastfeeding. When an infant is taken from the breast at 2 or 3 days of age because of jaundice, this interferes with the establishment of lactation at a critical time, especially for a primipara. Management of the jaundiced infant depends on adequate calories and the active passage of stools, which is the means by which the body excretes the bilirubin in meconium and stools.

"Breastfeeding jaundice," which is related to underfeeding or starvation, does not develop until the infant is 3 or more days old, so other causes must be sought. In addition, care must be taken to help the mother continue to stimulate production with manual expression or pumping to avoid inducing iatrogenic lactation failure. (See Chapter 14 for discussion of hyperbilirubinemia.)

Metabolic Screen. Most hospitals provide, often because the law mandates it, screening for metabolic disorders, including galactosemia, phenylketonuria, maple syrup urine disease, and disorders of metabolism of other amino acids. If these simple screening tests were not performed or their validity is in doubt, they should be done again. Usually the service is available in the state or county laboratory. Thyroid screening for abnormal thyroxine (T_4) or thyroid-stimulating hormone should also be performed. Mass screening programs for neonatal thyroid disease have identified cases of deficiency that, even in retrospect, were not in evidence; the infant showed none of the characteristic findings of hypothyroidism, such as thick coarse features, hoarse cry, slow pulse, macroglossia, umbilical hernia, and jaundice. In the neonate, hypothyroidism is often associated with failure to thrive if undiagnosed and untreated.

Galactosemia. Galactosemia, which is a hereditary disorder of the metabolism of galactose-1-phosphate, is manifest by renal disease and liver dysfunction after ingestion of lactose. The lack of galactose-1-phosphate uridyltransferase activity may be relative or partial. The clinical symptoms may be fulminating, with severe jaundice, hepatosplenomegaly, weight loss, vomiting, and diarrhea, or may be more subtle. Cataracts are not invariably present. In mild cases, failure to thrive may be the presenting symptom. A urine screen for reducing substances (by Clinitest and not Dextrostix, which will only identify glucose) should be done on all infants who fail to thrive, especially if there is hepatomegaly or jaundice.

The definitive diagnosis is the identification of absence or near absence of galactose-1-phosphate uridyltransferase activity in red blood cell hemolysates. Even though a routine initial metabolic screen for galactosemia was done on the second or third day of life, a urine screen should be considered. The treatment is a lactose-free diet, which would mandate prompt weaning from breast milk to prevent further insult to the liver, kidneys, and brain. This is one of the few indications for prompt weaning from human milk. A formula free of lactose (e.g., Isomil, Nutramigen) is indicated. No medical indications exist, however, to use a lactose-free formula for a normal breastfeeding infant either to supplement or to wean from breast milk, which contains lactose. (Refer to pediatric texts on neonatal metabolic disorders for a full description of galactosemia; see also Chapter 14.)

Vomiting and Diarrhea. Vomiting and diarrhea are unusual in a breastfed infant. Spitting up small amounts of milk after feedings is sometimes observed in otherwise normal infants and is of no consequence if it does not affect overall weight gain. Although pyloric stenosis is reportedly less common in breastfed infants, this phenomenon should be ruled out in any infant who vomits consistently after feeding, has diminished urine and stools, shows no weight gain or actually loses weight, and has reverse peristalsis. Usually these infants do well initially and then the vomiting becomes progressive.

Vomiting may be a presenting symptom for various metabolic disorders. Thus, metabolic disorders should be considered in the differential diagnosis. All possible metabolic disorders, such as congenital adrenal hyperplasia, are not routinely screened. These infants may present with vomiting and weight loss in the first week or two of life or with an acute episode of sepsis. The usual causes of vomiting, as well as the causes peculiar to breast milk, should be considered. Maternal diet should be checked for unusual foods. In families at high risk for allergy, intake by the mother of known family food allergens may cause symptoms in the infant. Diarrhea may be caused by foods in the mother's diet or her use of cathartics, such as phenolphthalein.

Chronic Infections. Chronic fetal infection in utero, which predisposes a SGA infant to intrauterine growth failure, may continue to cause growth problems in the presence of adequate kilocalories. Chronic viral infections include cytomegalovirus, hepatitis, acquired immunodeficiency syndrome (AIDS), or other less common viruses (see Chapter 13).

Acute Infections. An infant who is not growing well may have an infection in the gastrointestinal tract; therefore, the nature of the stools is important. The urinary tract may be another site of infection not readily identified. If, however, the initial evaluation includes a urinalysis with microscopic evaluation and a white blood cell count and differential count, this can usually be ruled out (see Chapter 13).

High Energy Requirements. When the metabolic rate of an infant is increased, weight gain will be diminished or absent. When the infant is hyperactive with a strong startle reflex and sleeps poorly, consideration should be given to stimulants present in the milk as well as to neurologic disorders. When a mother drinks coffee, tea (including herbal teas), cola, or other carbonated beverages with added caffeine, the accumulated caffeine may be sufficient to make the infant irritable and hyperactive. The best treatment is to replace the caffeine-containing beverages (see Chapter 12). Some disorders of the central nervous system are associated with hyperactivity. Infants with severe congenital heart disease are constantly exercising to breathe and oxygenate and have greatly increased metabolic rates. For management of these special infants at the breast, see Chapter 14.

Observation of Nursing Process

In addition to establishing that no obvious physical or metabolic reasons exist for the failure to gain weight, an infant should be observed suckling at the breast. Does the infant get a good grasp and suck vigorously? If not, what interferes? A receding chin, a weak suck, lack of coordination, the breast obstructing breathing, and mouthing of the nipple or other ineffectual sucking motions are some of the possibilities. If the problem is the suckling process, the infant may need assistance. This cause is more common with infants who have had some experience with bottles or rubber nipples or who use a pacifier. Small or slightly premature infants who were started on bottle feedings have trouble relearning the proper sucking motion with the tongue (see Chapter 8).

Bottle-feedings and pacifiers may have to be discontinued until the infant is more experienced at the breast. This will require a program of manually expressing milk to soften the areola, having milk at the nipple to entice the infant, and gently offering the nipple and areola well compressed between two fingers. If the infant has a receding chin or a relaxed jaw, it may help to have the mother hold the lower jaw forward by supporting the angle of the jaw with her thumb. The physician should examine the infant carefully to be sure the jaw is not dislocated, especially if a vertex delivery was done in the posterior position (sunny side up). The physician can easily move the jaw forward to relocate it.

Positioning the infant for the breast so the child directly faces the breast, straddling the mother's leg in a semiupright position, may work best. This is the position twins may assume when nursing simultaneously when they are 3 to 4 months old. Although it is not recommended routinely, for an infant with a receding chin or a cleft, having the mother lean slightly forward for latch-on may help. She should then bring the infant upward as she sits back for the feeding.

It may be necessary to assist both mother and baby. If the infant by 2 weeks of age cannot maintain the breast in the mouth without the mother holding it, it is an indication of improper suckling. In that situation, the infant may need to be repositioned with the ventral surface squarely facing the mother's chest wall—that is, tummy to tummy—and the breast presented by the mother with her hand positioned with thumb on top and fingers below the breast. (See discussion in Chapter 8.) The mother may have to maintain support throughout the feeding. Failure to maintain the breast in the mouth has neurologic implications for long-term follow-up.

When infants have trouble maintaining the latch when the flow of milk is excessive and causes choking, the mother may try lying flat on her back holding the infant over the breast, which she supports with her hand. The flow becomes manageable and the infant's mouth relaxes and draws the breast in.

A good check of adequate let-down is to observe the opposite breast as the baby nurses to see if milk flows. It can also be tested by seeing if milk is flowing when nursing is interrupted abruptly. If let-down was good, milk will continue to flow, at least drop by drop, for a few moments from the breast that had been suckled. A mother can be trained to listen for the infant's swallowing. During proper suckling, the masseter muscle in the jaw is in full view and is contracting visibly and rhythmically. Swallowing can be seen and heard. The ratio of suck to swallow is 1:1 or 2:1. Occasionally, infants do not suck vigorously at the breast but occasionally use rapid shallow sucks called "flutter sucking" with little or no swallowing. These infants can be gradually taught to suck effectively. Correct positioning of the breast directly in the infant's mouth and holding the breast firmly in position with all the fingers under the breast and only the thumb above allow the infant to grasp properly without sucking the tongue or lower lip. Nipple shields usually make the situation worse.

The most productive part of the diagnostic workup is often observation of the baby at the breast. For this reason, this critical responsibility should not be passed on to others but should be performed personally by the physician as well as an international board certified lactation consultant.

The five general types of nursing patterns described in Chapter 8 should be kept in mind. If the mother understands that it is acceptable for the infant to drop off to sleep and snack later, she may not hesitate to follow this lead, thus providing a more adequate feeding.

Some infants will not settle down and nurse well if there is too much activity or noise in the room. Some need to be tightly swaddled; others fall asleep and need to be unwrapped and stimulated to provide adequate suckling time. Frequent feedings, using both breasts, may be the answer in some cases. In others, there may be too many ineffective feedings, which are wearing the mother out; a change that lengthens the time between feedings but also lengthens the time at the breast may help, especially if it is quiet and the chair allows mother to nap while feeding. Concentrating on using one breast at a feeding to increase the fat content may be the most effective change.

PSYCHOSOCIAL FAILURE TO THRIVE

In the study of undernutrition in bottle-fed infants and infants beyond the suckling age, terminology has received more attention than the underlying issues. Thus, the emphasis has been on "organic" versus "nonorganic" failure to thrive. A disorder of maternal/infant bonding has become synonymous with maternal deprivation. *Reactive attachment disorder* has been the term substituted for psychosocial failure to thrive. When an infant does not have an organic disorder that explains the growth failure, the patient is diagnosed as having psychosocial failure to thrive. The typical psychosocial and nutritional pattern reported in psychosocial failure to thrive includes evidence of a chaotic family life, emotional deprivation, and inadequate nutrition.

Prolonged Exclusive Breastfeeding

Prolonged exclusive breastfeeding may occasionally result in a unique deficit in the developmental process of eating. Exclusive breastfeeding is not nutritionally adequate in the second half of the first year, especially beyond 12 months, although nursing can safely continue for several years when combined with adequate solids that provide protein, iron, and zinc.

The syndrome of the breastfed infant in the second 6 months of life with frequent breastfeedings, poor intake of complementary foods, and poor growth has been labeled a manifestation of "vulnerable child syndrome" by O'Connor and Szekely.[92] These children are described to have good weight gain for 5 to 6 months, but by 8 months their weight/height score has decreased dramatically. The intake of solid foods is minimal. These infants refuse solids, aggressively spitting food out. The breastfeeding pattern is usually every 1 to 2 hours during the day and frequently at night. Further investigation revealed numerous household stressors and usually the mother's need to maintain control by breastfeeding.

The growth of predominantly breastfed infants who live in underprivileged populations in developing countries falters between 4 and 6 months of age, but the reason has never been well understood. In developed countries, energy intake declines between 4 and 6 months but growth does not falter.

To determine whether growth faltering in this age-group was due to inadequate intake of human milk, the nutrient intakes of 30 Otami Indian infants from farms in Capulhuac, Mexico, were studied from 4 to 6 months. Growth velocities were not correlated with nutrient intakes. The children's growth faltered despite energy intakes comparable with those of children in more supportive and protected environments. The energy requirements of these children were significantly higher. Some infants in developed countries may live in equally challenging environments.

Parental misconception and health beliefs concerning what constitutes a normal diet for infants have been reported by Pugliese et al.[96] as a cause for failure to thrive as well. They reported seven infants from 7 to 22 months of age with poor weight gain and linear growth who received only 60% to 90% of minimum caloric intake for their age and sex. The parents explained that they wanted to avoid obesity, atherosclerosis, or junk food habits. It has also been shown that parental health beliefs and expectations have led to short stature and delayed puberty in older children.

Fruit Juice Excess

The custom of excessive use of fruit juices in recent decades has replaced the use of water for additional fluids after 6 months of life when the infant is learning to drink from a cup or a straw. The attractive packaging has contributed to this trend. Excessive fruit juice diminishes appetite, resulting in decreased dietary intake of nutrient-dense foods and a decrease in weight gain and ultimately in linear growth. An excess of fruit juice may be a cause of failure to thrive in older infants. Decrease in total high-energy intake is combined with malabsorption of fructose and diarrhea from sorbitol, thus compounding the problem.[101] Excessive fruit juice intake in infancy is a major nutrition problem because juice has low nutrient value but high calories. The AAP has developed a guideline with restrictions on the use of fruit juices. For older children, their high caloric content may be a contributor to obesity.

Maternal Causes

Questions about a mother's health, dietary habits, sleep pattern, smoking habits, medication intake, the events that occur during nursing, and the psychosocial atmosphere in the home are an important part of the history (Figure 11-2).

Anatomic Causes

Lactation failure from insufficient glandular development of the breast has been described by Neifert

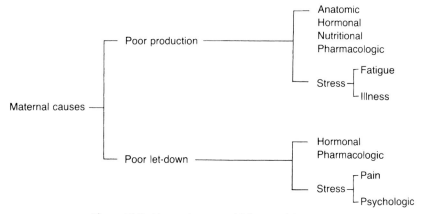

Figure 11-2. Maternal causes of failure to thrive.

and Seacat[90] and Neifert et al.,[89] who report three cases in which the breast tissue was asymmetric. Transillumination confirmed a minimally active gland. One family showed a history of similar failure. All three women benefited psychologically from the diagnosis and chose to continue to breastfeed and supplement. The authors have since identified 14 more women who had anatomic deficiency but normal prolactin levels and failed to respond to a thorough team approach to lactation support.[82] Retained placenta is also a cause of early lactation failure that is quickly identified by a complete history of postpartum breast change and patterns of lochia that an obstetrician associates with retained tissue (see Chapter 16). If prolactin response to stimulus is adequate, ultrasonography can determine the presence of adequate mammary tissue and ductal arborization.

One-Breast Versus Two-Breast Feeding

An infant whose failure to thrive was traced to inadequate fat intake associated with using both breasts, each feed resulting in low fat (and relatively high lactose by comparison), caused the debate regarding using one or two breasts during each feeding to be rekindled. When this infant was fed at one breast per feeding, the low-density feeding changed to high-fat feeding, resulting in decreased stooling and increased weight gain. Some women require more time to release fat into the milk, and limiting the feeding to one breast enhances fat content. In some cases this is true, and it is further verified by an infant fed at both breasts having many loose stools because of the high lactose and considerable gassy discomfort that also resolves with the change to single-breast feeds.

In early lactation, when milk supply is being established, mothers may be encouraged to nurse on both breasts at each feed to provide frequent stimulus. A clinician, however, should obtain a thorough history of feeding frequency and distribution between breasts, especially when the infant is well hydrated, has many stools, and may or may not be fussy but fails to gain weight, remaining less than birth weight for several weeks. The need for higher fat content in the feeding may be a consideration in the slow-gaining baby as well. An adjustment in feeding to enhance the fat content should be tried. Usually limiting each feeding to one breast will do that (see Chapter 8). However, some women have smaller storage capacity than others, as demonstrated with ultrasound imagery by Hartmann et al.[49] These women need to feed from both breasts at each feed. Storage capacity ranges from 100 to more than 250 mL per breast.[49]

Poor Milk Production

Diets. Although it has been demonstrated that malnourished mothers can produce milk for their infants, marginal diets in Western cultures do affect some mothers' ability to nourish an infant. A case of failure to thrive in a breastfed infant associated with maternal dietary protein and energy restriction was reported.[85] The mother, at 8 months postpartum, independently reduced her dietary energy to 20 kcal/kg/day and her protein to 0.7 g/kg/day to treat cholecystitis medically and avoid surgery. At 12 months, her infant's growth curves had fallen below the 5th percentile in both weight and length, although the infant had been receiving solid foods since 24 weeks of age. The authors concluded the failure to thrive was directly related to severe maternal restriction.[85]

Dietary analysis and maternal anthropometry showed that women who gained adequate weight and skin thickness during pregnancy had increased milk production and weight gain in their infants for the first 6 months of life.[30]

28. Ereman RR, Lönnerdal B, Dewey KG: Maternal sodium intake does not affect postprandial sodium concentrations in human milk, *J Nutr* 117:1154, 1987.
29. Fall C: Nutrition in early life and later outcome, *Eur J Clin Nutr* 46(Suppl 4):57, 1992.
30. Fawzi WW, Forman MR, Levy A, et al: Maternal anthropometry and infant feeding practices in Israel in relation to growth in infancy: the North African infant feeding study, *Am J Clin Nutr* 65:1731, 1997.
31. Fergusson DM, Beautrais AL, Silva PA: Breastfeeding and cognitive development in the first seven years of life, *Soc Sci Med* 16:1705, 1982.
32. Fergusson DM, Horwood LJ, Shannon FT: Breastfeeding and subsequent social adjustment in six- to eight-year-old children, *J Child Psychol Psychiatry* 28:379, 1987.
33. Finberg L, Kiley J, Luttrell CN: Mass accidental salt poisoning in infancy: a study of a hospital disaster, *JAMA* 184:187, 1963.
34. Fomon SJ, Rogers RR, Ziegler EE, et al: Indices of fatness and serum cholesterol at age eight years in relation to feeding and growth during early infancy, *Pediatr Res* 18:1233, 1984.
35. Forman MR, Lewando-Hundt G, Graubard BI, et al: Factors influencing milk insufficiency and its long term health effects: the Bedouin infant feeding study, *Int J Epidemiol* 21:53, 1992.
36. Frank DA, Silva M, Needleman R: Failure to thrive: mystery, myth and method, *Contemp Pediatr* 10:114, 1993.
37. Garza C, Frongillo E, Dewey KG: Implications of growth patterns of breastfed infants for growth references, *Acta Paediatr Suppl* 402:4, 1994.
38. Ghishan FK, Roloff JS: Malnutrition and hypernatremic dehydration in two breast-fed infants, *Clin Pediatr* 22:592, 1983.
39. Gibbs BG, Forste R: Socioeconomic status, infant feeding practices and early childhood obesity, *Pediatr Obes* 9:135–148, 2013.
40. Gilliman MW, Rifas-Shiman SI, Camargo CA, et al: Risk of overweight among adolescents who were breastfeeding as infants, *JAMA* 285:2461, 2001.
41. Gillman M: Breastfeeding and obesity, *J Pediatr* 141:749, 2002.
42. Grummer-Strawn LM: Does prolonged breastfeeding impair child growth? A critical review, *Pediatrics* 91:766, 1993.
43. Gunnarsdottir I, Thorsdottir I: Relationship between growth and feeding in infancy and body mass index at the age of 6 years, *Int J Obes* 27:1523, 2003.
44. Gupta AP, Gupta PK: Metoclopramide as a lactagogue, *Clin Pediatr* 24:269, 1985.
45. Habbick BF, Gerrard JW: Failure to thrive in the contented breastfed baby, *Can Med Assoc J* 131:765, 1984.
46. Hale TW: *Medications and mothers' milk*, ed 10, Amarillo, Tex., 2002, Pharmasoft Publications.
47. Hall DMB, Kay G: Effect of thyrotrophin-releasing factor on lactation, *Br Med J* 1:777, 1977.
48. Hamosh M: Does infant nutrition affect adiposity and cholesterol levels in the adult? *J Pediatr Gastroenterol Nutr* 7:10, 1988.
49. Hartmann PE, Regan MD, Ramsav DT, et al: Physiology of lactation in preterm mothers: initiation and maintenance, *Pediatr Ann* 32:351, 2003.
50. Heinig MJ, Nommsen LA, Peerson JM, et al: Energy and protein intakes of breastfed and formula fed infants during the first year of life and their association with growth velocity: the DARLING study, *Am J Clin Nutr* 58:152, 1993.
51. Hill ID, Bowie MD: Chloride deficiency syndrome due to chloride-deficient breast milk, *Arch Dis Child* 58:224, 1983.
52. Hilson JA, Rasmussen KM, Kjolhede CL: Maternal obesity and breast-feeding success in a rural population of white women, *Am J Clin Nutr* 66(6):1371, 1997.
53. Hoefer C, Hardy MC: Later development of breast-fed and artificially fed infants, *JAMA* 92:615, 1929.

54. Hopkinson JM, Schanler RJ, Fraley JK, et al: Milk production by mothers of premature infants: influence of cigarette smoking, *Pediatrics* 90:934, 1992.
55. Horwood LJ, Fergusson DM: Breastfeeding and later cognitive and academic outcomes, *Pediatrics* 101:e9, 1998. electronic article.
56. Jacobson SW, Jacobson JL: Breastfeeding and intelligence, *Lancet* 339:926, 1992.
57. Jakobsen MS, Sodemann M, Molbak K, et al: Reason for termination of breastfeeding and the length of breastfeeding, *Int J Epidemiol* 25:115, 1996.
58. Jelliffe DB, Jelliffe EFP: *Human milk in the modern world*, Oxford, 1978, Oxford University Press.
59. Juez G, Diaz S, Casado ME, et al: Growth pattern of selected urban Chilean infants during exclusive breastfeeding, *Am J Clin Nutr* 38:462, 1983.
60. Kramer KS, Oken E, Martin RM: Infant feeding and adiposity: scientific challenges in life-course epidemiology, *Am J Clin Nutr* 99:1281–1283, 2014.
61. Kramer M, Kakuman R: *The optimal duration of exclusive breastfeeding: a systematic review*, Geneva, Switzerland, 2001, World Health Organization.
62. Kramer MS, Barr RG, Leduc DG, et al: Determinants of weight and adiposity in the first year of life, *J Pediatr* 106:10–15, 1985.
63. Krebs NF, Westcott JE, Butler N, et al: Meat as a first complementary food for breastfed infants: feasibility and impact on zinc intake and status, *J Pediatr Gastroenterol Nutr* 42:207–214, 2006.
64. Kugyelka JG, Rasmussen KM, Frongillo EA: Maternal obesity and breastfeeding success among black and Hispanic women, *J Nutr* 134:1746, 2004.
65. Lampl M, Veldhuis JD, Johnson ML: Saltation and stasis: a model of human growth, *Science* 258:801, 1992.
66. Lawlor DA, Riddoch CU, Page AS, et al: Infant feeding and components of the metabolic syndrome: findings from the European youth heart study, *Arch Dis Child* 90:582–588, 2005.
67. Lawrence R: Maternal factors in lactation failure. In Hamosh M, Goldman AS, editors: *Human lactation. II. Maternal and environmental factors*, New York, 1986, Plenum.
68. Lawrence RA: Infant nutrition, *Pediatr Rev* 5:133, 1983.
69. Lawton ME: Alcohol in breast milk, *Aust N Z J Obstet Gynaecol* 25:71, 1985.
70. Lewis DS, Bertrand HA, McMahan CA, et al: Preweaning food intake influences the adiposity of young adult baboons, *J Clin Invest* 78:899, 1986.
71. Liese AD, Hirsch T, von Mutius E, et al: Inverse association of overweight and breastfeeding in 9 to 10 year old children in Germany, *J Hum Lact* 25:1644, 2001.
72. Little RE, Anderson KW, Ervin CH, et al: Maternal alcohol use during breastfeeding and infant mental and motor development at one year, *N Engl J Med* 321:425, 1989.
73. Lucas A, Fewtrell MS, Davies PSW, et al: Breastfeeding and catch-up growth in infants born small for gestational age, *Acta Paediatr* 86:564, 1997.
74. Lucas A, Morley R, Cole TJ, et al: Breast milk and subsequent intelligence quotient in children born premature, *Lancet* 339:261, 1992.
75. Lucas A, Morley R, Cole TJ, et al: Early diet in premature babies and developmental status at 18 months, *Lancet* 335:1477, 1990.
76. Lukefahr JL: Underlying illness associated with failure to thrive in breastfed infants, *Clin Pediatr* 29:468, 1990.
77. Mandel D, Lubetsky R, Dollberg S, et al: Fat and energy contents of expressed human breast milk in prolonged lactation, *Pediatrics* 116:e432–e435, 2005.
78. Marmot MG, Page CM, Atkins E, et al: Effect of breastfeeding on plasma cholesterol and weight in young adults, *J Epidemiol Community Health* 34:164, 1980.
79. Martin F-PJ, Moco S, Montoliu I, et al: Impact of breastfeeding and high and low protein formula on the metabolism and

growth of infants from overweight and obese mothers, *Pediatr Res* 75(4):535–543, 2014.

80. Martin RM, Smith GD, Mangtani P, et al: Association between breastfeeding and growth: the Boyd-Orr cohort study, *Arch Dis Child Fetal Neonatal Ed* 87: F193–F201, 2002.

81. Mennella JA, Beauchamp GK: The transfer of alcohol to human milk, *N Engl J Med* 325:981, 1991.

82. Michaelson KF, Larsen PS, Thomsen BL, et al: The Copenhagen cohort study on infant nutrition and growth: breast-milk intake, human milk macronutrient content, and influencing factors, *Am J Clin Nutr* 59:600, 1994.

83. Michaelson KF: Nutrition and growth during infancy: the Copenhagen cohort study, *Acta Paediatr* 86(Suppl 420):1, 1997.

84. Morley R, Cole TJ, Powell R, et al: Mother's choice to provide breast milk and developmental outcome, *Arch Dis Child* 63:1382, 1988.

85. Motil KJ, Sheng H-P, Montandon CM, et al: Case report: failure to thrive in a breast-fed infant is associated with maternal dietary protein and energy restriction, *J Am Coll Nutr* 13:203, 1994.

86. Motil KJ, Sheng H-P, Montandon CM, et al: Human milk protein does not limit growth of breast-fed infants, *J Pediatr Gastroenterol Nutr* 24:10, 1997.

87. Mott GE, Jackson EM, McMahan CA, et al: Cholesterol metabolism in juvenile baboons: influences of infant and juvenile diets, *Arteriosclerosis* 5:347, 1985.

88. Mott GE: Deferred effects of breastfeeding versus formula feeding on serum lipoprotein concentration and cholesterol metabolism in baboons, in *Report of the 91st Ross conference on pediatric research: the breastfed infant: a model performance*, Columbus, Ohio, 1986, Ross Laboratories.

89. Neifert MR, Seacat JM, Jobe WE: Lactation failure due to insufficient glandular development of the breast, *Pediatrics* 76:823, 1985.

90. Neifert MR, Seacat JM: Mammary gland anomalies and lactation failure. In Hamosh M, Goldman AS, editors: *Human lactation. II. Maternal and environmental factors*, New York, 1986, Plenum.

91. Nelson SE, Rogers RR, Ziegler EE, et al: Gain in weight and length during early infancy, *Early Hum Dev* 19:223, 1989.

92. O'Connor ME, Szekely LJ: Failure to thrive in breastfed 8-11 month olds: a manifestation of the "vulnerable child syndrome", *ABM News Views* 2(2):9, 1996.

93. Oliva-Rasbach J, Neville MC: Longitudinal growth patterns of a reference population of breastfed infants, *Fed Proc* 45:362, 1986.

94. Owen CG, Martin RM, Whineup PH, et al: Effect of infant feeding on the risk of obesity across the life course: a quantitative review of published evidence, *Pediatrics* 115:1367–1377, 2005.

95. Palmer MM, Crawley K, Blanco IA: Neonatal oral-motor assessment scale: a reliability study, *J Perinatol* 13:28, 1993.

96. Pugliese MT, Weyman-Daum M, Moses N, et al: Parental health beliefs as a cause of nonorganic failure to thrive, *Pediatrics* 80:175, 1987.

97. Ramsay M, Gisel EG, Boutry M: Non-organic failure to thrive: growth failure secondary to feeding skills disorder, *Dev Med Child Neurol* 35:285, 1993.

98. Richards M, Hardy R, Wadsworth ME: Long-term effects of breast-feeding in a national birth cohort: educational attainment and midlife cognitive function, *Public Health Nutr* 5:631, 2002.

99. Rousseaux J, Duhamel A, Turck D, et al: Breastfeeding shows a protective trend toward adolescents with higher abdominal adiposity, *Obes Facts* 7:289–301, 2014.

100. Savino F, Fissore MF, Liquori SA, et al: Can hormones contained in mother's milk account for the beneficial effect of breastfeeding on obesity in children, *Clin Endocrinol (Oxf)* 71(6):757–765, 2009.

101. Smith MM, Lifshitz F: Excess fruit juice consumption as a contributing factor in nonorganic failure to thrive, *Pediatrics* 93:436, 1994.

102. Strbák V, Skultétyová M, Hromadova M, et al: Late effects of breastfeeding and early weaning: seven-year prospective study in children, *Endocr Regul* 25:53, 1991.

103. Subcommittee on Nutrition During Lactation, Committee on Nutritional Status During Pregnancy and Lactation: *Nutrition during pregnancy and lactation: an implementation guide*, Washington, D.C., 1992, National Academy Press.

104. Subcommittee on Nutrition During Lactation, Committee on Nutritional Status During Pregnancy and Lactation, Food and Nutrition Board, et al: *Nutrition during lactation*, Washington, D.C., 1991, National Academy Press.

105. Taveras EM, Rifas-Shiman SL, Scanlon KS, et al: To what extent is the protective effect of breastfeeding on future over weight explained by decreased maternal feeding restriction? *Pediatrics* 118:2341–2348, 2006.

106. Taylor B, Wadsworth J: Breastfeeding and child development at five years, *Dev Med Child Neurol* 26:73, 1984.

107. The Endocrine Society: Clinical guidelines: prevention and treatment of pediatric obesity, *J Clin Endocrinol Metab* 93:4576–4599, 2008.

108. Toschke AM, Martin RM, vonKries R, et al: Infant feeding method and obesity: body mass index and dual energy X-ray absorptiometry measurements at 9-10 years of age from the Avon longitudinal study and children, *Am J Clin Nutr* 85:1578–1585, 2007.

109. von Kries R, Koletzko B, Sauerwald T, et al: Breastfeeding and obesity: cross sectional study, *BMJ* 319 (7203):147–150, 1999.

110. Wadsworth MEJ, Hardy RJ, Paul AA, et al: Leg and trunk length at 43 years in relation to childhood health, diet and family circumstance, *J Epidemiol Community Health* 52:142–152, 1998.

111. Weichert CE: Lactational reflex recovery in breastfeeding failure, *Pediatrics* 63:799, 1979.

112. Woo JG, Guerrero ML, Haye M, et al: Human milk adiponectin is associated with infant growth in two independent cohorts, *Breastfeed Med* 4(2):101, 2009.

113. World Health Organization Growth Reference Study Group: Reliability of anthropometric measurements in the WHO multicenter growth reference study, *Acta Paediatr Suppl*, 86–95, 2006.

114. World Health Organization Multicenter Growth Reference Study Group: Assessment of differences in linear growth among populations in the WHO multicenter reference study, *Acta Paediatr Suppl* 450:56–65, 2006.

115. World Health Organization Working Group on Infant Growth: An evaluation of infant growth: the use and interpretation of anthropometry in infants, *Bull World Health Organ* 73:165, 1995.

116. World Health Organization, Multicenter Reference Study Group: WHO motor development study: windows of achievements for six gross motor development milestones, *Acta Paediatr Suppl* 450:86–95, 2006.

117. World Health Organization/Centers for Disease Control: *Measuring change in nutritional status: guidelines for assessing the nutritional impact of supplementary feeding programmes for vulnerable groups*, Geneva, 1983, WHO.

118. Zheng J-S, Liu H, Li J, et al: Exclusive breastfeeding is inversely associated with risk of childhood overweight in a large Chinese cohort, *J Nutr* 144:1454–1459, 2014.

119. Zive MM, McKay H, Frank-Spohrer GC, et al: Infant feeding practices and adiposity in year old Anglo- and Mexican-Americans, *Am J Clin Nutr* 55:1104, 1992.

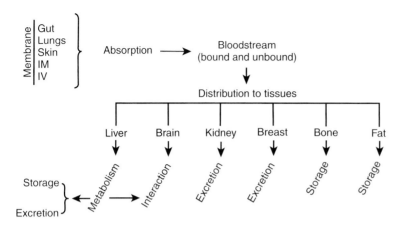

Figure 12-1. Distribution pathways for drugs once absorbed during lactation. (Modified from Rivera-Calimlim L: The significance of drugs in breast milk, *Clin Perinatol* 14:51, 1976.)

proteins (milk protein concentration is 0.9% in mature milk). Only those drug molecules that are free in solution can pass through the endothelial pores, either by diffusion or by reverse pinocytosis. *Pinocytosis* is the process whereby drug molecules dissolved in the interstitial fluid attach to receptors located at the surface of the cell membrane. The cell membrane invaginates at the site of the drug attachment, bringing the drug into the cell. The membrane is pinched off, and the drug, surrounded by membrane, remains in the cell. Then the membrane is dissolved, leaving the drug molecule free in the cell.

Reverse pinocytosis is the process by which the apical membrane evaginates after fusion of the intracellular membrane-bound secretion granules with the plasma membrane. The granules include lipids, proteins, lactose, drug molecules, and other cellular constituents. The evagination of the plasma membrane is pinched off and released into the alveolar lumen. Within the extravascular space, the drug may be bound to proteins in the interstitial fluid. Some agents in free solution can pass into the alveolar milk directly by way of the spaces between the mammary alveolar cells. These paracellular areas account for a major portion of the fluid changes across the epithelium. These spaces between adjacent alveolar cells serve to carry water-soluble drugs from the tissue into the milk.

The intercellular junctions are "open" at delivery as lactation is being established and gradually "tighten" over the next few days. The amount of drug passed into milk on day 1 is greater than on day 3 or later. The composition of the milk changes from colostrum to mature milk, altering the amount of protein and fat, which could also influence drug levels in the milk. It is always important to know when plasma and milk samples were measured in relationship to the onset of lactation. Furthermore, some studies have been done on nonlactating women by pumping

enough milk to measure the drug. These "weaning samples" provide only misinformation.

Ionization

Drugs that are nonionized are excreted in the milk in greater amounts than are ionized compounds. Depending on the pH of the solvent and the drug dissociation constant (pK_a), many weak electrolytes are more or less ionized in solution. Blood plasma and interstitial fluid are slightly alkaline (pH 7.4). Drugs that are weak acids are ionized to a greater extent in alkaline solution and are more extensively bound to protein. The amount of drug excreted from plasma (pH 7.4) to milk (pH 6.8 to 7.3, average 7.0) depends on the pH of the compound. Thus a weakly acidic compound has a higher concentration in plasma than in milk. Conversely, weakly alkaline compounds are in equal or higher levels in the milk than in the plasma.

The degree of drug ionization changes with the pH of the plasma and milk. Weak bases become more ionized with decreasing pH; thus the ionized component will increase in milk. The concentration in plasma and milk for the nonionized fraction will be the same, but the total amount of drug in the milk will be greater than in plasma. The sulfonamides demonstrate the effect of the pK_a on the concentration of drug that reaches the milk. Sulfacetamide, with a low pK_a (5.4), has a low milk/plasma (M/P) ratio (0.08), whereas sulfanilamide has a pK_a of 10.4 and an M/P ratio of 1.00 (Table 12-1).

The studies done in cows and goats with constant infusions demonstrate this principle more dramatically because the pH of bovine plasma is 7.4 to 7.5 and the pH of bovine milk is 6.5. Under normal circumstances, however, concentrations of drugs are rarely constant, and there is a delay in achieving a new equilibrium. During periods of rapidly decreasing blood levels, some back diffusion occurs into the plasma.

TABLE 12-1	Association Between Milk/Plasma (M/P) Ratios and Dissociation Constants (pKa) of Sulfonamides	
Sulfonamide	Milk/Plasma Ratio	pKa
Sulfacetamide	0.08	5.4
Sulfadiazine	0.21	6.5
Sulfathiazole	0.43	7.1
Sulfamethazine	0.51	7.4
Sulfapyridine	0.85	8.4
Sulfanilamide	1.00	10.4

Modified from Gaginella TS: Drugs and the nursing mother-infant, *US Pharm* 3:39, 1978.

Molecular Weight

The passage of molecules into the milk also depends on the size of the molecule, or the molecular weight (mol wt, in daltons). Water-filled membranous pores permit the movement of molecules of less than 100 mol wt. Because of action similar to the limitation of transport of certain large-molecular-weight chemicals across the placenta, insulin and heparin are not found in human milk either, presumably because of the molecule's size.

Solubility

The alveolar epithelium of the breast is a lipid barrier that is most permeable in the first few days of lactation, when colostrum is being produced. The solubility of a compound in water and in lipid is a determining factor in its transfer. Nonionized drugs, which are lipid soluble, usually dissolve and descend in the lipid phase of the membrane. The solubility is closely linked to the manner in which the drug crosses the membranes (Table 12-2). The membrane of the alveolar epithelial cells is composed of lipoprotein, glycolipid, phospholipid, and free lipids, as described in Chapter 4. The transfer of water-soluble drugs

TABLE 12-2	Predicted Distribution Ratios of Drug Concentrations in Milk and Plasma
General Drug Type	Milk/Plasma (M/P) Ratio
Highly lipid-soluble drugs	~1
Highly protein-bound drugs in maternal serum	<1
Small (mol wt <200) water-soluble drugs	~1
Weak acids	≤1
Weak bases	≥1
Actively transported drugs	>1

Modified from Gaginella TS: Drugs and the nursing mother-infant, *US Pharm* 3:39, 1978.

and ions is inhibited by this hydrophobic barrier. Water-soluble materials pass through pores in the basement membrane and paracellular spaces. Low lipid solubility of a nonionized compound will diminish its excretion into milk.

Lipid solubility affects the profile of the drug in the milk and plasma. A drug with high lipid solubility will have parallel elimination curves in the plasma and the milk. A drug with low lipid solubility will clear the plasma at a constant rate, but the clearance curve for the milk will peak lower and later, and the drug will linger in the milk. A prolonged terminal elimination phase may exist when time between feedings is long.

Mechanisms of Transport

Drugs pass into milk by simple diffusion, carrier-mediated diffusion, or active transport, as follows:

Simple diffusion: Concentration gradient decreases
Carrier-mediated diffusion: Concentration gradient decreases
Active transport: Concentration gradient increases

Pinocytosis

Reverse Pinocytosis. Pharmacokinetic principles relate to the specific variation with time of the drug concentration in the blood or plasma as a result of its absorption, distribution, and elimination. Ultimately, by extrapolation of these factors, one determines the effect of the drug. The most elementary kinetic model is based on the body as a single compartment. Distribution of the drug in the compartment is assumed to be uniform and rapidly equilibrated. In the single-compartment model, the volume of distribution of a drug is considered to be the same as that of the plasma, assuming a rapid uniform distribution.[43] The volume of distribution (V_d) is calculated as follows:

$$V_d = \frac{\text{Total amount drug in body}}{\text{Concentration of drug in plasma}}$$

The absorption and elimination are considered to be exponential or first-order kinetics. A two-compartment model of drug kinetics takes into account the phase of decreasing drug concentration as the drug distributes into the tissues. Initially, concentrations fall rapidly as the drug distributes, then first-order elimination follows. When considering the pharmacokinetics of drugs in breast milk, one must also consider that elimination in the breast is by two potential routes: excreted with the milk to the infant and back diffusion into the plasma to reequilibrate with the falling level in the plasma.

With access to the volume of distribution of the drug in question, the amount of the dose, and the weight of the mother, the concentration of drug in breast milk could be theoretically calculated as follows:

$$\text{Concentration in breast milk} = \frac{\text{Dose}}{\text{Volume of distribution}}$$

Other models have been developed for measuring the amount of drug that reaches the infant when the M/P ratio is not known. Using a stepwise linear regression for acidic and basic drugs, based on the drug's pK_a, the plasma protein binding value, and the octanol/water partition coefficient, an M/P ratio can be calculated. In a study of several proposed equations, the error is lowest for the drugs with the highest M/P ratio, that protein binding is the most important single predictor, and that the M/P ratios for basic drugs are more accurately predictable.

The concentration of the drug in the circulation of the mother depends on the mode of administration: oral, IV, IM, or TDDS. Absorption through the skin, the lungs (inhalants), or vaginally may also need to be considered.

The levels in the blood depend on the route of administration. The curves produced by bolus IV medication peak high and early and taper sharply, thus making avoiding peak plasma levels more feasible. Absorption from IM dosing is less rapid but follows a similar but less sharp curve. Oral dosing depends on other factors, such as whether the medication is taken between or during meals. Depending on the curve of uptake and removal of drug from the plasma, the area under the curve varies. Single doses are simple area-under-the-curve calculations, but calculations for multiple doses or chronic use vary with the steady state of the drug in the body. TDDS patches deliver the medication at a constant rate continuously.

Nonelectrolytes such as ethanol, urea, and antipyrine enter the milk by diffusion through the lipid membrane barrier and may reach the same concentrations in the milk as in the plasma, regardless of the pH. The main entrance site of molecules is at the basement laminal membrane, where water-soluble materials pass through the alveolar pores. Nonionized drugs cross the membrane more easily than ionized ones because of the structure of the membrane. The nonionized drugs pass through the membrane by diffusion. When simple diffusion takes place, the M/P ratio is 1.0. Passive diffusion provides the same ratio regardless of the plasma concentrations of the drug or the volume of milk secreted. Different M/P ratios depend on the binding to protein and are a measure of the protein-free fraction. The dissimilar ratios for the sulfa drugs

(see Table 12-1) partly result from the difference in protein binding and partly from ionization.

Large molecules depend on their lipid solubility and ionization to cross the membrane, because they pass in a lipid-soluble nonionized form. The M/P ratio is determined when equilibrium exists in the amount of nonionized drug in the aqueous phase on both sides of the membrane. When drugs are only partially ionized, the nonionized fraction determines the concentration that crosses the membrane. The drugs for which the nonionized fraction is not very lipid soluble will pass only in limited degree into breast milk.

Passive drug transport may occur in the form of *facilitated diffusion*. The active compound is transported across the cell membrane by a carrier enzyme or protein. The gradient is toward a lesser or equal concentration in both simple diffusion and facilitated diffusion and is controlled by chemical activity gradients. Facilitated diffusion usually involves a water-soluble substance too large to pass through the membrane pores.

Active transport mechanisms provide a process whereby the gradient is "uphill," or higher, in the milk. The process is similar to facilitated diffusion except that metabolic energy is required to overcome the gradient. Examples of substances actively transported include glucose, amino acids, calcium, magnesium, and sodium. Pinocytosis and reverse pinocytosis, as described previously, are involved in the transport of very large molecules and proteins. Chloride ions are secreted into milk via an active apical membrane pump, whereas sodium and potassium are diffused by electrical gradient. Because the level of sodium is kept low, an active return of sodium may occur into the plasma, referred to as a *reverse pump*. The TDDS depends on absorption of the drug through the skin at a steady rate; it has become a significant route of administration for certain medications. The delivery rate is determined by diffusion of drug from the reservoir matrix through the epidermis. This method offers some advantages, including convenience of dosing, reduced dosing frequency, ease of reaching a steady state, increased patient compliance, avoidance of first-pass hepatic biotransformation, avoidance of peaks and valleys in blood levels, and reduction of side effects through heightened selectivity of drug action.[71] The level in the plasma remains constant during the drug's anticipated life span while the patch is in place. The technology is limited to drugs with low molecular weight that are hydrophilic and can diffuse through the stratum corneum. The top molecular weight is 500 daltons. For patient compliance and economics the patch size is limited to 50 cm in diameter. Occasional patients experience skin irritation. Currently patches are limited to drugs that are potent in small

TABLE 12-3	Currently Available Transdermal Patches for Systemic Effects			
Generic Drug	**Brand Name**	**Strengths/Release Rate**	**Application Frequency**	**Total Drug Content per Patch**
Clonidine	Catapres-TTS	0.1, 0.2, 0.3 mg/24 h	7 days	2.5, 5, 7.5 mg
Estradiol	Alora	0.025, 0.05, 0.075, 0.1 mg/24 h	7 days	0.77, 1.5, 2.3, 3.1 mg
	Climara	0.025, 0.0375, 0.05, 0.06, 0.75, 0.1 mg/24 h	7 days	2, 2.85, 3.8, 4.55, 5.7, 7.6 mg
	Estraderm	0.05, 0.1 mg/24 h	3-4 days	4 mg, 8 mg
	Vivelle-Dot	0.025, 0.0375, 0.05, 0.075, 0.1 mg/24 h	3-4 days	0.62/2.7 mg, 0.51/4.8 mg
Estradiol/ Norelgestromin	Ortho Evra	20 mcg/150 mcg/24 h	7 days	0.75 mg/6 mg
Fentanyl	Duragesic	12.5, 25, 50, 100 mcg/h	72 hours	1.25, 2.5, 5, 7.5, 10 mg
Lidocaine	Lidoderm	35 mg/12 h	12 h/day	700 mg
Methylphenidate	Daytrana	10, 15, 20, 30 mg/9 h	9 h/day	27.5, 41, 3, 55, 82.5 mg
Nicotine	Habitrol	7, 14, 21 mg/24 h	16-24 h/day	17.5, 35, 52.5 mg
	NicoDerm CQ	7, 14, 21 mg/24 h	16-24 h/day	36, 78, 114 mg
Nitroglycerin	Nitro-Dur	0.1, 0.2, 0.3, 0.4, 0.6, 0.8 mg/h	12-14 h/day	20, 40, 60, 80, 120, 160 mg
	Minitran	0.1, 0.2, 0.4, 0.6 mg/h	12-14 h/day	Approx 8.6, 17, 34, 51.4 mg
Oxybutynin	Oxytrol	3.9 mg/24 h	24 h	36 mg
Rotigotine	Neupro	2, 4, 6 mg/24 h	24 h	4.5, 9, 13.5 mg
Scopolamine	Transderm-Scop	1.0 mg/72 h	3 days	1.5 mg
Selegiline	Emsam	6, 9, 12 mg/24 h	24 h	20, 30, 40 mg
Testosterone	Androderm	2.5, 5 mg/24 h	24 h	12.2, 24, 3 mg

amounts and highly diffusible through the skin. To maintain a constant rate, a surplus of drug must be present, often 20 to 30 times the amount that will be absorbed during the time of application. The potential for toxicity is great. If a patch is utilized while lactating it should be applied and covered so a nursing infant cannot accidently get to it.

TDDS patches are available for scopolamine, nicotine, clonidine, fentanyl, and other drugs (Table 12-3).

A summary of the steps in the passage of drugs into breast milk follows:

1. Mammary alveolar epithelium represents a lipid barrier with water-filled pores and is most permeable for drugs during the colostral phase of milk secretion (first week postpartum).
2. Drug excretion into milk depends on the drug's degree of ionization, molecular weight, solubility in fat and water, and relation of pH of plasma (7.4) to pH of milk (7.0).
3. Drugs preferably enter mammary cells basally in the nonionized, nonprotein-bound form by diffusion or active transport.
4. Water-soluble drugs less than 200 mol wt pass through water-filled membranous pores.

5. Drugs leave mammary alveolar cells apically by diffusion or active transport.
6. Drugs may enter milk via spaces between mammary alveolar cells.
7. Most ingested drugs appear in milk; drug amounts in milk usually do not exceed 1% of ingested dosage, and levels in the milk are independent of milk volume.
8. Drugs are bound much less to milk proteins than to plasma proteins.
9. Drug-metabolizing capacity of mammary epithelium is not understood.

Effect on Nursing Infant

ABSORPTION FROM GASTROINTESTINAL TRACT

Although concern surrounds the amount of a given agent in the breast milk, of greater importance is the amount absorbed into an infant's bloodstream. No accurate way exists to measure this because other factors also affect the level in an infant's bloodstream. The tolerance of the chemical to the pH of the stomach and the enzymatic activity of the intestinal tract are significant. The volume of milk consumed is a factor as well. Some drugs are not well absorbed with food (see later discussion of food-drug interactions). Oral bioavailability of a compound is a major factor of risk for an infant.

Infant's Ability to Detoxify and Excrete Agent

Any drug given to an infant by any route has to be evaluated according to the infant's ability to detoxify or conjugate the chemical in the liver and excrete it in the urine or stool. Some compounds that appear in milk in very low levels are not well excreted by infants and therefore accumulate in infants' systems to the point of toxicity.

Drugs that depend on the liver for conjugation, such as acetaminophen, are theoretic risks because of the limited reserve of the neonatal hepatic detoxification system. When actual measurements were made of neonates given acetaminophen, they were noted to handle it well because they conjugate it in the sulfhydryl system as an alternative pathway, which is used only to a small extent in adult metabolism of acetaminophen. When a single dose of a drug is given to a mother and the level is measured in her milk and in her infant, it does not give a clear picture of the potential for accumulation in the infant's system. The competition for binding a drug to protein is also important. Some drugs, such as sulfadiazine, compete for binding sites that might normally bind bilirubin in the first week or so of life. This puts an infant in jeopardy of kernicterus at a given bilirubin level because of an increase in the fraction of bilirubin left unbound for lack of binding sites. The indirect bilirubin level may even appear to be less than the dangerous level. Some other compounds that displace bilirubin from albumin-binding sites include salicylic acid (aspirin or acetylsalicylic acid breaks down to salicylic acid), furosemide, and phenylbutazone.

The maturity of an infant at birth is an extremely important factor during the first few months of life; thus the gestational age at birth should be established. Clearly, the less mature the infant, the less well tolerated drugs are, not only because of the immaturity of the organ systems but also because of differences in body composition (Figure 12-2). The less mature an infant, the greater the water content of the body and the proportion of extracellular water. Although the percentage of body weight that is protein is similar for all newborns (i.e., 12%), the absolute amount of protein for binding is less the smaller an infant is. The amount of

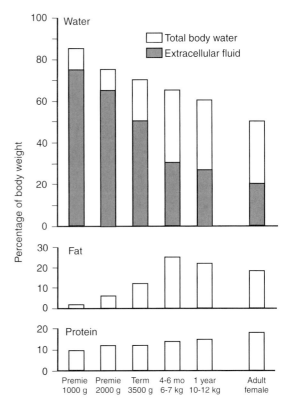

Figure 12-2. Comparative body composition of infants and adults. (Redrawn from Bechard LJ, Wroe E, Ellisk K: Body composition and growth. In Duggan C, Watkins JB, Walker WA, editors: *Nutrition in clinical practice*, ed 4, Hamilton, 2008, BC Decker.)

body fat is also low, by percentage of body weight and in absolute values. The distribution of highly lipid-soluble drugs therefore will be more apt to deposit in the brain of a 1000-g infant with 3% body fat by weight than in a 3500-g full-term infant with 12% body fat. This may explain the more sedating effect of a drug on the central nervous system (CNS) of a smaller, younger, and less mature infant. The relative lack of plasma protein-binding sites in a small, premature infant compared with a more mature, older infant results in more free (unbound) active drug in circulation. Complications of premature birth, such as acidosis and hypoxia, also contribute to the unavailability of albumin-binding sites and thus result in more unbound drug.

The inability of the liver to metabolize drugs effectively results in the accumulation of some compounds that might be readily cleared by an older infant. At about 42 weeks' conceptual age, an infant's liver is able to metabolize most drugs competently. Renal clearance similarly is less effective with decreasing maturity, which increases the risk for drug accumulation. The need to dose a premature infant only once or twice per day is common to many drugs, such as antibiotics, caffeine, and theophylline, and confirms that a small, premature infant does not clear drugs well.

Special problems in neonates in addition to the presence of jaundice or low serum albumin may require special consideration. Low Apgar scores at birth signifying some degree of stress, hypoxia, or acidosis may alter binding-site availability but may also alter metabolism and excretion of a drug. Continuing respiratory distress requiring ventilatory support, sepsis, and renal failure demand special consideration when determining if a sick neonate can receive the mother's milk when she is being treated with certain medications. Prescribing for such a mother should be done in consultation with the neonatologist if the woman is providing her milk for her infant.

The age of an infant makes a difference in the total volume of milk consumed; in an older child, the diet includes other items so that milk does not compose the total intake. Age makes a difference because the more mature infant can metabolize drugs more effectively; thus sulfa drugs, for instance, can be given to infants after the first month of life.

If the agent is fat soluble, the fat content of the milk may be a significant variable. The fat content at any feeding increases over time; thus the so-called foremilk is low in fat and the hindmilk is four to five times richer in fat toward the end of a feeding. Even though the total amount of fat will be about the same in each 24-hour period, the total amount of fat in a given feeding is less in the morning, peaks at midday, and drops off in the evening. The coefficient of lipid solubility for a nonionized drug determines both its penetration of the biologic membrane to gain entrance to milk and its concentration in milk fat. Sulfonamides with low fat solubility are in the aqueous and protein fraction of milk, whereas many barbiturates are in the lipid fraction. An inverse relationship exists between a drug's lipid solubility and the amount that appears in the skim fraction. The concentrations in fat differ for each member of the barbital family. Pentobarbital and secobarbital are found in the lipid phase, whereas phenobarbital is found in the aqueous phase.

The agent may appear in low levels in a mother's serum, but mammary blood flow during lactation is 500 mL/min and a mother produces between 60 and 300 mL of milk per hour. The agent that appears in minimal concentrations in the milk may present a significant problem when one considers that 1000 mL of milk may be consumed in a day by an infant. Even though the volume is low, during the colostral phase of lactation, the breast is more permeable to drugs.

Breast Milk/Plasma Ratio for Drugs Usually Not Useful

The M/P ratio for drugs has been measured and reported for many medications. By definition, M/P ratio is the concentration of the drug in the milk versus the concentration in maternal plasma (serum) at the same time. It presumes that the relationship between the two concentrations remains constant, which in most cases it does not. If it were a constant, it would allow the estimation of the amount of drug in the milk from any given plasma level in a mother.

An inaccurate ratio, or one determined under variable circumstances, produces erroneous estimates of the amount of drug in the milk, A pharmacokinetic model is a requisite foundation for studies of drugs in breast milk. A single-point-in-time M/P ratio, or an average ratio calculated with single-dose, area-under-the-curve data, does not work for all drugs. Neither ratio accounts for the importance of time-dependent variations of drug concentration in milk.

The M/P ratio is most valuable if obtained when an infant would be nursed. If the ratio is 1:0, it means only that the levels are equal. If the level is minimal in a mother's plasma because of the large volume of distribution, and if the milk level is also low, the M/P ratio is 1:0. If levels are drawn at peak plasma level and are equal, the M/P is still 1:0, but the infant receives a large dose. Thus the M/P ratio is valuable only when the time of the measurement is known in relationship to dosing of the mother. Dose strength, duration of dosing, maternal variation in drug disposition, maternal disease, drug interactions and competition of additional drugs for metabolism or binding sites, and racial variations in drug metabolism all influence the M/P interpretation. The M/P ratio may be greater than 1, which sounds alarming; however, a drug with a large volume of distribution will have low levels in the plasma and possibly high milk levels, but neither level may be therapeutically significant. The M/P ratio only confirms that the drug gets in the milk, and the safety cannot be measured.

Evaluating Drug Data

The paucity of carefully controlled studies on large enough samples to validate the results when such a large number of variables are active has been lamented by many authors. Some data collected are not pharmacokinetically sound. A clinician needs to understand these variables as well as pharmacokinetic principles to make a reasonable judgment about a given case.

Interethnic and racial differences in drug responsiveness are well established. The increased heterogeneity of national populations has brought increased awareness of genetic diversity. Plasma binding, especially with drugs dependent on glycoproteins for binding, often varies greatly between Caucasian and Chinese subjects, for example.[150] Such factors contribute to the differences in drug disposition and pharmacologic response.

It should be theoretically possible to determine how much of a specific drug reaches an infant in the mother's milk by knowing all the properties of the drug, including its volume of distribution, ionization, pK_a, lipid solubility, protein-binding activity, and rate of detoxification in the maternal system. Sufficient variation in the levels that reach an infant and in how the infant deals with the agent, however, makes it necessary to have specific data about a specific drug. Thus a few simple questions in the decision-making process are helpful in determining risk.

Safety for Infant

Ask, "Is this a drug that can be given to the infant directly if necessary?" Antibiotics (e.g., penicillin) that one could give an infant are in this category, whereas an antibiotic such as chloramphenicol, which one would not give an infant under ordinary circumstances, should be avoided in a nursing mother. The toxicity of chloramphenicol in an infant is dose related and associated with an unpredictable accumulation of the drug. Also, an idiosyncratic reaction occurs with chloramphenicol, which is unrelated to dose but is capable of causing pancytopenia.

If the drug in question can be given to an infant, does the amount in the milk create any risk to the infant? Phenobarbital can be given to infants for various reasons; thus the question is whether enough will reach the infant to cause difficulty. The infant should be watched for symptoms of lethargy or sleepiness, such as a change in feeding or sleeping pattern. If the infant is sleeping long periods and feeding less than usual (specifically, fewer than five or six times per day), the medication may be at fault. Phenobarbital is a significant drug for a mother with seizures; therefore a careful review of the risk/benefit ratio to both mother and infant should be undertaken. Barbiturates vary in their effect in young infants. A newborn does not handle the short-acting barbiturates well because they are dependent on detoxification in the liver, whereas phenobarbital depends more on the kidney for excretion.

If the drug was taken during pregnancy, as for epilepsy, an infant will already have the drug in his or her system via the placenta at a steady state and will have to begin to excrete it on his or her own after delivery.[104] Enzyme induction may have taken place in the neonate, however, because of exposure to the drug in utero; phenobarbital hastens maturation of the fetal liver.[109] Enzyme induction of the hepatic oxygenase system by phenobarbital, phenytoin, primidone, and carbamazepine is well established. Valproate, however, does not induce enzyme activity.

If one can safely give a drug to an infant, administration becomes a question of watching for any symptoms of excessive accumulation. The age of the infant affects the ability to clear the drug.

When the drug in question is one not normally given to an infant at that particular age, weight, or degree of maturity, decision-making is more difficult. Specific information about the amount of the drug that appears in the milk is essential in decision-making. Often, conflicting information is available. Many lists of drug-milk levels have perpetuated the same errors in calculation; thus having more than one reference report the same information may not provide confirmation of its accuracy.

If a medication will have to be taken for weeks or months, as with cardiovascular drugs, the drug has greater potential impact than when taken only for a few days. If the drug exposure has already occurred for 9 months in utero, some think it is less of a problem; however, it may compound the problem.

To determine the dose delivered to an infant, the following formula is used:

$$
\begin{aligned}
\text{Dose}/24\,\text{hours} \\
= \text{Concentration of drug in milk} \\
\times \text{Weight kg of infant} \\
\times \text{Volume of milk per kg ingested in 24 hours} \\
\text{Dose}/24\,\text{hours} = C_{milk} \times \text{Weight} \\
\times \text{Volume}/\text{kg}/24\,\text{hours}
\end{aligned}
$$

It has been recommended by Ito[60] and by Hale[47] that the calculation be the relative infant dose (RID), which is calculated as follows:

$$
\text{RID} = \frac{\text{Absolute infant dose mg/kg/day}}{\text{Maternal dose mg/kg/day}} \times 100
$$

It is also recommended that not more than 10% be acceptable for the calculated RID.

Sensitization

Is sensitization a risk, even in the small dosages of a drug that might pass into the milk? This question arises most frequently with the use of antibiotics, and use of penicillin is most frequently questioned. Certainly if a family has a strong history of drug sensitization, it should be considered. In that case, however, it should be questioned for a mother as well. Whether infants are put at risk for developing resistant strains of bacteria in their systems by small amounts of antibiotic in their feedings is a serious question. It also is as pertinent for the dairy and meat industries as for the humans who consume the food products that have a small amount of antibiotic because of administration to livestock.

Correlation of Drug Safety in Pregnancy and Lactation

Very rarely is valid information on the appearance of a drug in breast milk available on the package insert because pharmaceutical companies usually merely indicate that it should not be taken during pregnancy and lactation. To provide more information they would have to study it, which they typically choose not to do. Agents that may be safe during pregnancy may not be so during lactation. During pregnancy, the maternal liver and kidney are serving as detoxification and excretion resources for the fetus via the placenta, whereas during lactation an infant has to handle the drug totally on his or her own after it has reached his or her circulation. An infant in utero receives a drug in greater quantity via the circulation, whereas a nursing infant receives only what reaches the milk. One should be cautious about translating data pertaining to these two states back and forth. Drugs that are contraindicated in pregnancy may be acceptable during lactation.

Oral Bioavailability

The dose of a drug delivered via milk to an infant is significantly affected by oral bioavailability, which is the percentage of the drug absorbed into the infant's system via the gut.

Oral bioavailability is the rate and extent to which an active drug is absorbed and enters the general circulation. Absolute oral bioavailability compares the oral route with the IV route. To reach general circulation, an oral dose must pass through the wall of the gut, liver, or lungs.[125] First-pass metabolism or elimination in the tissues of these three organs may reduce a drug's bioavailability. It is possible for a drug to be 100% absorbed and be destroyed or eliminated and have 0% bioavailability because it is so rapidly metabolized.

If a compound is poorly absorbed, it is of less concern than one with 100% bioavailability. Most drugs administered by injection (e.g., insulin, heparin) only are not orally bioavailable.

Food-Drug Interactions

When drugs are taken with meals, numerous opportunities exist for food-drug interactions to occur.[103] Because a breastfed infant receives all maternal medications excreted in the milk "with food," this is an important consideration in the discussion of drugs in milk. The effects of food may reduce gastrointestinal (GI) absorption or irritation. Mechanisms of food-drug interactions can be summarized as follows.[103]

Physiologic
1. Changes in gastric emptying
2. Increased intestinal motility
3. Increased splanchnic blood flow
4. Increased bile, acid, and enzyme secretion
5. Induction and inhibition of drug metabolism
6. Competition in active transport

Physiochemical
1. Food as a mechanical barrier to absorption
2. Altered dissolution of drugs
3. Chelation and adsorption

Pharmacodynamic
1. Altered enzyme activity
2. Changes in homeostasis

Minimizing Effect of Maternal Medication

If a mother needs a specific medication and the hazards to the infant are minimal, the following important adjustments can be made to minimize the effects:

1. Do not use the long-acting form of the drug because the infant has even more difficulty excreting such an agent, which usually requires detoxification in the liver. Accumulation in the infant is then a genuine concern.
2. Schedule doses so the least amount possible gets into the milk. Check the usual absorption rates and peak blood levels of the drug. Having a mother take the medication immediately after breastfeeding is the safest time for the infant with most, but not all, drugs.
3. Watch the infant for any unusual signs or symptoms, such as change in feeding pattern or sleeping habits, fussiness, or rash whenever the mother takes medication.
4. When possible, choose the drug that produces the least amount in the milk (see Tables 12-1 and 12-2).

Classification Systems

The transfer of drugs and other chemicals into human milk also has been detailed in a statement by the AAP Committee on Drugs in 1983, 1989, 1994, and 2001.[23] The list includes only those drugs about which published information is available, and it does not provide the pharmacologic properties of the compounds. The 2001 list is divided into the same seven categories as the earlier lists, grouping drugs by their risk factors in relationship to breastfeeding. The categories are the following:

1. Cytotoxic drugs that may interfere with cellular metabolism of a nursing infant
2. Drugs of abuse
3. Radioactive compounds that require temporary cessation of breastfeeding
4. Drugs for which the effect on nursing infants is unknown but may be of concern
5. Drugs that have been associated with significant effects on some nursing infants and should be given to nursing mothers with caution
6. Maternal medications usually compatible with breastfeeding
7. Food and environmental agents: effect on breastfeeding

The list of more than 300 items is not inclusive. Further, the committee encourages physicians to report adverse effects in infants consuming milk of mothers taking specific drugs to the committee at the AAP.[23] Other rating systems have been suggested, but this system has been used consistently since 1983. A new edition of the list is in preparation and will appear in the journal *Pediatrics*.

As new texts regarding drugs in lactation are published, many authors have chosen their own scales to describe the status of a given drug, although AAP established one in 1983. Briggs et al.[17] use the AAP classification. Hale et al.[49] designed a new system—L1, safest; L2, safer; L3, moderately safe; L4, possibly hazardous; and L5, contraindicated—which is the reverse of the AAP system. Weiner and Buhimschi[141] published an additional system with only three categories: S, safe; NS, not safe; and U, unknown. To facilitate consistency this text will continue to use the AAP scale.

The Breastfeeding and Human Lactation Study Center at the University of Rochester continually updates its database on drugs, medications, and contaminants in human milk. More than 4000 references pertain to drugs in the database. In addition to information gleaned from reports of specific levels in breast milk, the tables include the ratings by the AAP,[23] Briggs et al.,[17] Hale et al.,[49]

Schaefer,[118] and Weiner and Buhimschi.[141] In addition, other drugs typically used by women in their childbearing years about which there are no specific milk levels are listed with their oral bioavailability for infants, peak serum time in the mothers, volume of distribution for the drugs, and other pharmacologic information (pH, solubility, protein binding, metabolism) obtained from a host of resources. With this information, a physician should be able to determine relative risk and thus select the best compound and adjust the dose and the time of, and association to, the breastfeeding.

Further information is available from the Finger Lakes Regional Poison and Drug Information Center, which has a specially equipped "Lactation line" to deal with questions about toxicity and lactation, at 585-275-3232. For hearing-impaired persons, TDD services (585-273-3854) are available 24 hours per day every day. This service is staffed by physicians, nurses, pharmacists, and clinical toxicologists. The Breastfeeding and Human Lactation Center is available during limited hours (8 AM to 4 PM EST, Monday to Friday) for more complex questions (585-275-0088).

Specific Drug Groups

ANALGESICS

Drugs such as heroin have been known for decades to appear in milk, and at one time withdrawal symptoms in neonates born to heroin-using mothers were prevented or treated by breastfeeding and then gradual weaning from the breast. Codeine and meperidine (Demerol) appear in milk at low levels. The pharmacokinetics of IV meperidine in neonates and infants younger than 5 months has shown great interindividual variability in elimination half-life, median clearance, and volume of distribution. Meperidine has been removed from many hospital pharmacies. A breastfed newborn was transferred to the special care nursery at Rochester because of unusual floppiness and poor muscle tone. His mother was taking dextropropoxyphene (Darvon) every 4 hours. Temporarily stopping breastfeeding until the mother's drug level dropped and discontinuing use of the drug produced dramatic improvement, which persisted when the infant went back to nursing.

Diazepam (Valium) taken in multiple doses by the mother has caused sleepiness, mild depression, and decreased intake in some infants and tends to accumulate in neonates, especially in the first weeks of life. However, an occasional dose of diazepam is not contraindicated.

The dose schedule for analgesics is usually a single dose, especially in the postpartum period.

A mother should not be subjected to great discomfort when a dose or two of analgesics would improve her well-being. Aspirin on a single-dose schedule is safe, although it is known to pass into the milk. The case of metabolic acidosis reported in a nursing infant occurred when the mother took 650 mg of aspirin every 4 hours for arthritis.[19] A serum salicylate level in the infant on the third day of hospitalization with no breastfeeding was still 24 mg/dL. This demonstrates the tendency of salicylate to accumulate in the neonate. Acetylsalicylic acid, not the metabolite salicylate, is responsible for the platelet aggregate abnormalities, so there should be no concern about aspirin in this regard because it is the metabolite salicylate that appears in the milk. Reye syndrome has also been a concern because of the association with aspirin. Again the breastfeeding neonate only gets salicylic acid, not acetylsalicylic acid. Acetaminophen is remarkably well tolerated by neonates and can be given to nursing mothers. Although it does reach the milk in small amounts, neonates metabolize it well.

Prescription ibuprofen has been extensively used in 600- to 800-mg doses as an antiinflammatory agent, especially in the treatment of arthritis. Since it became available in over-the-counter preparations of 200-mg tablets, ibuprofen has become widely used by the public for pain. Pediatricians are using it liberally for fever and myalgia and generalized aches and pains. It is widely used for postpartum pain of episiotomy or cesarean delivery.

Because of the initial concern about adverse effects of prostaglandin synthetase inhibiting drugs on neonates and a report of negligible (less than 0.05 mg/mL) levels in the milk of a woman after 17 days of therapy (400 mg twice per day), a careful study of ibuprofen was undertaken. After cesarean delivery, twelve women had serum and milk samples collected at intervals for 34 hours following 400 mg ibuprofen every 6 hours for five doses. Serum half-life was 1.5 hours. No measurable amounts (capable of detecting 1 mg/mL) of ibuprofen were found in breast milk. Under normal dosing, nursing infants would be exposed to less than 1 mg of ibuprofen per day. Ibuprofen is used to close the patent ductus in premature infants.

Fentanyl citrate is frequently used to provide analgesia or anesthesia to women during the postpartum period. It is a potent synthetic phenylpiperazine with extremely high lipid solubility and high pK_a but a large volume of distribution, suggesting a predisposition to appear in breast milk but clear rapidly. In a study of postpartum lactating women receiving fentanyl, concentrations were higher in colostrum than in the serum, probably due to the open intracellular junctions, peaked at 45 minutes after administration, and were undetectable 6 to 10 hours later. The oral bioavailability of less than 50% is reduced by food, which makes the risk to an infant minimal via the mother's milk, especially if peak serum time is avoided, which occurs within minutes depending upon the method of administering: IV, IM, or transdermally.

The use of epidural anesthesia during delivery and its continuation after cesarean delivery for pain has provided considerable relief to parturient women. Despite epidurals during labor becoming commonplace, the effects of this procedure on a neonate's ability to breastfeed continue to be disputed. The obstetric literature clearly shows that epidurals in early labor result in an increased rate of interventions, including forceps use, vacuum extraction, and cesarean delivery. These in turn result in increased postpartum complications and an increase in the length of hospital stay. When women who had cesarean delivery were followed prospectively, those who had epidural anesthesia breastfed sooner and continued longer than those women who had general anesthesia.

The challenging question, however, is whether epidurals affect infants' abilities to suckle and initiate breastfeeding in women who have a vaginal delivery (see infant suckling discussion in Chapter 8). Epidural medications vary by anesthesiologist but include fentanyl, sufentanil, morphine, bupivacaine, and rodocaine. The advantage of an epidural is that the anesthetic does not reach the general maternal circulation for about 6 hours. Ideally, a mother will deliver before 6 hours if the epidural was not administered too early in labor. Infants affected in ability to suckle had mothers who received more than one dose of medication via the epidural. A prospective cohort study following 1280 women who gave birth in the Australian capitol area was conducted by Torvaldsen et al.[138] They mailed questionnaires at 1, 8, 16, and 24 weeks. In the first week, 93% of women were breastfeeding fully or partially; 60% continued for 24 weeks. Intrapartum analgesia and type of delivery were associated with partial breastfeeding and breastfeeding difficulties. Women who had epidurals were more likely to stop breastfeeding before 24 weeks and to partially breastfeed than women who had other analgesia.

Although labor pain relief is superior with epidural analgesia compared with meperidine, labor is prolonged, risk for uterine infection increased, and the number of operative deliveries increased, all of which interfere with successful initiation of suckling in the neonate. Meperidine is no longer used during labor, but other short-acting analgesics such as nalbuphine (Nubain) are.[101,102] A study of butorphanol and nalbuphine demonstrated that receiving no medication or receiving a dose less than 1 hour before delivery was associated with earlier initiation of breastfeeding and establishment of effective feeding significantly earlier compared with mothers who received the drug more than an hour before delivery.[108] Righard and Alade[110] also observed the impact of meperidine on neonatal behavior. When they observed infants left on the maternal abdomen to find the breast and latch on, the nonmedicated infants were suckling in 20 minutes, but the medicated infants were unable to locate the breast and latch on and, in several cases, were unable to locate the breast after 40 minutes of trying.

Ketorolac tromethamine has been used for maternal pain in the first few days postpartum, especially in patients who had cesarean delivery. The concern has been the safety of breastfeeding during that time because ketorolac is an acidic pyrrolo-pyrrole prostaglandin synthetase inhibitor with a pK_a of 3.54 and 99.2% plasma protein binding. Would the drug get into the milk and interfere with the physiologic closing of an infant's ductus arteriosus? Wischnik et al.[145] examined this question in 10 women who received the drug 2 to 6 days after delivery. The mothers were pumping and discarding the milk because of illness in both mother and baby. Ketorolac 10 mg was given four times per day for 2 days. Plasma and milk samples were collected and levels measured; limits of detection were 10 mg/mL. The range was 5.9 mg/L to 7.9 mg/L in milk, although four patients never had measurable amounts in the milk. The M/P ratio was 0.015 to 0.037. The authors estimated that a maximum dose for an infant would be 3.16 to 7.9 mg/day. They assumed 400 to 1000 mL of milk was consumed, an improbable amount in the first few days. At maximum, the ketorolac level in milk was 0.16% to 0.40% of total daily maternal dose. Clinically, the authors concluded that significant sequelae from ketorolac are unlikely. The AAP rates ketorolac a category 6 drug, usually compatible with breastfeeding.[23]

ANTIBIOTICS

Levels of antibiotics in milk vary with the concentration of the drugs in plasma and their pK_a. The risks vary among groups of antibiotics. Penicillins are not usually toxic but theoretically can cause sensitivity. Sulfa drugs should not be used in the first month of life because they can interfere with the binding of bilirubin to albumen. The risk diminishes with age, and infants are given sulfa drugs directly at 4 to 6 weeks of age. Infants with glucose-6-phosphate dehydrogenase deficiency should never receive sulfa drugs directly or via breast milk. Chloramphenicol is contraindicated in nursing very young infants because of the risk for accumulation of the drug even from small amounts in milk and the potential for idiosyncratic reaction.

Tetracycline causes staining of teeth and abnormalities of bone growth when given directly to children for a week or more. Infants who are breastfed by mothers taking tetracycline for mastitis may have stained and mottled first and second teeth when therapy exceeds 10 days. The amount in milk is half that in the mother's plasma. Tetracycline should be given to mothers only for life-threatening infections.

Erythromycin appears in higher amounts in milk than in plasma. When given intravenously to the mother, the levels are 10 times higher. When an infant is old enough to receive erythromycin directly, the mother can take it as well. The major concerns regarding erythromycin pertain to its cross-effects with other medications. Erythromycin has the potential for decreasing the clearance of carbamazepine, cyclosporine, digoxin, triazolam, theophylline, anticoagulants, and drugs metabolized by the P-450 system.[17]

Aminoglycosides are common constituents of postpartum antibiotic therapy and are given parenterally. They readily appear in the milk but, as with kanamycin, are not readily absorbed from the GI tract; therefore under usual circumstances they pose no problem to a neonate, who will not absorb them. Newborns are given aminoglycosides directly.

Metronidazole (Flagyl) does appear in milk at levels equal to those in serum. Most researchers consider the risk to an infant insufficient to suggest alternative therapy for the mother. Symptoms in the mother include decreased appetite and vomiting and, occasionally, blood dyscrasia.

An alternative treatment regimen is 2 g metronidazole in a single dose. When milk concentrations are measured with a 2-g dose, the highest concentrations are found at 2 and 4 hours postingestion and decline over the next 12 hours to 19.1 mg/mL and to 12.6 mg/mL at 24 hours.[38,54] The dose to the infant is calculated to be 21.8 mg during the first 24 hours and only 3.5 mg in the second 24 hours. It has been recommended that a single-dose regimen be used in nursing mothers, which necessitates that a mother pump and discard milk for only 24 hours. Metronidazole in gel or cream form contains only 0.75% of the medication and is poorly absorbed because the purpose is to work on tissues locally. As a result, maternal plasma levels are 1/50 of levels from comparable oral dosing. Use of the drug in this form would probably result in undetectable amounts in the milk. Normally, the gel or cream is applied in small amounts twice daily. Peak absorption could be avoided. Metronidazole is often the only drug that works in a serious trichomoniasis, giardiasis, or amebiasis infection[38] when all other treatments have failed. It is now used directly in infants.

Amoxicillin, cephalexin, and cefadroxil, when given orally in a single dose, peak in the milk at 4 to 6 hours.[66] Cephalothin, cephapirin, and cefotaxime, when given in a bolus IV injection, peak at 2 hours. Cefadroxil reached the highest levels $(1.64 \pm 0.73 \text{ mg/mL})$ at 6 hours. Little gets into the milk. These drugs are also given to children.

Cephalosporins are weak acids with variable protein binding. Third-generation cephalosporins may affect the flora of the gut. Sterilization of the gut often leads to diarrhea. In general, cephalosporins are considered safe during lactation.[24] Breastfed infants rapidly recolonize the gut with lactobacillus. Oral absorption is poor and little reaches the milk, so they usually are considered safe.

The serum half-lives of parenterally administered cephalosporins are three to four times longer in neonates than the serum half-lives in mothers. The half-life of ceftriaxone in the milk is 12 to 17 hours compared with the maternal serum half-life of 6 hours. Neonates can be given cephalosporins directly. Ceftriaxone is given IM to infants once per day. Fluoroquinolones had been restricted in pediatric use because of early reports of arthropathy in immature animals and a single report of pseudomembranous colitis in a breastfeeding infant whose mother had self-medicated with ciprofloxacin.[52] More recently ciprofloxacin has been used in pediatric patients because it is valuable in gram-negative infections and also anthrax. Levels in milk are said to be low.[42] The AAP committee on drugs has designated it to be safe for breastfeeding women.[23]

Chloroquine, gentamicin, streptomycin, and rifampin (only 0.05%) are reported by the AAP[23] to be safe because they are not excreted in milk.

Because antibiotics are the medications most frequently prescribed for lactating women, it is noteworthy that compliance is low. Maternal noncompliance was measured by Ito[60] in 203 breastfeeding women who consulted the Motherisk Program for information about antibiotics. Despite reassuring advice, one in five women either did not initiate therapy or did not continue breastfeeding. This has serious implications for recurrent infections, especially mastitis. Mastitis represents another situation in which termination of breastfeeding is not indicated, or necessary.

ANTICHOLINERGICS

Anticholinergic drugs include atropine, scopolamine (hyoscine), and synthetic quaternary ammonium derivatives, some of which are available in over-the-counter medications. Some atropine does enter the milk. Infants are particularly sensitive to this drug; therefore an infant should be watched for tachycardia and thermal changes, which are more easily measured in infants. The most important consideration is that milk secretion may decrease in the mother. With repeat doses, constipation and urinary retention may occur in infants. The quaternary anticholinergics, however, should not appear in milk to any degree because, as anions, they do not pass into the acidic milk. Mepenzolate methylbromide (Cantil) does not appear in milk.

Scopolamine is available by dermal patch for motion sickness and causes maternal mucous membrane dryness, which could affect milk production as it restricts the secretions of other secretory glands. Only a small amount appears in milk. The AAP rates it and atropine as category 6, drugs usually compatible with breastfeeding, although the scopolamine patch, which provides a constant level, has not been tested per se.[23] Pressure point wristbands are reported to be effective for motion sickness in pregnancy and lactation and contain no medication.

GASTROINTESTINAL MEDICATIONS

Cimetidine (Tagamet), a potent H_2-receptor antagonist, is used for conditions associated with acid peptic digestion in the GI tract, especially elevated gastric acidity. Cimetidine excretion into breast milk has resulted in concentrations higher than in the corresponding plasma sample.[129] Levels were highest at 1 hour after a single dose (Table 12-4). Chronic-dose studies revealed variable M/P ratios, all of which were higher than the single-dose ratio. The authors suggest an active transport mechanism for this medication. The maximum amount of cimetidine ingested by an infant was calculated at 6 mg for 1 L of milk (or 1.5 mg/kg). It is rated category 6 by the AAP.[23]

The neonatal dose is 10 to 20 mg/kg/24 hours for severe gastroesophageal reflux or gastric ulcer, conditions that are rare in breastfed infants. The half-life in a neonate is 1.1 to 3.4 hours. It is contraindicated when either infant or mother is receiving cisapride because of the risk for precipitating cardiac arrhythmias.[129]

Caution is recommended with nursing when taking cimetidine until more is known of its side effects, especially antiandrogenic features. It is used in premature infants with reflux. Cimetidine does interfere with several drugs, including phenytoin, propranolol, warfarin, tricyclic antidepressants, diazepam, and cyclosporine.

Sulfasalazine treatment of ulcerative colitis and Crohn's disease during breastfeeding has been widely discussed on theoretic grounds because the compound splits to sulfapyridine and 5-aminosalicylic acid. The sulfapyridine is absorbed from the colon and is metabolized in the liver. The 5-aminosalicylic acid is partly absorbed and

TABLE 12-4 Antibiotic Selection for Bacterial Mastitis

Antibiotic	Spectrum	Dose	Safety	Comment
Dicloxacillin	Nonmethicillin-resistant Staphylococci	500 mg PO qid	Yes	Highest activity against MSSA
Clindamycin	Penicillin allergic Many CA-MRSA Test susceptibilities	300 mg PO qid	Probably safe	Excreted in milk; active against many strains of CA-MRSA
Erythromycin	Penicillin allergic	500 mg PO qid	Yes	GI intolerance
Azithromycin	Penicillin allergic	500-mg load, then 250 mg/day × 4 days	Probably safe	Limited *S. aureus* activity; less GI upset than erythromycin
Trimethoprim Sulfamethoxazole	Some CA-MRSA	One DS PO bid	Yes	Less effective when abscess present
Cephalexin	MSSA	500 mg PO qid	Yes	Relatively poor levels in breast tissue

bid, Twice per day; *CA-MRSA*, community-acquired methicillin-resistant *S. aureus*; *GI*, gastrointestinal; *MSSA*, methicillin-susceptible *S. aureus*; *PO*, by mouth; *qid*, four times per day.
From Nathan GG, Uhl K, Kennedy DL. Antibiotic use in pregnancy and lactation: what is and is not known about teratogenic and toxic risks, *Obstet Gynecol* 107:1120–1138, 2006.

rapidly excreted in the urine, so serum concentrations are low. The sulfapyridine and its metabolites do appear in the milk in lower concentrations than in the serum. A dose of 2 g/day of drug to a mother would produce 4 mg/kg of sulfapyridine in the milk, 40% of maternal levels. The oral absorption from the milk is low, so the actual amount in an infant's plasma is minimal. The risk for recurrent ulcerative colitis in the mother if medication is withdrawn outweighs the risk for sulfasalazine to the infant.[70]

Famotidine (Pepcid-AC) reduces gastric acidity. Milk levels are low and it has poor oral bioavailability so it is of little risk. Omeprazole (Prilosec), which also reduces gastric acidity, has milk levels that also are low. It is highly protein bound and only 40% orally bioavailable so should be safe. Levels are lower in the milk than cimetidine.

ANTICOAGULANTS

Heparin, regular or unfractionated, is a large-molecular-weight molecule that does not pass into breast milk. Because it is not absorbed from the GI tract, its use in the breastfeeding mother is acceptable.

Low-molecular-weight (LMW) heparins are glycosaminoglycans consisting of chains of alternating residues of D-glucosamine and uronic acid. Regular or unfractionated heparin is a heterogeneous mixture of polysaccharide chains ranging from 3000 to 30,000 mol wt. LMW heparin has a mean mol wt of 5000 daltons (2000 to 8000), with slight variation among brands: ardeparin (Normiflo), dalteparin (Fragmin), enoxaparin (Lovenox), nadroparin (Fraxiparine), reviparin (Clivarine), and tinzaparin

(Innohep). Both unfractionated and LMW heparins cause anticoagulation by activating antithrombin. LMW heparins produce a more predictable anticoagulant response because of their better bioavailability, longer half-life, dose-independent clearance, and decreased tendency to bind to plasma proteins and endothelium. They are less likely to interfere with platelets. They are considered safer and more effective in the treatment of venous thromboembolism, can be given subcutaneously without laboratory monitoring, carry less risk for thrombocytopenia and osteoporosis, and can be given at home.[142]

No studies are reported of LMW heparin use in pregnancy or lactation. Because mol wt is greater than 2000 and only a molecule of less than 1000 mol wt crosses the placenta or into the milk, these molecules are unlikely to cross. These LMW compounds are not orally bioavailable and would not be absorbed by an infant. They are considered safe during lactation.

Analysis of the milk of mothers using warfarin does not reveal any drug in the milk or in the infants. The infants' prothrombin times remained normal. This was demonstrated by McKenna et al.,[93] who followed two breastfed infants whose mothers were anticoagulated before delivery and maintained on warfarin postpartum. They found no immediate or delayed biologic effect on coagulation in 56 and 131 days of follow-up. From this, it has been suggested that warfarin is the drug of choice in lactating mothers who require anticoagulant therapy and want to continue breastfeeding. If surgery is contemplated or unusual trauma occurs, a review of an infant's coagulation status is indicated as a precautionary measure, and 1 mg vitamin K can be given orally or IM if there is concern.

ANTITHYROID DRUGS

Iodide has been known for generations to pass into the milk in levels higher than in the maternal plasma. It has been reported to cause symptoms in infants when used not only for hyperthyroidism but also in asthma preparations and cough medicines. Iodides have been noted to be goitrogenic and to sensitize the thyroid gland to other drugs, such as lithium, chlorpromazine, and methylxanthines.

Thiouracil is actively transported into the milk and appears in higher concentration in milk than in blood or urine, reported at levels 3 to 12 times higher in milk than in blood. It has the potential of causing goiter-suppressing thyroid activity or agranulocytes. Thiouracil is contraindicated during lactation.

Methimazole (Tapazole) presents risks to nursing infants similar to those seen with thiouracil (i.e., thyroid suppression, goiter). Giving 0.125 grain of thyroid extract may not adequately protect infants, and careful monitoring of neonatal thyroid function is mandatory. Measurements of amounts of methimazole in milk and serum when a mother received 2.5 mg every 12 hours were found to be similar. Tegler and Lindström[136] found 7% to 16% of the maternal dose in the milk; thus a dose of 5 mg four times daily might provide an infant with 3 mg daily. Studies of carbimazole using[35] S-labeled compound show a similar trend, with 0.47% of the dose appearing in the milk. Studies were done on a single dose of 10 mg carbimazole.

Propylthiouracil (PTU) has been investigated by several groups with similar results reported, showing that little of the compound is excreted in the milk (0.025% to 0.077% of total dose) in single-dose studies.[67] An infant who was followed 5 months on maternal doses of 200- to 300-mg PTU daily showed no neonatal thyroid symptoms and normal triiodothyronine (T_3), thyroxine (T_4), and thyroid-stimulating hormone. On the strength of these reports, others have proceeded to use PTU and permit breastfeeding. The availability of microdeterminations for T_3, T_4, and thyroid-stimulating hormone improves the quality of monitoring, and all infants given PTU via milk should be followed closely.[27] The AAP lists PTU in category 6, compatible with breastfeeding.[23]

CAFFEINE AND OTHER METHYLXANTHINES

Caffeine ingestion has been singled out for discussion because it is a frequent concern, but the data provided in most reviews are misleading. With a given dose of caffeine that is comparable with that in a cup of coffee, the level in the milk is low (1% of level in mother), and the level in an infant's plasma is also low. However, caffeine does accumulate in infants. This was learned when caffeine was introduced in neonatal intensive care units to treat apnea of prematurity.

Before the availability of the laboratory test for caffeine, cases were managed on clinical symptoms alone. Many clinicians recognized that wakeful, hyperactive infants were often the victims of caffeine stimulation. If a mother drank more than 6 to 8 cups of any caffeine-containing beverage in a day, her infant could accumulate symptomatic amounts of caffeine. Soft drinks such as colas and other carbonated drinks (e.g., Mountain Dew) often contributed to the caffeine buildup. When the situation was identified—a wide-eyed, active, alert infant who never slept for long—it was suggested that the mother try caffeine-free beverages, both hot and cold. Often the infant settled down to a reasonable sleep pattern after a few days with no caffeine.

Since information on milk and plasma levels has become available, researchers have identified three cases of caffeine excess in breastfed infants. The infants had measurable levels of caffeine in the plasma, which disappeared in a week after the caffeine was discontinued. The corresponding milk levels were as previously reported, about 1% of the mother's level, which supports the hypothesis that caffeine accumulates in infants. The infants do not need to be hospitalized, and verification of blood caffeine levels is helpful but not mandatory because a clinical trial will suffice. Smoking has been observed to augment the caffeine effect.

With an increasing number of women with asthma wanting to breastfeed, a question arises about the impact of methylxanthines that have also been used in apnea of prematurity. Information has been generated regarding dose, clearance, and toxicity in the neonate.[10] In addition, microdeterminations of blood levels are readily available.

Several studies of theophylline in mothers receiving regular doses have shown that the serum levels are lowest just before the oral dose and that M/P ratio is 0.60 to 0.73, with milk levels paralleling serum levels.[120,113,130] Infants receive an estimated 1% of the maternal dose. Data on IV and oral medication are similar in terms of M/P ratio. Maximum exposure was estimated at 7 to 8 mg/24 hours.

Dyphylline is a compound introduced clinically as a bronchodilator because of its lack of side effects.[64] It is excreted renally with little biotransformation. The M/P ratio was determined to be 2.08 ± 0.52, and the biologic half-life was 3.21 hours. Although this is considerably greater than that of

and safely.[15] When infant plasma level determinations are available, it might be advisable to check the plasma level after 1 or 2 weeks of nursing, providing an opportunity to evaluate possible accumulation.

Early childhood development was evaluated in children of women with epilepsy to determine the results of exposure to antiepileptic drugs during pregnancy and breastfeeding. The study had recruited 78,744 dyads, of which 223 were using antiepileptic drugs. Fine motor skills were noted to be reduced by 25% versus 4.8% in the reference group. Social skills were also diminished 23.5% compared to 10.2% in control. Continuous breastfeeding in children of women using antiepileptic drugs less often impaired development at 6 and 18 months compared with those not breastfeeding or breastfed less than 6 months. At 36 months, however, drug exposure was associated with adverse development regardless of breastfeeding. The authors thought that women should be encouraged to breastfeed regardless of need for drug treatment.

Psychotherapeutic Agents

Lithium is the one drug in the psychotherapeutic group with a clear risk for toxicity in the neonate and clear evidence that it reaches the breast milk. Lithium is contraindicated in pregnancy but has been used cautiously in lactation. Infants have been reported to be hypotonic, flaccid, and "depressed" when nursing mothers take lithium. Although rated a category 6 by the AAP at one time, it is now a 5, use with caution pending the dose used by the mother.

After a careful review of the clinical data, Schou[121] states that accumulating evidence points strongly to the beneficial effects of breastfeeding while taking lithium for both infants and mothers, mentally and physically. Lithium concentrations in breastfed infants have been measured at one tenth to one half of the concentration in the mothers' blood.[122] Such concentrations are considered harmless in adults, but the risk is unknown in children. A pitfall of measuring lithium levels in neonates was pointed out by Tanaka et al.[134] who describe two cases in which blood samples from the neonates were placed in tubes with lithium heparin as the anticoagulant. Schou[121] also states that, with support from her husband and physician, the mother should make her own choice. Initiating lithium therapy after delivery or when a breastfeeding infant is several months old greatly minimizes the theoretic risks. The Lactation Study Center has been contacted about several infants being breastfed by mothers taking lithium with the psychiatrist's and the pediatrician's consent. No

symptoms were apparent. No long-term follow-up is yet available on these children. In parts of the world where water supplies are not well controlled, lithium is a common contaminant—while lithium does appear in the milk of inhabitants, the levels in formula-fed infants are higher than the breastfed infants' levels because the formula is diluted with the water.[51]

Chlorpromazine or phenothiazine appears in the milk in small amounts, even at doses of 1200 mg, but apparently does not accumulate.[7] Doses of 100 mg/day do not appear to cause symptoms in infants. It is usually taken once per day, peaking in plasma 1 to 2 hours after dose, and breastfeeding should be timed to avoid peak. Diazepam (Valium) has been detected in milk and in breastfed infants' serum and urine. It has caused depression and poor feeding with weight loss in infants. In a single dose it should not present a problem. Shorter-acting lorazepam is safer for multiple dose therapy. Chlordiazepoxide (Librium) and clorazepate (Tranxene) do reach the milk and may cause drowsiness and poor suckling. These substances' metabolites are also active, and therefore the half-life of therapeutic activity is prolonged. Meprobamate (Miltown, Equanil) has an M/P ratio greater than 1 and has been identified in milk. Infants whose mothers are taking meprobamate may become drowsy, but dosage adjustment may be indicated if there is significant benefit for the mothers to breastfeed.[7] Usual dosing is three to four times per day, which makes avoiding peak plasma times difficult.

Tricyclic antidepressants, such as imipramine, are lipid soluble and have been identified in the breast milk; thus cautious use may be appropriate.[23] In an extensive study of tricyclic antidepressants in pregnancy and lactation, Misri and Sivertz[98] found that an attitude of informed and cautious encouragement may be appropriate regarding the growing information that suggests it is safe to breastfeed while taking such medication.[146] Consulting LactMed or a University of Rochester phone service may help in selecting the best drug for a given dyad (585-275-0088). When Yoshida et al.[149] investigated the pharmacokinetics and possible adverse effects in infants exposed to tricyclic antidepressants in breast milk, they found no reason to prevent mothers who are taking established tricyclic antidepressants from breastfeeding. The drugs were imipramine, amitriptyline, clomipramine, and dothiepin. They compared infants breastfed by mothers medicated with a tricyclic antidepressant with infants bottle fed by medicated mothers. In addition, they measured the drugs in all maternal plasma and urine and in the foremilk and hindmilk of the lactators. Infant plasma and urine levels were also measured. Levels in the mother and her milk were correlated with the dose. The daily dose of drug via the breast milk was 1% of the maternal dose per kilogram of weight. Amounts were barely detectable in infants' plasma and urine. The 30-month follow-up detected no differences in growth and development.[149]

The selective serotonin reuptake inhibitors are a class of drugs developed as antidepressants and used in the treatment of panic attacks, obsessive-compulsive disorder, obesity, substance abuse, sleep disorders, chemotherapy-induced nausea and vomiting, migraine, and appetite suppression. Serotonergic dysfunction has been implicated in these illnesses. This group of drugs has antidepressant actions and selectively blocks the reuptake of serotonin into presynaptic neurons (Box 12-2).

These agents undergo extensive metabolism to clinically inactive compounds, have large volumes of distribution, and are highly bound to maternal plasma proteins, suggesting little transfer into milk. The elimination half-lives in the mother range from 15 to 26 hours. Reports of isolated cases have recorded maternal plasma and milk levels of a few of the compounds, but no long-term follow-up of the nurslings. In general, no symptoms have been reported in the infants.

The clinician must weigh the risk/benefit ratio of each drug, keeping in mind that being cared for by depressed mothers is not beneficial for infants. Some mothers have been medicated with antidepressants during their pregnancies, and the withdrawal experienced when the infants are not breastfed may go undiagnosed and be attributed to colic, fussiness, or other disorders. If a mother is to begin medication during lactation, a baseline for the infant should be established by the pediatrician so that any effects of the medication received via the milk can be detected. The age of the infant and the feeding pattern are important issues in the decision (see Box 12-2).

Fluoxetine (Prozac), a common and usually effective therapy for depression and other neuropsychiatric disorders, is reported to have few side effects. Pharmacologically, it is chemically unrelated to antidepressants, has few autonomic effects,

and is considered an alternative to standard antidepressant therapy. Its peak plasma time is 6 to 8 hours, and it is highly protein bound.[18,60] Case studies on lactating women taking fluoxetine have reported no changes in the infants. Maternal blood and milk samples have one fifth to one quarter as much drug (i.e., M/P ratio = 0.20 to 0.25) when fluoxetine and the active metabolite norfluoxetine are measured.[60] Total ingestion by an infant per day was no more than 15 to 20 mcg/kg, a low exposure when the mother had received 20 mg at bedtime for 53 days. The reported levels in milk depend on sampling and lipid content of the milk and range from 47 to 469 ng/mL.[19] Hale et al.[50] report a case in which a mother took fluoxetine throughout pregnancy and while breastfeeding. At 11 days, the infant was somnolent, then unresponsive. Levels were measurable in milk and in the infant. Another case reports severe colic and crying until the drug was stopped.[83]

The AAP considers the psychotropic drugs to be of special concern because they are taken for a long time. Although no adverse effects have been published, the drugs do appear in milk and could conceivably alter short-term and long-term CNS function. These drugs clearly require a physician's careful consideration of the benefits of breastfeeding and the therapeutic risks in each case.[100] The peak plasma time varies from 1½ to 12 hours, so avoiding a peak is difficult. Giving a feeding of formula once daily would dilute the impact. Other selective serotonin reuptake inhibitors, such as sertraline (Zoloft), paroxetine (Paxil), and citalopram (Celexa), may be better choices. Neonatal paroxetine withdrawal syndrome has been described in four term infants who presented with jitteriness and necrotizing enterocolitis after paroxetine exposure in utero. Neonatal withdrawal from paroxetine in infants who did not breastfeed is 10 times higher (0.3/1000) than with sertraline and fluvoxamine and 100 times higher than with fluoxetine (0.002).[133]

Citalopram exposure in breastfeeding infants was examined prospectively in three groups: (a) depressed women treated with citalopram, (b) depressed women not treated with citalopram, and (c) normal women. The infants were no different in the three groups in feeding, medication, or adverse events.[83]

In a study of 78 infants[83] who were exposed to antidepressants through breast milk, the mothers' mood status was evaluated along with infants' weight gain.[55] Weights were not significantly different from the population of normal infants. The infants whose mothers relapsed to significant depression, however, did gain less weight. The authors concluded that the drugs did not decrease weight gain but maternal depression may influence

---

BOX 12-2. Serotonin (5-HT) Reuptake Inhibitors (Brand Names)

Fenfluramine (Ponderax, Pondimin)
Fluoxetine (Prozac)
Fluvoxamine (Faverin)
Nefazodone (Serzone)
Paroxetine (Paxil, Seroxat)
Sertraline (Lustral, Zoloft)
Trazodone (Desyrel)
Venlafaxine (Effexor)

behaviors that throughout 2 months could affect infants' weight gain. Bupropion (Wellbutrin, Zyban) is a well-known antidepressant and smoking deterrent that is unrelated to the tricyclics. No quantifiable amounts have been detected in infants nor were any adverse effects noted.[8] Peak milk levels have been observed 2 hours after dosing. Estimated dose to infant is only 2% of the maternal dose. Seizures were reported in a 6-month-old infant 4 days after administration of 150 mg per day of bupropion for the mother. The maternal drug was discontinued and no further seizures were observed although breastfeeding was continued.[21] The AAP rates bupropion a category 4, which is a drug for which the effect on nursing infants is unknown or may be of concern. Hale et al.[48] rate it moderately safe (L3), and Briggs et al.[17] say it has potential toxicity based on little data. Schaefer[118] point out that the relative dose, including metabolites, is 0.14%.

Methadone Maintenance and Risks of Breastfeeding

Methadone maintenance treatment for heroin and other addictions has had a significant impact on the recovery of many addicts. When first introduced, it was hoped it would be an ideal treatment for neonatal withdrawal syndrome. It was not. It was also hoped that withdrawal from methadone for an infant born to a woman receiving maintenance therapy would be negligible, but it is not. When pregnant women were maintained on 25 mg/day or less, neonatal withdrawal rarely required treatment. Present regimens during pregnancy typically are for maternal doses of more than 150 mg/day. Neonatal withdrawal from this level is substantial, requiring treatment.

The therapeutic use of methadone in opiate addiction has become a common concern in the childbearing years, especially during pregnancy and lactation. The recommended daily dose has been increased sharply from 25 mg/day to as high as 150 mg/day. Neonatal abstinence syndrome has become more common, often requiring 6 to 8 weeks of hospitalization for the neonate. The question of breastfeeding is frequently asked.

Two women had M/P ratios that remained constant at 0.32 and 0.61, and the infants received a calculated 0.01 to 0.03 mg of methadone per day. Kreek et al.[75] estimated daily infant intake from a mother taking 50 mg daily, assuming consumption of almost a liter of breast milk per day, with a maximum of 0.112 mg/day. Kreek et al.[75] also noted peak levels in the milk at 4 hours after dosing. Pumping and discarding the milk at 3 to 4 hours after dosing has been suggested as a method of reducing exposure.

A study of eight mother-baby pairs in which mothers were on at least 40 mg/dL methadone daily showed the infants received 2.8% of mothers' dose, not sufficient to prevent neonatal abstinence syndrome.[9] In a second study[93] of mothers on methadone who were receiving 25 to 180 mg/day, the methadone levels ranged from 27 to 260 ng/mL, with a mean of 95 ng/mL. No adverse events were associated with breastfeeding or weaning. It was estimated the infant received 0.05 mg/day, which parallels other estimates. An additional study of 12 methadone-maintained mothers found that the methadone concentrations were small, ranging from 21 to 314 ng/mL and unrelated to mothers' doses. The authors suggest that methadone-maintained women can breastfeed.[62] Five mothers who were methadone-maintained (doses 60 to 110 mg/day) were followed with breast milk and plasma samples for up to 6 months by Jansson et al.[63] Concentrations in the milk were small (daily dose to infant 0.15 to 0.30 mg/day). One child was still breastfeeding at a year and had methadone in low concentration in the plasma. A retrospective chart review of 190 drug dependent dyads grouped patients by feeding type—85 were breastfed, 105 were formula fed. Tracking by neonatal abstinence scores (Finnegan Scores), mean scores were significantly lower in the breastfed group. Fewer breastfed infants required withdrawal treatment and the median time to withdrawal was much later in this group. Controlling for type of drugs involved and prematurity still demonstrated reduced need for withdrawal therapy in breastfed infants.

Home-based detoxification for neonatal abstinence syndrome is associated with reduced hospital stays and increased rates of breastfeeding without prolonging therapy in selected dyads.

If the infant is weaned from the breast gradually, there should be no withdrawal, and breastfeeding should not be withheld. See Chapter 16 for discussion of smoking and marijuana (Table 12-10).

Pesticides and Pollutants

Since 1950 human milk has been used as a biomonitoring tool for assessing mothers' and infants' exposures to environmental chemicals. Since that time a solid database has been created on DDT, dioxins, furans, and polychlorinated biphenyls (PCBs) in various geographic areas. Consistency of analytic methods, sampling techniques, postpartum timing, and reporting chemical concentrations has been lacking. A technical workshop on Human Milk Surveillance and Research on Environmental Chemicals in the United States was held in 2002 and a published report appeared in the *Journal of Toxicology and Environmental Health*.[12] More and

TABLE 12-10	Maternal Methadone Dose, Milk Methadone Levels, and Infant Age		
Patient	Maternal Dose (mg/day)	Breast Milk Level (ng/mL)	Infant Age (days)
A	25	102	202
B1	96	100	60
B2	96	85	67
B3	96	82	68
C1	130	142	22
C2	130	91	22
C3	110	85	85
D	90	79	34
E	120	141	27
F	110	260	110
G1	80	19	3
G2	80	27	21
G3	80	83	33
H	180	32	173
Mean	102	95	66
SD	42	60	

From McCarthy JJ, Posey BL: Methadone levels in human milk, *J Hum Lact* 16:115, 2000.

more often, human milk is being used as the biologic marker of environmental exposures. The disturbing backlash is that the public interprets this to mean that breast milk is contaminated and the problem is getting worse.

Monitoring chemical exposure in a breastfed infant is the task of the epidemiologist and the chemist.[126] Human milk has been known to contain insecticides. Chlorinated hydrocarbons, such as DDT and its metabolites dieldrin, aldrin, and related compounds, are the best known. The major reason these compounds appear in breast milk is that they are deposited in body lipid stores and move with lipid. A fetus receives the greatest dose in utero, and adult body fat has approximately 30 times the concentration in milk. DEET has been shown to be absorbed through the skin in adult males within two hours of application and excreted from the plasma through the urine within 4 hours.

PCBs in heavily contaminated pregnant Japanese women produced small-for-gestational-age infants who had transient darkening of the skin ("cola babies"). Polybrominated biphenyls (PBBs) are similar compounds associated with a heavy exposure to farm animals and contaminated cattle in the lower Michigan peninsula. The women in the United States who have the greatest risk for high exposure to PCBs or PBBs are those who have extensively worked with, or eaten, the fish caught by sport fishing in contaminated waters.

Studies have refuted earlier observations of concern. No information is available in the United States on the levels of polychlorinated dibenzodioxins or polychlorinated dibenzofurans in anglers who consume a lot of fish.[71] Persons at high risk are those who live near a waste disposal site or have been involved in environmental spills. Unless there is heavy exposure, however, no contraindication exists to breastfeeding.

In most cases the levels of pesticides in human milk have been less than those in cow milk. The accumulated amounts have not usually exceeded safe allowable limits. Several extensive reviews explore the dilemma of pollutants in human milk.[112,113,144,147] In a 1997 review of world reports on occurrence and toxicity, Rogan[114] has reaffirmed that breastfeeding should be recommended despite the presence of chemical residues. He further states that the benefits of breastfeeding outweigh the risks of pollutants. It has been suggested that the body burden at birth can be added to by exposing an infant to small levels in the milk that may indeed exceed the exposure limits allowable for daily intake set by the WHO.[132] Human milk levels are used epidemiologically as markers of human exposure in community exposure because of a close correlation between milk levels and the levels in fat stores. Unselected mothers in the Great Lakes region were tested by the State of New York in 1978, and no chemical (PCB, PBB) was found in any milk in random sampling of residents. Thus unless the circumstances are unusual, breastfeeding should not be abandoned on the basis of insecticide contamination.

Chemicals that are lipophilic, biologically stable, nonionized at a physiologic pH, and of low molecular weight transfer easily into maternal milk. Ten to twenty times more of a mother's body burden of persistent organohalogens are transferred via the milk than via the placenta, according to Jensen and Slorach,[64] who published an extensive review of chemical contaminants in human milk. They further caution that the absolute amount transferred depends on the structure of the chemical. PCBs, for instance, are highly chlorinated and transfer more easily than less chlorinated PCBs. No difference was observed in placental and milk transfer of heavy metals.

If extractable fat is measured, the levels of persistent organohalogens are about the same in milk, blood, adipose tissue, and muscle. Mobilization from fat stores is greater than that from dietary intake during lactation.[65]

Agent Orange, the best known of the dioxins, was identified in Vietnam as a powerful teratogen. Dioxin has been found in human milk from pooled samples from high-risk women with known exposure. No evidence suggests that the population at large is at risk. Women working in dry-cleaning plants, viscose rayon plants, photographic laboratories, and chemical industries where proper precautions are not taken have been noted to absorb tetrachloroethylene, carbon disulfide, and bromides.[44]

Flame retardants, polybrominated diphenyl ethers, which are found in upholstery, electronics, automotive interiors, and plastics, have been banned in several states because of rising body burdens as reflected in several studies in breast milk. A fortyfold increase has been recorded since 1972. At high levels, polybrominated diphenyl ethers cause cognitive and behavior disorders. The risk is in utero. Risk is minimal from breastfeeding, so it is recommended that breastfeeding should take place.[45] Mother to child transfer of essential and toxic elements through breast milk in a mine-waste polluted area is reported by Castro and colleagues.[20] They reported that lower amounts of toxic elements are ingested by breastfed infants compared to infants who receive formula reconstituted with locally contaminated water. Extensive review of industrial chemicals and environmental contaminants in human milk is available in Schaefer, Peters, and Miller.[119]

Heavy Metals

Heavy metals that have been found in milk include lead, mercury, arsenic, cobalt, magnesium, and cadmium and are positively correlated with fish consumption.[14] Whenever maternal exposure occurs, a breastfed infant and the milk should be tested. The intake of lead and cadmium by breastfed infants, as reported by the WHO study, is the same as, or somewhat lower than, that of infants fed formula mixed with local water.[80] Levels of these heavy metals in milk, however, are lower than would be predicted from maternal levels.[118] Placental transfer is greater than by breastfeeding. Most common air pollutants are not found in human milk.

Although removal of lead from gasoline has been associated with a drop in blood lead levels in children from 15 mg/dL in 1978 to 2 mg/dL in 1999,[115] lead has become a significant issue because of the number of mothers testing positive for lead on routine screens for lead in family members of young infants. Release of lead from bone in pregnancy and lactation was studied by Manton et al.,[91] who concluded that the entire skeleton undergoes resorption and blood lead levels of nursing mothers continue to rise, reaching maximum at 6 to 8 months postpartum. They also noted that lead levels fall from pregnancy to pregnancy, suggesting that the greatest risk is with the first pregnancy.[91] The Centers for Disease Control and Prevention (CDC) has revised the standards for treatment downward (Table 12-11). Meta-analysis reflects a 2.6 to 5.8 point decline in IQ for an increase in lead level from 10 to 20 mg/dL.[115] Blood lead concentrations less than 10 mg/dL are inversely associated with children's IQ scores at 3 to 5 years of age according to studies by Canfield.[19] The first step is always to clean up the environment and identify the source. Lead abatement resources are available from the U.S. Department of Health. The level of lead in milk depends on its ionization and tight binding to red blood cells. The M/P ratio is 0.2. A lead level of 40 mg/dL or less in a nursing mother is considered below the level of transfer through the breast milk (Figure 12-3). In addition to environmental sources of lead (e.g., old paint, contaminated ground, lead batteries), diet should be reviewed. In some cities, the water supply is a significant source, especially in formula making. Herbs and herbal teas may also be a source. A long list of traditional and folk remedies contain lead, especially from China, Mexico, India, and Pakistan. A mother's diet should include extra calcium and iron to reduce the absorption of lead from the diet and mobilization from the bone. Newer lead removal medications are safer than the traditional

TABLE 12-11 Classes and Management of Lead Levels in Blood

Blood Lead Level (mcg/dL)	Class	Management
<10	I	Not considered lead poisoning
10-14	IIA	Many children (or a large proportion of children) with blood lead levels in this range should trigger community-wide childhood lead poisoning prevention activities. Children in this range may need to be rescreened more frequently.
15-19	IIB	Nutritional and educational interventions and more frequent screening; if level persists in this range, environmental investigation and intervention is recommended.
20-44	III	Environmental evaluation and remediation and a medical evaluation; possible pharmacologic treatment of lead poisoning
45-69	IV	Both medical and environmental intervention, including chelation therapy
>69	V	Medical emergency; immediate medical and environmental management

Modified from Centers for Disease Control and Prevention: Blood levels—United States, 1988-1991, *MMWR* 43:545, 1994.

Lead in blood and human milk

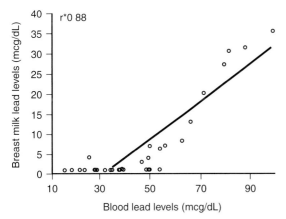

Figure 12-3. Graph showing regression line between blood lead levels and milk lead levels. (From Namihira D, Saldivar L, Pustilnik N, et al: Lead in human blood and milk from nursing women living near a smelter in Mexico City, *J Toxicol Environ Health* 38:225, 1993.)

British anti-lewisite. Succimer is believed safe during lactation and in infants older than 1 year if milk is pumped and discarded for 5 days.[12]

Arsenic is a heavy metal noted to contaminate some waterways and water supplies. It has been evaluated in several parts of the world, including Argentina, Germany, and India. The data are available from these regions on the levels in breast milk and the nursing infants. The arsenic level in drinking water in an Argentinean village was 200 mcg/L, the level in maternal blood 10 mcg/L, and the level in maternal urine 320 mcg/L. The average amount in the milk was 2.3 mcg/kg. Two infants were tested and levels in the urine were 17 and 47 mcg/L, considered very low. In India's West Bengal, an arsenic-affected area, 226 women were tested, some of whom had skin lesions and high levels in their hair. They had arsenic in the breast milk. Most of the arsenic in the milk was inorganic, but the infant levels ranged from 0.3 to 29 mcg/L; those infants who were partially breastfed and formula fed had levels from 0.4 to 1520 mcg/L. The authors conclude that little arsenic is excreted in breast milk, even when the exposure is high from contaminated water; thus exclusive breastfeeding appears to be protective and safer than formula feeding.

Organic mercury is another heavy metal that is being increasingly identified in food around the world. Fish is a major source, as are herbs and tonics. Levels of mercury in mothers' blood are about three times higher than levels in milk. Two major forms of mercury enter milk. Methylmercury is attached to red blood cells and so has limited access, although it is easily absorbed by infants. Inorganic mercury enters milk easily but is poorly absorbed by infants. When the source of the methylmercury is from breast milk, the developmental scores exceed those of formula-fed infants, suggesting that the advantages of breastfeeding are significant.[14] A similar, more extensive study in the Seychelles Islands of mothers and children followed from birth for 15 years suggests that the value of a fish diet over time and during breastfeeding is significant despite measurable mercury levels.[92] Almost all the infants in the Seychelles were breastfed for at least 6 months and meet or exceed international developmental scores.[92] Acute exposures to methylmercury from industrial or environmental sources should be evaluated on a case-by-case basis, although it appears breastfeeding is safe.

An increasing number of environmental chemicals are being measured in milk as a consequence of improved analytic capabilities and increased interest in biomonitoring.[78] The tolerable daily intake has been determined by the WHO. This intake is based on the lowest observed adverse effect levels based on laboratory studies from several species. Dioxin concentrations in the lipids of breastfed infants are higher than in formula-fed infants initially but the differences disappear with time. Subtle effects were associated with transplacental rather than lactational exposures in large epidemiological studies in Rotterdam, Amsterdam, and Duisburg. The conclusions supported the WHO position that the health significance of dioxin-like contamination does not reduce the value of promoting and supporting breastfeeding. In studies across time, according to the authors, even when environmental chemicals are high, beneficial effects associated with breastfeeding prevail.[78]

Well Water

Drinking well water has been a concern because of varying levels of minerals, especially nitrate. More than 18% of wells in the state of Iowa are reported to exceed the maximum contaminant level of 45 mg of nitrate/L or 10 mg NO_3/L. Infants younger than 6 months of age are especially susceptible to methemoglobinemia, which can lead to anoxic injury and death. It reportedly occurs at nitrate concentrations greater than 100 mg/L. Although this is a major issue for formula-fed infants, Dusdieker et al.[35] explored the question, "Does increased nitrate ingestion elevate nitrate levels in human milk?" Carefully studying 20 healthy mothers with breastfeeding infants older than 6 months subjected to 47, 168, and 270 mg of nitrate per day, they found that urine spot tests rose from 36 mg on day 1 to 66 mg on day 2 and 84 mg on day 3. Nitrate concentrations in the milk on days 1, 2, and 3 were 4.4, 5.1, and 5.2 mg/L, respectively. The authors concluded that "women who consume water with a nitrate concentration of 100 mg/L or less do not produce milk with elevated nitrate levels."[35]

Chemicals in the Workplace

An increasing number of women return to the workplace after the birth of an infant, and an increasing number are breastfeeding their infants. The need for information regarding the transfer of chemicals in the workplace to human milk is an increasing problem.

Volatile chemicals in the workplace represent an important but little understood hazard, especially in paint shops, repair shops, garages, and the chemical industry. Fisher et al.[39] developed a physiologically based pharmacokinetic model for lactating women to estimate the amount of chemical that their nursing infants ingest for a given nursing schedule and maternal occupational exposure. The two major factors are the blood/air partition coefficient, a thermodynamic factor that governs

the body burden that may be achieved from inhalation of a chemical, and the pharmacokinetics of the chemical, which determines the length of time a chemical remains in the systemic circulation and is available to transfer into milk. Because milk fat is available, preferential uptake of lipophilic chemicals occurs. Of the 19 chemicals simulated in the study, the authors consider bromochloromethane, perchloroethylene, and 1,4-dioxane exposure the highest risk to infants based on U.S. Environmental Protection Agency (EPA) drinking water guidelines (Table 12-12). Protective gear in the workplace is the most practical way of minimizing exposure to both mothers and infants.

The Occupational Health and Safety Act of the province of Quebec has mandated the establishment and maintenance of a Toxicological Index that provides information on chemical and biologic contaminants potentially present in the workplace.[44] Information can also serve as a basis for the protective reassignment of pregnant or breastfeeding employees. The Infotox database has

TABLE 12-12	Predicted Amount of Chemical Ingested by Nursing Infant (AMILK) During 24-Hour Period and EPA Drinking Water Health Advisory Values		
Chemical	**Threshold Limit Value (ppm)**	**AMILK (mg)**	**EPA Health Advisory Intake* (mg/day)**
Benzene	10	0.053	0.20[†]
Bromochloromethane	200	2.090	1.00
Carbon tetrachloride	5	0.055	0.07
Chlorobenzene	10	0.229	–
Chloroform	10	0.043	0.1
Methylchloroform	350	3.51	40.0
Diethylether	400	1.49	–
1,4-Dioxane	25	0.559	0.4[†]
Halothane	50	0.232	–
n-Hexane	50	0.052	4.0
Isoflurane	50[‡]	0.336	–
Methylene chloride	50	0.213	2.0[†]
Methyl ethyl ketone	200	12.08	–
Perchloroethylene	25	1.36	1.0
Styrene	50	0.650	2.0
Trichloroethylene	50	0.496	0.6[§]
1,1,1,2-Tetrachloroethane	100[‡]	4.31	0.9
Toluene	50	0.460	2.0
o,p,m-Xylenes	100	6.590	40.0

EPA, Environmental Protection Agency.

*Modified from EPA health advisory values for chronic ingestion of contaminated water by 10-kg (22-lb) children, assuming ingestion of 1 L of water per day. These health advisory concentrations for chemicals in water are thought to be protective of adverse health effects for chronic exposure.

[†]Modified from 10-day health advisory values for ingestion of contaminated water by 10-kg children, assuming ingestion of 1 L of water per day. These health advisory values for contaminated water are thought to be protective of adverse health effects for a 10-day period.

[‡]No threshold limit value; concentration value was assigned.

[§]Lifetime health advisory value for ingestion of 2 L water per day in adults.

From Fisher J, Mahle D, Bankston L, et al: Lactation transfer of volatile chemicals in breast milk, *Am Ind Hyg Assoc J* 58:429, 1997.

information about 5500 chemicals. Of the substances in the database, 2.2% (153 of 5736) show evidence of milk transfer and pose relative risks to breastfed infants.[44]

Psychologic Impact of Toxin in Milk

The psychologic reactions of a group of nursing mothers from the lower Michigan Peninsula whose breast milk was contaminated with a toxic fire-retardant chemical, PBB, were studied.[53] Every tenth woman who had had her milk tested for PBB was contacted for the study (a sample of 200 women); 139 responded and received a questionnaire, and 97 (70%) filled out the questionnaire. The subjects knew their own level and that the range for all mothers was from undetected to 0.46 ppm, with an average of 0.1 ppm. The testing was voluntary and cost $25. Of those tested, 96% had measurable amounts.

The data were collected in a six-page questionnaire. Two modes of coping emerged: denial and mastery. In general, the findings indicated that the greater the level of toxic contamination of PBB reported in a mother's milk, the greater the denial, to the point of not having correct information, even about her own level. Ambivalence toward nursing was correlated with guilt in both groups (only 15% discontinued breastfeeding). The "draw-a-baby" test showed an unusual amount (94%) of distortion and expressions of anguish. These findings were consistent throughout all test modalities; thus they were not thought to be a function of personality.[53]

Radioactive Materials

Because of the increasing number of diagnostic tests that use radioactive materials, a nursing mother may have such a procedure done, calculating the dose of radiation to the breastfed infant, as most radio pharmaceutical doses are estimated based on data from injected doses rather than oral exposure. Estimates assume the compound is absorbed from the stomach unchanged as in the adult.

Radioactive iodine (^{125}I and ^{131}I) passes into milk at levels as high as 5% of the dose. When this is used for diagnostic purposes, breastfeeding should be discontinued until milk is clear. The excretion by the breast may alter the validity of the test result. If radioactive iodine is to be used therapeutically, breastfeeding must be discontinued until the iodine has cleared the system, which may be 1 to 3 months. A carefully collected sample of milk can be tested for radioactivity so that the period that the infant is off the breast is not unnecessarily long. If a 30 mCi dose of ^{131}I is used, 24 hours may be adequate to pump and discard.

If an infant is older and receiving other foods, time can be altered accordingly. A lung scan (300-mCi dose) requires 7 days, and renography requires 2 days of pumping and discarding the milk.[69]

Gallium-67 citrate appears in significant amounts in the milk. It does clear the body quickly and is relatively safe for use in patients. Breastfeeding should be discontinued for at least 72 hours.

Technetium-99m (^{99m}Tc) is reported to clear the milk in 6 to 48 hours. The stage of lactation, whether the breast is emptied before receiving the dose, and the method of clearing the breast may be responsible for inconsistent results. Discontinuing breastfeeding for at least 24 hours is advisable.

The amount of radioactivity excreted in breast milk after administration of ^{99m}Tc hexakis 2-methoxyisobutyl isonitrile in a single dose was reported by Rubow et al.[116] The measurement was highest in the first sample at 3.3 hours, 0.488 kilobecquerel (kBq)/mL, with negligible amounts thereafter (less than 0.180 kBq/mL). Less than 2.96 kBq/mL is considered safe. Only the first sample needs to be discarded.[117]

The American College of Radiology (ACR) has recognized the need for good information about the administration of contrast medium to nursing mothers. When a conflict of opinion exists, one can refer to the 2010 edition of the *Contrast Manual* published by ACR.[3]

The ACR summarizes a review of the literature as follows:

1. Less than 1% of an administered maternal dose of contrast agent is excreted into breast milk.
2. Less than 1% of contrast medium in breast milk ingested by an infant is absorbed from the GI tract.

Iodinated x-ray media, both ionic and nonionic, when given intravenously, have a plasma half-life of approximately 2 hours, with nearly 100% clearance in 24 hours. Less than 1% is in the milk, and less than 1% is absorbed by an infant; therefore an infant receives less than 0.01% of the dose. The recommended dose for an infant receiving directly for a procedure is 2 mL/kg. Although not necessary, a mother may pump and discard her milk for 2 to 24 hours, if she chooses.

GADOLINIUM-BASED CONTRAST AGENTS

Free gadolinium is a neurotoxic, but it is safe when complexed with a variety of chelates. These hydrophilic agents behave much like the iodinated x-ray contrast media discussed previously with a plasma half-life of 2 hours and total clearance by 24 hours. In the case of gadolinium, only 0.04%

is excreted into the milk, and the expected dose absorbed by the infant is less than 0.0004% of the maternal dose.[76] The pediatric dose is 0.2 mmol/kg and breast milk dose would be less than 0.00008 mmol/kg. No untoward effects have been reported.

With the advent of ultrasound examination, computed tomography scanning, magnetic resonance imaging, and other techniques, in many situations alternatives to the use of radioactive material during lactation exist.

DERMATOLOGIC MEDICATION

The key issue involved with the dermatologic application of medications is whether or not they are absorbed through the skin. A small amount on the skin covering a few square inches may not be a problem from a dose standpoint. An important issue is the direct application to the nipple and areolar tissue because this area is in the baby's mouth during a feeding. Application to the breast should not be done until after the feeding in any case. Most prescription dermal medications indicate the percentage of active ingredient absorbed so the health care provider can determine the risk during lactation. Most antibiotics, antivirals, and antifungals applied dermally are safe because they could be given directly to the infant.

Scabies treatment should avoid lindane and malathion during lactation. Psoriasis therapy is a risk during lactation—anti-itch products are safe except doxepin. Acne treatments that include vitamins are a risk to an infant.

Immunizations

IMMUNIZING BREASTFED INFANTS

Questions often arise about whether breastfed infants should be immunized on a different schedule because of the protective maternal antibodies that might interfere with an infant's response to antigen stimulation. Following are some brief guidelines on the more common situations of concern.[25]

1. The AAP recommends that all infants should be vaccinated on the regular schedule regardless of the mode of feeding.
2. Vaccinations for diphtheria-pertussis-tetanus are not altered by breastfeeding, and the regular schedule should be followed for the infants.
3. Because oral poliovirus vaccine is a live virus vaccine, it was a concern that the maternal antibodies would inactivate it. However, the CDC recommendation is that the same schedule be followed. The current scientific literature

indicates that for infants older than 6 weeks, the earliest age of vaccination recommended, no indication exists for withholding breastfeeding in relationship to oral poliovirus vaccine administration, and no need exists for extra doses of vaccine. Furthermore, antibody responses to parenteral and oral vaccines are better in breastfed than formula-fed infants. The same is true for diphtheria and tetanus toxoid.[24]
4. Rubella, mumps, and measles vaccines should be given at the regularly scheduled times.[24]
5. A *Haemophilus influenzae* type B vaccine is available for infants. The *H. influenzae* type B conjugate vaccines should be given at 2 months of age or as soon as possible thereafter, following the AAP Red Book guidelines in the Report of the Committee on Infectious Disease. No modification of the immunization schedule is necessary for breastfed infants. Furthermore, data suggest breastfed infants ultimately have higher antibody titers than formula-fed infants.

IMMUNIZING THE NURSING MOTHER

There is no reason for concern about the potential presence of live viruses from vaccines in a mother's milk if she is vaccinated during the postpartum period. Breastfeeding women may follow the same schedule for adults that is followed for other adults for measles, mumps, rubella, tetanus, diphtheria, influenza, *Streptococcus pneumoniae* infection, hepatitis A, hepatitis B, and varicella. When traveling to an endemic area, inactivated poliovirus vaccine can be given.[25]

Smallpox

Smallpox vaccination is inadvisable for the mother of any infant younger than 1 year of age, nursing or not. The personal contact, not the breastfeeding, causes the risk; therefore no advantage exists to weaning if vaccination is necessary. This vaccination is not given routinely and is rarely indicated.

Rh Immune Globulin

Only rare trace amounts of anti-Rh are present in colostrum and none is found in the mature milk of women given large doses of Rh immune globulin immediately postpartum. No adverse response was noted, even with these high dosages. Any Rh antibodies in the mother's milk are thought to be inactivated by the gastric juices. Rh immune globulin or Rh sensitization is not a contraindication to breastfeeding.

Rubella

Following are the recommendations with respect to rubella:[25]

1. Approximately 85% to 90% of the adult female population are thought to have a high level of naturally acquired immunity, and only 10% to 15% are considered to be susceptible to rubella infection.
2. Vaccination of pregnant women is contraindicated under all circumstances.
3. No woman of childbearing age should be vaccinated without having been first tested for immunity.
4. If the test is negative, the woman may be vaccinated if there is reasonable assurance that she will not become pregnant for at least 2 months.

The rubella virus was found in the milk of 69% of the women immunized with live attenuated rubella (HPV-77 DE5 or RA 27/3 strains).[88] A virus-specific immunoglobulin A antibody response was seen in the milk of all the women. Infectious rubella virus or virus antigen was recovered from the nasopharynx and throat of 56% of the breastfed infants and none of the nonbreastfed infants. No infant had the disease in this study, but 25% of the breastfed group had seroconversion transiently. Infants given early strains of the virus via the milk were reported to develop mild symptoms.[72,79] Although the attenuated virus may appear in the milk, this should not dissuade one from vaccinating a breastfeeding mother at the safest time, that is, immediately postpartum.

REFERENCES

1. Abbott PJ: Comfrey: assessing the low-dose health risk, *Med J Aust* 149:678, 1988.
2. Academy of Breastfeeding Medicine. Protocol Committee, Jansson LM ABM Clinical Protocol #21: Guidelines for breastfeeding and the drug dependent woman, *Breastfeed Med* 4(4):225–228, 2009.
3. American College of Radiology (ACR) Contrast Manual 2010. http://www.act.org/mainmenucategories/about_us/committees/gpr-srg/administrationofcontrastmedium.
4. Amir LH, Donath SM: Does maternal smoking have a negative physiological effect on breastfeeding? The epidemiological evidence, *Breastfeed Rev* 11:L19, 2003.
5. Ang-Lee MK, Moss J, Yuan C-S: Herbal medicines and perioperative care, *JAMA* 286:208, 2001.
6. Aranda JV, Lambert C, Perez J, et al: Metabolism and renal elimination of furosemide in the newborn infant, *J Pediatr* 101:777, 1982.
7. Ayd F: Excretion of psychotropic drugs in human breast milk, *Int Drug Ther Newslett* 8:33, 1973.
8. Baab SW, Peindl KS, Piontek CM, et al: Serum bupropion levels in 2 breastfeeding mother-infant pairs, *J Clin Psychiatry* 63:910–911, 2002.
9. Bauer JH, Pape B, Zajicek J, et al: Propranolol in human plasma and breast milk, *Am J Cardiol* 43:860, 1979.
10. Berlin CM: Excretion of methylxanthines in human milk, *Semin Perinatol* 5:389, 1981.
11. Berlin CM, Daniel CH: Excretion of theobromine in human milk and saliva, *Pediatr Res* 15:492, 1981.
12. Berlin CM, LaKind JS, Selevan SG: Human milk monitoring for environmental chemicals: guidance for future research, *J Toxicol Environ Health* 66(22):1829, 2002.
13. Bichell RE: When edible plants turn their defenses on us. NPR.org/blogs/thesalt/2013/10/01/22822163.
14. Björnberg KA, Vahter M, Berglund B, et al: Transport of methylmercury and inorganic mercury to the fetus and breastfeeding infant, *Environ Health Perspect* 113:1381–1385, 2005.
15. Bossi L: Neonatal period including drug disposition in newborns: review of the literature. In Janz D, Dam M, Richens A, et al, editors: *Epilepsy, pregnancy and the child*, New York, 1982, Raven.
16. Boutroy MJ, Bianchetti G, Dubruc C, et al: To nurse when receiving acebutolol: is it dangerous for the neonate? *Eur J Clin Pharmacol* 30:737, 1986.
17. Briggs GG, Freeman RK, Yaffe S: *Drugs in pregnancy and lactation*, ed 9, Baltimore, 2011, Williams & Wilkins.
18. Burch KJ, Wells BG: Fluoxetine/norfluoxetine concentrations in human milk, *Pediatrics* 89:676, 1992.
19. Canfield RL, Henderson CR, Cory-Slechta DA, et al: Intellectual impairment in children with blood lead concentrations below 10 mg per deciliter, *N Engl J Med* 348:1517, 2003.
20. Castro F, Harari F, Lianos M, et al: Maternal-child transfer of essential and toxic elements through breast milk in a mine-waste polluted area, *Am J Perinatol* 31(11):993–1002, 2014.
21. Chaudron LH, Schonecker CJ: Bupropion and breastfeeding a case of possible infant seizure (Letter), *J Clin Psychiatry* 64:881–882, 2004.
22. Collaborative Group on Drug Use in Pregnancy: Medication during pregnancy: an intercontinental cooperative study, *Int J Gynaecol Obstet* 39(3):185, 1995.
23. Committee on Drugs, American Academy of Pediatrics: The transfer of drugs and other chemicals into human milk, *Pediatrics* 72:375, 1983. 84:924, 1989; 93:137, 1994; 108:776, 2001.
24. Committee on Infectious Disease: Report of the Committee on Infectious Disease. In *The red book*, Elk Grove, Ill., 2000, American Academy of Pediatrics.
25. Cooper DS: Antithyroid drugs: to breastfeed or not to breastfeed, *Am J Obstet Gynecol* 157:234–235, 1987.
26. daSilva VA, Malheiros LR, Moraes-Santos AR, et al: Ethanol pharmacokinetics in lactating women, *Braz J Med Biol Res* 26:1097, 1993.
27. daSilva OP, Knoppert DC, Angelini MM, et al: Effect of domperidone on milk production in mothers of premature newborns: a randomized, double-blind, placebo-controlled trial, *Can Med Assoc J* 164:17, 2001.
28. Davis EA, Morris DJ: Medicinal uses of licorice through the millennia: the good and plenty of it, *Mol Cell Endocrinol* 78:1, 1991.
29. Devlin RG, Fleiss PM: Captopril in human blood and breast milk, *J Clin Pharmacol* 21:110, 1981.
30. Devlin RG, Duchin KL, Fleiss PM: Nadolol in human serum and breast milk, *Br J Clin Pharmacol* 72:393, 1981.
31. Di Pierro F, Callegari A, Carotenuto D, et al: Clinical efficacy, safety and tolerability of Bio-C® (micronized silymarin) as a galactagogue, *Acta Biomed* 79:205–210, 2008.
32. Dugoua J-J, Mills E, Perri D, et al: Safety and efficacy of ginko during pregnancy and lactation, *Can J Clin Pharmacol* 13(3):e277–e284, 2006.
33. Dugoua J-J, Perri D, Seely D, et al: Safety and efficacy of blue cohosh during pregnancy and lactation, *Can J Clin Pharmacol* 15(1):e66–e73, 2008.
34. Dugoua J-J, Seely D, Perri D: Safety and efficacy of chaste-tree during pregnancy and lactation, *Can J Clin Pharmacol* 15(1):e74–e79, 2008.

35. Earth Mama. Angel Baby Herbs to Avoid During Breast-feeding 2014. EarthMamaAngelBaby.com.

36. Ellenhorn MJ: *Ellenhorn's medical toxicology: diagnosis and treatment of human poisoning,* ed 2, Baltimore, 1997, Williams & Wilkins.

37. Engels HJ, Wirth JC: No ergogenic effects of ginseng during graded maximal aerobic exercise, *J Am Diet Assoc* 97 (10):1110, 1997.

38. Erickson SH, Oppenheim GL, Smith GH: Metronidazole in breast milk, *Obstet Gynecol* 57:48, 1981.

39. Fisher J, Mahle D, Bankston L, et al: Lactational transfer of volatile chemicals in breast milk, *Am Ind Hyg Assoc J* 58:425, 1997.

40. Frey B, Schubiger G, Musy JP: Transient cholestatic hepatitis in a neonate associated with carbamazepine exposure during pregnancy and breastfeeding, *Eur J Pediatr* 150:136, 1990.

41. Giamarellou H, Kolokythas E, Petrikkos G, et al: Pharmaco-kinetics of three newer quinolones in pregnant and lactating women, *Am J Med* 87(Suppl):49s–51s, 1989.

42. Gilman AG, Rall TW, Nies AS, et al, editors: *Goodman and Gilman's the pharmacological basis of therapeutics,* ed 8, New York, 1990, Macmillan.

43. Giroux D, Lapointe G, Baril M: Toxicological index and the presence in the workplace of chemical hazards for workers who breastfeed infants, *Am Ind Hyg Assoc J* 53:471, 1992.

44. Greater Boston Physicians for Social Responsibility (GBPSR). In Harm's way: toxic threats to child development (May 2000). Accessed at http://ww.igc.org/psr/.

45. Grigg J: Environmental toxins: their impact on children's health, *Arch Dis Child* 89:244, 2004.

46. Grzeskowiak L: Use of domperidone to increase breast milk supply: are women really dying to breastfeed? *J Hum Lact* 30:498–499, 2014 (Letter-to the-Editor).

47. Hale TW, editor: *Medications and mother's milk,* 16 ed., Amarillo, Tex., 2014, Hale Publishing.

48. Hale TW, Shum S, Grossberg M: Fluoxetine toxicity in a breastfed infant, *Clin Pediatr* 40:681, 2001.

49. Hale TW, Kristensen JH, Ilett KF: The transfer of medications into human milk. In Hale TW, Hartmann P, editors: *Textbook of human lactation,* ed 1, Amarillo, Tex., 2007, Hale Publishing, pp 465–477.

50. Harari F, Ronco AM, Conch G, et al: Early-life exposure to lithium and boron from drinking water, *Reprod Toxicol* 34:552–560, 2012.

51. Harmon T, Burhart G, Applebaum H: Perforated pseudomembranous colitis in the breastfed infant, *J Pediatr Surg* 27:744–746, 1992.

52. Hatcher SL: The psychological experience of nursing mothers upon learning of a toxic substance in their breast milk, *Psychiatry* 45:172, 1982.

53. Healy M: Suppressing lactation with oral diuretics, *Lancet* 1:1353, 1961.

54. Heisterberg L, Branebjerg PE: Blood and milk concentrations of metronidazole in mothers and infants, *J Perinat Med* 11:114, 1983.

55. Ho E, Collantes A, Kapur BM: Alcohol and breastfeeding calculation of time to zero level in milk, *Biol Neonate* 80 (3):219–222, 2001.

56. Hogan RP III, : Hemorrhagic diathesis caused by drinking an herbal tea, *JAMA* 249:2679, 1983.

57. Horta BL, Kramer MS, Platt RW: Maternal smoking and the risk of early weaning: a meta-analysis, *Am J Public Health* 91:304, 2001.

58. Huxtable RJ: The myth of beneficent nature: the risks of herbal preparations, *Ann Intern Med* 117:165, 1992.

59. Illingworth RS, Finch E: Ethyl discoumacetate (Tromexan) in human milk, *J Obstet Gynaecol Br Emp* 66:487, 1959.

60. Ito S: Drug therapy for breastfeeding women, *N Engl J Med* 343:118–126, 2000.

61. Jansson LM, Choo RE, Harrow C, et al: Concentrations of methadone in breast milk and plasma in the immediate perinatal period, *J Hum Lact* 23:184–190, 2007.

62. Jansson LM, Choo R, Velez ML, et al: Methadone maintenance and long-term lactation, *Breastfeed Med* 3:34–37, 2007.

63. Jarboe CH, Cook LN, Malesic I, et al: Dyphylline elimination kinetics in lactating women: blood to milk transfer, *J Clin Pharmacol* 21:405, 1981.

64. Jensen AA, Slorach SA: *Chemical contaminants in human milk,* Boca Raton, Fla., 1991, CRC.

65. Jones AW: Alcohol in mother's milk, *N Engl J Med* 326:766, 1992.

66. Kafetzis DA, Siapas CA, Georgakopoulos PA, et al: Passage of cephalosporins and amoxicillin into breast milk, *Acta Paediatr Scand* 70:285, 1981.

67. Kaneko S, Suzuki K, Sato T, et al: The problems of antiepileptic medication during the neonatal period: is breastfeeding advisable?. In Janz D, Dam M, Richens A, et al, editors: *Epilepsy, pregnancy, and the child,* New York, 1982, Raven.

68. Karjalainen P, Penttilä IM, Pystynen P: The amount and form of radioactivity in human milk after lung scanning, renography and placental localization by ^{131}I labelled traces, *Acta Obstet Gynecol Scand* 50:357, 1971.

69. Khan AKA, Truelove SC: Placental and mammary transfer of sulphasalazine, *Br Med J* 2:1533, 1979.

70. Kimbrough RD: Consumption of fish: benefits and perceived risk, *J Toxicol Environ Health* 33:81, 1991.

71. Kirtschig C, Schaefer C: Dermatological medications and local therapeutics. In Schaefer C, Peters PWJ, Miller RK, editors: *Drugs during pregnancy and lactation,* ed 3, Amsterdam, London, 2014, Elsevier, pp 797–801.

72. Klier CM, Schmid-Siegel B, Schäfer MR, et al: St John's wort and breastfeeding: plasma and breastmilk concentrations of hyperforin for 5 mothers and 2 infants, *J Clin Psychiatry* 67:305–309, 2006.

73. Klotz U, Harings-Kaim A: Negligible excretion of 5-aminosalicylic acid in breast milk, *Lancet* 342:618–619, 1993.

74. Koren G, Randor S, Martin S, et al: Maternal ginseng use associated with neonatal androgenization, *JAMA* 264:2866, 1990.

75. Kreek MJ, Schecter A, Gutjahr CL, et al: Analyses of methadone and other drugs in maternal and neonatal body fluids: use in evaluation of symptoms in a neonate of mother maintained on methadone, *Am J Drug Alcohol Abuse* 1:409, 1974.

76. Kuhnz W, Koch S, Helge H, et al: Primidone and phenobarbital during lactation period in epileptic women: total and free drug serum levels in the nursed infants and their effects on neonatal behavior, *Dev Pharmacol Ther* 11:147, 1988.

77. Lakind JS, Berlin CM, Mattison DR: The heart of the matter on breastmilk and environmental chemicals: essential points for healthcare providers and new parents, *Breastfeed Med* 3:251–259, 2008.

78. Landes RD, Bass JW, Millunchick EW, et al: Neonatal rubella following postpartum maternal immunization, *J Pediatr* 97:465, 1980.

79. Larsson B, Slorach SA, Hagman U, et al: WHO Collaborative Breastfeeding Study. II. Levels of lead and cadmium in Swedish human milk, 1978-1979, *Acta Paediatr Scand* 70:281, 1981.

80. Lawrence RA, Parse M: Vaccines and immunoglobulins. In Schaefer C, Peters PWJ, Miller RK, editors: *Drugs during pregnancy and lactation,* ed 3, Amsterdam, London, 2014, Elsevier, pp 706–711.

81. Lee A, Minhas R, Matsuda N, et al: The safety of St. John's wort (*Hypericum perforation*) during breastfeeding, *J Clin Psychiatry* 64:966–968, 2003.

82. Lester BM, Cucca J, Andreozzi L, et al: Possible association between fluoxetine hydrochloride and colic in an infant, *J Am Acad Child Adolesc Psychiatry* 32:1253, 1993.

83. Levitan AA, Manion JC: Propranolol therapy during pregnancy and lactation, *Am J Cardiol* 32:247, 1973.

84. Liedholm H, Melander A, Bitzen PO, et al: Accumulation of atenolol and metoprolol in human breast milk, *Eur J Clin Pharmacol* 20:229, 1981.

85. Linde K, Ramirez G, Mulrow CD, et al: St. John's wort for depression: an overview and meta-analysis of randomised clinical trials, *Br Med J* 313:253, 1996.

86. Little RE, Anderson KW, Ervin CH, et al: Maternal alcohol use during breastfeeding and infant mental and motor development at one year, *N Engl J Med* 321:425, 1989.

87. Losonsky GA, Fishaut JM, Strussenberg J, et al: Effect of immunization against rubella on lactation products. I. Development and characterization of specific immunologic reactivity in breast milk, *J Infect Dis* 145:654, 1982.

88. Loughnan PM: Digoxin excretion in human breast milk, *J Pediatr* 92:1019, 1978.

89. Low-Dog T: The use of botanicals during pregnancy and lactation, *Altern Ther Health Med* 15:54–58, 2009.

90. Madachi P, Ross CJD, Hayden MR, et al: Pharmacogenetics of neonatal opioid toxicity following maternal use of codeine during breastfeeding: a case-controlled study, *Clin Pharmacol Ther* 85:31–35, 2009.

91. Marsh DO, Clarkson TW, Myers GJ, et al: Seychelles study of fetal methylmercury exposure and child development: introduction, *Neurotoxicology* 16(4):583, 1995.

92. Matheson I, Kristensen K, Lunde PKM: Drug utilization in breastfeeding women: a survey in Oslo, *Eur J Clin Pharmacol* 38:453, 1990.

93. McKenna R, Cole ER, Vasan U: Is warfarin sodium contraindicated in the lactating mother? *J Pediatr* 103:325, 1983.

94. Meador KJ: Breastfeeding and antiepileptic drugs, *JAMA Neurol* 70(11):1367–1374, 2013.

95. Mennella JA, Beauchamp GK: The transfer of alcohol to human milk, *N Engl J Med* 325:981, 1991.

96. Mennella JA, Gerrish CJ: Effects of exposure to alcohol in mother's milk on infant sleep, *Pediatrics* 101:e2, 1998.

97. Merbob P, Schaefer C: Psychotropic drugs. In Schaefer C, Peters PWJ, Miller RK, editors: *Drugs during pregnancy and lactation*, ed 3, Amsterdam, London, 2014, Elsevier, pp 743–769.

98. Misri S, Sivertz K: Tricyclic drugs in pregnancy and lactation: a preliminary report, *Int J Psychiatry Med* 21:157, 1991.

99. Mortola JF: The use of psychotropic agents in pregnancy and lactation, *Psychiatr Clin North Am* 12:69, 1989.

100. Namihira D, Saldivar L, Pustilnik N, et al: Lead in human blood and milk from nursing women living near a smelter in Mexico City, *J Toxicol Environ Health* 38:225, 1993.

101. Nau H, Rating D, Koch S, et al: Valproic acid and its metabolites: placental transfer, neonatal pharmacokinetics, transfer via mother's milk and clinical status in neonates of epileptic mothers, *J Pharmacol Exp Ther* 219:768, 1981.

102. Nau H, Rating D, Hauser I, et al: Placental transfer at birth and postnatal elimination of primidone and metabolites in neonates of epileptic mothers. In Janz D, Dam M, Richens A, et al, editors: *Epilepsy, pregnancy, and the child*, New York, 1982, Raven.

103. Neuvonen PJ, Kivistö KT: The clinical significance of food-drug interactions: a review, *Med J Aust* 150:36, 1989.

104. Nissen E, Matthiesen LG, Ransjo-Arvidsson A-S, et al: Effects of maternal pethidine on infant's developing breast-feeding behavior, *Acta Paediatr* 84:140, 1995.

105. Patil SP, Niphadkar PV, Bapat MM: Allergy to fenugreek (*Trigonelia foenum graecum*), *Ann Allergy Asthma Immunol* 78(3):297–300, 1997.

106. Pepino MY, Steinmeyer AL, Mennella JA: Lactational state modifies alcohol pharmacokinetics in women, *Alcohol Clin Exp Res* 31(6):909–918, 2007.

107. Pokela M-L, Olkkola KT, Koivisto M, et al: Pharmacokinetics and pharmacodynamics of intravenous meperidine in neonates and infants, *Clin Pharmacol Ther* 52:342, 1992.

108. Rasmussen F: Mammary excretion of benzylpenicillin, erythromycin and penethamate hydroiodide, *Acta Pharmacol Toxicol (Copenh)* 16:194, 1959.

109. Rating D, Jäger-Roman E, Koch S, et al: Enzyme induction in neonates due to antiepileptic therapy during pregnancy. In Janz D, Dam M, Richens A, et al, editors: *Epilepsy, pregnancy, and the child*, New York, 1982, Raven.

110. Righard L, Alade MO: Effect of delivery room routines on success of first breast-feed, *Lancet* 336(8723):1105, 1990.

111. Rogan WJ: Pollutants in breast milk, *Arch Pediatr Adolesc Med* 150:981, 1997.

112. Rogan WJ, Gladen B: Monitoring breast milk contamination to detect hazards from waste disposal, *Environ Health Perspect* 48:87, 1983.

113. Rogan WJ, Ware JH: Exposure to lead in children—how low is low enough? *N Engl J Med* 348:1515, 2003.

114. Rogan WJ, Bagniewska A, Damstra T: Pollutants in breast milk, *N Engl J Med* 302:1450, 1980.

115. Rossi M, Giorgi G: Domperidone and long Qt syndrome, *Curr Drug Saf* 5(3):257–262, 2010.

116. Rubow SM, Ellmann A, LeRoux J, et al: Excretion of technetium 99m hexakis methoxyisobutyl isonitrile in milk, *Eur J Nucl Med* 18:363, 1991.

117. Sakamoto M, Chan HM, Domingo JL, et al: Changes in body burden of mercury, lead, arsenic, cadmium, and selenium in infants during early lactation in comparison with placental transfer, *Ecotoxicol Environ Saf* 84:179–184, 2012.

118. Schaefer C: Industrial chemicals and environmental contaminants. In Schaefer C, Peters P, Miller RK, editors: *Drugs during pregnancy and lactation*, Amsterdam, London, 2014, Elsevier.

119. Schaefer C, Peters P, Miller RK: *Drugs during pregnancy and lactation*, ed 3, Amsterdam, London, 2014, Elsevier Academic Press.

120. Schou M: Lithium treatment during pregnancy, delivery and lactation: an update, *J Clin Psychiatry* 51:410, 1990.

121. Schou M, Amdisen A: Lithium and pregnancy. III. Lithium ingestion and children breastfed by women on lithium treatment, *Br Med J* 2:138, 1973.

122. Seely D, Dugoua J-J, Perri D, et al: Safety and efficacy of panax ginseng during pregnancy and lactation, *Can J Clin Pharmacol* 15(1):e87–e94, 2008.

123. Segelman AB, Segelman FP, Karliner J, et al: Sassafras and herb tea, *JAMA* 236:477, 1976.

124. Selim S, Hartnagel RE, Osimitz TG: Absorption, metabolism, and excretion of N,N-diethyl-m-toluamide (DEET) following dermal application to human volunteers, *Toxicol Sci* 25(1):95–100, 1995.

125. Sietsema WK: The absolute oral bioavailability of selected drugs, *Int J Clin Pharmacol Ther Toxicol* 27:179, 1989.

126. Skidmore-Roth L: *Mosby's handbook of herbs & natural supplements*, ed 3, St. Louis, 2006, Elsevier-Mosby.

127. Smirk CL, Bowman E, Doyle LW, et al: Home-based detoxification for neonatal abstinence syndrome reduces length of hospital admission without prolonging treatment, *Acta Paediatr* 103(6):601–604, 2014. http://dx.doi.org/10.1111/apa.12603.

128. Solomon GM, Weiss PM: Chemical contaminants in breast milk: time trends and regional variability, *Environ Health Perspect* 110:A339, 2002.

129. Somogyi A, Gugler R: Cimetidine excretion into breast milk, *Br J Clin Pharmacol* 7:627, 1979.

130. Stec GP, Greenberger P, Ruo TI, et al: Kinetics of theophylline transfer to breast milk, *Clin Pharmacol Ther* 28:404, 1980.

131. Stephens RD, Rappe C, Hayward DG, et al: World Health Organization international intercalibration study on

from breast milk is negligible, and *N. gonorrhoeae* does not seem to cause local infection of the breasts. Infection in neonates is most often ophthalmia neonatorum and less often a scalp abscess or disseminated infection. Mothers with presumed or documented gonorrhea should be reevaluated for other STDs, especially *Chlamydia trachomatis* and syphilis, because some therapies for gonorrhea are not adequate for either of these infections.

With the definitive identification of gonorrhea in a mother, empiric therapy should begin immediately, and the mother should be separated from the infant until the completion of 24 hours of adequate therapy. Treatment of the mother with ceftriaxone, cefixime, penicillin, or erythromycin is without significant risk for the infant. Single-dose treatment with spectinomycin, ciprofloxacin, ofloxacin, or azithromycin has not been adequately studied, but it would presumably be safe for the infant, given the 24-hour separation and a delay in breastfeeding without giving the infant the expressed breast milk (pump and discard). Doxycycline use in a nursing mother is not routinely recommended.

Careful preventive therapy for ophthalmia neonatorum should be provided, and close observation of the infant should continue for 2 to 7 days, the usual incubation period. Empiric or definitive therapy against *N. gonorrhoeae* may be necessary, depending on an infant's clinical status, and it should be chosen on the basis of the maternal isolate's sensitivity pattern. The mother should not handle other infants until after 24 hours of adequate therapy, and the infant should be separated from the rest of the nursery population, with or without breastfeeding.

HAEMOPHILUS INFLUENZAE

H. influenzae type B can cause severe invasive disease such as meningitis, sinusitis, pneumonia, epiglottitis, septic arthritis, pericarditis, and bacteremia. Shock can also occur. Because of the increased utilization of the *H. influenzae* type B conjugate vaccines, invasive disease caused by *Haemophilus* has decreased dramatically, with a greater than 95% reduction in the United States. Most invasive disease occurs in children 3 months to 3 years of age. Older children and adults rarely experience severe disease but do serve as sources of infection for young children. Children younger than 3 months of age seem to be protected because of passively acquired antibodies from the mothers, and some additional benefits may be received from breast milk.

Transmission occurs through contact with respiratory secretions, and droplet precautions are protective. No evidence suggests transmission through

breast milk or breastfeeding. Evidence supports that breast milk limits the colonization of *H. influenzae* in the throat.[203]

In the rare case of maternal infection, an inadequately immunized infant in a household is an indication to provide rifampin prophylaxis and close observation for all household contacts, including the breastfeeding infant. Expressed breast milk can be given to an infant during the 24-hour separation after the mother's initiation of antimicrobial therapy, or if the mother's illness prevents breastfeeding, it can be reinitiated when the mother is able (see Appendix F).

LEPROSY

Although uncommon in the United States, leprosy occurs throughout the world. This chronic disease presents with a spectrum of symptoms depending on the tissues involved (typically the skin, peripheral nerves, and mucous membranes of the upper respiratory tract) and the cellular immune response to the causative organism, *Mycobacterium leprae*. Transmission occurs through long-term contact with individuals with untreated or multibacillary (large numbers of organisms in the tissues) disease.

Leprosy is not a contraindication to breastfeeding, according to Jeliffe and Jeliffe.[222] The importance of breastfeeding and the urgency of treatment are recognized by experts who treat infants and mothers early and simultaneously. No mother-infant contact is permitted except to breastfeed. Dapsone, rifampin, and clofazimine are typically and safely used for infant and mother, regardless of the method of feeding (see Appendix D).

LISTERIOSIS

Listeriosis is a relatively uncommon infection that can have a broad range of manifestations. In immunocompetent individuals, including pregnant women, the infection can vary from being asymptomatic to presenting as an influenza-like illness, occasionally with GI symptoms or back pain. Severe disease occurs more frequently in immunodeficient individuals or infants infected in the perinatal period (pneumonia, sepsis, meningitis, and granulomatosis infantisepticum).

Although listeriosis during pregnancy may manifest as mild disease in a mother and is often difficult to recognize and diagnose, it is typically associated with stillbirth, abortion, and premature delivery. Transmission seems to occur through the transplacental hematogenous route, infecting the amniotic fluid, although ascending infection from the genital tract may occur.[134] Early and effective treatment of a woman can prevent fetal infection and sequelae.[227,286] Neonatal infection occurs as either early- or late-onset infection from transplacental spread late in pregnancy, ascending infection during labor and delivery, infection during passage through the birth canal, or, rarely, during postnatal exposure.

No evidence in the literature suggests that *Listeria* is transmitted through breast milk. Treatment of the mother with ampicillin, penicillin, or trimethoprim-sulfamethoxazole is not a contraindication to breastfeeding as long as the mother is well enough. Expressed colostrum or breast milk can also be given if the infant is able to feed orally. The management of lactation and feeding in neonatal listeriosis is conducted supportively, as it is in any situation in which an infant is extremely ill, beginning feeding with expressed breast milk or directly breastfeeding as soon as reasonable.

Meningococcal Infections

N. meningitidis most often causes severe invasive infections, including meningococcemia or meningitis, often associated with fever and a rash and progressing to purpura, disseminated intravascular coagulation, shock, coma, and death.

Transmission occurs via respiratory droplets. Spread can occur from an infected, ill individual or from an asymptomatic carrier. Droplet precautions are recommended until 24 hours after initiation of effective therapy. Despite the frequent occurrence of bacteremia, no evidence indicates breast involvement or transmission through breast milk.

The risk for maternal infection to an infant after birth is from droplet exposure and exists whether the infant is breastfeeding or bottle feeding. In either case, the exposed infant should receive chemoprophylaxis with rifampin, 10 mg/kg/dose every 12 hours for 2 days (5 mg/kg/dose for infants younger than 1 month of age), or ceftriaxone, 125 mg intramuscularly (IM) once, for children younger than 15 years of age. Close observation of the infant should continue for 7 days, and breastfeeding during and after prophylaxis is appropriate. The severity of maternal illness may prevent breastfeeding, but it can continue if the mother is able, after the mother and infant have been receiving antibiotics for 24 hours. A period of separation from the index case for the first 24 hours of effective therapy is recommended; expressed breast milk can be given during this period.

PERTUSSIS

Respiratory illness caused by *Bordetella pertussis* evolves in three stages: catarrhal (nasal discharge, congestion, increasing cough), paroxysmal (severe paroxysms of cough sometimes ending in an inspiratory whoop, i.e., whooping cough), and convalescent (gradual improvement in symptoms).

Transmission is via respiratory droplets. The greatest risk for transmission occurs in the catarrhal phase, often before the diagnosis of pertussis. The nasopharyngeal culture usually becomes negative after 5 days of antibiotic therapy. Chemoprophylaxis for all household contacts is routinely recommended. No evidence indicates transmission through breast milk, with similar risk to breastfed and bottle-fed infants.

In the case of maternal infection with pertussis, chemoprophylaxis for all household contacts, regardless of age or immunization status, is indicated. In addition to chemoprophylaxis of the infant, close observation and subsequent immunization (in infants older than 6 weeks of age) are appropriate. Prophylaxis for the infant should be azithromycin or erythromycin, although trimethoprim-sulfamethoxazole can be used when the infant is 6 weeks or older. Despite chemoprophylaxis, droplet precautions and the separation of mother and infant during the first 5 days of effective maternal antibiotic therapy are recommended. Expressed breast milk can be provided to the infant during this period.

Staphylococcal Infections

Staphylococcal infection in neonates can be caused by either *S. aureus* or coagulase-negative staphylococci (most often *Staphylococcus epidermidis*) and can manifest in a wide range of illnesses. Localized infection can be impetigo, pustulosis in neonates, cellulitis, or wound infection, and invasive or suppurative disease includes sepsis, pneumonia, osteomyelitis, arthritis, and endocarditis. *S. aureus* requires only a small inoculum (10 to 250 organisms) to produce colonization in newborns, most often of the nasal mucosa and umbilicus.[212] By the fifth day of life, 40% to 90% of the infants in the nursery will be colonized with *S. aureus*.[139] The organism is easily transmitted to others from mother, infant, family, or health care personnel through direct contact.

Outbreaks in nurseries were common in the past. Mothers, infants, health care workers, and even contaminated, unpasteurized, banked breast milk were sources of infection.[41a,337,366] Careful use of antibiotics, changes in nursery layout and procedures, standard precautions, and cohorting as needed decreased the spread of *S. aureus* in nurseries. Now the occurrence of methicillin-resistant *S. aureus* (MRSA) is again a common problem, requiring cohorting, occasional epidemiologic investigation, and careful infection-control intervention. There are numerous reports of MRSA outbreaks in NICUs.[37,159,231,282,322] The significance of colonization with *Staphylococcus* and the factors leading to development of disease in individual patients are not clear. The morbidity and mortality related to *S. aureus* infection in neonates is well described,[210,215,241] and the management of such outbreaks has been reviewed.[163,278] Little has been written about the role of breastfeeding in colonization with *S. aureus* in NICUs, well-baby nurseries, or at home.

MRSA is an important pathogen worldwide. Community-acquired MRSA is different from hospital-acquired MRSA. Community-acquired MRSA is usually defined as occurring in an individual without the common predisposing variables associated with hospital-acquired MRSA. Community-acquired MRSA also lacks an MDR phenotype (common with hospital-acquired MRSA); frequently carries multiple exotoxin virulence factors (such as Panton-Valentine leukocidin toxin), as well as the smaller type IV staphylococcal cassette cartridge for the *MecA* gene on a chromosome (hospital-acquired MRSA carries the types I-III staphylococcal cassette cartridge); and is molecularly distinct from the common nosocomial strains of hospital-acquired MRSA. Community-acquired MRSA is most commonly associated with skin and soft tissue infections and necrotizing pneumonia and less frequently associated with endocarditis, bacteremia, necrotizing fasciitis, myositis, osteomyelitis, or parapneumonic effusions. Community-acquired MRSA is so common that it is now being observed in hospital outbreaks.[26,159,182,401] Community-acquired MRSA transmission to infants via breast milk has been reported.[37,159,231,282,322] Premature or small-for-gestational-age infants are more susceptible to and at increased risk for significant morbidity and mortality due to MRSA, in part because of prolonged hospitalization, multiple courses of antibiotics, invasive procedures and intravenous (IV) lines, their relative immune deficiency related to prematurity and illness, and altered GI tract due to different flora and decreased gastric acidity. Therefore, colonization with MRSA may pose a greater risk to infants in NICUs in the long run. Full-term infants develop pustulosis, cellulitis, and soft tissue infections, but invasive disease has rarely been reported.[87,147,337] Fortunov et al.[147] from Texas reported 126 infections in term or late-preterm previously well infants, including 43 with pustulosis, 68 with celluliltis or

abscesses, and 15 invasive infections. A family history of soft tissue skin infections and male sex were the only variables associated with risk for infection; cesarean delivery, breastfeeding, and circumcision were not.[147] Nguyen et al.[337] reported MRSA infections in a well-infant nursery from California. The eleven cases were all in full-term boys with pustular-vesicular lesions in the groin. The infections were associated with longer length of stay, lidocaine injection use in infants, maternal age older than 30 years, and circumcision. Breastfeeding was not an associated risk factor for MRSA infection.[337] The question of the role of circumcision in MRSA outbreaks was addressed by Van Howe and Robson.[473] They reported that circumcised boys are at greater risk for staphylococcal colonization and infection.[473]

Others report that *S. aureus* carriage in infants (and subsequent infection) is most likely affected by multiple variables, including infant factors (antibiotics, surgical procedures [circumcision being the most common], duration of hospital stay as a newborn), maternal factors (previous colonization, previous antibiotic usage, mode of delivery, length of stay), and environmental factors (MRSA in the family or hospital, nursery stay versus rooming-in, hand hygiene).[57,96,210,221,368,400,401] Gerber et al.[163] from the Chicago area published a consensus statement for the management of MRSA outbreaks in the NICU. The recommendations, which were strongly supported by experimental, clinical, and epidemiologic data, included using a waterless, alcohol-based hand hygiene product, monitoring and enforcing hand hygiene, placing MRSA-positive infants in contact precautions with cohorting if possible, using gloves and gowns for direct contact and masks for aerosol-generating procedures, cohorting nurses for care of MRSA-positive infants when possible, periodic screening of infants for MRSA using nares or nasopharyngeal cultures, clarifying the MRSA status of infants being transferred into the NICU, limiting overcrowding, and maintaining ongoing instruction and monitoring of health care workers in their compliance with infection-control and hand-hygiene procedures. The evaluation of the outbreak could include screening of health care workers and environmental surfaces to corroborate epidemiologic data and laboratory molecular analysis of the MRSA strains if indicated epidemiologically. The use of mupirocin or other decolonizing procedures should be determined on an individual basis for each NICU.

S. aureus is the most common cause of mastitis in lactating women.[356,439,440,484] Recurrence or persistence of symptoms of mastitis is a well-described occurrence and an important issue in the management of mastitis. Community-acquired MRSA has been associated with mastitis as well[383,401,440] (see Chapter 16 for a complete discussion of mastitis).

Two studies, one from France and one from Brazil, investigated the occurrence of MRSA in expressed breast milk.[28,339] Barbe et al.[28] cultured 9171 expressed breast milk samples from 378 women and tested 2351 samples before pasteurization and 6820 samples after pasteurization. MRSA and methicillin-susceptible *S. aureus* were identified, respectively, in 8 samples (0.8%) from 3 mothers and 281 samples (19.3%) from 73 mothers, using the tested expressed breast milk before pasteurization. After pasteurization, *S. aureus* was not detected in any of the 6820 samples of expressed breast milk. Colonization of one infant with MRSA was identified, but no MRSA infections were identified in any of the hospitalized infants in the NICU during the 18 months of the study.[28] Novak et al.[339] identified MRSA in 57 of 500 samples (11%) of expressed fresh-frozen milk from 500 different donors from five Brazilian milk banks. Only 3 of the 57 samples were positive with high-level bacterial counts of MRSA (greater than 10,000 CFU/mL). These were the only samples that would not have been acceptable by bacteriological criteria according to Brazilian or American criteria for raw milk use. They did not investigate other epidemiological data to identify possible variables associated with low- or high-level contamination of expressed breast milk with MRSA.[339]

The management of an infant and/or mother with MRSA infection, relative to breastfeeding or use of breast milk, should be based on the severity of disease and whether the infant is premature, LBW, very low birth weight (VLBW), previously ill, or full term.

When full-term infants or their mothers develop mild to moderate infections (impetigo, pustulosis, cellulitis/abscess, mastitis/breast abscess, or soft tissue infection), those infants can continue breastfeeding after a short period of interruption (24 to 48 hours). During this time, pumping to maintain the milk supply should be supported, an initial evaluation for other evidence of infection should be done in the maternal-infant dyad, the infected child and/or mother should be placed on "commonly" effective therapy for the MRSA infection, and ongoing observation for clinical disease should continue. The mother and infant can "room-in" together in the hospital, if necessary, with standard and contact precautions. Culturing the breast milk is not necessary. Empiric therapy for the infant may be chosen based on medical concerns for the infant and the known sensitivity testing of the MRSA isolate. Appropriate antibiotic choices include short-term use of azithromycin (erythromycin use during

infancy [less than 6 weeks of age], or breastfeeding associated with an increased risk for hypertrophic pyloric stenosis), sulfamethoxazole-trimethoprim (in the absence of G6PD deficiency and older than 30 days of age), clindamycin, and perhaps linezolid for mild to moderate infections.

When infants in NICUs (premature, LBW, VLBW, and/or previously ill) or their mothers have a MRSA infection, those infants should have the breast milk cultured and suspend breastfeeding or receiving breast milk from their mothers until the breast milk is shown to be culture-negative for MRSA. The infant should be treated as indicated for infection or empirically treated if symptomatic (with pending culture results) and closely observed for the development of new signs or symptoms of infection. Pumping to maintain the milk supply and the use of banked breast milk are appropriate. The infant should be placed on contact precautions, in addition to the routine standard precautions. The infant can be cohorted with other MRSA-positive infants, with nursing care cohorted as well. The mother with MRSA infection should be instructed concerning hand hygiene; the careful collection, handling, and storage of breast milk; contact precautions to be used with her infant; and the avoidance of contact with any other infants. The mother can receive several possible antibiotics for MRSA that are compatible with breastfeeding when used for a short period. If the mother remains clinically well, including without evidence of mastitis, but her breast milk is positive for MRSA greater than 10^4 CFU/mL, empiric therapy to diminish or eradicate colonization would be appropriate. Various regimens have been proposed to "eradicate" MRSA colonization, but none has been proven to be highly efficacious. These regimens usually include systemic antibiotics with one or two medications (rifampin added as the second medication), as well as nasal mupirocin to the nares twice daily for 1 to 2 weeks with routine hygiene, with or without the usage of hexachlorophene (or similar topical agent or cleanser) for bathing during the 1- to 2-week treatment period. There is no clear information concerning the efficacy of using similar colonization-eradication regimens for other household members or pets in preventing recolonization of the mother or infant. Before reintroducing the use of the mother's breast milk to the infant, at least one negative breast milk culture should be obtained after the completion of therapy.

The routine screening of breast milk provided by mothers for their infants in NICUs for the presence of MRSA is not indicated in the absence of MRSA illness in the maternal-infant dyad, a MRSA outbreak in NICUs, or a high frequency of MRSA infection in a specific NICU.

TOXIN-MEDIATED *STAPHYLOCOCCUS* DISEASE

One case of staphylococcal scalded skin syndrome was reported by Katzman and Wald[229] in an infant breastfed by a mother with a lesion on her areola that did not respond to ampicillin therapy for 14 days. Subsequently, the infant developed conjunctivitis with *S. aureus*, which produced an exfoliative toxin, and a confluent erythematous rash without mucous membrane involvement or Nikolsky sign. No attempt to identify the exfoliative toxin in the breast milk was made, and the breast milk was not cultured for *S. aureus*. The child responded to IV therapy with nafcillin. This emphasizes the importance of evaluating mother and infant at the time of a suspected infection and the need for continued observation of the infant for evidence of a pyogenic infection or toxin-mediated disease, especially with maternal mastitis or breast lesions.

This case also raises the issue of when and how infants and their mothers become colonized with *S. aureus* and what factors lead to infection and illness in each. The concern is that *Staphylococcus* can be easily transmitted through skin-to-skin contact, colonization readily occurs, and potentially serious illness can occur later, long after colonization. In the case of staphylococcal scalded skin syndrome or toxic shock syndrome (TSS), the primary site of infection can be insignificant (e.g., conjunctivitis, infection of a circumcision, or simple pustulosis), but a clinically significant amount of toxin can be produced and lead to serious disease.

TSS can result from *S. aureus* or *Streptococcus pyogenes* infection and probably from a variety of antigens produced by other organisms. TSS-1 has been identified as a "superantigen" that affects the T lymphocytes and other components of the immune response, producing an unregulated and excessive immune response and resulting in an overwhelming systemic clinical response. TSS has been reported in association with vaginal delivery, cesarean delivery, mastitis, and other local infections in mothers. Mortality rates in mothers may be as high as 5%.

The case definition of staphylococcal TSS includes meeting all four major criteria: fever greater than 38.9° C, rash (diffuse macular erythroderma), hypotension, and desquamation (associated with subepidermal separation seen on skin biopsy). The definition also includes involvement of three or more organ systems (GI, muscular, mucous membrane, renal, hepatic, hematologic, or CNS); negative titers for Rocky Mountain spotted fever, leptospirosis, and rubeola; and lack of isolation of *S. pyogenes* from any source or *S. aureus* from the cerebrospinal fluid (CSF).[410] A similar case definition has been proposed for streptococcal TSS.[502]

Aggressive empiric antibiotic therapy against staphylococci and streptococci and careful supportive therapy are essential for decreasing illness and death. Oxacillin, nafcillin, first-generation cephalosporins, clindamycin, erythromycin, and vancomycin are acceptable antibiotics, even for a breastfeeding mother. The severity of illness in the mother may preclude breastfeeding, but it can be reinitiated when the mother is improving and wants to restart. Standard precautions, with breastfeeding, are recommended.

Staphylococcal enterotoxin F has been identified in breast milk specimens collected on days 5, 8, and 11 from a mother who developed TSS at 22 hours postpartum.[476] *S. aureus* that produced staphylococcal enterotoxin F was isolated from the mother's vagina but not from breast milk. Infant and mother lacked significant levels of antibodies against staphylococcal enterotoxin F in their sera. The infant remained healthy after 60 days of follow-up. Staphylococcal enterotoxin F is pepsin inactivated at pH 4.5 and therefore is probably destroyed in the stomach environment, presenting little or no risk to the breastfeeding infant.[39a] Breastfeeding can continue if the mother is able.

COAGULASE-NEGATIVE *STAPHYLOCOCCUS*

Coagulase-negative staphylococcal infection (*S. epidermidis* is the predominant isolate) produces minimal disease in healthy, full-term infants but is a significant problem in hospitalized or premature infants. Factors associated with increased risk for this infection include prematurity, high colonization rates in specific nurseries, invasive therapies (e.g., IV lines, chest tubes, intubation), and antibiotic use. Illness produced by coagulase-negative staphylococci can be invasive and severe in high-risk neonates but rarely in mothers. There are reports of necrotizing enterocolitis associated with coagulase-negative *Staphylococcus*. At 2 weeks of age, for infants still in the nursery, *S. epidermidis* is a frequent colonizing organism at multiple sites, with colonization rates as high as 75% to 100%. Serious infections with coagulase-negative staphylococci (e.g., abscesses, IV line infection, bacteremia/sepsis, endocarditis, osteomyelitis) require effective IV therapy. Many strains are resistant to penicillin and the semisynthetic penicillins, so that sensitivity testing is essential. Empiric or definitive therapy may require treatment with vancomycin, gentamicin, rifampin, teicoplanin, linezolid, or combinations of these for synergistic activity. Transmission of infection in association with breastfeeding appears to be no more common than with bottle feeding. As with *S. aureus*, infection control includes contact and standard precautions.

Occasionally, during presumed outbreaks, careful epidemiologic surveillance may be required, including cohorting, limiting overcrowding and understaffing, surveillance cultures of infants and nursery personnel, reemphasis of meticulous infection-control techniques for all individuals entering the nursery, and, rarely, removal of colonized personnel from direct infant contact.

S. epidermidis has been identified as part of the fecal microbiota of breastfed infants.[223] *S. epidermidis* has also been identified in the breast milk of women with clinical evidence of mastitis.[119] Nevertheless, *S. epidermidis* is rarely associated with infection in full-term infants. Conceivably, breast milk for premature infants could be a source of *S. epidermidis* colonization in the NICUs. The other factors associated with hospitalization in an NICU noted previously presumably play a significant role in both colonization and infection in premature infants. The benefits of early full human milk feeding potentially outweigh the risk for colonization with *S. epidermidis* via breast milk.[390] Ongoing education and assistance should be provided to mothers about the careful collection, storage, and delivery of human breast milk for their premature infants.[395]

Streptococcal Infections

Group A

S. pyogenes (β-hemolytic group A *Streptococcus* [GAS]) is a common cause of skin and throat infections in children, producing pharyngitis, cellulitis, and impetigo. Illnesses produced by GAS can be classified into three categories: (1) impetigo, cellulitis, or pharyngitis without invasion or complication; (2) severe invasive infection with bacteremia, necrotizing fasciitis, myositis, or systemic illness (e.g., streptococcal TSS); and (3) autoimmune-mediated phenomena, including acute rheumatic fever and acute glomerulonephritis. GAS can also cause puerperal sepsis, endometritis, and neonatal omphalitis. Significant morbidity and mortality rates are associated with invasive GAS infection; the mortality rate is 20% to 50%, with almost half the survivors requiring extensive tissue débridement or amputation.[389] Infants are not at risk for the autoimmune sequelae of GAS (rheumatic fever or poststreptococcal glomerulonephritis). Transmission is through direct contact (rarely indirect contact) and droplet spread. Outbreaks of GAS in the nursery are rare, unlike with staphylococcal infections. Either mother or infant can be initially colonized with GAS and transmit it to the other.

In the situation of maternal illness (extensive cellulitis, necrotizing fasciitis, myositis, pneumonia, TSS, and mastitis), it is appropriate to separate mother and infant until effective therapy (penicillin, ampicillin, cephalosporins, and erythromycin) has been given for at least 24 hours. Breastfeeding should also be suspended and may resume after 24 hours of therapy for the mother.

Group B

Group B *Streptococcus* (GBS, *Streptococcus agalactiae*) is a significant cause of perinatal bacterial infection. In parturient women, infection can lead to asymptomatic bacteriuria, urinary tract infection (often associated with premature birth), endometritis, or amnionitis. In infants, infection usually occurs between birth and 3 months of age (1 to 4 cases per 1000 live births). It is routinely classified by the time of onset of illness in the infant: early onset (0 to 7 days, majority less than 24 hours) and late onset (7 to 90 days, generally less than 4 weeks). Infants may develop sepsis, pneumonia, meningitis, osteomyelitis, arthritis, or cellulitis. Early-onset GBS disease is often fulminant, presenting as sepsis or pneumonia with respiratory failure; three-quarters of neonatal disease is early onset. Type III is the most common serotype causing disease.

Transmission is believed to occur in utero and during delivery. Colonization rates of mothers and infants vary between 5% and 35%. Postpartum transmission is thought to be uncommon, although it has been documented. Risk factors for early-onset GBS disease include delivery before 37 weeks of gestation, rupture of membranes for longer than 18 hours before delivery, intrapartum fever, heavy maternal colonization with GBS, or low concentrations of anti-GBS capsular antibody in maternal sera.[104] The common occurrence of severe GBS disease before 24 hours of age in neonates has led to prevention strategies. Revised guidelines developed by the AAP Committees on Infectious Diseases and on the Fetus and Newborn have tried to combine various variables for increased risk for GBS infection (prenatal colonization with GBS, obstetric and neonatal risk factors for early-onset disease) and to provide intrapartum prophylaxis to those at high risk[90,104] (CDCP Prev of Perinatal GBS Disease MMWR 2010 and Comm on Inf Dis and Comm on the Fetus and Newborn Pediatrics 2011) (Figure 13-1). The utilization of these guidelines, universal culture-based screening, and intrapartum prophylaxis across the United States have decreased the incidence of early-onset disease by approximately 80% from an estimated 1.4 cases of early-onset GBS disease (EOD) per 1000 live births in 1990 to 0.28 cases per 1000 live births in 2012 (Van Dyke et al.)[472]

The incidence of late-onset GBS disease (LOD) remains unchanged since 1990 (~0.3 to 0.4 cases

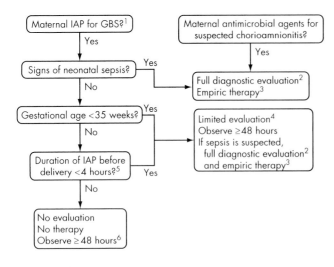

Maternal IAP for GBS?[1]
Yes
Signs of neonatal sepsis? —Yes→
No
Gestational age <35 weeks? —Yes→
No
Duration of IAP before delivery <4 hours?[5] —Yes→
No
No evaluation
No therapy
Observe ≥48 hours[6]

Maternal antimicrobial agents for suspected chorioamnionitis?
Yes
Full diagnostic evaluation[2]
Empiric therapy[3]

Limited evaluation[4]
Observe ≥48 hours
If sepsis is suspected,
  full diagnostic evaluation[2]
  and empiric therapy[3]

[1] If no maternal IAP for GBS was administered despite an indication being present, data are insufficient on which to recommend a single management strategy.

[2] Includes complete blood cell (CBC) count with differential, blood culture, and chest radiograph if respiratory abnormalities are present. When signs of sepsis are present, a lumbar puncture, if feasible, should be performed.

[3] Duration of therapy varies depending on results of blood culture, cerebrospinal fluid findings (if obtained), and the clinical course of the infant. If laboratory results and clinical course do not indicate bacterial infection, duration may be as short as 48 hours.

[4] CBC including WBC count with differential and blood culture.

[5] Applies only to penicillin, ampicillin, or cefazolin and assumes recommended dosing regimens.

[6] A healthy-appearing infant who was ≥38 weeks' gestation at delivery and whose mother received ≥4 hours of IAP before delivery may be discharged home after 24 hours *if* other discharge criteria have been met and a person able to comply fully with instructions for home observation will be present. If any one of these conditions is not met, the infant should be observed in the hospital for at least 48 hours and until criteria for discharge are achieved.

Figure 13-1. Empiric management of a neonate born to a mother who received intrapartum antimicrobial prophylaxis (IAP) for the prevention of early-onset group B streptococcal (GBS) disease. *CSF,* Cerebrospinal fluid; *CBC,* complete blood count. This algorithm is not an exclusive course of management. Variations that incorporate individual circumstances or institutional preferences may be appropriate. (From Committee on Infectious Diseases, American Academy of Pediatrics: *Red book report of the committee on infectious disease,* ed 26, Elk Grove, Ill., 2003, American Academy of Pediatrics, p 590.)

per 1000 live births) despite the implementation of screening and guidelines for preventing EOD (CDCP 2013 Active Bacterial Core Surveillance Report). LOD is thought to be the result of transmission during delivery or in the postnatal period from maternal, hospital, or community sources. Dillon et al.[124] demonstrated that 10 of 21 infants with late-onset disease were colonized at birth, but the source of colonization was unidentified in the others. Gardner et al.[157] showed that only 4.3% of 46 children who were culture-negative for GBS at discharge from the hospital had acquired GBS by 2 months of age. Anthony et al.[17] noted that many infants are colonized with GBS, but the actual attack rate for GBS disease is low and difficult to predict.

Acquisition of GBS through breast milk or breastfeeding is uncommon and remains a controversial topic.[38,143,275] Cases of LOD associated with GBS in the maternal milk have been reported.[65,236,352,408,485] Some of the mothers had bilateral mastitis, at least one had delayed evidence of unilateral mastitis, and the others were asymptomatic. It was not clear when colonization of the infants occurred or when infection or disease began in the infants. The authors discussed the possibility that the infants were originally colonized during delivery, subsequently colonized the

mothers' breasts during breastfeeding, and then became re-infected at a later time. Butter and DeMoor[63] showed that infants initially colonized on their heads at birth had GBS cultured from their throat, nose, or umbilicus 8 days later. Whenever they cultured GBS from the nipples of mothers, the authors also found it in the nose or throat of the infants.

Berardi et al.[37a] studied GBS colonization prospectively in 160 mother-infant dyads. They noted that few culture-positive women had GBS cultured from their milk through 60 days post hospital discharge. Neonates who were colonized at more than one site (throat, ear, or rectum) were most commonly born to culture-positive carrier mothers who were GBS positive at delivery. One of the three cases of neonatal GBS infection presented as LOD at 35 days of age, and one presented with EOD at birth. The third infant presented with EOD at 20 hours of age and was adequately treated. That same infant was retreated at 18 days of age for a GBS urinary tract infection. They concluded that there was no evidence that mother's milk was the cause of the neonatal infections and that the occurrence of GBS in human milk could have been contamination or colonization from infants who were already heavily colonized with GBS.[39] Filleron et al.[143] reviewed 48 cases in the literature of late-onset neonatal infection (LONI) associated with GBS and breast milk. They noted four cases of LONI that occurred in the absence of maternal GBS detection, in infants born by cesarean section and with GBS-positive mother's milk as the probable source of infection. Their analysis also demonstrated a high rate of recurrence of LONI (35% of the 48 neonates) had more than one LONI. They concluded,[143] as others have recommended (Berardi et al.,[39] Byrne et al.,[65] Lombard et al.,[288] and Davanzo et al.[117]), that additional attention should be given to the handling and use of raw human milk in "vulnerable" neonates and instances of GBS culture-positive human milk with or without maternal mastitis. Byrne et al.[65] presented a review of GBS disease associated with breastfeeding and made recommendations to decrease the risk for transmission of GBS to infants via breastfeeding or breast milk. Some of their recommendations included confirming appropriate collection and processing procedures for GBS cultures[412] in medical facilities to decrease false-negative cultures; reviewing proper hygiene for pumping, collection, and storage of expressed breast milk with mothers; reviewing the signs and symptoms of mastitis with mothers; and utilizing banked human milk as needed instead of mother's milk. Davanzo et al.[117] describe proposed "best practice guidance" for managing human milk feeding and group B *Streptococcus* in developed countries. This guidance includes the following: (1) Do not routinely perform microbial cultures of breast milk from the mother of the term or preterm infant. (2) Interruption of breastfeeding in most situations of maternal mastitis and healthy full term infants is unnecessary, but conservative management, including milk removal, supportive measures, and antibiotics for the mother, are appropriate if her symptoms persist or worsen. (3) In the case of mastitis in mothers of preterm infants, drain the affected breast, culture the milk, and treat the mother empirically. If the milk is GBS-positive, then the milk should either be pasteurized prior to giving it to the premature infant or discarded until there is a subsequent negative culture of the milk. (4) Prevention and management strategies for EOD GBS infection should follow the revised CDC guidelines from 2010 and the more recent recommendations for the prevention of perinatal GBS disease from the AAP's Committee on Infectious Diseases and Committee on Fetus and Newborn,[103] 2011 [CDCP Prev Perinatal GBS Dis Rev Guidelines 2010, Comm on ID and Comm on Fetus Newborn Policy Statement re GBS prevention 2011].[90] These documents do not recommend routine discontinuation of breastfeeding, discarding breast milk, or pasteurization of breast milk after EOD GBS, because there is no evidence that this is protective against LOD

GBS. (5) In the situation of LOD GBS disease and a positive breast milk culture for GBS, treat the mother to eradicate colonization (ampicillin or amoxicillin plus rifampin), pasteurize or discard breast milk until adequate therapy has been given to the mother or there is a negative breast milk culture, track breast milk cultures through hospitalization, and consider adding rifampin to the infant's antibiotic treatment to eradicate colonization in the infant, even though the "eradication" of colonization is difficult and inconsistent.

When a breastfed infant develops LOD, it is appropriate to culture the milk. (See discussion of culturing breast milk earlier in this chapter.) Consider treatment of the mother to prevent reinfection if the milk is culture positive for GBS (greater than 10^4 CFU/mL), with or without clinical evidence of mastitis in the mother. Withholding the mother's milk until it is confirmed to be culture negative for a pathogen is appropriate and should be accompanied by providing ongoing support and instruction to the mother concerning pumping and maintaining her milk supply. Serial culturing of expressed breast milk after treatment of the mother for GBS disease or colonization would be appropriate to insure the ongoing absence of a pathogen in the expressed breast milk. There are reports of reinfection of the infant from breast milk.[25,117,143,247,288] Eradication of GBS mucosal colonization in the infant or the mother may be difficult. Some authors have recommended using rifampin prophylactically in both the mother and infant at the end of treatment to eradicate mucosal colonization.[25,48] (See Chapter 16 for management of mastitis in the mother.) A mother or infant colonized or infected with GBS should be managed with standard precautions[102] while in the hospital. Ongoing close evaluation of the infant for infection or illness and empiric therapy for GBS in the infant are appropriate until the child has remained well and cultures are subsequently negative at 72 hours. Occasionally, epidemiologic investigation in the hospital will utilize the culturing of medical staff and family members to detect a source of LOD in the nursery. This can be useful when more than one case of LOD is detected with the same serotype. Cohorting in such a situation may be appropriate. Selective prophylactic therapy for colonized infants to eradicate colonization may be considered, but unlike GAS or *Staphylococcus* infection, GBS infection in nurseries has not been reported to cause outbreaks. No data support conducting GBS screening on all breastfeeding mothers and their expressed breast milk as a reasonable method for protecting against spread of GBS infection via expressed breast milk or LOD GBS infection. Selective culturing of expressed breast milk may be appropriate in certain situations.

TUBERCULOSIS

The face of TB is changing throughout the world. In the United States the incidence of TB rose from 1986 through 1993 and has been declining since then.[67] In 2013, the incidence rate was 3.0 cases per 100,000 population, which represents a decrease of 4.2% from 2012 (Alami et al.[3]).

TB during pregnancy has always been a significant concern for patients and physicians alike.[381] It is now clear that the course and prognosis of TB in pregnancy are less affected by the pregnancy and more determined by the location and extent of disease, as defined primarily by chest radiograph, and by the susceptibility of the individual patient. Untreated TB in pregnancy is associated with maternal and infant mortality rates of 30% to 40%.[407] Effective therapy is crucial to the clinical outcome in both pregnant and nonpregnant women. TB during pregnancy rarely results in congenital TB, although congenital TB has a mortality rate as high as 50%.[289]

Any individual in a high-risk group for TB should be screened with a tuberculin skin test (TST). No contraindication or altered responsiveness to the TST exists during pregnancy or breastfeeding. Interpretation of the TST should follow the most recent guidelines, using different sizes of induration in different-risk populations as cutoffs for a positive test, as proposed by the CDC.[75] Figure 13-2 outlines the evaluation and treatment of a pregnant woman with a positive TST.[443]

Treatment of active TB should begin as soon as the diagnosis is made, regardless of the fetus's gestational age, because the risk for disease to mother and fetus clearly outweighs the risks of treatment. Isoniazid, rifampin, and ethambutol have been used safely in all three trimesters. Isoniazid and pyridoxine therapy during breastfeeding is safe, although the risk for hepatotoxicity in the mother may be a concern during the first 2 months postpartum.[436]

Congenital TB is extremely rare, if one considers that 7 to 8 million cases of TB occur each year worldwide and that less than 300 cases of congenital TB have been reported in the literature. As with other infectious diseases presenting in the perinatal period, distinguishing congenital infection from perinatal or postnatal TB in infants can be difficult.

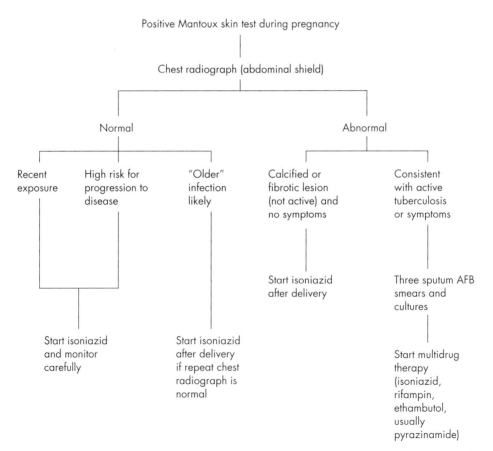

Figure 13-2. Evaluation and treatment of a pregnant woman with a positive tuberculin skin test. (From Starke JR: Tuberculosis, an old disease but a new threat to mother, fetus, and neonate, *Clin Perinatol* 24:107, 1997.)

Postnatal TB infection in infancy typically presents with severe disease and extrapulmonary extension (meningitis; lymphadenopathy; and bone, liver, spleen involvement). Airborne transmission of TB to infants is the major mode of postnatal infection because of close and prolonged exposure in enclosed spaces, especially in their own household, to any adult with infectious pulmonary TB. Potential infectious sources could be the mother or any adult caregiver, such as babysitters, day care workers, relatives, friends, neighbors, and even health care workers. Mittal et al. recently reviewed the management of the newborn infant exposed to their mother with TB.[318]

The suspicion of TB infection or disease in a household with possible exposure of an infant is a highly anxiety-provoking situation (Figure 13-3). Although protecting an infant from infection is foremost in everyone's mind, separation of the infant from the mother should be avoided when reasonable. Every situation is unique, and the best approach will vary according to the specifics of the case and accepted principles of TB management. The first step in caring for the potentially exposed infant is to determine accurately the true TB status of the suspected case (mother or household contact). This prompt evaluation should include a complete history (previous TB infection or disease, previous or ongoing TB treatment, TST status, symptoms suggestive of active TB, results of most recent chest radiograph, sputum smears, or cultures), physical examination, a TST if indicated, a new chest radiograph, and mycobacterial cultures and smears of any suspected sites of infection. All household contacts should be evaluated promptly, including history and TST with further evaluation as indicated.[75] Continued risk to the infant can occur from infectious household contacts who have not been effectively evaluated and treated.

An infant should be temporarily separated from the suspected source if symptoms suggest active disease or a recent TST documents conversion, and separation should continue until the results of the chest radiograph are seen. Because of considerable variability in the course of illness and the concomitant infectious period, debate continues without adequate data about the appropriate period of separation.[313] This should be individualized given the specific situation. HIV testing and assessment of the risk for MDR TB should be done in every case of active TB. Sensitivity testing should be done on every M. tuberculosis isolate. Table 13-1 summarizes the management of the newborn infant whose mother (or other household contact) has TB.

Initiation of prophylactic isoniazid therapy in the infant has been demonstrated to be effective in preventing TB infection and disease in the infant.

Therefore, continued separation of the infant and mother is unnecessary after therapy in both mother and child has begun.[107,126] The AAP recommends isoniazid (INH) prophylaxis for all infants whose mothers have been diagnosed with active pulmonary TB in the postpartum period. The real risk requiring infant separation is airborne transmission. Separation of the infant from a mother with active pulmonary TB is appropriate, regardless of the method of feeding. However, in many parts of the world, after therapy in the mother and prophylaxis with isoniazid in the infant has begun, the infant and mother are not separated. With or without separation, the mother and infant should continue to be closely observed throughout the course of maternal therapy to ensure good compliance with medication by both mother and infant and to identify, early on, any symptoms in the infant suggestive of TB. The mother should be followed to confirm that she is no longer considered infectious, with negative smears and cultures within 2 to 4 weeks of beginning TB therapy.

Tuberculous mastitis occurs rarely in the United States, but it does occur in other parts of the world[2,178,189,220,238,425] and can lead to infection in infants, frequently involving the tonsils. A mother usually has a single breast mass and associated axillary lymph node swelling and infrequently develops a draining sinus. TB of the breast can also present as a painless mass or edema. Involvement of the breast can occur with or without evidence of disease at other sites. Evaluation of the extent of the disease is appropriate, including lesion cultures by needle aspiration, biopsy, or wedge resection and milk cultures. Therapy should be with multiple anti-TB medications, but surgery should supplement this, as needed, to remove extensive necrotic tissue or a persistently draining sinus.[18] Neither breastfeeding nor breast milk feeding should be done until the lesion is healed, usually after 2 weeks or more. Continued anti-TB therapy for 6 months in the mother and prophylactic isoniazid for the infant for 3 to 6 months is indicated.

In the absence of tuberculous breast infection in the mother, the transmission of TB through breast milk has not been documented. Thus even though temporary separation of infant and mother may occur pending complete evaluation and initiation of adequate therapy in the mother and prophylactic isoniazid therapy (10 mg/kg/day as a single daily dose) in the infant, breast milk can be expressed and given to the infant during the short separation. Breastfeeding can safely continue when the mother, infant, or both are receiving anti-TB therapy. Anti-TB medications (isoniazid, rifampin, pyrazinamide, aminoglycosides, ethambutol, ethionamide, p-aminosalicylic acid) have been safely used in infancy, and therefore, the presence of

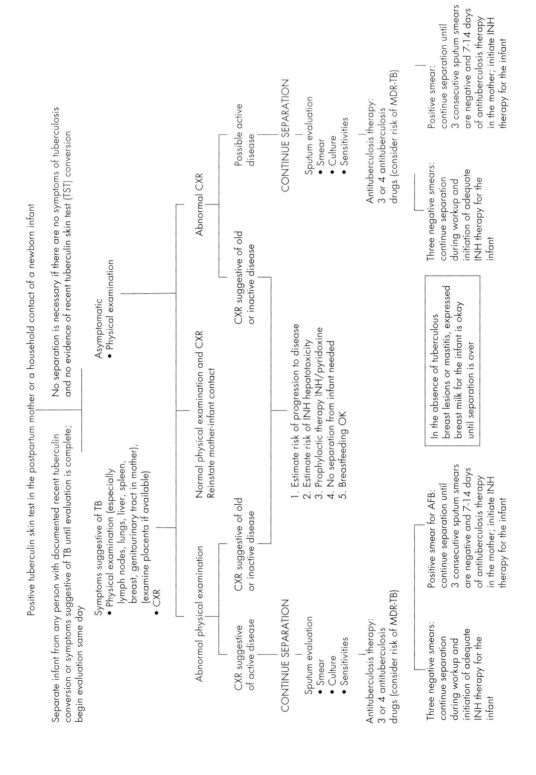

Figure 13-3. Management of a newborn infant exposed to tuberculin-positive household contact. *CXR*, Chest X-ray film; *INH*, isoniazid; *MDR*, multidrug-resistant; *TB*, tuberculosis.

TABLE 13-1 Management of a Newborn Whose Mother (or Other Household Contact) Has Tuberculosis (TB)

Mother/Infant Status	Additional Workup Recommended[1]	Therapy for Mother/Contact	Therapy for Infant	Separation[2]	Breast Milk[3]	Breastfeeding[3]
1. TB infection, no disease[4]	None for mother/contact	Prophylactic[5]	None	No	Yes	Yes
2. TB infection: Abnormal CXR not suggestive of active disease		Decide active vs. inactive disease				
a. Symptoms or physical findings suggestive of active TB	Aerosolized sputum (culture, smears)[6]	Active disease: empiric[5]	Isoniazid[7]	Yes	Yes	No[8]
		Inactive disease: prophylactic[5]	None	No	Yes	Yes
b. No symptoms or physical findings suggestive of active TB	Aerosolized sputum in select cases	Prophylactic[5]	None	No	Yes	Yes
3. TB infection: Abnormal CXR suggestive of active disease	Aerosolized sputum (culture, smears)[6]	Empiric therapy[5]	Isoniazid[7]	Yes	Yes	No[8]
4. Active pulmonary TB: Suspected MDR TB	Aerosolized sputum (culture, smears)[6]	Consult TB specialist for best regimen[9]	Consult pediatric TB specialist[9] Consider bacille Calmette-Guérin vaccine	Yes	Yes	No
5. TB disease: Suspected mastitis[10]	Aerosolized sputum (culture, smears)[6]	Empiric[5]	Isoniazid[7]	Yes	No[11]	No
6. TB infection: Status undertermined[12]	Perform/ interpret CXR within 24 hours			Yes, until CXR interpreted (see a and b)	Yes	No
a. Abnormal CXR not suggestive of active disease	Proceed as in 2		As in 2	As in 2	As in 2	
b. Abnormal CXR suggestive of active disease	Proceed as in 3		As in 3	As in 3	As in 3	

[1]Further workup should always include the evaluation of the TB status of all other household (or close) contacts by tuberculin skin testing (TST), review of symptoms, physical examination, and chest X-ray (CXR). Sputum smears and cultures should be done as indicated.

[2]Separation should occur until interpretation of CXR confirms the absence of active disease, or, with active disease, separation should continue until the individual is no longer considered infectious: three negative consecutive sputum smears, adequate ongoing empiric therapy, and decreased fever, cough, and sputum production. Separation means movement to a different house or location, not simply separate rooms in a household. The duration of separation should be individualized for each case, in consultation with the TB specialist.

[3]This assumes no evidence of breast involvement, suspected TB mastitis, or lesions (except in status 5, when breast involvement is considered). The risk to the infant is via aerosolized bacteria in the sputum from the lung. Expressed breast milk can be given even if separation of mother and infant is advised.

[4]TST positive, no symptoms or physical findings suggestive of TB, negative CXR.

[5]Prophylactic therapy: isoniazid 10 mg/kg/day, maximum 300 mg for 6 months; pyridoxine 25 to 50 mg/day for 6 months. Empiric therapy: standard three- or four-drug regimens for 2 months, and treatment should continue for total of 6 months with isoniazid and rifampin when the organism is shown to be sensitive. Suspected MDR TB requires consultation with a TB specialist to select the optimum empiric regimen and for ongoing monitoring of therapy and clinical response.

Continued

| TABLE 13-1 | Management of a Newborn Whose Mother (or Other Household Contact) Has Tuberculosis (TB)—cont'd |

[6]Sensitivity testing should be done on any positive culture.

[7]Isoniazid 10 mg/kg/day for 3 to 9 months, depending on the mother's or contact's status; repeat TST at 3 months and obtain a normal CXR in the infant before stopping isoniazid. Before beginning therapy, a workup of the infant for congenital or active TB may be appropriate. This workup should be determined based on the clinical status of the infant and the suspected potential risk, and it may include TST after 4 weeks of age, with CXR, complete blood count, and erythrocyte sedimentation rate, liver function tests, cerebrospinal fluid analysis, gastric aspirates, and sonography or computed tomography of liver, spleen, and chest, if congenital TB is suspected.

[8]Breastfeeding is proscribed when the separation of the mother and infant is indicated because of risk for aerosolized transmission of bacteria. Expressed breast milk given to the infant via bottle is acceptable in the absence of mastitis or breast lesions.

[9]Consult with a TB specialist about MDR TB. Empiric therapy will be chosen based on the most recent culture sensitivities of the index patient or perhaps the suspected source case, if known, as well as medication toxicities and other factors.

[10]TB mastitis usually involves a single breast with associated axillary lymph node swelling and, infrequently, a draining sinus tract. It can also present as a painless mass or edema of breast.

[11]With suspected mastitis or breast lesions caused by TB, even breast milk is contraindicated until the lesion or mastitis heals, usually after 2 weeks or more.

[12]Patient has a documented, recent TST conversion, but has not been completely evaluated. Evaluation should begin and CXR should be done and evaluated in less than 24 hours to minimize separation of this person from the infant. Further workup should proceed as indicated by symptoms, physical findings, and CXR results.

Data from the Committee on Infectious Diseases, American Academy of Pediatrics: *Red book: report of the committee on infectious diseases*, ed 26, Elk Grove Village, Ill., 2003, American Academy of Pediatrics.

these medications in smaller amounts in breast milk is not a contraindication to breastfeeding.

Although conflicting, reports indicate that breastfeeding by TST-positive mothers does influence infants' responses to bacille Calmette-Guérin vaccine, the TST, and perhaps the *M. tuberculosis* bacillus. Despite efforts to identify either a soluble substance or specific cell fractions (gamma/delta T cells) in colostrum and breast milk that affect infants' immune responsiveness, no unified theory explains the various reported changes, and no evidence has identified a consistent, clinically significant effect.[43,235,358,409]

Viral Infections

ARBOVIRUSES

Arboviruses were originally a large collection of viruses grouped together because of the common mode of transmission through arthropods. They have now been reclassified into several different families: Bunyaviridae, Togaviridae, Flaviviridae, Reoviridae, and others. They include more than 30 human pathogens.

These organisms primarily produce either CNS infections (encephalitis, meningoencephalitis) or undifferentiated illnesses associated with fever and rash, severe hemorrhagic manifestations, and involvement of other organs (hepatitis, myalgia, polyarthritis). Infection with this array of viruses may also be asymptomatic and subclinical, although how often this occurs is uncertain. Some of the notable human pathogens include Bunyaviridae (California serogroup viruses), *Hantavirus*,

Hantaan virus, *Phlebovirus* (Rift Valley fever), *Nairovirus* (Crimean-Congo hemorrhagic fever), *Alphavirus* (western, eastern, and Venezuelan equine encephalomyelitis viruses, chikungunya virus), *Flavivirus* (St. Louis encephalitis virus, Japanese encephalitis virus, dengue viruses, yellow fever virus, tick-borne encephalitis viruses, West Nile virus), and *Orbivirus* (Colorado tick fever). Other than for Crimean-Congo hemorrhagic fever and for reported cases of Colorado tick fever associated with transfusion, direct person-to-person spread has rarely been described. Outbreaks in 2005 and 2007 of chikungunya virus infection in Reunion Island and in India appear to have involved infection in young infants probably secondary to vertical spread from mother to infant transplacentally.[162,379,468] A few cases of early fetal deaths were associated with infection in pregnant women. The cases of vertical transmission occurred with near-term infection in the mothers, and the infants developed illness within 3 to 7 days of delivery.[162,379] No evidence for transmission via breast milk or breastfeeding is available.

Overall, little evidence indicates that these organisms can be transmitted through breast milk. The exceptions to this include evidence of transmission of three flaviviruses via breast milk: dengue virus, West Nile virus, and yellow fever vaccine virus. Standard precautions are generally sufficient. With any of these infections in a breastfeeding mother, the severity of the illness may determine the mother's ability to continue breastfeeding. Providing the infant with expressed breast milk is acceptable. (See the discussion of dengue virus, West Nile virus, and yellow fever vaccine virus later in this chapter.)

In general, treatment for these illnesses is supportive. However, ribavirin appears to decrease the severity of and mortality from *Hantavirus* pulmonary syndrome, hemorrhagic fever with renal failure, and Crimean-Congo hemorrhagic fever. Ribavirin has been described as teratogenic in various animal species and is contraindicated in pregnant women. No information is available concerning ribavirin in breast milk, with limited information available on the use of intravenous or oral ribavirin in infants.

ARENAVIRUSES

Arenaviruses are single-stranded ribonucleic acid (RNA) viruses that infect rodents and are acquired by humans through the rodents. The six major human pathogens in this group are (1) lymphocytic choriomeningitis virus, (2) Lassa fever virus, (3) Junin virus (Argentine hemorrhagic fever), (4) Machupo virus (Bolivian hemorrhagic fever), (5) Guanarito virus (Venezuelan hemorrhagic fever), and (6) Sabia virus. The geographic distribution of these viruses and the illness they cause are determined by the living range of the host rodent (reservoir). The exact mechanism of transmission to humans is unknown and hotly debated.[27,76,145] Direct contact and aerosolization of rodent excretions and secretions are probable mechanisms.

Lymphocytic choriomeningitis virus is well recognized in Europe, the Americas, and other areas. Perinatal maternal infection can lead to severe disease in the newborn, but no evidence suggests transmission through breast milk.[31,246] Standard precautions with breastfeeding are appropriate.

Lassa fever (West Africa) and Argentine hemorrhagic fever (Argentine pampas) are usually more severe illnesses, with dramatic bleeding and involvement of other organs, including the brain. These fevers more frequently lead to shock and death than do the forms of hemorrhagic fever caused by the other viruses in this group. Person-to-person spread of Lassa fever is believed to be common, and transmission within households does occur.[233] This may relate to prolonged viremia and excretion of the virus in the urine of humans for up to 30 days.[370] The possibility of persistent virus in human urine, semen, and blood after infection exists for each of the arenaviruses. The possibility of airborne transmission is undecided. Current recommendations by the CDC[76] are to use contact precautions for the duration of the illness in situations of suspected viral hemorrhagic fever. No substantial information describes the infectivity of various body fluids, including breast milk, for these different viral hemorrhagic fevers. Considering the severity of the illness in mothers and the risk to the infants, it is reasonable to avoid breastfeeding in these situations if alternative forms of infant nutrition can be provided for the short term.

As more information becomes available, reassessment of these recommendations is advisable. A vaccine is in trials in endemic areas for Junin virus and Argentine hemorrhagic fever.[237] Preliminary studies suggest it will be effective, but data are still being accumulated concerning the vaccine's use in children and pregnant or breastfeeding women.

CYTOMEGALOVIRUS

CMV is one of the human herpesviruses. Congenital infection of infants, postnatal infection of premature infants, and infection of immune-deficient individuals represent the most serious forms of this infection in children. The time at which the virus infects the fetus or infant and the presence or absence of antibodies against CMV from the mother are important determinants of the severity of infection and the likelihood of significant sequelae (congenital infection syndrome, deafness, chorioretinitis, abnormal neurodevelopment, learning disabilities).[258] About 1% of all infants are born excreting CMV at birth, and approximately 5% of these congenitally infected infants will demonstrate evidence of infection at birth (approximately 5 symptomatic cases per 10,000 live births). Approximately 15% of infants born after primary infection in a pregnant woman will manifest at least one sequela of prenatal infection.[106]

Various studies have detected that 3% to 28% of pregnant women have CMV in cervical cultures and that 4% to 5% of pregnant women have CMV in their urine.[132,190] Perinatal infection certainly occurs through contact with virus in these fluids, but it is not usually associated with clinical illness in full-term infants. The lack of illness is thought to result from the transplacental passive transfer of protective antibodies from the mother.

Postnatal infection later in infancy occurs via breastfeeding or contact with infected fluids (e.g., saliva, urine), but, again, it rarely causes clinical illness in full-term infants. Seroepidemiologic studies have documented the transmission of infection in infancy, with higher rates of transmission occurring in day care centers, especially when the prevalence of CMV in the urine and saliva is high. CMV has been identified in the milk of CMV-seropositive women at varying rates (10% to 85%), using viral cultures or CMV deoxyribonucleic acid (DNA) PCR.[190,340,442,478] CMV is more often identified in the breast milk of seropositive mothers than in vaginal fluids, urine, and saliva. The CMV isolation rate from colostrum is lower than that from mature milk.[190,441] The reason for the large degree of variability in the identification of CMV in breast milk in these studies probably relates to the intermittent nature of the reactivation and excretion of the virus, in addition to the variability, frequency, and duration of sampling of breast milk in the different studies. Some authors have hypothesized that the difference in isolation rates between breast milk and other fluids is caused by viral reactivation in cells (leukocytes or monocytes) in the breast leading to "selective" excretion in breast milk.[340] Vochem et al.[478] reported that the rate of virolactia was greatest at 3 to 4 weeks postpartum, and Yeager et al.[506] reported significant virolactia between 2 and 12 weeks postpartum. Antibodies (e.g., secretory IgA) to CMV are present in breast milk, along with various cytokines and other proteins (e.g., lactoferrin). These may influence virus binding to cells, but they do not prevent transmission of infection.[6,7,258,316,340,369,503]

Several studies have documented increased rates of postnatal CMV infection in breastfed infants (50% to 69%), compared with bottle-fed infants (12% to 27%), observed through the first year of life.[132,316,442,478] In these same studies, full-term infants who acquired CMV infection postnatally were only rarely mildly symptomatic at the time of seroconversion or documented viral excretion. Also, no evidence of late sequelae from CMV was found in these infants.

Postnatal exposure of susceptible infants to CMV, including premature infants without passively acquired maternal antibodies against CMV, infants born to CMV-seronegative mothers, and immunodeficient infants, can cause significant clinical illness (pneumonitis, hepatitis, thrombocytopenia).[64,115,187,186,271,301] In one study of premature infants followed up to 12 months, Vochem et al.[478] found CMV transmission in 17 of 29 infants (59%) exposed to CMV virolactia and breastfed, as compared with no infants among the 27 exposed to breast milk without CMV. No infant was given CMV-seropositive donor milk or blood. Five of the 12 infants who developed CMV infection after 2 months of age had mild signs of illness, including transient neutropenia, and only one infant had a short increase in episodes of apnea and a period of thrombocytopenia. Five other premature infants with CMV infection before 2 months of age had acute illness, including sepsis-like symptoms, apnea with bradycardia, hepatitis, leukopenia, and prolonged thrombocytopenia.[478] In a prospective study done in the United States, Josephson et al.[224] examined the role of transfusions and breastmilk causing CMV infection in VLBW infants. In the mothers, the seroprevalence of CMV was 76.2% (352/462). In 301 infants receiving 2061 transfusions of CMV-seronegative and leukoreduced blood, there were no CMV infections linked to transfusion. Postnatal CMV infection had a cumulative incidence at 12 weeks

post birth of 6.9% (95% CI, 4.2% to 9.2%), and 5 of 29 CMV-infected infants developed symptomatic disease or died. Twenty-seven of the 29 infants received CMV-positive breast milk. Factors associated with a higher risk of postnatal CMV infection were a higher CMV viral load in the breast milk and a higher number of breast milk-fed days. This study also demonstrated that the use of CMV-seronegative and leukoreduced blood products is effective at preventing transfusion-related CMV infection. In a systematic review and meta-analysis, Lanzieri et al.[268] utilized data from 17 studies published between 2001 and 2011. They reported on 299 infants who received untreated breast milk. Of these infants, 19% acquired CMV infection and 4% developed a sepsis-like syndrome related to CVM infection. Among the 212 infants included who received frozen breast milk (at various temperatures and durations in different studies—18° C to 20° C for over 24 hours or 72 hours), 13% developed CMV infection and 5% had an associated sepsis-like syndrome. Although the overall rate of CMV infection related to breast milk was slightly lower in the untreated breast milk group there was no difference in the occurrence of sepsis-like syndrome in the two groups.

Relative to long-term sequelae related to postnatal CMV infection in VLBW infants, Vollmer et al.[479] followed premature infants with early postnatal CMV infection acquired through breast milk for 2 to 4.5 years to assess neurodevelopment and hearing function. None of the children had sensorineural hearing loss. There was no difference between the 22 CMV-infected children and 22 matched premature control CMV-negative infants in terms of neurologic, speech and language or motor development.[479] Neuberger et al.[333] examined the symptoms and neonatal outcome of CMV infection transmitted via human milk in premature infants in a case-control fashion; 40 CMV-infected premature infants were compared with 40 CMV-negative matched premature infants. Neutropenia, thrombocytopenia, and cholestasis were associated with CMV infection in these infants. No other serious effects or illnesses were found directly associated with the infection, including intraventricular hemorrhage, periventricular leukomalacia, retinopathy of prematurity, necrotizing enterocolitis, bronchopulmonary dysplasia, duration of mechanical ventilation or oxygen therapy, duration of hospital stay or weight, gestational age, or head circumference at the time of discharge. More recent studies do not clarify the long-term effects on the neurodevelopmental status of premature or LBW infants with symptomatic postnatal CMV infection.[45,171,464] They present contradictory evidence concerning the occurrence of adverse neurologic outcomes or sensorineural hearing loss in these children.

Exposure of CMV-seronegative, premature, or VLBW infants to CMV-positive milk (donor or natural mother's) should be avoided.[422] Various methods of inactivating CMV in breast milk have been reported, including HP, freezing ($-20°C$ for 3 days), and brief high temperature ($72°C$ for 10 seconds).[132,150,173,438,506] One small prospective study suggests that freezing breast milk at $-20\ °C$ for 72 hours protects premature infants from CMV infection via breast milk. Sharland et al.[422] reported on 18 premature infants (less than 32 weeks) who were uninfected at birth and exposed to breast milk from their CMV-seropositive mothers. Only 1 of 18 (5%) infants became positive for CMV at 62 days of life, and this infant was clinically asymptomatic. This transmission rate is considerably lower than others reported in the literature. CM-seronegative and leukocyte-depleted blood products were used routinely. Banked breast milk was pasteurized and stored at $-20°C$ for various time periods, and maternal expressed breast milk was frozen at $-20°C$ before use whenever possible. The infants received breast milk for a median of 34 days (range: 11 to 74 days), and they were observed for a median of 67 days (range: 30 to 192 days). Breast milk samples pre- or postfreezing were not analyzed by PCR or culture for the presence of CMV.[422] Buxmann et al.[64] demonstrated no transmission of CMV in 23 premature infants receiving thawed frozen breast milk until 33 weeks (gestational age + postnatal age) (less than or equal to 31 weeks' gestational age) born to 19 mothers who were CMV-IgG negative. CMV infection was found in 5 premature infants of 35 infants born to 29 mothers who were CMV-IgG positive and who provided breast milk for their infants. Three of the five children remained asymptomatic. One child developed a respirator-dependent pneumonia, and the second developed an upper respiratory tract infection and thrombocytopenia in association with their CMV infections.[64] Yasuda et al.[505] reported on 43 preterm infants (median gestational age 31 weeks), demonstrating a peak in CMV DNA copies, detected by a real-time PCR assay, in breast milk at 4 to 6 weeks postpartum. Thirty of the 43 infants received CMV DNA-positive breast milk. Three of the 30 had CMV DNA detected in their sera, but none of the three had symptoms suggestive of CMV infection. Much of the breast milk had been stored at $-20°C$ before feeding, which the authors propose is the probable reason for less transmission in this cohort.[505] Lee et al.[276] reported on the use of maternal milk frozen at $-20\ °C$ for a minimum of 24 hours before feeding to premature infants in a NICU; 23 infants had CMV-seropositive mothers and 39 infants had CMV-seronegative mothers. Two infants developed CMV infection, which was symptomatic. They were both fed frozen and then thawed milk from CMV-seropositive mothers.[276] Others have reported individual cases of CMV infection in premature infants despite freezing and thawing breast milk.[302,353] More recent studies, including a prospective cohort study of breast milk transmission of CMV by Josephson et al.[224] and a systematic review and meta-analysis of breast milk-acquired CMV infection in VLBW and premature infants by Lanzieri et al.,[268] demonstrate that frozen-thawed breast milk provides minimal protection, at best, against breast milk-acquired CMV infection.[224,268] It is clear that the simple freezing and thawing of breast milk does not completely prevent transmission of CMV to premature and VLBW infants. The efficacy of freezing and thawing breast milk for varying lengths of time to prevent CMV infection in premature infants has not been studied prospectively in a randomized controlled trial. Eleven of 36 neonatal units in Sweden (27 of which have their own milk banks) freeze maternal milk to reduce the risk for CMV transmission to premature infants.[353]

A prominent group of neonatologists and pediatric infectious disease experts in California, who recognize the significant benefits of providing human milk to premature and LBW infants, recommend screening mothers of premature infants for CMV IgG at delivery and, when an infant's mother is CMV IgG positive at delivery, using either pasteurized banked human milk or frozen and then thawed maternal breast milk for premature infants until they reach the age of 32 weeks.[496] In consideration of the low rates of CMV virolactia in colostrum[186,442] and the predominant occurrence of virolactia between 2 and 12 weeks (peak at 3 to 4 weeks) postpartum,[478,506] they reasonably propose beginning colostrum and breast milk feedings for all infants until the maternal CMV-serologic screening is complete. They recommend close observation and follow-up of premature infants older than 3 weeks of age for signs, symptoms, and laboratory changes of CMV infection until discharge from the hospital or out to 32 weeks postconceptual age.[496] Additional research and discussion will be necessary to devise a protocol for the use of human milk in premature and VLBW infants to optimize their growth, development, and immune protection at the same time as preventing the risk of acquiring postnatal CMV infection.

There has been much discussion of the use of CMV immunoglobulin and/or antiviral medications (acyclovir, ganciclovir, valganciclovir) to treat women during pregnancy in order to protect against congenital CMV infection. Although these agents have also been used to treat infants with symptomatic congenital CMV and symptomatic acute postnatal CMV infection, they have not been studied as prophylaxis against postnatal CMV infection.

Full-term infants can be safely fed human milk from CMV-seropositive mothers because, despite a higher rate of CMV infection than in formula-fed infants observed through the first year of life, infection in this situation is not associated with significant clinical illness or acute or long-term sequelae.

DENGUE DISEASE

Dengue viruses (serotypes dengue 1 to 4) are flaviviruses associated primarily with febrile illnesses and rash; dengue fever, dengue hemorrhagic fever, and dengue shock syndrome. The mosquito *Aedes aegypti* is the main vector of transmission of dengue virus in countries lying between latitudes 35 degrees north and 35 degrees south. More than 2.5 billion people live in areas where transmission occurs; dengue virus infects over 100 million individuals a year and causes approximately 24,000 deaths per year.[177,181] Although dengue hemorrhagic fever and dengue shock syndrome occur frequently in children younger than 1 year of age, they are infrequently described in infants younger than 3 months of age.[185] There are also differences in the clinical and laboratory findings of dengue virus infection in children, as compared to adults.[244] Boussemart et al.[56] reported on two cases of perinatal/prenatal transmission of dengue and discussed eight additional cases in neonates from the literature. Prenatal or intrapartum transmission of the same type of dengue as the mother was confirmed by serology, culture, or PCR. Phongsamart et al.[373] described three additional cases of dengue virus infection late in pregnancy, with apparent transmission to two of the three infants and passive acquisition of antibody in the third infant. Sirinavin et al.[430] reported on 17 cases in the literature of vertical dengue infection, all presenting at less than 2 weeks of age, but no observations or discussion of breast milk or breastfeeding as a potential source of infection were published. Watanaveeradej et al.[487] presented an additional three cases of dengue infection in infants, documenting normal growth and development at follow-up at 12 months of age.

It has been postulated that more severe disease associated with dengue disease occurs when an individual has specific IgG against the same serotype as the infecting strain in a set concentration, leading to antibody-dependent enhancement of infection. The presence of preexisting dengue serotype-specific IgG in an infant implies either previous primary infection with the same serotype, passive acquisition of IgG from the mother (who had a previous primary infection with the same serotype), or perhaps acquisition of specific IgG from breast milk. Watanaveeradej et al.[487] documented transplacentally transferred antibodies

against all four serotypes of dengue virus in 97% of 2000 cord sera at delivery. Follow-up of 100 infants documented the loss of antibodies to dengue virus over time, with losses of 3%, 19%, 72%, 99%, and 100% at 2, 4, 6, 9, and 12 months of age, respectively.

No evidence is available in the literature about more severe disease in breastfed infants compared with formula-fed infants. There is no evidence of the interperson transmission of dengue virus in the absence of a mosquito vector. There is one case report of apparent transmission of dengue virus via breast milk to a 4-day-old infant, however. The mother had clinical illness consistent with dengue virus disease at delivery, and the infant developed disease on day 4 of life. The mother's blood was positive for dengue virus by RT-PCR on days 0 to 6 after delivery, and her breast milk was positive on days 2 and 4 after delivery. The infant's blood from days 0 and 2 and the cord blood were repeatedly negative by RT-PCR, but subsequently, the infant's blood was PCR positive for dengue virus on days 4 to 13 of life.[30] There is one report of a factor in the lipid portion of breast milk, which inhibits the dengue virus, but no evidence for antibody activity against the dengue virus in human breast milk is known.[140] Given the apparent rarity of the transmission of dengue virus via breast milk, breastfeeding during maternal or infant dengue disease should continue, as determined by the mother's or infant's severity of illness.

EPSTEIN-BARR VIRUS

Epstein-Barr virus (EBV) is a common infection in children, adolescents, and young adults. It is usually asymptomatic, but it most notably causes infectious mononucleosis and has been associated with chronic fatigue syndrome, Burkitt lymphoma, and nasopharyngeal carcinoma. Because EBV is one of the human herpesviruses, concern has been raised about lifelong latent infection and the potential risk for infection to a fetus and neonate from the mother. Primary EBV infection during pregnancy is unusual because few pregnant women are susceptible.[165,207] Although abortion, premature birth, and congenital infection from EBV are suspected, no distinct group of anomalies is linked to EBV infection in the fetus or neonate. Also, no virologic evidence of EBV as the cause of abnormalities was found in association with suspected EBV infection.

Culturing of EBV from various fluids or sites is difficult. The virus is detected by its capacity to transform B lymphocytes into persistent lymphoblastoid cell lines. PCR and DNA hybridization studies have detected EBV in the cervix and in breast milk. One study, which identified EBV DNA in breast milk cells in more than 40% of women donating milk to a breast milk bank, demonstrated that only 17% had antibodies to EBV (only IgG, no IgM).[225] EBV DNA was identified in 33% of 40 human milk samples from normal lactating women in a separate study.[169] However, a study by Kusuhara et al. examining serologic specimens from breastfed and bottle-fed infants showed similar seroprevalence of EBV at 12 to 23 months of age (36/66 [54.5%] and 24/43 [55.8%]) in the breastfed and bottle-fed children, respectively.[260] This suggests that early acquisition of EBV infection in infants is not significantly affected by the consumption of breast milk.

The question of the timing of EBV infection and the subsequent immune response and clinical disease produced requires continued study. Differences exist among the clinical syndromes that manifest at different ages. Infants and young children are asymptomatic, have illness not recognized as related to EBV, or have mild episodes of illness, including fever, lymphadenopathy, rhinitis, cough, hepatosplenomegaly, and rash. Adolescents or young adults who experience primary EBV infection more often demonstrate infectious mononucleosis syndrome or are asymptomatic. Chronic fatigue syndrome is more common in adolescents and young adults. Burkitt lymphoma, observed primarily in Africa, and nasopharyngeal carcinoma, seen in southeast Asia, where primary EBV infection usually occurs in young children, are tumors associated with early EBV infection.[273] These tumors are related to "chronic" EBV infection and tend to occur in individuals with persistently high antibody titers to EBV viral capsid antigen and early antigen. The questions of why these tumors occur with much greater frequency in these geographic areas and what cofactors (including altered immune response to infection associated with coinfections, immune escape by EBV leading to malignancy, or increased resistance to apoptosis secondary to EBV gene mutations) may contribute to their development remain unanswered.[23,326]

It also remains unknown to what degree breast milk could be a source of early EBV infection, as compared to other sources of EBV infection in an infant's environment. Similar to the situation of postnatal transmission of CMV in immunocompetent infants, clinically significant illness rarely is associated with primary EBV infection in infants. More data concerning the pathogenesis of EBV-associated tumors should be obtained before proscribing against breastfeeding is warranted, especially in areas where these tumors are common but the protective benefits of breastfeeding are high. In areas where Burkitt lymphoma and nasopharyngeal carcinoma are uncommon, EBV infection in mother or infant is certainly not a contraindication to breastfeeding.

FILOVIRIDAE

Marburg and Ebola viruses cause severe and highly fatal hemorrhagic fevers. The illness often presents with nonspecific symptoms (conjunctivitis, frontal headache, malaise, myalgia, bradycardia) and progresses with worsening hemorrhage to shock and subsequent death in 50% to 90% of patients. Person-to-person transmission through direct contact, droplet spread, or airborne spread is the common mode of transmission. However, the animal reservoir or source of these viruses in nature for human infection has not been identified. Attack rates in families are 5% to 16%.[370] No postexposure interventions have proved useful in preventing spread, and no treatment other than supportive is currently available.

One report documented the presence of Ebola virus in numerous body fluids, including breast milk. One acute breast milk sample on day 7 after the onset of illness in the mother and a "convalescent" breast milk sample on day 15 from the same woman were positive for Ebola virus by both culture and PCR testing.[33] In the same study, testing other body fluids in different persons, saliva remained virus positive for a mean of 16 days after disease onset, urine was positive for a mean of 28 days, and semen for a mean of 43 days after the onset of disease in survivors of Ebola infection.

No information is available concerning the risk for transmission of these viruses in breast milk or additional risks or benefits from breastfeeding in an area involved in an Ebola outbreak or with household members who are infected.

Contact precautions have been recommended for Marburg and Ebola virus infections and contact and airborne precautions for Ebola virus infection. The largest epidemic of EVD in West Africa (predominantly Guinea, Liberia, Sierra Leone), involving over 21,000 cases and over 8400 deaths, occurred through 2014 to 2015.[92] This outbreak has dramatically raised concerns about the transmission of Ebola to family members, close contacts, travelers, and health care personnel. To date, there are no newer publications for this epidemic on transmissibility from different body fluids and particularly from breast milk. The WHO and CDC have developed updated guidance for the use of personal protective equipment for health care workers (CDCP http://www.cdc.gov/vhf/ebola/hcp/procedures-for-ppe.html). This guidance continues to be updated (CDCP http://www.cdc.gov/media/releases/2014/fs1020-ebola-personal-protective-equipment.html). Both of these guidelines reinforce the high risk of Ebola virus infection without careful protection against contact with body fluids from a person with EVD. Given the high attack and mortality rates associated with EVD, these precautions should be carefully instituted within health care facilities, and breastfeeding should not be allowed if the mother has suspected EVD. If any other suitable source of nutrition can be found for an infant, expressed breast milk should also be proscribed for the infant of a mother with either of these infections for at least 3 weeks postrecovery.

Hepatitis in the Mother

The diagnosis of hepatitis in a pregnant woman or nursing mother causes significant anxiety. The first issue is determining the etiology of the hepatitis, which then allows for an informed discussion of risk to the fetus or infant. The differential diagnosis of acute hepatitis includes (1) common causes of hepatitis, such as hepatitis A, B, C, and D; (2) uncommon causes of hepatitis, such as hepatitis E and G, CMV, echoviruses, enteroviruses, EBV, HSV, rubella, varicella-zoster virus, yellow fever virus; (3) rare causes of hepatitis, such as Ebola virus, Junin virus, and Machupo virus (cause hemorrhagic fever), Lassa virus, and Marburg virus; and (4) nonviral causes, such as hepatotoxic drugs, alcoholic hepatitis, toxoplasmosis, autoimmune hepatitis, bile duct obstruction, ischemic liver damage, Wilson disease, α_1-antitrypsin deficiency, and metastatic liver disease. The following sections focus on hepatitis viruses A to G. Other infectious agents that can cause hepatitis are considered individually in other sections. Box 13-2 provides hepatitis terminology.

Martin et al.[299] outline a succinct diagnostic approach to a patient with acute viral hepatitis and chronic viral hepatitis (Figures 13-4 and 13-5). The approach involves using the four serologic markers (IgM anti-hepatitis A virus, hepatitis B surface antigen [HBsAg], IgM anti-HBcAg, anti-HCV) as the initial diagnostic tests. Simultaneous consideration of other etiologies of acute liver dysfunction is appropriate depending on a patient's history. If the initial diagnostic tests are all negative, subsequent additional testing for anti-hepatitis D virus (HDV), HCV RNA, hepatis G virus (HGV) RNA, anti-hepatitis E virus (HEV), or HEV RNA may be necessary. If initial testing reveals positive HBsAg, testing for anti-HDV, HBeAg, and HBV DNA is appropriate. These additional tests are useful in defining the prognosis for a mother and the risk for infection to an infant. During the diagnostic evaluation, it is appropriate to discuss with the mother or parents the theoretic risk for transmitting infectious agents that cause hepatitis via breastfeeding. The discussion should include an evaluation of the positive and negative effects of suspending or continuing breastfeeding until the exact etiologic diagnosis is determined. The relative risk for

BOX 13-2. Terminology for Hepatitis

Hepatitis A Virus (HAV)

IgM anti-HAV	Immunoglobulin M (IgM) antibody against HAV
HAV RNA	HAV ribonucleic acid

Hepatitis B Virus (HBV)

HBsAg	Hepatitis B surface antigen
HBeAg	Hepatitis Be antigen
HBcAg	Hepatitis B core antigen
Anti-HBe	Antibody against hepatitis Be antigen
IgM anti-HBcAg	IgM antibody against hepatitis B core antigen
HBV DNA	HBV deoxyribonucleic acid
HBIG	Hepatitis B immunoglobulin

Hepatitis C Virus (HCV)

Anti-HCV	Antibody against HCV
HCV RNA	HCV ribonucleic acid

Hepatitis D Virus (HDV)

Anti-HDV	Antibody against HDV

Hepatitis E Virus (HEV)

HEV RNA	HEV ribonucleic acid

Hepatitis G Virus (HGV)

HGV RNA	HGV ribonucleic acid

TT Virus (TTV)

TTV DNA	TT virus deoxyribonucleic acid

Other

NANBH	Non-A, non-B hepatitis
ISG	Immune serum globulin

transmission of infection to an infant can be estimated and specific preventive measures provided for the infant (Table 13-2).

HEPATITIS A

Hepatitis A virus (HAV) is usually an acute self-limited infection. The illness is typically mild, and it is generally subclinical in infants. Occasionally, HAV infection is prolonged or relapsing, extending 3 to 6 months, and rarely, it is fulminant, but HAV infection does not lead to chronic infection. The incidence of prematurity after maternal HAV infection is increased, but no evidence to date indicates obvious birth defects or a congenital syndrome.[415,517] HAV infection in premature infants may lead to prolonged viral shedding.[391] Transmission is most often person to person (fecal-oral), and transmission in foodborne or waterborne epidemics has been described. Transmission via blood products and vertical transmission (mother to infant) are

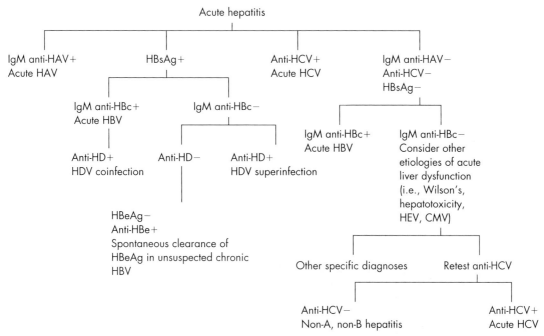

Figure 13-4. Diagnostic approach to a patient with acute viral hepatitis. See Box 13-2 for definitions of abbreviations. (From Martin P, Friedman L, Dienstag J: Diagnostic approach. In Zuckerman A, Thomas H, editors: *Viral hepatitis: scientific basis and clinical management,* Edinburgh, 1993, Churchill Livingstone.)

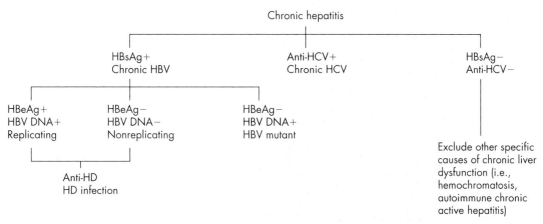

Figure 13-5. Diagnostic approach to a patient with chronic viral hepatitis. See Box 13-2 for definitions of abbreviations. (From Martin P, Friedman L, Dienstag J: Diagnostic approach. In Zuckerman A, Thomas H, editors: *Viral hepatitis: scientific basis and clinical management,* Edinburgh, 1993, Churchill Livingstone.)

rare.[488] Transmission in day care settings has been clearly described.

Infection with HAV in newborns is uncommon and does not seem to be a significant problem. The usual period of viral shedding and presumed contagiousness lasts 1 to 3 weeks. Acute maternal HAV infection in the last trimester or in the postpartum period could lead to infection in an infant. Symptomatic infection can be prevented by immunoglobulin (Ig) administration, and 80% to 90% of disease can be prevented by Ig administration within 2 weeks of exposure. HAV vaccine can be administered simultaneously with Ig without

affecting the seroconversion rate to produce rapid and prolonged HAV serum antibody levels.

The transmission of HAV via breast milk has been implicated in one case report, but no data exist on the frequency of isolating HAV from breast milk.[488] Because HAV infection in infancy is rare and usually subclinical without chronic disease and because exposure has already occurred by the time the etiologic diagnosis of hepatitis in a mother is made, no reason exists to interrupt breastfeeding with maternal HAV infection. The infant should receive Ig and HAV vaccine, administered simultaneously.

TABLE 13-2 Viral Hepatitis in Association With Breastfeeding*

Hepatitis	Virus	Identified in Breast Milk	Factors for Perinatal/Postnatal Transmission	Prevention	Breastfeeding†
A	Picornaviridae (RNA)	?	Vertical transmission uncertain or rare	ISG	Limited evidence of transmission via breastfeeding or of serious disease in infants
			HAV in pregnancy associated with premature birth	HAV vaccine	Breastfeeding OK after ISG and vaccine
B	Hepadnaviridae (DNA)	HBsAg	Increased risk for vertical transmission with	HBIG	Low theoretic risk
		HBV DNA	HBeAg+, in countries where HBV is endemic, or early in maternal infection, before Ab production	HBV vaccine	Virtually no risk after HBIG and HBV vaccine, breastfeeding OK after HBIG and vaccine
C	Flavivirus (RNA)	HCV RNA detected	Increased risk when mother HIV+ and HCV+ or with increased HCV RNA titers	None	Positive theoretic risk, inadequate data on relative risk, breastfeeding OK after informed discussion with parents
			Vertical transmission uncommon		
D	Delavirdine (RNA−strand, circular)	?	Requires coinfection/superinfection with HBV	None (except to prevent HBV infection, give HBIG/HBV vaccine)	Prevent HBV infection with HBIG and vaccine
			Vertical transmission rare		Breastfeeding OK after HBIG and vaccine
E	Caliciviridae (RNA)	+	Severe disease in pregnant women (20% mortality)	ISG and subunit vaccine being tested	Usually subclinical infection in children, breastfeeding OK
G	Related to calicivirus and flavivirus (RNA)	?	Vertical transmission occurs	None	Inadequate data
TT	TT virus (DNA, circular, single stranded)	TTV DNA detected	Vertical transmission occurs	None	Inadequate data

*See Box 13-2 for abbreviations. *Ab,* Antibody; *HIV,* human immunodeficiency virus.
†With any type of infectious hepatitis, discussion of what is known and not known concerning transmission should be related to the mother/parents, and an informed decision can then be made by the involved adults concerning breastfeeding.
  Data from Committee on Infectious Diseases, American Academy of Pediatrics: *Red book: report of the committee on infectious diseases,* ed 26, Elk Grove, Ill., 2003, American Academy of Pediatrics.

HEPATITIS B

HBV infection leads to a broad spectrum of illness, including asymptomatic seroconversion, nonspecific symptoms (fever, malaise, fatigue), clinical hepatitis with or without jaundice, extrahepatic manifestations (arthritis, rash, renal involvement), fulminant hepatitis, and chronic HBV infection. Chronic HBV infection occurs in up to 90% of infants infected via perinatal and vertical transmission and in 30% of children infected between 1 and 5 years of age. Given the increased risk for significant sequelae from chronic infection (chronic active hepatitis, chronic persistent hepatitis, cirrhosis, primary hepatocellular carcinoma), the prevention of HBV infection in infancy is crucial. Transmission of HBV is usually through blood or body fluids (stool, semen, saliva, urine, cervical secretions).[102]

Vertical transmission, either transplacentally or perinatally during delivery, has been well described throughout the world. Vertical transmission rates in areas where HBV is endemic (Taiwan and Japan) are high, whereas transmission to infants from HBV-carrier mothers in other areas where HBV carrier rates are low is uncommon.[444] The transmission of HBV to infants occurs in up to 50% of infants when the mothers are acutely infected immediately before, during, or soon after pregnancy.[514]

HBsAg is found in breast milk, but transmission by this route is not well documented. Beasley[34] and Beasley et al.[35] demonstrated that, although breast milk transmission is possible, seroconversion rates were no different between breastfed and non-breastfed infants in a long-term follow-up study of 147 HBsAg-positive mothers. Hill et al. [194] followed 101 breastfed infants and 268 formula-fed infants born to women who were chronically HBsAg positive. All infants received HBIg at birth and a full series of hepatitis B vaccine. None of the breastfed infants and nine of the formula-fed infants were positive for HBsAg after completion of the HBV vaccine series. Breastfeeding had occurred for a mean of 4.9 months (range: 2 weeks to 1 year). Transmission, when it does happen, probably occurs during labor and delivery. Another report from China followed 230 infants born to HBsAg-positive women. The infants received the appropriate dosing and timing of HBIG and HBV vaccine. At 1 year of age, anti-HBs antibodies were present in 90.9% of the breastfed infants and 90.3% of the bottle-fed infants.[486] Risk factors associated with immunoprophylaxis failure against vertical transmission of HBV include HBeAg-seropositive mothers and elevated HBV DNA "viral loads" in the mothers.[437] Zhang et al. also demonstrated in over 67,000 pregnant women and 1150 HBsAg-positive mothers that breastfeeding did not increase the risk of HBV mother-to-child transmission, as compared to formula-fed infants.[516] A systematic review and meta-analysis by Shi et al. including 10 controlled clinical trials reported an odds ratio for the development of hepatitis B surface antibodies in breastfeeding infants, compared with non-breastfeeding infants, of 0.98 (CI 0.69 to 1.40).[424] In 2009, the AAP Committee on Infectious Diseases stated "that breastfeeding of the infant by a HBsAg-positive mother poses no additional risk for acquisition of HBV infection by the infant with appropriate administration of hepatitis B vaccine and HBIG."[103]

Screening of all pregnant women for HBV infection is an essential first step to preventing vertical transmission. Universal HBV vaccination at birth and during infancy, with the administration of HBIg immediately after birth to infants of HBsAg-positive mothers, prevents HBV transmission in more than 95% of cases. Breastfeeding by HBsAg-positive women is not contraindicated, but the immediate administration of HBIG and HBV vaccine should occur. Two subsequent doses of vaccine should be given at appropriate intervals and dosages for the specific HBV vaccine product. This decreases the small theoretic risk for HBV transmission from breastfeeding to almost zero.

When acute peripartum or postpartum hepatitis occurs in a mother and HBV infection is a possibility, with its associated increased risk for transmission to the infant, a discussion with the mother or parents should identify the potential risks and benefits of continuing breastfeeding until the etiology of the hepatitis can be determined. If an appropriate alternative source of nutrition is available for the infant, breast milk should be withheld until the etiology of the hepatitis is identified. HBIG and HBV vaccine can be administered to the infant who has not already been immunized or has no documented immunity against HBV.[445] If acute HBV infection is documented in a mother, breastfeeding can continue after immunization has begun.

HEPATITIS C

Acute infection with HCV can be indistinguishable from hepatitis A or B infection; however, it is typically asymptomatic or mild. HCV infection is the major cause of blood-borne non-A, non-B hepatitis (NANBH). Chronic HCV infection is reported to occur 70% to 85% of the time regardless of age at time of infection. Sequelae of chronic HCV infection are similar to those associated with chronic HBV infection. Bortolotti et al.[54] described two groups of children with HCV infection who they observed for 12 to 48 months. The first group of 14 children, who acquired HCV infection early in life, presumably from their mothers, demonstrated biochemical evidence of liver disease in the first 12 months of life. Two of these children subsequently cleared the viremia and had normal liver function, an additional three children developed normal liver function despite persistent HCV viremia, and the remaining children had persistent viremia and abnormal liver function. The second group of 16 children, with chronic HCV infection, remained free of clinical symptoms of hepatitis, but 10 (62%) of them had mild alanine aminotransferase elevations, and 7 of the 16

(44%) who had liver biopsies had histologic evidence of mild to moderate hepatitis.

The two commonly identified mechanisms of transmission of HCV are transfusions of blood or blood products and IV drug use. However, other routes of transmission exist because HCV infection occurs even in the absence of obvious direct contact with significant amounts of blood. Other body fluids contaminated with blood probably serve as sources of infection. Transmission through sexual contact occurs infrequently and probably requires additional contributing factors, such as coinfection with other sexually transmitted agents or high viral loads in serum and other body fluids. Studies of transmission in households without other risk factors have demonstrated either low rates of transmission or no transmission.

The reported rates of vertical transmission vary widely. In mothers with unknown HIV status or known HIV infection, the rates of vertical transmission were 4% to 100%, whereas the rates varied between 0% and 42% in known HIV-negative mothers.[125] These same studies suggest that maternal coinfection with HIV, HCV genotype, active maternal liver disease, and the serum titer of maternal HCV RNA may be associated with increased rates of vertical transmission.[296,346,513] The correlation between HCV viremia, the HCV viral load in a mother, and vertical transmission of HCV is well documented.[325,397,451,507] The clinical significance and risk for liver disease after vertical transmission of HCV are still unknown. The timing of HCV infection in vertical transmission is also unknown. In utero transmission has been suggested by some studies,[138] whereas intrapartum or postpartum transmission was proposed by Ohto et al.[347] when they documented the absence of HCV RNA in the cord blood of neonates who later became HCV RNA positive at 1 to 2 months of age. More recently, Gibb et al.[166] reported two pieces of data supporting the likelihood of intrapartum transmission as the predominant time of vertical transmission: (1) low sensitivity of PCR for HCV RNA testing in the first month of life with a marked increase in sensitivity after that for diagnosing HCV infection in infants and (2) a lower transmission risk for elective cesarean delivery (without prolonged rupture of membranes) compared with vaginal or emergency cesarean delivery.[166] Another group, McMenamin et al.,[308] analyzed vertical transmission in 559 mother-infant dyads. The overall vertical transmission rate was 4.1% (18/441), with another 118 infants not tested or lost to follow-up. Comparison of the vertical transmission rate was no different for vaginal delivery or emergency cesarean in labor versus planned cesarean (4.2% vs. 3.0%). This held true even when mothers had hepatitis C RNA detected antenatally (7.2% vs.

5.3%). The authors did not support planned cesarean delivery to decrease vertical transmission of hepatitis C infection. No prospective, controlled trials of cesarean versus vaginal delivery and the occurrence of vertical hepatitis C transmission are available.

The risk for HCV transmission via breast milk is uncertain. Anti-HCV antibody and HCV RNA has been demonstrated in colostrum and breast milk, although the levels of HCV RNA in milk did not correlate with the titers of HCV RNA in serum.[40,180,285,397] Nevertheless, transmission of HCV via breastfeeding (and not in utero, intrapartum, or from other postpartum sources) has not been proven in the small number infants studied. Transmission rates in breastfed and nonbreastfed infants appear to be similar, but various important factors have not been controlled, such as HCV RNA titers in mothers, examination of the milk for HCV RNA, exclusive breastfeeding versus exclusive formula feeding versus partial breastfeeding, and duration of breastfeeding.[166,285,296,320,325,347,348,513] Zanetti et al.[513] documented the absence of HCV transmission in 94 mother-infant dyads when the mother had only HCV (no HIV) infection and no transmission in 71 mother-infant dyads who breastfed, including 23 infants whose mothers were seropositive for HCV RNA. Eight infants in that study were infected with HCV and their mothers had both HIV and HCV, and 3 of these 8 infants were infected with both HIV and HCV. The HCV RNA levels were significantly higher in the mothers coinfected with HIV than they were in mothers with HCV alone.

Overall, the risk for HCV infection via breastfeeding is low, the risk for HCV infection appears to be more frequent in association with HIV infection and higher levels of HCV RNA in maternal serum, no effective preventive therapies (Ig or vaccine) exist, and the risk for chronic HCV infection and subsequent sequelae with any infection is high. It is therefore appropriate to discuss the theoretic risk for breastfeeding in HCV-positive mothers with the mother or parents and to consider proscribing breast milk when appropriate alternative sources of nutrition are available for the infants. HIV infection is a separate contraindication to breastfeeding. Additional study is necessary to determine the exact role of breastfeeding in the transmission of HCV, including the quantitative measurement of HCV RNA in colostrum and breast milk, the relative risk for HCV transmission in exclusively or partially breastfed infants versus the risk in formula-fed infants, and the effect of duration of breastfeeding on transmission.

The current position of the CDC is that no data indicate that HCV virus is transmitted through breast milk.[88] Therefore, breastfeeding by an

HCV-positive, HIV-negative mother is not contraindicated.

Infants born to HCV RNA-positive mothers require follow-up through 18 to 24 months of age to determine the infants' HCV status, regardless of the mode of infant feeding. Infants should be tested for alanine aminotransferase and HCV RNA at 3 months and 12 to 15 months of age. Alanine aminotransferase and anti-HCV antibody should be tested at 18 to 24 months of age to confirm an infant's status: uninfected, ongoing hepatitis C infection, or past HCV infection.

HEPATITIS D

HDV is a defective RNA virus that causes hepatitis only in persons also infected with HBV. The infection occurs as either an acute coinfection of HBV and HDV or a superinfection of HBV carriers. This "double" infection results in more frequent fulminant hepatitis and chronic hepatitis, which can progress to cirrhosis. The virus uses its own HBV RNA (circular, negative-strand RNA) with an antigen, HDAg, surrounded by the surface antigen of HBV, HBsAg. HDV is transmitted in the same way as HBV, especially through the exchange of blood and body fluids. HDV infection is uncommon where the prevalence of HBV is low. In areas where HBV is endemic, the prevalence of HDV is highly variable. HDV is common in tropical Africa and South America, as well as in Greece and Italy, but it is uncommon in the Far East and in Alaskan Inuit despite the endemic occurrence of HBV in these areas.[434]

The transmission of HDV has been reported to occur from household contacts and, rarely, through vertical transmission. No data are available on the transmission of HDV by breastfeeding. HDV infection can be prevented by blocking infection with HBV; therefore, HBIG and HBV vaccine are the best protection. In addition to HBIG and HBV vaccine administration to the infant of a mother infected with both HBV and HDV, discussion with the mother or parents should include the theoretic risk for HBV and HDV transmission through breastfeeding. As with HBV, once HBIg and HBV vaccine have been given to the infant, the risk for HBV or HDV infection from breastfeeding is negligible. Therefore, breastfeeding after an informed discussion with the parents is acceptable.

HEPATITIS E

Hepatitis E virus (HEV) is a cause of sporadic and epidemic, enterically transmitted NANBH, which is typically self-limited and without chronic sequelae. HEV is notable for causing a high mortality rate in pregnant women. Transmission is primarily via the fecal-oral route, commonly via contaminated water or food. High infection rates have been reported in adolescents and young adults (ages 15 to 40 years). Tomar[461] reported that 70% of cases of HEV infections in the pediatric population in India manifest as acute hepatitis. Maternal-neonatal transmission was documented when the mother developed hepatitis E infection in the third trimester. Although HEV was demonstrated in breast milk, no transmission via breast milk was confirmed in this report. Five cases of transfusion-associated hepatitis E were reported.[461] In a review by Krain et al.,[249] vertical transmission was noted in reports from India and Ghana in the infants of pregnant women with acute viral hepatitis or fulminant hepatic failure.[249] Chibber et al.[98] reported on the presence of HEV RNA in the colostrum of HEV-infected mothers in significantly lower levels than in maternal serum. They also noted six infants who became infected within 2 weeks postpartum after being anti-HEV antibody and HEV RNA negative at birth. Four of these six infants were formula fed due to severe maternal illness. There was no transmission of HEV in 87 other infants who were exclusively breastfed and born to mothers positive for anti-HEV antibodies or HEV RNA in the third trimester.[98] Epidemics are usually related to contamination of water. Person-to-person spread is minimal, even in households and day care settings. Although Ig may be protective, no controlled trials have been done. Animal studies suggest that a recombinant subunit vaccine may be feasible.[385]

HEV infection in infancy is rare but does occur after maternal infection in the third trimester of pregnancy. Limited available data suggest that transmission of HEV by breastfeeding is rare. There is no evidence of clinically significant postnatal HEV infection or chronic sequelae in association with HEV infection in infants via breast milk. Currently no contraindication exists to breastfeeding with maternal HEV infection. Ig has not been shown to be effective in preventing infection, and no vaccine is available for HEV.

HEPATITIS G

Hepatitis G virus (HGV) has recently been confirmed as a cause of NANBH distinct from hepatitis viruses A through E. Several closely related genomes of HGV, currently named GBV-A, -B, and -C, appear to be related to HCV; the pestiviruses and the flaviviruses. Epidemiologically, HGV is most often associated with the transfusion of blood, although studies have identified nontransfusion-related cases. HGV genomic RNA has been detected in some patients with acute

The breast is a rare site of involvement.[123] HPV types 16 and 18 can immortalize normal breast epithelium in vitro.[489] HPV DNA has been detected in breast milk in 10 of 223 (4.5%) milk samples from 223 mothers, collected 3 days postpartum.[404] No attempt was made to correlate the presence of HPV DNA in breast milk with the HPV status of an infant or to assess the viral load of HPV in breast milk or its presence over the course of lactation. A second study found the DNA of cutaneous and mucosal HPV types in 2 of 25 human milk samples and 1 of 10 colostrum samples.[72] Yoshida et al. analyzed 80 maternal milk samples for HPV DNA, and HPV-16 nucleic acid was detected in 2 of 80 samples (2.5%), but there was no evidence of transmission to either of the infants.[510] No reports of HPV lesions of the breast or nipple and documented transmission to an infant secondary to breastfeeding are available.

No increased risk for acquiring HPV from breast milk is apparent, and breastfeeding is acceptable. Even in the rare occurrence of an HPV lesion of the nipple or breast, no data suggest that breastfeeding or the use of expressed breast milk is contraindicated.

MEASLES

Measles is another highly communicable childhood illness that can be more severe in neonates and adults. Measles is an exanthematous febrile illness following a prodrome of malaise, coryza, conjunctivitis, cough, and often Koplik spots in the mouth. The rash usually appears 10 to 14 days after exposure. Complications can include pneumonitis, encephalitis, and bacterial superinfection. With the availability of vaccination, measles in pregnancy is rare (0.4 in 10,000 pregnancies),[164] although respiratory complications (primary viral pneumonitis, secondary bacterial pneumonia), hepatitis, or other secondary bacterial infections often lead to more severe disease in these situations.

Prenatal infection with measles may cause premature delivery without disrupting normal uterine development. No specific group of congenital malformations have been described in association with in utero measles infection, although teratogenic effects of measles infection in pregnant women may rarely manifest in the infants.

Perinatal measles includes transplacental infection when measles occurs in an infant in the first 10 days of life. Infection from extrauterine exposure usually develops after 14 days of life. The severity of illness after the suspected transplacental spread of the virus to an infant varies from mild to severe and does not seem to vary with the antepartum or postpartum onset of rash in the mother. It is uncertain what role maternal antibodies play in the severity of an infant's disease. More severe disease seems to be associated with severe respiratory illness and bacterial infection. Postnatal exposure leading to measles after 14 days of life is generally mild, probably because of passively acquired antibodies from the mother. Severe measles in children younger than 1 year of age may occur because of declining passively acquired antibodies and complications of respiratory illness and rare cases of encephalitis.

Measles virus has not been identified in breast milk, whereas measles-specific antibodies have been documented.[1a] A report in 2014 examining measles in pregnancy in France during a resurgence of measles in the community did not demonstrate acquired measles in any of the 13 breastfed infants.[70] Infants exposed to mothers with documented measles while breastfeeding should be given immunoglobulin (Ig) and isolated from the mother until 72 hours after the onset of rash, which is often only a short period after diagnosis of measles in the mother. The breast milk can be pumped and given to the infant because secretory IgA begins to be secreted in breast milk within 48 hours of the onset of the exanthem in the mother. Table 13-3 summarizes the management of the hospitalized mother and infant with measles exposure or infection.[164]

MUMPS

Mumps is an acute transient benign illness with inflammation of the parotid gland and other salivary glands, and it often involves the pancreas, testicles, and meninges. Mumps occurs infrequently in pregnant women (1 to 10 cases in 10,000 pregnancies) and is generally benign. Mumps virus has been isolated from saliva, respiratory secretions, blood, testicular tissue, urine, CSF in cases of meningeal involvement, and breast milk. The period of infectivity is believed to be between 7 days before and 9 days after the onset of parotitis, with the usual incubation period being 14 to 18 days.

Prenatal infection with the mumps virus causes an increase in the number of abortions when infection occurs in the first trimester. A small increase in the number of premature births was noted in one prospective study of maternal mumps infection.[427] No conclusive evidence suggests congenital malformations are associated with prenatal infection, not even with endocardial fibroelastosis, as originally reported in the 1960s.

Perinatal mumps (transplacentally or postnatally acquired) has rarely if ever been documented. Natural mumps virus has been demonstrated to infect the placenta and infect the fetus, and live attenuated vaccine virus has been isolated from the placenta but not from fetal tissue in women

TABLE 13-3   Guidelines for Preventive Measures After Exposure to Measles in Nursery or Maternity Ward

Type of Exposure or Disease	Measles (Prodrome or Rash) Present*		Disposition
	Mother	Neonate	
A. Siblings at home have measles* when neonate and mother are ready for discharge from hospital	No	No	1. Neonate: Protective isolation and immunoglobulin (IG) indicated unless mother has unequivocal history of previous measles or measles vaccination†
			2. Mother: With history of previous measles or measles vaccination, she may either remain with the neonate or return to older children. Without previous history, she may remain with neonate until the older siblings are no longer infectious, or she may receive IG prophylactically and return to the older children
B. Mother has no history of measles or measles vaccination exposure 6 to 15 days antepartum‡	No	No	1. Exposed mother and infant: Administer IG to each and send home at the earliest date, unless siblings at home have communicable measles. Test mothers for susceptibility if possible. If susceptible, administer live measles vaccine 8 weeks after IG
			2. Other mothers and infants: Same approach, unless there is a clear history of previous measles or measles vaccination in the mother
			3. Hospital personnel: Unless there is a clear history of previous measles or measles vaccination, administer IG within 72 hours of exposure. Vaccinate 8 weeks or more later
C. Onset of maternal measles occurs antepartum or postpartum§	Yes	Yes	1. Infected mother and infant: Isolate together until clinically stable, then send home
			2. Other mothers and infants: Same as B-3, except infants should be vaccinated at 15 months of age
			3. Hospital personnel: Same as B-3.
D. Onset of maternal measles occurs antepartum or postpartum§	Yes	No	1. Infected mother: Isolate until no longer infectious§
			2. Infected mother's infant: Isolate separately from mother. Administer IG immediately. Send home when the mother is no longer infectious. Alternatively, observe in isolation for 18 days for modified measles,¶ especially if IG administration was delayed for more than 4 days
			3. Other mothers and infants: Same as C-2
			4. Hospital personnel: Same as B-3

*Catarrhal stage or less than 72 hours after the onset of exanthem.
†Vaccination with live attenuated measles virus.
‡With exposure less than 6 days antepartum, the mother would not be potentially infectious until at least 72 hours postpartum.
§Considered infectious from the onset of prodrome until 72 hours after the onset of exanthem.
¶Incubation period for modified measles may be prolonged beyond the usual 10 to 14 days.
From Gershon AA: Chickenpox, measles and mumps. In Remington JS, Klein JO, editors: *Infectious diseases of the fetus and newborn infant, ed 4*, Philadelphia, 1995, WB Saunders.

vaccinated 10 days before induced abortion. Antibodies to mumps do cross the placenta.

Postnatal mumps in the first year of life is typically benign. No epidemiologic data suggest that mumps infection is more or less common or severe in breastfed infants compared with formula-fed infants. Although mumps virus has been identified in breast milk and mastitis is a rare complication of mumps in mature women, no evidence indicates that breast involvement occurs more frequently in lactating women. If mumps occurs in the mother, breastfeeding can continue because exposure has already occurred throughout the 7 days before the development of symptoms in the mother, and secretory IgA in the milk may help to mitigate the symptoms in the infant.[164]

PARVOVIRUS

Human parvovirus B19 causes a broad range of clinical manifestations, including asymptomatic infection (most frequent manifestation in all ages), erythema infectiosum (fifth disease), arthralgia and arthritis, red blood cell (RBC) aplasia (and, less often, decreased white blood cells or platelets), chronic infection in immunodeficient individuals, and rarely myocarditis, vasculitis, or hemophagocytic syndrome.

Intrauterine vertical transmission can lead to severe anemia and immune-mediated hydrops fetalis, which can be treated, if accurately diagnosed, by intrauterine transfusion. Inflammation of the liver or CNS can be seen in the infant, along with vasculitis. If the child is clinically well at birth, hidden or persistent abnormalities are rarely identified. No evidence indicates that parvovirus B19 causes an identified pattern of birth defects.[462]

Postnatal transmission usually occurs person to person via contact with respiratory secretions, saliva, and rarely blood or urine. The seroprevalence in children at 5 years of age is less than 5%, with the peak age of infection occurring during the school-age years (5% to 40% of children infected). The majority of infections are asymptomatic or undiagnosed seroconversions.[462] Severe disease, such as prolonged aplastic anemia, occurs in individuals with hemoglobinopathies or abnormal RBC maturation. Attack rates have been estimated to be 17% to 30% in casual contacts and up to 50% among household contacts. In one study of 235 susceptible pregnant women, the annual seroconversion rate was 1.4%.[245]

No reports of transmission to an infant through breastfeeding are available. Excretion in breast milk has not been studied because of limitations in culturing techniques. Rat parvovirus has been demonstrated in rat milk. IgE antiparvovirus antibodies have been detected in human breast milk in one study.[435]

The very low seroconversion rate in young children and the absence of chronic or frequent severe disease suggest that the risk for parvovirus infection via breast milk is not significant. The possibility of antibodies against parvovirus or other protective constituents in breast milk has not been systematically studied. Breastfeeding by a mother with parvovirus infection is acceptable.

POLIOVIRUSES

Poliovirus infections (types 1, 2, and 3) cause a range of illness, with 90% to 95% subclinical, 4% to 8% abortive, and 1% to 2% manifesting as paralytic poliomyelitis. A 1955 review by Bates[32] of 58 cases of poliomyelitis in infants younger than 1 month of age demonstrated paralysis or death in more than 70% and only one child without evidence of even transient paralysis. More than half the cases were ascribed to transmission from the mothers, although no mention was made of breastfeeding. Breastfeeding rates at the time were approximately 25%.

Prenatal infection with polioviruses does cause an increased incidence of abortion. Prematurity and stillbirth apparently occur more frequently in mothers who developed paralytic disease versus inapparent infection.[206] Although individual reports of congenital malformations in association with maternal poliomyelitis exist, no epidemiologic data suggest that polioviruses are teratogenic. Also, no evidence indicates that live attenuated vaccine poliovirus given during pregnancy is associated with congenital malformations.[97,188]

Perinatal infection has been noted in several case reports of infants, infected in utero several days before birth, who had severe disease manifesting with neurologic symptoms (paralysis) but without fever, irritability, or vomiting. Additional case reports of infection acquired postnatally demonstrate illness more consistent with poliomyelitis of childhood. These cases were more severe and involved paralysis, which may represent reporting bias.[97]

No data are available concerning the presence of poliovirus in breast milk, although antibodies to poliovirus types 1, 2, and 3 have been documented.[304] In this era of increasing worldwide poliovirus vaccination, the likelihood of prenatal or perinatal poliovirus infection is decreasing. Maternal susceptibility to poliovirus should be determined before conception and poliovirus vaccine offered to susceptible women. An analysis of the last great epidemic of poliovirus infection in Italy in 1958 was done using a population-based case-control study.[376] In 114,000 births, 942 infants were reported with paralytic poliomyelitis. A group of matched control subjects was selected from infants admitted to the hospital at the same time. Using the dichotomous variable of never breastfed and partially breastfed, 75 never-breastfed infants were among the cases and 88 among the control group. The authors determined an odds ratio of 4.2, with 95% confidence interval of 1.4 to 14, demonstrating that the risk for paralytic poliomyelitis was higher in infants never breastfed and lowest among those exclusively breastfed. Because by the time the diagnosis of poliomyelitis is made in a breastfeeding mother, the exposure of the infant to poliovirus from maternal secretions has already occurred, and because the breast milk already contains antibodies that may be protective, no reason exists to interrupt breastfeeding. Breastfeeding also does not interfere with successful immunization against poliomyelitis with oral or inactivated poliovirus vaccine.[77]

RETROVIRUSES
Human T-Cell Leukemia Virus Type I

The occurrence of human T-cell leukemia virus type I (HTLV-I) is endemic in parts of southwestern Japan,[74,228,501] the Caribbean, South America,[174] and sub-Saharan Africa. HTLV-I is associated with adult T-cell leukemia/lymphoma and a chronic condition with progressive neuropathy. The progressive neuropathy is called HTLV-I-associated myelopathy or tropical spastic paraparesis.[151] Other illnesses have been reported in association with HTLV-I infection, including dermatitis, uveitis, arthritis, Sjögren syndrome in adults, and infective dermatitis and persistent lymphadenitis in children. Transmission of HTLV-I occurs most often through sexual contact, via blood or blood products, and via breast milk. Infrequent transmission does occur in utero or at delivery and with casual or household contact.[328]

Seroprevalence generally increases with age and varies widely in different regions and in populations of different backgrounds. In some areas of Japan, seropositivity can be as high as 12% to 16%, but in South America, Africa, and some Caribbean countries, the rates are 2% to 6%. In Latin America seropositive rates can be as high as 10% to 25% among female sex workers or attendees to STD clinics.[174] In blood donors in Europe, the seroprevalence of HTLV-I has been reported at 0.001% to 0.03%. The seroprevalence in pregnant women in endemic areas of Japan is as high as 4% to 5% and in nonendemic areas as low as 0.1% to 1.0%. HTLV-I is not a major disease in the United States. In studies from Europe, the seroprevalence in pregnant women has been noted to be up to 0.6%. These pregnant women were primarily of African or Caribbean descent.[153]

HTLV-I antigen has been identified in breast milk of HTLV-I-positive mothers.[242] Another report shows that basal mammary epithelial cells can be infected with HTLV-I and can transfer infection to peripheral blood monocytes.[283] Human milk from HTLV-I-positive mothers caused infection in marmosets.[243,504] HTLV-I infection clearly occurs via breastfeeding, and a number of reports document an increased rate of transmission of HTLV-I to breastfed infants compared with formula-fed infants.[15,14,11–13,196,199,197,452] Ando et al.,[12,13] in two separate reports, demonstrated a parallel decline in antibodies against HTLV-I in both formula-fed and breastfed infants to a nadir at approximately 1 year of age and a subsequent increase in antibodies from 1 to 2 years of age. The percentage of children seropositive at 1 year of age in the breastfed and formula-fed groups was 3.0% and 0.6%, respectively; at 1.5 years of age, it was 15.2% and 3.9%; and at 2 years of age, it was 41.9% and 4.6%. A smaller group of children, followed through 11 to 12 years of age, demonstrated no newly infected children after 2 years of age and no loss of antibodies in any child who was seropositive at 2 years of age.[12,13]

TABLE 13-4 HTLV-I Transmission Related to the Duration of Breastfeeding

Author (Reference)	Duration (month)	Seroconversion Rate (%)	Number of Children*
Takahashi[385]	≤6	4.4	4/90
	≥7	14.4	20/139
	(bottle-fed)	5.7	9/158
Takezaki[387]	≤6	3.9	2/51
	>6	20.3	13/64
Wiktor[423]	<12	9.0	8/86
	≥12	32	19/60

HTLV, Human T-cell leukemia virus.
*Number of children positive for HTLV-I over the number of children examined.

Transmission of HTLV-I infection via breastfeeding is also clearly associated with the duration of breastfeeding.[452,453,497,498] It has been postulated that the persistence of passively acquired antibodies against HTLV-I offers some protection through 6 months of life (Table 13-4).

Other factors relating to HTLV-I transmission via breast milk have been proposed. Yoshinaga et al.[512] presented data on the HTLV-I antigen-producing capacity of peripheral blood and breast milk cells and showed an increased mother-to-child transmission rate when the mother's blood and breast milk produced large numbers of antigen-producing cells in culture.[512] Hisada et al.[201] reported on 150 mothers and infants in Jamaica, demonstrating that a higher maternal provirus level and a higher HTLV-I antibody titer were independently associated with HTLV-I transmission to the infant. Ureta-Vidal et al.[467] reported an increased seropositivity rate in children of mothers with a high proviral load and elevated maternal HTLV-I antibody titers.

Various interventions have been proposed to decrease HTLV-I transmission via breastfeeding. Complete avoidance of breastfeeding was shown to be an effective intervention by Hino et al.[197,198] in a large population of Japanese in Nagasaki. Avoiding breastfeeding led to an 80% decrease in transmission. Breastfeeding for a shorter duration is another effective alternative. Ando et al.[11] showed that freezing and thawing breast milk decreased the infectivity of HTLV-I. Sawada et al.[405] demonstrated in a rabbit model that HTLV-I immunoglobulin protected against HTLV-I transmission via milk. It is reasonable to postulate that any measure that would decrease the maternal provirus load or increase the anti-HTLV-I antibodies available to infants might decrease the risk for transmission. The overall prevalence of HTLV-I infection during childhood is unknown because the majority of with breastfeeding and two different infant prophylaxis regimens. At 9 months of age, they observed a 10.6% occurrence of HIV transmission for infants receiving a single dose of NVP plus 1 week of ZDV, compared with 5.2% in the group receiving a single dose of NVP plus 1 week of ZDV plus 14 weeks of daily NVP, and 6.4% in the group receiving a single dose of NVP plus 1 week of ZDV plus 14 weeks of NVP and ZDV.[259] In the Mitra Study in Tanzania in which the median time of breastfeeding was 18 weeks, the HIV transmission rate at 6 months in the infants who received ZDV plus 3TC for 1 week plus 3TC alone for breastfeeding through 6 months of age was less than 50% of the transmission rate for those infants receiving only 1 week of ZDV plus 3TC.[239] A summary of three trials in Ethiopia, India, and Uganda compared a single dose of NVP at birth for infants with 6 weeks of daily NVP in predominantly breastfed infants whose mothers were counseled regarding feeding per the WHO/UNICEF guidelines.[465] At 6 months, 87 of 986 infants in the single-dose group and 62 of 901 in the extended-dose group were HIV infected, which was not statistically significant. The authors suggested that a longer course of infant antiretroviral prophylaxis might be more effective.[432] A Cochrane review by White et al.[492] examined seven studies of antiretroviral interventions relative to preventing transmission of HIV via breast milk. The trials considered maternal and infant prophylaxis, and the authors conclude that antiretroviral prophylaxis for the mother or infant while breastfeeding is effective in the prevention of mother-to-child HIV transmission. There remains research to be done, which documents the safety of antiretroviral therapy for the mother and infant and achieves the goals of optimizing maternal health and survival and optimizing infant health and survival at the same time.[336,492]

Human Immune Deficiency Virus in Maternal Health and Breastfeeding. The potential effect of breastfeeding on the HIV-positive mother needs to be adequately assessed in relation to the mother's health status. From Uganda and Zimbabwe, Mbizvo et al.[305] reported no difference in the number of hospital admissions or mortality between HIV-positive and HIV-negative women during pregnancy. In the 2 years after delivery, the HIV-positive women had higher hospital admission (approximately two times increased risk) and death rates (relative risk greater than 10) than HIV-negative women.[305] Chilongozi et al.[99] reported on 2292 HIV-positive mothers from four sub-Saharan sites followed for 112 months. Serious adverse events occurred in 166 women (7.2%); 42 deaths occurred in the HIV-positive women,

and no deaths occurred in 331 HIV-negative women.[99]

Several studies have examined breastfeeding relative to mothers' health and reported conflicting results. The first study from Kenya demonstrated a significantly higher mortality rate in breastfeeding mothers compared with a formula-feeding group in the 2 years after delivery. The hypothesized explanation offered by the authors for this difference was increased metabolic demands, greater weight loss, and nutritional depletion.[331] A second study from South Africa showed an overall lower mortality rate in the two groups with no significant difference in mortality rate in the 10 months of observation.[111] Kuhn et al.[253] reported no difference in mortality at 12 months after delivery between 653 women randomly assigned to a short breastfeeding group (4.93%, with 95% CI of 2.42 to 7.46. Out of 326 women, with a median breastfeeding duration of 4 months, 21% were still breastfeeding at 12 months) and a long breastfeeding group (4.89%, with 95% CI of 2.38 to 7.40. Out of 327 women, 90% were breastfeeding at 5 months, and 72% were breastfeeding at 12 months, for a median of 15 months). The HIV-related mortality rates were high but not associated with prolonged lactation.[253] Walson et al.[481] followed 535 HIV-positive women for 1 to 2 years in Kenya. The mortality risk was 1.9% at 1 year and 4.8% at 2 years of follow-up. Although less than 10% of women reported a hospitalization during the 2 years, they experienced various common infections (pneumonia, diarrhea, TB, malaria, STDs, urinary tract infections, mastitis). Breastfeeding was a significant cofactor for diarrhea and mastitis but not for pneumonia, TB, or hospitalization.[481]

HIV Child-to-Breastfeeding Woman Transmission

HIV child-to-breastfeeding woman transmission (CBWT) has been a theoretical concern since the beginning of the HIV epidemic. There have been rare cases where this has been suspected but not sufficiently investigated to document its occurrence. Little et al. reviewed the topic in 2012, examining a number of published accounts in a systematic review.[287] Two larger studies from the Russian Federation and Libya examined outbreaks of nosocomial HIV spread in pediatric hospitals. The infants became infected through blood products, unsterilized needles, or injection equipment. The epidemiologic investigations tried to exclude the other possible sources of HIV infection in the women and delineate the character and timing of the exposures of the mothers to their infants. In Russia, 12 mothers of 152 infected infants were documented to be HIV positive, and the odds of breastfeeding were greater in the HIV-infected group. Infant stomatitis and cracked nipples in the mothers seemed to also correlate, although the duration of breastfeeding did not seem to be a significant factor. In Libya, there were 20 infected mothers associated with 402 children (5.0%) found to be HIV infected. A substudy of 118 mother-infant dyads documented HIV infection in the 118 infants and 18 mothers, while at the same time confirming the HIV-negative status of the remaining 100 women and all 75 of the fathers tested. Fourteen of the 18 HIV-positive women had no other risk factors identified except breastfeeding their HIV-positive infants. Breastfeeding was an independent predictor of maternal HIV infection. Three other published reports in the same paper[287] were discussed, documenting the occurrence of CBWT via breastfeeding in Kazakhstan, Kyrgyzstan, and Romania. The authors raise the concern that many parts of the world where wet-nursing and cross-nursing are socially acceptable and more common may overlap with higher HIV-prevalence areas and raise the risk of CBWT. They discuss the very high rates of orphanhood in areas with high HIV prevalence and perinatal HIV transmission. They recognize the greater likelihood that female relatives of the orphaned children are wet- or cross-nursing without knowing that there is a risk of transmission of HIV to themselves in this practice. The authors conclude that, in addition to optimizing the ongoing efforts of HIV transmission prevention in adults and children, the WHO guidelines on infant feeding should include information about the risks of wet-nursing or cross-nursing HIV-infected infants. Women should be counseled about the possibility of CBWT, and the infants and women should be provided HIV testing in order to offer women the necessary knowledge and information to make informed feeding decisions.[287]

In summary, the breastfeeding of infants by HIV-positive mothers does lead to an increased risk for HIV infection in the infants. Much remains to be understood about the mechanisms of HIV transmission via breast milk and the action and efficacy of different interventions to prevent such transmission. The complete avoidance of breastfeeding is a crucial component for the prevention of perinatal HIV infection in the United States and many other countries.[492]

For resource-poor settings, where breastfeeding is the norm and where it provides vital nutritional and infection protective benefits, the WHO, UNICEF, and the Joint United Nations Programme on HIV/AIDS (UNAIDS) made updated recommendations in 2010: *Guidelines on HIV and infant feeding: Principles and recommendations for infant feeding in the context of HIV and a summary of evidence*[493] (http://www.who.int/maternal_child_adolescent/documents/9789241599535/en/). Although most of the recommendations are in line with previous WHO recommendations, this publication supports national authorities deciding on their own country's plan for infant-feeding practice to optimize the health of the mother and infant, to limit the mother-to-child transmission of HIV, and to accomplish this by incorporating the policy and interventions in the country's maternal and child health services. There are nine key principles proposed to guide national authorities (see Box 13-3).

Mothers choosing to breastfeed should receive additional education, support, and medical care to minimize the risk for HIV transmission and to optimize their own health status during and after breastfeeding. Mothers choosing to use replacement feedings should receive parallel education, support, and medical care for themselves and their infants to minimize the effect of the lack of breastfeeding.[492]

Good evidence now shows that antiretroviral prophylactic regimens for mothers or infants, while continuing breastfeeding, do decrease postnatal HIV transmission. Early weaning is associated with increased morbidity and mortality for the infants. Further carefully controlled research is indicated in order to adequately assess the risks and benefits

---

BOX 13-3. Nine Key Principles for the Current Guidelines on HIV and Infant Feeding From the WHO

1. Balancing HIV prevention with protection from other causes of child mortality
2. Integrating HIV interventions into maternal and child health services
3. Set national and sub-national recommendations for infant feeding in the context of HIV
4. Provide breastfeeding to infants born to HIV-infected mothers with a greater chance of HIV-free survival even if antiretroviral drugs are not immediately available
5. Inform mothers known to be HIV-infected about infant feeding alternatives
6. Provide services to specifically support mothers to appropriately feed their infants
7. Avoid harm to infant feeding practices in the general population
8. Advise mothers who are HIV uninfected or whose HIV status is unknown about infant feeding alternatives
9. Invest in improvements in infant feeding practices in the context of HIV

World Health Organization/UNAIDS/UNICEF. Infant Feeding Guidelines. http://www.unicef.org/programme/breastfeeding/feeding.htm (accessed 18.01.15)

Exclusive breastfeeding may decrease the likelihood of severe rotavirus-related diarrhea by as much as 90%.[101,420] Although breastfeeding does not prevent infection with rotavirus, it seems to decrease the severity of rotavirus-induced illness in children younger than 2 years old.[101,135,202] At least one study suggested that this may simply represent the postponement of severe rotavirus infection until an older age.[101] Another study suggested that protection against rotavirus rapidly declines upon discontinuation of breastfeeding.[399] This delay in rotavirus infection until the child is older may be beneficial in that the older child may be able to tolerate the infection or illness with a lower likelihood of becoming dehydrated or malnourished. Continuing breastfeeding during an episode of rotavirus illness, with or without vomiting, is appropriate and often helpful to the infant. No reason to suspend breastfeeding by a mother infected with rotavirus is apparent.

Two rotavirus vaccines (RotaTeq and Rotarix) have been licensed for use in more than 90 countries, but fewer than 20 countries have routine immunization programs. Additional types of rotavirus vaccines are undergoing study in various countries, specifically examining the efficacy of the vaccines in low- and medium-income countries.[495] Some of the explanations for the slow global implementation of an effective vaccine include differences in protection with specific vaccines in high-income countries compared with low- or medium-income countries, the unfortunate association with intussusception in the United States, the delayed recognition of the significant rotavirus-related morbidity and mortality, and the cost of the new vaccines. The question of the variable efficacy of the specific rotavirus vaccines in developed and developing countries remains an important one.[281] Several trials are examining this issue and attempting to address factors such as transplacentally transferred maternal antibodies, breastfeeding practices (especially immediately before immunization with a live oral rotavirus vaccine), stomach acid, micronutrient malnutrition, interfering gut flora, and differences in the epidemiology of rotavirus in different locations.[367] Evidence indicates that maternal immunization with rotavirus vaccine can increase both the transplacental acquisition of antibodies and secretory IgA in breast milk.[374] Additionally, oral rotavirus vaccines have been able to stimulate a good serologic response in both formula-fed and breastfed infants, although the antigen titers may need to be modified to create an optimal response in all infants.[93] The actual protective effect of these vaccines in different situations and strategies will require measurement in ongoing prospective studies.

RUBELLA VIRUS

Congenital rubella infection has been well described, and the contributing variables to infection and severe disease have been elucidated. The primary intervention to prevent congenital rubella has been to establish the existence of maternal immunity to rubella before conception, including immunization with rubella vaccine and reimmunization if indicated. Perinatal infection is not clinically significant. Postnatal infection occurs infrequently in children younger than 1 year of age because of passively acquired maternal antibodies. The predominant age of infection is 5 to 14 years old, and more than half of those with infections are asymptomatic. Postnatal rubella is a self-limited, mild viral infection associated with an evanescent rash, shotty adenopathy, and low-grade transient fever. It most often occurs in the late winter and spring. Infants with congenital infection shed the virus for prolonged periods from various sites and may serve as a source of infection throughout the year. Contact isolation is appropriate for suspected and proven congenital infection for at least 1 year, including exclusion from day care and avoidance of pregnant women, whereas postnatal rubella infection requires droplet precautions for 7 days after the onset of rash.

Rubella virus has been isolated from breast milk after natural infection (congenital or postnatal) and after immunization with live attenuated vaccine virus. Both IgA antibodies and immunoreactive cells against rubella have been identified in breast milk. Breastfed infants can acquire vaccine-virus infection via milk but are asymptomatic. Because postpartum infection with this virus (natural or vaccine) is not associated with clinically significant illness, no reason exists to prevent breastfeeding after congenital infection, postpartum infection with this virus, or maternal immunization with rubella vaccine.[102]

SEVERE ACUTE RESPIRATORY SYNDROME

Severe acute respiratory syndrome (SARS) is a term that could be applied to any serious acute respiratory illness caused by or associated with a variety of infectious agents. Since 2003, it has been linked with SARS-associated coronavirus (SARS-CoV). In the global outbreak of 2002 to 2003, more than 8400 probable cases of SARS and more than 800 deaths occurred. More than the actual number of affected individuals or its associated mortality rate (approximately 10% mortality overall, and closer to 50% mortality in persons older than 65 years of age), the lack of data on this new unusual illness and the tremendous publicity surrounding it made SARS such a sensation. We now know the cause of this illness, known as the SARS-CoV. SARS-CoV was shown not to be closely related to the previously characterized coronavirus groups.[298,392] Despite intense international collaboration to study the illness and the virus, many things are not known, such as the degree of infectiousness, the actual period of transmissibility, all the modes of transmission, how many people have an asymptomatic infection as compared to those with symptoms or severe illnesses, how to make a rapid diagnosis of confirmed cases, and where the virus originated.

At least 21 cases of probable SARS in children have been described in the literature.[49,205,423,431] In general, the illness in children is a mild, nonspecific respiratory illness, but in adolescents and adults, it is more likely to progress to severe respiratory distress. It has been reported that children are less likely to transmit SARS than adults.[205] The overall clinical course, the radiologic evolution, and the histologic findings of this illness are consistent with the host's immune response playing a significant role in disease production.

Five infants were born to mothers with confirmed SARS. The infants were born prematurely (26 to 37 weeks), presumably due to maternal illness. Although two of the five infants had serious abdominal illnesses (other coronaviruses have been associated with reported outbreaks of necrotizing enterocolitis), the presence of SARS-CoV could not be demonstrated in any of these infants.[423] No evidence of vertical transmission of SARS is available. The mode of feeding for any of the reported cases of young children with SARS or the infants born to mothers with SARS was not mentioned.

Since 2012, a second coronavirus (CoV) has been associated with epidemic SARS: Middle East respiratory syndrome (MERS-CoV), named after the initial outbreak described in Saudi Arabia. This illness has an estimated incubation period of 5 to 14 days and manifests similarly to SARS-CoV with a variety of extrapulmonary manifestations, and it seems to affect individuals with comorbid conditions.[211] It also appears to be transmitted primarily by respiratory droplets.

As with other respiratory viruses predominantly transmitted by droplets, transmission via breast milk is an insignificant mode of transmission, if it occurs at all. The benefits of breastfeeding being what they are, mothers with SARS or MERS should continue breastfeeding if they are able, or expressed breast milk can be given to an infant until the mother is able to breastfeed.

SMALLPOX

In this era of worry about biologic terrorism, smallpox is an important concern. The concern for infants (breastfed or formula-fed) is direct contact with mothers or household members with smallpox. Smallpox is highly contagious in the household setting due to person-to-person spread via droplet nuclei or aerosolization from the oropharynx and direct contact with the rash. Additional potential exposures for infants include the release of a smallpox aerosol into the environment by terrorists, contact with a smallpox-contaminated space or the clothes of household members exposed to an aerosol, and infection via contact with a mother's or a household member's smallpox vaccination site. These risks are the same for breastfed and formula-fed infants. No evidence for the transmission of the smallpox virus via breast milk exists.

A contact is defined as a person who has been in the same household or had face-to-face contact with a patient with smallpox after the onset of fever. Patients do not transmit infection until after progression from the fever stage to the development of the rash. An exposed contact does not need to be isolated from others during the postcontact observation period (usually 17 days) until that person develops fever. The temperature of the exposed contact should be monitored daily. Personal contact and breastfeeding between mother and infant can continue until the onset of fever, when immediate isolation (at home) should begin. Providing expressed breast milk for the infant of a mother with smallpox should be avoided because of the extensive nature of the smallpox rash and the possibility of contamination (from the rash) of the milk during the expression process. No literature documents transmission of the smallpox virus via expressed breast milk.

The other issue for breastfeeding infants is the question of maternal vaccination with smallpox in a preexposure-event vaccination program. Children older than 1 year of age can be safely and reasonably vaccinated with smallpox in the face of a probable smallpox exposure. The smallpox vaccination of infants younger than 1 year of age is contraindicated. Breastfeeding is listed as a contraindication to vaccination in the preevent vaccination program. It is unknown whether the vaccine virus or antibodies are present in breast milk. The risk for infection due to contact or aerosolization of virus from a mother's smallpox vaccination site is the same for breastfed and formula-fed infants. The Advisory Committee on Immunization Practices also does not recommend preventing the smallpox vaccination of children younger than 18 years old.[491]

One report documents tertiary-contact vaccinia in a breastfeeding infant.[155] A United States military person received a primary smallpox vaccination and developed a local reaction at the inoculation site. Despite reportedly observing appropriate precautions, the individual's wife developed vesicles on both areolae (secondary-contact vaccinia). Subsequently, the breastfeeding infant developed lesions on her philtrum, cheek, and tongue. Both the mother and infant remained well, and the infections resolved without therapy. Culture and PCR testing confirmed vaccinia in both the mother's and the infant's lesions. The breast milk was not tested.[155]

In a review of the literature from 1931 to 1981, Sepkowitz[418] reported on 27 cases of secondary vaccinia in households. The CDC reported 30 suspected cases of secondary/tertiary vaccinia, with 18 of those cases confirmed by culture or PCR. The 30 cases were related to 578,286 vaccinated military personnel. This is an incidence of 5.2 cases per 100,000 vaccinees and 7.4 cases per 100,000 primary vaccinees.[85] In a separate report on the civilian smallpox-prevention vaccination program, 37,802 individuals were vaccinated between January and June 2003, and no cases of contact vaccinia were reported.[83]

The risk for contact vaccinia is low. The risk is from close or intimate contact. In the mentioned case, the risk for the infant was contact with the mother's breasts, the inadvertent site of her contact vaccinia. Breastfed and formula-fed infants are equally at risk from close contact in the household of a smallpox vaccinee or a case of secondary vaccinia, and separation from the individual is appropriate in both situations. If the breast of the nursing mother is not involved, expressed breast milk can be given to the infant.

Another orthopoxvirus that has emerged in the past decade is monkeypox. Most commonly it is a zoonotic pathogen, spreading to humans though direct contact with infected animals. There are reports of transmission from person to person, but this seems to be an uncommon event.[146] Similar to smallpox, the likelihood of spread is probably similar for formula-fed or breastfed infants, and as long as the breast of a mother with monkeypox is not involved, then expressed breast milk can be given to the infant.

TT VIRUS

TT virus (TTV) is a recently identified virus found in a patient (TT) with posttransfusion hepatitis not associated with the other hepatitis-related viruses, A through G. TTV has been described as an unenveloped, circular, single-stranded DNA virus.[350] This virus is prevalent in healthy individuals, including healthy blood donors, and it has been identified in patients with hepatitis. TTV DNA has been detected in infants of TTV-positive and TTV-negative mothers. Ohto et al.[349] reported no TTV DNA was detected in cord blood from 38 infants, and it was detected in only 1 of 14 samples taken at 1 month of age. They noted an increasing prevalence from 6 months (22%) to 2 years (33%), which they ascribed to acquisition via nonparenteral routes. In comparisons of the TTV DNA in TTV-positive mothers and their TTV-positive infants, 6 of 13 showed high-level nucleotide sequence similarity, and 7 of 13 differed by greater than 10%.[349]

Schröter et al.[413] reported on TTV DNA in breast milk examined retrospectively. Notably, TTV DNA was detected in 22 of 23 serum samples of infants at 1 week of age, who were born to 22 women viremic for TTV DNA. Twenty-four women who were negative for TTV DNA gave birth to 24 children who were initially negative for TTV DNA and remained negative throughout the observation period (mean 7.5 months, range 1 to 28 months). TTV DNA was detected in 77% of breast milk samples from TTV-viremic women and in none of the breast milk samples from TTV-negative women. No clinical or laboratory evidence of hepatitis was found in the 22 children who were observed to be TTV DNA positive during the period of the study.[413] Other authors have reported TTV in breast milk, as detected by PCR. They describe the absence of TTV DNA in infants at 5 days and 3 months of age, and 4 of 10 infants were positive for TTV DNA at 6 months of age, suggesting the late acquisition of infection via breastfeeding.[217]

The TTV is transmitted in utero and is found in breast milk.[349] No evidence of clinical hepatitis in infants related to TTV infection and no evidence for a late chronic hepatitis exist. Given the current available information, no reason to proscribe breastfeeding by TTV-positive mothers is compelling. Certainly, more needs to be understood concerning the chronic nature of this infection and the possible pathogenesis of liver disease.[413]

TUMOR VIRUS IN BREAST MILK

No documented evidence indicates that women with breast cancer have RNA of tumor virus in their milk. No correlation between RNA-directed DNA polymerase activity has been found in women with a family history of breast cancer. RNA-directed DNA polymerase activity, a reserve transcriptase, is a normal feature of the lactating breast.[100,142,394]

Epidemiologic data conflict with the suggestion that the tumor agent is transmitted through the breast milk. The incidence of breast cancer is low among women who nursed their infants, including lower economic groups, foreign-born groups, and those in sparsely populated areas.[294] The frequency of breast cancer in mothers and sisters of a woman with breast cancer is two to three times that expected by chance. This could be genetic or environmental. In actuality, cancer is equally common on both sides of the family of an affected woman. If breast milk were the cause, it should be transmitted from mother to daughter. When the mother-daughter incidence of cancer was studied, no relationship was found to breastfeeding.

Sarkar et al.[403] reported that human milk, when incubated with mouse mammary tumor virus, caused degradation of the particular morphology or the virions, while decreasing infectivity and reversing transcriptase activity. They suggest that the significance of this destructive effect of human milk on mouse mammary tumor virus may account for the difficulty in isolating the putative human mammary tumor agent. Sanner[402] showed that the inhibitory enzymes in milk can be removed using a special sedimentation technique. He ascribes the discrepancies in isolating virus particles in human milk to these factors, which inhibit RNA-directed DNA polymerase. Human mammary tumor virus (HMTV) sequences were detected in the breast milk of women who had had a history of breast biopsy for suspicion of cancer, as compared to a reference group of women who had not been biopsied. Of the eight women who had breast cancer (8/73), only one had HMTV sequences detected in her breast milk.[329] Melana et al. identified viral particles within human breast cancer cells that had a sequence homology of 95% with the HMTV proviruses as potential etiologic agents in human breast cancer pathogenesis.[312]

The fear of cancer in breastfed female offspring of a woman with breast cancer does not justify avoiding breastfeeding. Breastfed women have the same breast cancer experience as nonbreastfed women, and no increase is seen in benign tumors. Daughters of breast-cancer patients have an increased risk for developing benign and malignant tumors because of their heredity, not because of their breastfeeding history.[314,323]

Unilateral breastfeeding (limited to the right breast) is a custom of Tanka women of the fishing villages of Hong Kong. Ing et al.[213] investigated the question, "Does the unsuckled breast have an altered risk for cancer?" They studied breast cancer data from 1958 to 1975. Breast cancer occurred equally in the left and the right breasts. A comparison of patients who had nursed unilaterally with nulliparous patients and with patients who had borne children but not breastfed indicated a highly significantly increased risk for cancer in the unsuckled breast. The authors conclude that, in postmenopausal women who have breastfed unilaterally, the risk for cancer is significantly higher in the unsuckled breast. They propose that breastfeeding may help protect the suckled breast against cancer.[213]

Others[307] have suggested that Tanka women are an ethnically separate people and that left-sided breast cancer may be related to their genetic pool and not to their breastfeeding habits. No mention has been made of other possible influences, such as the impact of their role as "fishermen" or any inherent trauma to the left breast.[307]

In 1926, Lane-Claypon[266] stated that a breast that had never lactated was more liable to become cancerous. Nulliparity and absence of breastfeeding had been considered to be important risk factors for breast cancer. MacMahon et al.[294] reported in 1970 that age at first full-term pregnancy was the compelling factor, and the younger the mother, the less the risk.

In a collective review of the etiologic factors in cancer of the breast in humans, Papaioannou concludes, "Genetic factors, viruses, hormones, psychogenic stress, diet, and other possible factors, probably in that order of importance, contribute to some extent to the development of cancer of the breast."[364]

In her 1977 review on human milk and health, Wing[500] concluded that "in view of the complete absence of any studies showing a relationship between breastfeeding and increased risk of breast cancer, the presence of virus-like particles in breast milk should not be a contraindication to breastfeeding." Henderson et al.[191] made a similar statement in 1974, whereas Vorherr[480] concluded in 1979 that the roles of pregnancy and lactation in the development and prognosis of breast cancer had not been determined.

Gradually, additional studies have appeared, challenging the dogma. Brinton et al.,[59] McTiernan and Thomas,[309] and Layde et al.[272] showed the clearly protective effects of breastfeeding. Another example is a study conducted to clarify whether lactation has a protective role against breast cancer in an Asian people, regardless of the confounding effects of age at first pregnancy, parity, and closely related factors.[509] In a hospital-based case-control study of 521 women without breast cancer, statistical adjustment for potential confounders and a likelihood ratio test for a linear trend were done by unconditional logistic regression. Total months of lactation regardless of parity was the discriminator. Regardless of age of first pregnancy and parity, lactation had an independent protective effect against breast cancer in Japanese women.[509] Although breast cancer incidence is influenced by genetics, stress, hormones, and pregnancy, breastfeeding clearly has a protective effect. "There is a reduction in the risk of breast cancer among premenopausal women who have lactated. No reduction in the risk of breast cancer occurred among postmenopausal women with a history of lactation," according to Newcombe et al.,[335] reporting a multicenter study in 1993. Ip et al. conducted a systematic review and analysis on breastfeeding and maternal and infant health in developed countries for the Agency of Healthcare Research and Quality, and they reported on two previously done meta-analyses that concluded that there was a reduced risk of breast cancer in women who breastfed their infants.[214] The original meta-analyses were evaluated as fair quality, estimating the reduced risk of breast cancer as 4.3% for each year of breastfeeding, and the second study estimated a decrease in breast cancer risk of 28% for 12 or more months of breastfeeding.[41]

There is good evidence that a longer duration of breastfeeding does decrease the risk of developing breast cancer, and there are no direct data suggesting that the presence of HMTV in breast milk is a reason to stop breastfeeding.

VARICELLA-ZOSTER VIRUS

Varicella-zoster virus infection (varicella/chickenpox, zoster/shingles) is one of the most communicable diseases of humans, in a class with measles and smallpox. Transmission is thought to occur via respiratory droplets and virus from vesicles. Varicella in pregnancy is a rare event, although disease can be more severe with varicella pneumonia, and it can be fatal.

Congenital varicella-zoster virus infection occurs infrequently, causing abortion, prematurity, and congenital malformations. A syndrome of malformations has been carefully described with congenital varicella-zoster virus infection, typically involving limb deformity, skin scarring, and nerve damage, including to the eye and brain.[164]

Perinatal infection can lead to severe infection in infants if maternal rash develops 5 days or less before delivery and within 2 days after delivery. Illness in infants usually develops before 10 days of age and is believed to be more severe because of the lack of adequate transfer of antibody from the mother during this period and the transplacental spread of virus to the fetus and infant during viremia in the mother. Varicella in a mother occurring before 5 days before delivery allows the sufficient formation and transplacental transfer of antibodies to the infant to ameliorate disease, even if the infant is infected with varicella-zoster virus. Mothers who develop varicella rash more than 2 days after delivery are less likely to transplacentally transfer the virus to the infant. Such mothers do pose a risk to their infants from postnatal exposure, which can be diminished by the administration of varicella-zoster Ig to the infant. Postnatal transmission is believed to occur through aerosolized virus from skin lesions or the respiratory tract entering the susceptible infant's respiratory tract. Airborne

precautions are therefore appropriate in the hospital setting. Infants infected with varicella-zoster virus in utero or in the perinatal period (younger than 1 month of age) are more likely to develop zoster (reactivation of latent varicella-zoster virus) during childhood or as young adults. Table 13-5 summarizes the management of varicella in the hospitalized mother or infant.[164]

Postnatal varicella from nonmaternal exposure can occur, but it is generally mild when it develops after 3 weeks of age or when a mother has passed on antibodies against varicella-zoster virus via the placenta. Severe postnatal varicella does occur in premature infants or infants of varicella-susceptible mothers. When a mother's immune status relative to varicella-zoster virus is uncertain and the measurement of antibodies to varicella-zoster virus in the mother or infant cannot be performed promptly (less than 72 hours), the administration of VZIG[86] or IVIG to the infant exposed to varicella or zoster in the postnatal period is indicated. Ideally, a mother's varicella status should be known before pregnancy, when the varicella virus vaccine could be given if indicated.

The varicella-zoster virus has not been cultured from milk, but varicella-zoster virus DNA has been identified in breast milk.[511] Antibodies against varicella-zoster virus have also been found in breast milk.[304] Breast milk from mothers who had received the varicella vaccine in the postpartum period was tested for varicella-zoster virus DNA. Varicella DNA was not detected in any of the 217 breast milk samples from the 12 women, all of whom seroconverted after vaccination.[52] One case of suspected transfer of varicella-zoster virus to an infant via breastfeeding has been reported, but the virus may have been transmitted by respiratory droplets or exposure to rash before the mother began antiviral therapy.[511]

The isolation of an infant from the mother with varicella and interruption of breastfeeding should occur only while the mother remains clinically infectious, regardless of the method of feeding. As soon as the infant has received the varicella-zoster Ig, expressed breast milk can be given to an infant if no skin lesions involve the breasts. Persons with varicella rash are considered noninfectious when no new vesicles have appeared for 72 hours and all lesions have crusted, usually in 6 to 10 days. Immunocompetent mothers who develop zoster can continue to breastfeed if the lesions do not involve the breast and can be covered because antibodies against varicella-zoster virus are provided to the infant via the placenta and breast milk, and these antibodies will diminish the severity of disease, even if not preventing it. Conservative management in this scenario would include giving an infant varicella-zoster Ig as well (see Table 13-5).

	Chickenpox Lesions Present		
Type of Exposure or Disease	**Mother**	**Neonate**	**Disposition**
A. Siblings at home have active chickenpox when the neonate and mother are ready for discharge from hospital	No	No	1. Mother: If she has a history of chickenpox, she may return home. Without a history, she should be tested for the varicella-zoster virus antibody titer.* If the test is positive, she may return home. If the test is negative, varicella-zoster Ig† is administered and she is discharged home
			2. Neonate: May be discharged home with mother if the mother has a history of varicella or is varicella-zoster virus-antibody positive. If the mother is susceptible, administer varicella-zoster Ig to the infant and discharge home or place in protective isolation
B. Mother has no history of chickenpox; exposed during period 6-20 days antepartum‡	No	No	1. Exposed mother and infant: Send home at the earliest date, unless siblings at home have communicable chickenpox.§ If so, may administer varicella-zoster Ig and discharge home, as above
			2. Other mothers and infants: No special management indicated
			3. Hospital personnel: No precautions indicated if there is a history of previous chickenpox or zoster. In absence of a history, immediate serologic testing is indicated to determine immune status.* Nonimmune personnel should be excluded from patient contact until 21 days after an exposure
			4. If the mother develops varicella 1 to 2 days postpartum, the infant should be given varicella-zoster Ig
C. Onset of maternal chickenpox occurs antepartum‡ or postpartum	Yes	No	1. Infected mother: Isolate until no longer clinically infectious. If seriously ill, treat with acyclovir¶
			2. Infected mother's infant: Administer varicella-zoster Ig† to neonates born to mothers with onset of chickenpox less than 5 days before delivery and isolate separately from mother. Send home with the mother if no lesions develop by the time the mother is noninfectious.
			3. Other mothers and infants: Send home at the earliest date. Varicella-zoster Ig may be given to exposed neonates
			4. Hospital personnel: Same as B-3
D. Onset of maternal chickenpox occurs antepartum§			1. Mother: Isolation unnecessary
			2. Infant: Isolate from other infants but not from the mother
			3. Other mothers and infants: Same as C-3 (if exposed)
			4. Hospital personnel: Same as B-3 (if exposed)
E. Congenital chickenpox	No	Yes	1. Infected infant and mother: Same as D-1 and D-2
			2. Other mothers and infants: Same as C-3
			3. Hospital personnel: Same as B-3

TABLE 13-5 Guidelines for Preventive Measures After Exposure to Chickenpox in the Nursery or Maternity Ward

ELISA, Enzyme-linked immunosorbent assay; *FAMA,* fluorescent antibody to membrane antigen; *LA,* latex agglutination.

*Send serum to virus diagnostic laboratory for determination of antibodies to varicella-zoster virus by a sensitive technique (e.g., FAMA, LA, ELISA). Personnel may continue to work for 8 days after exposure, pending serologic results because they are not potentially infectious during this period. Antibodies to varicella-zoster virus greater than 1:4 are probably indicative of immunity.

†Varicella-zoster Ig is available as VariZIG under an investigational new drug (IND) application from the Food and Drug Administration. It is obtainable through FFF Enterprises at 800-843-7477. The dose for a newborn is 1.25 mL (1 vial). The dose for a pregnant woman is conventionally 6.25 mL (5 vials).

‡If exposure occurred less than 6 days antepartum, the mother would not be potentially infectious until at least 72 hours postpartum.

§Considered noninfectious when no new vesicles have appeared for 72 hours and all lesions have crusted.

¶The dosage of acyclovir for a pregnant woman is 30 mg/kg/day; for a seriously ill infant with varicella, 750 to 1500 mg/m^2/day.

From Gershon AA: Chickenpox, measles and mumps. In Remington JS, Klein JO, editors: *Infectious diseases of the fetus and newborn infant,* ed 4, Philadelphia, 1995, WB Saunders.

WEST NILE VIRUS

West Nile virus disease in the United States is one of the best examples of an emerging infectious disease taking on new importance in public awareness about health issues. In 2003, 9136 human cases of West Nile infection were reported to the CDC (through 2/11/2004). Cases were reported from 45 states, including 6256 cases (68%) of West Nile fever (milder cases), 2718 cases (30%) of West Nile meningoencephalitis, and 228 deaths related to West Nile disease.[84] West Nile virus is endemic in Israel and parts of Africa. Outbreaks have been reported from Romania (1996), Russia (1999), Israel (2000), and Canada (2002), as well as the United States (1999 to 2003).[371] In 2013, there were 2469 reported cases of West Nile virus illness reported, including 1267 cases with neuroinvasive disease.[79-81]

It is estimated that 150 to 300 asymptomatic cases of West Nile infection occur for every 20 febrile illnesses and for every one case of meningoencephalitis associated with West Nile virus. West Nile fever is usually a mild illness of 3 to 6 days' duration. The symptoms are relatively nonspecific, including malaise, nausea, vomiting, headache, myalgia, lymphadenopathy, and rash. West Nile disease is characterized by severe neurologic symptoms (e.g., meningitis, encephalitis, or acute flaccid paralysis, and occasionally optic neuritis, cranial nerve abnormalities, and seizures). Children are infrequently sick with West Nile virus infection, and infants younger than 1 year of age have rarely been reported.[371] The case-fatality rate for 2003 in the United States was approximately 2.5%, but the rate has been reported to be as high as 4% to 18% in hospitalized patients. The case-fatality rate for persons older than 70 years of age is considered to be higher, 15% to 29%, as documented among hospitalized patients in outbreaks in Romania and Israel.[371]

The primary mechanism of transmission is via a mosquito bite. Mosquitoes from the genus *Culex* are primary vectors. The bird-mosquito-bird cycle serves to maintain and amplify the virus in the environment. Humans and horses are incidental hosts. The pathogenesis of the infection is believed to occur via replication of the virus in the skin and lymph nodes, leading to a primary viremia that seeds secondary sites before a second viremia causes the infection of the CNS and other affected organs.[66,122] Transmission has been reported in rare instances during pregnancy,[8,79] via organ transplant,[219] and percutaneously in laboratory workers.[81]

A study of West Nile virus infection in pregnancy documented four miscarriages, two elective abortions, and 72 live births. Cord-blood samples were tested in 55 infants, and 54 of 55 were negative for anti-West Nile virus IgM. Three infants had West Nile virus infection, which could have been acquired congenitally. Three of seven infants had congenital malformations that might have been caused by maternal West Nile virus infection based on timing in pregnancy, but no evidence of West Nile virus etiology was conclusively demonstrated.[351] West Nile virus transmission occurs via blood and blood-product transfusion,[204] and the incidence has been estimated to be as high as 21 per 10,000 donations during epidemics in specific cities.[46] No evidence of direct person-to-person transmission without the mosquito vector has been found.

One case of possible West Nile virus transmission via breastfeeding has been documented.[80] The mother acquired the virus via packed RBC transfusions after delivery. The second unit of blood she received was associated with other blood products from the same donation causing West Nile infection in another transfusion recipient. Eight days later, the mother had a severe headache and was hospitalized with fever and a CSF pleocytosis on day 12 after delivery. The mother's CSF was positive for West Nile virus-specific IgM antibody. The infant had been breastfed from birth through the second day of hospitalization of the mother. Samples of breast milk were West Nile virus-specific IgG and IgM positive on day 16 after delivery and West Nile virus-specific IgM positive on day 24. The same milk was West Nile virus RNA positive by PCR testing on day 16 but not on day 24 after delivery. The infant tested positive for West Nile virus-specific IgM in serum at day 25 of age but remained well without fever. No clear-cut exposure to mosquitoes for the infant were reported. The cord blood and placenta were not available to be tested. IgM antibodies can be found in low concentrations in breast milk, but this is not common or as efficient as the transfer of IgA, secretory IgA, or IgG into breast milk.[80]

A review of West Nile virus illness during breastfeeding identified six occurrences of breastfeeding during maternal West Nile virus illness.[195] Five of the six infants had no illness or detectable antibodies to West Nile virus in their blood. One infant developed a rash and was otherwise well after maternal West Nile virus illness, but was not tested for West Nile virus infection. Two infants developed West Nile virus illness while breastfeeding, but no preceding West Nile virus infection was demonstrated in their mothers. Two other breastfeeding infants developed West Nile virus-specific antibodies after their mothers acquired West Nile virus illness in the last week of pregnancy, but congenital infection could not be ruled out. Live virus was not cultured from 45 samples of breast milk from mothers infected with West Nile virus during pregnancy, but West Nile virus RNA was detected in two samples and 14 samples had IgM antibodies to West Nile virus. [195]

The mentioned data suggest that West Nile virus infection through breastfeeding is rare. To date, evidence of significant disease due to West Nile virus infection in young breastfeeding children is lacking. At this time, no reason exists to proscribe breastfeeding in the case of maternal West Nile virus infection if a mother is well enough to breast-feed. As with many other maternal viral illnesses, by the time the diagnosis is made in a mother, the infant may have already been exposed during maternal viremia and possible virolactia. The infant can and should continue to receive breast milk for the potential specific and nonspecific antiviral immunologic benefits.

YELLOW FEVER VIRUS

Yellow fever virus is a flavivirus that is transmitted to humans by infected *Aedes* and *Haemogogus* mosquitos in tropical areas of South America and Africa. Large outbreaks occur when mosquitos in a populated area become infected from biting viremic humans infected with yellow fever virus. Transmission from the mosquitos to other humans occurs after an incubation period in the mosquito of 8 days. Direct person-to-person spread has not been reported. Illness due to yellow fever virus usually begins after an incubation period of 3 to 6 days, with acute onset of headache, fever, chills, and myalgia. Photophobia, back pain, anorexia, vomiting, and restlessness are other common symptoms. The individual is usually viremic for the first 4 days of illness until the fever and other symptoms diminish. Liver dysfunction and even failure can develop, as can myocardial dysfunction. CNS infection is uncommon, but symptoms can include seizures and coma. Medical care should include intensive supportive care and fluid management.

One case of congenital infection after immunization of a pregnant woman with the attenuated vaccine strain has been reported. One of 41 infants whose mothers had inadvertently received the yellow fever virus vaccine during pregnancy developed IgM and elevated neutralizing antibodies against the yellow fever virus without any evidence of illness or abnormalities. [463] A more recent study [449] from Brazil examined inadvertent yellow fever virus immunization during pregnancy during a mass vaccination campaign in 2000; 480 pregnant women received the yellow fever virus at a mean of 5.7 weeks' gestation, the majority of whom did not know their pregnancy status at the time. Seroconversion occurred in 98.2% of the women after at least 6 weeks after vaccination. Mild

postvaccination illness (headache, fever, or myalgia) was reported by 19.6% of the 480 women. The frequency of malformations, miscarriages, stillbirths, and premature deliveries was similar to that found in the general population. At the 12-month follow-up point, 7% of the infants still demonstrated neutralizing antibodies against yellow fever virus, but after 12 months, only one child was still seropositive. [449]

Transmission of the yellow fever vaccine virus through breastfeeding was reported from Brazil in 2009. [91] The mother was immunized during a yellow fever epidemic in a nonendemic area in Brazil; 15 days after delivering a healthy female infant (39 weeks' gestational age) the mother received the 17DD yellow fever vaccine, and 5 days later, the mother reported headache, malaise, and low-grade fever that persisted for 2 days. The mother continued breastfeeding and did not seek medical care for herself. At 23 days of age the infant became irritable, developed fever, and refused to nurse. The infant developed seizures and subsequent evaluation of the infant demonstrated an abnormal CSF, and a CT of the brain showed bilateral areas of diffuse low density suggestive of inflammation and consistent with encephalitis. Yellow fever-specific IgM antibodies were identified in the infant's serum and CSF. Reverse-transcriptase polymerase chain reaction (RT-PCR) testing of the CSF also demonstrated yellow fever virus RNA identical to the 17DD yellow fever vaccine virus. Breast milk and maternal serum were not tested for yellow fever virus. [91] A second similar case of possible transmission of the vaccine strain of yellow fever virus was described in Canada. [257] Yellow fever virus, wild or vaccine type, has not been identified in human breast milk, although another flavivirus, West Nile virus, has been detected in milk from a few lactating women with West Nile virus infection. [195] (See the section on West Nile virus.) Yellow fever vaccine-associated neurologic disease occurs at different rates in different age-groups, including 0.5 to 4.0 cases per 1000 infants younger than 6 months of age. [321] The 17D-derived yellow fever vaccines are contraindicated in infants younger than 6 months of age.

Since 2002, the Advisory Committee on Immunization Practices has recommended, based on theoretical risk, that yellow fever vaccine be avoided in nursing mothers, except when exposure in high-risk yellow fever endemic areas is likely to occur. [82]

No case of transmission of yellow fever virus from an infected mother to her infant via breastfeeding or breast milk has been reported. Published information on the severity of yellow fever virus infection in infants younger than 1 year of age, potential protection from passively acquired antibodies, or protection from breast milk is limited.

No information on the differential risk for infection in breastfed versus formula-fed infants is available. Given the well-documented method of transmission of yellow fever virus via mosquitos, and the lack of evidence of transmission via breast milk, it makes more sense to protect all infants against mosquito bites than to proscribe breastfeeding, even when the mother is infected with yellow fever virus. Continued breastfeeding or use of expressed breast milk will depend on a mother's health status and ability to maintain the milk supply while acutely ill. If another source of feeding is readily available, then temporarily discarding expressed breast milk for at least 4 days of acute illness in the mother is a reasonable precaution.[82,91]

SPIROCHETES

Lyme Disease

Lyme disease, as with other human illnesses caused by spirochetes, especially syphilis, is characterized by a protean course and distinct phases (stages) of disease. Lyme borreliosis was described in Europe in the early twentieth century. Since the 1970s, tremendous recognition, description, and investigation of Lyme disease have occurred in the United States and Europe. Public concern surrounding this illness is dramatic.

Lyme disease is a multisystem disease characterized by involvement of the skin, heart, joints, and nervous system (peripheral and central). Stages of disease are identified as early localized (erythema migrans, often accompanied by arthralgia, neck stiffness, fever, malaise, and headache), early disseminated (multiple erythema migrans lesions, cranial nerve palsies, meningitis, conjunctivitis, arthralgia, myalgia, headache, fatigue, and, rarely, myocarditis), and late disease (recurrent arthritis, encephalopathy, and neuropathy). The varied manifestations of disease may relate to the degree of spirochetemia, the extent of dissemination to specific tissues, and the host's immunologic response.

The diagnosis of Lyme disease is often difficult, in part, because of the broad spectrum of presentations, inapparent exposure to the tick, and the lack of adequately standardized serologic tests. Culturing of the spirochete, Borrelia burgdorferi, is not readily available. Enzyme-linked immunosorbent assay (ELISA), immunofluorescent assay, and immunoblot assay are the usual tests. PCR detection of spirochetal DNA requires additional testing in clinical situations to clarify and standardize its utility.

Gardner[156] reviewed infection during pregnancy, summarizing a total of 46 adverse outcomes from 161 cases reported in the literature. The adverse outcomes included miscarriage and stillbirth (11% of cases), perinatal death (3%), congenital anomalies (15%), and both early- and late-onset progressive infection in the infants. Silver[428] reviewed 11 published reports and concluded that Lyme disease during pregnancy is uncommon, even in endemic areas. Although the spirochete can be transmitted transplacentally, a significant immune response in the fetus is often lacking, and the association of Lyme infection with congenital abnormalities is weak.[446,499]

Little published information exists on whether B. burgdorferi can be transmitted via breast milk. One report showed the detection of B. burgdorferi DNA by PCR in the breast milk of two lactating women with untreated erythema migrans, but no evidence of Lyme disease or transmission of the spirochete in the one infant followed for 1 year.[411] No attempt to culture the spirochete was made, so it is not possible to determine if the detectable DNA was from viable spirochetes or noninfectious fragments. In that same study of 56 women with untreated erythema migrans who had detectable B. burgdorferi DNA in the urine, 32 still had detectable DNA in the urine 15 to 30 days after starting treatment, but none had it 6 months after initiating therapy. Ziska et al.[519] reported on the management of nine cases of Lyme disease in women, associated with pregnancy; seven of the nine women were symptomatic at conception, and six received antibiotics throughout pregnancy. Follow-up of the infants showed no transmission of Lyme disease, even in the seven infants who had been breastfed.[519]

The lack of adequate information on the transmission of B. burgdorferi via breast milk cannot be taken as proof that it is not occurring. If one extrapolates from data on syphilis and the Treponema pallidum spirochete, it would be prudent to discuss the lack of information on the transmission of B. burgdorferi via breast milk with the mother or parents and to consider withholding breast milk at least until therapy for Lyme disease has begun or has been completed. If the infection occurred during pregnancy and treatment has already been completed, an infant can breastfeed. If infection occurs postpartum or the diagnosis is made postpartum, infant exposure may have already occurred. Again, discussion with the mother or parents about withholding versus continuing breastfeeding is appropriate.

After prenatal or postnatal exposure, an infant should be closely observed and empiric therapy considered if the infant develops a rash or symptoms suggestive of Lyme borreliosis. The treatment of mother and infant with ceftriaxone, penicillin, or amoxicillin is acceptable during breastfeeding relative to the infant's exposure to these medications. Doxycycline should not be administered for more than 14 days while continuing breastfeeding because of possible dental staining in the neonate. Continued surveillance for viable organisms in breast milk and evidence of transmission through breastfeeding is recommended.

A large body of information is available on various "Lyme vaccines" used in mouse models and dogs, but these vaccines are only partially protective and must be repeated yearly. Preliminary information suggests that a vaccine for use in humans safely produces good serologic responses, but protective efficacy has not been demonstrated, and no information exists on its use during pregnancy or breastfeeding.

Syphilis

Syphilis is the classic example of a spirochetal infection that causes multisystem disease in various stages. Both acquired syphilis and congenital syphilis are well-described entities. Acquired syphilis is almost always transmitted through direct sexual contact with open lesions of the skin or mucous membranes of individuals infected with the spirochete, *T. pallidum*. Congenital syphilis occurs by infection across the placenta (placentitis) at any time during the pregnancy or by contact with the spirochete during passage through the birth canal. Any stage of the disease (primary, secondary, tertiary) in a mother can lead to infection of the fetus, but transmission in association with secondary syphilis approaches 100%. Infection with primary syphilis during pregnancy, without treatment, leads to spontaneous abortion, stillbirth, or perinatal death in 40% of cases. Similar to acquired syphilis, congenital syphilis manifests with moist lesions or secretions from rhinitis (snuffles), condylomata lata, or bullous lesions. These lesions and secretions contain numerous spirochetes and are therefore highly infectious.

Postnatal infection of an infant can occur through contact with open, moist lesions of the skin or mucous membranes of the mother or other infected individuals. If the mother or infant has potentially infectious lesions, isolation from each other and from other infants and mothers is recommended. If lesions are on the breasts or nipples, breastfeeding or using expressed milk is contraindicated until treatment is complete and the lesions have cleared. Spirochetes are rarely identified in open lesions after more than 24 hours of appropriate treatment. Penicillin remains the best therapy.

The evaluation of an infant with suspected syphilis should be based on the mother's clinical and serologic status, history of adequate therapy in the mother, and the infant's clinical status. Histologic examination of the placenta and umbilical cord, serologic testing of the infant's blood and CSF, complete analysis of the CSF, long bone

and chest radiographs, liver function tests, and a complete blood cell count are all appropriate, given the specific clinical situation. Treatment of the infant should follow recommended protocols for suspected, probable, or proven syphilitic infection.[105]

No evidence indicates transmission of syphilis via breast milk exists in the absence of a breast or nipple lesion. When a mother has no suspicious breast lesions, breastfeeding is acceptable as long as appropriate therapy for suspected or proven syphilis is begun in the mother and infant.

PARASITES

Giardia lamblia

Giardiasis is a localized infection limited to the intestinal tract, causing diarrhea and malabsorption. Immunocompetent individuals show no evidence of invasive infection, and no evidence indicates fetal infection from maternal infection during pregnancy. Giardiasis is rare in children younger than 6 months of age, although neonatal infection from fecal contamination at birth has been described.[24] Human milk has an in vivo protective effect against *Giardia lamblia* infection, as documented by work from central Africa, where the end of breastfeeding heralds the onset of *Giardia* infection.[160] This has been reaffirmed in undeveloped countries around the world.

The protective effect of breast milk has been identified in the milk of noninfected donors.[167] The antiparasitic effect does not result from specific antibodies but rather from lipase enzymatic activity. The lipase acts in the presence of bile salts to destroy the trophozoites as they emerge from their cysts in the GI tract. Hernell et al.[193] demonstrated that free fatty acids have a marked giardiacidal effect, which supports the conclusion that lipase activity releasing fatty acids is responsible for killing *G. lamblia*.

G. lamblia has also been reported to appear in the mother's milk, and the parasite has been transmitted to newborns via that route. The exact relationship of breastfeeding to the transmission of *G. lamblia* and the effect on infants continue to be studied, even though symptomatic infection in breastfed infants is rare.[167] One report from the Middle East suggests that even partial breastfeeding is protective against infection with intestinal parasites, including *Cryptosporidium* and *G. lamblia*.[47] A second report from Egypt suggests that breastfeeding has a protective effect against infantile diarrhea caused by intestinal protozoa.[1] The affected organisms included *Cryptosporidium* sp., *Entamoeba histolytica*, *Giardia*, and *Blastocytis*, although the number of infants studied was too small to demonstrate significant protection against each individual protozoon.

Breastfeeding by mothers with giardiasis is problematic mainly because of the medications used for therapy. Metronidazole's safety in infants has not been established, although it is commonly used in premature neonates and infants. Little information is available on quinacrine hydrochloride and furazolidone in breast milk. Paromomycin, an orally nonabsorbable aminoglycoside, is a reasonable alternative recommended for treatment of pregnant women. Breastfeeding by a mother with symptomatic giardiasis is acceptable when consideration is given to the presence of the therapeutic agents in the breast milk.

Hookworm Infection

Hookworm infection, most often caused by *Ancylostoma duodenale* and *Necator americanus*, is common in children younger than the age of 4 years, and there is at least one report on infantile hookworm disease from China.[417] This publication from the Chinese literature reports hundreds of cases of infantile hookworm disease that include the common symptoms of bloody stools, melena, anorexia, listlessness, and edema. Anemia, eosinophilia, and even leukemoid reactions occur as part of the clinical picture in young children. They also note at least 20 cases of hookworm diseases in newborn infants younger than 1 month of age. In the discussion of infantile hookworm infection, they note four routes of infection: direct contact with contaminated soil, "sand-stuffed" diapers, contaminated "washed/wet" diapers, and vertical transmammary transmission or transplacental transmission. They postulated that infection of infants before 40 to 50 days of age would most likely be due to transplacental transmission, and infection before environmental contact would most likely be due to transmammary transmission. Ample evidence is available in veterinary medicine of transmammary spread of helminths.[341,426] At least two reports suggest the possibility of transmammary transmission of hookworms in humans. Setasuban et al.[419] described the prevalence of *N. americanus* in 128 nursing mothers as 61% and identified *N. americanus* in breast milk in one case. Nwosu[342] documented stool samples positive for hookworms in 33 of 316 neonates (10%) at 4 to 5 weeks of age in southern Nigeria. The majority of neonatal infections were due to *A. duodenale*, although *N. americanus* is more prevalent in that area of Nigeria. Examination of colostral milk did not demonstrate any hookworm larvae.[342]

Additional epidemiologic work is necessary to determine the potential significance of the transmammary spread of helminths in humans, and more careful examination of breast milk as a source of hookworm infection is required before reasonable recommendations are possible.

Malaria

Malaria is recognized as a major health problem in many countries. The effect of malaria infection on pregnant and lactating women and thus on the developing fetus, neonate, and growing infant can be significant. The four species of malaria, *Plasmodium vivax*, *P. ovale*, *P. malariae*, and *P. falciparum*, vary in the specific aspects of the disease they produce. *P. vivax* exists throughout the world, but *P. falciparum* predominates in the tropics and is most problematic in its chloroquine-resistant form. Malaria in the United States is most often seen in individuals traveling from areas where malaria is endemic. The parasite can exist in the blood for weeks, and infection with *P. vivax* and *P. malariae* can lead to relapses years later. Transmission occurs through the bite of the anopheline mosquito and can occur via transfusion of blood products and transplacentally.

Congenital malaria is rare but seems to occur more often with *P. vivax* and *P. falciparum*. It usually presents in the first 7 days of life (range: 1 day to 2 months). It may resemble neonatal sepsis, with fever, anemia, and splenomegaly occurring in the most neonates and hyperbilirubinemia and hepatomegaly in less than half.

Malaria in infants younger than 3 months of age generally manifests with less severe disease and death than it does in older children. Possible explanations include the effect of less exposure to mosquitoes, passive antibody acquired from the mother, and the high level of fetal hemoglobin in infants at this age.[24] The variations in the infection rates in children younger than 3 months of age during the wet and dry seasons support the idea that postnatal infection is more common than congenital infection. No evidence indicates that malaria is transmitted through breast milk. The greatest risk to infants is exposure to the anopheline mosquito infected with malaria.

The main issues relative to malaria and breastfeeding are how to protect both mothers and infants effectively from mosquitoes and what drugs for treating malaria in mothers are appropriate during lactation. Protection from mosquito bites includes screened-in living areas, mosquito nets while sleeping, protective clothing with or without repellents on the clothes, and community efforts to eradicate the mosquitoes. Chloroquine, quinine, and tetracycline are acceptable during breastfeeding. Sulfonamides should be avoided in the first month of an infant's life, but pyrimethamine-sulfadoxine (Fansidar) can be used later.

Mefloquine is not approved for infants or pregnant women. However, the milk-to-plasma ratio for mefloquine is less than 0.25, there is a large volume of distribution of the drug, high protein-binding of the drug limits its presence in breast milk, and the relative importance of breastfeeding in areas where malaria is prevalent shifts the risk-to-benefit ratio in favor of treatment with mefloquine. The single dose recommended for treatment or the once-weekly dose for prevention allows for continued breastfeeding with discarding of the milk for short periods after a dose (1 to 6 hours). Maternal plasma levels of primaquine range from 53 to 107 ng/mL, but no information is available on levels in human milk. Primaquine is used in children, and once daily dosing in the mother would allow for discarding milk with peak levels of drug. Therefore, breastfeeding during maternal malaria even with treatment is appropriate with specific medications.

Strongyloides

Strongyloides stercoralis is a nematode (roundworm). Most infections are asymptomatic, but clinically significant infections in humans can include larval skin invasion, tissue migration, intestinal invasion with abdominal pain and GI symptoms, and a Loeffler-like syndrome due to migration to the lungs. Immune-compromised individuals can develop dissemination of larvae systemically, causing various clinical symptoms. Humans are the principal hosts, but other mammals can serve as reservoirs. Infection via the skin by filariform larvae is the most common form of transmission, and ingestion is an uncommon occurrence. The transmammary transmission of *Strongyloides* species has been described in dogs, ewes, and rats.[232,341,426] Only one report of transmammary passage of *Strongyloides* larvae in humans is available. In 76 infants younger than 200 days of age, 34% demonstrated the presence of *S. fuelleborni* on stool examination. The clinical significance of this was not elucidated. *Strongyloides* larvae were identified in only one sample of milk from 25 nursing mothers.[60]

In the absence of an understanding of the clinical significance of *Strongyloides* in the stools of young infants, given the lack of exclusion of the most common mechanism of transmission (through the skin) in the single report and the apparent infrequent evidence of these larvae in human milk, it is difficult to make any recommendations concerning breastfeeding and *Strongyloides*.

Toxoplasmosis

Toxoplasmosis is one of the most common infections of humans throughout the world. The infective organism, *Toxoplasma gondii*, is ubiquitous in nature. The prevalence of positive serologic test titers increases with age, indicating past exposure and infection. The cat is the definitive host, although infection occurs in most species of warm-blooded animals.

Postnatal infection with toxoplasmosis is usually asymptomatic. Symptomatic infection typically manifests with nonspecific symptoms, including fever, malaise, myalgia, sore throat, lymphadenopathy, rash, hepatosplenomegaly, and occasionally a mononucleosis-like illness. The illness usually resolves without treatment or significant complications.

Congenital infection or infection in an immunodeficient individual can be persistent and severe, causing significant morbidity and even death. Although most infants with congenital infection are asymptomatic at birth, visual abnormalities, learning disabilities, and mental retardation can occur months or years later. The syndrome of congenital toxoplasmosis is clearly defined, with the most severe manifestations involving the CNS, including hydrocephalus, cerebral calcifications, microcephaly, chorioretinitis, seizures, or simply isolated ocular involvement. The risk for fetal infection is related to the timing of primary maternal infection, although transmission can occur with preexisting maternal toxoplasmosis.[267] In the last months of pregnancy, the protozoan is more readily transmitted to the fetus, but the infection is more likely to be subclinical. Early in pregnancy the transmission to a fetus occurs less frequently, but it does result in severe disease. Treatment of documented congenital infection is currently recommended, although the duration and optimal regimen have not been determined, and reversal of preexisting sequelae generally does not occur.[384]

The prevention of infection in susceptible pregnant women is possible by avoiding exposure to cat feces or the organism in the soil. Pregnant or lactating women should not change cat litter boxes, but if they must, it should be done daily and while wearing gloves. The oocyst is not infective for the first 24 to 48 hours after passage. Mothers can avoid ingestion of the organism by fully cooking meats and carefully washing fruits, vegetables, and food preparation surfaces.[102]

In various animal models, *T. gondii* has been transmitted through the milk to the suckling young. The organism has been isolated from colostrum as well. The newborn animals became asymptomatically infected when nursed by an infected mother whose colostrum contained *T. gondii*. Only one report has identified *T. gondii* in human milk, and some question surrounds the reliability of that report.[267] Transmission during breastfeeding in humans has not been demonstrated. Breast milk may contain appropriate antibodies against *T.*

gondii. Given the benign nature of postnatal infection, the absence of documented transmission in human breast milk, and the potential antibodies in breast milk, no reason exists to proscribe breastfeeding by a mother known to be infected with toxoplasmosis.

Trichomonas vaginalis

Trichomonas vaginalis is a flagellated protozoan that can produce vaginitis (see Chapter 16 for a discussion of vaginitis), but it frequently causes asymptomatic infection in both men and women. The parasite is found in 10% to 25% of women in the childbearing years. It is transmitted predominantly by sexual intercourse, but it can be transmitted to the neonate by passage through the birth canal. This parasite often coexists with other STDs, especially gonorrhea.

Infection during pregnancy or while taking oral contraceptives is more difficult to treat. Some evidence suggests that infection with and growth of the parasite are enhanced by estrogens or their effect on the vaginal epithelium. No evidence indicates adverse effects on the fetus in association with maternal infection during pregnancy. Occasionally, female newborns have vaginal discharge during the first weeks of life caused by *T. vaginalis.* This is thought to be influenced by the effect of maternal estrogen on the infant's vaginal epithelium and the acquisition of the organism during passage through the birth canal. The organism does not seem to cause significant disease in a healthy infant. No documentation exists on transmission of *T. vaginalis* via breast milk.

The difficulty encountered with maternal infection during lactation stems from concerns regarding the use of metronidazole, the drug of choice. There are data on the use of metronidazole in premature infants and neonates without difficulty. Although topical agents containing povidone-iodine (Betadine) or sodium lauryl sulfate (Trichotine) can be effective when given as douches, creams, or suppositories, metronidazole remains the treatment of choice. The AAP advises using metronidazole only with a physician's direction and considers its effect on a nursing infant unknown but possibly a concern. The potential concerns are metronidazole's disulfiram-like effect in association with alcohol, tumorigenicity in animal studies, and leukopenia and neurologic side effects described in adults. On the other hand, metronidazole is given to neonates and children beyond the neonatal period to treat serious infections with various bacteria or other parasites, such as *E. histolytica.*

The current recommendation for lactating women is to try local treatments first, and if these fail, then to try metronidazole. A 2-g single-dose treatment produces peak levels after 1 hour, and discarding expressed breast milk for the next 12 to 24 hours is recommended. If this treatment also fails, a 1-g twice-daily regimen for 7 days or a 2-g single daily dose for 3 to 5 days is recommended, with the discarding of breast milk close to the dose and timing of feedings distant from the dose.

Strongyloides

Strongyloides, one of the intestinal nematodes with both skin and diffuse organ dissemination, is found worldwide in tropical and temperate environments. Its true prevalence is probably significantly underestimated because of subclinical infection and the resulting difficulty of diagnosing it. Acute infection can cause a cutaneous eruption. In more chronic infection, it is associated with the GI tract and malabsorption, chronic diarrhea, failure to thrive, fever, cachexia, abdominal pain, cramping, and alternating diarrhea and constipation. Hyperinfection and invasive disease are most often evident in the lungs, but *Strongyloides* can include many organs, such as the lymph nodes, skeletal muscle, heart, liver, and brain. There is a syndrome of infantile strongyloidiasis caused by *S. fuelleborni* affecting the infant in the first months of life with prolonged diarrhea, abdominal distention, failure to thrive, and malnutrition. Due to the timing, it is suspected that this syndrome appearing in early infancy is due to vertical transmission. *Strongyloides* is passed in the milk of a number of animal species.[60] Nevertheless, *Strongyloides* was detected in human milk of only one sample out of 113 samples tested by Brown and Girardeau.

Costa-Macedo and Rey reported that, although they identified a variety of intestinal parasites in 208 children less than 2 years of age in Rio de Janeiro, 12.7% of the children had one or more parasites in stool studies. *Ascaris lumbricoides* was the parasite most frequently detected in children less than 1 year of age. The presence of parasites was statistically less in the breastfed infants, and no exclusively breastfed child presented with infection.[110] Mota-Ferreira et al. identified IgA and IgG antibodies specific against *S. stercoralis* in breastmilk by ELISA (IgA in 28.9%, and IgG in 25.5% of the samples) and indirect fluorescent antibody test (IFAT) (IgA in 42.25%, and IgG in 18.9% of the samples, with over 90% concurrence).

Given the uncommon association of parasites with breastfed infants, the limited evidence of *Strongyloides* in human milk, and the presence of antibodies against specific antigens of *S. stercoralis,* there is no reason to proscribe breastfeeding relative to *Strongyloides* infection.

Trypanosoma cruzi

Chagas disease, caused by the protozoa *Trypnosoma cruzi*, is a major cause of disease in the Americas, and it is endemic in many parts of South America. Pregnant or breastfeeding women can be chronically infected (often asymptomatic) or acutely infected. Infection in pregnancy is associated with an increased risk of preterm birth, low birth weight, or stillbirth. There is a clinical picture of congenital Chagas disease that includes hepatosplenomegaly, myocarditis, anemia, anasarca, and meningoencephalitis in the severest form, but it is most commonly an asymptomatic infection. A systematic review and meta-analysis reported a prevalence ranging from 0.1% to 8.5% in pregnant women in Brazil, with congenital transmission rates of 0% to 5.2%.[300] In congenital infection, the treatment success is close to 90%. In Spain, a nonendemic country, Ramos et al. reported a seroprevalence rate in pregnant immigrant women from South America as 1.28%, but they were unable to identify a case of congenital Chagas disease in 545 infants.[380]

A recent review of Chagas disease and breastfeeding noted that *T. cruzi* has been identified in the milk of chronically infected mice, but transmission through breast milk has been uncommon, and histologic examination of the breasts did not reveal any parasites.[338] They summarized eight reports in the literature of possible transmission of *T. cruzi* via breastfeeding in humans. In the majority of cases, the parasite could not be identified in the human milk, the exact mechanism could not be effectively pinpointed, and contamination of the breast milk with blood or another mechanism of transmission could not be excluded. They also noted that the "blood-form trypomastigotes" that would be expected to be found in the human milk would potentially have different surface receptors than "infectious metacyclic trypomastigotes" and therefore have altered infectious capability across mucous membranes. They also discussed acute Chagas disease, with probable parasitemia, noting that in only one case was the *T. cruzi* identified in the breast milk and that infant was not breastfed.

In light of the very rare occurrence of possible transmission of *T. cruzi* through human milk, it is not reasonable to proscribe breastfeeding by women with chronic Chagas disease. Even in women with acute Chagas and an increased likelihood of a transient parasitemia, by the time the diagnosis is made in the mother, the infant has probably already been exposed. Treating the mother and continuing breastfeeding is appropriate. The medications benznidazole and nifurtimox have been used to treat congenital infection in infants.

CANDIDA INFECTIONS

Candida consists of multiple species. The most common species affecting humans include *C. albicans*, as the dominant agent, and *C. tropicalis*, *C. krusei*, and *C. parapsilosis*, as well as many other uncommon species. In general, *Candida* exists as a commensal organism colonizing the oropharynx, GI tract, vagina, and skin without causing disease until some change disrupts the balance between the organism and the host. Mild mucocutaneous infection is the most common illness, which can lead to vulvovaginitis, mastitis, or, uncommonly, oral mucositis in a mother, and thrush (oral candidiasis) and candidal diaper rash in an infant.

Invasive candidal infection occurs infrequently, usually when a person has other illness, impaired resistance to infection (HIV, diabetes mellitus, neutropenia; decreased cell-mediated immunity in premature infants or LBW or VLBW infants), or disrupted normal mucosal and skin barriers and has received antibiotics or corticosteroids. Invasive disease can occur through local spread, and it may present more often in the genitourinary tract (urethra, bladder, ureters, kidneys), although it usually develops in association with candidemia. The bladder and kidney are more frequently involved, but when dissemination occurs via candidemia, a careful search for other sites of infection should be made (e.g., retina, liver, spleen, lung, meninges).[315]

Transmission usually occurs from healthy individuals colonized with *Candida* through direct contact or contact with their oral or vaginal secretions. Intrauterine infection can occur through ascending infection through the birth canal, but it is rare. This can cause congenital cutaneous candidiasis usually evident on the first day of life. Most often, an infant is infected in passing through the birth canal and remains colonized. Postnatal transmission can occur through direct contact with caregivers.

The mother and infant serve as an immediate source of recolonization for each other, especially during the direct contact of breastfeeding. For this reason, an infant and breastfeeding mother should be treated simultaneously when treating thrush, vulvovaginitis, diaper candidiasis, or mastitis. Colonization with this organism usually occurs in the absence of any clinical evidence of infection. Simultaneous treatment should occur even in the absence of any clinical evidence of *Candida* infection or colonization in the apparently uninvolved individual of the breastfeeding dyad.

No well-controlled clinical trials define the most appropriate or most effective method(s) of treatment for candidal infection in breastfeeding mother-infant dyads. The list of possible treatment products is extensive and includes many anecdotal and empirical regimens. In the face of this absence

181. Guzman MG, Kouri G: Dengue: an update, *Lancet Infect Dis* 2:33–42, 2002.

182. Haas J, Larson E, Ross B, et al: Epidemiology and diagnosis of hospital acquired conjunctivitis among neonatal intensive care unit patients, *Pediatr Infect Dis* 24:586–589, 2005.

183. Hale TW, Bateman TL, Finkelman MA, et al: The absence of *Candida albicans* in milk samples of women with clinical symptoms of ductal candidiasis, *Breastfeed Med* 4(2):57–61, 2009.

184. Hall CB, Caserta MT, Schnabel KC, et al: Congenital infections with human herpes virus 6 (HHV6) and human herpes virus 7 (HHV7), *J Pediatr* 145:472–477, 2004.

185. Halstead SB, Lan NT, Myint TT, et al: Dengue hemorrhagic fever in infants: research opportunities ignored, *Emerg Infect Dis* 8(12):1474, 2002.

186. Hamprecht K, Maschmann J, Jahn G, et al: Cytomegalovirus transmission to preterm infants during lactation, *J Clin Virol* 41:198–205, 2008.

187. Hamprecht K, Maschmann J, Vochem M, et al: Epidemiology of transmission of cytomegalovirus from mother to preterm infant by breastfeeding, *Lancet* 357(9255):513, 2001.

188. Harjulhto T, Aro T, Hovi T, et al: Congenital malformations and oral poliovirus vaccination during pregnancy, *Lancet I* 771:1989.

189. Harris SH, Khan MA, Khan R, et al: Mammary tuberculosis: analysis of thirty-eight patients, *ANZ J Surg* 76:234–237, 2006.

190. Hayes K, Danks DM, Gibas H, et al: Cytomegalovirus in human milk, *N Engl J Med* 287:177, 1972.

191. Henderson BE, Powell D, Rosario I, et al: An epidemiologic study of breast cancer, *J Natl Cancer Inst* 53:609, 1974.

192. Heneine W, Woods T, Green D, et al: Detection of HTLV-II in breast milk of HTLV-II infected mothers, *Lancet* 340:1157, 1992.

193. Hernell O, Ward H, Blackberg L: Killing of *Giardia lamblia* by human milk lipases: an effect mediated by lipolysis of milk lipids, *J Infect Dis* 153:715, 1986.

194. Hill JB, Sheffield JS, Kim MJ, et al: Risk of hepatitis B transmission in breast-fed infants of chronic hepatitis B carriers, *Obstet Gynecol* 99:1049–1052, 2002.

195. Hinckley AF, O'Leary DR, Hayes EB: Transmission of West Nile virus through human breast milk seems to be rare, *Pediatrics* 119:E666–E671, 2007.

196. Hino S: Milk-borne transmission of HTLV-I as a major route in the endemic cycle, *Acta Paediatr Jpn* 31:428, 1989.

197. Hino S, Katamine S, Miyata H, et al: Primary prevention of HTLV-I in Japan, *J Acquir Immune Defic Syndr Hum Retrovirol* 13S:515, 1996.

198. Hino S, Katamine S, Miyata H, et al: Primary prevention of HTLV-1 in Japan, *Leukemia* 11:S57, 1997.

199. Hino S, Sugiyama H, Doi H, et al: Breaking the cycle of HTLV-I transmission via carrier mothers milk, *Lancet* 2:158, 1987.

200. Hira SK, Mangrola UG, Mwale C, et al: Apparent vertical transmission of human immunodeficiency virus type 1 by breast-feeding in Zambia, *J Pediatr* 117(3):421, 1990.

201. Hisada M, Maloney EM, Sawada T, et al: Virus markers associated with vertical transmission of human T lymphotropic virus type 1 in Jamaica, *Clin Infect Dis* 34: 1551, 2002.

202. Hjelt K, Granbella PC, Haagen O, et al: Rotavirus antibodies in the mother and her breastfed infant, *J Pediatr Gastroenterol Nutr* 4:414, 1985.

203. Hokama T, Sakamoto R, Yara A, et al: Incidence of *Haemophilus influenzae* in the throats of healthy infants with different feeding methods, *Pediatr Int* 41(3):277, 1999.

204. Hollinger FB, Kleinman S: Transfusion transmission of West Nile virus: a merging of historical and contemporary perspectives, *Transfusion* 43:992, 2003.

205. Hon K, Leung CW, Cheng W, et al: Clinical presentations and outcomes of severe acute respiratory syndrome in children, *Lancet* 361:1701, 2003.

206. Horn P: Poliomyelitis in pregnancy: a twenty-year report from Los Angeles County, California, *Obstet Gynecol* 6:121, 1955.

207. Horowitz CA, Henle W, Henle G, et al: Long-term serologic follow-up of patients for Epstein-Barr virus after recovery from infectious mononucleosis, *J Infect Dis* 151:1150, 1985.

208. Horsburgh CR, Holmberg SC: The global distribution of human immunodeficiency virus type 2 (HIV-2) infection, *Transfusion* 28:192, 1988.

209. Horvath T, Madi BC, Iuppa IM, et al: Interventions for preventing late postnatal mother-to-child transmission of HIV, *Cochrane Database Syst Rev* 21, 2009. CD006734.

210. Huang YC, Chou YH, Su LH, et al: Methicillin-resistant *S. aureus* colonization and its association with infection among infants hospitalized in neonatal intensive care units, *Pediatrics* 118:469–474, 2006.

211. Hui DS, Memish ZA, Zumla A: Severe acute respiratory syndrome vs. the Middle East respiratory syndrome, *Curr Opin Pulm Med* 20(3):233–241, 2014. http://dx.doi.org/10.1097/MCP.0000000000000046.

212. Hurst V: *S. aureus* in the infant upper respiratory tract. I. Observations on hospital-born babies, *J Hyg (Lond)* 55:299, 1957.

213. Ing R, Ho JHC, Petrakis NL: Unilateral breast feeding and breast cancer, *Lancet* 2:124, 1977.

214. Ip S, Chung M, Raman G, et al: A summary of the Agency for Healthcare Research and Quality's evidence report on breastfeeding in developed countries, *Breastfeed Med* 4 (Suppl 1):S17–S30, 2009. http://dx.doi.org/10.1089/bfm.2009.0050.

215. Isaacs D, Fraser S, Hogg G, et al: *S. aureus* in Australasian neonatal nurseries, *Arch Dis Child Fetal Neonatal Ed* 89: F331–F335, 2004.

216. Ishak R, Harrington WJ, Azeuedo VN, et al: Identification of human T-cell lymphotropic virus type IIa infection in the Kayapo, an indigenous population of Brazil, *AIDS Res Hum Retroviruses* 11(7):813, 1995.

217. Iso K, Suzuki Y, Takayama M: Mother-to-infant transmission of TT virus in Japan, *Int J Gynaecol Obstet* 75:11, 2001.

218. Italian Register for HIV Infection in Children: HIV-1 infection and breast milk, *Acta Paediatr Suppl* 400:51, 1994.

219. Iwamoto W, Jernigan DB, Guasch A, et al: Transmission of West Nile virus from an organ donor to four transplant recipients, *N Engl J Med* 348:2196, 2003.

220. Jalali U, Rasul S, Khan A, et al: Tuberculosis mastitis, *J Coll Physicians Surg Pak* 15:234–237, 2005.

221. James L, Gorwitz RJ, Jones RC, et al: Methicillin-resistant *S. aureus* infections among healthy full-term newborns, *Arch Dis Child Fetal Neonatal Ed* 93:F40–F44, 2008.

222. Jeliffe DB, Jeliffe EFP: *Human milk in the modern world*, Oxford, 1978, Oxford University Press.

223. Jimenez E, Delgado S, Maldonado A, et al: *Staphylococcus epidermidis*: a differential trait of the fecal microbiota of breast-fed infants, *BMC Microbiol* 8:143, 2008.

224. Josephson CD, Caliendo AM, Easley KA, et al: Blood transfusion and breast milk transmission of cytomegalovirus in very low-birth-weight infants: a prospective cohort study, *JAMA Pediatr* 168(11):1054–1062, 2014. http://dx.doi.org/10.1001/jamapediatrics.2014.1360.

225. Junker AK, Thomas EE, Radcliffe A, et al: Epstein-Barr virus shedding in breast milk, *Am J Med Sci* 302:220–223, 1991.

226. Kafulafula G: Post weaning gastroenteritis and mortality in HIV-1 uninfected African infants receiving antiretroviral prophylaxis to prevent MTCT of HIV-1. In *Program and abstracts of the 14th conference on retroviruses and opportunistic*

infections, 25-28 *Feb* 2007, Los Angeles, California, Alexandria, Virginia, 2007, Conference of Retroviruses and Opportunistic Infections, http://www.retroconference.org/2007/Abstracts/28294.htm (abstract 773) (accessed 19.12.07).

227. Kalstone C: Successful antepartum treatment of listeriosis, *Am J Obstet Gynecol* 164:57, 1991.

228. Kaplan JE, Abrams E, Shaffer N, et al: Low risk for mother-to-child transmission of human T lymphotropic virus type II in non-breastfed infants, *J Infect Dis* 166:892, 1992.

229. Katzman DK, Wald ER: Staphylococcal scalded skin syndrome in a breastfed infant, *Pediatr Infect Dis J* 6:295, 1987.

230. Kaufman D, Boyle R, Hazen KC, et al: Fluconazole prophylaxis against fungal colonization and infection in preterm infants, *N Engl J Med* 345:1660, 2001.

231. Kawada M, Okuzumi K, Shigemi H, et al: Transmission of *Staphylococus aureus* between healthy lactating mothers and their infants by breastfeeding, *J Hum Lact* 19:411, 2003.

232. Kawanabe M, Nojima H, Uchikawa R: Transmammary transmission of *Strongyloides ratti*, *Parasitol Res* 75:50–56, 1988.

233. Keelyside RA, McCormick JB, Webb PA, et al: Case-control study of *Mastomys natalensis* and humans in Lassa virus-infected households in Sierra Leone, *Am J Trop Med Hyg* 32:829, 1983.

234. Keim SA, Hogan JS, McNamara KA, et al: Microbial contamination of human milk purchased via the Internet, *Pediatrics* 132(5):e1227–e1235, 2013. http://dx.doi.org/10.1542/peds.2013-1687 (Epub 2013 Oct 21).

235. Keller MA, Rodriguez AI, Alvarez S, et al: Transfer of tuberculin immunity from mother to infant, *Pediatr Res* 22:277, 1987.

236. Kenny JF, Zedd AJ: Recurrent group B streptococcal disease in an infant associated with the ingestion of infected mother's milk, *J Pediatr* 91:158, 1977.

237. Kerber R, Reindl S, Romanowski V, et al: Research efforts to control highly pathogenic arenaviruses: a summary of the progress and gaps, *J Clin Virol*, 2014 http://dx.doi.org/10.1016/j.jcv.2014.12.004 pii: S1386-6532(14)00466-1 (Epub ahead of print).

238. Khanna R, Prasanna GV, Gupta P, et al: Mammary tuberculosis: report on 52 cases, *Postgrad Med J* 78:422–424, 2002.

239. Kilewo C, Karlsson K, Massawe A, et al: Prevention of mother-to-child transmission of HIV-1 through breast feeding by treating infants prophylactically with lamivudine in Dar es Salaam, Tanzania, *J Acquir Immune Defic Syndr* 48:315–323, 2008.

240. Kilewo C, Karlsson K, Ngarina M, et al: Prevention of mother-to-child transmission of HIV through breastfeeding by treating mothers with triple antiretroviral therapy in Dar es Salaam, Tanzania: the Mitra Plus study, *J Acquir Immune Defic Syndr* 52:406–416, 2009.

241. Kim YH, Chang SS, Kim YS, et al: Clinical outcomes in methicillin-resistant *S. aureus* colonized neonates in the neonatal intensive care unit, *Neonatology* 91:241–247, 2007.

242. Kinoshita K, Hino S, Amagasaki T, et al: Demonstration of adult T-cell leukemia virus antigen in milk from three seropositive mothers, *Gann* 75:103, 1984.

243. Kinoshita K, Yamanouchi K, Ikeda S, et al: Oral infection of a common marmoset with human T-cell leukemia virus type I (HTLV-I by fresh human milk of HTLV-I carrier mothers), *Jpn J Cancer Res* 76:1147, 1985.

244. Kittigul L, Pitakarnjanakul P, Sujirarat D, et al: The differences of clinical manifestations and laboratory findings in children and adults with dengue virus infection, *J Clin Virol* 39:76–81, 2007.

245. Koch WC, Adler SP: Human parvovirus B19 infection in women of childbearing age and within families, *Pediatr Infect Dis J* 8:83, 1989.

246. Komrower GM, Williams BL, Stones PB: Lymphocytic choriomeningitis in the newborn, *Lancet* 1:697, 1955.

247. Kotiw M, Zhang GW, Daggard G, et al: Late-onset and recurrent neonatal group B streptococcal disease associated with breast-milk transmission, *Pediatr Dev Pathol* 6:251–256, 2003.

248. Kourtis A: Diarrhoea in uninfected infants of HIV-infected mothers who stop breastfeeding at 6 months: the BAN study experience. In *Program and abstracts of the 14th conference on retroviruses and opportunistic infections*, 25-28 Feb 2007, Los Angeles, California, Alexandria, Virginia, 2007, Conference of Retroviruses and Opportunistic Infections, http://www.retroconference.org/2007/Abstracts/28294.htm (abstract 772) (accessed 19.12.07).

249. Krain LJ, Atwell JE, Nelson KE, et al: Fetal and neonatal health consequences of vertically transmitted hepatitis E virus infection, *Am J Trop Med Hyg* 90(2):365–370, 2014. http://dx.doi.org/10.4269/ajtmh.13-0265 (Epub 2014 Jan 13).

250. Kuhn L, Aldrovandi GM, Sinkala M, et al: High uptake of exclusive breastfeeding and reduced postnatal HIV transmission; prospective results from the Zambia exclusive breastfeeding study. In *Program and abstracts of the 4th international AIDS society conference on HIV pathogenesis, treatment and prevention*, 22-25 July 2007; Sydney, Australia, Geneva, Switzerland, 2007, http://www.iasociety.org/Default.aspx?pageId=11&abstractid=200701784 (abstract TUAX 103) (accessed 19.12.07).

251. Kuhn J, Aldrovandi GM, Sinkala M, et al: Effect of early, abrupt weaning on HIV-free survival of children in Zambia, *N Engl J Med* 359:130–141, 2008.

252. Kuhn L, Aldrovandi GM, Sinkala M, et al: Differential effects of early weaning for HIV-free survival of children born to HIV-infected mothers by severity of maternal disease, *PLoS ONE* 4, 2009. e6059.

253. Kuhn L, Kasonde P, Sinkala M, et al: Prolonged breastfeeding and mortality up to two years postpartum among HIV positive women in Zambia, *AIDS* 19:1677–1681, 2005.

254. Kuhn L, Reitz C, Abrams EJ: Breastfeeding and AIDS in the developing world, *Curr Opin Pediatr* 21:83–93, 2009.

255. Kuhn L, Sinkala M, Thea DM, et al: HIV prevention is not enough: child survival in the context of prevention of mother to child HIV transmission, *J Int AIDS Soc* 12:36, 2009.

256. Kuhn L, Trabattoni D, Kankasa C, et al: HIV specific secretory IgA in breast milk of HIV-positive mothers is not associated with protection against HIV transmission among breast-fed infants, *J Pediatr* 149:611–616, 2006.

257. Kuhn S, Twele-Montecinos L, MacDonald J, et al: Case report: probable transmission of vaccine strain of yellow fever virus to an infant via breast milk, *CMAJ* 183(4):E243–E245, 2011. http://dx.doi.org/10.1503/cmaj.100619 (Epub 2011 Feb 7).

258. Kumar ML, Nankervis GA, Jacobs IB, et al: Congenital and postnatally acquired cytomegalovirus infections: long-term follow-up, *J Pediatr* 104:674, 1984.

259. Kumwenda NI, Hoover DR, Mofenson LM, et al: Extended antiretroviral prophylaxis to reduce breast milk HIV-1 transmission, *N Eng J Med* 359:119–129, 2008.

260. Kusuhara K, Takabayashi A, Ueda K, et al: Breast milk is not a significant source for early Epstein-Barr virus or human herpes virus 6 infection in infants: a seroepidemiologic study in 2 endemic areas of human T-cell lymphotropic virus type I in Japan, *Microbiol Immunol* 41:309–312, 1997.

261. Lal RB, Owen SM, Segurado AAC, et al: Mother-to-child transmission of human T-lymphotropic virus type II (HTLV-II), *Ann Intern Med* 120:300, 1994.

262. Lal RB, Renan A, Gongora-Biaanchi A, et al: Evidence for mother-to-child transmission of human T-lymphotropic virus type II, *J Infect Dis* 168:586, 1993.

263. Lamprecht CL, Krause HE, Mufson MA: Role of maternal antibody in pneumonia and bronchiolitis due to respiratory syncytial virus, *J Infect Dis* 134:211, 1976.

503. Wu J, Tang ZY, Wu YX, et al: Acquired cytomegalovirus infection of breast milk in infancy, *Chin Med J* 102:124, 1989.

504. Yamanouchi K, Kinochita K, Moriuchi R, et al: Oral transmission of human T-cell leukemia virus type 1 into a common marmoset as an experimental model for milk-borne transmission, *Jpn J Cancer Res* 76:481, 1985.

505. Yasuda A, Kimura H, Hayakawa M, et al: Evaluation of cytomegalovirus infections transmitted via breast milk in preterm infants with a real-time polymerase chain reaction assay, *Pediatrics* 111:1333, 2003.

506. Yeager AS, Palumbo PE, Malachowski N, et al: Sequelae of maternally derived cytomegalovirus infections in premature infants, *J Pediatr* 102:918, 1983.

507. Yeung LTF, King SM, Roberts EA: Mother-to-infant transmission of hepatitis C virus, *Hepatology* 34(2):223, 2001.

508. Yolken RH, Peterson JA, Vonderfecht SL, et al: Human milk mucin inhibits rotavirus replication and prevents experimental gastroenteritis, *J Clin Invest* 90(5):1984–1991, 1992.

509. Yoo K-Y, Tajima K, Kuroishi T, et al: Independent protective effect of lactation against breast cancer: a case-control study in Japan, *Am J Epidemiol* 135:726, 1992.

510. Yoshida K, Furumoto H, Abe A, et al: The possibility of vertical transmission of human papillomavirus through maternal milk, *J Obstet Gynaecol* 31(6):503–506, 2011. http://dx.doi.org/10.3109/01443615.2011.570814.

511. Yoshida M, Yamagami N, Tezuka T, et al: Case report: detection of varicella-zoster virus DNA in maternal breast milk, *J Med Virol* 38:108, 1992.

512. Yoshinaga M, Yashiki S, Fujiyoshi T, et al: A maternal factor for mother-to-child transmission: viral antigen-producing capacities in culture of peripheral blood and breast milk cells, *Jpn J Cancer Res* 86:649, 1995.

513. Zanetti AR, Tanzi E, Paccagnini S, et al: Mother-to-infant transmission of hepatitis C virus, *Lancet* 345:289, 1995.

514. Zeldis JB, Crumpacker CS: Hepatitis. In Remington JS, Klein JO, editors: *Infectious diseases of the fetus and newborn infant*, ed 4, Philadelphia, 1995, WB Saunders.

515. Zerr DM, Huang ML, Corey L, et al: Sensitive method for detection of human herpes viruses 6 and 7 in saliva collected in field studies, *J Clin Microbiol* 38:1981–1983, 2000.

516. Zhang L, Gui X, Wang B, et al: A study of immunoprophylaxis failure and risk factors of hepatitis B virus mother-to-infant transmission, *Eur J Pediatr* 173(9):1161–1168, 2014. http://dx.doi.org/10.1007/s00431-014-2305-7 (Epub 2014 Apr 5).

517. Zhang RJ, Zeng JS, Zhang HZ: Survey of 34 pregnant women with hepatitis A and their neonates, *Chin Med J* 103:552, 1990.

518. Ziegler JB, Cooper DA, Johnson RO, et al: Postnatal transmission of AIDS-associated retrovirus from mother to infant, *Lancet* 1:896, 1985.

519. Ziska MH, Giovanello T, Johnson MJ, et al: Disseminated Lyme disease and pregnancy. In 9th annual international scientific conference on Lyme disease and other tick-borne disorders, Boston, MA, April 19-20. 1996.

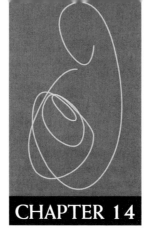

CHAPTER 14

Breastfeeding Infants with Problems

|||||||||||||||||||||||||||||||||||||||||||||||||||||||||||||||||||||

Breastfeeding is the ideal and preferred feeding method for a newborn. Occasionally infant problems interfere with breastfeeding and require the attention of the infant's physician to diagnose and treat the problem.

Breastfeeding is a natural behavior for infants and provides the ideal nourishment, but some infants with complicating issues may need special assistance or adjustments.[7] Prematurity is discussed in Chapter 15. Infants with structural abnormalities, metabolic challenges or neurologic difficulties, stressed infants, and twins and triplets will be discussed in this chapter.

Procedural Pain Relief

Systematic review and meta-analysis of procedural pain relief for neonates was reported by Shah et al. Infants with congenital, developmental, and environmental problems in the newborn period are often subjected to multiple procedures. Compared to placebo, positioning, or no intervention, breastfeeding is best. Glucose and sucrose are a substitute of necessity when mother's milk is not available.

Perinatal Issues: Postmature Infants

Postmature infants are full-grown, mature infants who have stayed in utero beyond the full vigor of the placenta and have begun to lose weight in utero.[37] They are usually "older looking" and have a wide-eyed countenance. Their skin is dry and peeling, and subcutaneous tissue is diminished; thus the skin appears too large. These infants have lost subcutaneous fat and lack glycogen stores. Initially they may be hypoglycemic and require early feedings to maintain blood glucose levels of 40 mg/dL or higher. If breastfed, the infants should go to the breast early, taking special care to maintain body temperature, which is labile in postmature infants who lack the insulating fat layer. Blood sugar levels should be followed. Initially, these infants may feed poorly and require considerable prodding to suckle. If the infant becomes hypoglycemic despite careful management, a feeding of 10% glucose in water should be considered. In extreme cases of hypoglycemia, an intravenous (IV) infusion may be necessary, and management should follow guidelines for any infant who has hypoglycemia that is resistant to routine early feedings. Because the infants lack glycogen stores, hypoglycemia may persist, and glucagon is contraindicated because no glycogen stores are present to be stimulated. Calcium problems, on the other hand, although common in these infants, generally are rare if the infant is adequately breastfed early because of the physiologic calcium/phosphorus ratio in breast milk. After postmature infants begin to feed well, they tend to catch up quickly and adapt well. Problems with hyperbilirubinemia seldom occur because their livers are mature. Postmature infants gain well at the breast once they stabilize.

FETAL DISTRESS AND HYPOXIA AND LOW APGAR SCORES

Infants who have been compromised in utero or during delivery because of insufficient placental reserve, cord accidents, or other causes of intrauterine hypoxia have very low Apgar scores at birth and need special treatment.[131] An asphyxiated infant cannot be fed for at least 48 hours, and, depending on associated findings, it may be 96 hours or more before it is safe to put food in the gastrointestinal (GI) tract, which has been poorly perfused during the hypoxia. The infant must be maintained on IV fluids. If the mother is to breastfeed or donor milk is available, human milk can be started sooner. Her colostrum will be valuable to the infant and will be better tolerated by the infant's intestinal tract, which has usually suffered hypoxic damage in these circumstances. Small amounts of colostrum can be given in 24 hours. Hypoxia decreases the motility of the gut and decreases stimulating hormones. The colostrum should be pumped and become the first oral feedings drop by drop.

Mothers will need help initiating lactation and understanding the pathophysiology of the infants' disease. These infants often have a poor suck that does not coordinate with the swallow, making nursing at the breast and bottle equally difficult. The mother may need to hold her breast in place and hold the infant's chin as well. These infants are especially susceptible to "nipple confusion," so means of sustaining nourishment other than a bottle should be sought. Cup feeding has been well tolerated using a soft plastic one-ounce medicine cup. Even infants who will not be breastfed but feed poorly from a bottle for neurologic reasons will do better with a cup.[69,70,90] Weaning slowly from the IV hyperalimentation fluids while introducing breastfeeding is helpful. Using a dropper and employing the nursing supplementer are options if milk supply from the breasts is low. These infants

may continue to feed poorly for neurologic reasons. They do not do better with a bottle. If the mother is taught to cope with the problem, nursing should progress satisfactorily. She may always need to hold her breast in place, which would be the best evidence of residual damage from the hypoxia.

Infants can be held in positions that may help an individual baby adapt better. The "football hold" is a popular but poorly named position in which an infant is held close to the mother's body with the feet to her side. The head and face are squarely in front of the breast and steadied by the mother's arm and hand on that side. Cupping the breast and the jaw in one hand facilitates the infant's seal around the breast with the mouth (Figure 14-1). This position has been called the "dancer hold."[104] One of the most valuable suggestions is the use of a sling or pleat-seat to hold an infant's body in a flexed position, thus giving the mother both hands free to hold the head and the breast in position for feeding (Figure 14-2).

Pacing the feedings and pumping after feedings will increase a mother's milk supply when the infant is unable to suck vigorously enough. Giving the pumped milk by lactation supplementer, small cup, or dropper ensures proper weight gain in the early weeks.[104] Holding an infant in a flexed position that mimics the fetal position relaxes an infant who is hypertonic or arching away from the breast.

In a study of energetics and mechanics of nutritive sucking in preterm and term neonates, Jain et al.[80] compared 38-gestational-week infants with 35-gestational-week infants and noted that preterm infants use less energy to suck the same volume of milk. The preterm infant took only up to 0.5 mL per

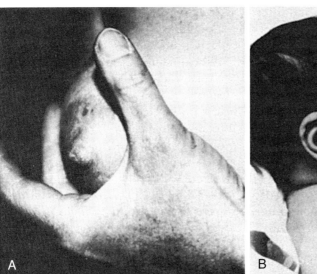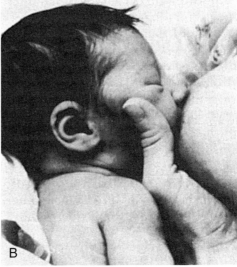

Figure 14-1. Dancer hold. **A,** Hand position of mother. **B,** Infant in position at breast with support. (From McBride MC, Danner SC: Sucking disorders in neurologically impaired infants: assessment and facilitation of breastfeeding, *Clin Perinatol* 14:109, 1987.)

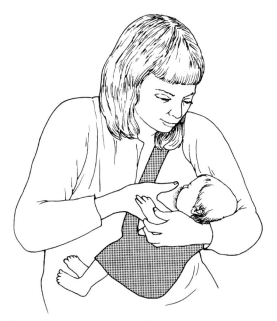

Figure 14-2. Pleat-seat or sling baby carrier holds the infant in a flexed position that facilitates infant suckling, leaving the mother's hands free to support her breast and the infant. (Redrawn from McBride MC, Danner SC: Sucking disorders in neurologically impaired infants: assessment and facilitation of breastfeeding, *Clin Perinatol* 14:109, 1987.)

suck and generated lower pressures and a lower frequency.

Exploring the hypothesis that milk flow achieved during feeding contributes to ventilatory depression during rubber-nipple feeding, Mathew[103] compared nipples with different flow rates. Decreases in minute ventilation and breathing frequency were significantly greater with high-flow nipples, thus confirming that milk flow influences breathing in premature infants who are unable to self-regulate the flow.

Tracings were made from the first oral feeding to time of discharge in term and premature infants. Serial oxygen pressure values showed small undulations across baseline (above and below) while breastfeeding. Substantial dips while bottle feeding were shown with recovery, but not above baseline. The quality and quantity of variation were different in the two modes of sucking (i.e., breast or bottle), with large drops in oxygen saturation occurring during actual sucking of the bottle but only during burping or repositioning while breastfeeding. Meier[106,107] concludes that the findings do not support the widely held view that breastfeeding is more stressful. The comparative data suggest that both pacifier and bottle feeding are more stressful than suckling at the breast. For further discussion of the stress of breastfeeding versus bottle feeding see Chapter 15, feeding the 28 to 32 week premature infant. If an infant has significant motor tone

disabilities or lacks the usual oral reflexes in response to stimulus of the rooting and sucking reflexes, a neonatal neurologist should assess the infant before any routine exercises are initiated.

It has been suggested that perioral stimulation enhances an immature or neurologically impaired infant's ability to suck and to coordinate suck and swallow.[91] Perioral stimulation, consisting of stimulating the skin overlying the masseter and buccinator muscles by manually applying a quick-touch pressure stimulus lasting 1 second, was studied. This is accomplished by simultaneously squeezing the buccal fat of both cheeks. Suck-monitoring equipment revealed that perioral stimulation increased the sucking rate, suggesting that this may facilitate sucking.[91] Exercising the mouths of infants who already have excessive mouth stimulation may not be appropriate. Many infants in a neonatal intensive care unit (NICU) are being suctioned, tube fed, and orally stimulated for other reasons, which may lead to oral aversion.

Kangaroo care is recommended for full-term infants who are neurologically or metabolically impaired. It involves holding the infant skin to skin inside the parent's shirt. It can stabilize temperature, respirations, and heart rate and be neurologically calming. For a mother who is to breastfeed, it facilitates milk production and helps a mother learn to handle her infant.[72] Kangaroo care is further discussed in Chapter 15.

GALACTAGOGUES: MEDICATION-INDUCED MILK PRODUCTION WHEN PUMPING

Stimulating milk production pharmacologically in mothers of LBW infants who are pumping to provide milk for their infants has been recommended by several authors, as reported by Ehrenkranz and Ackerman.[48] They used 10-mg metoclopramide orally every 8 hours for 7 days, tapering during 2 days more. Milk production increased within 2 days, but after therapy decreased, milk production decreased. Prolactin levels also increased during the treatment. Extensive use (more than 2 weeks) may cause cardiovascular symptoms in the mother.

Improved lactation occurred in 67% of mothers with no breast milk at onset and in 100% of mothers with poor supply given metoclopramide (10 mg three times per day for 10 days) by Gupta and Gupta.[61] They reported that the improvement persisted when the drug was discontinued. None of the 32 women had any symptoms or side effects. This drug is a substituted benzamide, which has selective dopamine-antagonist activity.

Although growth hormone has been observed to enhance milk supply, no recommended protocol exists for its clinical use.[60] In one study, 20 healthy mothers with insufficient milk who delivered between 26 and 34 weeks were given growth hormone, 0.2 international units/kg/day subcutaneously for 7 days. A group of 10 mothers received a placebo. Milk volume increased in the treated mothers. No change was noted in plasma growth hormone levels, but an increase was seen in insulin-like growth factor. No other changes were noted during this short-term therapy.[60]

Other drugs have been noted to enhance milk production. Domperidone (Motilium) is currently unavailable in the United States because the FDA banned its distribution. It is widely available in Canada, Europe, and Australia. It is fully discussed in Chapter 12. A dosage of 10 mg three times per day is reported to increase milk supply in some women. The drug is not without side effects, however. Other galactagogues are discussed in Chapter 12.

Breastfeeding Twins and Triplets

Many case reports support that a mother can nurse twins and triplets. It has been documented for centuries that an individual mother can provide adequate nourishment for more than one infant. In seventeenth-century France, wet nurses were allowed to nurse up to six infants at one time. Foundling homes provided wet nurses for every three to six infants.

The key deterrent to nursing twins is not usually the milk supply but time. If a mother can nurse both infants simultaneously, the time factor is reduced (Figure 14-3). Many tricks have been suggested to achieve this. As the infants become larger and more active, it may be difficult to keep them simultaneously nursing with only two hands to cope. However, twins trained from birth to nurse simultaneously will often continue to nurse in a position that allows both to nurse when they are older, even if the other is not nursing at the moment. If a

mother has help at home to assist with feedings, breastfeeding can be accomplished. The first year of life for a mother of a set of twins is an extremely busy one and really requires additional help, particularly if the mother is going to breastfeed. She will need time for adequate rest and nourishment. She often benefits from suggestions from other mothers of twins. The incidence of prematurity with twins is 3 in 10, with triplets 9 of 10, and with singletons just 1 in 10 pregnancies.

The challenge of breastfeeding twins was investigated by questionnaire of mothers who were members of the Mothers of Twins Clubs of Southern California, a national organization that offers help and advice to mothers of twins. No other socioeconomic information was available. Of the respondents, 41 mothers (23.7%) breastfed from birth, although 30% of the infants were premature. Of those who did not breastfeed, 9% were told not to do so by their physician, 11% did not think it was possible, and 11% did not think they would have enough milk for two. Of multiparas who had breastfed their first child, an equal number breastfed and bottle fed. Of the mothers who breastfed, 39 breastfed more than 1 month and 12 breastfed more than 6 months.

Eight healthy women who were breastfeeding twins and one breastfeeding triplets participated in a study by Saint et al.[128] to determine the yield and nutrient content of their milk at 2, 3, 6, 9, and 12 months postpartum. At 6 months, they fed an average 15 feeds per day. Fully breastfeeding women produced 0.84 to 2.16 kg of milk in 24 hours. Those partially breastfeeding produced 0.420 to 1.392 kg in 24 hours. The mother feeding triplets at 2½ months produced 3.08 kg/day, and the three infants were fed a total of 27 times per day. At 6 months the twins received 64% to 100% of total energy from breastfeeding and at 12 months received 6% to 13%. This further demonstrates that breasts are capable of responding to nutritional demands.

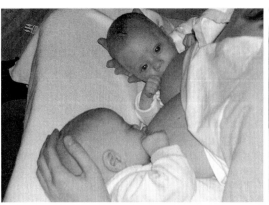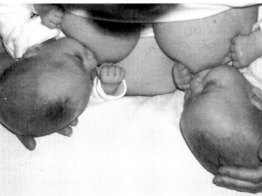

Figure 14-3. Premature twins nursing simultaneously, resting on a nursing pillow.

Guidelines for success in breastfeeding twins reported by Hattori and Hattori[66] admit that many obstacles exist but suggest that health care professionals should provide extended support to mothers of multiples to promote successful breastfeeding.[66] An extra pair of helpful hands provide significant assistance and relieve some of the fatigue. The initiation and duration of breast milk feedings by mothers of multiples compared with mothers of singletons were studied by a mailed questionnaire to 555 women.[57] The 358 mothers with multiples who answered were older, had higher incomes, were married, and were less likely to return to work by 6 months postpartum. Initiation of breastfeeding was comparable between mothers of multiples and singletons, but mothers of multiples provided milk for a shorter period of time, and mothers of preterm multiples breastfed the shortest period of time. At 6 months, 33% of mothers of term singletons were breastfeeding partially compared with 37% of mothers of term multiples. For preterm singletons, 31% were breastfed compared with 16% of preterm multiples.[57]

The medical literature on nursing twins or triplets or multiples in general is lean. It is well established that mothers can make enough milk. On the other hand, books, pamphlets, and websites supply personal stories and advice for mothers, fathers, and families. LaLeche League International, mothers of twins, pregnancytoday.com, parentingweb.com, multiplebirthsfamilies.com, and others have copious commentaries for mothers. Coping strategies can be helpful. Wisdom from Gromada[59] is shared with mothers in her book *Mothering Multiples, Breastfeeding and Caring for Twins or More*. A case of a mother successfully nursing quadruplets is reported by Berlin.[23] A helpful device is the "breastfeeding pillow," which is a pillow that wraps around the mother as she sits to nurse. The two infants can be supported by the pillow.

Full-Term Infants with Medical Problems

Infants who have self-limited acute illnesses, such as fever, upper respiratory infection, colds, diarrhea, or contagious diseases such as chickenpox, do best if breastfeeding is maintained. Because of breast milk's low solute load, an infant can be kept well hydrated despite fever or other increased fluid losses. If respiratory symptoms are significant, an infant seems to nurse well at the breast and poorly with a bottle. This observation has been documented many times when nursing mothers have roomed-in with their sick infants in the hospital. The studies of Johnson and Salisbury[82] on the synchrony of respirations in breastfeeding in contrast to the periodic breathing or gasping apnea pattern of the normal bottle-fed infant may well provide the underlying explanation for the phenomenon of an acutely ill infant continuing to nurse at the breast.

In addition to the appropriateness of human milk for a sick infant, nursing and closeness with the mother provide comfort. If an infant is suddenly weaned, psychologic trauma is added to the stress of the illness.[8] The American Academy of Pediatrics (AAP) Committee on Nutrition has reversed its recommendation and does not recommend replacing breastfeeding in a sick child.

It may be difficult to distinguish the effect of trauma of acute weaning from the symptoms of the primary illness, such as poor feeding or lethargy, if the acutely weaned infant fails to respond to adequate treatment. Returning to breastfeeding may be the treatment because the stress of acute weaning will be removed.

It is not appropriate to give a mother medicine intended to treat the infant, especially antibiotics. This has been tried to the detriment of the child because variable amounts of the drug reach the infant depending on the dose, dosage schedule, and amount of milk consumed. Maternal drugs can produce symptoms in an infant in some cases,[76] and thus maternal history of ingestants is important in assessing symptoms in a breastfed infant (see Chapter 12).

BUCCAL SMEARS IN BREASTFEEDING INFANTS

Guidelines for buccal smear collection in breastfed infants should be followed when genetic review is indicated. A buccal smear is a noninvasive, fast, and relatively inexpensive diagnostic method for collecting genetic material. It is used for sex determination as well as aneusomy, microdeletion syndromes, and a variety of polymerase chain reaction-based molecular genetic tests. Maternal cells can contaminate smears taken from breastfed infants. The recommendation is to wait at least 1 hour after a feeding. Buccal mucosa should be cleansed thoroughly with a cotton swab applicator. These procedures apply to both neonates and older nursing children.[16]

GASTROINTESTINAL DISEASE

Bouts of diarrhea and intestinal tract disease are less common in breastfed infants than in bottle-fed infants, but when they occur, the infant should be maintained on the breast if possible.[8,130] Human milk is a physiologic solution that normally causes neither dehydration nor hypernatremia. Occasionally, an infant will have diarrhea or an intestinal upset because of something in the mother's diet. It is usually self-limited, and the best treatment is to continue to nurse at the breast. If a mother has been taking a laxative that is absorbed or has been eating laxative foods, such as fruits, in excess, she should adjust her diet. Intractable diarrhea should be evaluated as it would be in any infant. Allergy to mother's milk is extremely rare and would require substantial evidence to support the diagnosis. Allergy to a foreign protein passed into the milk, such as bovine β-globulin, as in cow milk, however, can cause severe allergic symptoms in an infant (see Chapter 17).

COLITIS WHILE BREASTFEEDING

Severe colitis in a totally breastfed infant, usually with onset in the neonatal period, suggests an intrinsic metabolic disorder in the infant or an exquisite intolerance to something in mother's milk, such as cow milk protein.[89] Six infants with protein-induced enterocolitis presenting in the first month of life with severe bloody diarrhea responded to weaning and use of hydrolyzed protein formula. Other cases have been reported, requiring long periods of hyperalimentation and utilization of special formulas such as Nutramigen.

Induced colitis in infants is usually caused by some dietary insult, such as exposure to cow milk.[89,135] It has been reported in breastfed infants, most of whom responded to removal of cow milk from the maternal diet. Several had been given formula at birth, which is believed to have sensitized them. The symptoms included bloody diarrhea, and sigmoidoscopy revealed focal ulcerations, edema, and increased friability of the intestinal mucosa. On relief of symptoms by dietary change, the intestinal tract biopsy returns to normal. Removal of all bovine protein, not just cow milk, from the mother's diet may be required to ensure recovery while returning to breastfeeding. It may take 10 to 14 days to clear the bovine protein from the mother's milk.

A prospective study examined 35 consecutive infants who had fresh blood mixed with stools at approximately 4 weeks of age.[96] The infants were otherwise asymptomatic and had no infection, bleeding diathesis, or necrotizing enterocolitis (NEC); 31 had histopathologic evidence of colitis characterized by marked eosinophilic infiltrate (more than 20 eosinophils per high-power field) compared with control subjects and low mean serum albumin. Ten of these 31 were exclusively breastfed, nine were fed cow milk formula, nine soy formula, two mixed breast milk and formula, and one Nutramigen. The low serum albumin and high peripheral eosinophil count suggested the diagnosis of allergic colitis. All cases cleared with

dietary change. The breastfed infants were weaned, unfortunately, and not managed by dietary adjustment in the mother in this series.[96]

Protein-induced colitis can follow a benign course with proper treatment. Israel et al.[75] studied 13 infants with blood from the rectum, negative stool cultures, and colonoscopic and histologic evidence of colitis. The infants were all less than 3½ months of age, and six were breastfed and five had been supplemented. All were gaining weight well. The mothers of the breastfed infants restricted cow milk in their diet, and the infants were able to return to exclusively breastfeeding. All recovered.

Dietary protein-induced proctocolitis in exclusively breastfed infants should be taken into consideration as a cause of rectal bleeding or blood-streaked stool in the neonatal period and early infancy (hematochezia). Benign eosinophilic proctocolitis diagnosed by colonoscopy the is best treated by the exclusion of the allergen from the mother's diet. Resolution has taken place within 72 to 96 hours of elimination of the offending protein so temporarily stopping breastfeeding may not be necessary in some cases.[122]

An 8-week-old infant boy presented with irritability and projectile vomiting for an ultrasound to rule out pyloric stenosis. The ultrasound revealed colitis, and further history revealed bloody stools. He responded to removing bovine protein from his mother's diet and continuing to breastfeed.[115]

Harmon et al.[65] described a case of perforated pseudomembranous colitis in a breastfed infant. Other cases had been associated with giving antibiotics to an infant. The infant's stool was *Clostridium difficile* toxin positive, and the child required bowel resection for abscess and perforation. The mother had taken ciprofloxacin without consulting a physician for days before the infant's admission.

The Lactation Study Center has been notified of other cases of bloody diarrhea with a diagnosis of colitis that did appear to respond to maternal dietary restrictions. One infant showed brief improvement when all cow milk products were removed from the mother's diet and then had a relapse. Removing all bovine (both meat and milk) products from the maternal diet resulted in recovery without relapse with exclusive breastfeeding. In retrospect the mother recalled switching from a vegetarian diet to high meat, especially beef, intake throughout pregnancy.

A case of fucose intolerance is reported in a breastfed infant who was not intolerant of lactose but of the by-product of the oligosaccharides in human milk, passing large amounts of fucose in the stool.[18] The infant tolerated Pregestimil and then was weaned to regular formula.

It has been recommended by Haight[63] that severe cases of allergic colitis and also severe GI colic can be alleviated by treating the mother with pancreatic enzymes, 25 mg three times per day. It is safe for the mother and often dramatic for the infant. This is especially effective when eliminating cow protein has not solved the problem.

A formal study of this therapy was reported by Repucci[124] who described four term infants who were exclusively breastfeeding between 1 and 3 months of age who had positive family history for atopy. Elimination of bovine protein had not relieved the blood in the stools. Mothers were prescribed pancreatic enzymes (Pancrease MT4 USP units: 4000 lipase, 12,000 amylase, and 12,000 protease), two capsules with each meal and one capsule for snacks. Blood cleared within 2 days. One mother had to increase the dose to three capsules per meal and two with snacks. Mothers experienced no side effects due to this therapy. Anecdotal reports continue to confirm this therapy.

The management of protracted diarrhea in infants never breastfed is reported by many human milk banks on a case-by-case basis. Eleven of 24 children managed by MacFarlane and Miller[96] in a hyperalimentation referral unit recovered when fed banked human milk orally without protracted IV therapy. All the infants had been tried on all the available special formulas first. A study of oral rehydration in 26 children younger than the age of 2 years showed that the children who continued to breastfeed while receiving rehydration fluid had fewer stools and recovered more rapidly than those receiving only rehydration fluid.[84] The Pima Infant Feeding Study clearly showed that in less developed and more disadvantaged communities in the United States, exclusive breastfeeding protected against severe diarrhea and other GI disorders.[53]

LACTOSE INTOLERANCE

Suckling milk is the defining characteristic of mammals. Lactose, the major carbohydrate in milk, is hydrolyzed by lactase-phlorhizin hydrolase, an enzyme of the small intestine. Lactase plays a critical role in the nutrition of mammalian neonates. Congenital lactase deficiency, present from birth, is extremely rare and is inherited as an autosomal recessive gene.[108] Most humans (except Northern Europeans) and other adult mammals do not drink milk beyond infancy; it causes indigestion and mild to severe GI symptoms because of an adult's inability to digest lactose. Low lactase levels result from injury or genetic expression of lactase. The enzyme hydrolyzes lactose, phlorhizin, and glycosyl ceramides. A decline in lactase-specific activity occurs at the time of weaning in most mammalian species. In humans it may occur as early as 3 to 5 years of age; in other species the elevated juvenile levels of lactase-specific activity persist.

The developmental patterns of lactase expression are regulated at the level of gene transcription.[108]

Premature infants and those recovering from severe diarrhea have transient lactose intolerance. The only treatment is a temporary lactose-free diet. Reports of lactose-hydrolyzed human milk suggest that banked human milk can be treated with lactase (Keralac), which will hydrolyze the lactose (900 enzyme activity units to 200 mL breast milk degraded 82% of the lactose).[136] In one case the reason for using human milk was that the infant became infection prone when he was weaned from the breast at the time the initial diagnosis was made. He showed marked improvement with treated human milk. In a breastfed infant, lactase deficiency may be manifest by chronic diarrhea and marked failure to thrive.

An additional clinical syndrome related to slow gaining or failure to thrive is excessive lactose, resulting when the fat level in the milk is low and an excessive amount of milk is consumed because of the low-calorie content. The first documented case was reported by Woolridge and Fisher.[157] Lactose production drives the milk-making capacity. When a feeding at one breast does not last long enough for the fat to let down, the result is low-calorie high-lactose milk. The authors recommend in such cases that an entire feeding be taken at one breast.[157] (For further discussion of this phenomenon, see Chapter 8.)

CELIAC DISEASE, CROHN'S DISEASE, AND INFLAMMATORY BOWEL DISEASE

Some chronic diseases are better controlled by keeping an infant on breast milk, as symptoms usually become more severe with weaning. If an infant is weaned and does poorly on formula, relactation of the mother should be considered. With the availability of the nursing supplementer, this possibility is no longer remote (see Chapter 19).

Celiac disease or permanent gluten-sensitive enteropathy is an immunologic disease dependent on the exposure to wheat gluten or related proteins in rye and barley.[77]

A case-control study[120] was done on the effect of infant feeding on celiac disease to investigate the association between duration of breastfeeding and age at first gluten introduction into the infant diet and the incidence and age of onset of celiac disease. A significant protective effect on the incidence of celiac disease was related to the duration of breastfeeding after 2 months. It was not related to the age of first gluten in diet, although the age of first exposure did affect the age of onset of symptoms.[120]

The risk for celiac disease was reduced in children younger than 2 years old in a study of 2000

Swedish children if they were still being breastfed when dietary gluten was introduced. The effect was more pronounced if breastfeeding continued after gluten was introduced. The authors conclude that gradual introduction of gluten-containing foods into the diet while breastfeeding reduces the risk for ever getting celiac disease.[77] The declining incidence of celiac disease and transient gluten intolerance has been associated with changing feeding practices, which include later introduction of dietary gluten, the use of gluten-free foods for weaning (rice), and the increased initiation and duration of breastfeeding.[29]

The risk for celiac disease autoimmunity and timing of gluten introduction into the diet of infants at increased risk for the disease was determined by Norris et al.[115] who studied 1560 children prospectively. They had been determined to be at increased risk because they possessed either HLA-DR3 or DR4 alleles or had a first-degree relative with type 1 diabetes. Diagnosis of celiac disease was based on positive small bowel biopsy and positive for tissue transglutaminase autoantibody. Children exposed to gluten in the first 3 months of life or not until after 7 months of age developed the disease; 4 to 6 months of age appeared to be a safe period when gluten was tolerated. Breastfeeding may offer protection against the development of celiac disease. Breastfeeding during the introduction of gluten in the diet (wheat, barley, or rye) and increasing the duration of breastfeeding was associated with reduced risk for developing the disease, as reported by Akobeng et al.[4] who did a systematic review and meta-analysis.

The discussion is not over and the guidelines are not confirmed. It is agreed that celiac disease is an immune-mediated disease that is not uncommon. An estimated 1% of the population is affected. It negatively influences the quality of life of affected individuals. Prevention strategies focusing on early infant feeding practices (i.e., breastfeeding) and timing of introduction of gluten into the infant's diet have had conflicting results. Large multiple country prospective studies are underway. Although breastfeeding in multiple smaller studies has shown to be protective, there may prove to be limitations to that. Because risk can be anticipated by family history and testing for HLA-DQ2 or HLA-DQ8, dietary management appears to at least postpone the onset of symptoms if not prevent it.

A window of opportunity has been suggested to reduce the risk of celiac disease by introducing gluten no sooner than 4 months and no later than seven months of age and exclusive breastfeeding until 12 months of age but not beyond. In progress is a multicentered, randomized, double blind, placebo controlled dietary intervention study involving 944 HLA positive children; the Norwegian mother and child cohort study of 324 cases out of a cohort of 82,167, and a systematic review of available data from a large randomized controlled trial in 10 European countries.

The current consensus is that gluten should be added to the diet between 4 and 7 months and breastfeeding should continue until 12 months in at-risk infants. The AAP states that breastfeeding reduces the risk of celiac disease by 52%.

A family with two sons at ages 33 months and 8 months came to the attention of the Lactation Study Center. Both were breastfed. They developed an inability to sleep comfortably after having slept well previously. They cried and thrashed about, needing constant attention and motion around the clock. At age 27 months, the older son had x-rays, biopsies, and genetic testing. Endoscopy was inconclusive with moderate inflammation and smoothing. He was positive for one of the three genetic markers for celiac disease. He had been weaned at 18 months and was started on a gluten-free diet, which "cured" him. At the center, the mother was recommended a gluten-free diet while she continued to breastfeed the 8-month-old child. In 48 hours he was remarkably improved and is now symptom free, breastfeeding, and eating gluten-free solids. With the availability of gluten-free foods in supermarkets, the diet for mothers is more accessible. The public interest in gluten-free food has increased and many are trying it at random.

The development of Crohn's disease later in life has increased in recent decades. Because it has been suggested that breast milk is essential for the development of the normal immunologic competence of the intestinal mucosa, investigators have studied the association between breastfeeding and later Crohn's disease. Bergstrand and Hellers[21] studied 826 patients who developed Crohn's disease between 1955 and 1974 and their matched control subjects. Mean length of breastfeeding was 4.59 months among patients and 5.76 among control subjects ($p < 0.01$). Patients with Crohn's disease were overrepresented among those with no, or short, periods of breastfeeding. The role of infant feeding practices in the development of Crohn's disease in childhood was reported by Koletzko et al.[87] in a study of 145 families with similar results. Although Crohn's disease may develop in genetically susceptible people as a result of an immunologic response to unidentified antigen in the mucosa, early feeding practices are significant.

Early determinants of inflammatory bowel disease have pointed toward infectious diseases in childhood, especially measles, and even in utero infections as possible causative factors.[19] It has become a major disease of adults in Europe with 5.12 cases per 1000 individuals older than 43 years

(National Survey of Health and Development of 1946) and 2.02 to 2.54 cases per 1000 adults by age 33 years (1958 National Child Development Study). In examining early determinants, these cohorts did not show a protective effect of breast-feeding. The authors comment, however, that the study recorded "ever breastfed" with no distinction for length of breastfeeding.[143]

A systematic review with meta-analysis of breastfeeding and risk for inflammatory bowel disease was conducted by Klement et al.[86] who concluded that breastfeeding is associated with lower risks of Crohn's disease and ulcerative colitis. The reports that were included were published between 1961 and 2000. A report was published in 2005 of a pediatric case-control study of inflammatory bowel disease and 60 cases of ulcerative colitis in children younger than 17 years of age. The results did not support a protective effect of breastfeeding and suggested an association with the disease.[81] When these data were included in the meta-analysis by Klement,[86] however, the results still showed a protective effect of breastfeeding for these two bowel diseases.[85]

Breastfeeding is associated with a 31% reduction for childhood inflammatory bowel disease according to the AAP. It is thought that the reduction results from the interaction of the immunomodulating effect of human milk and the underlying genetic susceptibility of the infant. The abnormal colonization of the gut in formula-fed infants may increase risk.

The severity of GI infection is attenuated if not prevented in breastfeeding infants according to the AAP. Infections due to enteric pathogens such as *Rotavirus, Giardia, Shigella, Campylobacter* and entero toxigenic *Escherichia coli*. The risk of these illnesses is reduced by 64% for infants who are breastfeeding.

RESPIRATORY ILLNESS AND OTITIS MEDIA

Infants who develop respiratory illnesses should be maintained at the breast. The added advantages of antibodies and antiinfective properties are valuable to infants. Sick infants can nurse more easily than they can cope with a bottle. Furthermore, the comfort of having the mother nearby is important whenever the infant has a crisis; weaning during illness may be devastating to infants.

Wheezing and lower respiratory tract disease and other respiratory illnesses are lower in frequency and duration when the infant is breastfed. Recovery is accelerated if breastfeeding is maintained. The AHRQ reported a 72% reduction in the risk of hospitalization for respiratory infections in children under a year of age who were exclusively breastfed for at least 4 months.

Otitis media in infants occurs less frequently in breastfed infants because of the infection protection properties of human milk and the protective effect of suckling at the breast. Recurrent otitis media is associated with bottle feeding in a study of 237 children, in contrast to prolonged breastfeeding, which had a long-term protective effect up to 3 years of age.[126]

A regional birth cohort of 5356 children was followed prospectively regarding the occurrence of infectious disease in the first year of life.[83] One third developed otitis media. Median age of onset was 8 months, and 10% had had three episodes by 1 year of age. Breastfeeding for 9 months or longer had a significant impact on otitis, as did the number of siblings and daycare. Otitis media in 3- to 8-year-old children in Greenland was studied as a national concern for the incidence and associated deafness. Children who were breastfed were spared, especially if nursed a long time.[117]

A protective effect of breastfeeding in otitis media was shown in a large prospective study. The AHRQ reported that exclusive breastfeeding for 3 to 6 months provided a 50% reduction in otitis media compared to formula feeding even when controlling for socioeconomic status, parental smoking, and the presence of siblings.

Young infants who have older siblings may well be exposed to some virulent viruses and bacteria. Developing croup, for instance, may make an infant seriously ill. Hydration can be maintained by frequent, short breastfeedings. Studies have shown that respirations are maintained more easily when feeding on human milk than on cow milk, even from a bottle. Nursing at the breast permits regular respirations, whereas bottle feeding is associated with a more gasping pattern. Thus breastfed infants should continue to nurse when they are ill. If an infant is hospitalized, every effort should be made to maintain breastfeeding or to provide expressed breast milk if the infant can be fed at all. Staff should provide rooming-in for the mother if a care-by-parent ward is not available.

Colostrum and milk contain large amounts of IgA antibody, some of which is respiratory syncytial virus (RSV) specific. Breastfed but not bottle-fed infants have IgA in their nasal secretions. Neutralizing inhibitors to RSV have been demonstrated in the whey of most samples of human milk tested.[144] IgG anti-RSV antibodies are present in milk and in reactive T-lymphocytes. Breastfeeding-induced resistance to RSV was associated with the presence of interferon and virus-specific lymphocyte transformation activity, suggesting that breastfeeding has unique mechanisms for modulating the immune response of infants to RSV infection.[32] Clinical studies indicating a relative protection from RSV in breastfed infants were clouded by other factors.[145] The populations were unequal because of socioeconomic factors and smoking (i.e., bottle-feeding mothers were in lower socioeconomic groups and smoked more). In general, if breastfed infants become ill, they have less severe illness.[144,145] Although breastfeeding protects, parental smoking and daycare are important negative factors in the incidence of respiratory infection. Respiratory illness in either infant or mother should be treated symptomatically and breastfeeding continued. If the infant has nasal congestion, nasal aspiration and saline nose drops just before a feed are helpful.

GALACTOSEMIA

Galactosemia, caused by deficiency of galactose-1-phosphate uridyltransferase, is a rare circumstance in which an infant is unable to metabolize galactose and must be placed on a galactose-free diet. The disease can be rapidly fatal in the severe form. The infant may have severe and persistent jaundice, vomiting, diarrhea, electrolyte imbalances, cerebral signs, and weight loss. This is a medical emergency. This does necessitate weaning from the breast to a special formula because human milk, as with all mammalian milks, contains high levels of lactose, which is a disaccharide that splits into glucose and galactose. The condition is suspected when reducing substances are found in the urine in the newborn, and the diagnosis is confirmed by measuring the enzyme uridyltransferase in the red and white blood cells. The several forms can be distinguished by genetic testing, but except for the mild form, the infant must be weaned to a lactose-free diet. An infection with E. coli in the newborn period may be the trigger that precipitates serious symptoms associated with this or other metabolic disorders. Galactosemia is screened for in most states in the United States along with phenylketonuria (PKU) and other metabolic disorders.

When the diagnosis is made, genetic testing should be done. The Duarte variant of the disease is mild; some enzyme is available. Breastfeeding is permitted but the infant should be followed closely initially. Some infants can only be partially breastfed, with some lactose-free formula in addition for necessary calories. An endocrinologist should make the decision for the exact balance of milks. Classic galactose-1-phosphate uridyltransferase deficiency makes breastfeeding contraindicated.

INBORN ERRORS OF METABOLISM

Other metabolic deficiency syndromes are usually only apparent as mild failure-to-thrive syndrome until the infant is weaned from the breast and the symptoms become severe. This particularly applies to inborn errors of metabolism caused by an inability to handle one or more of the essential amino acids that are in higher concentration in cow milk than human milk. Infection is often a complication early in the lives of these infants, with inborn errors most commonly due to E. coli bacteria. While the acute infection is being treated, the infant may be weaned from the breast, and the metabolic disorder then becomes apparent precipitously.

Certain amino acids, including phenylalanine, methionine, leucine, isoleucine, and others associated with metabolic disorders, have significantly lower levels in human milk than in cow milk. Management of an amino acid metabolic disorder while breastfeeding depends on careful monitoring of blood and urine levels of the specific amino acids involved. Because these are essential amino acids, a certain amount is necessary in the diet of all infants, including those with disease. An appropriate combination of breastfeeding and milk free of the offending amino acid should be developed. The care of such infants should be in consultation with a pediatric endocrinologist. Transient neonatal tyrosinemia, which has been reported to occur in a high percentage (up to 80%) of neonates fed cow milk, is associated with blood tyrosine levels 10 times those of adults. Wong et al.[156] have associated severe cases with learning disabilities in later years. Tyrosine appears in human milk at low levels. Tyrosinemia type I is an inherited autosomal recessive trait. Symptoms are caused by accumulation of tyrosine and its metabolites in the liver. It is treated by dietary control consisting of low protein with limited phenylalanine and tyrosine. Some breastfeeding is possible combined with protein-free supplements. 2-(2-Nitro-4-trifluoromethylbenzyl)-1-3-cyclohexanedione reduces the production of toxic metabolites. Liver failure is common. Dietary restrictions are lifelong.

Screening programs that test all newborns have identified many victims early. Almost all programs test for PKU, galactosemia, and hypothyroidism, and increasingly maple syrup urine disease, homocystinuria, biotinidase deficiency, tyrosinemia, and now cystic fibrosis are included. Most cases can be managed with continued breastfeeding and diet modification. Congenital adrenal hyperplasia requires corticosteroids but the feeding can be breast milk. If it is the salt wasting variety, an infant must have added salt.

PHENYLKETONURIA

The most common of the amino acid metabolic disorders is PKU, in which the amino acid accumulates for lack of an enzyme. The treatment has

been phenylalanine-free formula, available from Abbott Laboratories and Bristol-Myers, combined with added standard formula or breast milk to provide a little phenylalanine because every infant needs a small amount. If an infant is breastfed, the mother is usually willing to continue on an adjusted schedule. An infant may supplement the Lofenalac or Analog XP with breast milk. With careful monitoring of the blood levels and control of the amount of breastfeeding, a balance can be struck that permits optimal phenylalanine levels and breastfeeding. The infant will require some phenylalanine-free formula to provide enough calories and nutrients. A detailed outline of management called *Guide to Breast Feeding the Infant with PKU*, prepared by Ernest et al.,[50a] is available from the Superintendent of Documents, U.S. Government Printing Office, Washington, DC 20402.

Literature values for phenylalanine range from 29 to 64 mg/dL in human milk. The amount for Lofenalac or Analog XP and human milk for a given baby is calculated by weight, age, blood levels, and needs for growth. As an example, a 3-week-old baby weighing 3.7 kg whose blood level was 52.5 mg/dL when he was ingesting an estimated 570 mL of breast milk would receive 240 mL Lofenalac and 360 mL breast milk (four breastfeedings per day with before and after weighing). The details of every step of management are available in the guide to assist a physician in planning treatment.[48] Test weighing, which is now a simple home procedure with a digital scale, greatly facilitates the accuracy of this management.

As soon as the diagnosis is made, an infant should be placed on a low-phenylalanine formula to reduce the levels in the plasma promptly. The mother should pump her breasts to maintain her milk supply. Human milk has less phenylalanine than formula, but it exceeds the tolerance of most infants with PKU. The breastfed infant is offered a small volume of special formula (10 to 30 mL) first and then completes the feeding at the breast. As long as the blood phenylalanine levels can be maintained between 120 and 300 mmol/L, exact intake need not be measured. Initially, weight checks to ensure adequate growth are essential because poor intake leading to a catabolic state will interfere with control. Because human milk is low in phenylalanine, the offending amino acid, more than half the diet can be breast milk.

Another protocol for breastfeeding an infant with PKU was studied by van Rijn et al. The feeding schedule was based on alternating breastfeeding and phenylalanine-free formula by bottle. Each child had a separate schedule convenient for the mother-baby dyad depending on tolerance and age. At the beginning of treatment, the mother breastfed once daily allowing the infant to feed

until satiated, and the mother pumped the rest of the day. Breastfeedings were increased while monitoring phenylalanine plasma levels. Ultimately breast and bottle feeding were alternated and equal. At all feedings, the infant drank until satisfied. The breastfed infants did well on this protocol and plasma levels were stable. An essential member of the management team is a board certified licensed lactation consultant to assist the mother in managing her milk supply.

The weaning of this special infant should be similar to that of other infants. Adding solid foods can be initiated at 6 months.[34] The liquid part of the diet continues as before, that is, two feeding components of low-phenylalanine formula and breastfeeding plus solids with little or no phenylalanine (fruits, vegetables, low-protein foods). Rice and wheat contain too much phenylalanine. When the decision is made to wean from the breast, solid foods can be used to replace the phenylalanine in the breast milk as needed. Growth should be followed closely. When weaning is complete, the infant should be given other less bulky sources of protein free of phenylalanine. This stage will be carefully orchestrated by the endocrinologist and nutritionist. Because infants with PKU are more prone to thrush infection, the mother should be alerted to watch for symptoms in the infant and the onset of sore nipples that could be caused by *Candida albicans*. Treatment is nystatin for both the mother and baby initially. (See discussion in Chapter 16.)

The other benefits of human milk make the effort to breastfeed valuable for the infant and for the mother, who usually wants to continue to contribute to her infant's nurturing and nourishment. The prognosis for intellectual development is excellent if treatment is initiated early and the blood levels maintained at less than 10 mg/dL phenylalanine (120 to 300 mmol/L).

A retrospective study of 26 school-age children who had been breastfed or formula fed for 20 to 40 days before dietary intervention was conducted by Riva et al.[125] The children who had been breastfed had a 14-point IQ advantage, which persisted at 12.9 points when corrected for maternal social and educational status. The age of treatment onset for PKU was not related to IQ scores. This study strongly supports the belief that breastfeeding in the prediagnostic stage has an impact on the long-range neurodevelopmental performance of patients with PKU (Figure 14-4).

Nutrition management of infants with organic acidemias involves limiting the intake of the offending amino acid(s) to the minimum necessary for normal growth and development and suppressing amino acid degradation during catabolic periods by providing alternative fuels such as glucose. In some disorders, including isovaleric

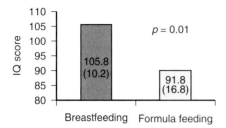

Figure 14-4. Intellectual quotient (IQ) in patients with phenylketonuria, evaluated by Wechsler Intelligence Scale for Children score, in relation to the type of feeding in the first weeks of life. (From Giovannini M, Verduci E, Salvatici E, et al: Phenylketonuria: dietary and therapeutic challenges, *J Inherit Metab Dis* 30:145–152, 2007.)

acidemia, specific treatment is included to increase the excretion of toxic metabolites by enhancing the body's capacity to make isovalerylglycine, an acyl-carnitine translocase. As more specific amino acid-free formulas are made available, a recipe for combining breastfeeding with the special formula can be engineered to specific infants' needs. The endocrinologist and the nutritionist can provide such a recipe. Dietary precautions for the mother of a breastfeeding child with PKU are to avoid the artificial sweetener aspartame (NutraSweet), which metabolizes to phenylalanine.

Other Metabolic Disorders

Pompe disease (acid maltase deficiency or glycogen storage disease type II) is an inborn error of metabolism caused by a complete or partial deficiency of the enzyme acid α-glucosidase that normally breaks down lysosomal glycogen into glucose. Glycogen accumulates in the tissues, especially muscles. The disease takes various forms. Infantile onset has a poor prognosis and treatment is supportive. Because of the frequency of respiratory infection and difficulty feeding, breastfeeding would be palliative because liver disease is rapidly progressive.

Ornithine transcarbamylase deficiency is a rare life-threatening genetic disorder. It is one of six urea cycle disorders named for the specific enzyme deficiency present.

A lack of enzyme results in excessive and symptomatic accumulation of ammonia in the blood (hyperammonemia). Symptoms vary but can occur within 72 hours of birth and include poor suck, irritability, vomiting, and progressive lethargy followed, if untreated, by hypotonia, seizures, respiratory distress, and coma. Infant onset disease is more common in males. Treatment involves limiting nitrogen intake and assisting nitrogen excretion with phenylbutyrate (Buphenyl). Infants can be breastfed and receive nonprotein caloric supplement. The advantage of human milk is not only

dietary but the infection protection and immune protective qualities. An essential amino acid formula is available for those not breastfeeding.

There are many other variations of these enzyme deficiency diseases. Without treatment, they all lead to deterioration, mental retardation, and often organ failure, especially liver failure.[155] The National Organization for Rare Disorders Inc. (NORD) provides information for professionals, the lay public, and support groups regarding more than 1000 rare diseases. It lobbies for development of specific treatments (orphan drugs). (Specific treatment information is available at their website, http://www.rarediseases.org.)

CYSTIC FIBROSIS

Cystic fibrosis is an autosome recessive disease caused by mutations in the cystic fibrosis transmembrane conductance regulator (CFTR) gene. The CFTR protein is in the epithelia of tissues including lung, sweat glands, pancreas, and GI tract.

Screening tests for cystic fibrosis (CF) have been initiated in many state-mandated metabolic screening programs for newborns, so a greater number will be identified early. Meconium plug, especially large plugs and full-blown meconium ileus, have a high correlation with pancreatic enzyme deficiency and CF. As clinicians are alerted to meconium plugs, early tests for CF can be carried out and management adjusted. Breastfeeding is optimal not only for the nutrition but for the presence of enzymes to facilitate digestion and absorption of nutrients. Because infection is a significant morbidity in these children, the infection protection properties of human milk make a critical impact. A study of infants exclusively breastfed or formula fed showed that breastfeeding does not compromise growth and is associated with fewer infections and respiratory problems in infants with CF.[79]

The first symptom in infants with CF is often failure to thrive. If an infant is breastfed, the mother may be forced to wean, yet the infant feeds even less well and has no weight gain on formula. Infants do better if placed back on the breast. Pumping to increase the mother's milk supply will help the child's hunger. In a study of CF centers, 77% recommended breastfeeding either alone or with pancreatic enzyme supplements.[93] The recommended breastfeeding duration was 3 to 6 months by 43% of the centers (Tables 14-1–14-3A and 14-3B). If supplementation is required, hydrolyzed formula is recommended. Generic and name-brand enzymes are not biologically equal, and some formulas were more frequently associated with greasy stools and abdominal cramping. Use of enzymes may be a way to improve tolerance and weight gain

TABLE 14-1	Recommendations about Breastfeeding by Cystic Fibrosis Center Directors for CFIM		
Recommendations		**Response***	**%**
Breastfeeding only		3	2.6
Plus pancreatic enzymes		39	34.2
Plus hydrolyzed formula		7	6.1
Plus pancreatic enzymes and hydrolyzed formula		39	34.2
Hydrolyzed formula with pancreatic enzymes		18	15.8
Hydrolyzed formula only		2	1.8
Not applicable and/or other category		6	5.3
Total		114	100

CFIM, Mothers of infants with cystic fibrosis.
 *Many centers chose more than one answer; therefore, response rate for each answer is calculated as a percentage of total responses.
 Modified from Luder E, Kattan M, Tanzer-Torres G, et al: Current recommendations for breast feeding in cystic fibrosis centers. *Am J Dis Child* 144:1153, 1990.

TABLE 14-2	Factors for Discontinuation of Breastfeeding According to Cystic Fibrosis Center Directors for CFIM		
Factors for Discontinuation		**Response***	**%**
Protein-energy malnutrition		69	51.1
Marked steatorrhea		29	21.5
Meconium ileus		16	11.9
Carrier of chronic bacterial pathogen(s)		8	5.9
Not applicable and/or other category		13	9.6
Total		135	100

CFIM, Mothers of infants with cystic fibrosis.
 *Many centers chose more than one answer; therefore, response rate for each answer is calculated as a percentage of total responses.
 Modified from Luder E, Kattan M, Tanzer-Torres G, et al: Current recommendations for breastfeeding in cystic fibrosis centers, *Am J Dis Child* 144:1153, 1990.

in these special breastfed infants rather than weaning to formula.[28] Prescribing pancreatic enzymes for a mother while breastfeeding, as described earlier, is also a consideration.[63]

ALPHA₁-ANTITRYPSIN DEFICIENCY

Alpha$_1$-antitrypsin is a serum protease inhibitor that inactivates a number of proteases. More than 24 genetic variants of this disease are designated B through Z, with the M variant being most

TABLE 14-3A	Duration of Breastfeeding as Reported by Cystic Fibrosis Center Directors for CFIM		
Duration (mo)		**Centers***	**%**
<3		34	40
3-6		37	43
>6		5	5.8
Not applicable and/or other category		10	12
Total		86	100

CFIM, Mothers of infants with cystic fibrosis.
 *Many centers chose more than one answer; therefore, response rate for each answer is calculated as a percentage of total responses.
 Modified from Luder E, Kattan M, Tanzer-Torres G, et al: Current recommendations for breastfeeding in cystic fibrosis centers, *Am J Dis Child* 144:1153, 1990.

| TABLE 14-3B | Number of Infective Episodes and Hospital Admissions (Mean ± SD) in the First 3 Years of Life in Patients with Cystic Fibrosis, Subdivided According to Breastfeeding Duration* |

	No BF (n = 56)	BF 1-4 Mo (n = 56)	BF >4 Mo (n = 34)	p Value
Infections†	8 ± 5.5	7.5 ± 5	5 ± 4	0.015
Admissions†	2 ± 2	2 ± 2	1 ± 2	0.424

BF, Breastfeeding.
 *Different superscripts indicate between-group differences (p < 0.05) after Bonferroni correction.
 †Numbers are approximated at the nearest 0.5 unit.

common. Children with α_1-antitrypsin deficiency are at increased risk for liver disease, which occurs most often during infancy and often progresses to cirrhosis and death. Udall et al.[147] investigated the relationship between early feedings and the onset of liver disease. Severe liver disease was present in eight (40%) of the bottle-fed and one (8%) of the breastfed infants (breastfed for only 5 weeks). Of the 32 infants, 24 were still alive at the end of the study; 12 had been breastfed and 12 bottle fed during their first month of life. All eight of the deceased children had been bottle fed; small-for-gestational-age (SGA) and preterm infants had been excluded from the study so that all infants were equally stable at birth and capable of breastfeeding. A bottle-fed infant was seven times more likely to develop liver disease.

With the increasing early diagnosis of α_1-antitrypsin deficiency, encouraging a mother to breastfeed if her infant is affected would appear to have a significant impact on reducing the chance of long-range liver disease in her infant.

ACRODERMATITIS ENTEROPATHICA (DANBOLT-CLOSS SYNDROME)

Acrodermatitis enteropathica is a rare and unique disease in which feeding an infant with human milk may be lifesaving. It is an autosomal recessive disorder with an onset as early as 3 weeks old.[132] It is inherited as an autosomal recessive trait and is characterized by a symmetric rash around the mouth, genitalia, and periphery of the extremities. The rash is an acute vesicobullous and eczematous eruption often secondarily infected with *C. albicans*. It may be seen by the third week of life or not until late in infancy and has been associated with weaning from the breast. Failure to thrive, hair loss, irritability, and chronic severe intractable diarrhea are often life threatening. The disease has been associated with extremely low plasma zinc levels. Oral zinc sulfate has produced remission of the syndrome. Zinc deficiency was seen frequently in premature infants on peripheral alimentation until zinc was added to the solution.

Human milk contains less zinc than does bovine milk, with zinc concentrations of both decreasing throughout lactation. Eckert et al.[47] studied the zinc binding in human and cow milk and noted that the low-molecular-weight binding ligand isolated from human milk may enhance absorption of zinc in these patients. Gel chromatography indicated that most of the zinc in cow milk was associated with high-molecular-weight fractions, whereas zinc in human milk was associated with low-molecular-weight fractions. The copper/zinc ratio may also be of significance because the ratio is lower in cow milk.

The zinc-binding ligand from human milk was further identified as prostaglandin E by chromatography, ultrafiltration, and infrared spectroscopy by Evans and Johnson.[51] Patients also have low arachidonic acid levels. Arachidonic acid is a precursor of prostaglandin. The efficacy of human milk in the treatment of acrodermatitis enteropathica results from the presence of the zinc-prostaglandin complex. The primary deficiency in an infant is an inability to absorb zinc except in this complex form.

The clinical significance of the relationship of human milk to onset of the disease and its treatment is in developing lactation in the mother of such an infant, rare as the disease may be. Delayed lactation or relactation is possible and should be offered as an option to the mother of such an infant (see Chapter 19).

Several reports of isolated cases of zinc deficiency during breastfeeding have appeared in the literature.[2,3] In some cases, zinc levels in the milk were low; in others, they were not measured.[158] One child had a classic "zinc-deficient" rash that responded to oral zinc therapy. One should keep in mind that any deficiency is possible and consider intake deficiency when symptoms occur in a breastfed infant. The basic defect is presumed to be related to GI malabsorption of zinc.

The treatment of choice is oral administration of zinc in the sulfate or gluconate form. It is usually well tolerated, safe, inexpensive, effective, and expedient. When zinc deficiency occurs in a breastfed infant, the possibility of zinc deficiency in the milk, although a rare disorder, should be considered.[132] Treating the mother would be the appropriate therapy in such a case.

Premature infants have a negative zinc balance associated with inadequate mineral stores and high requirement associated with rapid growth.[35] Transient zinc deficiency in breastfed infants has been described as manifest by the classic zinc deficiency rash and was treated by oral zinc to the infant because milk levels are normal in the mother.

The regulation of iron, zinc, and copper in breast milk and the transport of these minerals across the mammary gland epithelium is poorly understood. Milk values at 9 months postpartum were not associated with maternal mineral status.[45] This suggests an active transport mechanism according to the investigators.[45] Milk zinc levels increase at weaning time while iron levels decrease.

NEUROLOGICALLY IMPAIRED INFANTS

In addition to infants who have been neurologically impaired by perinatal hypoxia or asphyxia and low Apgars, a rare infant may have an inherited neurologic problem as in a trisomy or a congenital abnormality such as spina bifida. These infants can be breastfed in most cases but it requires patience and perseverance. Holding the infant in a flexed position is an essential element of breastfeeding. A sling works well.

Down syndrome is one of the more common syndromes, occurring in 1 of 800 to 1000 births. Hypotonia is a major feature that, along with small mouth and large tongue, make breastfeeding a challenge. At first, the infant may quickly drift off to sleep at the breast and weight gain is slow. The mother learns to hold her breast in place as the infant's grasp is not strong enough to overcome gravity. The sling works also to hold the infant in place and free both the mother's hands to hold both the breast and infant jaw.

When the suckling is weak initially, mother should pump between feedings to stimulate production of milk. If supplements are required, it is best to provide them with a Lact-Aid or a cup as the infant with Down syndrome is easily confused.

DOWN SYNDROME

Infants with Down syndrome or other trisomies may be difficult to feed. When they are breastfed, mothers need patience to teach the infants to suck with sufficient vigor to initiate the let-down reflex and to stimulate adequate production of milk. Using manual expression to start flow and holding the breast firmly for the infant so that the nipple does not drop out of the mouth when the infant stops suckling will assist the process.

Initially however, an infant with Down syndrome may have surprisingly good tone and may even suck well at the breast, only to develop problems after mother and infant have been discharged home. Providing support for the head, the jaw, and the general body hypotonia will require considerable coordination by the mother. Propping the baby firmly with a pillow in the mother's lap or supporting the infant in a sling frees a much-needed hand for steadying the jaw and breast (see Figure 14-2).[103]

A nurse clinician in the hospital who is knowledgeable and experienced in dealing with neurologically impaired infants should be available to the parents. The initial goals for the mother-infant pair are developing confidence in handling the infant, adjusting to the infant's problem, and dealing with the parental grief and sense of loss—loss of the normal infant that was expected. If the mother has breastfed other children, the emphasis on breastfeeding modifications are more successful, and milk supply usually responds to manual expression and pumping. Initiating sufficient stimulus to the breast to increase milk production is critical in the first few days to induce good prolactin response, especially in primiparas. Renting an electric breast pump is a good investment, justifiable for reimbursement from health insurance by physician prescription.

With ultrasound and amniocentesis, the diagnosis is often known before birth so that the family can be prepared. In developing a discharge plan for an infant with Down syndrome, a pediatrician will need to coordinate a team to avoid the fragmented care that develops with a multiproblem situation, which may require the consultation of a geneticist, genetic counselor, cardiologist, and other medical experts to deal with the problems. Ideally a pediatrician and an office nurse practitioner can provide the additional support and counsel necessary. Many families prefer to leave the hospital early to retreat to the comfort and privacy of their home and the health care provider they selected. Home visits by the pediatrician's staff can provide the necessary monitoring of weight gain and nutrition and counseling by someone capable of handling all the problems that arise, including breastfeeding. No referrals should be made without the pediatrician's knowledge and agreement. The pediatrician or family physician has the advantage of knowing both the family and the child.

In a study of 59 breastfed infants with Down syndrome, Aumonier and Cunningham[14] reported that 31 had no sucking difficulty, 12 were successfully nursing within a week, and 16 required tube feeding initially, which was associated with other medical problems, including low birth weight (LBW), cardiac lesions, and jaundice. Hyperbilirubinemia is common in trisomy and was seen in 49% of the infants in this study. Eighteen babies had multiple medical conditions, and 11 of them sucked poorly. The authors[14] point out that the initial sucking ability of the infants did not appear to be a major cause for nonmaintenance of breastfeeding; 10 of the 13 mothers who discontinued breastfeeding cited insufficient milk as a contributing cause, which might have been prevented by early pumping of the breasts between feedings. With amniocentesis, genetic testing, and screening in older mothers (older than 35 years), many are diagnosed prenatally. Parents are then partly prepared before birth.

The birth of an infant with a major genetic abnormality is a shock, even to the strongest parents. If the mother wants to breastfeed, she should be offered all the encouragement and support necessary. Usually she needs to talk with someone to express her anguish about the infant, not the feeding per se. A sympathetic nurse practitioner in the pediatric office can be invaluable in providing support and the expertise to help with the various management problems. If the mother chooses not to breastfeed, appropriate support can also be provided without disrupting treatment continuity.

It is especially important that these infants be breastfed if possible because they are particularly prone to infection, especially otitis media. Before the advent of antibiotics, they often died of overwhelming infection and rarely survived past 20 years of age. These infants and most other infants with developmental disorders do better with stimulation and affection, so the body contact and communication while at the breast are especially important. Those who have associated cardiac lesions not only can suckle, swallow, and breathe with less effort at the breast, but also can receive a fluid more physiologic for their needs. Breastfed or bottle fed, these infants gain poorly; thus switching to a bottle does not solve the problem. The recommendation that children with Down syndrome receive extra vitamins was tested in a controlled study in children 5 to 13 years of age, and no sustained improvement in the children's appearance, growth, behavior, or development was seen with added vitamins.[20]

Growth charts from birth to 18 years illustrate the deficient growth through the growing periods. In infancy they fall behind, so this observation should not be used to discontinue breastfeeding. Breastfed infants remain healthier. Children with Down syndrome are usually overweight throughout life, beginning in infancy.[38]

Down syndrome is a lifelong condition. Having a support system is important for a family. Support groups of other families in the community serve as vital peer support.

HYPOTHYROIDISM

Bode et al.[25] reported that an infant with congenital cretinism was spared the severe effects of the disease because he was breastfed. This was attributed to significant quantities of thyroid hormone in the milk. In a prospective study of 12 cases of hypothyroidism in breastfed infants, however, no protective effect against the disease was found, nor was the onset of the disease delayed. Anthropometric measurements, biochemical values, and psychologic testing at 1 year of age did not differ from those in the 33 bottle-fed hypothyroid infants. Abbassi and Steinour[1] also reported successful diagnosis of congenital hypothyroidism in four breastfed neonates.

Sack et al.[127] measured thyroxine (T_4) concentrations in human milk and found it to be present in significant amounts. Varma et al.[149] studied T_4, triiodothyronine (T_3), and reverse T_3 concentrations in human milk in 77 healthy euthyroid mothers from the day of delivery to 148 days postpartum. From their data, they calculated that if infants received 900 to 1200 mL of milk per day, they would receive 2.1 to 2.6 mg of T_4 per day, based on 238.1 ng/dL of milk after the first week. This amount of T_4 is much less than the recommended dose for the treatment of hypothyroidism (18.8 to 25 mg/day of levo-T_3). T_4 was essentially immeasurable in the milk sampled. In another study, however, comparing 22 breastfed and 25 formula-fed infants who were 2 to 3 weeks old, the levels of T_3 and T_4 were significantly higher in the breastfed infants.[62] No definite relationship between the levels of T_3 and reverse T_3 could be found.

A 6-week-old girl was diagnosed to have congenital hypothyroidism by routine neonatal screening when T_4 was reported at 3 mg/dL (normal greater than 7 mg/dL).[40] The mother gave a history of multiple applications of povidone-iodine during pregnancy and continuing during lactation. Further testing revealed thyroid-stimulating hormone levels of 0.9 mU/mL (normal 0.8 to 5 μ/mL). Iodine treatment was stopped and breastfeeding continued while treatment of thyroid replacement was begun. At 1 year, growth and development were normal. It is, therefore, suggested that neonatal screening for thyroid disease may be even more urgent if the clinical symptoms are apt to be masked in a breastfed infant. No contraindication exists to breastfeeding when the infant is hypothyroid, and it would be beneficial.[95] Appropriate therapy should also be instituted promptly. Mandatory screening for hypothyroidism is available to newborns in developed countries. Many infants that screen positive do not have at birth the characteristic signs and symptoms associated with cretinism, but therapy is just as urgent. Breastfeeding is ideal for these infants as well.

ADRENAL HYPERPLASIA

In an analysis of 32 infants with salt-losing congenital adrenal hyperplasia who were in adrenal crisis, eight had been breastfed, five had been breastfed with formula supplements, and 19 had been formula fed. Infants who were breastfed were admitted to the hospital later than the formula-fed infants, although the breastfed infants had lower serum sodium levels on admission. The breastfed infants did not vomit and remained stable longer, although they had severe failure to thrive.[39] Weaning initiated vomiting and precipitated crises in the breastfed infants. The authors suggest that congenital adrenal hyperplasia should be considered in a breastfed infant with failure to thrive. Electrolytes should be obtained before weaning to make the diagnosis and avoid precipitating a crisis by weaning. Then breastfeeding can continue as treatment is initiated.

HYPERNATREMIC DEHYDRATION ASSOCIATED WITH BREASTFEEDING

The consequences of inadequate intake of breast milk range from hyperbilirubinemia, infant hunger, and low weight gain to life-threatening dehydration and starvation. The number of reported cases of hypernatremic dehydration has significantly increased because more infants have been breastfed and more infants are managed outside the hospital by lactation experts without pediatric oversight.[136] Term breastfed infants with serum sodium levels of 150 mEq/L or higher were found to be 4.1% of the 4136 term infants hospitalized and reviewed by Unal et al.[148] in the Children's Research Hospital in Ankara, Turkey. These children had lost 15.9% birth weight (range 5.4% to 32.7%). The presenting symptom in 47.3% of cases was hyperbilirubinemia and poor suck in 29.6%. Other complications included acute renal failure in 82.8%, elevated liver enzymes in 20.7%, disseminated intracranial hemorrhage in 3.6%, and thromboses in 1.8%. Ten patients developed seizures and two died. In another study, 60 term infants were readmitted to the hospital with ketoacidosis with plasma serum sodium levels greater than 145 mmol/L. The hospital had recently upgraded its newborn discharge policy to include weights by trained midwives at 72 to 96 hours and at 7 to 10 days of age. Voiding, stooling, and breastfeeding were also checked, and infants who lost more than 10% of birth weight were sent to the hospital. The incidence of hypernatremia with plasma serum sodium levels greater than 145 mmol/L was 7.4 and 5.0 per 10,000 live births before and after the new policy, respectively, but the percentages of cases with plasma serum sodium levels greater than 150 mmol/L was 56.5% versus 18.9%. It was concluded that weighing and lactation support resulted in less dehydration and less severe hypernatremia and better breastfeeding rates.[78] Hypernatremic dehydration in neonates due to inadequate breastfeeding is serious, a well-recognized cause of permanent neurologic abnormality, and life threatening. Sodium levels in breast milk vary, and highly elevated levels impair lactogenesis and cause failure to breastfeed. The etiology can be associated initially with poor milk production. As milk decreases in volume in the normal weaning process the sodium level increases. With lactation failure the sodium level is usually elevated. When levels in the infant reach 145 mEq/L urgent therapy is required. Serum osmolarity is also elevated, urine output is low, and the specific gravity elevated. Sodium levels in early milk are 300 to 400 mEq/L, and as volume increases the levels drop to 120 to 250 mEq/L. The problem is seen more commonly in primiparas. Loss of weight of over 10% deserves evaluation. It is recommended that these dyads be seen by the pediatrician within 2 days of hospital discharge. Treatment not only includes aggressive rehydration of the infant but skilled intense establishment of a full milk supply. Follow-up of infants with proper medical care by pediatricians is essential.

NEONATAL BREASTS AND NIPPLE DISCHARGE

A newborn may have swelling of the breasts for the first few days of life, whether male or female; this is unrelated to being breastfed. If the infant's breast is squeezed, milk can be obtained. This has been called *witch's milk*. The constituents of neonatal milk were studied in the milk of 18 normal newborns and infants with sepsis, adrenal hyperplasia, CF, and meconium ileus.[22] Electrolyte values were similar

to those in adult women in all infants except one with mastitis in whom the sodium level was elevated and the potassium decreased. Total protein and lactose were also similar to those in adult women. The fat was different, increasing with postnatal age and being higher in short-chain fatty acids. It was indeed true milk.

Two infants, one female and one male, were reported to have bilateral bloody discharge from the nipples at 6 weeks of age. Cultures and smears were unrevealing.[22] No biopsy was done. The female infant's swelling and discharge cleared after 5 months; the male infant's was present at 10 weeks when he was lost to follow-up. Galactorrhea or persistent neonatal milk has been reported in association with neonatal hyperthyroidism. In another report, a 21-day-old female infant was seen because of a goiter and galactorrhea. The infant had 50% 24-hour[105] I uptake and elevated prolactin levels, which slowly responded to Lugol solution treatment for hyperthyroidism.[94]

NEONATAL MASTITIS

Neonatal mastitis occurs infrequently, although it was a common event in the 1940s and 1950s, when staphylococcal disease was rampant in nurseries. It occurs in full-term infants 1 to 5 weeks of age and in as many girls as boys, usually unilaterally.[151] It is unrelated to maternal mastitis and usually occurs in bottle-fed infants. Before IV antibiotic therapy, surgical incision and drainage were common. Prognosis for cure is excellent. In recent years the rare cases that occur are seen in conjunction with manipulation of the neonatal breast to express the natural secretion when the newborn breast is engorged (witch's milk). In some primitive cultures expressing milk from swollen newborn breasts is done and often leads to mastitis.

HYPERBILIRUBINEMIA AND JAUNDICE

Jaundice in newborns has become a source of considerable misinformation, confusion, and anxiety. Incidence of jaundice is higher in full-term infants than a decade ago. From 1994 to 2002 11.9% of newborns were hospitalized for hyperbilirubinemia; rates rose to 20.0% in 2003 to 2005. The incidence of kernicterus dropped from 5.8 per 100,000 live births to 1.6 per 100,000 live births as a result of aggressive preventive measures in these years according to Burke et al.[27] More physicians are paying attention to the development of hyperbilirubinemia in newborns. These two factors serve to increase the frequency of the question of the role of breastfeeding in the development of hyperbilirubinemia.

Some of the confusion and inconsistencies associated with the management can be attributed to indecisive terminology. This discussion attempts to clarify the issues and outlines the causes and effects of hyperbilirubinemia.

Why the Concern about Jaundice?

Bilirubin is a cell toxin, as can be demonstrated dramatically by adding a little bilirubin to a tissue culture, which will be quickly destroyed. Excessive bilirubin causes concern because when free, unbound, unconjugated bilirubin is in the system, it can be deposited in various tissues, ultimately causing necrosis of the cells. The brain and brain cells, if destroyed by bilirubin deposits, do not regenerate.[64] The full-blown end result is bilirubin encephalopathy, or kernicterus, which is essentially a pathologic diagnosis that depends on identifying the yellow pigmentation and necrosis in the brain, especially in the basal ganglion, hippocampal cortex, and subthalamic nuclei. At autopsy, 50% of infants with kernicterus also have other lesions caused by bilirubin toxicity. Necrosis of renal tubular cells, intestinal mucosa, or pancreatic cells or associated GI hemorrhage may be seen.

The classic clinical manifestations of bilirubin encephalopathy are characterized by progressive lethargy, rigidity, opisthotonos, high-pitched cry, fever, and convulsions. The mortality rate is 50%. Survivors usually have choreoathetoid cerebral palsy, asymmetric spasticity, paresis of upward gaze, high-frequency deafness, and mental retardation.[42] Premature infants are particularly susceptible to bilirubin-related brain damage and may have kernicterus at autopsy without the typical clinical syndrome. A significant correlation exists between level of bilirubin and hearing impairment in newborns when other risk factors are present. Classic full-blown kernicterus rarely occurs today, but mild effects on the brain may be manifested clinically in later life in the form of lack of coordination, hypertonicity, and mental retardation or learning disabilities, symptoms sometimes collectively called minimal brain damage.[64] Bilirubin encephalopathy is the appropriate term for conditions in which bilirubin is thought to be the cause of brain toxicity.

Mechanism of Bilirubin Production in the Neonate

A normal full-term infant has a hematocrit in utero of 50% to 65%. Because of the low oxygen tension delivered to the fetus via the placenta, the fetus requires more hemoglobin (Hb) to carry the oxygen. As soon as an infant is born and begins to breathe room air, the need is gone. The infant bone marrow does not make more cells, and excess cells are destroyed and not replaced. The life span of a fetal red blood cell (RBC) is 70 to 90 days instead of an adult's 120 days. Normally, when RBCs are destroyed, the released Hb is broken down to heme in the reticuloendothelial system. The reticuloendothelial system cells contain a microsomal enzyme, heme oxygenase, which is capable of oxidizing the α-methene bridge carbon of the heme molecule after the loss of the iron and the globin to form biliverdin, a green pigment. Biliverdin is water soluble and is rapidly degraded to bilirubin. A gram of hemoglobulin will produce 34 mg of bilirubin.

The reticuloendothelial cell releases the bilirubin into the circulation, where it is rapidly bound to albumin. Indirect bilirubin is essentially insoluble (less than 0.01 mg% soluble) and is a yellow pigment. Adult albumin can bind two molecules of bilirubin, the first more tightly than the second. Newborn albumin has reduced molar binding capacities that vary with maturity and other factors, such as pH, infection, and hypoglycemia.

Unconjugated bilirubin is removed from the circulation by the hepatocyte, which converts it by conjugation of each molecule of bilirubin with two molecules of glucuronic acid into direct bilirubin. Direct bilirubin is water soluble and is excreted via the bile to the stools. The balance between hepatic cell uptake of bilirubin and the rate of bilirubin production determines the serum unconjugated bilirubin concentration. Laboratory measurements include both bound and unbound indirect bilirubin. The amount of unconjugated bilirubin that exceeds the binding capacity of an infant's albumen is the unbound unconjugated bilirubin available to deposit in the brain.

Evaluation and Management

Normal full-term newborns have serial bilirubin tests to determine the range of values. The cord bilirubin level may be as high as 2 mg% and rise in the first 72 hours to 5 to 6 mg%, which is barely in the visible range, and gradually taper off, assuming normal adult levels of 1 mg% after 10 days. Less than 50% of normal infants are visibly jaundiced in the first week of life. This would suggest that visible jaundice is idiopathic, not physiologic. The level of bilirubin that is acceptable depends on a number of factors. In some premature infants, even bilirubin levels under 10 mg/dL may be of concern because of the limited albumen binding sites in premature infants.

Factors That Influence Significance. For a given level of bilirubin, several associated factors may need to be considered. If an infant has acidosis, anoxia, asphyxia, hypothermia, hypoglycemia, or infection, even lower levels of bilirubin may have significant risk for causing deposition of bilirubin in the brain cells. The most important factor is prematurity, which affects liver and brain metabolism and albumin binding sites. An increased incidence of elevated bilirubin levels occurs in certain races and populations. Asian populations, including Chinese, Japanese, and Korean, and Native Americans may have bilirubin levels averaging 10 to 14 mg%. A higher incidence of autopsy-identified kernicterus also is seen in these populations. Glucose-6-phosphate dehydrogenase deficiency, a genetic disorder, is also common in these groups. Infants who carry the 211 and 388 variants, respectively, in the *UGTIA1* and *OATP2* genes and are breastfed were found to be at high risk to develop severe hyperbilirubinemia according to Huang et al.,[71] who investigated infants born in Cathay Hospital in Taipei, Taiwan, where glucose-6-phosphate dehydrogenase is prevalent. They also noted that glucose-6-phosphate dehydrogenase is the most common genetic defect and urge more frequent screening. Infants with these genetic variants who were not breastfed had hyperbilirubinemia that was less responsive to phototherapy; thus it is recommended that breastfeeding not be discontinued.[71]

Determination of Cause of Jaundice

Following the chain of events from the destruction of RBCs in newborns through the final excretion of conjugated bilirubin in the stools simplifies understanding the cause of a specific case of jaundice. Causes include (1) increased destruction of RBCs, (2) decreased conjugation in the glucuronidase system, (3) decreased albumin binding, and (4) increased reabsorption from the GI tract and decreased excretion. To be excreted from the body, unconjugated bilirubin has to be conjugated with glucuronic acid in the hepatocyte, which becomes water-soluble bilirubin glucuronide. The enzyme involved is a specific hepatic enzyme isoform (1A1) belonging to the uridine diphosphoglucuronate glucuronosyltransferase (UGT) family of enzymes. Much has been learned about these enzymes and their relationship to bilirubin metabolism.[83] UGTs catalyze the conjugation of not only bilirubin but steroids, bile acids, drugs, and other xenobiotics. The two separate families of genes, *UGT1* and *UGT2*, have different actions. Gilbert syndrome, an uncommon genetic anemia associated with persistent hyperbilirubinemia in neonates, is associated with a mutation in the coding area of the *UGT1A1* gene. Similar genetic variations are present in Crigler-Najjar syndrome. These genetic variations are probably the cause of most persistent hyperbilirubinemia.

Ethnic background, risk factors, previous infants with hyperbilirubinemia, and family history of anemia and jaundice are important to the correct diagnosis and management, the preservation of breastfeeding, and the safety of the infant.

When albumin binding is altered, the visibility of the jaundice is not affected. The bilirubin level may not be very high, but the substance is not bound to albumin and is available at lower levels to pass into the brain cells.[99] Premature infants have much lower albumin levels and thus have fewer binding sites. Drugs that also bind to albumin (e.g., aspirin, sulfadiazine) compete for the same binding sites. A lower level of bilirubin puts infants who have these medications in their system at risk because the bilirubin is unbound and available to enter tissue cells, including brain cells.

Reabsorption of bilirubin from stool in the GI tract can increase the bilirubin level. This occurs when the conjugated bilirubin that was excreted into the colon and the stool is slow to pass. It is unconjugated by the action of intestinal bacteria and reabsorbed, which happens when stools are decreased or slowed in passage. Poor feedings, pyloric stenosis, and other forms of intestinal obstruction are common causes of this type of jaundice. Some bacteria are more likely than others to unconjugate conjugated bilirubin.

Sepsis, on the other hand, was not found in more than 300 infants readmitted for hyperbilirubinemia while healthy and breastfeeding. Lower total bilirubin and direct bilirubin levels greater than 2.0 mg% in a sick baby have a high correlation with sepsis.

Safe Levels of Bilirubin. Safe levels of bilirubin depend on a number of factors, including acidosis, hypoxia or anoxia, and sepsis. A handy rule of thumb is the correlation of birth weight in a premature infant and the indirect bilirubin level, using a value 2 to 3 mg lower when an infant has multiple problems. The risk for elevated bilirubin is related to the availability of albumin to bind the indirect bilirubin and prevent it from entering the brain cells. The amount of albumin is related to the degree of prematurity, and thus the rule of thumb is based on birth weight and/or gestational age. When an infant is sick, fewer albumin-binding sites are available, and the bilirubin level of concern is even lower.

Any value of 20 mg/dL or greater warrants consideration of aggressive treatment. Jaundice visible when an infant is younger than 24 hours of age is of special concern because it is usually associated with an incompatibility or infection. Rapidly rising bilirubin levels are also of concern, and a 0.5-mg/dL rise per hour is an indication for treatment.

The AAP has published a practice parameter for the management of hyperbilirubinemia in healthy term newborns.[139] Term infants who are visibly jaundiced at or before 24 hours of life are not considered healthy and require a diagnostic work up regardless of feeding method.

The AAP also addresses jaundice associated with breastfeeding in healthy term infants. The AAP discourages the interruption of breastfeeding in healthy term newborns and encourages continued and frequent breastfeeding (at least 8 to 10 times every 24 hours). Supplementing nursing with water or dextrose water does not lower the bilirubin level in jaundiced, healthy, breastfeeding infants.[134]

Early Jaundice while Breastfeeding. Many studies of bilirubin levels in normal newborn nurseries have been conducted that look at method of feeding. Unfortunately, few have detailed frequency of feeds, supplementation, and stool pattern.[98] A review summarizing results in 13 studies covering more than 20,000 infants showed a relationship between breastfeeding and jaundice. A pooled analysis of 12 studies showed 514 of 3997 breastfed infants to have total serum bilirubin (TSB) levels of 12 mg/dL or higher versus 172 of 4255 bottle-fed infants. In a smaller group of studies, 54 of 2655 breastfed infants had bilirubin levels of 15 mg/dL or greater versus 10 of 3002 bottle-fed infants. Eleven of 13 studies reported that breastfed infants had higher mean bilirubin levels. In a series of more than 12,000 infants, the risk for a breastfed infant becoming jaundiced was 1:8. The risk for becoming jaundiced for a premature infant was 3:6; for an infant of Asian race, 3:56; and with prolonged rupture of membranes, 1:91.[139]

Relationship of Bilirubin Level to Passage of Stools. There are 450 mg of bilirubin in the intestinal tract meconium of an average newborn infant. Passing this meconium is critical to avoid the deconjugation and reabsorption of unconjugated bilirubin from the gut into the serum. Failure to pass meconium is correlated with elevated serum bilirubin. Time of first stool is also correlated with level of serum bilirubin. Bottle-fed infants excrete more stool (82 g) and more bilirubin (23.8 mg) in the first 3 days than breastfed infants, who excreted 58 g of stool and 15.7 mg bilirubin. The serum bilirubin levels were 6.8 mg/dL in bottle-fed and 9.5 mg/dL in breastfed infants. Furthermore, when the breastfed infants excreted more stools and more bilirubin, they had lower bilirubin levels. This relationship has been confirmed in multiple studies.

Clinical Risk Factors in Hyperbilirubinemia

Clinical examination by visual assessment of jaundice in newborns is not reliable in a study comparing visual estimates with laboratory values by Moyer et al.[111] They suggested bilirubin testing should be based on risk factors. Clinical risk factors significantly improve prediction of hyperbilirubinemia compared with the use of early total bilirubin levels, as reported by Newman et al.[114] based on a study of almost 54,000 infants older than 36-weeks' gestational age and at least 2000 g birth weight. From this group, 207 cases were found with elevated bilirubins drawn before 48-hour discharge. The authors found the risk index was the best predictor of elevated bilirubin (Table 14-4). Clearly, prematurity carries the greatest risk. The TSB before 48 hours was an accurate predictor of reaching a bilirubin of 20 mg/dL (Figure 14-5).

When the number of feedings at the breast in the first 3 days of life is related to bilirubin levels, there is a significant relationship. The greater the number of breastfeedings, the lower the bilirubin. Infants with more than eight feedings per day were not significantly jaundiced. Water and dextrose supplements were associated with higher bilirubin levels. Sugar-water intake in the first 3 days negatively affects the volume of breast milk available on the fourth day. The infants with high glucose intake have higher bilirubin levels.

Caloric Deprivation and Starvation. Elevated bilirubin does not impede sucking ability. Reduced caloric intake or starvation has been associated with hyperbilirubinemia in adult humans and in many animals. The association between starvation and early

TABLE 14-4	Modified Risk Index for Predicting Hyperbilirubinemia in Infants Who Do Not Have Early Jaundice
Variable	**Points**
Exclusive breastfeeding at hospital discharge	6
Bruising noted	4
Asian race	4
Cephalohematoma	3
Mother's age ≥ 25 years	3
Male sex	1
Black race	−2
Gestational age	$2 \times (40 -$ gestational age)

Modified from Newman TB, Liljestrand P, Escobar GJ: Combining clinical risk factors with serum bilirubin levels to predict hyperbilirubinemia in newborns, *Arch Pediatr Adolesc Med* 159:113, 2005.

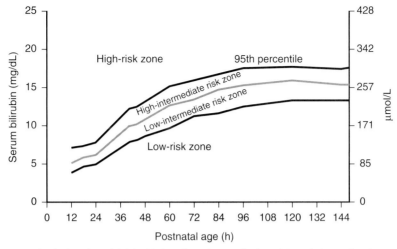

Figure 14-5. Nomogram for designation of risk in 2840 well newborns of at least 36 weeks' gestational age with birth weight of 2000 g or greater or of at least 35 weeks' gestational age with birth weight of 2500 g or greater based on the hour-specific serum bilirubin values. The serum bilirubin level was obtained before discharge, and the zone in which the value fell predicted the likelihood of a subsequent bilirubin level exceeding the 95th percentile (high-risk zone). (From American Academy of Pediatrics Subcommittee on Hyperbilirubinemia: Management of hyperbilirubinemia in the newborn infant 35 or more weeks of gestation, *Pediatrics* 114:297, 2004.)

neonatal jaundice has been described. Gartner[54] has postulated that starvation may increase bilirubin production, shift bilirubin pools, reduce hepatic bilirubin uptake, diminish hepatic bilirubin conjugation, or increase enteric bilirubin reabsorption. Adequate caloric intake may simply diminish intestinal bilirubin absorption. Infants with intestinal obstruction (pyloric stenosis) at birth or in the early weeks of life are often jaundiced.

Treatment of Early Hyperbilirubinemia. Serum bilirubin levels in newborns and the relationship to breastfeeding were measured, and 8 of 10 infants with serum bilirubin greater than 12.9 mg/dL were breastfed.[99] It is the process of altered nourishment that is the cause of relative starvation. The amount of stress for a mother generated by separation from her infant for phototherapy was measured by urine cortisol levels and compared with levels in mothers who roomed-in with their jaundiced infants during phototherapy. The separated mothers were more stressed and were more likely to discontinue breastfeeding than those who remained with their infants.[50]

In a controlled trial of four interventions,[114] 125 of 1685 infants in the birth cohort whose bilirubin levels reached 17 mg/dL (291 mmol/L) were randomly assigned to treatment. The four interventions were (1) continue breastfeeding and observe; (2) discontinue breastfeeding and substitute formula; (3) discontinue breastfeeding, substitute formula, and use phototherapy; and (4) continue breastfeeding and use phototherapy. The bilirubin reached

20 mg/dL (342 mmol/L) in 24% of group 1, 19% of group 2, 3% of group 3, and 14% of group 4. Phototherapy clearly adds to the decline in bilirubin, and the authors[114] suggest that the parents can be offered the management of their choice. Newman and Maisels recommend that because jaundiced infants are rarely sick, the only laboratory work necessary is a blood type and Coombs test; only when jaundice is excessive should bilirubin levels be followed closely. Infants with incompatibilities should be treated aggressively.

An evaluation of the transcutaneous bilirubinometer demonstrated that it correlated well with TSBs done in the laboratory.[97] The correlation in black infants was not as close but levels erred on the high side so that underdiagnosing is not a risk. Multiple checks with the meter are easily done to establish trends so that a breastfed infant can be followed closely without painful sticks. Blood levels are essential if phototherapy is needed and after it is initiated.[97]

Hyperbilirubinemia results from unphysiologic management of breastfeeding, expressed largely through insufficient frequency of breastfeeding. To treat the actual cause, that is, failed breastfeeding or inadequate stooling or underfeeding, breastfeeding should be reviewed for frequency, length of suckling, and apparent supply of milk, adjusting the breastfeeding to improve any deficits. If stooling is the problem, an infant should be stimulated to stool. If starvation is the problem, the infant should receive additional calories (formula) while the milk supply is being increased by better breastfeeding techniques.

The same would apply to bottle-feeding jaundice (i.e., any infant with idiopathic jaundice who is being bottle fed and has a bilirubin level greater than 12.9 mg/dL). Stooling, frequency of feeds, and kilocalories would be improved. Box 14-1 provides a management schema for preventing or treating jaundice in the breastfed infant. All infants must have the appropriate laboratory studies performed.[98]

Guidelines for the management of hyperbilirubinemia of a newborn who is at least 35 weeks' gestational age have been developed by the Subcommittee on Hyperbilirubinemia of the AAP (see Box 14-1).[139] The key elements of their recommendations appear in Table 14-5. The nomogram for designation of risk for jaundice is illustrated in Figure 14-5. Guidelines for phototherapies are illustrated in Figure 14-6.

The Academy of Breastfeeding Medicine developed a protocol for hyperbilirubinemia which is on its website: http://www.AcademyofMedicine.com. Jaundice in LVW infants at less than 35 weeks' gestation also results from increased bilirubin production, decreased hepatic conjugation in an immature liver, and inadequate excretion via the stool. Hyperbilirubinemia in preterm infants is more prevalent, more severe, and more protracted. The risk for kernicterus is greater as well. Its management is the purview of a neonatologist.[153] In most cases, if human milk is provided it is maintained. Maisels et al.[98] add the following recommendations: management and follow-up plans should be based on gestational age, predischarge bilirubins, and risk factors for subsequent hyperbilirubinemia (Box 14-2). They begin with suggesting lactation evaluation and support for all breastfeeding mothers. They also recommend that timing of repeat bilirubin measurements after discharge depend on age at time of measurement and on degree the level is above the

TABLE 14-5	Risk Factors for Development of Severe Hyperbilirubinemia in Infants of 35 Weeks' Gestation or Older (in Approximate Order of Importance)

Major risk factors

Predischarge TSB or TcB level in the high-risk zone

Jaundice observed in the first 24 hours

Blood group incompatibility with positive direct antiglobulin test, other known hemolytic disease (e.g., glucose-6-phosphate dehydrogenase deficiency), elevated ETCOc

Gestational age 35 to 36 weeks

Previous sibling received phototherapy

Cephalohematoma or significant bruising

Exclusive breastfeeding, particularly if nursing is not going well and weight loss is excessive

East Asian race*

Minor risk factors

Predischarge TSB or TcB level in the high intermediate-risk zone

Gestational age 37 to 38 weeks

Jaundice observed before discharge

Previous sibling with jaundice

Macrosomic infant of a mother with diabetes

Maternal age 25 years or older

Male sex

Decreased risk

(These factors are associated with decreased risk for significant jaundice, listed in order of decreasing importance.)

TSB or TcB level in the low-risk zone

Gestational age 41 weeks or more

Exclusive bottle feeding

Black race*

Discharge from hospital after 72 hours

ETCOc, End tidal carbon monoxide corrected for ambient air; *TcB,* transcutaneous bilirubin; *TSB,* total serum bilirubin.
  *Race as defined by mother's description.
  From American Academy of Pediatrics Subcommittee on Hyperbilirubinemia: Management of hyperbilirubinemia in the newborn infant 35 or more weeks of gestation, *Pediatrics* 114:297, 2004.

BOX 14-1. Management Outline for Early Jaundice while Breastfeeding

1. Monitor all infants for initial stooling. Stimulate stool if no stool in 24 hours.
2. Initiate breastfeeding early and frequently. Frequent short feeding is more effective than infrequent prolonged feeding, although total time may be the same.
3. Discourage water, dextrose water, or formula supplements.
4. Monitor weight, voidings, and stooling in association with breastfeeding pattern.
5. When bilirubin level approaches 15 mg/dL, stimulate stooling, augment feeds, stimulate breast milk production with pumping, and, if this aggressive approach fails and bilirubin approaches 20 mg/dL, use phototherapy.

95th percentile. Follow-up recommendations can be modified according to the level of risk. Infants should have a predischarge bilirubin, which has been the recommendation to improve the chances of preventing kernicterus. Universal predischarge bilirubin screening using TSB or transcutaneous bilirubin (TcB) measurements, which help to assess the risk of subsequent severe hyperbilirubinemia, is recommended. A more structured approach to management and follow-up according to the predischarge TSB/TcB, gestational age, and other risk factors for hyperbilirubinemia are essential.

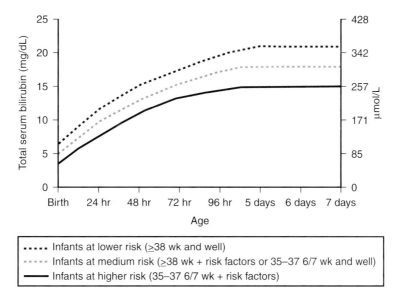

Figure 14-6. Guidelines for phototherapy in hospitalized infants of at least 35 weeks' gestation. Note: These guidelines are based on limited evidence and the levels shown are approximations. The guidelines refer to the use of intensive phototherapy, which should be used when the total serum bilirubin exceeds the line indicated for each category. Infants are designated as "higher risk" because of the potential negative effects of the conditions listed on albumin binding of bilirubin, the blood-brain barrier, and the susceptibility of the brain cells to damage by bilirubin. (From American Academy of Pediatrics Subcommittee on Hyperbilirubinemia: Management of hyperbilirubinemia in the newborn infant 35 or more weeks of gestation, *Pediatrics* 114:297, 2004.)

Kernicterus in Late Preterm Infants Cared for as Term Healthy Infants

Late prematurity (34 6/7 to 36 6/7 weeks' gestational age) has not been recognized as a risk factor for hazardous hyperbilirubinemia by practitioners according to Bhutani and Johnson,[24] who report cases of acute and chronic posticteric sequelae. Large-for-gestational-age and late preterm infants are disproportionately represented in the group with kernicterus. Unsuccessful and suboptimal lactation experience was the most frequent associated factor. The authors urge attention to early bilirubin values, additional risk factors, and the success of breastfeeding in these infants. These infants require close monitoring by the pediatrician.

Breast Milk Jaundice. Apart from the frequent but low level (usually less than 12 mg/dL) hyperbilirubinemia, breastfeeding rarely is associated with delayed but prolonged hyperbilirubinemia, which,

if unchecked, may exceed 20 mg/dL. This syndrome has been called breast milk jaundice, late-onset jaundice, and breast milk jaundice syndrome.[54] It occurs in less than 1 in 200 births; the numbers are imprecise because not all mothers breastfeed. This syndrome is associated with the milk of a particular mother and will occur with each pregnancy in varying degrees, depending on each infant's ability to conjugate bilirubin (i.e., a premature sibling might be more severely affected).[54] Early-onset jaundice is related to the process of breastfeeding, not the milk itself. It is essential to rule out other causes of prolonged or excessive jaundice, especially hemolytic disease, hypothyroidism, glucose-6-phosphate dehydrogenase deficiency, inherited hepatic glucuronyl transferase deficiency (Gilbert syndrome, etc.), and intestinal obstruction.

The pattern of this jaundice is distinctly different. Normally, idiopathic jaundice peaks on the third day and then begins to drop. Breast milk jaundice, however, becomes apparent or continues to

BOX 14-2. Key Elements to Hyperbilirubinemia Management

1. Promote and support successful breastfeeding.
2. Establish nursery protocols for the identification and evaluation of hyperbilirubinemia.
3. Measure the total serum bilirubin or transcutaneous bilirubin level in infants jaundiced in the first 24 hours.
4. Recognize that visual estimation of the degree of jaundice can lead to errors, particularly in darkly pigmented infants.
5. Interpret all bilirubin levels according to an infant's age in hours.
6. Recognize that infants born at less than 38 weeks' gestation, particularly those who are breastfed, are at higher risk for developing hyperbilirubinemia and require closer surveillance and monitoring.
7. Perform a systematic assessment on all infants before discharge for the risk of severe hyperbilirubinemia.
8. Provide parents with written and verbal information about newborn jaundice.
9. Provide appropriate follow-up based on the time of discharge and the risk assessment.
10. Treat newborns, when indicated, with phototherapy or exchange transfusion.

rise after the third day, and bilirubin levels may peak any time from the seventh to the tenth day, with untreated cases being reported to peak as late as the fifteenth day. Values have ranged from 10 to 27 mg/dL during this time. No correlation exists with weight loss or gain, and stools are normal.

The syndrome of breast milk jaundice was attributed by Arias et al.[12] to a substance in the milk of some mothers that inhibits the hepatic enzyme glucuronyl transferase, preventing the conjugation of bilirubin. The substance has been identified as 5β-pregnane-3α,20α-diol, a breakdown product of progesterone and an isomer of pregnanediol that is not usually found in milk but occurs normally in 10% of the lactating population. Although this substance had also been isolated from the milk and serum of mothers whose infants were not jaundiced, this work has not been duplicated.

In a definitive study of breast milk β-glucuronidase, Wilson et al. examined 55 mother-infant pairs. No correlation was found between serum bilirubin levels and breast milk β-glucuronidase between days 3 and 6 postpartum.

The role of lipoprotein lipase and bile salt-stimulated lipase in breast milk jaundice continues under investigation. The role of free fatty acids and the possibility of abnormal lipases are unresolved. The undisputed cause of breast milk jaundice continues to elude investigators.

As in early jaundice associated with breastfeeding, jaundiced infants at 3 weeks do not produce more bilirubin than their unjaundiced breastfed peers or bottle-fed infants.

Diagnosis depends on circumstantial evidence, because no easy, rapid laboratory test exists. All other causes, including infection, should be ruled out in the usual manner and a thorough history taken, including medications and family history and ethnic background. If the mother has nursed other infants, were they jaundiced? Usually 70% of the previous children of a given mother whose infant has breast milk jaundice have been jaundiced. The difference may be related to the greater maturity of the liver of a given infant who then is able to handle the increased demands on the glucuronyl transferase system. Genetic variations in *UGTIA1* and *OATP2* genes may hold answers. To establish the diagnosis firmly, and this is necessary when the bilirubin level is greater than 16 mg/dL for more than 24 hours, a bilirubin reading should be obtained 2 hours after a breastfeeding and then breastfeeding discontinued for at least 12 hours.[113] The infant must be fed fluids and calories. The infant's mother should be assisted in pumping her breasts to maintain her supply. Even more urgent is providing the mother with a sympathetic explanation of the problem and the process. After at least 12 hours without mother's milk, the bilirubin level should be measured. If a significant drop of more than 2 mg/dL occurs, it is diagnostic. When the level is less than 15 mg/dL, the infant can be put to the breast. Bilirubin levels should be obtained to determine if the bilirubin rises again and, if so, how much. In most cases, in the time not breastfeeding, the infant's body equilibrates the levels sufficiently, so only a slight increase in bilirubin occurs on return to breastfeeding followed by a slow but steady drop. If that is the case, breastfeeding can continue. The bilirubin level should be checked at 10 to 14 days to be certain the bilirubin is truly clearing.

If the bilirubin has not dropped significantly after 12 hours without breast milk, the time off the breast should be extended to 18 to 24 hours, measuring bilirubin levels every 6 hours. If the bilirubin rises while the infant is off the breast, the cause of jaundice is clearly not the breast milk; breastfeeding should be resumed and other causes for the jaundice reevaluated.

Phototherapy and Breast Milk Jaundice. If the bilirubin is substantially greater than 20 mg/dL in a full-term infant (or proportionately lower in a preterm infant), it is important to lower the bilirubin promptly; thus phototherapy should be initiated as soon as the blood work is drawn (Figure 14-7). The relationship to breastfeeding can be established later. Often IV fluids are also necessary.

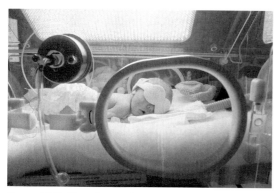

Figure 14-7. Phototherapy for a premature infant with two overhead banks of lights while lying on a fiberoptic blanket.

If one is attempting to establish the diagnosis of breast milk jaundice, phototherapy should not be used while breast milk is being discontinued. If establishing the diagnosis is not necessary (perhaps because of the same diagnosis in older siblings), phototherapy can be used to bring the values to a more acceptable range (i.e., less than 12 mg/dL). When phototherapy is discontinued, it is most important to establish that no rebound hyperbilirubinemia occurs. In addition, it is important to follow the infant at home after discharge through at least 14 days of life or longer if the values are not less than 12 mg/dL. It should not be assumed that the diagnosis is breast milk jaundice when breastfeeding has been stopped and phototherapy initiated simultaneously.

Late Diagnosis of Breast Milk Jaundice

With the frequency of early discharge from the hospital, especially for families enjoying the birthing center concept, breastfed infants are often discharged before jaundice for any reason has developed. Because breast milk jaundice is likely to be delayed to the fourth or fifth day, peaking at 10 to 14 days of age, most normal infants are already home. Occasionally, an infant is observed in a pediatrician's office at 10 days of age or older with a bilirubin level greater than 20 mg/dL, often 23 to 25 mg/dL. This necessitates the immediate admission of the infant to the hospital for a complete bilirubin work up. It is important to recognize that other causes of hyperbilirubinemia must be ruled out, including blood-type incompatibilities. At this age, it is also necessary to rule out biliary obstruction and hepatitis, which might have a high direct or conjugated bilirubin level.

Phototherapy is used for 4 to 6 hours to establish whether this therapy will be effective in dropping the level sufficiently. When bilirubin is substantially greater than 20 mg/dL and if a possible association with breast milk exists, it is necessary to stop

breastfeeding temporarily and start phototherapy immediately on admission while the diagnostic work up is being performed. Otherwise, breastfeeding may continue even though IV fluids may also be necessary.

The Agency for Health Care Research and Quality, through its Evidence-Based Practice Centers, published a report on management of neonatal hyperbilirubinemia in 2003 after an extensive review of more than 4560 abstracts from which 241 articles were examined and 138 included in the report.[74] In contrast, Chou et al.[33] proposed a management of hyperbilirubinemia using a benchmarking model in a 3-year prospective cohort study. They found association of high bilirubin with lower gestational age, older mother, and exclusive or partial breastfeeding. The authors recommend assessing breastfeeding and promoting breastfeeding, supplementing if necessary but never with water, in combination with phototherapy as most efficacious.[33] The natural history of jaundice in predominantly breastfed infants is described by Maisels et al. They point out after measuring TcBs in 1044 breastfed infants of at least 35 weeks' gestation, that 20% to 30% of predominantly breastfed infants will be jaundiced by transcutaneous measurement at 3 to 4 weeks. Levels of 5 mg/dL or more will be found in 30% to 40%. When drawn, a TcB of zero was highly predictive that the bilirubin was less than 12.9 mg/dL and could be used for screening purposes at 1 month.

Infants discharged early (less than 30 hours of age) were more likely to be rehospitalized for hyperbilirubinemia within 7 days of discharge in a study of 310,000 newborns in the State of Washington, when compared to children discharged from 30 to 78 hours after birth. Of the children readmitted, 94% were breastfed.[58] Bilirubins at discharge are recommended. Prolonged breast milk jaundice has not been studied in follow-up when the association of the bilirubin elevation has been made with breast milk. A pediatric practice may see only a few in a lifetime. The safe level for chronic indirect bilirubin has not been established. The lactation study center recommends greater than or equal to 10 mg/dL. Others allow a level of 12 mg/dL. This is accomplished most easily with phototherapy; usually having an infant sleep under phototherapy 12 hours per day, utilizing home devices such as the "bilirubin blanket," will control the levels. This is not a casual arrangement. The eyes must be protected and the bilirubin monitored. As the liver matures, the problem disappears and phototherapy can be discontinued. The infant must be under the care of an experienced pediatrician. In some cases, the bilirubin can be controlled with partial breastfeeding with the addition of formula in sufficient amounts to maintain the bilirubin at less than 10 mg/dL. Children with Gilbert syndrome, Crigler-Najjar syndrome, glucose-6-phosphate dehydrogenase, and other genetic variations must be managed individually by a genetic specialist and the pediatrician. These children have chronic hyperbilirubinemia and usually need to sleep under phototherapy.

SUCKLING PROBLEMS RELATED TO ANATOMY AND NEURAL DISORDERS

Most problems with latch-on during breastfeeding can be solved with adjustment of position and approach, but a few cannot because an infant has an anatomic variation of the mouth or a neurodevelopmental problem. A thorough examination is required to evaluate the mouth and cheek for potential associated lesions and syndromes. Premature infants are more often identified with suckling problems because they not only are immature but also have been suctioned, intubated, and perhaps ventilated. Much has been put in their mouths. They may also have a high arched or grooved palate from the endotracheal tube used to ventilate.

When the mouth is carefully examined, an infant may have cysts on the dental ridge or under the tongue, the tongue may have limited range of motion, or the palate may be abnormal. A number of observations are being reported in the literature, such as "bubble palate" or variation in infant palatal structure. Schneider et al.[132] recommend alternative positioning and repatterning oral behavior to increase the transfer of milk and reduce the trauma to the maternal nipple. Breastfeeding in the supine position with the infant prone encourages the infant's tongue to fall down and forward and keeps the nipple from being abraded by "the bubble." Marmet and Shell[101] describe a bubble palate as a concavity in the hard palate, usually about $\frac{3}{8}$ to $\frac{3}{4}$ inch (1 to 2 cm) in diameter and $\frac{1}{4}$ inch (0.5 cm) deep. Similar adjustments to positioning would be appropriate for high arched palates.

Macroglossia presents a problem of too much tongue for the oral cavity. These infants do better at the breast than with a bottle. The main problem is to have the infant bring the tongue forward to avoid gagging.

Abnormal oral motor patterns are more common in premature infants and those who have been asphyxiated at birth. These movements include exaggerated tongue thrust (often from bottle feeding and nipple confusion), tonic bite, jaw thrust, jaw clenching, and lip pursing. Some of these behaviors are associated with postural muscle tone abnormalities.[152] Normal muscle tone and strength throughout breastfeeding, especially alignment of the head and neck, are required to form a stable base to anchor the oral and pharyngeal musculature. Hypertonic

and hypotonic infants may pose problems. Hypertonic infants are usually overflexed or overextended and have hypertonic mouths with tonic bite, jaw thrusting, and clenching. Inducing relaxation, minimizing handling, and using gentle strokes to calm the infant can be effective. If the infant is extended, flexion may be achieved with a pleat-seat carrier (see Figure 14-2) or pillows. Flexed position in these infants relaxes the jaw and mouth and allows latching to take place. Finger feeding may help train these infants. If done just before a feed, the infant can be transferred to the breast smoothly.

Oral tactile hypersensitivity is often seen in infants who have had oral tubes, especially feeding tubes. Touching around the mouth causes feeding rejection. Decreased oral awareness may result in drooling and poor suckling. These infants may respond to stroking the oral area gently. Most infants have a strong arching reflex, which is elicited by touching or applying pressure on the back of the head, causing the infant to arch back away from the breast. Positions that require the mother to hold the head (e.g., "football hold") may trigger this reflex. Infants prefer to be swaddled but always respond better to a firm supportive hold of the body, slightly flexing the arms, legs, and trunk. Pillows can be used for support of the baby or the mother's arms.

The development of an infant's oral motor and feeding skills parallels general physical development, especially gross and fine motor skills. When an infant is having persistent feeding problems, the infant needs total neuromotor assessment. Minor problems may be solved by the firm supportive hold of a swaddled infant who is gently handled and encouraged.

Illingworth and Lister[73] first put forth the concept of a critical or sensitive period for the development of a skill. Conditioned dysphagia is a learned disorder, acquired and maintained through a behavioral conditioning process that occurs when a noxious stimulus is paired with the act of swallowing.[44] This is noted with suctioning of the mouth or nasopharynx and nasogastric feeding tubes in a NICU.

An infant with a true feeding disorder requires an assessment with a neonatal oral-motor review by a trained physical therapist. Training the infant to suckle will be required. These infants ultimately do best if sucking is limited to the breast. Cup feedings are more effective than bottle feeding.

Infants with Problems Requiring Surgery

Human milk should be the food of choice for surgical infants, in other words, all newborns who undergo surgery early in life. Their own mother's

TABLE 14-6	Comparison of Early and Late Jaundice Associated with Hyperbilirubinemia while Breastfeeding	
Early Jaundice	**Late Jaundice**
Occurs 2-5 days of age	Occurs 5-10 days of age
Transient: 10 days	Persists >1 month
More common in primiparas	All children of a given mother
Infrequent feeds	Milk volume not a problem May have abundant milk
Stools delayed and infrequent	Normal stooling
Receiving water or dextrose water	No supplements
Bilirubin peaks ≤15 mg/dL	Bilirubin may be >20 mg/dL
Treatment: None or phototherapy	Treatment: Phototherapy Discontinue breastfeeding temporarily Rarely: Exchange transfusion
Associations: Low Apgar scores, water or dextrose water supplement, prematurity	Associations: None identified

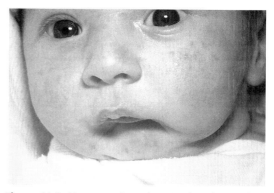

Figure 14-8. Demonstration of a significantly receding-chin. (From Biancuzzo M: *Breastfeeding the newborn, clinical strategies for nurses*, ed 2, St. Louis, 2003, Mosby.)

milk is the best option, a donor milk program is the first alternative.[13,129,138] The UNICEF 10 steps can be modified and adopted for a neonatal surgical unit as recommended by Salvatori (Table 14-6).

IMMEDIATE NEONATAL PERIOD

First-Arch Disorders

Feeding of any sort may be greatly hindered by abnormalities of the jaw, nose, and mouth. A receding chin may seem to be a minor problem and require only positioning the jaw forward. It is essential to establish that the jaw is not dislocated (Figure 14-8). A mother can hook the angle of the jaw with her finger and draw it forward. If the tongue is too large for the jaw, the infant will actually nurse better at the breast than at the bottle because the human nipple fits into the mouth with less bulk. Infants with first-arch abnormalities usually require considerable help in feeding. A cleft palate may also be present. If choanal atresia is present, because infants are obligatory nose breathers it may be necessary to insert semipermanent nasal tubes so that the infant can be fed orally until older; definitive surgery may be necessary later. Once the nasal tubes are in place, the infant can manage at the breast. Feeding by any technique, however, is never easy.

CLEFT LIP

A solitary cleft lip is usually repaired in the first few weeks of life. Before surgery, an infant will need some help, but the infant can nurse at the breast if a seal around the areola can be developed. Actually the breast may fill the defect, and suckling will go well. The mother may be able to put her thumb in the cleft to create a seal as she holds the breast to the infant's mouth. It is important to encourage the infant to suck to strengthen the tongue and jaw muscles. If all else fails, a breast shield can be tried, affixing a special cleft lip nipple to the shield. The mother will need to pump after feedings to increase milk supply. In some cases, the mother may have to express or pump milk and offer it by dropper or other means if sucking is ineffective. The pediatrician, plastic surgeon, and parents should work together as a team from the time of birth to determine a coordinated plan of treatment. Some surgeons have special protocols before and after surgery to ensure optimal healing. It is important to make all plans for feeding around the surgical plan. The literature reports individual mothers' experiences nursing infants with lip defects. The major caution in sharing these experiences is to consider that the supportive surgical approach may differ from those reported in the literature.[68] In these cases, a plastic surgeon is the captain of the team, working with the pediatrician and support staff. As breastfeeding has increased, lactation consultants have joined the surgical repair team, working directly with the surgeon. Ideally this lactation consultant is a skilled nurse.

CLEFT PALATE

The prognosis for successful feeding of an infant with a cleft palate depends on the size and position of the defect (soft palate, hard palate) as well as the associated lesions. Masera et al.[102] and Reid et al.[123] recommend the application of an orthopedic appliance to the neonatal maxilla to close the gap, thus aiding nursing, stimulating orofacial development, developing the palatal shelves, preventing tongue distortions, preventing nasal septum irritation, and decreasing the number of ear infections. This will make it easier for the plastic surgeon and help the mother psychologically as well. A cleft involving the secondary palate can interfere with normal nursing. For the infant to suckle, the nose must be sealed off from the mouth, creating a negative pressure in the oral cavity. The milk may also run out the nose. The absence of palatal tissue can prevent expulsion of milk from the nipple. The orthodontic appliance prosthetically restores the anatomy of the palate, permitting normal suckling.

Because the purpose of the negative pressure in the mouth is to hold the nipple and areola in place and not to extract milk from the breast, a seal is needed to keep the pressure. A mother may be able to perform the positioning task by holding the breast to her infant's mouth firmly between two fingers, as shown in Figures 8-13, 14-1, 14-2, and 14-9. The infant is then able to milk the areola and nipple with the tongue pressing it against the roof of the mouth, even with the cleft. The breast must be held in position just as a bottle must be held throughout the feeding.

An infant's ability to generate negative intraoral pressure and to move the tongue against the nipple is important to effective feeding techniques. These findings were summarized in relation to the possibility of breastfeeding (Table 14-7). Normal children with a cleft can swallow normally. A defect in the bony structure of the palate, however, creates a hole that is difficult to plug; thus these children are more difficult to feed by any method.[116]

Problems with intraoral muscular movements are associated with bilateral cleft lip, which causes severe anterior projection of the premaxilla that precludes stabilizing the nipple, with wide palatal clefts, which offer no back guard for tongue movements, and retroplaced tongues that cannot compress the nipple effectively. When neurologic problems are causing dysrhythmic tongue movements, a weak tongue, or grinding of the gum on the nipple, it is more than a simple anatomic problem and is usually part of a syndrome (e.g., first-arch syndrome). These children usually have swallowing problems as well (e.g., Pierre Robin syndrome).

Feeding procedures for each infant vary.[102,123] Early assessment of infant and mother can usually lead to successful feeding within 1 to 2 days. The infant should not go hungry, and the mother should not spend hours struggling with a system that is not successful for her child. The Lact-Aid or the lactation supplementer can be helpful because the mother can control the flow by squeezing the reservoir, and the infant can have some suckling experience, which will strengthen the oral structure and avoid the trauma of invasive devices. The mother will need to pump to increase her milk supply.

Weatherley-White et al.[154] reported a program of early repair in breastfeeding infants with cleft lip. Repair has been initiated earlier and earlier, but these authors present 100 consecutive repairs: 51 infants were older than 3 weeks, and 49 were younger, of whom 26 underwent surgery at age 1 week or less. No increase in complication rate and no increase in need for revision of repair was observed. Sixty mothers were offered the opportunity to breastfeed immediately postoperatively; 38 began within hours. Of these, 16 infants breastfed more than 6 weeks, 22 converted by 6 weeks, and 22 were fed by cup or syringe. Breastfed infants gained more weight, and hospital stay was a day shorter. A prospective randomized

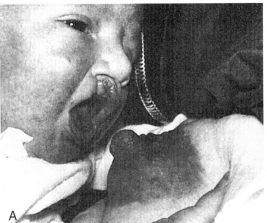 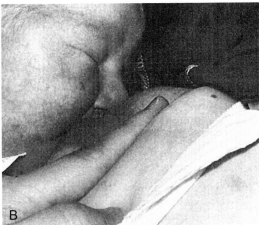

Figure 14-9. A, Infant with cleft lip and palate opening wide to latch on for a feeding. **B,** Same infant suckling at breast. Defect in lip and palate is comfortably filled by breast tissue. (Photos obtained with assistance of Marie Biancuzzo, RN, MSN.)

TABLE 14-7 Assessment of Sucking and Feeding Techniques for Infants with Clefts of Lip and Palate

Condition	Assessment		Feeding Techniques
	Generation of Negative Pressure	Ability to Make Mechanical Movements	
Cleft lip and palate	−	±	Breastfeeding is unlikely. Deliver milk into infant's mouth.
Cleft palate only	±	+	Breastfeeding sometimes succeeds. Soft artificial nipples with large openings are effective. Infant may need delivery of milk into the mouth.
Cleft of soft palate	±	+	Breastfeeding or normal bottle feeding usually works well.
Pierre Robin syndrome	±	−	Breastfeeding is unlikely. Nipple position is critical. Many infants need delivery of milk into mouth.
Cleft lip only	±	+	Breastfeeding works well. Artificial nipple with large base works well.

+, Present; −, absent; ±, partial.

From Clarren SK, Anderson B, Wolf LS: Feeding infants with cleft lip, cleft palate, or cleft lip and palate, *Cleft Palate J* 24:244, 1987.

trial of 40 infants showed that early postoperative breastfeeding after cleft lip repair is safe and results in more weight gain by 6 weeks after surgery when compared with infants randomized to be spoon-fed postoperatively.[41]

A position that is particularly effective is to have the infant straddle the mother's leg so he is directly facing the breast. If mother leans back slightly and the infant has to lean forward, structures fall in place to facilitate suckling. The breast needs to be held throughout the feeding.

Similar experience with early surgery and breastfeeding is confirmed by Fisher,[52] who reported performing reconstructive surgery in the Third World, where breastfeeding is undisputed and is very successful. He also reported greater success rate with breastfeeding but noted that it requires the conviction not only of the surgeon and pediatrician but also of the nurse, nutritionist, mother, and grandmother. It takes the presence of all these elements for success, but the absence of only one for failure.

As noted previously, breastfed infants have fewer bouts with otitis media, which has been attributed to the position of the infant while feeding at the breast and the antiinfective properties of the milk. This is an important consideration in infants with cleft palates, who have been identified as having more ear infections in general than other infants.[44]

Children with cleft palates may also fail to thrive, not only as a function of their feeding difficulty but also because they may have an underlying increased metabolic need. In a study of 37 children with cleft palates and no other anomalies, the median birth weight was at the 30th percentile.[15] By 1 to 2 months, weights had dropped to the 20th percentile and did not recover to the 30th until 6 months of age.

It is important to have a plastic surgeon involved promptly after birth so that management plans can be developed with the family immediately. This also avoids conflicting information from others.

The Academy of Breastfeeding Medicine has developed protocol No. 17, Guidelines for Breastfeeding Infants with cleft lip, cleft palate, or cleft lip and palate.

Oral Defects: Feeding Recommendations

Feeding infants with oral defects requires extra effort. Each infant is slightly different. Usually mothers learn to feed their own infants more effectively, even when bottle feeding, than the skilled professional can advise them. This amplifies that it requires a special patience and knack. Breastfeeding can be successful. Infants with cleft lip or palate should be managed as normal infants. Cupping of the infant's jaw and filling the defect with the mother's thumb while supporting the breast in place for suckling will allow effective breastfeeding in the infant with cleft lip. This has been referred to as the "dancer hold" (see Figure 14-1).[100] As with any infant, the infant should be taken to the mother to feed and for rooming-in. Reinforcing that the infant is normal and merely needs some reconstructive surgery is important in helping parents adjust. Parent-to-parent programs are most helpful. The primary care physician coordinates care with the specialist and the rest of the health care team.

Pediatric reconstructive surgeons usually have a team of professionals, including otolaryngologists, audiologists and affiliated therapists, social

their severity. The mother should be counseled about the prognosis and encouraged to express milk manually and by pump to provide her milk for her infant postoperatively. The decision should be made among the parents, surgeon, neonatologist, and pediatrician. Frequently, infants with atresias are also small or premature and have protracted recovery periods because of the removal of considerable intestinal tract. If the infant will be breastfed, breast milk can be introduced earlier than formula. Short gut syndrome requires special management, but human milk is usually tolerated and donor milk should be obtained if the mother is unable to lactate.

Disorders of the Colon. Disorders of the colon occur more often in full-term infants. Hirschsprung's disease, or congenital aganglionic megacolon, is the most common lesion. Passage of meconium is usually delayed; however, only 10% to 15% of all children with delayed passage of meconium have Hirschsprung's disease. Constipation and abdominal distention are the most frequent initial symptoms. They may begin during the first few days of life and gradually progress to include bilious vomiting. The clinical picture may be indistinguishable from meconium ileus, ileal atresia, or large bowel obstruction. In any infant with perforation of the colon, ileum, or appendix, Hirschsprung's disease should be considered. A breastfed infant may have milder symptoms and delayed onset of real stress because the breast milk stools are normally loose and seedy and easily passed.[79] The pH and flora of the intestinal tract are also different, leading to less distention. Enterocolitis may occur at any age and is the major cause of death.

No data have been found to distinguish the incidence of this complication in breastfed and bottle-fed infants, although an argument could be mounted regarding the projected value of secretory

IgA and intestinal flora of the breastfed infant. The treatment depends on the symptoms, x-ray findings, and biopsy results for the identification of the aganglionic segment. Colostomy is usually done at the time of diagnosis, with definitive surgery later in the first year of life. Feedings can be resumed as soon as the infant is stable, after the colostomy has healed sufficiently to permit bowel activity. Human milk has the same advantages for early postoperative feeding in this disease as well because of its antiinfective properties and easy digestibility.

Meconium Plug Syndrome and Meconium Ileus. Meconium plug syndrome and meconium ileus are less common and less severe in breastfed infants who have received a full measure of colostrum, which has a cathartic effect and stimulates the passage of meconium. If either disorder is diagnosed, an infant should continue to nurse in addition to any other treatment, which should include an assessment for CF and pancreatic insufficiency.

Congenital Chylothorax. Congenital chylothorax, although uncommon, is the most common cause of pleural effusion in the newborn period. It affects the respiratory, nutritional, and immunologic systems and is potentially life-threatening. Most cases are single abnormalities, but may be associated with other anomalies, lymphangiectasia, or neuroblastoma. Management is controversial. Parenteral nutrition and mechanical ventilation have improved the outcome. If diagnosed prenatally, transabdominal thoracocentesis can be done and delivery initiated after 32 weeks. The chest can be tapped or put to continuous drainage (Tables 14-8A and 14-8B).

Nutrition starts with total parenteral nutrition (TPN). Enteral feedings are started as soon as

TABLE 14-8A	Clinical Summary of Infants with Chylothorax					
Patient	Gestation (wks)	Birth Weight (g)	Diagnosis	Age FFM Started	Duration of FFM	Supplements Used
1	37	2780	Congenital	5 wks	11 days	Pregestimil
2	31	1681	Congenital	5 mo	34 days	Pregestimil MCT
3	36	2050	Acquired CHD repair	7 wks	14 days	TPN + Intralipid
4	40	3040	Acquired CHD repair	8 mo	21 days	Portagen ProMod
5	39	3430	Acquired CHD repair	2 mo	11 days	MCT glucose polymers
6	33	2750	Congenital	2 mo	7 days	MCT glucose polymers
7	39	3293	Acquired CDH repair	1 mo	14 days	TPN + Intralipid

CDH, Congenital diaphragmatic hernia; *CHD,* congenital heart disorder; *FFM,* fat-free milk; *MCT,* medium-chain triglycerides; *TPN,* total parenteral nutrition.

TABLE 14-8B	Composition of Human Milk Before and after Fat Removal (Mean ± SD)	
	Before	**After**
Fat (g/dL)	5 ± 1	0
Sodium (mEq/L)	40 ± 9	42 ± 9
Potassium (mEq/L)	15 ± 3	14 ± 3
Calcium (mg/dL)	25 ± 4	27 ± 2
Zinc (mcg/dL)	294 ± 135	385 ± 130
Total volume (mL)	100 ± 1	95 ± 1

SD, Standard deviation.

possible (5 to 7 days) using breast milk or regular formula. If the chylothorax worsens, oral feeds are stopped for another 3 to 7 days and then restarted with special medium-chain triglyceride-rich formula (e.g., Pregestimil) and then in 2 to 4 weeks breast milk or regular formula. In a retrospective study by Al-Tawil et al.,[5] 19 infants were reviewed; 18 were followed for 7 years and were successfully managed after 7 weeks with breastfeeding or regular formula. In another study, infants managed with TPN (*n* = 9) recovered more rapidly (mean 10 days) than those treated with medium-chain triglycerides (*n* = 8; mean 23 days). TPN treatment permitted progression to earlier oral feeds and earlier breastfeeding.[6] Iatrogenic chylothorax management is not as simple and may take weeks of TPN and then the use of defatted breast milk. Defatted human milk was used in seven infants with chylous pleural effusion.[30] Mother's milk was placed in a clear 240-mL container and centrifuged at 3000 rotations per minute for 15 minutes at 2° C in a Beckman J2-21 High Speed Floor Model Centrifuge. The solidified-fat top layer was separated from the liquid portion. The liquid portion was poured into clean cups and frozen for later use. Before and after samples were tested for fat, sodium, potassium, calcium, and zinc. Mean fat removal was 5 g/dL. The infants started on the milk after a month of age for an average of 16 days (7 to 34 days). No reaccumulation of the chylous pleural effusion was observed.[30]

Intensivists and neonatologists have recognized the value of human milk and have reported the practice of defatting human milk for infants with congenital as well as iatrogenic chylothorax.[31] One of the first reports described spinning the breast milk at 3000 rpms for 15 minutes using a cold centrifuge. The milk was successfully used in seven infants. Children's Hospital of Philadelphia (CHOP) opened a Human Milk Management Center.[137] Skim milk is prepared by their milk technicians utilizing a cold centrifuge (Thermo Fisher Scientific I ST 16). Milk is spun at 4000 rpms for 20 minutes. They report 29 infants in 23 months of use. Chylothorax was due to congenital

diaphragmatic hernia and congenital cardiac defects that were repaired surgically. Skim milk was used an average of 16 days (range 1 to 85 days). All milk used had a creamatocrit of less than 1%. It was concluded that a standard skim milk protocol allowed infants to continue the additional benefits of their mother's own milk.

Necrotizing Enterocolitis. Although NEC has been known for 100 years, only since 1960 has it been identified with any frequency, which suggests an iatrogenic component. It is most common in premature infants and infants compromised by asphyxia. It has been associated with umbilical catheters, exchange transfusions, polycythemia, hyperosmolar feedings, and infection. Its cause is not clear. Work with animals has suggested that human breast milk, specifically colostrum, provides protection against the disease. A "dose or two" of human milk may not be enough. Reported cases of NEC have occurred so early in life that no feedings had been given. Present regimens of treatment call for cessation of all oral feedings and use of oral and systemic antibiotics, gastric decompression, plasma or blood transfusions, and rigorous monitoring for progression or perforation with serial x-ray studies as well as a septic work up. The organisms generally associated with NEC are gram-negative organisms such as bacteroides, *E. coli*, and especially *Klebsiella*. Eighty-nine percent of infants with NEC had received cow milk formulas, and gram-negative bacteria and endotoxins were present in the stool. Colonization of breastfed infants with *Klebsiella* does not usually occur, and *Lactobacillus bifidus* predominates. The rare occurrence of NEC in Helsinki, at the University of Helsinki Children's Hospital intensive care nursery, is significant. All the premature infants are routinely fed colostrum and breast milk in Helsinki.

The role of bacterial colonization in NEC was further explored by Newburg and Walker,[113] who suggest that the beneficial effects of suppression of colonization of harmful bacteria and the stimulation of bifidobacterial growth with human milk is a valuable approach to the prevention and treatment of NEC. In a systemic review of the question of the value of donor milk versus formula for preventing NEC, the authors suggest that donor milk reduces the incidence of NEC in preterm or LBW infants.[113] Continued discussion of NEC appears in Chapter 15 on prematures.

Imperforate Anus. Defects in the rectum and anal sphincter are usually diagnosed in the first few hours of life on physical examination. When the blind pouch is more generous, diagnosis may depend on the evaluation of failure to pass stool. Depending on associated lesions and fistulas to the bladder or vagina, surgical decompression can be performed. Until this time, oral feedings are withheld. High lesions require an immediate colostomy with later final repair, whereas low lesions may be repaired at the primary procedure through a perineal approach. Infants may be breastfed as soon as any bowel activity can be permitted, often 2 to 3 days postoperatively.

Gastrointestinal Bleeding. The most common cause of vomiting blood or passing blood via the rectum in a breastfed infant is a bleeding nipple in the mother, which may or may not be painful. Any time fresh blood is found in the vomitus or stool of any newborn, the blood should be tested for adult or fetal Hb. If adult Hb, it indicates the source is maternal. This is done by a qualitative test, the Apt test.

Mix red blood with 2 to 3 mL normal saline solution, and add this mixture to 3 mL of 10% NaOH (0.25 M). Mix gently. Observe for color change. Fetal Hb is stable in alkali and will remain pink, whereas adult Hb turns brown. Use a known adult sample as a color control. If the blood is adult Hb in a breastfed infant, the possibility of a cracked and bleeding nipple should be ruled out by examining the sample of expressed milk for color and guaiac, and inspection of the maternal breast (see Chapter 8).

If the blood is fetal Hb, the differential diagnosis for bleeding in any neonate should be followed. Breastfeeding can be maintained, unless a lesion requiring surgery is identified. More than 50% of cases of GI bleeding in the neonate go undiagnosed. Anorectal fissure is an uncommon cause in breastfed infants. Allergy to human milk itself has been reported as a cause of intestinal bleeding.[118] The distribution of causes of intestinal bleeding in the neonate, without selection for type of feeding, follows: idiopathic, 50%; hemorrhagic disorders, 20%; swallowed maternal blood, 10%; anorectal fissures, 10%; intestinal ischemia, 5%; and colitis, 5%. When the bleeding occurs beyond the newborn period, colitis (see previous discussion) becomes a more frequent cause, as does Meckel's diverticulum. Sullivan[140] has reviewed the subject of cow milk-induced intestinal bleeding in infancy.

Otitis Media

Acute otitis media is a common affliction among young children that has increased in incidence, paralleling increasing attendance at daycare facilities.[119] Population density and air pollution have also been identified as factors. In a Finnish study of 471 2- to 3-year-old children, 188 had three or more attacks of otitis media, 76 had one to two attacks, and 207 had none.[121] Incidence was increased in those who attended day care or had several siblings. Prolonged breastfeeding (longer than 6 months) was associated with a decreased risk.

Any breastfeeding reduces the incidence of otitis media by 23%, exclusive breastfeeding for more than 3 months reduces the risk by 50%, and exclusive breastfeeding for 6 months decreases the risk of respiratory infections and otitis by 63%.[46]

With daycare exposure and other environmental risk factors, it does have a measurable effect. Breastfeeding is also more comfortable for an infant with a painful otitis than bottle feeding because of the physiologic suck/swallow mechanism. If an infant is having difficulty feeding, providing a dose of acetaminophen or ibuprofen before the feeding can be helpful.

Congenital Dislocation of Hip

When procedures or treatments need to be initiated for an infant previously thought to be normal, breastfeeding may not go smoothly. Using congenital dislocation of the hip as a prototype, Elander[49] looked at overall breastfeeding success. Compared with a randomly chosen control group of 113 infants, the 30 study infants who required the von Rosen splint were less successfully fed. However, a higher incidence of cesarean deliveries was seen in the study group (30% vs. 4%). The groups had equal numbers of primiparas (50% vs. 48%). After breastfeeding was established, the long-range success rate was no different. Mothers were pleased to be able to do something special for their splinted children (i.e., breastfeed). This would suggest that special support and guidance regarding breastfeeding issues may be needed, along with details on how to apply the splint and how to cope with the splint while positioning for breastfeeding.

Malformations of Central Nervous System

Malformations of the central nervous system diagnosed at birth include the clinical spectrum from anencephaly and complete craniorachischisis to dermal sinuses. Defects of the spinal column range from complete spinal rachischisis to spina bifida occulta. A mother who had planned to breastfeed an infant with an inoperable condition or for whom breastfeeding is incompatible with life is presented with the additional problem of coping with her desire to nurse her infant. If an infant is to be given normal newborn care and the mother desires to nurse this infant, breastfeeding should be discussed by the pediatrician and parents together. It has been well demonstrated that parents grieve more physiologically if they have contact with their abnormal infant, but their imaginations are more vicious than some abnormalities of development. A professional's personal bias for how to deal with the infant should not overshadow the discussion with the parents. If a mother wants to nurse an infant who has no life expectancy and the infant is to be fed at all by mouth, she should have that choice. This includes infants with trisomy 13 and 15.

Infants with central nervous system abnormalities requiring surgery can be breastfed until the procedure and postoperatively as soon as oral intake is permitted. When the GI tract is not involved, breastfeeding can be initiated 6 to 8 hours postoperatively at the surgeon's discretion. The risk for lung irritation from breast milk is minimal. The rapid emptying time of the stomach and presence of antiinfective factors serve as advantages in the postoperative course. The placing of a shunt for hydrocephalus is a common procedure, and breastfeeding is an ideal feeding mode for this infant.

Surgery or Rehospitalization Beyond Neonatal Period

Anesthesia is a main concern when any patient is scheduled for surgery. Traditionally, a patient has been ordered "nothing by mouth" after midnight or 6 to 8 hours preoperatively. Young infants used to feeding every 4 hours are frantic when ready for the operating room.

Recommendations for fasting intervals preoperatively have changed with the belief that clear liquids are safe to within 2 hours of anesthesia, with similar gastric volumes and pH at 2 and 8 hours.[10] Children younger than 1 year had not been studied until the report by Litman et al.,[92] who evaluated 77 infants between 2 weeks and 1 year of age. Bottle-fed infants had no solids within 6 hours and only clear liquids up to 8 oz within 2 hours of surgery. Breastfed infants had no solids but were permitted to breastfeed to within 2 hours of surgery. After 0.02 mg/kg oral atropine 30 to 45 minutes before surgery, induction anesthesia, and tracheal intubation, gastric fluid was aspirated by a blinded researcher who measured volume and pH. The study was discontinued when an unacceptable number of infants in the breastfed group had gastric volumes greater than 1 mL/kg (7 of 24 breastfed and 2 of 46 bottle fed). The pH of the gastric contents of bottle-fed infants was less than 2.5 in 9 of 10 infants (90%) with measurable fluid, whereas pH greater than 2.5 in breastfed infants was found in three of eight (38%). Low pH is probably a greater risk than volume, but the residual in breastfed infants is much greater than with clear fluids.[92] Instructions to breastfeeding mothers should limit the amount

of breastfeeding after 4 hours and permit feeding on a prepumped breast (i.e., empty breast), predominantly for comfort, to 2 hours before surgery. According to the American Society of Anesthesiologists, adhering to these guidelines is essential for safety of the anesthesia.[10]

An infant who requires surgery or rehospitalization can and should be breastfed postoperatively in most cases. The gravity of the surgery and the length of the recovery phase will determine the time necessary for the mother to pump and manually express her milk to keep her supply available. The infant who is hospitalized is already traumatized by the separation, the strange surroundings and people, and the underlying discomfort of the disease process itself. If the infant is to be fed orally, feeding should be at the breast as often as possible. If the mother can room-in or the hospital has a care-by-parent ward, this works well. If obligations to other family members make it impossible for the mother to stay, she can pump her milk and bring it in fresh day by day or frozen if the time interval between visits is longer than a day. Freezing will destroy the cellular content, but this is not a major problem beyond the immediate neonatal period. The infant should not be subjected to the added trauma of being weaned from the breast when the infant needs the security and intimacy of nursing most, unless weaning is absolutely unavoidable.

The medical profession needs to be aware of these infants and mothers and their special needs for support. An opportunity to discuss the breastfeeding aspect of the infant's management should be offered by the physician. The pediatrician should assume the advocacy role. The parents should not have to fight for the right to maintain breastfeeding. Plans for pumping and saving milk should be discussed and provided. If the infant is recovering in an open ward or a room with other infants and their parents without adequate privacy, a separate room should be provided for the mother to nurse or pump her milk. This room should be clean, neat, adequately illuminated, and equipped with a sink for washing hands. Storerooms, broom closets, and staff dressing rooms are inappropriate. If a mechanical pump is to be used, it should be kept clean and operable with disposable tubing and attachments that come in contact with the milk or the breast. If a breast pump is not provided in the pediatric department, it should be available from the newborn or NICU.

Arrangements for providing sterile containers for collecting milk and storing it will be discussed (see Chapter 21). Occasionally a mother may become so concerned about the adequacy of her milk for her infant that she may nurse much too frequently. Actually her child will need much more nonnutritive cuddling and holding than usual. A physician may need to reassure the mother when pointing this out. The father should also be encouraged to understand all the tubes, bandages, and appliances the infant may have attached. He is an important member of the parenting team and should provide some of the soothing and especially the nonnutritive cuddling.

Congenital Heart Disease

When an infant who is diagnosed with congenital heart disease is already feeding at the breast, it is usually not a medical indication to interrupt the process unless surgery is imminent. Even infants with cyanotic heart disease, if they can be fed orally, can be breastfed. The "work" required to breastfeed is less than the "work" required to bottle feed. Heart and respiratory rates remain stable during feeding at the breast. The misconception that it is more work to breastfeed is incorrect. A study compared oxygen saturation levels (SaO_2) as an indicator of cardiorespiratory effort during breast versus bottle feeding.[100] The SaO_2 levels were higher and less variable during breastfeeding than the SaO_2 levels during bottle feeding, especially when the infant had congenital heart disease. A second study compared growth patterns of breastsfed and bottle-fed infants with cardiac defects. The breastfed infants gained weight more quickly and had shorter hospital stays.[36] Breastfeeding is less strenuous as seen in these and other studies.

If the infant is unable to generate enough sucking stimulus to the breast to increase the milk supply, an electric pump can be used between feedings to increase the mother's supply.

Not all infants with congenital heart disease are diagnosed at birth. When an infant is failing to thrive in spite of good breastfeeding, it is time to consider a work up for cardiac or renal disease.[112] Clinicians may focus on the breastfeeding and miss the "elephant in the room."

Cardiac surgeons frequently plan surgery for a certain weight or age. A mother can be assisted in helping the infant reach the goal. Human milk is low in sodium and easily digested, thus permitting frequent feedings. The nurse practitioner or lactation consultant should assist the mother in increasing her production and increasing fat content at each feeding. Feeding at one breast per feeding usually increases fat. In the case of a cardiac-compromised infant, using one breast also diminishes the stress of switching to the other side. The mother may need extra support and encouragement. Providing one's milk for one's sick infant may be extremely important. The breastfeeding relationship may be important for the infant as well. Research has shown that infants have important

cardiovascular responses to nutrient intake.[110] These responses are regulated by changes in autonomic activity to the heart and vasculature. These early life-shaping interactions that occur when the offspring is fed by the mother have been demonstrated in the animal model. Interactions between mothers and their young serve as hidden regulators of physiologic function. The program at CHOP is very successful in having mothers breastfeeding and pump their milk. Of mothers of infants with CHD, 89% initiate lactation.[146]

If oral intake must be restricted preoperatively or immediately postoperatively, "nonnutritive" suckling at the previously pumped breast can be calming and comforting for the infant.

Sudden Infant Death Syndrome

SIDS is the leading cause of death in infants after 1 month of age, accounting for one third of all deaths in the first year. Healthy, full-term infants account for 85% of the deaths.

In a 3-year, multicenter, controlled study of SIDS in New Zealand reported in 1993,[133] the National Cot Death Prevention Programme[106] sought to reduce the rising incidence of infant death by determining associated factors. Sleeping prone, maternal smoking, lack of breastfeeding, and the infant sharing a bed were the four modifiable risk factors. New Zealand launched a major prevention program to educate the public about these risk factors.[109] The AAP launched a similar program focusing only on sleeping prone. A case-control study in the United States by Frederickson et al. analyzed births of infants weighing more than 2000 g between 1988 and 1989. The study included 7102 control infants and 499 SIDS and 584 non-SIDS deaths. Breastfeeding offered dose-response protection against SIDS across races and socioeconomic levels. For white infants, the risk for SIDS increased 19% for every month of not breastfeeding and 100% for every month of nonexclusive breastfeeding. For black infants, the risk was 19% and 113%, respectively. Whether breastfeeding reduces the risk for SIDS was explored by Vennemann et al.[150] in a German study of SIDS that included 333 deaths and 998 matched controls. Being exclusively breastfed and even partially breastfed in the previous month reduced the risk by 50% throughout infancy. The authors recommend breastfeeding be included in the prevention messages.[150]

Numerous studies have been conducted to define further the associations with SIDS. Prone sleeping position continues to be the most important correlation, and the AAP continues the "back to sleep" campaign. The protective influence of breastfeeding is actually strongest among infants of smoking mothers. SIDS rates are higher among infants of mothers who smoke, but breastfeeding by a smoking mother lowers that to a rate equal to that of bottle-fed infants with nonsmoking mothers. An association has also been suggested with pacifier use in bottle-fed infants. Pacifiers are not known to lower SIDS rates among breastfed infants beyond normal breastfeeding rates. Should pacifiers be recommended to prevent SIDS, use should be limited to bottle feeders because pacifiers are associated with decreased duration of breast-feeding. Although some studies show a protective effect of bed sharing in breastfeeding, the AAP Task Force on SIDS has campaigned against bed sharing because of the reported risk for roll-over deaths and the need for additional studies.[142]

MOUTH PROBLEMS

Alveolar lymphangiomas are elevations along the alveolar ridge that are isolated, bluish, firm cysts 3 to 10 mm in diameter. More than one may be present. They may interfere with suckling. They contain no dental tissue and gradually disappear in the first year. Breastfeeding is less influenced than bottle and pacifier sucking.

ORAL HEALTH

Oral health risk assessment has been recommended by the Section on Pediatric Dentistry of the AAP with the establishment of a dental home by 1 year of age.[9] Visits are recommended to begin at 7 to 9 months. Recommendations include systematic examination and oral fluoride, elimination of simple sugars in the diet, and initiation of oral hygiene early. The infant is not colonized until the eruption of the primary teeth. Caries are associated with *Streptococcus mutans* and usually occur at the age of 2 years. High caries rates run in families, usually passed mother to child; 70% of caries occur in 20% of children. Children who sleep with the mother and nurse throughout the night are at higher risk, especially if the mother is prone to caries.

Nursing Bottle Caries in Breastfed Infants

The development of rampant dental caries can occur in breastfed infants.[26] Usually the children have been nursed for 2 or 3 years, spending long stretches at the breast. One infant had early signs at 9 months, and by 18 months she required full mouth reconstruction.

A physician should be alert to the potential for dental decay when infants nurse frequently, especially through the night. Family history of dental enamel problems is worth investigating. Certainly these children are candidates for fluoride treatment.

The levels of mutant streptococci in saliva and plaque are higher in children with rampant cavities than in control subjects.[102] All breastfed infants have mutant streptococci and lactobacilli on their teeth. Tooth susceptibility is genetically programmed. Children with a strong family history of caries may need fluoride supplements while breastfeeding.[43] They are at special risk if they suckle all night beyond 1 year of age. The most cariogenic solutions are soda, fruit juice, sweetened cow milk, chocolate milk, and sugar water. If a mother is prone to caries, it increases the risk to the infant, not just because of family history but by sharing cariogenic bacteria.

Ankyloglossia is a short lingual frenulum that results in restricted range of tongue movement, especially forward protrusion and lateral mobility. The incidence is estimated at between 3% and 10%. It is discussed in Chapter 8, but the concern for breastfeeding infants has precipitated controversy about the frequency of feeding difficulties, later speech problems, and concerns about swallowing. Nipple pain is the most common cause for considering frenulotomy. In addition to maternal pain, the infant may have trouble with latching and suboptimal weight gain; 24 mother-infant dyads with these symptoms received submental ultrasound scans of the oral cavity before and 7 days after frenulotomy.[56] Milk transfer, pain, latch, swallowing, shape of nipple, and comfort were recorded. Milk intake was also measured by test weighing. Significant improvement was recorded by all dyads. The infants demonstrated less compression of the nipple by ultrasound after frenulotomy. The diagnosis was confirmed by ultrasound before the surgery.

Use of the Hazelbaker Assessment Tool for Lingual Frenulum Function has been reviewed by many clinicians.[67] More than 3000 patients were examined by Ballard et al.[17] who found 123 dyads who fit the description by Hazelbaker criteria. They received frenulotomies with latch improvement in all cases and pain reduced in most. Amir et al.[11] also used the Hazelbaker scoring tool and found that using part of the tool worked well in assessing 58 dyads.

REFERENCES

1. Abbassi V, Steinour TA: Successful diagnosis of congenital hypothyroidism in four breast-fed neonates, *J Pediatr* 97:259, 1980.
2. Aggett PJ, Atherton DJ, More J, et al: Symptomatic zinc deficiency in a breast-fed preterm infant, *Arch Dis Child* 55:547, 1980.
3. Ahmed S, Blair AW: Symptomatic zinc deficiency in a breast-fed infant, *Arch Dis Child* 56:315, 1981.
4. Akobeng AK, Ramanan AV, Bucan I, et al: Effect of breast-feeding on risk of celiac disease: a systematic review and

meta-analysis of observational studies, *Arch Dis Child* 91:39–43, 2006.

5. Al-Tawil K, Ahmed G, Al-Hathal M: Congenital chylothorax, *Am J Perinatol* 17:121, 2000.

6. Alvarez JRF, Kalache KD, Grauel EL: Management of spontaneous congenital chylothorax: oral medium-chain triglycerides versus total parenteral nutrition, *Am J Perinatol* 16:415, 1999.

7. American Academy of Pediatrics: Policy statement: breastfeeding and the use of human milk, *Pediatrics* 129(3):e827–e841, 2012.

8. American Academy of Pediatrics. In: Kleinman RE, editor: *Pediatric nutrition handbook*, ed 7, Elk Grove, Ill., 2014, American Academy of Pediatrics.

9. American Academy of Pediatrics Section on Pediatric Dentistry AAP: Oral health risk assessment timing and establishment of the dental home, *Pediatrics* 111:1113–1116, 2003.

10. American Society of Anesthesiology Task Force on Preoperative Fasting: *Practice guidelines for pre-operative fasting in elective surgery*, Park Ridge, Ill., 2000, ASA.

11. Amir LH, James JP, Donath SM: Reliability of the Hazelbaker Assessment Tool for Lingual Frenulum Function, *Int Breastfeed J* 1:3, 2006.

12. Arias IM, Gartner LM, Seifter S, et al: Prolonged neonatal unconjugated hyperbilirubinemia associated with breast feeding and steroid pregnane-3α,20β-diol in maternal milk that inhibits glucuronide formation in vitro, *J Clin Invest* 43:2037, 1964.

13. Arslanoglu S, Corpeleijn W, Moro G, et al: Donor human milk for preterm infants. Current evidence and research directions, *J Pediatr Gastroenterol Nutr* 57:535–542, 2013.

14. Aumonier ME, Cunningham CC: Breastfeeding in infants with Down's syndrome, *Child Care Health Dev* 9: 247, 1983.

15. Avedian LV, Ruberg RL: Impaired weight gain in cleft palate infants, *Cleft Palate J* 17:24, 1980.

16. Babovic-Vuksanovic D, Michels VV, Law ME, et al: Guidelines for buccal smear collection in breast-fed infants, *Am J Med Genet* 84:357, 1999.

17. Ballard JL, Auer CE, Khoury JC: Ankyloglossia: assessment, incidence and effect of frenuloplasty on the breastfeeding dyad, *Pediatrics* 110:e63–e69, 2002.

18. Barfoot RA, McEnery G, Ersser RS, et al: Diarrhea due to breast milk: a case of fructose intolerance? *Arch Dis Child* 63:311, 1988.

19. Barons TD, Leplat C, et al: Environmental risk factors in pediatric inflammatory bowel disease: a population-based case-control study, *Gut* 54:357–363, 2005.

20. Bennett FC, McClelland S, Kriegsmann EA, et al: Vitamin and mineral supplementation in Down's syndrome, *Pediatrics* 72:707, 1983.

21. Bergstrand O, Hellers G: Breastfeeding during infancy in patients who later develop Crohn's disease, *Scand J Gastroenterol* 18:903, 1983.

22. Berkowitz CD, Inkelis SH: Bloody nipple discharge in infancy, *J Pediatr* 103:755, 1983.

23. Berlin C: Breastfeeding quadruplets, *Breastfeed Med* 4:149, 2007.

23a. Bhatia J, Parish A: GERD or not GERD: the fussy infant, *J Perinatol* 29:S7–S11, 2009.

24. Bhutani VK, Johnson L: Kernicterus in late preterm infants cared for as healthy term infants, *Semin Perinatol* 30:89–97, 2006.

25. Bode HH, Vanjonack WJ, Crawford JD: Mitigation of cretinism by breastfeeding, *Pediatrics* 62:13, 1978.

26. Brams M, Maloney J: "Nursing bottle caries" in breast-fed children, *J Pediatr* 103:415, 1983.

27. Burke BL, Robbins JM, MacBird T, et al: Trends in hospitalizations for neonatal jaundice and kernicterus in the United States, 1988-2005, *Pediatrics* 123:524–532, 2009.

28. Cannella PC, Bowser EK, Guyer LK, et al: Feeding practices and nutrition recommendations for infants with cystic fibrosis, *J Am Diet Assoc* 93:297, 1993.

29. Challacombe DN, Mecrow IK, Elliott K, et al: Changing infant feeding practices and declining incidence of celiac disease in West Somerset, *Arch Dis Child* 77:206, 1997.

30. Chan GM, Lechtenberg E: The use of fat-free human milk in infants with chylouspleural effusion, *J Perinatol* 27:434–436, 2007.

31. Chang PF, Lin Y-C, Liu K, et al: Indentifying term breastfed infants at risk of significant hyperbilirubin, *Pediatric Research* 74(4):408–412, 2013.

32. Chiba Y, Minagawa T, Mito K, et al: Effect of breastfeeding on responses of systemic interferon and virus-specific lymphocyte transformation in infants with respiratory syncytial virus infection, *J Med Virol* 21:7, 1987.

33. Chou S-C, Palmer RH, Ezhuthachan S, et al: Management of hyperbilirubinemia in newborns: measuring performance by using a benchmarking model, *Pediatrics* 112:1264, 2003.

34. Clark BJ: After a positive Guthrie—what next? Dietary management for the child with phenylketonuria, *Eur J Clin Nutr* 46(Suppl I):S33, 1992.

35. Coelho S, Fernandes B, Rodrigues F, et al: Transient zinc deficiency in a breastfed premature infant, *Eur J Dermatol* 16:193–195, 2006.

36. Combs VL, Marino BL: Comparison of growth patterns in breast- and bottle-fed infants with congenital diseases, *Pediatrics Nursing* 19(2):175–179, 2011.

37. Committee on Obstetric Practice: *American College of Obstetricians and Gynecologists, Committee on the Fetus and Newborn, American Academy of Pediatrics: guidelines for perinatal care*, ed 5, Elk Grove, Ill., 2002, American Academy of Pediatrics.

38. Cronk C, Crocker AC, Pueschel SM, et al: Growth charts for children with Down syndrome: 1 month to 18 years of age, *Pediatrics* 81:102–110, 1988.

39. Curtis JA, Bailey JD: Influence of breastfeeding on the clinical features of salt-losing congenital adrenal hyperplasia, *Arch Dis Child* 58:71, 1983.

40. Danziger Y, Pertzelan A, Mimouni M: Transient congenital hypothyroidism after topical iodine in pregnancy and lactation, *Arch Dis Child* 62:295, 1987.

41. Darzi MA, Chowdri NA, Bhat AN: Breast feeding or spoon feeding after cleft lip repair: a prospective, randomized study, *Br J Plast Surg* 49:24, 1996.

42. DeVries LS, Lary S, Whitelaw AG, et al: Relationship of serum bilirubin levels and hearing impairment in newborn infants, *Early Hum Dev* 15:269, 1987.

43. Deyano MP, Degana RA: Breastfeeding and oral health, *N Y State Dent J* 59:30, 1993.

44. DiScippio W, Kaslon KR: Conditioned dysphagia in cleft palate children after pharyngeal flap surgery, *Psychol Med* 44:247, 1982.

45. Domellöf M, Lönnerdal B, Dewey KG, et al: Iron, zinc, copper concentrations in breast milk are independent of maternal mineral status, *Am J Clin Nutr* 79:111–115, 2004.

46. Duijts I, Jadd VW, Hoffman A, et al: Prolonged and exclusive breastfeeding reduces the risk of infectious diseases in infancy, *Pediatrics* 126(1):e18–e25, 2010.

47. Eckert CD, Sloan MV, Duncan JR, et al: Zinc binding: a difference between human and bovine milk, *Science* 195:789, 1977.

48. Ehrenkranz RA, Ackerman BA: Metoclopramide effect on faltering milk production by mothers of premature infants, *Pediatrics* 78:614, 1986.

49. Elander G: Breastfeeding of infants diagnosed as having congenital hip joint dislocation and treated in the von Rosen splint, *Midwifery* 2:147, 1986.

50. Elander G, Lindberg T: Hospital routines in infants with hyperbilirubinemia influence the duration of breastfeeding, *Acta Paediatr Scand* 75:708, 1986.

50a. Ernest AE, McCabe ERB, Neifert MR, et al: Guide to breast feeding the infant with PKU, Washington, DC, 1980, U.S. Government Printing Office.

51. Evans GW, Johnson PE: Defective prostaglandin synthesis in acrodermatitis enteropathica, *Lancet* 1:52, 1977.

52. Fisher JC: Early repair and breastfeeding for infants with cleft lip, *Plast Reconstr Surg* 79:886, 1987.

53. Forman MR, Graubard BI, Hoffman HJ, et al: The PIMA infant study: breastfeeding and gastroenteritis in the first year of life, *Am J Epidemiol* 119:335, 1984.

54. Gartner LM: Hyperbilirubinemia and breastfeeding. In Hale TW, Hartman PE, editors: *Textbook of human lactation*, Amarillo, Tex., 2007, Hale Publishing.

55. Garza JJ, Morash D, Dzakovic A, et al: Ad libitum feeding decreases hospital stay for neonates after pyloromyotomy, *J Pediatr Surg* 37:493–495, 2002.

56. Geddes DT, Langton DB, Gollow I, et al: Frenulatomy for breastfeeding infants with ankyloglossia: effect on milk removal and sucking mechanism as imaged by ultrasound, *Pediatrics* 122:e188–e194, 2008.

57. Geraghty SR, Kalkwarf HJ, Pinney SM, et al: The initiation and duration of breast milk feedings by mothers of multiples compared to mothers of singletons, *ABM News Views* 9:21, 2003.

58. Gourley GR: Breastfeeding, diet and neonatal hyperbilirubinemia, *Neoreviews* 1:e25–e31, 2000.

59. Gromada KK: *Mothering multiples*, ed 3, Schaumberg, Ill., 2007, La Leche International.

60. Gunn AJ, Gunn TR, Rabone DL, et al: Growth hormone increases breast milk volumes in mothers of preterm infants, *Pediatrics* 98:279, 1996.

61. Gupta AP, Gupta PK: Metoclopramide as a lactagogue, *Clin Pediatr (Phila)* 24:269, 1985.

62. Hahn HB, Spiekerman AM, Otto WR, et al: Thyroid function tests in neonates fed human milk, *Am J Dis Child* 137:220, 1983.

63. Haight M: Personal correspondence [editor: incompleted reference].

64. Hansen TWR, Bratlid D: Bilirubin and brain toxicity, *Acta Paediatr Scand* 75:513, 1986.

65. Harmon T, Burkhart G, Applebaum H: Perforated pseudomembranous colitis in the breastfed infant, *J Pediatr Surg* 27:744, 1992.

66. Hattori R, Hattori H: Breastfeeding twins: guidelines for success, *Birth* 26:37, 1999.

67. Hazelbaker AK: The Assessment Tool for Lingual Frenulum Function (ATLFF): use in a lactation consultant private practice. Thesis: Pasadena, CA Pacific Oaks College, 1993.

68. Hemingway L: Breastfeeding a cleft-palate baby, *Med J Aust* 2:626, 1972.

69. Howard CR, de Blieck EA, ten Hoopen CB, et al: Physiologic stability of newborns during cup-and bottle-feeding, *Pediatrics* 104:1204–1207, 1999.

70. Howard CR, Howard FM, Lamphear B, et al: Randomized clinical trial of pacifier use and bottle feeding or cup feeding and their effect on breastfeeding, *Pediatrics* 111:511–518, 2003.

71. Huang MJ, Kua L-E, Teng H-C, et al: Risk factors for severe hyperbilirubinemia in neonates, *Pediatr Res* 56:682–689, 2004.

72. Hurst NM, Valentine CJ, Renfro L, et al: Skin-to-skin holding in the neonatal intensive care unit influences maternal milk volume, *J Perinatol* 17:213–217, 1997.

73. Illingworth RS, Lister J: The critical or sensitive period, with special reference to certain feeding problems in infants and children, *J Pediatr* 65:839, 1964.

74. Ip S, Glicken S, Kulig J, et al: *Management of neonatal hyperbilirubinemia, evidence report/technology assessment. No. 65, AHRQ Pub. No. 03-E011*, Rockville, Md., 2003, U.S. Department of Health and Human Services, Agency for Health Care Research and Quality.

75. Israel D, Levine J, Pettel M, et al: Protein induced allergic colitis (PAC) in infants, *Pediatr Res* 25:116A, 1989.

76. Ito S, Blajchman A, Stephenson M, et al: Prospective follow-up of adverse reactions in breast-fed infants exposed to maternal medication, *Am J Obstet Gynecol* 168:1393, 1993.

77. Ivarsson A, Hernell O, Stenlund H, et al: Breast-feeding protects against celiac disease, *Am J Clin Nutr* 75:914, 2002.

78. Iyer NP, Srinivasan R, Evans K, et al: Impact of an early weighing policy on neonatal hypernatremic dehydration and breastfeeding, *Arch Dis Child* 93:297–299, 2008.

79. Jadin SA, Wu GS, Zhang Z, et al: Growth and pulmonary outcomes during the first 2 years of life of breastfeeding and formula fed infants diagnosed with cystic fibrosis through the Wisconsin Newborn Screening Program, *Am J Clin Nutr* 93(5):1038–1047, 2011.

80. Jain L, Sivieri E, Abbasi S, et al: Energetics and mechanics of nutritive sucking in the preterm and term neonate, *J Pediatr* 111:894, 1987.

81. Jantchou P, Turek D, Balde M, et al: Breastfeeding and risk of inflammatory bowel disease: results of a pediatric, population based, case-controlled study (Letter), *Am J Clin Nutr* 90(4):887–888, 2009.

82. Johnson P, Salisbury DM: Breathing and sucking during feeding in the newborn. In Hofer MA, editor: *Ciba Foundation Symposium No. 33. Parent-infant interaction*, Amsterdam, 1975, Elsevier Scientific.

83. Kaplan M, Hammerman C, Maisels MJ: Bilirubin genetics for the nongeneticist: hereditary defects of neonatal bilirubin conjugation, *Pediatrics* 111:886–893, 2003.

84. Kero P, Piekkala P: Factors affecting the occurrence of acute otitis media during the first year of life, *Acta Paediatr Scand* 76:618, 1987.

85. Klement E, Reifs S: Breastfeeding and risk of inflammatory bowel disease, *Am J Clin Nutr* 81:486, 2005 (letter).

86. Klement E, Cohen RV, Boxman J, et al: Breastfeeding and risk of inflammatory bowel disease: a systemic review with meta-analysis, *Am J Clin Nutr* 80:1342–1352, 2004.

87. Koletzko S, Sherman P, Corey M, et al: Role of infant feeding practices in development of Crohn's disease in childhood, *Br Med J* 298:1617, 1989.

88. Krogh C, Biggar RJ, Fischer TK, et al: Bottle-feeding and the risk of pyloric stenosis, *Pediatrics* 130(4):e1–e7, 2012.

89. LaGamma EF, Ostertag SG, Birenbaum H: Failure of delayed oral feedings to prevent necrotizing enterocolitis: results of studying very low birth weight neonates, *Am J Dis Child* 139:385, 1985.

90. Lang S, Lawrence CJ, L'eormc R: Cup-feeding: an alternative method of infant feeding, *Arch Dis Child* 71:365–369, 1994.

91. Leonard EL, Trykowski LE, Kirkpatrick BV: Nutritive sucking in high-risk neonates after perioral stimulation, *Phys Ther* 60:299, 1980.

92. Litman RS, Wu CL, Quinlivan JK: *Gastric volume and pH in infants fed clear liquids and breast milk prior to surgery*, Washington, D.C., 1993, Abstract for presentation to the American Society of Anesthesiology.

93. Lucas A, Cole TJ: Breast milk and neonatal necrotising enterocolitis, *Lancet* 336:1519, 1990.

94. Luder E, Kattan M, Tanzer-Torres G, et al: Current recommendations for breastfeeding in cystic fibrosis centers, *Am J Dis Child* 144:1153, 1990.

95. Macaron C: Galactorrhea and neonatal hypothyroidism, *J Pediatr* 101:576, 1982.

96. MacFarlane PI, Miller V: Human milk in the management of protracted diarrhea of infancy, *Arch Dis Child* 59:260, 1984.

97. Maisels MJ, Ostrea EM, Touch S, et al: Evaluation of a new trancutaneous bilirubinometer, *Pediatrics* 113:1628–1635, 2004.

98. Maisels MJ, Bhutani VK, Bogen D, et al: Hyperbilirubinemia in the newborn infant ≥ 35 weeks gestation: an update with clarifications, *Pediatrics* 124:1195–1198, 2009.

99. Maisels MJ, Clune S, Coleman K, et al: The natural history of jaundice in predominantly breastfed infants, *Pediatrics* 134:e340–e345, 2014.

100. Marino BL, O'Brien P, Lore H, editor: Incompleted reference.

101. Marmet C, Shell E: *Lactation forms: a guide to lactation consultant charting,* Encino, Calif., 1993, Lactation Institute and Breastfeeding Clinic.

102. Masera AG, Sell D, Habel A, et al: The nature of feeding in infants with unrepaired cleft lip and/or palate compared with healthy no cleft patients, *Cleft Palate Craniofac J* 44:321–328, 2007.

103. Mathew OP: Breathing patterns of preterm infants during bottle feeding: role of milk flow, *J Pediatr* 119:960, 1991.

104. McBride MC, Danner SC: Sucking disorders in neurologically impaired infants: assessment and facilitation of breastfeeding, *Clin Perinatol* 14:109, 1987.

105. McDonagh AF: Is bilirubin good for you? *Clin Perinatol* 17:359, 1990.

106. Meier P: Bottle- and breast-feeding: effects on transcutaneous oxygen pressure and temperature in preterm infants, *Nurs Res* 37:36, 1988.

107. Meier P, Anderson GC: Responses of small preterm infants to bottle- and breast-feeding, *Matern Child Nurs J* 12:97, 1987.

108. Mitchell EA, Aley P, Eastwood J: The national COT death prevention programme in New Zealand, *Aust J Public Health* 16:158, 1992.

109. Mitchell EA, Taylor BJ, Ford RPK, et al: Four modifiable and other major risk factors for cot death: the New Zealand study, *J Paediatr Child Health* 28(Suppl 1):53, 1992.

110. Montgomery RK, Buller HA, Rings EHHM, et al: Lactose intolerance and the genetic regulation of intestinal lactase-phlorizin hydrolase, *FASEB J* 5:2824, 1991.

111. Moyer VA, Ahn C, Sneed S: Accuracy of clinical judgment in neonatal jaundice, *Arch Pediatr Adolesc Med* 154:391–394, 2000.

112. Myers MM, Shair HN, Hofer MA: Feeding in infancy: short- and long-term effects on cardiovascular function, *Experientia* 48:322, 1992.

113. Newburg DS, Walker WA: Protection of the neonate by the innate immune system of developing gut and of human milk, *Pediatr Res* 61:2–8, 2007.

114. Newman TB, Liljestrand P, Escobar GJ: Combining clinical risk factors with serum bilirubin levels to predict hyperbilirubinemia in newborns, *Arch Pediatr Adolesc Med* 159:113–119, 2005.

115. Norris JM, Barriga K, Hoffenberg EJ, et al: Risk of celiac disease autoimmunity and timing of gluten introduction in the diet of infants at increased risk of disease, *JAMA* 293:2343–2351, 2005.

116. Palmer MM, Crawley K, Blanco IA: Neonatal oral-motor assessment scale: a reliability study, *J Perinatol* 13:28, 1993.

117. Paludetto R, Robertson SS, Hack M, et al: Transcutaneous oxygen tension during nonnutritive sucking in preterm infants, *Pediatrics* 74:539, 1984.

118. Patenaude Y, Bernard C, Schreiber R, et al: Cow's milk-induced allergic colitis in an exclusively breast-fed infant: diagnosed with ultrasound, *Pediatr Radiol* 30:379, 2000.

119. Pedersen CB, Zachau-Christiansen B: Otitis media in Greenland children: acute, chronic and secretory otitis media in three to eight year olds, *J Otolaryngol* 15:332, 1986.

120. Peters U, Schneeweiss S, Trautwein EA, et al: A case-control study of the effect of infant feeding on celiac disease, *Ann Nutr Metab* 45:135, 2001.

121. Pukander J, Luotonen J, Timonen M: Risk factors affecting the occurrence of acute otitis media among 2- to 3-year-old urban children, *Acta Otolaryngol* 100:260, 1985.

122. Pumberger W, Pomberger G, Geissler W: Proctocolitis in breast fed infants: a contribution to differential diagnosis of haematochezia in early childhood, *Postgrad Med J* 77:252, 2001.

123. Reid J, Reilly S, Kilpatrick N: Sucking performance of babies with cleft conditions, *Cleft Palate Craniofac J* 44:312–320, 2007.

124. Repucci A: Resolution of stool blood in breast-fed infants with maternal ingestion of pancreatic enzymes, *J Pediatr Gastroenterol Nutr* 29:500, 1999 (abstract).

125. Riva E, Agostoni C, Biasucci G, et al: Early breastfeeding is linked to higher intelligence quotient scores in dietary treated phenylketonuric children, *Acta Paediatr* 85:56, 1996.

126. Saarinen UM: Prolonged breast feeding as prophylaxis for recurrent otitis media, *Acta Paediatr Scand* 71:567, 1982.

127. Sack J, Amado O, Lunenfeld B: Thyroxine concentration in human milk, *J Clin Endocrinol Metab* 45:171, 1977.

128. Saint L, Maggiore P, Hartman PE: Yield and nutrient content of milk in eight women breastfeeding twins and one woman breastfeeding triplets, *Br J Nutr* 56:49, 1986.

129. Salvatori G, Foligno S, Occasi F, et al: Human milk and breastfeeding in surgical infants, *Breastfeed Med* 9(10): 491–493, 2014.

130. Sazawal S, Bhan MK, Bhandari N: Type of milk feeding during acute diarrhea and the risk of persistent diarrhea: a case control study, *Acta Paediatr Suppl* 381:93, 1992.

131. Schanler RJ, Lau C, Hurst NM, et al: Randomized trial of donor human milk versus preterm formula as substitutes for mother's own milk in the feeding of extremely premature infants, *Pediatrics* 116:400–406, 2005.

132. Schneider JR, Fischer H, Feingold M: Acrodermatitis enteropathica, *Am J Dis Child* 145:212, 1991.

133. Scragg LK, Mitchell EA, Tonkin SL, et al: Evaluation of the cot death prevention programme in South Auckland, *N Z Med J* 106:8, 1993.

134. Shah PS, Aliwalas L, Shah V: Breastfeeding or breast milk to alleviate procedural pain in neonates: a systematic review, *Breastfeed Med* 2(2):74–82, 2007.

135. Shmerling DH: Dietary protein-induced colitis in breastfed infants, *J Pediatr* 103:500, 1983.

136. Similä S, Kokkonen J, Kouvalainen K: Use of lactose-hydrolyzed human milk in congenital lactase deficiency, *J Pediatr* 101:584, 1982.

137. Spatz DL, Schmidt K, Kinzler S: Implementation of a human milk management center, *Adv Neonatal Care,* 14(4):253–261, 2014.

138. Strand H, Blomqvist YT, Gradin M, et al: Kangaroo mother care in the neonatal intensive care unit, *Acta Paediatr* 103:373–378, 2014.

139. Subcommittee on hyperbilirubinemia in the newborn infant 35 or more weeks of gestation, *Pediatrics* 114: 297–316, 2004.

140. Sullivan PB: Cows' milk induced intestinal bleeding in infancy, *Arch Dis Child* 68:240, 1993.

141. Suri S, Eradi B, Chowdhary SK, et al: Early postoperative feeding and outcome in neonates, *Nutrition* 18:380, 2002.

142. Task Force on Infant Positioning and SIDS: American Academy of Pediatrics: positioning and sudden infant death syndrome (SIDS): update, *Pediatrics* 98:1216, 1996.

143. Thompson NP, Montgomery SM, Wadsworth ME, et al: Early determinants of inflammatory bowel disease: use of two national longitudinal birth cohorts, *Eur J Gastroenterol Hepatol* 12:25, 2000.

144. Toms GL, Scott R: Respiratory syncytial virus and the infant immune response, *Arch Dis Child* 62:544, 1987.

145. Toms GL, Gardner PS, Pullan CR, et al: Secretion of respiratory syncytial virus inhibitors and antibody in human milk through lactation, *J Med Virol* 5:351, 1980.

146. Torowicz DL, Seelhorst A, Froh EB, et al: Human milk and breastfeeding outcomes in infants with congenital heart disease, *Breastfeed Med* 10(1):31–37, 2015.

147. Udall JN, Dixon M, Newman AP, et al: Liver disease in α-1-antitrypsin deficiency, *JAMA* 253:2679, 1985.

148. Unal S, Arhan E, Kara N, et al: Breastfeeding-associated hypernatremia: retrospective analysis of 169 term newborns, *Pediatr Int* 50:29–34, 2008.

149. Varma SK, Collins M, Row A, et al: Thyroxine, tri-iodothyronine, and reverse tri-iodothyronine concentrations in human milk, *J Pediatr* 93:803, 1978.

150. Vennemann MM, Bajanowski T, Brinkmann B, et al: Does breastfeeding reduce the risk of sudden infant death syndrome, *Pediatrics* 123:e406–e410, 2009.

151. Walsh M, McIntosh K: Neonatal mastitis, *Clin Pediatr (Phila)* 25:395, 1986.

152. Walter RS: Issues surrounding the development of feeding and swallowing. In Tuchman DN, Walter RS, editors: *Disorders of feeding and swallowing in infants and children:* *pathophysiology, diagnosis, and treatment,* San Diego, 1994, Singular.

153. Watchko JF, Maisels MJ: Jaundice in low birth weight infants: pathobiology and outcome, *Arch Dis Child Fetal Neonatal Ed* 88:F455–F458, 2003.

154. Weatherley-White RC, Kuehn DP, Mirrett P, et al: Early repair and breastfeeding for infants with cleft lip, *Plast Reconstr Surg* 879–887, 1987.

155. Winter S, Buist N: Clinical guide to inborn errors of metabolism, *J Rare Dis* IV:18, 1998.

156. Wong PWK, Lambert AM, Komrowe GM: Tyrosinaemia and tyrosinuria in infancy, *Dev Med Child Neurol* 9:551, 1967.

157. Woolridge MW, Fisher C: Colic, "overfeeding" and symptoms of lactose malabsorption in the breastfed baby: a possible artifact of feed management, *Lancet* 2:382, 1988.

158. Zimmerman AW, Hambridge KM, Lepow ML, et al: Acrodermatitis in breastfed premature infants: evidence for a defect of mammary gland zinc secretion, *Pediatrics* 69:176, 1982.

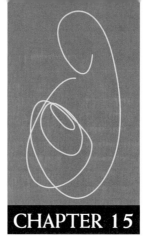

CHAPTER 15

Premature Infants and Breastfeeding

Premature Infants

The data are overwhelming. Even the most reluctant of neonatologists have accepted the tremendous importance of human milk to all infants large and small.

Research in the science of nutrition for low-birth-weight (LBW) infants and micropremature infants has advanced tremendously as the technology to study the important questions has improved. Neonatologists meanwhile have spent the past decades studying the physiology of respiration. Their advances have contributed to the survival of smaller and smaller infants. The edge of viability is 24 weeks and a weight of 500 g; however, infants have survived under these values. One of the key points learned retrospectively about survival, generation after generation, has been the critical impact of fluid and nutrition. Although human milk has gained prominence in these studies, the early use of unsupplemented drip milk and some donor milks produced poor growth patterns. Drip milk is low in fat and, therefore, low in calories. The protein levels in donor milk from women late in lactation (i.e., beyond 6 to 8 months, when the levels have dropped) parallel a child's decreased biologic needs with the addition of solid foods. These factors contributed to the abandonment of human milk until supplements were developed and studies of the milk of women who had delivered prematurely sparked new investigations.

This discussion highlights only the important issues; the reader is referred to reviews such as the exhaustive summary of human milk for the premature infant in the technical review of the optimal feeding of LBW infants for the World Health Organization (WHO) by Edmond and Bahl[36] that was released in 2006. Policy statements from WHO, UNICEF, and other international and national organizations confirm the importance of providing a mother's own milk to preterm and small-for-gestational-age (SGA) infants. Standard practice in neonatal units is to promote mother's own milk as the food of choice for all LBW infants.[130] Edmond and Bahl state that their review confirms this position worldwide. *Nutritional Needs of the Preterm Infant* by Tsang et al.[132] is an international collaboration that involved many major premature infant centers in discussions to create unity out of a tremendous disparity of practice and various recipes for nutritional support in 1993. This collaboration also produced a consensus on individual nutrient requirements for infants of less than 1000-g birth weight, for 1000- to 1750-g infants, and for post-discharge management. In spite of these strong statements, however, neonatologists have not reached a consensus on the feeding of premature infants.[69] The absolute standard for evaluating the nutritional outcome of preterm infants remains undefined. A strategy to minimize mobilization of endogenous nutrient stores is moving from a focus on intrauterine-based, short-term growth and nutrient retention rates to a system that considers long-term growth achievement.[102] The optimal time to initiate oral feedings in the smallest and sickest preterm infants is under revision.[97] Prolonged exclusive parenteral nutrition is being replaced with minimal amounts of oral feedings with parenteral nutrition to preserve and maintain intestinal function. As nutritional markers shift, a preterm infant's own mother's milk may well be recognized, even by the most skeptical clinicians, as the "gold standard" to prevent short-term morbidities and enhance long-term outcome. With this change comes the recognition that even fortified donor milk is superior to artificial feeds.

LBW has been defined by WHO as a weight at birth of less than 2500 g. The global incidence of LBW is 15.5%, which includes 20.6 million infants born each year, only 35% of which occur in developed countries. LBW infants form a heterogeneous group, some born early, some who are born at term but are SGA, and some both early and small. LBW infants account for 60% to 80% of all neonatal deaths and are at high risk for early growth retardation, infectious disease, developmental delay, and death in infancy and childhood.

A normal full-term infant can usually be breastfed with only minor adjustments, even without the support of medical expertise. When an infant cannot nurse directly at the breast, is providing mother's milk appropriate? What is the overall prognosis for ever feeding at the breast or, perhaps, for survival itself? Parents are so awed by the medical staff of special and intensive care nurseries that they are often afraid to bring up the subject of breastfeeding. In addition, the nursery staff may be so busy balancing electrolytes and adjusting ventilators and monitors that they have not thought to ask what plans the mother might have had for feeding before the infant developed a problem (Table 15-1).

The birth of an extremely LBW (ELBW) premature infant is a nutritional emergency. Even with parenteral nutrition from the first day, weight loss exceeds 10%, and it takes at least 10 days to regain birth weight. The long-term consequences of early nutrition have a great impact on neurodevelopment and may well reduce the risk for perinatal brain lesions. Fetal and postnatal events affect gut development.

Gastrointestinal Tract Development

The gastrointestinal (GI) tract is one of the first structures defined in the developing embryo. Gut length proceeds rapidly throughout fetal life and for the first years of life. The proton pump is present at 13 weeks of gestation. Intrinsic factor and pepsin are identifiable a few weeks later (Figure 15-1). Even in ELBW premature infants, the gastric pH can be lowered to 4.0. Digestive enzymes are capable of intraluminal digestion of fat, protein, and carbohydrates. Although pancreatic lipase and bile salts are minimal in ELBW infants, the introduction of mother's milk will stimulate maturation and also provide lipases and other digestive enzymes.

The intestinal villi and cellular differentiation occur at about 10 to 12 weeks' gestation and begin a complex interrelationship with developing epithelium and the mesoderm, according to Newell.[111] Lactase and other carbohydrate enzymes begin to appear. Gut motility is believed to appear first as irregular GI activity at 23 weeks progressing to organized motility at approximately 28 weeks. Most studies of nutritive sucking and swallowing are done with artificial feeding with a bottle. Suckling at the breast, which begins with peristaltic motion of the tongue and continues down the esophagus, has been initiated by breastfeeding as early as 28 weeks or sooner.

TABLE 15-1	Risks of Neonatal Mortality According to Timing of Initiation of Breastfeeding in Singletons Who Initiated Breastfeeding and Survived to Day 2			
Initiation of Breastfeeding	No. of Infants (%)	No. of Deaths (% risk)*	aOR 1 (95% CI)[†]	aOR 2 (95% CI)[‡]
Within 1 h	4763 (43)	34 (0.7)	1	1
From 1 h to end of day 1	3105 (28)	36 (1.2)	1.45 (0.90-2.35)	1.43 (0.88-2.31)
Day 2	2138 (20)	48 (2.3)	2.70 (1.70-4.30)	2.52 (1.58-4.02)[§]
Day 3	797 (7.3)	21 (2.6)	3.01 (1.70-5.38)	2.84 (1.59-5.06)[§]
After day 3	144 (1.3)	6 (4.2)	4.42 (1.76-11.09)	3.64 (1.43-9.30)[§]
Total	10,947 (100)	145 (1.3)		
			$p_{LRT} < 0.0001$	$p_{LRT} = 0.0001$
			$p_{trend} < 0.0001$	$p_{trend} < 0.0001$

*% risk, number of deaths/number of infants in exposure category.
[†]Adjusted for sex, birth size, gestational age, presence of a congenital anomaly, health on the day of birth, health at the time of interview, mother's health at the time of delivery, age of mother, parity, educational level of mother, mother having cash income, household water supply, place of defecation, number of antenatal visits, place of birth, and birth attendant.
[‡]Adjusted for all factors mentioned previously plus established breastfeeding pattern.
[§]The combined aOR for initiation of breastfeeding after 1 day was 2.88 (95% CI, 1.87 to 4.42).
aOR, Adjusted odds ratio; *CI*, confidence interval; *LRT*, likelihood ratio test.
Edmond KM, Zandoh C, Quigley MA, et al: Delayed breastfeeding initiation increases risk of neonatal mortality, *Pediatrics* 117:e380, 2006.

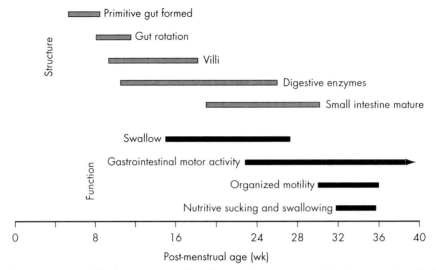

Figure 15-1. The ontogenic timetable showing structural and functional gastrointestinal development. (Modified from Newell SJ: Enteral feeding of the micropremie, *Clin Perinatol* 27:221, 2000.)

BOX 15-1. Factors Affecting Gastric Emptying

Faster gastric emptying	No effect	Slower gastric emptying
Breast milk	Phototherapy	Prematurity
Glucose	Feed	Formula milk
polymers	temperature	Caloric density
Starch	Nonnutritive	Fatty acids
Medium-	sucking	Dextrose
chain		concentration
triglycerides		Long-chain
Prone position		triglycerides
		Osmolality
		Illness

Gastric emptying in premature infants is slow, generating the impression that feedings are not tolerated. Gastric emptying is enhanced by human milk and slowed by formula and increased osmolarity (Box 15-1). Half emptying time with human milk is reported to be as rapid as 20 to 40 minutes.[70] Ultrasound studies have assessed small volume feeds. Some premature infants show delayed antral distention after a nasogastric feeding with emptying that follows a curvilinear pattern after an initial rapid phase.

Maturation of the small intestinal motility, and hence tolerance of feeds, is enhanced by previous exposure of the gut to nutrition. Early feeding precipitates preferential maturation and thus a more mature response to feeds. Total gut transit time in premature infants varies from 1 to 5 days and is more rapid in those who have received food.[12] In those younger than 28 weeks, it takes 3 days to pass meconium. Breast milk feedings, however, increase motility and stool passage.

When prematurity is complicated by intrauterine growth failure, the resultant cascade of events includes decreased splanchnic circulation and oligohydramnios, poor gut perfusion, decreased growth of the small intestine and pancreas culminating in a fetal echogenic gut, and poor intestinal motility resulting in poor tolerance to milk feeds. It is not uncommon for this to result in necrotizing enterocolitis (NEC). These events require careful consideration, including the choice to use mother's milk, especially beginning with colostrum.

Although feeding regimens vary, evidence is strong and consistent that feeding mother's own milk to preterm infants at any gestation is associated with a lower incidence of infections and NEC and improved neurodevelopmental outcome compared with the use of bovine milk products.[36] The challenge is to increase the availability of mother's milk (Figure 15-2).

GI Priming

When feedings are delayed in any newborn, luminal starvation results in epithelial cell atrophy. Lung injury may aggravate this because of multiorgan system dysfunction, increasing the risk for intestinal mucosal injury and associated barrier dysfunction. The ultimate injury would be the invasion of bacteria from the gut lumen.[21] Initiating feeds is a delicate balance between insufficient feeds that fail to trigger gut maturation and excessive feeds that overwhelm the digestive capacity. Also, excessive feeds can result in bacterial overgrowth and injury to the brush border.[21] When internal nutrients are absent, the intestinal size and weight are

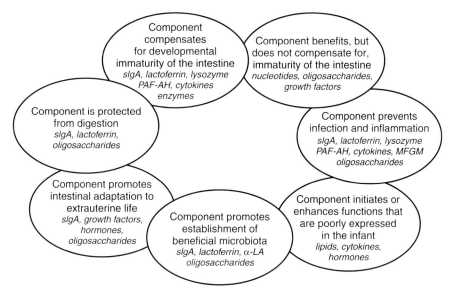

Figure 15-2. Strategies for beneficial effects of bioactive agents in human milk. Human milk contains bioactive agents with overlapping and synergic effects on intestinal development of neonates. *MFGM,* Milk fat globule membrane; *PAF-AH,* platelet-activating factor-acetylhydrolase. (Modified from Goldman AS: Modulation of the gastrointestinal tract of infants by human milk. Interface and interactions. An evolutionary perspective, *J Nutr* 130:426S, 2000.)

diminished; atrophy of the mucosa, delayed maturation of intestinal enzymes, and increased permeability and bacterial translocation may occur. Intestinal motilities, perfusion, and reactions to the usual GI tropic hormones are also affected by lack of nutrients. Trophic hormone levels in the plasma are significantly altered by starvation.

In the words of Lucas,[83] "It is fundamentally unphysiological to deprive an infant of any gestation of enteral feeding since the deprivation would never normally occur at any stage." This statement is based on the fact that a fetus normally makes sucking motions and swallows amniotic fluid from early gestation. This may even have a trophic effect on the gut. By the third trimester, a fetus is swallowing up to 150 mL/kg/day, which actually provides as much as 3 g/kg of protein per day. The secretion of GI hormones is believed to occur in response to the first postdelivery feedings.[132] In animals, after only a few days of deprivation of enteral feeds, atrophic changes take place in the gut.[85] In human infants who have never received enteral feedings, no gut peptide surges occur, not even those of the trophic hormones enteroglucagon, gastrin, and gastric inhibitory polypeptide. These hormones are believed to be key to the activation of the enteroinsular axis[85] (Box 15-2). Clinical trials of early priming in premature infants showed that infants primed in the first few days or first week had better feeding tolerance to advancing feeds and were weaned from parenteral nutrition promptly. It was also associated with lower serum alkaline phosphatase activity and significant stimulation of GI

BOX 15-2. Biology of the Gut in VLBW Infants

- Swallows amniotic fluid daily, up to 150 mL/kg/day
- Potential for gut atrophy if not fed
- All of gastrointestinal track is immature
- Enzymes and nutrients in human milk enhance maturation
- Higher total body water, muscle mass, growth accretion rates, and oxygen consumption
- Higher evaporative water loss due to greater surface area
- Prone to hyperglycemia due to poor insulin response
- Lower brown fat reserves and glycogen stores
- Immature thyroid control of metabolic rate

  VLBW, Very low-birth-weight.

hormones such as gastrin. It also resulted in more mature intestinal motility patterns, greater absorption of Ca and P, increased lactase activity, increased bone mineral content (BMC), and reduced intestinal permeability. Tyson and Kennedy[133] reviewed the studies of early priming and found shorter times to full feeding, fewer days when feedings were held, a shorter duration of hospitalization, and no increase in NEC. Many of the involved infants were actually at high risk for complications by virtue of their own morbidities, including mechanical ventilation, umbilical catheterization, and patent ductus arteriosus. Schanler[123] recommended that ELBW infants who are ill be

BOX 15-6. Milk of Mothers Who Deliver Preterm

Level increased in preterm	Level unchanged in preterm
Total nitrogen	Volume
Protein nitrogen	Calories
Long-chain fatty acids	Lactose (? less)
Medium-chain fatty acids	Fat (?) by "creamatocrit"
Short-chain fatty acids	Linolenic acid
Sodium	Potassium
Chloride	Calcium
Magnesium (?)	Phosphorus
Iron	Copper
	Zinc
	Osmolality
	Vitamin B_{1-12}

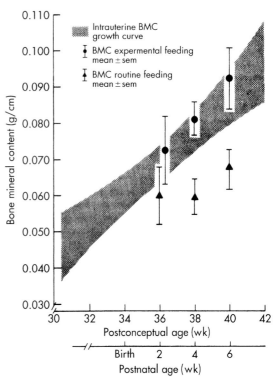

Figure 15-4. Postnatal bone mineral content (BMC) in 33- to 35-week-old appropriate-for-gestational-age or preterm infants compared with intrauterine bone mineralization curve. Regression curve and 95th percentile confidence limits for regression for BMC of infants born at different gestational ages (30 to 42 weeks' gestational age) represent intrauterine bone mineralization curve. Infants fed routine cow milk formula *(solid triangles)* had significantly lower BMC than infants fed standard formula supplemented with calcium and phosphorus *(solid circles).* In these infants, BMC was not different from intrauterine bone mineralization curve at 4 and 6 weeks' postnatal age. (From Steichen JJ, Gratton TL, Tsang RC: Osteopenia of prematurity: the cause and possible treatment, *J Pediatr* 96:528, 1980.)

and fats,[119] and the low renal solute load. The presence of active enzymes enhances maturation and supplements the enzyme activity of this underdeveloped gut. The antiinfective properties and living cells protect immature infants from infection and protect against NEC. The psychological benefit to the mother who can participate in her infant's care by providing her milk is a less tangible but no less important advantage.

The disadvantages are the possible gaps in certain nutrients that have been estimated to be required for adequate growth, which include the volume of total protein and macrominerals, especially calcium and phosphorus.[43–45] Much of the attention to the shortcomings has been based on work done using pooled milk samples collected from women whose infants are full term and many months old, resulting in the impression that mother's milk is inadequate. The sources of the human milk and processing—freezing or pasteurizing—are significant to the question of nutritional adequacies. Many laboratory and clinical scientists have studied the questions posed here with new techniques and provided hundreds of reports regarding the nutrition and nurturance of LBW and VLBW infants. Only a fraction of the resources can be referenced here.[13,44]

Optimal Growth for Premature Infants

Optimal growth for infants born prematurely is considered to be the growth curve they would have followed had they remained in utero[45] (Figure 15-4

and Tables 15-3 and 15-4). Achieving this goal utilizing the immature intestinal tract requires that the nutrients be digestible and absorbable and not impose a significant metabolic stress on the other immature organs, especially the kidney. Although human milk provides the ideal nutrients, it would require an inordinate nonphysiologic volume to achieve adequate amounts of some nutrients without calculated supplementation. To fill these growth needs, one can use an artificial or chemical formula or use human milk as a base, with all its advantages, and add the deficient nutrients to it.

Special Properties of Preterm Milk

The identification of special quantitative differences in nutrients in the milk of mothers who

TABLE 15-3	Estimated Requirements and Advisable Intakes for Protein by Infant's Weight as Derived by Factorial Approach							
Birth Weight Range (g)	Tissue Increment (g/day)	Dermal Loss (g/day)	Urine Loss (g/day)	Intestinal Absorption (% intake)	Estimated Requirement (g/day)	Advisable Intake		
						g/day	g/kg*	g/100 kcal[†]
800-1200	2.32	0.17	0.68	87 g[†]	3.64	4.0	4.0	3.1
1200-1800	3.01	0.25	0.90	87 g	4.78	5.2	3.5	2.7

*Assuming body weight of 1000 and 1500 g for 800- to 1200-g infant and 1200- to 1800-g infant, respectively.
[†]Assuming calorie intake of 120 kcal/day.
Adapted from Ziegler EE, Biga RL, Fomon SJ: Nutritional requirements of the premature infant. In Suskind RM, editor: *Textbook of pediatric nutrition*, New York, 1981, Raven, pp 29–39.

TABLE 15-4	Accumulation of Various Components During Last Trimester of Pregnancy				
	Accumulation During Various Stages of Gestation (wk)				
Component	26-31	31-33	33-35	35-38	38-40
Body weight (g)*	500	500	500	500	–
Water (g)	410	350	320	240	220
Fat (g)	25	65	85	175	200
Nitrogen (g)	11	12	12	6	7
Calcium (g)	4	5	5	5	5
Phosphorus (g)	2.2	2.6	2.8	3.0	3.0
Magnesium (mg)	130	110	120	120	80
Sodium (mEq)	35	25	40	40	40
Potassium (mEq)	19	24	26	20	20
Chloride (mEq)	30	24	10	20	10
Iron (mg)	36	60	60	40	20
Copper (mg)	2.1	2.4	2.0	2.0	2.0
Zinc (mg)	9.0	10.0	8.0	7.0	3.0

*Body weight of 26-week fetus is 1000 g and of 40-week fetus is 3500 g.
  Modified from data of Widdowson from Heird WC, Anderson TL: Nutritional requirements and methods of feeding low birth weight infants. In Gluck L et al., editors: *Current problems in pediatrics,* vol. 7, no. 8, Chicago, 1977, Year Book, pp 1–4.

delivered prematurely created new interest in the use of human milk for premature infants (see Box 15-6). Many investigators have contributed to the pool of knowledge after the initial revelations in 1980 by Atkinson et al.,[8] who reported the nitrogen concentration of milk from mothers of premature infants to be greater than that of milk from mothers delivering at term.[9,14]

Preterm milk is higher in protein content during the first months of lactation, containing between 1.8 and 2.4 g/dL. Preterm milk contains similar fat in quality and quantity, although Anderson et al.[5] reported increased values for preterm milk over term milk. Lactose in preterm milk averages 5.96 g/dL and up to 6.95 g/dL at 28 days, whereas the values in term milk are 6.16 and 7.26 g/dL, respectively. Preterm milk has higher energy than term milk, 58 to 70 kcal/dL, compared with 48 to 64 kcal/dL in the first month postpartum (Figure 15-5).

The macronutrients calcium and phosphorus are slightly higher in preterm milk (14 to 16 mEq/L vs. 13 to 16 mEq/L calcium and 4.7 to 5.5 m/L vs. 4.0 to 5.1 m/L phosphorus). Neither term nor preterm milk has adequate calcium and phosphorus for the VLBW infant. Magnesium levels in preterm milk are 28 to 31 mg/L, dropping to 25 mg/L at 28 days, and term milk levels are 25 to 29 mg/L. Zinc levels are higher in preterm milk, beginning at 5.3 mg/L and dropping to 3.9 mg/L, whereas term milk begins at 5.4 mg/L and drops to 2.6 mg/L. Sodium levels in preterm milk are higher (26.6 mEq/L, dropping to 12.6 mEq/L), whereas term milk is 22.3 mEq/L, decreasing to 8.5 mEq/L at 28 days.[106] Chloride has a similar average (preterm 31.6 mEq/L, decreasing to 16.8 mEq/L, and term 26.9 mEq/L, decreasing to 13.1 mEq/L).

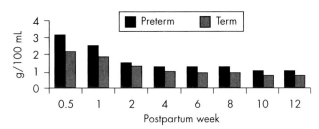

Figure 15-5. Protein content of human milk. (Data from Butte NF, Garza C, Johnson CA, et al: Longitudinal changes in milk composition of mothers delivering preterm and term infants, *Early Hum Dev* 9:153, 1984; Gross SJ, David RJ, Bauman L, Tomarelli RM: Nutritional composition of milk produced by mothers delivering preterm, *J Pediatr* 96:641, 1980.)

of the entire microbiome, including some microbes not culturable at this time. Early gut microbiota play a major role in intestinal health and disease. The human milk glycans, especially the oligosaccharides and human microbes, are a major component of the immune system by which breastfeeding mothers protect their infants from disease, especially their micropremature.

Use of Human Milk for Premature Infants

A clear distinction must be made between an infant's own mother's milk and pooled human milk for the feeding of LBW infants. The mother's premature milk has some higher levels of nutrients but never lower levels than term milk. Mothers who donate to milk banks are also feeding their own infants, who may be any age from birth to 6 months or older. Donor milk must also be prepared by sterilization. An infant's own mother's milk may be fed fresh or fresh-frozen and is rarely heat treated. Chapter 21 discusses milk storage and milk banking.

When the volume of milk produced by a mother is not sufficient to meet the infant's needs each day, providing additional nourishment by donor milk is clearly needed. There are several choices for human milk supplementation.

A 2001- to 2500-g infant without complications may be weaned from the incubator to an open crib within 24 hours. Although the suck reflex may be poor, the infant can usually be breastfed. The infant is ready to breastfeed even if he or she takes a bottle poorly. If the infant can stimulate the breast briefly and obtain the rich, antibody-containing, cell-filled colostrum, the infant will be protected against infection while receiving nutrition. Inadequate stimulation of the breast by the infant will require mechanical pumping after the feeding. If the infant cannot suck and must be tube fed, any colostrum the mother can manually express or pump from the breast can be given by gavage tube along with donor milk or, if human milk is not available, the prescribed formula necessary for nourishment. Chapter 5 reviews the protective value of colostrum to the infant.

Intestinal permeability is another parameter of great importance to LBW infants. The GI tract development provides an important barrier to infectious materials and a path for protective and nourishing substances. A precarious balance of intestinal permeability is required to promote infant growth and to avoid severe preterm infant diseases.[131] Decreasing intestinal permeability is associated with gut maturation. In a study of 62 preterm infants ($\leq$32 weeks' gestation), the children were

evaluated utilizing enteral lactulose and mannitol administration and urinary measurements at three points in the first month postnatally while assessing their feeding type.[131] Those infants receiving predominantly human milk (>75%) had significantly lower intestinal permeability compared with those receiving formula and little or no human milk. The portion of human milk received increased in importance over time, with more than 25% required by 30 days of age to see a significant advantage.

A study in Guatemala that was repeated in the special care nursery of the Rainbow Children's Hospital in Cleveland showed that the infection rate among sick and premature newborns was greatly diminished by providing 15 mL of human colostrum contributed by random donors daily.[32] These findings were especially dramatic in Guatemala, where the mortality rate from infection in the nursery was extremely high. It has been suggested that mixed feedings of an infant's own mother's milk and formula to necessary volume be calculated over a 24-hour period so that the infant receives some mother's milk at each feeding and a supplement of formula, in contrast to alternating feedings or using all mother's milk until it runs out and finishing the day with formula. The reasoning is based on the concept of "inoculating" every feeding with human milk to provide the enzymes and immunologic properties with each feeding. Generous levels of active enzymes in the milk will also assist in the digestion and absorption of the formula. The immunologic properties are less measurable, but the only known interference with function is the addition of iron, which blocks the effectiveness of lactoferrin. Therefore, the nutritional and infection-protective properties are also spread throughout each feeding around the clock. Now that donor milk is more readily available, it is recommended to make up the deficit in volume of mother's milk with donor milk.

The quantities of direct-acting antimicrobial factors in human milk vary according to the method of collection, processing, and storage.[39] The ability of donor milk to protect against infection in premature infants is being tested in multiple clinical studies.[48]

Supplementation of Mother's Own Milk or Pooled Human Milk

No supplement to human milk is usually needed if the infant is more than 1500 g at birth.

The options for supplementing an infant's own mother's milk depend on need for additional volume or for specific nutrients, especially protein, calcium, and phosphorus, based on birth weight and growth rates.[65,66]

The ideal supplementation is one using human milk nutrients and is referred to as *lacto engineering*, in which nutrient concentration is increased by adding specific nutrients derived from human milk. Techniques involve use of donor milk and separating the cream and protein fractions, reducing the lactose content, and heat-treating the product with a high-temperature, short-time process of pasteurization. This completely human milk product provides higher protein and energy needs so that weight gains and nitrogen retention are similar to intrauterine rates.

Using a feeding prepared from human milk protein and medium-chain triglyceride supplementation of human milk for VLBW infants was reported by Rönnholm et al.[119] Forty-four infants averaging 30 weeks' gestation with birth weights ranging from 710 to 1510 g were nourished by one of four protocols: plain human milk, human milk and protein, human milk and triglycerides, or human milk and protein and triglycerides. The triglycerides did not influence weight and length, but the two groups receiving added protein gained along a curve comparable with the intrauterine growth for their birth weight, gaining faster from 4 to 6 weeks than the unsupplemented infants. The protein-supplemented groups also grew more in length; however, head circumference growth was similar in all groups.

Total protein is usually calculated by determining the total nitrogen content (Kjeldahl method) and multiplying the number by the protein factor (6.25). Total protein corrected for nonprotein nitrogen, which is high in human milk, is true protein.[10] True protein is a heterogeneous mixture of casein and whey proteins. Whey proteins include lactoferrin, immunoglobulin, and lysozyme. True protein minus those more or less indigestible proteins is called *digestible protein*. Analysis of preterm milk by Beijers et al.[10] demonstrated that nonprotein nitrogen was dependent on the degree of prematurity and averaged 20% to 25%, increasing during the time of lactation. Only 30% to 60% of total protein is available for synthesis. However, in absolute amounts over lactation time, it remains stable.

Schanler et al. compared plasma amino acid levels in VLBW infants (mean age 16 days, mean birth weight 1180 g, mean gestation 29 weeks) fed either human milk fortified with human milk or whey-dominant cow milk formula. The infants received continuous enteral infusions of isonitrogenous, isocaloric preparations. Taurine and cystine were significantly higher in the infants fed human milk, and threonine, valine, methionine, and lysine were significantly higher in the infants fed formula.

Mother's own milk shows a wide variability in nutrient components when being pumped for a

---

BOX 15-10. Steps to Preserve the Nutrient Value of Mother's Milk

I. Most variable component: Fat
  A. Lost in collection and storage
  B. Settles out on standing
  C. In one report fat content ranged from 2.2 to 4.7 g/dL
  D. Steps to enhance fat
    (1) Avoid separation of fat
    (2) Avoid continuous feeds
    (3) Utilize intermittent bolus feeds
    (4) Orient syringe of milk upward
    (5) Use short length of tubing
    (6) Empty syringe completely at end of infusion
  E. Use hind milk preferentially if volume is adequate
II. Protein content declines from transitional to mature milk
  A. Nutrient needs for premature are higher
III. Mineral content has increased bioavailability but content is lower than needs of premature infants. Vitamins A, C, and riboflavin levels decrease with collection, storage, and delivery.

---

hospitalized premature infant. Nutrient supplementation is necessary to maintain adequate growth and good nutritional status. According to Herman and Schanler,[58] extraordinary efforts should be made to use mother's own milk because the advantages of nonnutrient components in human milk are significantly diminished by storage and heat processing. The most variable constituent is fat (Box 15-10). Protein does not meet the needs of a small premature. Although levels of minerals (Ca, P) are stable, the needs of VLBW infants require supplementation. Substantial benefits of mother's own milk include reduced infection, enhanced neurodevelopmental outcome, and healthy postnatal growth. The minimum dose of mother's milk when given with various fortifications has been found to be more than 50 mL/kg/day to protect against infection, especially late-onset sepsis.[47] A systemic review looking at multinutrient fortification for human milk involved 10 trials and a total of more than 600 infants weighing less than 1800 g.[73] It clearly showed improvement in weight gain increments in length, head circumference, and BMC compared with unsupplemented milk. Neurodevelopmental outcomes were significantly improved with mother's milk. The magnitude of the effect was seen as mother's milk intake increased to 110 mL/kg/day; the developmental scales showed an increase of five points, an important gain for these ELBW infants. Preterm infants have lower energy expenditure when they are fed breast milk than when they are fed preterm infant formula.

Preterm infants with birth weights from 750 to 1250 g were randomly assigned to a cream or control group. The cream group received a human milk-derived cream supplement if the energy density of the human milk tested below 20 kcal/oz, measured using a near infrared human milk analyzer. The control group received their mother's own milk or donor human milk with donor human milk-derived fortifier. Premature infants who received human milk-derived cream as a fortifier had improved weight and length compared to the control group. Cream can be used as an adjunctive supplement to an exclusive human milk-based diet to improve growth rates (see Figure 15-6 Prolact CR[TM] Human Milk Caloric Fortifier).

All preterm infants should receive human milk fortified with protein, minerals, and vitamins when birth weight is less than 1500 g according to the American Academy of Pediatrics' section on breastfeeding.

Artificial Fortification of Human Milk

No longer is supplementing an infant's own mother's milk with specially prepared formula supplements necessary. Available commercial preparations for such supplementation were intended to complement human milk and not to be used as an exclusive formula. When multicomponent fortified human milk product for promoting growth in preterm infants was examined in a Cochrane Review,[74] the authors found short-term increases in weight gain, linear growth, and head circumference. No effect was seen on serum alkaline phosphatase levels, and the effect on BMC was unclear. Nitrogen retention and blood urea levels were increased. Conclusions about long-term neurodevelopmental and growth outcomes were limited by insufficient data after 1 year. The significance of increased blood urea nitrogen and blood pH levels was unclear. Preparations are different and are used differently (Table 15-9). The powdered supplement is intended to add special nutrients to an adequate volume of mother's own milk (Enfamil human milk fortifier or Similac human milk fortifier), or it can be used to enhance pooled donor human milk. Neither fortifier contains fat. Milk fortification extends the mother's milk and provides additional nitrogen, calcium, phosphorus, and vitamins for an LBW infant. If an infant is fed the mother's milk, pooled donor milk, and a fortifier, the sum total should meet the infant's daily requirements (Table 15-10). Any addition of artificial formula interferes with the infection protection qualities and other benefits of human milk so use of formula-based supplementation should be

avoided unless human milk-based formula is not available. Preventing one case of NEC saves $100,000.

Studies comparing fortified mother's milk with premature infant formulas have shown comparable growth in weight, length, and head circumference. This makes it possible to lose many advantages of a mother's milk, while providing the additional nutrients for appropriate accretion rates.[127]

When powdered fortifier was added to a mother's milk, the supplemented infants had significantly greater weight gain, linear growth, and head circumference growth than those not supplemented. The supplemented infants also had higher blood urea nitrogen levels (Table 15-11).[53] The loss of human milk benefits is of significant concern.

When a preterm infant's own mother's milk was fortified with protein (0.85 g/dL), calcium (90 mg/dL), and phosphorus (45 mg/dL), the rate of weight gain was greater than that of the unfortified group and comparable with that of the Similac Natural Care formula group.[50–52] Bone mineralization improved during the 6 weeks of the study but did not reach the intrauterine accretion rate of 150 mg/kg/day. A relative phosphorus deficiency occurred in the human milk groups, both with and without supplementation. Fortifying preterm mother's milk permits biochemically adequate growth comparable with that provided by special care formula (Table 15-12).

The effect of calcium supplementation on fatty acid balance studies in LBW infants fed human milk or formula has been shown to be significant. A decrease in total fatty acid absorption both in LBW infants fed their own mother's milk and in formula-fed infants was seen when calcium was added. Fecal output of fat and fatty acid excretion was higher in the formula-fed infants. In mother's milk-fed infants, the total fat absorption and the coefficient of absorption were higher.

Preterm milk with routine multivitamin supplementation (providing 4.1 mg of tocopherol) uniformly resulted in vitamin sufficiency in VLBW infants in a control study by Gross and Gabriel.[54] This was true when they received iron, as well as when they were not iron supplemented. VLBW infants were fed preterm milk, bank milk, or formula, utilizing 2 mg/day of iron. Vitamin E content of preterm milk does not differ significantly from that of term human milk from days 3 to 36.[56]

Jocson et al.[68] studied the effects of nutrient fortification and varying storage conditions on host-defense properties of human milk. Total bacterial colony counts and immunoglobulin A (IgA) were not affected by the addition of fortifier.

The effect of powdered human milk fortifiers on the antibacterial actions of human milk were

TABLE 15-9 — Composition of Infant Feeding Using Human Milk With and Without Various Supplements

	Preterm Human Milk		Similac Natural Care	50:50 Mix Similac Natural Care and Preterm Human Milk*		Enfamil Human Milk Fortifier (four packets)	Enfamil Human Milk Fortifier (four packets) Added to Preterm Human Milk*	
Weeks postpartum	1	4		1	4		1	4
Kilocalories	67	70	81	72	76	14	81	84
Protein (g)	2.44	1.81	2.1	2.27	1.96	0.7	3.14	2.5
Carbohydrate (g)	6.05	6.95	8.6	7.3	7.8	2.7	8.75	9.65
Fat (g)	3.81	4.00	3.6	3.7	3.8	0.04	3.85	4.04
Vitamin A (IU)[†]	330	230	550	440	390	780	1110	1010
Vitamin E (mg)[†]	0.9	0.25	3	2.0	1.61	3.4	4.3	3.65
Vitamin K (mcg)[†]	NA	1.5	10	NA	5.8	9.1	NA	10.6
Vitamin D (IU)[†]	NA	2.5	120	NA	61	260	NA	262
Thiamin (mcg)	5.4	8.9	200	103	104	187	192	196
Riboflavin (mcg)	36.0	26.6	500	268	263	250	286	277
Niacin (mg)	0.11	0.21	4.0	2.1	2.1	3.1	3.2	3.3
Pyridoxine (mcg)	2.6	6.2	200	101	103	193	196	199
Folate (mcg)	2.1	3.1	30	16.1	16.6	23	25	26
Vitamin B$_{12}$ (mcg)	NA	0.1	0.45	NA	0.27	0.21	NA	0.3
Vitamin C (mg)[†]	7	5	30	19	18	24	31	29
Calcium (mg)	25	22	170	98	96	60	85	82
Phosphorus (mg)	14	14	85	50	50	33	47	47
Magnesium (mg)	3	2.5	10	6.5	6.3	4	7	6.5
Iron (mg)	0.1	0.1	0.3	0.2	0.2	0	0.1	0.1
Sodium (mEq)	2.2	1.3	1.7	2.0	1.5	0.3	2.5	1.6
Potassium (mEq)	1.8	1.7	2.9	2.4	2.3	0.4	2.2	2.1
Chloride (mEq)	2.5	1.6	2.0	2.3	1.8	0.5	3.0	2.1
Zinc (mg)	0.48	0.39	1.2	0.84	0.80	0.31	0.79	0.70
Copper (mg)	0.08	0.06	0.2	0.14	0.13	0.08	0.16	0.14
Manganese (mcg)[†]	NA	0.4	NA	NA	NA	9	NA	9.4
Biotin (mcg)	0.15	0.54	NA	NA	NA	0.8	0.95	1.34
Pantothenic acid (mg)	0.16	0.23	1.5	0.83	0.87	0.79	0.95	1.02
Osmolality (mOsm/kg H$_2$O)[†]	302	305	300	301	303	+60	362	365

*Volume 100 mL (1 dL).

[†]Listed values for 1 and 4 weeks reflect reported values for full-term transitional and mature human milk, respectively.

IU, International units; NA, not available.

TABLE 15-10 — Protein, Calcium, and Sodium Requirements by Growing Premature Infants and Composition of Banked Human Milk

	Protein (g/100 kcal)	Calcium (mg/100 kcal)	Sodium (mEq/100 kcal)
Estimated requirements for hypothetic, growing premature infants*	2.54	132[†]	2.3
Composition of banked human milk	1.50	43	0.8

*Assumed body weight is 1200 g; weight gain, 20 g/day; energy intake, 120 kcal/kg/day. The basis for estimating requirements is described in the text.

[†]This estimate does not apply to infants fed formulas from which calcium absorption is less than 65% of intake.

From Fomon SJ, Ziegler EE, Vazquez HD: Human milk and the small premature infant, Am J Dis Child 131:463, 1977.

TABLE 15-11 — Fortified Versus Unfortified Human Milk

Growth	Fortified
*13 studies, 596 infants; randomized**	
Weight gain	+3.7 g/kg/day
Length	+0.13 cm/wk
Head circumference	+0.12 cm/wk
Bone mineral content	+8.3 mg/cm
Nitrogen balance	+66 mg/kg/day
BUN	+5.8 mg/dL
Necrotizing enterocolitis	No significant difference
Feeding tolerance	No significant difference

*Some comparisons with partial supplements.

BUN, Blood urea nitrogen.

From Kuschel CA, Harding JE: Multicomponent fortified human milk for promoting growth in preterm infants (Cochrane Review). In The Cochrane Library, Issue 4, Chichester, 2004, John Wiley and Sons.

TABLE 15-12 Comparison of Selected Fortifiers for Human Milk (Prepared per 100 mL Milk)

Fortifier	PrHM	EHMF	SNC	Eoprotin*	S-26/SMA HMF	FM85†	SHMF
Energy (kJ) (kcal)	298 (71)	357 (85)	319 (76)	357 (85)	361 (86)	374 (89)	357 (85)
Fat (g)	3.6	3.6‡	4.0	3.6‡	3.65	3.6	4.0
Carbohydrate (g)	7.0	9.7	7.8	9.8	9.4	10.6	8.8
Protein (g)	1.8	2.5	2.0	2.6	2.8	2.6	2.8
Calcium (mg)	22	112	97	72	112	73	139
Phosphorus (mg)	14	59	50	48	59	48	81
Magnesium (mg)	2.5	3.5	6.3	5.3	4.0	4.5	9.5
Sodium (mEq)	0.7	1.0	1.1	1.9	1.1	1.9	1.35
Zinc (mcg)	320	1030	760	320‡	450	320‡	1320
Copper (mcg)	60	122	1045	60‡	60‡	60‡	230
Vitamins	Yes	Multi§	Multi§	A, C, E, K	Multi§	Multi§	Multi§

*Milupa, Friedrichsdorf, Germany.
†Nestle, Vevey, Switzerland.
‡Nutrient not contained in fortifier.
§Multivitamins: A, D, E, K, B_1, B_2, B_6, C, B_{12}, niacin, folate, pantothenate, and biotin.
EHMF, Enfamil Human Milk Fortifier (Mead Johnson Nutritionals, Evansville, Ind.); *HMF*, human milk-fed; *PrHM*, preterm human milk; *S-26/SMA HMF*, SMA Human Milk Fortifier (Wyeth Nutritionals, Philadelphia, Pa.); *SHMF*, Similac Human Milk Fortifier (Ross Laboratories, Columbus, Ohio); *SNC*, Similac Natural Care (Ross Laboratories, Columbus, Ohio) mixed 1:1 (vol: vol) with PrHM.
From Schanler RJ: The use of human milk for premature infants, *Pediatr Clin North Am* 48:207, 2001.

explored by Chan.[24] Human milk inhibited the growth of *Escherichia coli, Staphylococcus aureus, Enterobacter sakazakii,* and group B *Streptococcus* when Enfamil and Similac human milk fortifiers were mixed with human milk, along with medium-chain triglycerides and 1.09 mg ferrous sulfate (in 25 mL milk). The fortifiers containing iron and the iron alone inhibited the protective effect of human milk against the bacteria. The probable explanation is the interference of iron with the protective action of lactoferrin in human milk. The ferrous iron in the fortifier is changed to a ferric state in human milk, which readily binds with lactoferrin.

Concerns over the nutrient content of supplemented human milk have been expressed by many authors since the early work on premature infants from the Houston group.[125] After noting growth failure in some premature infants, it was discovered that some mother's milk was lower in calories than 20 kcal/oz. This has been reported by Prolacta Biologicals, which tests the protein and caloric content of all donations. This is a major issue for premature infants who have a restricted fluid intake in the early months of life. Preterm infants fed a commercially prepared, bovine-based human milk fortifier receive less protein than they need, according to Arslanoglu et al.[7] They tested the actual nutrient intakes observed in a previously reported study, with assumed nutrient intakes based on the usual assumptions about the composition of human milk. Actual protein intakes were significantly and consistently lower than the levels assumed based on the standard protein content of human milk. Actual

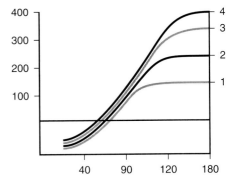

Figure 15-7. WHO technical report on optimal feeding for LBW infants.

intakes of protein by preterm infants fed bovine-fortified human milk were significantly lower, especially after 3 weeks postpartum when the mother's milk no longer had the higher protein content of the milk of a mother who delivers prematurely. Calorie content was not significantly lower (Figure 15-7).

The Committee on Nutrition of the AAP has outlined requirements for the premature infant who is less than 27 weeks' gestation and less than 1000 g at birth, regarding calcium and vitamin D. Bone mineral status should be started by 4 to 5 weeks after birth. Alkaline phosphatase above 800 to 1000 IU/L or clinical evidence of fractures require radiographic evaluation. A persistent serum phosphorus concentration less than 4 mg/dL should be monitored and supplementation with phosphorus considered. Postdischarge monitoring

BOX 15-11. Protein Recommendations

- Categorized by life stage and gender, because among healthy individuals, these are the two parameters responsible for variations in the body's need for protein
  - The Pediatrics Stage has been subdivided into six groupings: *infancy*, 0 to 6 months of age; *infancy*, 7 to 12 months of age; *toddlers*, 1 to 3 years of age; *early childhood*, 4 to 8 years of age; *puberty*, 9 to 13 years of age; and *adolescence*, 14 to 18 years of age
- Optimal food for full-term infants is human milk
  - Recommended that it be the sole source of nutrition for infants during the first 6 months of life
  - On average, infants to 6 months of age consume 0.78 L of milk per day
- Average value of 11.7 g/L used to calculate adequate intake for protein
- Nonprotein nitrogen component of human milk contains substantial quantities of taurine, which is virtually absent from cow milk
- Human milk proteins have a high nutritional quality and are digested and absorbed more efficiently than cow milk proteins
- Breastfed infants' protein intakes appear to satisfy the infant requirements for maintenance and growth without an amino acid or solute excess

Data from Rigo J, Senterre J: Nutritional needs of premature infants: current issues, *J Pediatr* 149:880, 2006; Kleinman RE, editor: *Pediatric nutrition*, ed 7, 2013, American Academy of Pediatrics; and World Health Organization: *Protein and amino acid requirements in human nutrition*, Geneva, 2007, World Health Organization.

is also necessary if exclusively breastfed. When the infant reaches 1500 g, vitamin D intake should be 400 IU/day minimum and up to a maximum of 1000 IU/day. A mineral intake between 100 and 166 mg/kg/day of highly absorbed calcium and 60 to 75 mg/kg/day of phosphorus is recommended to provide appropriate mineralization. Protein requirement is considered to be a matter of some debate, as human milk protein is readily absorbed, and bovine protein is less well absorbed. The revised recommendations for protein appear in Box 15-11. These adjustments were an effort to reduce metabolic stress from protein overload and unbalanced amino acid supply. Human milk has the ideal balance of casein and whey.

Fortification of Human Milk with Human Milk

The problem of adding nutrients to mothers' milk to meet the increased nutrient needs of premature infants, especially ELBW premature infants, has

challenged neonatologists for years. The commercial products developed from a bovine milk base have been widely used and have improved the nutrient intake of these infants. The theoretical concern about the impact of bovine milk on the infection protection properties of human milk has been argued.[62] A minimum of 50 mL/kg/day of the mother's milk is deemed necessary to maintain the protection provided by the mother's milk. A number of investigators have explored the possibility of a fortifier made out of human milk, so the feeding would meet needs with entirely human constituents. The antibacterial activity inherent in human milk was inhibited when a bovine-based fortifier containing added iron was mixed with human milk. Chan et al.[25] tested the same antibacterial activity when a newly derived human milk-based product became available (Prolacta Bioscience, Monrovia, Calif.). Human milk samples from 10 fully lactating mothers were utilized to test the effect on the antimicrobial activity of human milk, milk plus bovine fortifier, and milk plus human milk fortifier against *Ent. sakazakii, E. coli, Clostridium difficile,* and *Shigella soneii.* Human milk inhibited the growth of all the test organisms. The antibacterial activity was almost completely inhibited by the addition of the bovine-based fortifier. The activity was unaffected by the addition of human milk-based fortifier. Further studies of human milk-based fortifier (H²MF) have been conducted at national and international sites. The fortifier (H²MF) is available from Prolacta Bioscience. Preliminary results from University of Florida, Schneider's Children's Hospital, Baylor College of Medicine, and Yale-New Haven Medical Center were reported on 207 extremely premature infants whose mothers intended to provide their milk. The infants were randomized to one of three groups: mother's milk plus (HUM40) or 100 mL/kg/day (HUM100); the third group received mother's milk plus 100 mL/kg/day of the bovine-based product (Table 15-13). The groups had similar lengths of stay and rates of growth, chronic lung disease, and sepsis. However, significantly lower rates of NEC, surgical NEC, and combined deaths were observed with the human-based fortifier. Further results are available from other participating centers and all involved patients.

Long-Term Follow-Up of Growth Parameters in VLBW Infants

Weight gain and growth in length and head circumference are similar in VLBW infants who are breastfed or given standard formula after discharge. BMC was also followed at 10, 16, and 25 postnatal

TABLE 15-13 Use of Human Milk Fortifier Made from Human Milk

	BOV	HUM40	HUM100	p value*
N	69	71	67	
Gestation (wk)[†]	27.3±2.0	27.2±2.3	27.2±2.2	NS
Birth weight (g)[†]	922±197	921±188	945±202	NS
OMM consumed, mL (% of enteral intake)[‡]	5676 (82%)	4539 (70%)	4048 (73%)	NS
Days of PN[‡]	22	20	20	NS
NEC, n (%)	11 (15.9)	5 (7.0)	3 (4.5)	0.05
Surgical NEC, n (%)	8 (11.6)	1 (1.4)	1 (1.5)	0.007
Death, n (%)	5 (7.2)	2 (2.8)	1 (1.5)	NS
Death or NEC, n (%)	14 (20.3)	6 (8.5)	5 (7.5)	0.04

Results: The groups had similar lengths of stay and rates of growth, CLD, and sepsis. Other results are shown.

BOV, Bovine; *CLD*, central line day; *HUM40*, human milk (mother's milk) plus fortifier (Prolacta Bioscience); *HUM100*, human milk (mother's milk) 100 mL/kg/day; *OMM*, own mother's milk; *PN*, parenteral nutrition; *NEC*, necrotizing enterocolitis.

*Chi-square, Kruskal-Wallis, log-rank test.

[†]Mean±SD.

[‡]Median.

From Sullivan S, Schanler R, Abrams S, et al: Abstract at PAS 2009. #2155.1 Neonatal nutrition and follow up 5/2/09. Sullivan S, Schanler R, Abrams S, et al: *A randomized controlled trial of human versus bovine-based human milk fortifier in extremely preterm infants*, Baltimore, Md., 2009, PAS Meetings.

weeks in those graduates from the NICU who had formerly received fortified human milk. At 16 and 25 weeks, the breastfed infants had lower BMC and BMC/bone width ratio, as well as serum phosphorus concentration and higher alkaline phosphate activity than the formula-fed group. These data suggest a need to carefully monitor this select group of VLBW infants for suboptimal bone accretion while receiving their mother's milk. However, human milk-based fortifier should solve this problem.[57]

Reduced bone mineralization is common in preterm infants and has been associated with growth stunting at 18 months of age and dietary insufficiency of calcium and phosphorus. Bishop et al.[16] evaluated 54 children at a mean age of 5 years who were born prematurely and had been part of a longitudinal dietary growth study. The diets included were either banked donor milk or preterm formula as a supplement to the mothers' own milk. Increased human milk intake was strongly associated with better BMC. Those children who had the greater proportion of human milk had greater BMC than children born at term. That is, supplementing with donor milk produced a better outcome at age 5 years than supplementing with infant formula, even though the nutrient content of formula was greater. The later skeletal growth and mineralization of an infant can be calculated and feeding adjusted to add necessary mineralization with human milk-based supplements.

Iron status has also been studied in LBW infants at 6 months' chronologic age. The incidence of iron deficiency was 86% in the breastfed group of LBW infants and only 33% in those receiving iron-fortified formula.[2] The breastfed group had significantly lower serum ferritin and hemoglobin values at 4 months of age. Abouelfettoh et al.[1] recommended that these special breastfed infants should receive iron from 2 months of age, because they were developed.

The AAP recommends that infants less than 1500 g birth weight receive 4 mg/kg/day of iron. There were no studies to test this until Taylor and Kennedy compared the effect of 2 mg/kg/day in a multivitamin on the hematocrit at 36 weeks' postmenstrual age. It was concluded that this iron therapy for infants under 1500 g at birth, in addition to dietary intake, did not improve the hematocrit or the number of transfusions required compared to the controls who received no additional iron.

The feeding of these special VLBW infants after discharge and for the next 6 to 9 months is an important consideration. Breastfeeding with added supplementation has been studied. Some important results came from a randomized, double-blind trial of the effect of supplementary standard formula feedings.[84] Growth and clinical status of infants receiving nutrient-enriched "postdischarge" formula were significantly affected, without vomiting, gas, or stool problems. The group receiving the enriched formula ingested volumes similar to those receiving regular formula.

A large multicenter follow-up study of more than 1000 ELBW infants who had extensive nutritional data collected was reported by Vohr et al.[136] Birth weight, gestational age, intraventricular hemorrhage status, sepsis, bronchopulmonary dysplasia, and hospital stay were similar between those never receiving human milk and those for whom variables of socioeconomic status, race, ethnicity, educational attainment, and parity were adjusted. Effects of human milk intake on mental and motor development were significantly positive. The impact of receiving 110 mL/kg/day of human milk was correlated with a 5-point increase on the Bayley scales. Human milk feedings affect scores even when donor milk is used, compared with term formula.[19]

Infants fed breast milk were found to have faster brainstem maturation, compared to those infants who received formula. This was determined by an analysis of the rate of maturation of the BAERs (auditory evoked response). Components of human milk improved cognitive and neurological outcomes in a series of studies on VLBW infants. Lack of breastfeeding was a major predictor of poor cognitive outcome in very preterm infants, compared to low social status and cerebral lesions by ultrasound.

The association of human milk feedings with a reduction in retinopathy of prematurity among VLBW infants compared to formula-fed infants, after adjusting for confounding variables, is significant. It can be considered as available intervention.

Box 15-12 lists recommendations modified from the work of Tsang et al.[123a] and Schanler and Hurst.

Antimicrobial Properties of Preterm Breast Milk

The infection-protective properties of human milk have been considered to be a key reason to provide human milk to high-risk infants who are prone to devastating infections such as NEC, sepsis, and meningitis and viral infections such as respiratory syncytial virus and rotavirus. The antimicrobial properties of milk produced by mothers who deliver preterm have been studied by several investigators.

The antiinfective factors in preterm human colostrum were studied by Mathur et al.,[95] who compared the colostrum values of a comparable group of postpartum mothers. The mean concentrations of IgA, lysozyme, and lactoferrin were significantly higher than in full-term colostrum. IgG and IgM were similar in both groups. The absolute counts of total cells, macrophages, lymphocytes, and neutrophils were significantly higher in preterm colostrum. The mean percentage of IgA in the premature colostrum was also significantly higher. The degree of prematurity had no effect, although the study group ranged in gestation from

---

> **BOX 15-12. Feeding Schedule for Human Milk in Low-Birth-Weight Infants**
>
> 1. Use refrigerated milk from the preterm infant's mother when it is available and has been collected within 48 hours of feeding.
> 2. When fresh milk is not available, use frozen human milk from the infant's mother. This milk should be provided in the sequence that it was collected to provide the greatest nutritional benefit.
> 3. When the preterm infant is tolerating human milk at greater than 100 mL/kg/day, supplementation using a human milk fortifier is started.
>   a. If it requires more than 1 week to reach 100 mL/kg/day intake, fortifier is added even though volume tolerance has not been achieved.
>   b. Milk volumes should increase to 150 but not exceed 200 mL/kg/day. Weight gain is optimally 15 g/kg/day and length increment 1 cm/wk. Urinary excretion of calcium should be less than 6 mg/kg/day and phosphorus greater than 4 mg/kg/day.
>   c. If weight gain is less than 15 g/kg/day, hind milk is used if mother's milk production exceeds the infant's requirements by 30%.
> 4. If the mother's milk supply is inadequate to meet her infant's feeding needs, an infant formula designed for preterm feeding is used as described.
> 5. Fortification of human milk is recommended until the infant is taking all feedings from the breast directly or weighs 1800 to 2000 g, depending on nursery policy on infant discharge weight. During the transition from feeding human milk by gavage or bottle and nipple to feeding at the breast, only those feedings given by gavage or bottle require fortification.
> 6. Multivitamin supplementation is started once feeding tolerance has been established. This supplementation varies depending on the composition of human milk fortifier.
> 7. Iron supplementation providing 2 mg/kg/day is started by the time the infant has doubled birth weight.

---

28 to 36 weeks (mean 33 ± 2.1 weeks), compared with the control infants, who were at 38 to 40 weeks (mean 39.1 ± 0.8 weeks). The colostrum of preterm mothers had an even greater potential for preventing infection than term colostrum and are an additional reason to begin early enteral feeds with human colostrum.[95] Table 15-14 lists the specific antiinfective components.

The cells of preterm milk were compared with those of term milk and found to be similar in number and in capacity to phagocytose and kill staphylococci.[108] The ability of the preterm cells to produce interferon on stimulation with mitogens was marginally better than that of term cells. The cells survived 24 hours refrigerated at 4°C (39.2°F);

TABLE 15-14	Comparison of Antiinfective Properties in Colostrum of Preterm Versus Term Mothers	
	Preterm Colostrum	**Term Colostrum**
Total protein (g/L)	0.43±1.3	0.31±0.05
IgA (mg/g protein)	310.5±70	168.2±21
IgG (mg/g protein)	7.6±3.9	8.4±1
IgM (mg/g protein)	39.6±23	36.1±16
Lysozyme (mg/g protein)	1.5±0.5	1.1±0.3
Lactoferrin (mg/g protein)	165±37	102±25
Total cells (mL^{-3})	6794±1946	3064±424
Macrophages	4041±1420	1597±303
Lymphocytes	1850±543	954±143
Neutrophils	842±404	512±178

Modified from Mathur NB, Dwarkadas AM, Sharma VK, et al.: Anti-infective factors in preterm human colostrum, *Acta Paediatr Scand* 79:1039, 1990.

at 48 hours, cell number, but not function, was reduced. Passing the milk through a feeding tube did not diminish the number or function of the cells. The levels of lactoferrin and lysozyme were greater in preterm milk than in term milk from the 2nd to 12th weeks postpartum.[49]

Secretory IgA is the predominant form of IgA, and values increased from the 6th to 12th weeks in preterm milk. The increase in IgA is not dependent on method of collection, rate of flow, or time of day, but the concentration varied inversely with the milk volume. Thus some investigators think that total production of IgA in 24 hours is comparable for the two groups.[26] Preterm infants (31 to 36 weeks' gestation) were fed human milk and compared with a matched group of premature infants fed infant formula. The serum levels of IgA at 9 to 13 weeks were higher in the human milk-fed infants.[121] Those infants who received at least 60% of their own mother's milk had higher IgA levels at 3 weeks of age than those receiving less than 30% of the feedings from their mother's milk.

Serum IgG levels were higher in the breast milk group, and serum IgM levels were similar in the two feeding groups. Samples of precolostrum collected from undelivered mothers were assayed and found to contain equal or greater amounts of IgA, IgG, IgM, lactoferrin, and lysozyme as mature colostrum.[79]

When the impact on actual prevention of infection among premature infants is reviewed, significantly less infection is found in infants receiving human milk compared with those receiving formula (9 of 32 receiving breast milk, 28.1%; 24 of 38 receiving formula, 63.3%). In a prospective evaluation of the antiinfective property of varying quantities of

expressed human milk for high-risk LBW infants, infections were found to be significantly less frequent in the groups that received human milk.[128] This has been documented for decades.

NEC is a major cause of morbidity and death in preterm and other high-risk infants. The absolute cause has eluded neonatologists, although many theories have been put forth and associations suggested[86] (Box 15-13). When researchers investigate its prevention, the role of human milk is prominent. In a large prospective multicenter study of 926 infants, 51 infants (5.5%) developed NEC. The mortality rate was 26% (Figure 15-8). In exclusively formula-fed infants, the incidence was 6 to 10

BOX 15-13. Issues and Risk Factors Associated with Enteral (Oral) Intake and the Causation of NEC

- Initiation of oral fluids too early
- Excessively rapid increases in volume or concentration of oral fluids
- Nutritional and nonnutritive sucking
- Hyperosmolar fluids
- Formula compared with human breast milk
- Feeding intolerance (cannot advance, residuals)
- Transpyloric compared with gastric gavage
- Bolus compared with continuous gavage
- Malabsorption of carbohydrates (lactose)—low luminal pH and ischemia
- Malabsorption of protein—low luminal pH
- Differences in gut bacterial or viral flora (epidemic NEC)
- Labile or inadequate gut blood flow (e.g., diving reflex, apnea, asphyxia)
- Increased work of gut muscle (increased oxygen consumption) because of gut motility

NEC, necrotizing enterocolitis.

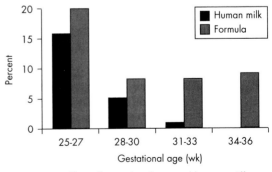

Figure 15-8. Effect of gestational age and human milk versus formula feeding on necrotizing enterocolitis (NEC). In infants fed formula, incidence of NEC decreases after 27 weeks and then remains the same. In infants fed human milk, incidence of NEC continues to decline. (From Lucas A, Cole TJ: Breast milk and neonatal necrotising enterocolitis, *Lancet* 336:1519, 1990.)

times more common than in those who received human milk exclusively. In those who received human milk and formula, it was three times more common than in the exclusively breastfed group. Pasteurization did not diminish the effect of human milk in these studies.[86,128] The comparison was more dramatic at more than 30 weeks' gestation, when formula-fed infants were 20 times more apt to develop NEC than human milk-fed infants. Early enteral feeding did not change the risk in those receiving breast milk, whereas delaying feedings of formula did lower the rate of NEC.[75] In a study of the prevention of NEC in LBW infants, with feedings higher in IgA and IgG, none of the infants in the study group or the breastfeeding comparison group developed NEC. Six cases developed among the 91 infants in the untreated group.[37]

It is notable that human milk also affects the incidence of other infections in the premature infant, including upper respiratory infections (Figure 15-9).

When stool colonization and incidence of sepsis in human milk-fed and formula-fed infants were studied in an intensive care nursery, a protective effect was seen against nosocomial sepsis, which was unrelated to GI flora. It was concluded that human milk feeding is associated with a significantly decreased incidence of nosocomially acquired sepsis that cannot be explained by the effect of human milk feeding on the GI flora. In a retrospective review of a group of premature infants fed fortified human milk, a 26% incidence of infection was seen. Those fed all formula had an infection rate of 49%.[87] Infants fed predominantly human milk (i.e., more than 50 mL/kg/day) had significantly less late-onset sepsis and NEC and shorter hospital stays compared with those receiving preterm formula. This dose of at least 50 mL/kg/day as protective was confirmed in another study.[47] The greater the dose of human milk, the greater the effect was.[102] A large multicenter study in Norway[118] reported that early feeding of extremely

premature infants with human milk and subsequent fortified human milk was associated with significantly less late-onset sepsis and improved survival. Probiotics for the prevention of NEC in preterm infants were subjected to a Cochrane Review. Milk feeding and bacterial growth play a role. Dietary supplements containing potentially beneficial bacteria reduce the occurrence of NEC and death in premature infants under 1500 g. However, this review did not find support for probiotics in infants under 1000 g at birth.

The impact of postnatal antibiotics on the preterm intestinal microbiome was studied in a group of premature infants between 24 and 31 weeks' gestation. They received at least 50% or more of breast milk per day and had received only 2 days of antibiotics or 7 days of antibiotics. The results showed that antibiotics disturbed the acquisition of bacteria in the gut.

Dysbiosis in the first week of life is related to later onset of NEC. Neuregulin-4 (NRG4) is an ErbB4-specific ligand that has been shown to help epithelial cells survive. Epithelial cell death is a major pathologic feature of NEC. Studies of ErbB4, which is found in the developing human intestine, as well as NRG4 (its receptor), which is found in human milk, suggest that NRG4-ErbB4 signaling may be a special pathway for therapeutic intervention to prevent NEC. Perhaps this explains the role of human milk.

An exclusively human milk-based diet is associated with a lower rate of NEC than a diet of human milk and bovine milk-based product. This was demonstrated by a multicentered study involving 207 infants.[130] A human milk diet with human milk-based fortification allows the neonatologist to feed premature infants on totally human milk, meeting nutritional needs and preventing NEC.

NEC has historically had a variable rate in nurseries but the etiology has remained elusive. Patel et al. developed an NEC QI initiative when their NEC rates went from 4% in 2005 to 2006 to

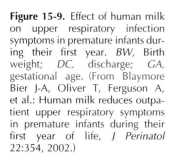

Figure 15-9. Effect of human milk on upper respiratory infection symptoms in premature infants during their first year. *BW,* Birth weight; *DC,* discharge; *GA,* gestational age. (From Blaymore Bier J-A, Oliver T, Ferguson A, et al.: Human milk reduces outpatient upper respiratory symptoms in premature infants during their first year of life, *J Perinatol* 22:354, 2002.)

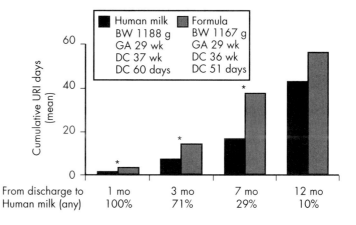

10% in 2007 to 2008. A change in feeding protocol had no effect. However, NEC rates did change significantly when nasogastric tube management was redesigned to include more frequent NG tube changes, as well as reeducation of parents about pump cleaning and storage. This project demonstrated the need for ongoing evaluation of routines and protocols.

Changing to an exclusively human milk diet for infants under 33 weeks' gestational age was tested to reduce the incidence of NEC. The diet was limited to the mother's milk and human milk-based fortifier and excluded any trace of bovine protein. It was compared to the incidence of NEC during the years that formula was used, and human milk was fortified with bovine-based supplements. It reduced the incidence of NEC from 3.4% down to 1%.[59]

When donor milk was compared to the mother's own milk, it provided no short-term advantage in infection rates over premature formula. The mother's own milk appears to protect the premature infant from infectious morbidity[58] (Table 15-15). Further investigation into pasteurization techniques is important. High-temperature short-time techniques appear to protect more infectious protection properties than the Holter technique.

In South Africa, where mothers remain with and help care for their premature babies, a study compared feeding an infant its own mother's milk with feeding pooled pasteurized breast milk. Birth weights were between 1000 and 1500 g. Babies who were not on ventilators began feedings by 96 hours of age. Weight gain was significantly greater using untreated mother's milk, both for regaining birth weight and reaching 1800 g sooner. Both SGA and AGA infants did better on their own mothers' milk. This diet decreased hospital stays and decreased hospital-acquired infection. The authors attribute the advantages to the milk being fed fresh, with early initiation of feeding at the breast, compared to the pasteurization of the bank milk.[127]

Kangaroo Care and Skin-to-Skin Care

Kangaroo care and skin-to-skin care are important constituents of the support program for milk production by mothers who are pumping to produce milk, without the benefit of the infant suckling at the breast. The conduction of heat from parent to infant is sufficiently high to compensate for the increase in evaporative and conductive heat loss.

Extensive studies have been carried out to substantiate not only the safety, but also the benefits of the skin-to-skin contact for fragile prematures, including microprematures, at 24 weeks' gestation. All the reports recommend initiation directly after birth, even when the infant requires ventilator care. Stability of heart rate, respirations, and oxygen saturation during skin-to-skin care is remarkably calm.[42] This technique was started initially in resource-poor countries but has been so effective in calming stabilizing infants that it has become universal. It is particularly effective when the mother is initiating breastfeeding and pumping to start milk production. The Kangaroo Mother Care (KMC) method is a standardized, protocol-based system for preterm and/or LBW infants. The cardiorespiratory instability seen in separated infants during the first hours is consistent with the mammalian "protest-despair" biology and with a hyperarousal and dissociation response.[11] The aim is to empower the mother (and father, if possible) by gradually transferring the skills and responsibility for becoming the child's primary caregiver. It has been formally organized internationally.[18,112] See Boxes 15-14 and 15-15.

Skin to skin has been evaluated by utilizing a number of measurements to demonstrate the physiologic benefits of this close contact with a parent for prematures. Measurements of salivary cortisol showed that the infant's cortisol reactivity decreased in response to handling. In addition, skin to skin improves the symmetry between the mother's and the infant's salivary cortisol levels.[103] It also helps

TABLE 15-15	Effects of Refrigeration Versus Freezing on Pasturized STHT Milk			
Component		Refrigerated	40°C Frozen	Pasteurized STHT
Vitamin C	40%			
Lysozyme	40%	20%	0-65%	20-40%
Lactoferrin	30%	NC	0-65%	0-85%
Lipase	25%		100%	
Secretory IgA	40%		20-50%	0-20%
Specific IgH	Variable	?		

STHT, Short time high temperature.

Modified with permission from Schanler RJ, Anderson D: The low-birth weight infant in patient care. In Duggan C, Watkins JB, Walker WA, editors: *Nutrition in pediatrics,* ed 4, Hamilton, 2008, BC Decker.

BOX 15-14. Kangaroo Mother Care

There is sufficient evidence to make the following general statements about KMC:

- The kangaroo position provides a neutral thermal environment that provides immature infants with optimal thermal regulation, which is the same or better than provided by an incubator.
- KMC enhances bonding and attachment, universal human needs that apply to all preterm and low-birth-weight infants, their parents, and families.
- Avoiding unwarranted mother-infant separation and initiating the kangaroo position as early as possible helps repair a bonding process that is disrupted by delivering a preterm or ill infant.
- KMC helps reduce maternal postpartum depression symptoms and increases parental sensitivity to infant cues.
- Initiation of KMC as soon as possible is essential for the establishment of breastfeeding and for increasing the duration of exclusive and any breastfeeding.
- KMC has positive effects on infant/parent psychological development and the development of mutual communication, understanding, and social recognition; reduces parenting stress; and contributes to an optimal family home environment.

KMC, Kangaroo Mother Care.

From Nyqvist KH, Anderson GC, Bergman N, et al.: Towards universal Kangaroo Mother Care: recommendations and report from the first European conference and Seventh International Workshop of Kangaroo Mother Care, *Acta Paediatr* 99:820, 2010.

BOX 15-15. Kangaroo Mother Care Principles

The following guiding principles should pervade all components in KMC protocols:

- All intrapartum and postnatal care should adhere to a paradigm of nonseparation of infants and their mothers/families.
- Preterm/low-birth-weight infants should be regarded as extero-gestational fetuses needing skin-to-skin contact to promote maturation.
- KMC should begin as soon as possible after birth and continue as often and for as long as appropriate (depending on circumstances).

KMC, Kangaroo Mother Care.

From Nyqvist KH, Anderson GC, Bergman N, et al.: Towards universal Kangaroo Mother Care: recommendations and report from the first European conference and Seventh International Workshop of Kangaroo Mother Care, *Acta Paediatr* 99:820, 2010.

allay the father's fears of spousal relationship problems, as he feels abandoned when the mother is totally consumed by the infant's needs. Breastfeeding was more common and more exclusive in the skin-to-skin group than in the control group at 1 and 4 months (all 18 dyads vs. 16 of 19).[103]

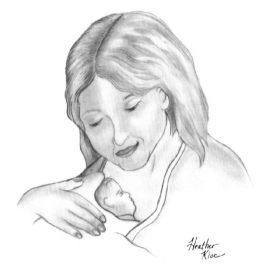

Figure 15-10. Kangaroo care method.

KANGAROO CARE

Kangaroo care was first introduced in 1979 in a hospital in Bogota, Colombia, because of a shortage of incubators, high death rate from infection, and abandonment of premature infants by their mothers. Since that time, many investigators have carefully evaluated kangaroo care and found it to be beneficial to mother and infant.[71] Dressed only in a diaper, an infant is held skin to skin against the mother's chest between her breasts, snug inside the mother's clothing, often for hours. The father can do the same. Many advantages have been noted, including more stable respirations, heart rates, and temperatures. The infants spend less time crying and more time in a quiet, alert state and deep sleep.[82] Some studies suggest better weight gain and earlier discharge. Hurst et al.[61] also reported an increase in milk volume during pumping (Figure 15-10).

Mothers who give kangaroo care breastfeed longer and more frequently. They also report greater confidence in caring for their fragile infant than those who experience traditional care.[6] NICU nurseries should encourage kangaroo care. All parents should be assisted in providing it whenever they are in the nursery to benefit both the mother and the infant. This skin-to-skin contact enhances milk production, especially when the infant is too immature to suckle.

Milk Production by Mothers of Premature Infants

The Committee on Nutrition at the AAP[28] published a handbook in 2014 that included a section on nutritional needs of LBW infants. They suggest that the mother's own milk and new special formulas for those babies who need breast milk substitutes are promising alternatives.

A joint effort of the AAP Committee on the Fetus and Newborn and the American College of Obstetricians and Gynecologists Committee on Obstetric Practice states that "human milk has a number of special features that make its use desirable in feeding preterm babies."[29]

The production of milk by a mother who is not actively nursing her infant, as is frequently the case in LBW infants and other neonates in NICUs, is a challenge to the resources of the NICU and the postpartum staff. Insufficient milk production is a common problem that becomes more critical as time passes. As production continues to drop, an infant's needs increase. Evaluation of various protocols has been undertaken by investigators who looked at onset of pumping postpartum, frequency of pumping, and duration in total minutes per day and length of time when no pumping occurred.

Hopkinson et al.[60] enrolled 32 healthy mothers, 19 of whom had no previous breastfeeding experience, into a study protocol. Their infants were 28 to 30 weeks' gestation. All of the mothers initiated pumping between days 2 and 6. The day of initiation was correlated with the volume of milk at 2 weeks, but not at 4 weeks, with mothers who had nursed previously and initiated pumping sooner. Parity, gravidity, age, and previous nursing experience were not correlated with volumes at 2 weeks. Parity and previous nursing experience were associated with milk volume at 4 weeks, with multiparas producing 60% greater volumes. The investigators found no significant relationship between 24-hour milk volume and frequency, duration, or maximal night interval. The change in milk volume from 2 to 4 weeks was correlated with frequency and duration of pumping but not to maximal night intervals. The range in number of pumpings per day was four to nine. The authors[60] concluded that optimal milk production occurs with at least five expressions per day and pumping durations that exceed 100 min/day.

The frequency of milk expression was evaluated by de Carvalho et al.[32] in a crossover design study of 25 mothers who delivered at 28 to 37 weeks' gestation. Frequent expression of milk was significantly associated with greater milk production (342 ± 229 mL) than with infrequent expression (221 ± 141 mL). They compared three or fewer pumpings per day to four or more. The mean numbers were 2.4 versus 5.7, neither equaling the frequency that a mother would usually feed her infant in the first few weeks.

Minimum frequency and duration figures have been provided. However, it is advisable to increase the frequency of pumping as the need to raise production increases and as the time for discharge and feeding the infant exclusively at the breast approaches. Consideration for increasing nighttime pumpings is also important as discharge approaches. Some mothers experience a dread of the pump when demands are increased for "more milk production." The management of the mother producing milk for her hospitalized infant should be coordinated by a neonatologist and a primary care physician. She should be assisted by a primary care nurse and the unit's lactation coordinator and lactation consultants to maximize support and minimize stress.

Peer counselors have become important members of the lactation support teams in the NICU, as they have been in birth centers and in the community. Peer support was originated by the LaLeche League. Anthropologist Dana Raphael coined the expression "a friend from across the street." Health departments and WIC programs have developed peer counselor programs, where women (peers) with breastfeeding experience are trained to provide support and counsel but not practice medicine.[114] Very successful programs have been developed in NICUs. A combination of a lactation consultant and a peer counselor provides the most effective breastfeeding support in the NICU[100] (see Figure 15-11 and Chapter 22).

The NICU at Rush University Medical Center developed a lactation support program that included peer counselors who were former NICU parents.[120] They work directly with NICU mothers and babies, in collaboration with the NICU nurses, to promote successful breastfeeding. The health care providers in a study of 17 university NICUs thought the peer counselors improved the care of the infants by empowering the mothers to provide milk and modeling good infant care for the mothers.

When the physiology of lactation is applied to the practical management of inducing milk supply without the benefit of an infant's participation, it is apparent that mimicking natural breastfeeding is more effective. The breast can be prepared with massage and manual expression. Although some women succeed with manual expression alone, it is rare, and a good pump should be recommended. None of the hand pumps can truly duplicate the milking action of the infant, and all are essentially vacuum extractors. They should be used only as a stopgap measure when the electric pump is unavailable (see Chapter 21). A pump that can be used on both breasts simultaneously saves time and generates higher levels of prolactin. These pumps also generate a greater total milk volume than pumping each breast separately for the same length of

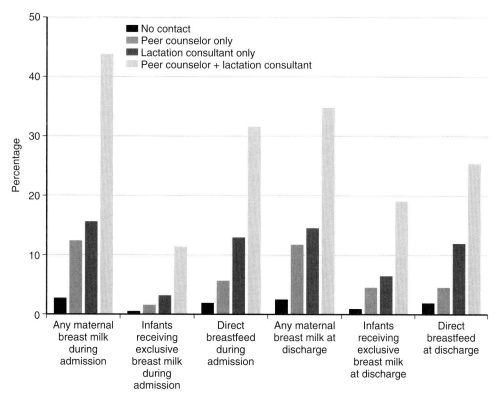

Figure 15-11. Breastfeeding outcomes during hospital stay by lactation staff type. χ^2 tests for overall differences within each outcome were significant at $p < 0.001$. Breastfeeding outcomes were classified as any maternal breast milk (infant receiving *any* maternal breast milk via direct breastfeeding and/or pumping regardless of supplementation with formula), *exclusive* breast milk (infant receiving exclusive maternal milk via direct breastfeeding and/or pumping without any formula supplementation), and any direct breastfeeding during NICU admission and at discharge (infant fed directly at the breast for at least one feeding with or without subsequent formula supplementation) during NICU admission and at discharge. Estimates do not include exclusive donor milk. (From Oza-Frank R, Bhatia A, Smith C: Combined peer counselor and lactation consultant support increases breastfeeding in the NICU, *Breastfeed Med* 8:509, 2013.)

time.[103] Subsequent studies have produced variable observations. Groh-Wargo et al.[52] studied 32 women who were randomly assigned to single or double pumping for 6 weeks. No difference was found in prolactin levels or total volume of milk produced by these investigations, although the time-saving effect was considered important.

Jones et al.[69] reported a randomized, controlled trial that was designed to compare methods of milk expression after preterm delivery. It involved 36 women: 19 used simultaneous pumping and 17 used sequential pumping by random assignment. A crossover design was used to evaluate the effect of breast massage on milk volume and fat content (estimated by creamatocrit). The authors reported that the results were unequivocal, showing that pumping both breasts simultaneously produced more milk—125.1 g with massage and 87.7 g without. This was compared with sequential volumes of 78.7 g with massage and 51.3 g without.

Pumping should be initiated as soon as a mother's condition permits. Offering this opportunity to the mother should be part of the supportive care offered by postpartum staff. All the points of preparation for pumping should be included: comfortable position, tranquil atmosphere, preparation of the breast with gentle stroking and warmth, massage during pumping, confidence, and reassurance from the staff. The obstetrician is in an important position to initiate the offer to pump, because he or she should know whether or not the mother intends to breastfeed from conversations during the mother's prenatal care. The mother may not know it is appropriate to ask for a pump. Providing knowledgeable, accurate, consistent, and sensitive support should be the rule in every perinatal center, especially for mothers of high-risk infants who choose to breastfeed.[100,103] The opportunity to pump should be offered to all women, regardless of previous feeding choice. Often a mother changes her mind when her infant is high risk and would receive many additional benefits from her milk.

Providing an appropriate room for pumping after the mother has been discharged is critical to individual success and is an expression of commitment to breastfeeding by the NICU. This room should be clean, bright, and cheerful and accommodate more than one mother and companion at a time, unless several rooms are available. It should have a sink for washing hands and storage for equipment and supplies. A nurse call button or other alarm system is also essential. Additional features are soft music, a telephone, and reading material. The hospital should have a supply of approved electric pumps and individual disposable attachment packets for each mother. A place should be available to store her properly labeled and dated milk in a freezer or refrigerator. Sterile storage containers should be readily available.

A mother should be encouraged to rent a pump for home use and around-the-clock pumping. These are available from medical supply stores, pharmacies, home care services, hospitals, and some lactation consultants. Insurance companies reimburse for the cost of the rental when the milk is prescribed for a high-risk infant. A neonatologist can provide an appropriate letter of support. The hospital support staff who are coordinating the mother's care or the NICU staff should be sure that the mother understands how to use the equipment effectively. Ideally, NICUs have at least one staff member who is a licensed, certified lactation consultant who will coordinate this effort under the direction of the obstetrician, pediatrician, and neonatologist. One lactation consultant per 15 infants in the NICU is ideal. The mother should not be subjected to pressures of pump equipment entrepreneurs and unsolicited advice. The best remedy is for the NICU to provide on-staff, up-to-date experience and support to the mother in her efforts to provide milk and breastfeed her high-risk infant. Box 15-16 outlines key strategies for successful

> **BOX 15-16. Guidelines for Initiating Milk Supply Without Infant Suckling**
>
> 1. Begin as soon after delivery as maternal condition permits.
> 2. Initiate use of electric pump while in hospital.
> 3. Begin slowly, increasing time over first week.
> 4. Pump on more regular basis as soon as engorgement is evident.
> 5. Pump at least five times in 24 hours.
> 6. Allow a rest period for uninterrupted sleep of at least 6 hours.
> 7. Pump a total of at least 100 min/day.
> 8. Use "double" pump to pump both breasts simultaneously, which can cut total time proportionately.
> 9. Prepare breast with warm soaks, gentle stroking, and light massage to maximize production of milk.
> 10. Encourage skin-to-skin care (kangaroo care).

pumping when an infant is unable to suckle the breast. All neonatal nurses should be familiar with the available pumps and their use and be supportive of mothers who are pumping.[100]

Who Produces Milk for LBW or SGA Infants?

Nationwide, mothers who give birth to infants who are admitted to special care nurseries are less likely to initiate lactation than mothers of healthy term infants, according to Meier.[97] The profile of mothers who give birth to these high-risk infants includes a higher percentage of low-income, low-education, young mothers, who do not breastfeed in great numbers. Postpartum and NICU staff should work to encourage these women to initiate lactation.

Maternal choice to breastfeed or provide milk for an LBW infant is influenced by many factors beyond those that affect most feeding decisions of normal full-term infants.[92] Lucas et al.[88,89] sought to answer two major questions in a study of 925 mother-infant pairs in five hospitals. Do health care professionals in neonatal units exert a major influence on a mother's feeding preference and availability of her milk for her infant? Are there population differences between mothers who do and do not provide their milk? In this study of five centers, the demographic characteristics of the mother were important, not those of the staff. This study did not look at success rates, however.

Mothers in a study by Verronen[135] had delivered infants at a mean of 31 weeks' gestation; the infants weighed less than 1850 g with a mean of 1370 g. More educated mothers provided their milk (98%) than uneducated (40%). Factors of higher socioeconomic class, lower parity or fewer living children, being married, and being older than 20 years of age were associated with providing milk. Boys were more apt to receive mother's milk, as shown in other studies. Birth weight and extreme immaturity were not a determinant, nor was transfer of the infant to another center. The Rush Mother's Milk Club, which is a breastfeeding intervention for mothers of VLBW infants in Chicago, was developed and directed by Meier and colleagues.[98,99] In the 52-bed urban NICU, the staff provided facilitated learning. Transportation was provided for mothers from home, as well as a weekly interactive social luncheon. They employ five peer counselors and provide a 24-hour, toll-free pager information line. The peer counselors also contact mothers at home. Low milk supply is aggressively managed with record keeping, encouragement, and counseling. The lactation initiation rate among these predominantly low-income African-American women was

72.9%. Exclusive mother's milk was attained by 57.2% and some mother's milk by 72.5%.[101] Skin-to-skin and kangaroo care are important features of this program and many others.[91]

Feeding the Near-Term Infant (35 to 37 Weeks' Gestation) at the Breast

Near-term infants (i.e., 35 0/7 weeks to 36 6/7 weeks) may be nursed at the breast if otherwise stable. Breastfeeding should be initiated by one hour of age if mother and infant are stable. Health care professionals should monitor to ensure that frequent ongoing feedings are occurring "on demand" at least 10-12 times a day. Communication among staff and with the parents is key to success. Involvement of lactation-trained staff who are also skilled neonatal nurses mitigates confusion and conflicting messages to the family. Particular care should be given to assist a mother in getting the infant to suckle, especially if the breast and nipples are large or engorged.[107,110] Weight should be followed closely to prevent excessive weight loss. Infants who receive sugar water and formula supplements lose more weight than those who are nursed frequently at the breast without supplementation. If breastfeeding is going well, the infant could be discharged with the mother from the hospital as soon as the infant begins to gain substantially, with close follow-up at home. Poor weight gain, less than 20 g/day, is usually the result of inadequate intake. Average weight gain should be 26 to 31 g/day (see Appendix J). A mother may need to pump between feedings if the infant does not stimulate the breasts adequately. The milk can be provided by cup or lactation aide device (see Appendix J and Figure 14-10). Difficulties with latch should be investigated with a careful examination of the infant's mouth and the mother's breast and nipples. Before discharge, the physician, as well as the nurse, should observe the dyad.[116] If a mother is a low producer, galactagogues can be considered. (See Chapter 11 and Protocol #9 in Appendix J.) Follow-up should include frequent weighings and growth measurements (length and head circumference should increase approximately 0.5 cm/wk). Home visits or office checks are crucial to monitor progress. An extensive review of practice guidelines for the care of the late preterm infant has been prepared by the National Perinatal Association.

Premature Infants of 28 6/7 Weeks to 32 6/7 Weeks

Infants of gestational age more than 28 weeks but less than 35 weeks are frequently breastfed in

NICUs, because the value of human milk has been recognized by most neonatologists.

Feeding at the breast when an infant is less than 1500 g is considered too strenuous by many neonatologists, even though it has been proved that it takes less energy and less impact on vital signs to breastfeed than bottle feed.[81] When the feeding of infants of less than 1500 g was examined, however, the growth of those fed at the breast was comparable with that of matched control infants fed expressed human milk by bottle.[69] Breastfeeding was started when sucking movements were observed. Initially, they received supplementary human milk by tube plus 800 units of vitamin D and 60 mg of vitamin C daily. Unrestricted visiting of parents to the neonatal unit, an optimistic and knowledgeable attitude of the nursing staff toward breastfeeding, and the avoidance of a bottle for the infants are important to success.[93,94] Encouraging the expression of milk by the mothers early in the postpartum period is essential. The main deterrent to successful breastfeeding was lack of maternal interest and commitment.

Blaymore Bier et al.[17] undertook a clinical study of breast feeding and bottle feedings in ELBW infants (birth weight 800 g or less) when they were considered ready to bottle feed. This was at a mean age of 35 weeks since conception (corrected gestational age). One breastfeeding and one bottle feeding were monitored each day for 10 days. Prefeeding and postfeeding weights, oxygen saturation, respiratory and heart rates, and axillary temperature were recorded. Higher oxygen saturation and higher temperatures during breastfeeding and less likelihood of desaturation below 90% were noted in the breastfed infants. The weights reflecting intake were higher in the bottle-fed infants. The authors concluded that it was physiologically safe and less stressful for infants to breastfeed. The lower intake requires monitoring, however.[17]

The ontogenic and temporal organization of nonnutritive sucking during active sleep was studied by Hack et al.[55] in preterm infants. One of the six infants studied had recognizable rhythmic sucking bursts at 28 weeks, and all had bursts by 31 to 32 weeks. The number of bursts increased and the interval between bursts decreased as the infants matured, with the earliest indications of intrinsic rhythm beginning at 30 weeks.

Nonnutritive sucking has become a subject of controversy in NICUs. Allowing premature infants to suck on a pacifier during gavage feedings was initially reported to be associated with increased weight gain and shorter hospitalization. When nutrient intake and other parameters were controlled, however, no advantages to nonnutritive sucking were observed in somatic growth, serum proteins, energy absorption, or feeding tolerance, nor was any increase in tropic hormones or growth promoters seen.[33,40,93] Infants have been observed to have transcutaneous oxygen saturation measurements increase by 3% to 4% during nonnutritive sucking.[32] Nonnutritive sucking does not appear to carry risk for infants destined for further bottle feeding. However, it should be avoided for infants destined to breastfeed, in order to avoid interference with normal sucking. Unfortunately, most studies have been done with bottles.[35]

Of greater significance is the value of having these infants placed at the "emptied" breast during gavage tube feedings. When Narayanan et al.[109] studied this practice, they found no change in weight gain or length of hospital stay. The practice did, however, result in more successful and longer duration of breastfeeding after discharge. This technique was originally designed in our nursery to improve the mother's milk production and encourage mothers who were becoming discouraged. As the infant matures and begins swallowing with sucking, it becomes unnecessary to pump the breast "empty" before presenting it to the infant. This is because any milk provided could be suckled and swallowed. Suckling at the breast initiates a peristaltic action that also triggers swallowing and the physiologic response of the entire GI tract (see Chapter 8). Suckling the breast also improves the mother's success when pumping. Readiness to wean from tube feedings to oral feeding is poorly defined and based on observations utilizing a bottle and/or a pacifier. Stable cardiopulmonary status at 33 to 34 weeks is associated with sucking patterns that resemble term infants (i.e., rhythmic alteration of suction and expression and the positive pressure generated by compression). Mature sucking pattern is not necessary for safe, successful feeding at the breast.[76] Infants can feed orally without suction. The undulating motion of the tongue does trigger let-down and the swallowing of fluid. An infant's behavioral state and organization during feeding, as well as the nursery environment (especially light and sound), and a caretaker's approach to oral feeding all affect an infant's performance.[76] This is another point supportive of early breastfeeding. Avoidance of bottles during the establishment of breastfeeding in premature infants has been evaluated in a Cochrane Review.[27] Small premature infants begin with tube feedings of their mother's milk. As they mature, they have breastfeedings added. But in many nurseries, the bottle with the mother's milk is introduced. Its impact on successful breastfeeding is challenged. Five studies of 543 infants were included in a Cochrane Review by Collins et al.[27] Four of the studies substituted cup feeding when mother was not available to breastfeed. The cup feedings increased the probability of successful breastfeeding and continuation of breastfeeding. Cup feedings, however, prolonged hospitalizations by 10 days. Noncompliance was

an issue as well. A study in Egypt, after this review, reported 30 cup-fed premature infants compared with 30 bottle-fed infants who were breastfed on discharge because mothers did not provide their milk or breastfeed before discharge. The cup-fed infants breastfed for longer durations and in greater numbers.[1] The crucial role of adequate nutrition to brain growth, especially in the premature infant, is generally acknowledged. Although nutrition may not overcome all the problems of extreme prematurity and its impact on the immature brain, it does reduce infections and NEC and has immunomodulatory properties when it includes over 50% human milk. The impact of human milk constituents on the white matter and its development is remarkable. This is being attributed to the gut-immune brain axis.[71] The nutritional adjustments to use human milk and human milk supplements are considered safe, inexpensive, cause few side effects, and are easily implemented.

Breastfeeding the Extremely Premature Infant

Evaluations of feeding strategies are rarely conducted or published, in spite of rigid protocols in some nurseries. Early initiation of feedings has been thought valuable and safe. In a study of 171 premature infants between 26 and 30 weeks' gestation, Schanler et al.[124] tested the validity of GI priming and continuous infusion, versus intermittent bolus tube feeding with human milk or preterm formula. Infants were randomized to four treatment combinations in a balanced two-way design. Investigators compared the presence or absence of GI priming for 10 days and continuous infusion versus intermittent bolus tube feeding. Time to full feeding was similar in all groups. GI priming had no adverse effects and improved calcium/phosphorus retention and shorter intentional transient times. Bolus feeding was associated with less feeding intolerance and greater weight gain than the continuous method. The more human milk fed, the lower the morbidity rate was. The authors concluded that early GI priming with human milk and bolus feedings provided the best advantage for premature infants. Very preterm infants, born at 26 to 31 weeks' gestation, have the capacity for the early development of oral motor competence that is sufficient for establishment of full breastfeeding at a low postmenstrual age, according to Nyqvist.[112] Using the Preterm Infant Breastfeeding Behavior Scale (Table 15-16), designed for use by mothers and professionals to observe levels of competence in oral motor behavior during breastfeeding, the author studied 15 infants born at 26 to 31 weeks'

TABLE 15-16   The Preterm Infant Breastfeeding Behavior Scale (PIBBS)

Scale Items	Levels of Competence
Rooting	Did not root
	Showed some rooting behavior (mouth opening, tongue extension, hand-to-mouth/face movements, head turning)
	Showed obvious rooting behavior (simultaneous mouth opening and head turning)
Areolar grasp (how much of the breast was inside the baby's mouth)	None, the mouth only touched the nipple
	Part of the nipple
	The whole nipple, not the areola
	The nipple and some of the areola
Latched on and fixed to the breast	Did not latch on at all so the mother felt it
	Latched on for <1 min
	Latched on for 1-15 min or more, recorded by marking a cross along a line graded 1-15 min
Sucking	No sucking or licking
	Licking and tasting, but no sucking
	Single sucks, occasional short sucking bursts (2-9 sucks)
	Repeated (2 or more consecutive) short sucking bursts, occasional long bursts (10 sucks or more before a pause)
	Repeated long sucking bursts
Longest sucking bursts	Maximum number of consecutive sucks, recorded by marking a cross along a line graded 1-30
Swallowing	Swallowing was not noticed
	Occasional swallowing was noticed

From Nyqvist KH: Early attainment of breastfeeding competence in very preterm infants, *Acta Paediatr* 97:776, 2008, p 778, Figure 1.

gestational age. The author made daily assessments. Semidemand feeding was utilized with a prescribed total daily income volume. Breastfeeding was initiated at 29 weeks. Rooting, efficient areolar grasp, and repeated short sucking bursts were noted at 29 weeks. At 31 weeks, long sucking bursts and repeated swallowing were observed. Sucking rates ranged from 5 to 24 with a median of 17. Full breastfeeding was reached between 32 and 38 weeks with a median of 35 weeks. Weight gain was described as adequate. Alternative techniques were described in a report from a nursery in Brazil,[31] in which they placed infants in groups trying techniques of relactation, translactation, and breast-orogastric tubes. They described 432 infants who, at discharge, were breastfeeding 85%, 100%, and 100% in each group, respectively. All attained good weight gain, with only 1.6% feeding-related problems. The definition of relactation and translactation resembles other nurseries' use of lactation aide devices for additional nutrition.

Transpyloric tube feeding in VLBW infants with suspected gastroesophageal reflux has been used successfully by Malcolm et al.[92] They described 72 VLBW infants with a median birth weight of 870 g (a range of 365 to 1435 g) and a gestational age of 26 weeks (range 23 to 31 weeks) who received transpyloric feedings. They observed a reduction in apneic episodes and a decrease in bradycardia. Five infants developed NEC, none of

whom were receiving human milk. The authors concluded that transpyloric feedings, when limited to human milk, may safely reduce episodes of apnea and bradycardia in preterm infants suspected of gastroesophageal reflux. They suggest confirmation of this work in other NICUs, with the potential of changing hospital procedures.

SGA Infants

Infants who are below the 10th percentile (or 2 SDs) in weight for their gestational age are termed *SGA*. These infants may also be shorter in length and have smaller heads, depending on when in gestational life the insult to their growth occurred. The more general the growth failure is, the earlier the intrauterine effect appears. For example, rubella in the first trimester causes total growth retardation, whereas hypertension in the mother in the third trimester predominantly affects weight. The more profound the growth retardation is, the more difficult the nutritional problems are.

SGA infants are prone to be hypocalcemic; however, if they can be provided with adequate breast milk early, this complication may be avoided. This is because the calcium/phosphorus ratio is more physiologic in human milk than formula. Other problems, including hypothermia and hypoglycemia, which lead to a vicious circle of acidosis and associated problems, can be triggered by

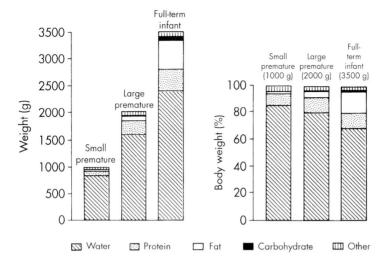

Figure 15-13. Absolute and relative body composition of infants weighing 1000, 2000, and 3500 g at birth. (From Heird WC, Anderson TL: Nutritional requirements and methods of feeding low-birth-weight infants. In Gluck L et al., editors: *Current problems in pediatrics*, vol. 7, no. 8, Chicago, 1977, Year Book.)

a large volume of milk by pumping. It can be done, however, with supportive counseling by staff and the initiation of kangaroo care. Milk volumes usually increase when an infant begins to actually breastfeed, not unlike relactation (see Chapter 19) or increasing milk volume in other situations (see Chapter 8).

When nipple feeding is possible, an infant can be put to the breast. It requires less energy to suckle at the breast than to feed from a bottle. The peristaltic motion of the tongue, which is the normal innate suckling mode, initiates the peristaltic motion of the GI tract and triggers the swallow. If no pacifiers or rubber nipples have been given, an infant may be able to suckle at the breast well before he reaches 1500 g. Figure 19-3 illustrates an infant who first nursed at 1100 g. If little or no breastfeeding has been done in the hospital and the mother has been unable to pump enough to sustain the daily needs, then an infant may be frustrated at the breast when sent home from the hospital unless intervention is provided.

One can see that the reserves of premature infants are limited if one studies the absolute and relative body compositions of infants at birth (Figure 15-13). If one considers how little time it takes to starve a premature infant compared with a full-term infant, the risks of starving a premature infant while the infant adapts to nursing at the breast are real[126] (Figure 15-14). The solution to the problem is to provide nourishment while the infant stimulates maternal milk production by suckling at the breast. A piece of equipment called a nursing supplementer provides this setup very effectively (see Figure 19-4). It was developed to provide nourishment for an adopted infant who is being nursed by a mother who has not been pregnant or has never lactated. It sustains the infant while the mother's milk supply develops (see

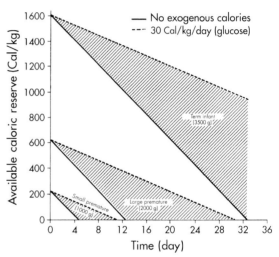

Figure 15-14. Estimated survival of starved and semistarved infants weighing 1000, 2000, and 3500 g at birth. (From Heird WC, Anderson TL: Nutritional requirements and methods of feeding low-birth-weight infants. In Gluck L et al., editors: *Current problems in pediatrics*, vol. 7, no. 8, Chicago, 1977, Year Book.)

Chapter 19). The same effect can be provided for premature or sick infants who have not nursed at the breast since birth and need nourishment while the mothers' supply develops, even though she has been pumping.

The infant can continue to gain weight while stimulating the breast if a supplementer is used. The volume required from the nursing supplementer drops continually in a week or so. Occasional infants require the supplementer for a month. The mother should continue to pump after breastfeedings until her volume increases.

The nursing supplementer provides a simple means of ensuring adequate nourishment while adapting to the breast. It is preferable to using

TABLE 15-17	Postdischarge Nutritional Screening Assessment
	Action Values
Growth	
Weight gain	<20 g/day
Length growth	<0.5 cm/wk
Head circumference	<0.5 cm/wk
Biochemical test	
Phosphorus	<4.5 mg/dL
Alkaline phosphatase	>450 IU/L
Urea nitrogen	<5 mg/dL

IU, International units.

Modified from Hall, RT: Nutritional follow-up of the breastfeeding premature infant after hospital discharge, *Pediatr Clin North Am* 48:435, 2001.

supplemental bottles because the infant is not confused by the rubber nipple, which requires a different mechanism of sucking than the human nipple. Furthermore, the suckling of the breast provides the continued stimulus necessary for increasing milk production. Cup feeding is an alternative to the bottle if the infant needs additional nourishment.

The parameters that are to be met before discharge home from the hospital include sustained weight gain, growth in length and head circumference, and stable biochemical parameters[49] (Table 15-17). After discharge from the hospital, these same parameters should be met. If faltering is persistent, fortifying breastfeeding may be indicated. This can be accomplished without interfering with the breastfeeding process again by using a lactation supplementer containing enriched breast milk that had been previously pumped or donor milk, which is preferable to formula.

Posthospitalization breastfeeding patterns of moderately preterm infants (30 to 35 weeks) were studied by Wooldridge and Hall[138] using daily feeding diaries in 55 women for the first month after discharge. Those women who were able to exclusively breastfeed before the end of the first week at home were able to maintain their supply. In general, those women who did not have an adequate supply during the first week were unlikely to achieve it by week 4. The proportion of breastfeeds increased during the 4 weeks of observation, but only 56% achieved exclusive breastfeeds by 4 weeks in this study. Proper preparation prior to discharge and adequate support at home assures success.

REFERENCES

1. Abouelfettoh AM, Dowling DA, Elguindy SR, et al: Cup versus bottle feeding for hospitalized late preterm infants in Egypt: a quasi-experimental study, *Neonatal Intensive Care* 22:33–38, 2009.
2. Abrahms SA, Schanler RJ, Garza C: Bone mineralization in former very low birth weight infants fed either human milk or commercial formula, *J Pediatr* 112:956, 1988.
3. Alfaleh K, Anabrees J: Probiotics for prevention of necrotizing enterocolitis in preterm infants (review), *Cochrane Libr* (4)2014.
4. American Academy of Pediatrics, Section on Breastfeeding: Breastfeeding and the use of human milk, *Pediatrics* 129:e527–e544, 2012.
5. Anderson DM, William FH, Merkatz RB, et al: Length of gestation and nutritional composition of human milk, *Am J Clin Nutr* 37:810, 1983.
6. Anderson GC: Touch and the kangaroo care method. In Field TM, editor: *Touch in early development*, Mahwah, N.J., 1995, Erlbaum Associates.
7. Arslanoglu S, Moro GE, Ziegler EE: Preterm infants fed fortified human milk receive less protein than they need, *J Perinatol* 29:489–492, 2009.
8. Atkinson SA, Anderson GH, Bryan MH: Human milk: comparison of the nitrogen composition in milk from mothers of premature and full-term infants, *Am J Clin Nutr* 33:811, 1980.
9. Atkinson SA, Radde IC, Chance GW, et al: Macromineral content of milk obtained during early lactation from mothers of premature infants, *Early Hum Dev* 4:5, 1980.
10. Beijers RJW, Graaf FVD, Schaafsma A, et al: Composition of premature breast milk during lactation: constant digestible protein content (as in full term milk), *Early Hum Dev* 29:351, 1992.
11. Bergman NJ, Linley LL, Faucus SR: Randomized controlled trial of skin-to-skin contact from birth versus conventional incubator for physiological stabilization in 1200 to 2199 gram newborns, *Acta Paediatr* 93:779–785, 2004.
12. Berseth CL: Gastrointestinal motility in the neonate, *Clin Perinatol* 23:179, 1996.
13. Bigger HR, Fogg LJ, Patel A, et al: Quality indicators for human milk use in very low-birthweight infants; are we measuring what we should be measuring? *J Perinatol* 34:287–291, 2014.
14. Billeaud C, Senterre J, Rigo J: Osmolality of the gastric and duodenal contents in low birth weight infants fed human milk or various formulae, *Acta Paediatr Scand* 71:799, 1982.
15. Birch DG, Birch EE, Hoffman DR, et al: Retinal development in very-low-birth-weight infants fed diets differing in omega-3 fatty acids, *Invest Ophthalmol Vis Sci* 33:2365, 1992.
16. Bishop NJ, Dahlenburg SL, Fewtrell MS, et al: Early diet of preterm infants and bone mineralization at age five years, *Acta Paediatr* 85:230, 1996.
17. Blaymore Bier JA, Oliver T, Ferguson AE, et al: Human milk improves cognitive and motor development of premature infants during infancy, *J Hum Lact* 18:361, 2002.
18. Blomqvist YT, Ewald V, Grandin M, et al: Initiation and extent of skin-to-skin at two Swedish neonatal intensive care units, *Acta Paediatr* 102:22–28, 2013.
19. Boyd CA, Quigley MA, Brocklehurst P: Donor breast milk versus infant formula for preterm infants: a systematic review and meta analysis, *Arch Dis Child Fetal Neonatal Ed* 92:F169, 2006.
20. Brownell EA, Lussier MM, Hagadorn JI, et al: Independent predictors of human milk receipt at NICU discharge, *Am J Perinatol* 31(10):891–898, 2014.
21. Brumberg H, LaGamma EF: Perspectives on nutrition: enhance outcomes for premature infants, *Pediatr Ann* 32 (9):617, 2003.
22. Carey DE, Rowe JC, Goetz CA, et al: Growth and phosphorus metabolism in premature infants fed human milk, fortified human milk, or special premature formula, *Am J Dis Child* 141:511, 1987.

23. Cavell B: Gastric emptying in preterm infants, *Acta Paediatr Scand* 68:725, 1979.

24. Chan GM: Effects of powdered human milk fortifiers on anti bacterial actions of human milk, *J Perinatol* 23:620–623, 2002.

25. Chan GM, Lee ML, Rechtman DJ: Effects of a human milk-derived human milk fortifier on the antibacterial actions of human milk, *Breastfeed Med* 2(2):205–208, 2007.

26. Chandra RK: Immunoglobulin and protein levels in breast milk produced by mothers of preterm infants, *Nutr Res* 2:27, 1982.

27. Collins CT, Makrides M, Gillis J, et al: Avoidance of bottles during the establishment of breastfeeds in preterm infants, *Cochrane Database Syst Rev* 1, 2004.

28. Committee on Nutrition, American Academy of Pediatrics: Nutritional needs of the preterm infant, *Pediatric nutrition handbook*, ed 7, Elk Grove, Ill., 2014, American Academy of Pediatrics.

29. Committee on Obstetric Practice, American College of Obstetricians and Gynecologists, Committee on the Fetus and Newborn, et al: *Guidelines for perinatal care*, ed 4, Elk Grove, Ill., 2007, American Academy of Pediatrics.

30. Davey AM, Wagner CL, Phelps DL, et al: Do premature infants with umbilical artery catheters tolerate oral feeds? *Pediatr Res* 31:199A, 1992.

31. de Aquino RR, Osorio MM: Relactation, translactation and breast-orogastric tube as transition methods in feeding preterm babies, *J Hum Lact* 25:420, 2009.

32. de Carvalho M, Anderson DM, Giangreco A, et al: Frequency of milk expression and milk production by mothers of non-nursing premature neonates, *Am J Dis Child* 139:483–485, 1985.

33. DeCurtis M, McIntosh N, Ventura V, et al: Effect of non-nutritive suckling on nutrient retention in preterm infants, *J Pediatr* 109:888, 1986.

34. Domany KA, Mandel D, Kedem MH, et al: Breast milk fat content of mothers to small-for-gestational-age infants, *J Perinatol* 34:1–3, 2014.

35. Dowling (deMonterice) D: Physiologic responses of breastfeeding and bottle feeding, *Nurs Res* 48:78, 1999.

36. Edmond K, Bahl R: *Optimal feeding of low-birth-weight infants: technical review*, Geneva, 2006, WHO Library.

37. Eibl MM, Wolf HM, Furnkranz H, et al: Prevention of necrotizing enterocolitis in low-birth-weight infants by IgA-IgG feeding, *N Engl J Med* 319:1, 1988.

38. Eidelmann AI, Hoffman NW, Kaitz M: Cognitive deficits in women after childbirth, *Obstet Gynecol* 81:764, 1993.

39. El-Mohaneles AE, Picard MB, Simmens SJ, et al: Use of human milk in the intensive care nursery decreases the incidence of nosocomial sepsis, *J Perinatol* 17:130, 1997.

40. Ernst JA, Rickard KA, Neal PR, et al: Lack of improved growth outcome related to non-nutritive sucking in very low birth weight premature infants fed a controlled nutrient, *Pediatrics* 83:706, 1989.

41. Feldman R, Eidelman AI: Direct and indirect effects of breast milk on the neurobehavioral and cognitive development of premature infants, *Dev Psychobiol* 43:109, 2003.

42. Fischer CB, Sontheimer D, Scheffer F, et al: Cardiorespiratory stability of premature boys and girls during kangaroo care, *Early Hum Dev* 52:145–153, 1998.

43. Forbes GB: Nutritional adequacy of human breast milk for premature infants. In Lebenthal E, editor: *Textbook of gastroenterology and nutrition*, New York, 1981, Raven.

44. Forbes GB: Human milk and the small baby, *Am J Dis Child* 136:577, 1982.

45. Forbes GB: Fetal growth and body composition: implications for the premature infant, *J Pediatr Gastroenterol Nutr* 2 (Suppl):552, 1983.

46. Ford JE, Zechalko A, Murphy J, et al: Comparison of the B vitamin composition of milk from mothers of preterm and term babies, *Arch Dis Child* 58:367, 1983.

47. Furman L, Taylor G, Minich N, et al: The effect of maternal milk on neonatal morbidity of very low-birth-weight infants, *Arch Pediatr Adolesc Med* 157:66–71, 2003.

48. Goldman AS, Chheda S, Keeney SE, et al: Immunologic protection of the premature newborn by human milk, *Semin Perinatol* 18:495, 1994.

49. Goldman AS, Garza C, Nichols B, et al: Effects of prematurity on the immunologic system in human milk, *J Pediatr* 101:901, 1982.

50. Greer FR, McCormick A: Improved bone mineralization and growth in premature infants fed fortified own mother's milk, *J Pediatr* 112:961, 1988.

51. Greer FR, Tsang RC: Calcium, phosphorus, magnesium, and vitamin D requirements for preterm infants. In Tsang RC, editor: *Vitamin and mineral requirements for preterm infants*, New York, 1985, Marcel Dekker.

52. Groh-Wargo S, Toth A, Mahoney K: The utility of a bilateral breast pumping system for mothers of premature infants, *Neonatal Netw* 14:31, 1995.

53. Gross SJ: Bone mineralization in preterm infants fed human milk with and without mineral supplementation, *J Pediatr* 111:450, 1987.

54. Gross SJ, Gabriel E: Vitamin E status in preterm infants fed human milk or infant formula, *J Pediatr* 106:635, 1985.

55. Hack M, Estabrook MM, Robertson SS: Development of sucking rhythm in preterm infants, *Early Hum Dev* 11:133, 1985.

56. Haug M, Laubach C, Burke M, et al: Vitamin E in human milk from mothers of preterm and term infants, *J Pediatr Gastroenterol Nutr* 6:605, 1987.

57. Heine W: Is mother's milk the most suitable food for low birth weight infants? *Early Hum Dev* 29:345, 1992.

58. Herman H, Schanler RJ: Benefits of maternal and donor human milk for premature infants, *Early Hum Dev* 82:781, 2006.

59. Herrmann K, Carroll K: An exclusively human milk diet reduces necrotizing enterocolitis, *Breastfeed Med* 9 (4):184–190, 2014.

60. Hopkinson JM, Schanler RJ, Garza C: Milk production by mothers of premature infants, *Pediatrics* 81:815, 1988.

61. Hurst NM, Valentine CJ, Renfro L, et al: Skin-to-skin holding in the neonatal intensive care unit influences maternal milk volume, *J Perinatol* 17:213, 1997.

62. Hylander MA, Strobino DM, Dhanireddy R: Human milk feedings and infection among very low birth weight infants, *Pediatrics* 102e:38, 1998.

63. Itabashi K, Hayashi T, Tsugoshi T, et al: Fortified preterm human milk for very low birth weight infants, *Early Hum Dev* 29:339, 1992.

64. Iwai Y, Takanashi T, Nakao Y, et al: Iron status in low birth weight infants on breast and formula feeding, *Eur J Pediatr* 145:63, 1986.

65. Jävenpää AL: Feeding the low-birth-weight infant. IV. Fat absorption as a function of diet and duodenal bile acids, *Pediatrics* 72:684, 1983.

66. Jävenpää AL, Raiha NCR, Rassin DK, et al: Preterm infants fed human milk attain intrauterine weight gain, *Acta Paediatr Scand* 72:239, 1983.

67. Jensen RG, Jensen GL: Specialty lipids for infant nutrition. I milks and formulas, *J Pediatr Gastroenterol Nutr* 15:232–245, 1992.

68. Jocson MAL, Mason EO, Schanler RJ: The effects of nutrient fortification and varying storage conditions on host defense properties of human milk, *Pediatrics* 100:240, 1997.

69. Jones E, Dimmock PW, Spencer SA: A randomised controlled trial to compare methods of milk expression after

preterm delivery, *Arch Dis Child Fetal Neonatal Ed* 85:F91, 2001.

70. Kelly EJ, Newell SJ: Gastric ontogeny: clinical implications, *Arch Dis Child* 71:F136, 1994.
71. Keunen K, VanElburg RM, VanBel F, et al: Impact of nutrition on brain development and its neuroprotective implications following preterm birth (review), *Pediatr Res* 77(1):148–155, 2015.
72. Klein CJ: Nutrient requirements for preterm infant formulas, *J Nutr* 132:1395S–1577S, 2002.
73. Kuschel CA, Harding JE: Multicomponent fortified human milk for promoting growth in preterm infants, *Cochrane Database Syst Rev* 8(4)2004.
74. Kuschel CA, Harding JE: Multicomponent fortified human milk for promoting growth in preterm infants (Cochrane review). In *The Cochrane Library, issue 4*, Chichester, 2004, John Wiley and Sons.
75. LaGamma EF, Browne LE: Feeding practices for infants weighing less than 1500 g at birth and the pathogenesis of failure of delayed oral feedings to prevent necrotizing enterocolitis, *Clin Perinatol* 21:271–306, 1994.
76. Lau C: Oral feeding in the preterm infant, *Neoreviews* 7: e19–e27, 2006.
77. Lebenthal E, Leung YK: The impact of development of the gut on infant nutrition, *Pediatr Ann* 16:211, 1987.
78. Letarte J, Guyda H, Dussault JH, et al: Lack of protective effect of breastfeeding in congenital hypothyroidism: report of 12 cases, *Pediatrics* 65:703, 1980.
79. Lewis-Jones DI, Reynolds GI: A suggested role for precolostrum in preterm and sick newborn infants, *Acta Paediatr Scand* 72:13, 1983.
80. Lubetsky R, Mandel D, Mimouni FB, et al: Diurnal variations in creamatocrits from expressed breast milk of preterm infants. Neonatal Fetal Nutr Metab abstract no. 644, *Pediatr Res* 55:644, 2003.
81. Lubetsky R, Vaisman N, Mimouni FB, et al: Energy expenditure in human milk versus formula-fed preterm infants, *J Pediatr* 143:750–753, 2003.
82. Lubit EC: Cleft palate orthodontics: why, when, how? *Am J Orthod* 69:562, 1976.
83. Lucas A: Enteral nutrition. In Tsang RC, Lucas A, Uauy R, et al, editors: *Nutritional needs of the preterm infant*, Baltimore, 1993, Williams & Wilkins.
84. Lucas A, Bishop NJ, King FL, et al: Randomized trial of nutrition for preterm infants after discharge, *Arch Dis Child* 67:324, 1992.
85. Lucas A, Bloom SR, Aynsley-Green A: Gut hormones and "minimal enteral feeding," *Acta Paediatr Scand* 75:719, 1986.
86. Lucas A, Cole TJ: Breast milk and neonatal necrotising enterocolitis, *Lancet* 336:1519, 1990.
87. Lucas A, Fewtrell MS, Morley R, et al: Randomized outcome trial of human milk fortification and developmental outcome in preterm infants, *Am J Clin Nutr* 64:142, 1996.
88. Lucas A, Morley R, Cole TJ, et al: Early diet in preterm babies and developmental status in infancy, *Arch Dis Child* 64:1570, 1989.
89. Lucas A, Morley R, Cole TJ, et al: Early diet in preterm babies and developmental status at 18 months, *Lancet* 335:1477, 1990.
90. Lucas A, Morley R, Cole TJ, et al: Breast milk and subsequent intelligence quotient in children born premature, *Lancet* 339:261, 1992.
91. Maastrup R, Greisen G: Extremely preterm infants tolerate skin-to-skin contact during first weeks of life, *Acta Paediatr* 99:1145–1149, 2010.
92. Malcolm WF, Smith PB, Mears S, et al: Transpyloric tube feeding in very low birth weight infants with suspected gastroesophageal reflux: impact on apnea and bradycardia, *J Perinatol* 29:372–375, 2009.

93. Mathew OP: Science of bottle feeding, *J Pediatr* 119:511, 1991.
94. Mathew OP, Bhatia J: Sucking and breathing patterns during breast- and bottle-feeding in term neonates: effects of nutrient delivery and composition, *Am J Dis Child* 143:588, 1989.
95. Mathur NB, Dwarkadas AM, Sharma VK, et al: Anti-infective factors in preterm human colostrum, *Acta Paediatr Scand* 79:1039, 1990.
96. Meerlo-Habing ZE, Koster-Boes EA, Klip H, et al: Early discharge with tube feeding at home for preterm infants is associated with longer duration of breast feeding, *Arch Dis Child Fetal Neonatal Ed* 94:F294–F297, 2009.
97. Meier PP: Supporting lactation in mothers with very low birth weight infants, *Pediatr Ann* 32:317–325, 2003.
98. Meier PP, Brown LP, Hurst NM: Breastfeeding the preterm infants. In Riordan J, Auerbach K, editors: *Breastfeeding and human lactation*, ed 4, Boston, 2014, Jones & Bartlett, p 449.
99. Meier PP, Brown LP, Hurst NM, et al: Nipple shields for preterm infants: effects on milk transfer and duration of breastfeeding, *J Hum Lact* 10:63–68, 1994.
100. Meir PP, Engstrom JL, Rossman B: Breastfeeding peer counselors as direct lactation care providers in the neonatal intensive care unit, *J Hum Lact* 29:313–322, 2013.
101. Meier PP, Engstrom JL, Spanier S, et al: The Rush Mothers' Milk Club: breastfeeding interventions for mothers with very-low-birth weight infants, *J Obstet Gynecol Neonatal Nurs* 33:164–174, 2004.
102. Meinzen-Derr J, Poindexter BB, Donovan EF, et al: The role of human milk feedings in risk of late onset sepsis, *Pediatr Res* 55:393A, 2004.
103. Morelius E, Ortenstrand A, Theodoresson E, et al: A randomized trial of continuous skin-to-skin contact after preterm birth and the effects on salivary cortisol, parental stress, depression and breastfeeding, *Early Hum Dev* 91:63–70, 2015.
104. Morley R, Fewtrell MS, Abbott RA, et al: Neurodevelopment in children born small for gestational age: a randomized trial of nutrient-enriched versus standard formula and comparison with a reference breastfed group, *Pediatrics* 113:515, 2004.
105. Morton J, Hall JY, Wong RJ, et al: Combining hand techniques with electric pumping increases milk production in mothers of preterm infants, *J Perinatol* 289:757–764, 2009.
106. Mortensen EL, Michaelsen KF, Sanders SA, et al: The association between duration of breastfeeding and adult intelligence, *JAMA* 287:2365, 2002.
107. Morton JA: The role of the pediatrician in extended breastfeeding of the preterm infant, *Pediatr Ann* 32:308, 2003.
108. Murphy JF, Neale ML, Matthews N: Antimicrobial properties of preterm breast milk cells, *Arch Dis Child* 58:198, 1983.
109. Narayanan I, Mehta R, Choudhury DK, et al: Sucking on the "emptied" breast: non-nutritive sucking with a difference, *Arch Dis Child* 66:241, 1991.
110. Neifert MR, Seacat JM: Practical aspects of breastfeeding the premature infant, *Perinat Neonatal* 12:24, 1988.
111. Newell SJ: Enteral feeding of the micro preemie, *Clin Perinatol* 27:221, 2000.
112. Nyqvist KH: Early attainment of breastfeeding competence in very preterm infants, *Acta Paediatr* 97:776–781, 2008.
113. Omarsduttir S, Casper C, Akerman A, et al: Breast milk handling routines for preterm infants in Sweden: a national cross-sectional study, *Breastfeed Med* 3:165–170, 2008.
114. Orza-Frank R, Bhatia A, Smith C: Combined peer counselor and lactation consultant support increases breastfeeding in the NICU, *Breastfeed Med* 8(6):509–510, 2013.
115. Oski FA: Iron requirements of the premature infant. In Tsang RC, editor: *Vitamin and mineral requirements in preterm infants*, New York, 1985, Marcel Dekker.

116. Phillips RM, Goldstein M, Houglan K, et al: Multidisciplinary guidelines for the care of the late preterm infants, *J Perinatol* 33:S5–S22, 2013.

117. Picciano MF: Nutrient composition of human milk, *Pediatr Clin North Am* 48:53, 2001.

118. Ronnestad A, Abrahamsen TG, Medbo S, et al: Late-onset septicemia in a Norwegian national cohort of extremely premature infants receiving very early full human milk feeding, *Pediatrics* 115:269–276, 2006.

119. Rönnholm KAR, Perheentupa J, Siimes MA: Supplementation with human milk protein improves growth of small premature infants fed human milk, *Pediatrics* 77:649, 1986.

120. Rossman B, Engstrom JL, Meier PP: Healthcare providers' perceptions of breastfeeding peer counselors in the neonatal intensive care unit, *Res Nurs Health* 35 (5):460–474, 2012.

121. Savilahti E, Järvenpää A-L, Räihä NCR: Serum immunoglobulin in preterm infants: comparison of human milk and formula feeding, *Pediatrics* 72:312, 1983.

122. Schanler RJ, Abrams SA: Postnatal attainment of intrauterine macro mineral accretion rates in low birth weight infants fed fortified human milk, *J Pediatr* 126:441, 1995.

123. Schanler RJ, Anderson D: The low-birth weight infant. In Duggan C, Watkins JB, Walker WA, editors: *Nutrition in pediatrics*, ed 4, Hamilton, 2008, BC Decker.

123a. Schanler RJ, Hurst NM: *Semin Perinatol*, 18:476, 1994.

124. Schanler RJ, Shulman RJ, Lau C, et al: Feeding strategies for premature infants: randomized trial of gastrointestinal priming and tube-feeding method, *Pediatrics* 103:434–439, 1999.

125. Schanler RJ, Shulman RN, Lau C, et al: Feeding strategies for premature infants: randomized trial of gastrointestinal priming and tube-feeding method, *Pediatrics* 103:434–439, 1999.

126. Senterre J, Patel G, Salle B, et al: Beneficial outcomes of feeding fortified human milk versus preterm formula, *J Pediatr* 103:1150–1157, 1983.

127. Stein H, Cohen D, Herman AAB, et al: Pooled pasteurized breast milk and untreated own mother's milk in the feeding of very low birth weight babies: a randomized controlled trial, *J Pediatr Gastroenterol Nutr* 5:242, 1986.

128. Stevenson DK, Yang C, Kerner JA, et al: Intestinal flora in the second week of life in hospitalized preterm infants fed stored frozen breast milk or a proprietary formula, *Clin Pediatr (Phila)* 24:338, 1985.

129. Sturman JA, Rassin DK, Gaull GE: A mini review: taurine in development, *Life Sci* 21:1, 1977.

130. Schanler RJ, et al: Subcommittee on Nutrition during Lactation, Institute of Medicine: *Nutrition during lactation*, Washington, D.C., 1991, National Academies Press.

131. Taylor SN, Basile LA, Ebeling M, et al: Intestinal permeability in preterm infants by feeding type: mother's milk versus formula, *Breastfeed Med* 4:11–15, 2009.

132. Tsang RC, Lucas A, Uauy R, et al: *Nutritional needs of the preterm infant*, Baltimore, 1993, Williams & Wilkins.

133. Tyson JE, Kennedy KA: Trophic feedings for parenterally fed infants, *Cochrane Database Syst Rev* 2005, http://dx.doi.org/10.1002/14651858.CD000504. Art. No.: CD000504.

134. Uauy RD, Birch DG, Birch EE: Effect of dietary omega-3 fatty acids on retinal function of very low birth weight neonates, *Pediatr Res* 28:245, 1990.

135. Verronen P: Breastfeeding of low birth weight infants, *Acta Paediatr Scand* 74:495, 1985.

136. Vohr BR, Poindexter BB, Dusick AM, et al: Beneficial effects of breast milk in the neonatal intensive care unit on the developmental outcome of extremely low birth weight infants at 18 months, *Pediatrics* 118:115–123, 2006.

137. Wagner CL, Greer FR, AAP Section on Breastfeeding and Committee on Nutrition: Prevention of rickets and vitamin D deficiency in infants, children, and adolescents, *Pediatrics* 122:1142–1152, 2008.

138. Wooldridge J, Hall WA: Post hospitalization breastfeeding patterns of moderately preterm infants, *J Perinat Neonatal Nurs* 17:50, 2003.

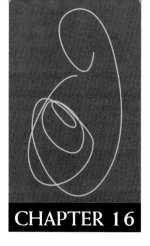

CHAPTER 16

Medical Complications of Mothers

Suboptimal breastfeeding has been shown to take its toll on women's health. The U.S. maternal health burden from current breastfeeding rates has been calculated in terms of premature death, as well as economic costs, by Bartick et al.[27] Working with a cohort of women between 15 and 70 in 2002, involving 1.88 million, they modeled cases of breast cancer, premenopausal ovarian cancer, hypertension, type 2 diabetes, and myocardial infarction. They considered direct costs, indirect costs, and the cost of premature death (before age 70) expressed in 2011 dollars. They calculated that suboptimal breastfeeding costs 17.4 billion dollars to U.S. society, in premature death and poor health. Breastfeeding and maternal disease is discussed in this chapter.

Obstetric Complications

ENGORGEMENT ASSOCIATED WITH DRUGS FOR PRETERM LABOR

Breast engorgement and galactorrhea have been reported to be associated with the use of ritodrine for tocolysis. Evaluations were done in 11 women, with measurements of serum prolactin, progesterone, estradiol, and estriol excretion. No differences were noted in association with the ritodrine. Apparently, the effect is unrelated to hormone changes.[236]

Reports of breast engorgement and galactorrhea have also been reported with other tocolytics. One case was associated with the use of intravenous (IV) magnesium sulfate in a 24-year-old woman at 30 weeks' gestation.[172] Plasma magnesium levels ranged between 4.1 and 6.4 mg/mL. On day 4 of treatment, engorgement and dripping of milk developed. Prolactin level was 83.6 ng/L; normal range in pregnancy is up to 200 ng/L. Magnesium was replaced with nifedipine, and the symptoms gradually subsided. Another case report describes tocolysis, in which thyrotropin-releasing hormone 400 mcg every 8 hours for four doses was used with corticosteroids to enhance fetal lung maturity. This has been associated with an increase in prolactin. The patient also received magnesium sulfate initially, followed by oral terbutaline. Thirty-six hours after the last dose of thyrotropin-releasing hormone, the patient experienced painful bilateral engorgement, tender masses in both axillae, and lactation. Prolactin level was 55.4 ng/mL. Symptoms subsided in 96 hours.[107]

CESAREAN DELIVERY

When birth takes place by cesarean delivery, a mother becomes a surgical patient with all the inherent risks and problems. If the procedure is anticipated because of a previous cesarean delivery, cephalopelvic disproportion, or some other identifiable reason, a mother can prepare herself psychologically for the event and usually tolerates the process better. When the procedure is unplanned and done during the process of labor, it is psychologically more traumatic, and the mother tends to feel as if she has failed in her role. In addition to this unexpected disappointment, medical emergencies such as a long, difficult labor, abruptio placentae, blood loss, toxemia, or infection may also have an impact on the mother's well-being.

A mother who plans to breastfeed after cesarean delivery should be able to do so if the infant is well enough. The method of delivery makes no significant difference to the timing of the milk coming in or the changes in the concentration of the major milk constituents in the first 7 days postpartum.[156] Depending on the type of anesthesia and the associated circumstances, the mother may feel alert enough to put the infant to breast within the first hour. The obstetrician, surgeon, and the operating room nurses are key in making it happen.

Bupivacaine is being used as an epidural block for cesarean or vaginal delivery because it does not result in the decrease in muscle tone and strength reported in neonates whose mothers have received lidocaine or mepivacaine.[174,229] Bupivacaine and tetracaine are highly protein bound and appear in milk in low concentrations, in contrast to lidocaine and mepivacaine, which are nonionized and unbound in serum. Because most local or regional anesthetics are used with epinephrine, which causes local vasoconstriction, thus slowing the rate of absorption, the anesthetic effects are prolonged and the amount secreted into the milk is minimal.

Epidural morphine is used for more prolonged analgesia and is used in cesarean delivery because it can then be continued postpartum for the relief of postoperative pain. Bernstein et al.[34] showed that epidurally administered morphine enters the breast milk in low levels compared with the levels in maternal urine, which were several thousand times higher. Most of the morphine in colostrum is in the conjugated form, and thus pharmacologically inactive. Other studies report a milk/plasma ratio of 2:45; the amount received via the milk is calculated to be less than 50 mcg/dL of milk, causing no untoward symptoms in any of the cases reported. At birth, infants may have morphine in their system from transplacental transfer of intrapartum maternal dosing. Transplacental medication has depressed some infants and may interfere with early attempts to suckle.

In a scheduled cesarean delivery under controlled circumstances, the procedure is initiated using local anesthesia to the skin and facial layers. Systemic anesthesia is given as soon as the cord is clamped, sparing the transfer of anesthetics to the newborn.

Regional anesthesia permits the mother to remain awake, and she may be ready to nurse as soon as the IV lines and urinary catheter are stabilized. The mother will need considerable help from nursing staff. She should remain flat if she has had a spinal anesthetic to prevent developing a spinal headache. She can turn to one side and offer the breast by placing the infant on his or her side and stroking the infant's perioral area with the nipple. The normal full-term infant who has not been depressed by maternal medication should do well. If the mother can be turned to the other side, the infant may nurse on both sides. In this first encounter, the emphasis is on some suckling, not switching. The bedside rails will help the mother turn and provide safety for her.

Maternal fluids and medications in the first 48 hours postoperatively should not affect the infant adversely. Pain medication is usually required for approximately 72 hours. It is best given immediately after breastfeeding to permit the level to peak before the next feeding. The medication used should be limited to short-acting drugs that an adult eliminates quickly (i.e., within 4 hours) and that the newborn is able to excrete. Ibuprofen and acetaminophen are in that category; codeine is also acceptable (see Chapter 11). Low-grade fever may occur and should not interrupt lactation.

Some positive factors are associated with breastfeeding for the mother who has had a cesarean delivery. Lactation is advantageous to the postoperative uterus, in that the oxytocin production stimulated by suckling will assist in its involution. In addition, the traumatized psyche of a mother, whose delivery did not occur naturally as planned, is more quickly healed when she can demonstrate her maternal capabilities by breastfeeding.

Whether breastfeeding can be introduced early, or must await stabilization of medical problems in mother or infant, when the section was done emergently, it is a reasonable goal for the mother to seek in most cases. Supportive nursing care is critical to establishing successful lactation. None of this can take place, however, unless a physician has carefully assessed the condition of the mother and the infant in light of the great advantages and possible disadvantages of breastfeeding to both.

The management should include the following:

1. A postoperative care plan that includes sufficient rest. Most postpartum wards are not scheduled to include adequate rest for postoperative patients.
2. The family must be instructed on the needs for rest at home and assistance with the household chores. With shorter hospital stays, this is even more critical.
3. The impact on the infant should be considered when writing the mother's medication orders.
4. If the infant cannot be put to breast, arrangements should be made to pump the mother's breasts on a regular basis with a quality hospital-grade double electric pump. This should be done at least every 3 hours during waking hours, and at least once at night, even if separation will last only a day or two. Milk should be given to the infant if the infant is able to feed.
5. If the mother is in intensive care, pumping can still be done by a skilled bedside nurse or lactation consultant.

Hypergalactia or Over-Supply While Breastfeeding

Hypergalactia or overproduction of milk while breastfeeding is the problem of producing excessive amounts of milk, which is then associated with discomfort. It often leads to the mother pumping and storing milk beyond her infant's needs. The real clinical issues early in lactation, however, are rapid let-down, excessive flow, and choking and gasping by the infant. In the long range, it leads to acute mastitis, plugged ducts, chronic breast pain, pumping, and early weaning, especially due to soaked under clothing and wet stains of the outer clothing. During actual breastfeeding, the latch is often shallow, causing nipple pain, milk leakage, and continually engorged and leaking breasts. The infant may also have increased weight gain, fogginess, excessive flatus, and explosive green stools. This is associated with high lactose, low-fat milk. It may also be associated with loose stools resembling mucus.

If simple adjustments to feeding do not help, the mother's thyroid function should be checked as both hyper- and hypothyroidism can be associated with prolactinemia. Prolactin levels can be measured using the standard protocol (see Chapter 8). It requires two levels of prolactin. The mother has a small butterfly needle with a stop cock and attached IV with a heparin lock. After recovery from the needle stick (10 minutes), a sample of blood is drawn and the system turned to the heparin lock. The infant is fed, or the breasts are pumped, for 10 minutes, and a second blood sample is drawn. The baseline level should be 100 or less, and the second level should be about twice the first measurement.

Management that has been effective is called block feeding. This is a process by which the mother nurses from one breast only for a block of 3 to 4 hours, and then from the other breast exclusively for a block of time. Feedings last 30 to 60 minutes. Usually the mother's milk supply drops within 48 hours. If further therapy is necessary, the mother can try pseudoephedrine (available in nose drops), or birth control pills containing estrogen, or herbs such as sage, parsley, or peppermint. Bromocriptine or cabergoline should only be used with the physician's involvement.

The mothers have trouble again when it is time to wean, so efforts should be made to avoid mastitis, plugged ducts, and other complications. An extensive review of hypergalactia is available by Eglash.[76]

PREGNANCY RELATED HYPERTENSION

The terminology regarding hypertension has been redesigned by the Working Group on High Blood Pressure in Pregnancy of the National Institutes of Health and is available worldwide. The term toxemia has been replaced with the terms preeclampsia, eclampsia, and HELLP (hemolysis, elevated liver enzymes, and low platelets). In all of these situations, the mother is monitored closely. In preeclampsia, the patient is at risk for cerebral edema, microscopic liver involvement, and glomerular lesion, pathognomonic of preeclampsia. The mother is seriously ill and at risk for serious complications of all these organs, including seizures.

Complications of hypertension usually begin after 32 weeks' gestation, but have also been observed to occur 24 to 48 hours or later postpartum. Close fetal monitoring is essential. Convulsions, renal disease, and cerebral hemorrhage in a mother are complications that can be prevented by careful management. Because serious hypertension in the mother may necessitate delivery of a premature infant, or an infant compromised by a poorly perfused placenta or maternal medications, a number of contraindications to immediate breastfeeding exist in the early postpartum period.

Initial treatment of a patient with preeclampsia includes bed rest, preferably lying on her side in a quiet room that is darkened to prevent photic and auditory stimuli. Blood pressure and proteinuria should be carefully monitored.[59] Magnesium sulfate is superior to phenytoin and diazepam. Treatment also includes salt restriction, and diuretics, such as thiazide or furosemide, may be used. Hydralazine (Apresoline) and methyldopa (Aldomet) or other antihypertensives may be indicated to lower blood pressure. Magnesium sulfate is safest for a breastfeeding infant. Many patients recover quickly after the infant and placenta are delivered, requiring only 24 to 48 hours of postpartum sedation.[59]

Often the infant is small for gestational age, or premature, and may require special or intensive care; therefore, the decision of when to initiate breastfeeding depends on the infant's condition. If the infant is full term and well, breastfeeding is initiated when toxemia precautions are discontinued. Magnesium can be closely monitored if the mother continues to receive it. It may be necessary to wait until the other medications can be discontinued, especially the diuretics, hydralazine, and methyldopa.

After the risk for convulsions is past, some attention can be given to manual expression or pumping, even if an infant cannot be nursed yet. If medications are a problem temporarily, the milk may have to be discarded, but the expression of milk will serve to stimulate the breast and initiate lactation.

Diminution of stress is a critical factor in hypertensive therapy, so maternal anxiety about being able to nurse must be managed with open discussion of the overall plan and the role of the bedside nurse. On the other hand, the stress of early feedings that do not go well because the infant has been confused by initial bottle-feedings may also present a hazard in the course of maternal management. This can be minimized by cup feedings. The most important element in every case is communication with the patient about her expectations or needs regarding breastfeeding. A physician's therapeutic management design can put this in appropriate perspective. Because of the calming effects of oxytocin and prolactin, it may be therapeutic to breastfeed.

RETENTION OF PLACENTA AND LACTATION FAILURE

Three cases of failed onset of lactation were reported by Neifert et al.[197] Although the original association of the placenta with delayed lactation was made a century ago, most reports of retained placenta merely discuss persistent hemorrhage as a recognized symptom. In each of the three cases the failure of breast engorgement and leakage of milk was evident from delivery. However, the hemorrhage and emergency curettage occurred at 1 week, 3 weeks, and 4 weeks postpartum, respectively. In each case, spontaneous milk flow began immediately postoperatively, after the removal of placental fragments. The authors suggest that failure of lactogenesis may be an early sign of retained placenta that should not be ignored.[197]

VENOUS THROMBOSIS AND PULMONARY EMBOLISM

Venous thrombosis and pulmonary embolism are the most common serious vascular complications associated with pregnancy and the postpartum period. Pulmonary embolism has assumed relatively greater importance because of the decline in morbidity and mortality rates from sepsis and eclampsia. Varicose veins also present more problems during pregnancy than at any other time. These vascular complications all represent common features in vein physiology, as associated with the perinatal period.

In addition to the well-being of the mother, major concerns during lactation include procedures that might be necessary to establish a diagnosis and the systemic medications necessary for treatment that could have an impact on the nursing infant via the milk. Accurate diagnosis is urgent and is far more complex than therapy. Besides the health of a mother in this life-threatening state, any program of contraception after childbirth is fundamentally affected by the established diagnosis of thromboembolism. Thus the diagnosis must be precise.

Diagnosis

Laboratory procedures, such as evaluation of arterial blood gases, liver function studies, and fibrin/fibrinogen derivatives, are not a problem to breastfeeding. The absence of fibrin split products in plasma and serum virtually excludes the diagnosis of embolism, although their presence does not confirm it. The most definitive diagnosis is made with radioactive scanning procedures and angiography.

Contrast venography is the most definitive method available for diagnosing deep vein thrombosis. The perfusion lung scan is the pivotal test for the investigation of patients with suspected pulmonary embolism. The radiopharmaceuticals used are technetium-99m-microaggregated albumin or microspheres (usual dose 3 mCi), which clear the milk promptly, thus requiring pumping and discarding the milk for 8 hours.[93] Pulmonary angiography, the most definitive test for pulmonary embolism, requires fluoroscopy, which is not a risk to a breastfeeding infant. The total dose is approximately 400 mrad, and thus should not interfere with lactation. In deep vein thrombosis of the leg, fibrinogen leg scanning uses iodine-125 (^{125}I) fibrinogen, which requires 2 weeks of pumping and discarding the milk. Radioactive materials vary in their half-lives and disappearance time from breast milk. They all appear in breast milk (see Chapter 11).

Another diagnostic technique is duplex ultrasonography. It consistently visualizes the iliac veins. Impedance plethysmography is noninvasive, but not reliable for calf thromboses, and is contraindicated in lactating mothers.[89] At present, computed tomography and ultrasound are effective in diagnosing major arterial aneurysms only.

Magnetic resonance imaging (MRI) is a safe procedure while lactating. Radiocontrast agents, however, may be required. Gadolinium-containing contrast agents are tightly bound to the molecule and are not free in the plasma. They penetrate into milk only slightly and are not absorbed orally. The half-life is short (1.1 to 2.0 hours). They are safe for breastfeeding infants. They should clear a mother's system completely in 5 to 10 hours, depending upon the compound.

TREATMENT

Anticoagulant therapy is the treatment of choice for established venous thrombosis with or without embolism. Heparin must be given parenterally and is destroyed by gastric juices. Because this large molecule does not cross the placenta or appear in breast milk, it can be used during lactation. This therapy is adequate for a hospitalized patient, where constant monitoring of coagulation is possible. Warfarin has been considered the best replacement for heparin for home use, but it is secreted in the breast milk (see Chapter 11). The amount transmitted is minuscule, and it is considered safe to breastfeed while taking warfarin. In long-term therapy the prothrombin time should be monitored at least monthly in the infant, and vitamin K can be given if necessary.

The low-molecular-weight heparins are still large molecules. They do not pass into the milk and are orally poorly absorbed.

Medical Problems

MASTITIS

Mastitis is an infectious process in the breast that produces localized tenderness, redness, and heat, together with systemic reactions of fever, malaise, and sometimes nausea and vomiting. It no longer occurs in epidemics, as was once seen in hospitals before the common use of antibiotics and when hospital stays were prolonged for normal childbirth. The infection, however, may be hospital acquired if mother or infant is colonized with virulent bacteria before leaving the hospital, especially methicillin-resistant *Staphylococcus aureus* (MRSA).

Prospective studies estimate the incidence to be between 3% and 20%, depending on the definition and the length of follow-up postpartum. The common onset is within the first 6 weeks postpartum, but can occur anytime during lactation. Technically, mastitis is an inflammation of the breast, which may or may not involve an infection. It is not uncommon for the problem to start with engorgement, then become noninfective mastitis, followed by infective mastitis, and then to abscess if treatment is not introduced promptly (Figure 16-1).

The current definition of mastitis includes fever of 38.5°C (101°F) or more, chills, flulike aching, systemic illness, and a pink, tender, hot, swollen, wedge-shaped area of the breast[199] (Figure 16-2). Table 16-1 lists the significant differential points among mastitis, engorgement, and plugged duct.

The portal of entry of the disease is through the lactiferous ducts to a secreting lobule, through a nipple fissure to periductal lymphatics, or through hematogenous spread. The common organisms involved include *S. aureus*, including MRSA, *Escherichia coli*, and (rarely) Streptococcus. Tuberculous mastitis does occur, and the infant often develops tuberculosis of the tonsils. In populations in which tuberculosis is endemic, it occurs in approximately 1% of cases of mastitis.[101]

Factors predisposing a woman to mastitis include poor drainage of a duct and then of an alveolus, presence of an organism, and lowered maternal defenses such as those associated with stress and fatigue (Figures 16-2 and 16-3). Insufficient emptying and obstruction of ducts by tight clothing can cause plugged ducts, which can be prevented from becoming mastitis if identified early and treated vigorously with local massage, moist heat, and rest. Missing a feeding or having an infant suddenly sleep through the night may cause engorgement, plugging, and then mastitis. Cracked or painful nipples may herald a problem, more because the mother avoids complete emptying on the painful side than because bacteria suddenly gain access. If a mother has cracked, fissured, sore nipples, then the breast pain and redness is more than likely mastitis.

Devereux[67] described 20 years of experience with 53 lactating patients who experienced 71 acute attacks of mastitis. The highest incidence was in the second and third weeks postpartum. No infant was weaned because of the mastitis. No infants were sick in association with the mastitis. All but five mothers nursed subsequent infants. Six patients had mastitis with other pregnancies. Eight of 71 patients (11.1%) developed abscesses, six of which required incision and drainage. The bacterial cause was not stated. When antibiotic treatment was delayed beyond 24 hours, the abscess rate increased.[67]

Studies by Fetherston et al.[82] observed increased breast permeability, reduced milk synthesis, and increased concentration of immune components sIgA and lactoferrin, with increasing severity and systemic symptoms. They also observed increased sodium and decreased glucose in milk of the involved breast compared with the uninvolved breast and normal breasts (which is suggestive of weaning milk).

Although breastfed infants usually remain well during bouts of acute mastitis in their mothers, there is reported a case of scalded skin syndrome in an infant fed by a mother with mastitis that did not respond to ampicillin for 14 days. The child responded to IV nafcillin.

Using leukocyte counts and microbiologic counts, Thomsen et al.[261] have separated breast inflammations into three clinical states: milk stasis (counts less than 106 leukocytes and less than 103 bacteria per milliliter of milk), noninfectious inflammation (counts greater than 106 leukocytes and less than 103 bacteria), and infectious mastitis (counts greater than 106 leukocytes and greater than 103 bacteria) (Tables 16-2 and 16-3). The authors concluded that no treatment was needed in stasis, but lack of treatment led to recurrence and lactation failure in noninfectious inflammation and abscess in mastitis. Emptying the breast (frequent feedings and pumping or hand-expressing three times per day after a feed) was sufficient in

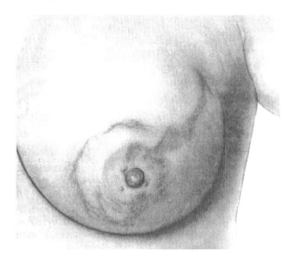

Figure 16-4. Inflammation of lymphatics of breast demonstrating drainage of breast. Generalized infection of breast, especially Staphylococcal, occasionally presents as lymph duct infection.

slept through the night, or the mothers left the babies for many hours and did not pump, was a prominent feature. Apart from mastitis, one third of mothers reported nipple cracks and sores in the first week postpartum; 64% of cases were diagnosed by telephone (physicians 59%, nurses 23%, and others 18%). The most common symptoms were breast tenderness (98%), fever (82%), malaise (87%), chills (78%), redness (98%), and hot spots (62%).[75] The most frequent treatment was cephalexin (46%), amoxicillin (7%), ampicillin (7%), and amoxicillin clavulanate (Augmentin; 7%).[24]

The use of oral administration of lactobacilli isolated from the milk of healthy mothers for the treatment of infectious mastitis was compared with standard antibiotic therapy.[20] Three groups were formed from 352 women with mastitis. One group ingested colony-forming units of *Lactobacillus fermentum* (CECT 5716) daily, a second group ingested *L. salivarius* (CECT 5713) for 3 weeks, and the third group received antibiotics prescribed by their health care centers. Women who received the probiotics improved more rapidly and had fewer recurrences than the antibiotic group.[20]

Most series of acute mastitis clearly demonstrate that the cases that result in unfavorable outcomes, including abscess and recurrent disease, had significant delay between onset of symptoms and request for medical advice. Recurrence rates run from 14% to 20%.[24] When proper treatment is initiated promptly, the course of the disease is usually brief; if treatment is delayed, prolonged antibiotics become necessary. Treatment with less than 10 days of antibiotics is also associated with recurrence and/or more virulent bacteria. Thus cultures are appropriate in the case of recurrence (Table 16-4).

Recommended Management Regimen

1. Advise patient to continue to nurse on both breasts, but start the infant on the unaffected side, while the affected side "lets down" to reduce the pain. Be sure to empty the affected side by feeding or pumping.

TABLE 16-4	Antibiotic Selection for Bacterial Mastitis			
Antibiotic	**Spectrum**	**Dose**	**Safety***	**Comment**
Dicloxacillin	Nonmethicillin-resistant staphylococci	500 mg PO qid	Yes	Highest activity against MSSA
Clindamycin	Penicillin allergic Many CA-MRSA test susceptibilities	300 mg PO qid	Probably safe	Excreted in milk; active against many strains of CA-MRSA
Erythromycin	Penicillin allergic	500 mg PO qid	Yes	GI intolerance
Azithromycin	Penicillin allergic	500 mg load, then 250 mg/day for 4 days	Probably safe	Limited *S. aureus* activity; less GI upset than erythromycin
Trimethoprim-sulfamethoxazole	Some CA-MRSA	100 mg PO bid	Yes	Less effective when abscess present
Cephalexin	MSSA	500 mg PO qid	Yes	Relatively poor levels in breast tissue

CA-MRSA, Community-acquired methicillin-resistant *S. aureus*; *GI,* gastrointestinal; *MSSA,* methicillin-susceptible *S. aureus.*
*Data are relatively limited for many antibiotics, but the relative safety is based upon the following review: Nahum GG, UI K, Kennedy DL: Antibiotic use in pregnancy and lactation: what is and is not known about teratogenic and toxic risks, *Obstet Gynecol* 107:1120, 2006.

2. Insist on bed rest (mandatory). The mother can take the infant to bed and obtain assistance for the care of other family members.

3. Choose an antibiotic that can be tolerated by the infant, as well as the mother (avoid sulfa drugs when the infant is younger than 1 month). The decision should be based on local sensitivities and length of time since delivery or exposure to resistant flora.

4. Apply ice packs or warm packs to the breast, whichever provides the most comfort. Experience indicates that heat provides drainage and pain relief.

5. Provide plenty of fluids for the mother.

6. Give an analgesic such as acetaminophen or ibuprofen.

7. The mother should wear a supporting brassiere that does not cause painful pressure.

Empiric therapy without cultures should consider the common organisms causing mastitis: *S. aureus* (50%), *E. coli* or other gram-negative organisms, group A streptococci, *Streptococcus pneumoniae* species, and Bacteroides species (especially with abscesses). Less common organisms include *Candida albicans* and *Mycobacterium tuberculosis*. First-line antibiotics that are safe for mothers and infants include first-generation cephalosporins or dicloxacillin/oxacillin. Treatment of suspected gram-negative organisms includes first-generation cephalosporins or amoxicillin clavulanate (Augmentin). Treatment of abscesses should include some anaerobic coverage with Augmentin or clindamycin. Therapy for women with penicillin or cephalosporin allergy can include erythromycin or clindamycin. Suspected MRSA can be treated with vancomycin, clindamycin, or rifampin, considering organism sensitivity.

An unusual case of *S. pneumoniae* mastitis was reported in a 38-year-old woman who was partially breastfeeding her 9-month-old infant. Cultures of breast milk had more than 106 *S. pneumoniae* bacteria per milliliter of milk. Cultures of the infant's nose and throat also grew *S. pneumoniae*, although he was asymptomatic. Treatment was flucloxacillin. C-reactive protein was 177 mg/L at onset and 18.6 mg/L on day 6. The infant was presumed to have infected the mother.[274]

Regardless of the disease course, the antibiotic should be given for at least 10 to 14 days. Shorter courses are associated with a high incidence of relapse. Once relapsed, it can become chronic until the infant is weaned. A Cochrane Review of antibiotics for mastitis failed to identify the best antibiotic, but it did confirm antibiotics were better than supportive care for length of illness and abscess formation.[124]

COMMUNITY-ACQUIRED METHICILLIN-RESISTANT *STAPHYLOCOCCUS AUREUS*

A relative increase in MRSA is being reported, manifesting as cases of postpartum mastitis. Reviewing all cases of postpartum mastitis from 1998 through 2005, Reddy et al.[220] noted MRSA and methicillin-susceptible *S. aureus* (MSSA) increased dramatically from 1 case of MRSA in 1998 to 18 in 2005 and 17 cases of MSSA. Rates were not related to artificial rupture of membranes, epidural anesthesia, vaginal lacerations, episiotomy, cesarean delivery, or intrapartum antibiotics. In another series, 127 women from 136,459 deliveries were admitted for postpartum mastitis. This calculates to 7.8 to 11.1 per 10,000 deliveries with an incidence of abscess of 2.6 per 10,000 deliveries. Community-acquired MRSA was cultured in 18 of the cases (67%). Most did not receive antibiotic therapy to which their bacteria were sensitive.[247] The most common organism cultured in nonpuerperal breast abscesses was MRSA (58%), which was sensitive to clindamycin, trimethoprim-sulfamethoxazole, and linezolid, according to Moazzez et al.[188] Clinicians should be aware of the likelihood of MRSA in the community and the effective therapies. Breast milk culture and sensitivities should be obtained when the patient is unresponsive to the first-line treatment. A full discussion of MRSA appears in Chapter 17.

See also Appendix P, Protocol 4 (Revised 2014) for further information on management of mastitis.

RECURRENT OR CHRONIC MASTITIS AND CANDIDAL INFECTION

Recurrent mastitis is usually caused by delayed or inadequate treatment of the initial disease. If antibiotics are started, they should be continued for a minimum of 10 to 14 days. Often, because a mother feels better, she discontinues them on her own. At the first recurrence, cultures should be sent of the midstream clean-catch specimen of breast milk and the infant's nasopharynx and oropharynx. The patient should be seen and the circumstances completely reviewed. An aggressive course of rest, nourishment, stress management, and complete drainage of the breast by suckling or pumping should be initiated. The antibiotics should be carefully selected by culture sensitivities and maintained for 2 weeks. Fluids should be increased. Failure of the second treatment is usually caused by failure to complete the entire treatment, which may also mean failure to get adequate rest and build up maternal resistance. The clinical protocol from ABM, MASTITIS, is available in Appendix P, revised in 2014.

find that they have a strong let-down reflex with an initially soaking spray of milk. This is not hypergalactia and usually diminishes in 1 or 2 weeks.

If this phenomenon persists for more than 1 or 2 weeks, an evaluation for prolactinoma is in order. A baseline level and a stimulus-associated level of prolactin, after 10 minutes of suckling or pumping with a breast pump, should be obtained. If the patient has associated symptoms of headache or visual disturbances, further work up for pituitary adenoma would be appropriate. The phenomenon, however, may not be associated with any identifiable pathology. Idiopathic hypergalactia may diminish throughout months of breastfeeding. It occurs more often with first pregnancies and may not recur with subsequent pregnancies.

Treatment is palliative, including a tight, well-fitting brassiere that is well padded between feedings. A trial of low-dose estrogen, as available in oral contraceptives, may be effective. A careful history to identify any medications or herbs that are galactagogues or any form of stimulus other than breastfeeding is essential to management. Although bromocriptine would theoretically be effective, it would only be indicated in patients with hyperprolactinemia associated with pituitary adenoma. In such patients the diagnosis should be established first. Bromocriptine has potentially serious side effects and should not be used casually. Cabergoline is preferred as a treatment for pituitary adenoma and may be used cautiously during lactation to control the tumor. Excessive milk production has also been associated with hyperthyroidism and postpartum thyroiditis.

HYPERACTIVE LET-DOWN REFLEX

Hyperactive let-down reflex may occur, especially among primiparas. It is characterized by a spray of milk on initiation of a feeding. If the other breast is checked, it also is flowing. The infant is often overwhelmed by the rate of flow and begins to choke or is gulping frantically to keep up. Milk runs out the corners of the mouth. When the milk is high volume but low fat, it may be accompanied by increased gas formation and colic.[272]

Treatment involves controlling the flow. Initially, expressing a little milk (and saving it in the freezer) until the flow slows and then putting the infant to the breast usually solves the problem. If the fat of hindmilk is slow to come, additional milk can be expressed until the fat begins to be secreted. The high-fat milk, or hindmilk, will decrease the relative volume of lactose and the relative amount of gas produced, reducing the colic, thrashing about during feedings, and green stools.

Mothers may reduce the flow from the opposite breast during feedings by folding the nipple down and wearing a firm brassiere. Pressing her arm across the breast can also diminish flow.

DIABETES MELLITUS

Interest in lactation among women with diabetes is high, and clinical research on the topic is gradually increasing.[22,47] The laboratory has been the site of considerable study of the disease in the animal model and of the role of insulin.[22] The breast is known to be a target organ for insulin, and insulin receptors are in the mammary gland acini. The mammary gland is an insulin-sensitive tissue, where acute changes in insulin concentration result in a rapid alteration in the rate of lipogenesis and the utilization of glucose. Cultures of mammalian breast tissue serve as ideal laboratory models for the exploration of insulin activity.

It is significant to note that the longer the duration of breastfeeding, the greater the reduction in the incidence of type 2 diabetes. The study was from two large cohorts of women. The authors suggest that lactation may reduce risk of type 2 diabetes in young and middle-aged women by improving glucose homeostasis.[252]

Pregnancy has become a more common event in women with well-controlled diabetes, and fertility rates compare with those of women without diabetes. Much has been said about labor and delivery in mothers with diabetes and almost nothing about lactation in these mothers. Mothers with diabetes should be offered the same opportunity to breastfeed that is offered to all patients, unless the disease is so incapacitating that any metabolic stress is contraindicated. When the progress of the infant of a mother with diabetes is uneventful and the infant can be treated normally, no contraindication exists to breastfeeding. The timely onset of stage II lactogenesis is important for the ultimate success of breastfeeding. Gestational diabetes and/or obesity were reported to be associated with delayed lactogenesis.[178] Therefore, early breastfeeding support is essential for mothers with diabetes. Lactation may be more difficult in mothers with diabetes, perhaps as a result of cesarean delivery or the need to keep an infant in a special care unit for the first few days of life. Congenital malformations in infants of mothers with diabetes are more common (two to six times the normal rate), occurring in 8% to 10% of births of mothers with insulin-dependent diabetes mellitus (IDDM). They cover all organ systems. Congenital cardiac disease continues to be most common. At birth, the major problems are macrosomia, complicating delivery, hypoglycemia, respiratory distress syndrome, hypocalcia, and hypomagnesemia, polycythemia, and hyperbilirubinemia. Thus close monitoring is mandatory while providing as "normal" an experience as possible.

Cordero et al.[54] reported 530 infants born to 332 women with diabetes and 177 women with IDDM; 36% were large for gestational age, 76 (14%) were born at less than 34 weeks' gestation, 115 (22%) were born at 34 to 37 weeks' gestation, and 339 (64%) were born at term. Almost half (47%) were admitted to the NICU due to respiratory distress syndrome, prematurity, hypoglycemia, or congenital malformation. Hypoglycemia occurred in 137 (27%) and more commonly among mothers with severe types of diabetes; 182 (34%) had respiratory distress syndrome. Although 244 infants were admitted to normal newborn care, 43 had to be transferred for hypoglycemia. Routine care failures were less frequent among breastfed infants. The authors recognize the improvements in care of the mother; however, they caution about hypoglycemia and respiratory distress syndrome in infants who are overstressed. They recommend observation of the infant in a special care nursery, especially when the mother's disease is advanced. They further say breastfeeding should be encouraged in these mothers. Rates of breastfeeding in women with diabetes are lower than in nondiabetics, despite the greater advantages to both mother and infant.[83]

In a retrospective study of 25 mothers who were insulin dependent before pregnancy, breastfeeding was both successful (13) and unsuccessful (12).[81] The successful ones were slightly older and better educated and had diabetes longer (13.7 years vs. 8.2 years). The infants were half a week more mature and spent less time in the intensive care nursery (1.8 days vs. 7.2 days). Delay to first breastfeeding and introduction of a bottle in the intensive care nursery were no different, and both groups of mothers experienced an adjustment period. Observations about diet, insulin, and control of diabetes were similar in the two groups and paralleled the observations made in the study by Ferris et al.[81]

During the last stages of pregnancy in normal women, a more or less constant excretion of lactose occurs in the urine, with the peak reached on the day of delivery. After delivery the lactose excretion immediately drops to a low level, where it remains for 2 to 5 days, followed by a sudden large excretion of lactose.[237] Lactosuria in a mother with diabetes may lead to diagnostic confusion. It normally occurs late in pregnancy and in the postpartum period before the infant takes much milk, if the mother does not nurse, or if the supply of milk exceeds the infant's requirement. Lactose reabsorbed from the breasts is excreted in the urine. Urine sugar tests are not reliable during lactation.

The sparing effect of lactation on the insulin requirement has been observed by many, beginning with Joselin et al.[129] The depression of the level of the blood sugar in normal nursing women with

diabetes may lead to hypoglycemic symptoms. The simultaneous lactosuria may be misdiagnosed as glucosuria and excessive insulin taken. The improved tolerance has been explained by the transference of sugar from the blood to the breast for conversion to galactose and lactose. Joselin et al.[129] reported that the majority of patients at the Joselin Clinic, as well as those at Johns Hopkins Hospital, breastfed in whole or in part. They recommended the increased administration of the B vitamins for the mother with diabetes during lactation.

Milk composition in diabetes has been studied by Butte et al.[46] in a group of moderately well controlled insulin-dependent women (type 1) at 3 months postpartum. Women with diabetes in pregnancy and postpartum have been observed to have low levels of prolactin, placental lactogen, and parathyroid hormone. Whether the observed decreased placental blood flow is associated with diminished mammary blood flow in lactation has not been established.

In this small sample size, no significant difference was seen in the values for total nitrogen, lactose, fat, and calories, given the normally wide variations found among control subjects as well. Mineral content was not different except for sodium, which averaged 140 mg/g compared with reference milk's 100 mg/g. The glucose concentrations were significantly higher in the milk of women with diabetes, and this varied greatly without any pattern throughout the 24-hour collections, although lactose fluctuated little. The mean glucose value was 0.70 ± 0.11 mg/g in women with diabetes and 0.32 ± 0.08 mg/g in the reference women. During the collections the women with diabetes were noted to have periods of hyperglycemia. Total milk volumes were not measured in the study by Butte et al., but the infants were noted to gain weight appropriately.[38] Measurements of glycosylated hemoglobin within a month of the milk collections were noted to be $8.1 \pm 0.6\%$, which is above the normal range of 4.0% to 7.6%. It is appropriate for clinicians to be aware of the slightly elevated sodium levels, especially if mastitis develops. The glucose elevations probably have little clinical significance to the infants because glucose makes up only about 0.4% of the total energy content of the milk.

When milk volume and composition were measured serially, on days 3 to 7 postpartum, in a woman with diabetes by Bitman et al.,[35] sodium, potassium, chloride, lactose, protein, calcium, magnesium, and citrate were within the limits of a reference population without diabetes. Unlike Butte et al.,[46] Bitman et al.[35] found that fat content was lower, with free fatty acids 2% of total lipid on day 3 but 23% on days 4 through 7. Lipoprotein fatigue, and antibiotics for at least 10 days when indicated, mastitis should not pose a threat. Candidal infections are more common because of the glucose-rich vaginal secretions, and most women with diabetes are alert to the early signs of a fungal vaginitis. When the infant is born by cesarean delivery, no exposure occurs in the birth canal. Infection of the nipples can also occur from *C. albicans*, even though the infant does not have obvious thrush. Early specific treatment with nystatin ointment or gentian violet to the breast and mouth of the infant whenever sore nipples do not respond to the usual nonspecific treatment is recommended. Treatment of both mother and infant simultaneously is necessary or they will reseed each other (see Chapter 8).

Infants of women with diabetes present a special problem in breastfeeding because they are often premature, frequently have respiratory distress syndrome and hyperbilirubinemia, and may be poor feeders at first. Hypoglycemia is the immediate problem, and its management may initially preclude dependency on breast milk as the sole source of nourishment. Because less than half of the infants develop problems, many need not be separated from their mothers. For those that require special or intensive care, lactation may have to be postponed briefly depending on the infant's status.

Providing an electric breast pump and assistance in pumping is essential if the infant is too ill to be fed. Attention to this detail is important, regardless of the reason for separation of the mother and infant.[22]

The hypoglycemia of the infant of a woman with diabetes occurs early and is proportional to the level of hyperglycemia in the mother at delivery. Cord blood sugar and microsugar levels at 30 minutes and 1 hour of age provide the curve of glucose disappearance and potential for hypoglycemia. If lactation can be established, the glucose can be managed by breastfeeding. It must be closely monitored, however, so that intervention can be initiated when necessary. Incidence of hypocalcemia in infants of mothers with diabetes is high, which is believed to result from functional hypoparathyroidism, because phosphorus and calcitonin levels are normal.[184] The role of magnesium in this balance has not been clearly defined but needs to be monitored.

Hyperbilirubinemia occurs more frequently in infants of mothers with diabetes. β-Glucuronidase and bilirubin measurements were made on 10 breastfed infants of women with diabetes and 10 normal breastfed control infants by Sirota et al.[240] The concentrations of β-glucuronidase were higher in the serum of the milk of mothers with diabetes, and the bilirubin levels were higher in their infants. None of the control infants required phototherapy, whereas 50% of the infants of the women with IDDM did. Other investigators compared β-glucuronidase and bilirubin levels in a group of normal breastfed infants on the third and fifth days of life and found no correlation between the values. Although infants of women with diabetes are clearly more prone to hyperbilirubinemia, the central cause remains elusive.

Antenatal breast milk expression by women with diabetes for improving infant outcomes is a controversial procedure.[244] Small studies all express alarm regarding outcomes,[86] but the Cochrane Review expressed concern about lack of evidence and controlled studies.[73] It is being done in many countries per the Internet without benefit of study.

Women with diabetes in pregnancy are being encouraged to express colostrum before birth and store it for use immediately after birth to avoid their infant receiving artificial formula or intravenous dextrose for hypoglycemia in the neonate. The concerns include reports of stimulation of premature labor in multiple cases. Breast stimulus has been used to initiate labor in select cases; in other situations, an increase in the number of infants requiring care in intensive care units or special care nurseries is also observed. There are still no published, randomized, controlled trials, according to the Cochrane report.[73] No benefits have been reported to date either. To avoid use of bovine protein formula at birth, donor milk should be readily available or special non-bovine formula. Of additional concern is the evaluation of the amount of colostrum still available after delivery. This has not been studied. The total amount available to the infant may be diminished.

Breastfeeding and Onset of Diabetes

Breastfeeding has been associated with the prevention of type 2 diabetes mellitus in women who experience gestational diabetes during pregnancy. Gestational diabetes occurs in 4% of pregnancies and represents 90% of diabetes seen in pregnancy. Breastfeeding is associated with reduced blood glucose levels, postpartum weight loss, reduced long-term obesity, and a lower prevalence of metabolic syndrome, according to Bentley-Lewis et al.[32] Improvement in glucose and insulin homeostasis was seen in lactation in a study of type 2 diabetes mellitus in the Nurses' Health Study I and II reported by Stuebe et al.[252] The longer the duration of breastfeeding was, the lower the incidence of type 2 diabetes documented in this large cohort of more than 2 million person-years. For each additional year of lactation, normal women, without gestational diabetes but with a birth in the previous 15 years, had a 15% decrease in the risk for diabetes (Tables 16-6A and 16-6B).

TABLE 16-6A Duration of Breastfeeding and Diabetes: Comparison of Nurses' Health Study and Nurses' Health Study II Cohorts

	Nurses' Health Study	Nurses' Health Study II
Total number of participants	121,700	116,671
Year of birth	1921-1945	1946-1965
Timing of questionnaires	Every 2 years, beginning in 1976	Every 2 years, beginning in 1989
Assessment of lactation	1986: "How many months in total (all births combined) did you breastfeed?" Response options: did not breastfeed, <1, 1-3, 4-6, 7-11, 12-17, 18-23, 24-35, 36-47, ≥48, cannot remember	1993: "How many months in total (all births combined) did you breastfeed?" Response options: did not breastfeed, <1, 1-3, 4-6, 7-11, 12-17, 18-23, 24-35, 36-47, ≥48, cannot remember 1997: For each of first 4 pregnancies, detailed questions regarding return of menses, use of medication to suppress lactation, timing of introduction of infant formula/solid food, pumping, more than 6 h at night without breastfeeding Response options: 0-2, 3, 4-5, 6-7, 8-11, or ≥12 mo. Cessation of breastfeeding Response options: 1-2, 3-5, 6-8, 9-11, 12-18, or ≥19 months 2003: Supplemental questionnaire sent to women reporting births since 1997; same information gathered as on 1997 lactation questionnaire
Pregnancies	Baseline parity in 1976, additional pregnancies reported in 1978, 1980, 1982, 1984	Baseline parity in 1989, additional pregnancies reported every 2 yr thereafter
Weight	Baseline weight in 1976, update on weight every 2 yr thereafter	Baseline weight in 1989, update on weight every 2 yr thereafter
Weight at age 18 yr	1980	1989
Diabetes	Assessed on questionnaires every 2 yr, confirmed by supplemental questionnaire	Assessed on questionnaires every 2 yr, confirmed by supplemental questionnaire
Gestational diabetes	Not assessed	Assessed on questionnaires every 2 yr

JAMA, November 23/30, 2005-Vol. 294, No. 20 (Reprinted) ©2005 American Medical Association. All rights reserved, Stuebe AM, Rich-Edwards JW, Willett WC, et al: Duration of lactation and incidence of type 2 diabetes, *JAMA* 294:2601, 2005.

Epidemiologic reports[37,87] continue to accumulate, suggesting that being breastfed has a protective effect on the onset of diabetes in childhood. Children in Western Australia who were studied to the age of 14 years revealed an incidence of 0.59 children with diabetes per 1000.[94] No significant trends or associations with illness were made, except that breastfeeding beyond 1 week of age was less frequent in diabetic than nondiabetic cohorts. In a study of 95 children of women with diabetes and their siblings and peers without diabetes, the incidence of breastfeeding was only 18% but was comparable in all three groups. Twice as many children with diabetes had received soy formula as the other children. In a study of IDDM in Scandinavian populations, fewer children with childhood-onset diabetes were breastfed, and those who were breastfed were breastfed for shorter periods.[37] The authors suggest that insufficient breastfeeding of genetically susceptible newborn infants may lead to B-cell infection and IDDM in later

life. The prevalence of diabetes in black populations throughout Africa, where breastfeeding is common, is usually considerably lower than in Western countries among those of African descent.[153]

The Colorado IDDM Registry was studied retrospectively to determine the possible relationship between breastfeeding and development of childhood diabetes, in comparison with randomly selected control subjects.[179] Incidence of IDDM was less frequent among breastfed infants, and the longer the breastfeeding, the greater the effect. The population percentage with attributable risk ranged from 2% to 26%. Because of the increasing incidence of childhood diabetes throughout Scandinavia, a prospective study followed children for 7 years. Results demonstrate a clear relationship between lack of breastfeeding and IDDM in the first 7 years of life, or, conversely, a protective effect of breastfeeding. This effect is strongest with at least 4 months of exclusive breastfeeding.[37]

TABLE 16-6B Hazard Ratios for Type 2 Diabetes, Parous Women Only, in Analyses Restricted to Women Reporting a Birth in the Past 15 Years

	None	Cumulative Duration of Lactation (mo)					p Value for Trend*	HR per Additional Year of Lactation
		>0 to 3	>3 to 6	>6 to 11	>11 to 23	>23		
No. of cases, Nurses' Health Study†	68	30	18	18	28	24		
Person-years of follow-up	23,419	12,400	8669	9415	15,251	15,023		
Age-adjusted HR (95% CI)	1.00	0.76 (0.48-1.18)	0.76 (0.45-1.31)	0.61 (0.35-1.05)	0.63 (0.40-0.99)	0.41 (0.25-0.67)	<0.001	0.80 (0.70-0.93)
Covariate-adjusted HR (95% CI)‡	1.00	0.68 (0.42-1.09)	0.67 (0.39-1.18)	0.61 (0.34-1.08)	0.67 (0.42-1.08)	0.44 (0.26-0.74)	0.008	0.84 (0.73-0.98)
Covariate-adjusted HR (95% CI), including current BMI‡	1.00	0.72 (0.44-1.18)	0.74 (0.42-1.32)	0.64 (0.35-1.17)	0.70 (0.42-1.15)	0.47 (0.27-0.81)	0.02	0.85 (0.73-0.99)
No. of cases, Nurses' Health Study II§	117	116	69	112	147	110		
Person-years of follow-up	72,041	70,354	62,386	116,228	155,323	143,430		
Age-adjusted HR (95% CI)	1.00	1.07 (0.83-1.39)	0.73 (0.54-0.99)	0.62 (0.48-0.81)	0.57 (0.44-0.72)	0.40 (0.31-0.53)	<0.001	0.76 (0.70-0.82)
Covariate-adjusted HR (95% CI)‡	1.00	1.03 (0.80-1.35)	0.78 (0.57-1.06)	0.76 (0.58-0.99)	0.76 (0.59-0.98)	0.53 (0.40-0.70)	<0.001	0.82 (0.76-0.89)
Covariate-adjusted HR (95% CI), including current BMI‡	1.00	0.98 (0.75-1.28)	0.98 (0.75-1.28)	0.76 (0.55-1.03)	0.74 (0.56-0.96)	0.59 (0.44-0.79)	<0.001	0.86 (0.79-0.93)

BMI, Body mass index; CI, confidence interval; HR, hazard ratio.
*p value for trend across categories, based on category midpoint.
†Nurses' Health Study: prospective analysis using cases from 1986 to 2002.
‡Adjusted for parity, BMI at age 18 years. Dietary score quintile, physical activity, family history of diabetes, smoking status, birth weight of participant, and multivitamin use.
§Nurses' Health Study II: retrospective analysis using lactation data from 1997 and 2003, cases from 1989 to 2001, parous women only.
JAMA, November 23/30, 2005–Vol. 294, No. 20 (Reprinted) ©2005 American Medical Association. All rights reserved.

Other investigators are exploring the possible relationship of early exposure to cow milk and the onset of diabetes. It is suggested that the etiology of the disease has both a genetic and an environmental component. Karjalainen et al.[135] report the identification of a bovine albumin peptide as a possible trigger of IDDM. The antibodies to this peptide are said to react with P69, a B-cell surface protein that may represent the target antigen for milk-induced B-cell-specific immunity. The antibodies decline in 1 to 2 years to normal values. Much lower values were found in all the control children.

Utilizing the Colorado IDDM Registry, Kostraba et al.[152] compared children with high and low genetic risk for IDDM with a group of matched normal control subjects. They used a HLA-DQB1 molecular marker. Early exposure to cow milk and solid foods was strongly associated with IDDM in genetically high-risk individuals. The authors suggest that the inclusion of the HLA-encoded risk in the analyses demonstrates the combined effect of genetic and environmental factors.

The association of serum immunoglobulin A (IgA) antibodies with milk antigens in patients with severe arteriosclerosis is under review. The presence of antibodies against dietary antigens is well documented. Its relevance is under study by Muscari et al.[193] and others.

Rennie[221] showed a relationship between the consumption of cow milk and the incidence of diabetes, between the ages of 0 to 14 years, in countries around the world (Figure 16-6). The association between IDDM and early exposure to cow milk may be explained by the generation of a specific immune response to β-casein. A cellular and humoral anti-β-casein immune response is triggered by exposure to cow milk and may cross-react with B-cell antigen. Sequential homologies exist between β-casein and several B-cell molecules.[49] The systemic review of published studies indicated that breastfeeding did influence risk for type 2 diabetes in later life. Maternal type 1 diabetes is not an independent risk factor for being overweight in childhood in these children. However, lack of being breastfed is a risk factor, as well as their higher birth weight.[62,120] The introduction of cereal younger than 6 months of age was shown to increase the incidence of diabetes in at-risk children. Much work remains to be done. In the meantime, this may be one more reason for mothers to consider breastfeeding, especially in families at high risk for diabetes, and delaying the introduction of solid food until 6 months of age, as recommended by WHO/UNICEF for all children.[64,70]

THYROID DISEASE

The thyroid gland is intimately involved with hormone activity of pregnancy. The metabolic and hormonal demands of pregnancy alter the thyroid gland. Conversely, the outcome of pregnancy may be altered by changes in the thyroid gland. Thyroxine-binding globulin increases secondary to the increased estrogens. The normal pregnant woman may be euthyroid, but changes occur in the basal metabolic rate, radioactive iodine uptake, and thyroid size.

Thyroid disease is four times more common in women than men, and thyroid abnormality is common in pregnancy. The diagnosis is more difficult to make during pregnancy because of problems with the interpretation of thyroid function tests. Treatment must take into account the presence of the fetus once the management decision is made. During the postpartum period, autoimmune thyroid disease is exacerbated. New-onset autoimmune thyroid disease occurs in 10% of postpartum women but is often overlooked when mothers are dismissed as depressed. More than 60% of patients with Graves disease trace the onset to their postpartum period. Most of the immune changes of pregnancy gradually return to normal by 12 months. An explanation for the postpartum autoimmune exacerbation is that a reduction of feral cells is associated with a reduction in maternal tolerance of the remaining microchimeric cells and a loss of major placental peptide complexes associated with T-cell energy during pregnancy (Figure 16-7).

Thyroid disease is increasingly common postpartum and often presents as depression. No postpartum woman should be started on antidepressive drugs without a thyroid screen, especially if she has not been symptomatic before pregnancy. Unfortunately, most textbooks that discuss thyroid disease

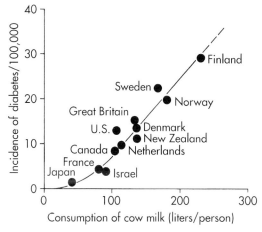

Figure 16-6. Annual consumption of cow milk and incidence of diabetes (ages 0 to 14). (Modified from Rennie J: Formula for diabetes? *Sci Am* 267:24, 1992.)

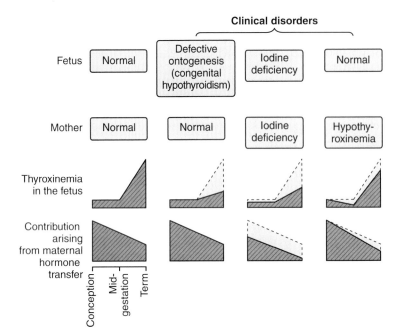

Figure 16-7. Thyroid function disorders. Schematic representation of the three sets of clinical conditions that can affect thyroid function in the mother alone, in the fetus alone, or in the fetomaternal unit shows the relative contributions of impaired maternal or fetal thyroid function that may eventually lead to alterations in fetal tyrosinemia. (Reprinted by permission from Glinoer D, Delange F: The potential repercussions of maternal, fetal, neonatal hypothyroxinemia on the progeny, *Thyroid* 10: 871, 2000.)

in pregnancy and postpartum do not discuss breastfeeding or lactation, except Creasy et al.[59]

POSTPARTUM THYROIDITIS

Postpartum thyroiditis is diagnosed when abnormal levels of thyroid-stimulating hormone (TSH) are documented, either elevated or suppressed during the first year postpartum, and Graves disease has been excluded by positive thyroid-stimulating immunoglobulins, or a toxic nodule is present. Usually a transient hyperthyroid phase lasts 6 weeks to 6 months after delivery. This is followed by a hypothyroid phase that lasts up to a year after delivery (Figure 16-8). The incidence of this autoimmune disease is as high as 6% to 9%, and is higher in individuals with type 1 diabetes. The hyperthyroid phase is characterized by fatigue, palpations, heat intolerance, and nervousness. It is of limited duration, a few weeks to a few months. Antithyroid drugs should be used, although beta blockers may help with symptoms. The hypothyroid phase follows with marked fatigue, hair loss, depression, poor concentration, and dry skin. Treatment with thyroxine (T_4) (Synthroid) is appropriate. Postpartum thyroiditis, which is a destructive process, is characterized by positive antithyroid antibodies (antithyroglobulin and antithyroid peroxidase). The TSH levels are suppressed, and T_4 levels are high in the hyperthyroid phase. This is in addition to extremely suppressed radioactive iodine uptake, which should not be done during lactation. The diagnosis can be confirmed by the absence of thyroid-stimulating immunoglobulins, which rules

out Graves disease. Distinguishing postpartum thyroiditis and postpartum depression can be done by measuring thyroid antibodies, which will be negative in most cases of clinical postpartum depression. The two postpartum diseases can coexist. These patients deserve endocrinologist and psychiatrist consultation. Lactation will and can continue if already established. Any faltering in supply can be managed with the usual protocol of increased stimulus and galactagogues.

MATERNAL HYPOTHYROIDISM

It has long been held that hypothyroidism is associated with infertility. The incidence of hypothyroidism during pregnancy is low. Because of the difficulty in maintaining pregnancy in individuals with hypothyroidism, the number of women who are truly hypothyroid at delivery is also low. Some women who are maintained on thyroid treatment for one reason or another do bear children. If hypothyroidism is diagnosed, it should be treated with full replacement therapy, 75 to 125 mcg of desiccated thyroid daily. The medication should be continued after delivery. The mother should be permitted to breastfeed without question. There is measurable thyroid hormone in the milk of normal women. Breastfeeding is not contraindicated because proper treatment makes her euthyroid.

If a mother is truly hypothyroid, particular care should be used to rule out hypothyroidism in the infant, using neonatal screening with T_4 and TSH if necessary. Diagnosis can be performed by evaluating maternal blood values and is not a hazard to

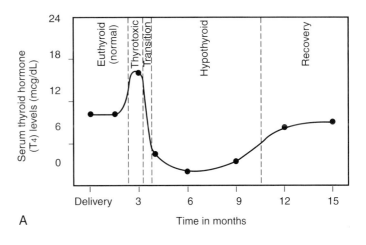

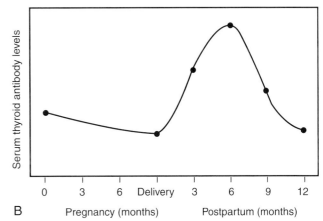

Figure 16-8. Postpartum thyroiditis and changes in thyroid antibody concentrations. **A,** Postpartum thyroiditis manifests with a transient hyperthyroid phase, during which serum levels of thyroxine (T4) are elevated. A hyperthyroid phase follows. **B,** Serum thyroid antibody levels fluctuate during and after pregnancy. (From Smallridge RC, Fein HC, Hayship CC: Postpartum thyroiditis, *Bridge Newslett* (Thyroid Foundation America) 3:3, 1988.)

the nursling. Thyroiditis may well be the cause and should be considered. Because of the small amount of thyroid hormone in breast milk, a breastfed child with hypothyroidism may be undiagnosed unless laboratory values are carefully reviewed.

An increase in hypothyroidism is being identified postpartum, especially when normal women have prolonged "baby blues" and fatigue or appear to have new-onset depression. Screening for thyroid disease is appropriate before prescribing antidepressants. Self-medication has led women to initiate treatment with St. John's wort, thus masking the thyroid disease. Obtaining a thorough history is always important, including self-medication with other drugs and herbs. Herbal treatments are being recommended by paraprofessionals during lactation. Therefore, a physician should be especially vigilant when taking a history, and include specific questions about herbal use.

MATERNAL HYPERTHYROIDISM

The diagnostic procedures and therapeutic management of the mother with possible hyperthyroidism present some hazards to the breastfed infant.

The diagnosis can be made without radioactive material. The combination of an elevated serum T_4 level and a normal resin triiodothyronine (T_3) uptake is helpful. These two determinations can be combined to obtain a free-T_4 index, which reflects these determinations in a single value. The possibility of thyroiditis should be considered. Whether the patient eventually has a thyroidectomy or not, her thyrotoxicosis must first be medically stabilized. Surgery is usually not indicated in postpartum thyrotoxicosis.

Postpartum thyroiditis has also increased in frequency to 1 in 20 women. It is characterized by symptoms of hyperthyroidism with pounding tachycardia, rapid weight loss, insatiable appetite, and excessive milk production.[134] One case reported to the lactation center was notable for a stimulating reaction to prenatal vitamins (possible iodine effect), caffeine, and high-protein beverages.

A distinction between postpartum thyroiditis and Graves disease should be made (Table 16-7). Those with postpartum thyroiditis initially appear to suffer from hyperthyroidism but develop hypothyroidism at approximately 6 weeks and usually require thyroid replacement indefinitely.

Michael and Mueller[186] reviewed five women with CF and their infants. Evaluations indicating their need for enzyme therapy and their pulmonary disease status classified these women as mild cases. The infants averaged 37.4 ± 1.5 weeks' gestation with birth weights of 3.0 ± 0.5 kg. Sweat tests were negative for all the infants. Duration of breastfeeding ranged from 3 to 30 weeks. Four of the five infants maintained good growth during breastfeeding. Four of the five mothers were at or above their standard body weight throughout lactation. The authors conclude that women with mild CF can not only sustain a pregnancy, but also support the growth of a healthy infant through breastfeeding while maintaining their own weight.[186]

Current recommendations for breastfeeding by mothers with CF were published by Luder et al.,[171] after a survey of CF centers (Tables 16-8 and 16-9).

TABLE 16-8 Recommendations About Breastfeeding by Cystic Fibrosis Center Directors for Mothers with Cystic Fibrosis*

Recommendation	Response, No. (%)
Recommend breastfeeding	14 (11.2)
Do not recommend breastfeeding	10 (8.0)
Recommendation made according to each patient's health status	52 (41.6)
Recommendation made according to each patient's personal wishes	40 (32.0)
Not applicable and/or other category	9 (7.2)
Total	125 (100)

*Many centers chose more than one answer; therefore the response rate for each answer is calculated as a percentage of total responses.

Modified from Luder E, Kaltan M, Tanzer-Torres G, et al: Current recommendations for breastfeeding in cystic fibrosis centers, *Am J Dis Child* 144:1153, 1990.

TABLE 16-9 Duration of Breastfeeding as Reported by Cystic Fibrosis Center Directors for Mothers With Cystic Fibrosis

Duration (mo)	Centers, No. (%)
<3	35 (41)
3-6	9 (10)
>6	1 (1.2)
Not applicable and/or other category	41 (48)
Total	86 (100)

Modified from Luder E, Kaltan M, Tanzer-Torres G, et al: Current recommendations for breastfeeding in cystic fibrosis centers, *Am J Dis Child* 144:1153, 1990.

For mothers with CF, 11% of centers recommend breastfeeding, 8% do not recommend it, 42% tailor their recommendations to the mother's health, and 32% make recommendations on the basis of the mother's wishes. Of the centers, 41% report breastfeeding duration of less than 3 months. Table 16-9 lists factors that preclude breastfeeding and factors contributing to discontinuation, as reported by directors of CF centers. 81 centers (94%) have support services available throughout the course of lactation.

As the survival of patients with CF continues to improve and more women reach the childbearing years, an increasing number will choose to breastfeed.[171] Additional research is necessary to help mothers with CF maintain their health while lactating and to monitor growth in infants with CF, and their general health status, while breastfeeding. Breastfeeding usually enhances the health of an infant with CF, because it helps to protect against infection and provide active enzymes (see Chapter 15).

Studies demonstrate that mothers with pulmonary and pancreatic disease of CF can breastfeed and that their infants do well. It is appropriate, however, to test milk samples occasionally for sodium, chloride, and total fat, and to follow the infant's growth pattern critically.

CELIAC DISEASE

All the clinical and epidemiologic evidence suggests breastfeeding is protective against celiac disease, delaying the onset and reducing the severity. The milk of mothers with celiac disease is characterized by a reduced abundance of immunoprotective compounds (TGF-β1 and sIgA) and bifido bacteria. It is possible this could somewhat reduce the protective effects of breastfeeding.[205] However, these constituents are still present in significant amounts. Trace amounts of gluten (α-gliadin) can be found in breast milk. No evidence shows that gluten in breast milk triggers celiac disease in susceptible babies. Mothers of at-risk infants or infants who have been diagnosed can go on a gluten-free diet while breastfeeding.[18] In a case, a 6-month-old breastfeeding infant, whose older brother had been diagnosed with celiac disease at 18 months of age after months of crying, colic, abdominal pain, and gas, began developing similar symptoms. The mother began a gluten-free diet and within 48 hours the infant was dramatically better and continued to breastfeed.[18] See the discussion of when to initiate change in diet of an infant in Chapter 14.

HYPERLIPOPROTEINEMIA

The effect of pregnancy and lactation on lipoprotein and cholesterol metabolism was studied in the rat model by Smith et al.[241] It is well established that cholesterol levels are elevated in normal women during pregnancy and lactation. These new findings further defined the process. The origins of this hyperlipidemia and cholestasis were traced through plasma and hepatic cholesterol metabolism during pregnancy, lactation, and postlactation. The activities of hepatic enzymes were significantly lower for SR-B$_1$, which was elevated. Once lactation began the enzymes increased, except for SR-B, which was decreased compared with nonpregnant nonlactating normal women. In later stages of lactation, most hepatic elements returned to near-normal levels. Plasma cholesterol levels were higher at birth and during lactation with an increase in low-density lipoprotein (LDL)-sized particles. Twenty-four hours after lactation ceased (i.e., suckling ceased), plasma triglycerides were 3.7-fold higher, but cholesterol was unchanged. Very large lipoproteins were present, but LDL-sized particles were absent. Hepatic cholesterol acyltransferase was only 27% of control levels, while diacylglycerol acyltransferase increased three times and LDL lipoprotein receptors doubled. Three weeks after weaning, most values were normal except for lipoprotein receptors, which were still elevated.[241]

The study of a mother with type I hyperlipoproteinemia nursing her second child is reported by Steiner et al.[248] The milk and plasma were carefully analyzed, and it appeared that the deficit of lipoprotein lipase extended to the mammary gland. The milk had low total lipids and a bizarre composition of fatty acids. Her milk differed greatly from her plasma triglycerides in comparison to normal mothers, whose fatty acid profile in the milk matched the plasma. Low concentrations of essential linoleic ($C_{18.2,20.4}$) and arachidonic ($C_{20:4}$) acids in her milk made it inadequate for her infant. Other women in the literature with hyperlipoproteinemia have been reported to develop pancreatitis during pregnancy. Lactation is not advisable when the milk has major deficiencies.

GALACTOSEMIA

The case of a 25-year-old woman, who had been diagnosed with galactosemia, herself, at the age of 3 weeks, was reported by Forbes et al.[85] at the time of her first baby, whom she breastfed. The woman had blood transferase activity that hovered from zero to 1.9 U (normal 18 to 25 U/g hemoglobin). Despite irregular menses, she conceived and delivered a normal girl who thrived on breastfeeding exclusively. Solid foods were added at 5 months. The analysis of her milk at 4½ weeks postpartum revealed protein 1.42 g/dL, lactose 7.5 g/dL, fat 4.25 g/dL, and calculated energy content 74 kcal/dL. The fatty acid profile was normal, except for 18:3, which was low. Macrominerals were all within normal range. Glucose was 26 mg/dL and galactose

less than 15 mg/dL. The authors point out that, because lactose can be found from uridine diphosphogalactose (by means of epimerase) and glucose (a reaction stimulated by lactalbumin) in the absence of transferase enzyme, one could have predicted that lactose would be present in her milk.[85]

PHENYLKETONURIA

The success of newborn screening and early treatment has resulted in a population of adolescents with phenylketonuria (PKU) moving into the childbearing years with normal intelligence. Matalon et al.[176] reported a pregnancy and lactation experience in a woman who had stopped her diet and did not seek medical care until 16 weeks' gestation. They also reported their experience with 32 young adults who had discontinued their diets. The authors make the following recommendations:

1. Diet restrictions for PKU should not be discontinued at any age, especially in women.
2. Strict control should begin before conception to bring blood phenylalanine levels to 4 mg/dL or lower.
3. Breastfeeding is permitted.

Matalon et al.[176] report that the milk of mothers with PKU controlled by diet is normal (Table 16-10).

RADIATION EXPOSURE AND INTERVENTIONAL RADIOLOGY

The diagnosis and treatment of a lactating woman with malignancy may well necessitate the use of radioactive compounds or antimetabolites. Because the breast is a minor route of excretion for most of these compounds, it is probably inappropriate to continue nursing during such exposure. Although the dose of the material drug in a single aliquot of milk may be small, the effects are cumulative. No long-range studies indicate the outcome of offspring exposed in utero. In addition, a mother with malignancy should be encouraged to spare all her resources to overcome the disease. Lactation is as draining in such a situation as pregnancy.

TABLE 16-10	Amino Acid Levels (mmol/dL) in Milk of Mothers With Phenylketonuria (PKU)	
Amino Acid	**PKU Milk**	**Reference Values**
Phenylalanine	0.5	0.62
Tyrosine	0.5	1-2
Taurine	36.7	41-45

Iron, zinc, copper, magnesium, and selenium were also within normal range.

Diagnostic or therapeutic measures using radioactive materials are contraindicated in pregnancy and lactation because they tend to accumulate in the fetal and neonatal thyroid gland and the maternal breast. If radioactive testing is deemed essential before treatment can be carried out, a test dose of iodine-123 (^{123}I) can be given and breastfeeding discontinued for 66 hours. (The half-life of ^{123}I is 13.2 hours; $5 \times 13.2 = 66$ hours.) The validity of the test during lactation has been questioned because the mammary gland may divert a disproportionate amount of ^{123}I to the milk. The milk should be expressed during the 66-hour period and discarded.[39] The milk should be scanned for radioactivity before breastfeeding is resumed.

Breast interventions beyond the diagnosis of pathology are becoming more common and may be urgent. Acute breast situations are those specifically related to breastfeeding such as abscesses, extreme plugged duct, and breast swelling requiring irrigation. Cannulation of a duct can be done by an interventional radiologist.[121] Trauma to the breast may require an invasive technique. See Figure 16-9, an abscess irrigated with saline, and Figure 16-10, hemorrhage following biopsy.

BREAST CANCER

In the young patient with cancer, another concern is what risk lactation adds to the mother's long-range prognosis. The automatic response tends to be not to become pregnant and, in any event, not to breastfeed. This question was examined by Hornstein et al.,[118] who indicate that "the current data suggest that pregnant women with early breast carcinoma may be treated in the same way as nonpregnant women without affecting the pregnancy."

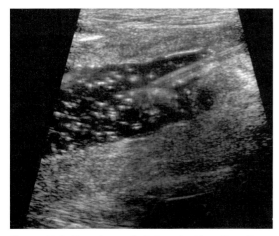

Figure 16-9. The abscess is irrigated with saline. (From Ingram AD, Mahoney MC: An overview of breast emergencies and guide to management by interventional radiologists, *Tech Vasc Interv Radiol* 17:55, 2014 (Figure 12).)

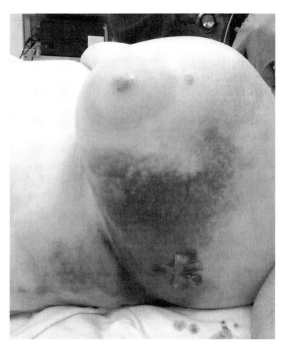

Figure 16-10. Postbiopsy hemorrhage has led to significant asymmetric enlargement of the left breast and bruising extending over the left breast and down the side and flank. (From Ingram AD, Mahoney MC: An overview of breast emergencies and guide to management by interventional radiologists, *Tech Vasc Interv Radiol* 17:55, 2014 (Figure 13).)

Disease that is detected toward the end of pregnancy may be treated with surgery immediately, and then the patient may receive adjuvant therapy if indicated after delivery. Advanced disease should be treated aggressively, and the infant delivered and not breastfed. During lactation, the diagnosis of breast carcinoma requires the immediate suppression of lactation by medications other than estrogens. The carcinoma is then treated by standard methods. When a woman has already had a radical mastectomy for breast cancer, she can have subsequent pregnancies, but they should be delayed until the period of greatest risk is over (i.e., at least 3 to 5 years). She may also breastfeed.

Kalache et al.[130] report that 7% of fertile women have one or more pregnancies after mastectomy; 70% of these pregnancies have occurred within 5 years after treatment. Women who have pregnancies after potentially curative mastectomy have survival rates of 5 to 10 years—as good or better than those who do not become pregnant. The patients with the best prognosis, however, may be a function of selection, because they are healthier and thus able to become pregnant. Uneventful pregnancy does not guarantee cure, although the highest rate of recurrence is in the first 3 years, and gradually declines. It is never zero. Metastases to the axilla increase the risk. Recurrence in the chest wall during pregnancy can be treated with local shielded radiation, but anything more extensive requires aggressive intervention.

The importance of careful monitoring during pregnancy is obvious. One of the major contributors to a more grave prognosis of the original disease that appears during pregnancy and lactation is not the underlying disease. Rather, it is the difficulty of detecting the lesion during pregnancy and lactation, and the reluctance of patient and physician to make a diagnosis and initiate treatment. The greatest risk for neoplastic growth occurs in the first 20 weeks of pregnancy, when the immune system is suppressed, and growth of the mammary tissues is at its peak under the stimulus from estrogen, progesterone, and prolactin levels.[167,223] No data were provided on the influence of postmastectomy lactation on long-range survival. Some women have wanted to nurse with the remaining breast. The decision would necessitate consideration of the individual situation. It represents a different risk/benefit ratio than pregnancy itself. Extensive epidemiologic studies of large populations of women do not indicate that breastfeeding has any relationship to the overall risk for breast cancer. Epidemiologic data about breastfeeding on the remaining breast are not available.[167]

The incidence of cancer in the remaining breast has fueled the question of prophylactic contralateral mastectomy. The women who are at the greatest risk for cancer in the second breast are those who have a family history of breast cancer in their mother or sister, who have had onset in childbearing years, or whose original cancer involved multiple lesions in the primary breast. In their discussion of the other breast, Leis and Urban[167] state that if a postmastectomy patient were to become pregnant and deliver, "it would be rare indeed that the patient would allow or the attending physician would condone the use of the remaining breast for nursing." Although some women cherish the remaining breast, most, in the experience of Leis and Urban,[167] are ashamed of it and keep it hidden.

Lactation after primary radiation therapy for carcinoma of the breast was reported in a major literature search by Burns[45] to have occurred successfully in one patient, whose primary lesion was in the tail of Spence. One year after radiation, she became pregnant and successfully breastfed. She had less milk on the treated side. Her malignancy had not recurred. Another patient received radiotherapy after biopsy for an invasive duct carcinoma known to be present for a year. She had a week of boost therapy 8 weeks later. She became pregnant a year later, delivering a full-term infant 22 months after the original radiation. She successfully established lactation on the uninvolved side but was unable to obtain any response from the irradiated breast. No comment was made about the radiated breast's response to pregnancy. She weaned her infant at 6 weeks.[63] Two years after treatment the patient had no evidence of recurrence.

The incidence of breast cancer diagnosed during pregnancy in a large series was 3 per 10,000 pregnancies, or 1% to 2% of breast cancer cases. Delay in diagnosis is the primary reason for the seemingly worse overall prognosis for breast cancer diagnosed during pregnancy and lactation, with the duration of symptoms averaging 5 to 15 months. The incidence of spread to the axilla is 70% to 80% in the perinatal period, compared with a 40% to 50% node-positive rate in nonpregnant women.[116]

Breast cancers continue to be reported in the literature during lactation. The case of a 33-year-old lactating woman presented with a 10-cm breast abscess.[6] Biopsy of the abscess wall was done following IV antibiotics and drainage of 300 mL of pus.[6] The woman had been treated with multiple rounds of antibiotics for mastitis, and then the abscess was diagnosed by ultrasound. After several months of antibiotics, she was referred for evaluation and treatment. Biopsy is standard treatment for abscesses in this surgical clinic. The biopsy revealed an adenosquamous carcinoma requiring surgery, chemo, and radiation. The authors recommend biopsy for all breast abscesses that require surgical drainage.[6] In another case, a 29-year-old women was lactating when a mass was noted in the right breast.[218] She was diagnosed with a granular cell tumor, which was difficult to diagnose and finally to surgically remove and treat. Breastfeeding had to be discontinued.

Any dominant mass during pregnancy or lactation should be evaluated promptly. Ultrasound is effective and safe during pregnancy and lactation. A fine-needle biopsy will distinguish cystic from solid lesions. A solid mass can be biopsied during pregnancy or lactation.[226] The risk for milk fistulas is very low. Suppression of lactation is not necessary. After the diagnosis of cancer is made, staging is essential before treatment is begun. Staging during pregnancy is more difficult because of the need for ionizing radiation.

Further surgery, including mastectomy, can be done during pregnancy and lactation. Because radiation and chemotherapy will also be necessary, breastfeeding is not recommended. When breast cancer is diagnosed during lactation, treatment should be initiated promptly and the infant weaned when chemotherapy is begun. Newer chemotherapy drugs have short half-lives so that it may only be necessary to pump and discard for 10 to 12 hours (5 × half-life = clearance time). The half-life of the specific drug can be obtained on Lact-Med (see Chapter 12).

When young patients are treated with breast-conserving therapy and radiation for early-stage breast cancer, they may experience full-term pregnancies subsequently. Successful breastfeeding on the untreated breast as well as the treated breast is possible after conservative lumpectomy and radiation in some patients. The volume and the duration of lactation are less on the treated side. When the incision is circumareolar, successful lactation is less likely. Usually the function of the untreated breast is unaffected.[113]

Treatment with chemotherapy is changing as new protocols are developed. Mothers determined to breastfeed can indeed pump and discard for the required time and then resume breastfeeding. It takes a flexible infant for this schedule as well. Each chemotherapeutic agent is being evaluated for half-life and clearance time.

African-American women have a disproportionately high incidence of estrogen receptor-negative breast cancer, a subtype of unexplained etiology. A study by Palmer et al.[208] looked at parity and breastfeeding, in relationship to cancer. African-American women had more pregnancies and little or no breastfeeding. They stated that lactation might be an effective tool for reducing the occurrence of the subtypes of cancer that contribute disproportionately to breast cancer mortality.

AUTOIMMUNE THROMBOCYTOPENIC PURPURA

Reports are conflicting regarding the passage of antibodies to platelets via the breast milk in mothers with autoimmune thrombocytopenic purpura.[106,183] Laboratory efforts to demonstrate absorption of these antibodies from the breast milk failed. One case report detailed the successful breastfeeding of a severely affected premature infant who had required exchange transfusion and multiple platelet transfusions at birth.[175] No relapses occurred with introduction of maternal milk at 5 days of age. Steroids were discontinued at 2 weeks, and the infant thrived at the breast.

RHEUMATOID ARTHRITIS AND OTHER CONNECTIVE TISSUE DISORDERS

The influence of lactation on the development and progression of rheumatoid arthritis (RA) has been the subject of several epidemiologic studies. Previous observations noted an increased risk for RA developing postpartum, particularly after the first pregnancy. The contribution of hormonal factors occurring before onset of RA, such as age of menarche, parity, age at first birth, breastfeeding, use of oral contraceptives, irregular menstrual cycles, and postmenopausal hormone use, to the development

of RA was examined by Karlson et al.[136] in the 121,700 women enrolled in the Nurses' Health Study. RA was diagnosed in 674 women between 1976 and 2002, confirmed by connective disease screening questionnaire and blinded medical record review using the American College of Rheumatology criteria. Rheumatoid factor was positive in 60% of the patients. Using Cox proportional hazard risk models, a strong trend was found for a decreasing risk for RA with increasing duration of breastfeeding ($p = 0.001$). Only irregular menses and onset of menses at less than 10 years were weakly associated with RA risk. Other parameters were not associated. The authors concluded that there was a dose-dependent protective effect of breastfeeding duration against RA.[222] Several additional series have shown similar results where rheumatoid arthritis onset was reduced or delayed with breastfeeding, and the effect was does dependent. Long-term breastfeeding is associated with significant reduction in the risk of RA. This was shown in a population involving 121,700 women from the Nurses' Health Study, 7349 Chinese women in the Guangzhou Biobank Cohort Study, and 18,326 women linked to regional registers.[1] RA is two to four times more common in women, suggesting the protection of androgens. Protection from oral contraceptives has been suggested in some studies[128] and refuted in others.

A national cohort of 187 women who developed RA within 12 months of pregnancy was studied. Of the 88 women who developed the disease after their first pregnancy, 71 breastfed (81%), compared with only half of control mothers. A smaller risk was noted after the second pregnancy. No added risk with the third pregnancy was associated with breastfeeding. The increase in risk was highest in those women whose disease was erosive and rheumatoid factor positive. Other investigators, who reviewed a cohort of 176 women with RA who had at least one child and a mean age of 46 years at diagnosis, concluded that parity and, to a lesser degree, breastfeeding before RA onset worsened the prognosis for severe disease. Oral contraceptive use had a protective effect.[128]

The evidence regarding reproductive events as risk factors for RA is conflicting. A population-based study of 63,090 women, followed from 1961 to 1989, examined reproductive factors and mortality rates. The role of parity, age at first and last birth, or age at menarche and menopause showed no relationship to RA. A protective effect of lactation was noted, however, with total time of lactation associated with decreased mortality rate from RA with a dose-response relationship.[42]

Rheumatic disease may necessitate treatment of pregnant and lactating patients with disease-modifying active rheumatic disease drugs or immunosuppressive drugs. Nonsteroidal antiinflammatory drugs (NSAIDs), in general, are passed into the milk in low doses. Shorter acting drugs are safer. The immediate postpartum period is usually associated with a flare up. Medications need to be selected carefully. The benefits of breastfeeding are significant for these infants. Safe drugs are short-acting NSAIDs, prednisone and prednisolone, antimalarials, and sulfasalazine. AZA and anti-TNF-α inhibitors are also safe. The newer small molecule UAK-inhibitors methotrexate and leflunomide are not recommended. Cyclosporine is not recommended as a therapy during breastfeeding.

Prolactin levels are greatly elevated during pregnancy in women with systemic lupus erythematosus.[125] Most patients with systemic lupus erythematosus have elevated prolactin levels, as do patients with RA, osteoarthritis, fibromyalgia, and polymyalgia. A dysregulation of pituitary response has been suggested as the etiology in RA. The role of prolactin in other autoimmune disorders is not understood, but supports the concept that a close relationship exists between neuroendocrine and immune systems.

If symptoms can be controlled with NSAIDs, such as acetaminophen, ibuprofen, hydroxychloroquine (Plaquenil), ketorolac, and piroxicam, which are all acceptable according to the American Academy of Pediatrics (AAP) list, treatment is not a problem during lactation. The use of corticosteroids (prednisone 120 mg/day) is considered safe. Injections of steroids into the joint, even the more potent triamcinolone, provide only low doses in the serum and can be tolerated for brief courses. The disease-modifying active rheumatic disease drugs, which include methotrexate, gold salts, and azathioprine, are critical to management. They cannot be delayed in a patient with a confirmed diagnosis and joint pain with an elevated sedimentation rate. They are toxic and breastfeeding is contraindicated. Gold salts, which differ from gold, have been found in milk and in a nursing infant.[268]

Postpartum flare of inflammatory polyarthritis may be induced by breastfeeding, according to a prospective study of over 100 women with RA.[13] The first-time breastfeeders had increased disease activity 6 months postpartum based on symptoms, joint counts, and C-reactive protein levels. Not all women had flares, and long-term implications were not investigated. It was less frequent and less severe in those who had breastfed previously. The authors relate it to prolonged, elevated levels of prolactin.[25]

Karlson et al. reported that women who breastfeed more than a total of 24 months reduce their risk for rheumatoid arthritis by 50%. This finding was part of a study of more than 120,000 women.[136]

Primary Sjögren syndrome, which involves the glands of secretion (sweat, salivary), is known to be associated with hyperprolactinemia. However, because of the characteristic abnormalities of secreting glands, lactation may not be successful.[14] Sjögren syndrome has also been seen in association with Raynaud phenomenon[123] (see later discussion). Breastfeeding is not contraindicated.

HYPERTENSION AND CARDIOVASCULAR DISEASE

Hypertension is a major public health problem. Successful management of hypertension, however, is pharmacologic. Before one considers the drugs involved, it is appropriate to consider that lactation may present some therapeutic advantages. The high levels of prolactin may be physiologically soothing to the mother, and it has been shown in animals that females given high levels of prolactin respond with nesting and mothering behavior. The breast is also an organ of secretion, and a liter or so of fluid is produced per day. In dehydrated women, lactation continues while urine production diminishes. The appropriate use of low-dose diuretics may control hypertension, whereas high-dose thiazides can cause suppression of lactation. Chlorothiazide, hydrochlorothiazides, and chlorthalidone are minimally excreted in milk (see Chapter 11), as are spironolactone and its metabolite canrenone, according to single-dose kinetics.

Propranolol has been widely studied and is probably the safest of the beta blockers during lactation. This is due to its low level in milk compared with other beta blockers, which are weak bases with an average pKa of 9.2 to 9.5, predisposing them to appear in slightly acidic human milk. Methyldopa appears in low amounts in milk, but its direct action on the pituitary to suppress prolactin release presents a theoretic risk for suppressing milk production. An obstetrician should be aware of this potential if lactation is going poorly. Reserpine poses a recognized risk to infants during delivery and postpartum. Other drugs appropriate to hypertension management are discussed in Chapter 11.

Maternal risk for cardiovascular disease is reduced by breastfeeding during the reproductive years. Data from 139,681 postmenopausal women in the Women's Health Initiative were reviewed by Schwarz et al.[233] to determine the dose-response relationships between the cumulative number of months of lactation and disease. More than 12 months of breastfeeding provided a reduced risk for hypertension, diabetes, hyperlipidemia, and cardiovascular disease, which is now the leading cause of death for women in developed countries.

Never breastfeeding or limited breastfeeding has been correlated with increased incidence of chronic disease, including hypertension. An observational cohort study of 55,636 parous women in the US Nurses' Health Study II was conducted by Steube et al.[249] Never breastfeeding, or curtailed breastfeeding, was associated with an increased risk of incident hypertension. Women who never breastfed were more likely to develop hypertension than those women who breastfed their first child at least 12 months.

Primary prevention of hypertension is a major public health priority.

Breastfeeding has been reported to affect the cardiovascular function of a woman, but some of the studies have been conflicting. Two separate studies examined the effects of breastfeeding on cardiovascular function. The first study[185] compared the pre-ejection period (PEP), heart rate, cardiac output (CO), and total peripheral resistance (TPR) in groups of breastfeeding women and bottle-feeding women. Breastfeeding women had higher cardiac output throughout the session. When the mothers fed their infants, both groups increased blood pressure and decreased heart rate. Blood pressure was increased more in the breastfeeding women. The authors reported that both arms of the study supported the theory that breastfeeding alters maternal cardiovascular function, possibly due to the action of oxytocin.[252]

Orthostatic reflex tachycardia is tachycardia, extreme weakness, and hypertension and is often associated with pregnancy and delivery. It tends to dissipate, but if it lasts more than 6 months it is referred to as postural orthostatic tachycardia syndrome. Provided the medications are compatible, breastfeeding is not contraindicated. Any condition that leads to worsening the tachycardia should be avoided, such as dehydration and other symptoms of fever, anxiety, or bleeding. Postural orthostatic tachycardia syndrome is difficult to diagnose accurately and difficult to treat. Treatment is symptomatic, chiefly with antihypertensives. Breastfeeding in a semireclined position (i.e., not totally flat or sitting at 90°) is helpful. Elastic stockings are essential.

CARDIAC, LIVER, AND RENAL TRANSPLANTATION

The number and survival times of patients receiving heart transplants are increasing, as is their quality of life. In young recipients, childbearing becomes important. Teratogenicity has not been reported with traditional immunosuppressive agents, such as prednisone and azathioprine, or with cyclosporine. Osteoporosis prophylaxis is important in pregnancy and lactation associated with chronic use of prednisone. A successful pregnancy after cardiac transplantation is reported with the birth of a normal infant who had normal growth and development for the 3 years of follow-up. The infant was not breastfed.[141]

Successful pregnancy after liver transplant has been reported in at least six patients.[239] Immunosuppression was maintained throughout pregnancy, and the infants were normal. Breastfeeding was not recommended because of the cyclosporine therapy.

Of infants born to mothers with renal transplants, 60% to 70% have uncomplicated neonatal courses. Thymic atrophy, leukopenia, anemia, thrombocytopenia, chromosome aberrations in lymphocytes, and certain abnormalities of the immune system have been seen.[141]

Breastfed infants of mothers with renal transplants have normal blood counts and show no increase in infection and above-average growth rates.[151] The immunosuppressants azathioprine, 6-mercaptopurine, and 6-methylprednisolone have been found in milk in very low levels. Cyclosporine, however, has been detected in breast milk at levels approximating maternal concentrations. The advice when cyclosporine is the drug has been not to breastfeed, with varying decisions about 6-mercaptopurine and azathioprine.

Pregnancy after renal transplant is relatively safe when renal function is adequate before conception and when maintenance immunosuppressive therapy is instituted. Most patients receive azathioprine and prednisone or methylprednisolone. When the actual levels of these compounds were studied in two patients, one of whom breastfed her infant,[51] measurements of IgA were also done because of the concept that immunosuppressed women might produce immunoincompetent milk.

The levels of 6-mercaptopurine in the milk averaged 3.4 ng/mL in one patient and 18 ng/mL in the other. The therapeutic level is 50 ng/mL, with the use of the normal daily dose. The levels of methylprednisolone in the milk (daily dose 6 mg) were at or below the levels measured in normal drug-free control subjects. The IgA determination in the milk was similar in both transplant and control mothers. The breastfed infant whose mother had a transplant had normal blood cell counts, no increase in infections, and an above-average growth rate.[55] Improved outcome of allogeneic bone marrow transplantation, due to breastfeeding-induced tolerance to maternal antigens, has been demonstrated by Aoyama et al.[17] Exposure of offspring to noninherited maternal antigens through breast milk reduced the graft-versus-host disease in the experimental model.

BREASTFEEDING AND MATERNAL DONOR RENAL ALLOGRAFTS

With the advent of renal transplants, a new mode of investigation with the role of human milk in the host-graft relationship has developed.[22] Large numbers of living maternal lymphocytes are present in human milk. Campbell et al.[48] investigated the question of whether exposure of an infant to maternal lymphocytes during breastfeeding would affect the subsequent reactivity of a patient to a maternal donor-related renal transplant. They studied the posttransplant course of 55 patients with a primary maternal donor transplant, 27 of whom were breastfed and 28 of whom were not. The 1-year graft-function rate was 82% for those breastfed and 57% for the bottle-fed ($p \leq 0.05$) infants. Five-year follow-up did not sustain the statistically significant difference. Paternal donor relationship in a small group of patients did not reveal significant difference.

The same group of investigators[150] reported that a history of breastfeeding was associated with improved results in a different patient population (HLA-semiidentical sibling donors). Breastfed patients in whom both donor and recipient were breastfed by the same mother showed dramatic improvements in graft-function rates, compared with nonbreastfed counterparts, at all intervals studied up to 9 years ($p \leq 0.001$). The authors[150] concluded that the breastfeeding effect is not entirely specific for maternal antigens because transplantation was improved for both sibling donor and maternal donor. They consider a history of being breastfed an important variable in clinically related renal transplantation.

Because these studies used retrospective questionnaires, they did not take into account the length of time breastfeeding took place, which included all cases "ever breastfed." Although this is potentially important, studies of graft recipients' donors are another means of understanding more about the role of breast milk for humans.

In a study of renal transplants, 45 breastfed subjects with maternal donor transplants were compared with 43 bottle-fed subjects with maternal donor transplants and 62 subjects with paternal donor transplants.[84] No statistically significant differences were seen in graft survival between the groups. Length of breastfeeding was not stated.

Since women who have had transplants have been experiencing pregnancy in greater numbers, the number who have been breastfed has also increased from a rate of ±5% of infants in 1994 to over 35% in 2012. Breastfeeding is recommended, except in the rare situation that the immunosuppressant medications are contraindicated. Prednisone, AZA, CSA, and tacrolimus are acceptable. Infant blood levels can always be checked. On the other hand, sirolimus, everolimus, and belatacept (MPA product) are a concern, and there are no data to prove their safety.

GLOMERULAR DISEASE AND LACTATION

A high percentage of pregnant patients show their first evidence of renal disease, probably not because pregnancy precipitates the disease, but because it is the first time these young women have had urinalysis and blood pressure studies. The series of glomerular disease in pregnancy published by Surian et al.[253] reported that, in most cases, the disease is not made worse by pregnancy. A disease with a poor prognosis such as membranoproliferative glomerulonephritis is neither worsened nor bettered by pregnancy. When the nonpregnant serum creatine and urea nitrogen levels exceed 3 mg/dL and 300 mg/dL, respectively, normal pregnancy is uncommon. Lupus nephropathy, however, has a poor prognosis in pregnancy, with considerable fetal loss and morbidity.[55] Eclampsia, however, increases the future risk of cardiovascular and renal disease.

Hypertension, as a complication, influences the obstetric complication rate and the fetal outcome. The infant may be premature, small for gestational age, or both. The option to breastfeed is a matter of the risk/benefit ratio.[22] It involves not only the medical status of the mother, but also that of the infant and the drugs that must be used to keep the mother stable. The obstetrician, nephrologist, and neonatologist must determine the appropriateness of breastfeeding on a case-by-case basis.

OSTEOPOROSIS

Tremendous attention has been focused on osteoporosis in women, particularly following childbirth and lactation. Clearly the demands for calcium and phosphorus during the perinatal period are great, but they can be met by diet with any degree of attention. In addition to dairy products and other supplemented foods, such as orange juice, other sources of calcium exist (Box 16-2). Modern advertising in the wave of the calcium hysteria has suggested women take various medicinal forms of calcium. The incidence of calcium-containing renal calculi has increased as a result.

BOX 16-2. Calcium Content of Foods (mg per serving)

100±	150±	200±	250±
10 Brazil nuts	1 cup ice cream	1 cup beet greens	1 cup almonds
1 medium stalk broccoli	1 cup oysters	1 oz cheddar or Muenster cheese	1 oz Swiss or Parmesan cheese
1 cup instant Farina	1 cup cooked rhubarb		1 cup cooked collard greens
3 oz canned herring	3 oz canned salmon with bones		1 cup cooked dandelion greens
1 cup cooked kale	1 cup cooked spinach		4 oz self-rising flour
1 Tbsp blackstrap molasses	1 oz feta or mozzarella cheese		1 cup milk
3 Tbsp light (regular) molasses	½ cup cooked chopped collard greens		3 oz sardines
1 cup cooked navy beans			½ cup cooked ricotta cheese
3.5 oz soybean curd (tofu)			
3.5 oz sunflower seeds			
5 Tbsp maple syrup			
1 cup cottage cheese, regular or low fat			

Modified from Kleinman RE, editor: *Pediatric nutrition handbook*, ed 6, Elk Grove, Ill., 2009, American Academy of Pediatrics.

A syndrome of severe osteoporosis is associated with pregnancy and lactation. Three cases are reported by Gruber et al.[99] These young women had vertebral fractures and skeletal complications, but most of their studies were normal except for their bony structure. They had no osteomalacia, however. They apparently recovered after lactation ceased and had no residual high-turnover osteoporosis. This suggests an association with low calcium in the diet. A rare cause of postpartum low back pain was found to be due to pregnancy and lactation-associated osteoporosis after exclusion of other causes.[259]

Bone density changes during pregnancy and lactation in active women were followed in a longitudinal study by Drinkwater and Chesnut.[71] The variations at the femoral neck, radial shaft, tibia, and lumbar spine were attributed to mechanical stress of weight gain and changes in posture in pregnancy and lactation. Further studies have confirmed that lactation-associated bone-mineral mobilization does not require parathyroid hormone or parathyroid tissue.[114]

Extended lactation (70% or more of infant energy intake provided for 6 months or more) is associated with bone loss; however, evidence exists of return to baseline by 12 months.[246] Those who breastfed a month or less lost no bone mass. Age, diet, body size, and physical activity were not correlated in these healthy white women. A return to normal bone densities was observed 6 months after weaning. A systematic review of maternal bone health to determine the influence of pregnancy and lactation was under taken. Osteoporosis is considered an important public health problem in postmenopausal women. There was no consensus, despite controversial results regarding the protective effect that pregnancy has been considered to have on bone, especially if followed by lactation.[227]

HYPOMAGNESEMIA CAUSED BY LACTATIONAL LOSSES

As magnesium sulfate is used more frequently in obstetrics, it is important to understand its action. Magnesium acts by competition with calcium either at the motor end plate or at the cell membrane. Myometrial contractility is inhibited when maternal serum levels of magnesium are 5 to 8 mg/dL. Deep tendon reflexes may be lost when levels rise to 9 to 13 mg/dL. At 14 mg/dL, respirations are depressed. Magnesium sulfate is excreted by the kidneys, and almost 90% is gone in the first 24 hours. Increases in magnesium result in hypocalcinemia. Magnesium ions cross the placenta, rapidly increasing parallel to maternal levels. The half-life in the fetus or neonate may be as long as 40 hours, however.[59] An infant born to a woman on a magnesium drip may be hypotonic, requiring calcium therapy immediately.

When 10 preeclampic patients received magnesium sulfate, 1 g/hour IV in the first 24 hours after delivery, magnesium levels in the breast milk were 64 mcg/mL, as compared to only 48 mcg/mL in untreated controls. Twenty-four hours after stopping the magnesium levels were 38 mcg/mL in the cases, and 32 mcg/mL in the controls. By 48 hours the levels were equal.[40] There is a normal concentrating mechanism for magnesium in the milk. Oral magnesium absorption is very poor, so little would be absorbed from the milk. Studies of women taking over-the-counter laxatives containing magnesium showed no change in the stools of their breastfed infants.[103]

A case of hypomagnesemic tetany caused by excessive lactation was reported by Greenwald et al.[98] The 20-year-old patient had been fully nursing her own 3-month-old infant and contributing 50 oz per day to the local milk bank. She was hospitalized with painful muscle spasms of her hands and feet that improved slightly but did not clear with calcium (serum level 9.6 mg/dL). Serum magnesium levels were low (0.4 mEq/L).

Kamble and Ookalka[131] reported on a 24-year-old woman who was breastfeeding a 15-day-old full-term infant. She presented with the sudden onset of rapidly progressive weakness of all her limbs. She had successfully breastfed two previous children. Electrocardiogram showed "hypokalemia" and multiple ventricular premature beats. Serum magnesium was 0.5 mmol/L (normal 0.8 to 1.7 mmol/L); milk magnesium was 4.9 mmol/L (normal 1.6 mmol/L). Serum calcium was 2.8 mmol/L, phosphate 1.1 mmol/L, and parathyroid hormone normal. Urinary potassium was 36 mmol/L. After treatment with potassium and magnesium, the electrocardiogram and muscle tone returned to normal. This woman continued to breastfeed. She had three times the normal level of magnesium in her milk.

Lactational hypomagnesemia is well described in the bovine model.

CROHN DISEASE AND ULCERATIVE COLITIS

Inflammatory bowel disease (IBD) includes both ulcerative colitis and Crohn disease. They are similar, involving inflammatory conditions of the luminal gastrointestinal tract. They differ in terms of the layer of the intestinal wall involved and the part of the intestinal tract involved (colitis only involves the colon). There is a genetic component. There is increased inflammatory response against the tissues of the gastrointestinal tract. A meta-analysis, systematically reviewing breastfeeding and the risk of IBD, showed that breastfeeding was protective against the diseases.[146]

The preferred treatments during pregnancy and lactation are sulfasalazine, 5-amino salicylates, and corticosteroids, which are considered safe during lactation as well as pregnancy. It is important to note that there is a case reported of early vitamin K deficiency bleeding in a neonate, associated with maternal Crohn disease. Possible repeat dosing of vitamin K is recommended if the infant is breastfed. Close monitoring in such cases is essential.[204]

Ulcerative colitis and Crohn disease (and recently rheumatoid arthritis) are treated with salazosulfapyridine (SASP). Because of the concern about exposing the fetus to sulfisoxazole at the end of pregnancy or during lactation (owing to the suggestion that sulfa drugs, even at low levels, predispose to kernicterus), this therapy has been discontinued in the third trimester. Recently, it was noted that sulfapyridine (SP), the main split product of SASP, has a low affinity for albumin-binding sites.

Esbjorner et al.[78] studied the binding capacities in both mothers and babies and found them low. They measured cord blood levels in the mothers of 11.5 mmol/L and in the infants of 20 mmol/L. Follow-up infant blood levels showed a clearance in 70 to 90 hours. Infants who were being breastfed did not increase their levels of SASP or SP. The milk/serum levels for SP were 0.4 to 0.6, and those for SASP were undetectable. Infant serum samples were 10% of maternal SP levels, and only one infant had detectable SASP. No children had complications of hyperbilirubinemia or kernicterus. All the infants were term infants without major complications. The authors[67] concluded that it is safe to continue the SASP throughout pregnancy and lactation in full-term infants. The effect on premature infants is under study. Prednisone therapy is usually safe because levels in milk are low.[4]

Irritable Bowel Syndrome

Irritable bowel syndrome is recognized more frequently in modern medicine, and more women with the disease are achieving pregnancy. It affects young women more commonly. It is characterized by chronic abdominal pain and altered bowel habits without obvious organic cause. It is the most common gastrointestinal disease. The pain is persistent, crampy, and relieved by defecation. The patient alternates between constipation and diarrhea. Patients also have GERD, dyspepsia, and nausea. All symptoms are made worse with stress. Treatment is nonspecific and symptomatic and is made better when the physician is sympathetic and understanding. Dietary changes can be effective. Medications are needed only by a few patients. Low-dose antispasmodics in the belladonna family, such as hyoscyamine, are sometimes used, causing drying of secretions, constipation, and dilated pupils. They are excreted into milk in only trace amounts. The drug should be safe for the infant if it is taken after breastfeeding and breastfeeding does not begin again until 2 hours after dosing. Chronic use can decrease milk supply, just as it decreases production in the other secreting glands (dry mouth and decreased sweat). The diarrhea and constipation can be mitigated with drugs that act directly on the gut and are not absorbed.

EPILEPSY

A history of epilepsy in a mother is of concern for an obstetrician during pregnancy, and much has been written on the topic. Seizures in pregnancy are more dangerous to the fetus than the medication is. Antiepileptic drugs (AEDs) include phenobarbital, primidone, phenytoin, carbamazepine, ethosuximide, valproic acid, diazepam, and topiramate (Topamax). The concern regarding lactation includes the effect of the disease on the fetus in terms of major and minor malformations, the level of drugs in the infant's serum at birth, and the state of the mother postpartum. Breastfeeding may provide a means of gradually withdrawing the infant from maternal medication and avoiding the syndrome of withdrawal (i.e., hyperirritability, tremor, vomiting, poor sucking, hyperventilation, sleep disturbances). A good mother-infant relationship is important for a mother with epilepsy. Brodie[41] recommends alternating the breast with an occasional bottle (once per day or more) if the infant is sedated by maternal medication to reduce the effect and dilute the blood levels.

Table 16-11 lists the half-lives of various AEDs. These compounds have a sedating effect and may prevent the infant from suckling adequately in the first few days. Attention must be paid to the infant's behavior to avoid not only under nutrition, but also failure to provide sufficient stimulus to the breast. The infant may need some supplementation and the mother some stimulus with an electric pump, carefully coordinated with support.

Whether an infant is breastfed or bottle fed, it is necessary to establish that the mother will remain seizure free and be able to care for the infant. Kaneko et al.[133] studied 42 infants of 32 epileptic mothers for harmful side effects of AEDs while breastfeeding. The duration of poor sucking was correlated with the drug and the levels. The poor

weight gain of the mixed-fed infants (breast/bottle) was associated with vomiting and infant drowsiness during feeding. These authors recommend mixing feedings (breastfeeding and formula) early postpartum to reduce the medication to the infant until levels in infant serum taper a little and the infant's metabolism increases to promote drug clearance. Full breastfeeding can then proceed if care has been taken to establish a good milk supply with supplementary pumping.

Topiramate is used most frequently with much success in the treatment of seizures. It is excreted in breast milk, which is not surprising as it is of low molecular weight, minimal protein binding (15%), and prolonged plasma elimination. In three mother/baby dyads, who were breastfeeding and were tested at 3 months, the weight adjusted doses for the infants were 0.1 to 0.7 mg/kg/day or 3% to 23% of the maternal dose.[40] No adverse effects were detected at 3 months of age. Breastfed infants whose mothers are taking topiramate should be closely monitored for alertness, changes in behavior, or diminished feeds due to sleepiness.

NEUROPATHIES ASSOCIATED WITH BREASTFEEDING/NUMBNESS AND TINGLING OF THE ARM

A number of neurologic symptoms have been described in association with lactation. During periods of engorgement, pressure on nerves in the axilla, especially from an engorged tail of Spence (see Chapter 2), has caused numbness and tingling down the arms on the flexor surface to the ulnar distribution of the hands, similar to crutch palsy. The numbness and tingling usually abate as soon as the infant nurses and then gradually return as the breast fills again. Symptoms gradually disappear after several weeks, as engorgement disappears.

TABLE 16-11	Pharmacokinetic Data on Antiepileptic Drugs (AEDs) in Newborns				
AED	Free Fraction (% Unbound)	Volume Distribution (L/kg)	Half-Life (h)	AAP Rating	Hale Rating
Phenobarbital	57-72	0.6-1.5	40-500	5	L3
Primidone	?	?	7-60	5	L3
Phenytoin	15-30	0.7-2.0	15-105	6	L2
Carbamazepine	?	1.1-2.6	8-28	6	L2
Ethosuximide	?	?	40	6	L4
Valproic acid	~15	0.2-0.4	14-88	6	L2
Diazepam	~14	1.8-2.1	40-400	4	L3
Topiramate	85	0.7	18-24	Not rated	L3

TENNIS ELBOW WITH HAND PUMPING

Symptoms similar to those associated with tennis elbow—pain and tingling with flexion of the fore-arm—have developed in nursing women who are pumping milk with a Kaneson-style hand pump.[271] Similar symptoms have been experienced by mothers just holding a newborn over time, especially primiparas and especially heavy infants.

Carpal tunnel syndrome has been described in pregnancy, causing paresthesia of the hands. Two cases were reported by Yagnik,[275] in which symptoms developed 1 month postpartum in breastfeeding women. The diagnosis was confirmed by electromyography and nerve conduction studies. The second case was bilateral. Symptoms disappeared after the infants were weaned. Five other cases are described in the literature: all the women were breastfeeding, all showed improvement with temporary suspension of breastfeeding, and all recovered completely within a month of complete weaning.[243]

A retrospective study of 27 women who had developed carpal tunnel syndrome postpartum was carried out by mail.[266,267] The women affected were older (mean age 31.5 years) and were primiparous, and 24 of 27 were breastfeeding. The three women who were bottle-feeding had less severe symptoms that cleared in less than 1 month. Symptoms (predominantly paresthesias, clumsiness, and pain) began at a mean of 3.5 weeks postpartum and lasted 6.5 months. Resolution began after 2 weeks of beginning to wean. Two women required surgical intervention. All were symptom free within a year.[266] The recommended treatment for carpal tunnel syndrome is conservative, with rest, diuretics, hand splint, and local corticosteroid injection, because it is usually reversible. No woman had residual signs or symptoms, so perseverance with lactation and symptomatic treatment is appropriate.

RAYNAUD PHENOMENON

Raynaud phenomenon was first described by Maurice Raynaud in 1862 as episodic digital ischemia provoked by cold and emotion. The true cause remains obscure, despite elaborate efforts to identify it. It is widely thought to be a cutaneous manifestation of a generalized vascular disorder, often associated, in complex cases, with scleroderma and vasoconstriction of the kidneys, heart, and lungs. Patients with Raynaud phenomenon have significantly more migraine headaches. The basic research on the subject does not mention vasospasm of the nipples. The digital vessels of patients are more sensitive to the cold. Not all vasospasm is Raynaud phenomenon and is limited to individuals with other signs and symptoms compatible with the diagnosis.[273]

Five cases of Raynaud phenomenon of the nipple are described in the literature as severe blanching and debilitating pain.[163] Several women had white, blue, and red color changes, but only of the nipple. All were treated with nifedipine (10 mg three times per day or 30 mg by slow-release tablet). Nifedipine (Adalat, Procardia) is an antihypertensive calcium channel blocker. It does pass into the milk and is estimated to provide about 7.0 mg/kg/day (5%) of the pediatric dose. The AAP rates nifedipine a category 6 and Hale rates it an L2, which are equivalent, suggesting it is safe during lactation (see Table 19-18). All the women responded with a decrease or obliteration of the painful blanching. Oral bioavailability is only 50%, which reduces the risk to the breastfeeding infant.

The clinical parameters used to diagnose this disease are important.[75] Some history or other evidence of Raynaud phenomenon is essential when associating it with nipple blanching.[273] The patient should have some history of sensitivity to cold. Hands and feet are common sites of blanching and pain.[26] It is questionable that it is Raynaud's of the nipples, unless it occurs elsewhere, associated with cold. Before prescribing a medication, the other therapeutic first options should be initiated.[162] Discontinuing smoking or avoiding secondhand smoke is imperative. Steady ambient temperature and warm clothing are important. Adding fish oil to the diet has helped some patients, as has evening primrose oil, which is a rich source of essential polyunsaturated fatty acid, especially γ-linoleic acid.[13] Evening primrose oil has been used effectively in patients with mastalgia of unknown origin.

Peripheral tissue ischemia in neonates has been treated with topical nitroglycerin ointment, which is well absorbed through intact skin. Effects are usually seen within 30 to 60 minutes and last 6 to 8 hours. Because of the risk for hypotension, constant observation is necessary. Although this is theoretically an effective therapy for blanched nipples, no studies report on its safety. No data are available on its secondary effect on the infant, who would receive it through the milk or directly from the nipple. When mothers ingest nitrates, which have a short half-life, little is found in the milk and it is rapidly cleared from serum. Other medications that have been used for Raynaud phenomenon include angiotensin-converting enzyme inhibitors (e.g., captopril, enalapril) and prostaglandins for severe prolonged attacks.

Restless Leg Syndrome/Willis-Ekbom Disease

Restless leg syndrome (RLS), or Willis-Ekbom disease, is common in pregnancy and lactation. It is estimated to involve one in five pregnant women

Breast cytologic examination is an important part of an evaluation during pregnancy and lactation, as well as any other time. During pregnancy, the ductal lobular system undergoes marked hyperplasia with rapid proliferation of the epithelial linings as they form new ductules.[207] Lymphocytes, plasma cells, and eosinophils infiltrate during the proliferation process. After 16 weeks, colostrum-like fluid is present in the ducts. Cytologic appearance of the breast during pregnancy is cellular; the cell types are the same as in the resting breast, although the proportions differ.[115] Epithelial cells are numerous and suggest a papillary structure. Neutrophils are abundant as well. The most common cell types are foam cells, leukocytes, histiocytes, and gland epithelial cells consisting of single cells and cell clusters.[115] The foam cells in pregnant patients exhibit nuclear enlargement, binucleation, multinucleation, and increased cytoplasmic vacuolization, compared with those of nonpregnant women. Unexpectedly large numbers of ductal epithelial cells are present in pregnancy and lactation. Groups of cells are papillary in structure and similar to the papillary fronds of an intraductal papilloma. In the immediate postpartum period, a lactating woman's secretions are virtually acellular at the end of the first week; nonlactators exhibited cellularity characteristics of pregnancy, according to work by Holmquist and Papanicolaou.[115]

Biopsies during the third trimester of pregnancy, as described by Kline and Lash,[148] had "tufts of cells forming spurs or invaginations into duct and alveolar lumens and similar structures that were desquamated into lumens and groups of cells found in the breast secretions." The investigators also commented that the "spurs" were closely associated with the formation of new alveoli, suggesting their origin. Delicate capillary networks within these tufts of cells might easily be traumatized and result in the bloody secretion described in pregnancy and early lactation. Kline and Lash[127] reported the persistence of the antepartum cellular findings in 31 of 72 postpartum women. The correlation to lactation or its suppression was not made. Biopsies, however, demonstrated findings similar to those in pregnancy; these changes lasted up to 2 months.

Conclusions drawn from multiple studies by King and Goodson[143] are that breast-fluid cytologic examination during pregnancy and lactation reveals the following:

1. Increased cellularity is seen and is most marked in late pregnancy.
2. Cellularity is variable postpartum.
3. Increased numbers of duct epithelial cells in groups are similar to intraductal papilloma or papillary hyperplasia.

4. Blood may be found in pregnancy and lactation in the absence of clinical lesion.
5. Interpretation of secretions in pregnancy and lactation justifies caution.

Cytologic findings referred to as "hyperplasia" in lactation have no apparent association with increased risk for breast cancer. Lesions usually not associated with increased risk for cancer are apocrine metaplasia, cyst, duct ectasia, fibroadenoma, fibrosis, mastitis, periductal mastitis, squamous metaplasia, and milk hyperplasmia.

Milky Discharge

Persistent bilateral lactation is the presentation following breastfeeding and, as noted, may represent pituitary disease. If no surgical disease (e.g., adenoma) exists, medical treatment to suppress prolactin (e.g., estrogens, bromocriptine) is no longer employed, and involution is left to take place naturally. In a nonlactating woman, this finding is called galactorrhea and is a spontaneous, milky, multiductal, bilateral discharge (see earlier discussion).[214]

Multicolored and Sticky Discharge

Multicolored, sticky, spontaneous bilateral discharges from multiple ducts usually show only normal skin flora when cultured.[167] This discharge is usually green, but may be yellow, brown, red-brown, or gray; it is Hemastix or guaiac negative. The discharge can occur from puberty to the postmenopausal years and is most common in parous women. It is often associated with nipple manipulation, especially when seen in the third trimester or early lactation. Simple cases can be treated with good hygiene and discontinuing nipple manipulation. If it occurs at delivery, lactation can be initiated after cleansing and removal and discarding of early secretion. Normal colostrum usually follows.

Duct ectasia, or comedomastitis, is the most common cause of multicolored sticky discharge.[214] It begins as a dilatation of the terminal ducts and may occur during pregnancy, although it is most common between the ages of 35 and 40. It is rare in virgins and most common in women who have lactated. An irritating lipid forms in the ducts, producing an inflammatory reaction and nipple discharge. Cytologic examination shows debris and epithelial cells. Duct ectasia may be associated with burning pain, itching, and swelling of the nipple and areola. Palpation reveals a wormlike tube, once called a varicocele tumor of the breast. As the disease progresses, a mass may develop that mimics cancer, and chronic inflammation leads to fibrosis.

Surgery is not indicated unless the discharge becomes bloody. The disease is usually treated with thorough cleansing with pHisoHex or povidone-iodine (Betadine) daily and avoidance of nipple manipulation. Lactation would aggravate preexisting diseases but would not be an absolute contraindication. When the nipple becomes inflamed and clogged with a thick, sticky, gray-green discharge with no apparent cause, especially nearing menopause, treatment is warm compresses, antibiotics, and, if necessary, surgical removal of the duct. Pink milk observed while pumping has been detected to be due to *Serratia marcescens* contaminating the pump and breast.[198]

Purulent Discharge

Purulent discharge is caused by acute puerperal mastitis, chronic lactation mastitis, central breast abscess, or plasma cell mastitis. It is usually unilateral, involving one or two ducts. Once diagnosed, the treatment is antibiotics. When an abscess does not clear after withholding of lactation and adequate treatment, a biopsy should be done to rule out secondary necrosis and infection of an underlying lesion. Ultrasound or other imaging may assist in the diagnosis.

Watery, Serous, Serosanguineous, and Bloody Discharges

A volunteer survey among members of the Nursing Mothers Association of Australia resulted in a report of 37 cases in 32 women who had bloody or serosanguineous secretion in either pregnancy or lactation. The condition usually occurred in the first pregnancy (27 of 37) or was a recurrence in a second pregnancy (five cases), with one case occurring in the third pregnancy. It was usually bilateral, although onset might be unilateral. The earliest case started in the fourth month of pregnancy, although most began at delivery and in early lactation. More than 50% of the women had practiced prenatal nipple "exercising." Most cases cleared within 3 to 7 days of onset of lactation. These cases were distinct from trauma, cracked nipple, or mastitis.

The Lactation Study Center frequently receives calls regarding pink (guaiac positive) or frankly bloody milk, referred to by some as "rusty-pipe syndrome." It is painless and may go unnoticed unless the mother is pumping her milk or her infant vomits blood that is positive for adult hemoglobin (Apt test). This eliminates cases of bleeding of the newborn GI tract, which is positive for fetal blood by Apt test. If the infant tolerates the milk, breastfeeding can continue and the blood usually disappears in 3 to 7 days.

The explanation for this phenomenon is probably the increased vascularization of the breast coupled with the rapid development of the alveoli.[149] If the blood persists or is recurrent, the breast should be evaluated by mammography.

The cytology of breast secretions obtained during the third trimester from 50 pregnant women aged 16 to 39 years was reported by Kline and Lash.[149] Cellularity was increased with epithelial cell clusters and capillary groupings forming "spurs" or invaginations into duct and alveolar lumina. The authors noted that the spurs were closely associated with the formation of new alveoli; the delicate capillary networks within these tufts could be easily traumatized and result in blood escaping into the breast secretions.

The other cells found in secretions during pregnancy and lactation, when breast secretions were aspirated, were foam cells, leukocytes, histiocytes, and gland epithelial cells. Foam cells are also referred to as colostrum bodies and have large nuclei or are binuclear or multinucleated. When lactation is suppressed postpartum, the secretion is almost acellular by the seventh day.[149]

Nipple discharges are primarily of surgical significance. They are the second most common indication for breast surgery. Watery or colorless, serous or yellow, serosanguineous or pink, and sanguineous discharges are more common in women older than the age of 50 years, but younger women do not escape them.[214] Bloody discharge in pregnancy and lactation is most often caused by vascular engorgement or breast trauma. The next most common causes in pregnancy and lactation are intraductal papilloma (50%) and fibrocystic disease (31%). Because the type of discharge does not identify the malignant or nonmalignant nature of the problem, all patients with unusual discharge should be seen by an appropriate surgeon for diagnosis.

Nipple discharges with blood visible, or detected by cytologic examination, are common during pregnancy and lactation. Lafreniere[158] estimated that 15% of asymptomatic lactating women have blood in their early secretions when they are examined cytologically. An intraductal papilloma is a small, usually noncancerous growth protruding into a duct near the nipple in women 35 to 45 years old.

In intraductal papilloma the discharge is usually spontaneous, unilateral, and from a single duct. It is occasionally associated with a nontender lump in the subareolar area. Symptoms may include bleeding, which is usually painless, during pregnancy. It is possible to excise the involved duct and wedge of tissue, leaving the rest intact to preserve mammary function, when surgery is required for intraductal papilloma. Painless bleeding during pregnancy may be bilateral or unilateral and may cease after delivery. After serious disease has been ruled out by physical examination and cytologic evaluation, lactation is possible.[158]

To be significant, a discharge should be true, persistent, spontaneous, and nonlactational. Single-duct unilateral discharges are more apt to be surgically significant. A true discharge comes from a duct to the surface of the nipple. Pseudodischarges occur on the surface and may be associated with inverted nipples, eczematoid lesions, trauma, herpes simplex, infections of the Montgomery glands, and mammary duct fistulas. Discharges are more common in women taking oral contraceptives, tranquilizers, or rauwolfia alkaloids and in those who are postmenopausal and menopausal. Cytologic examination should be part of any examination for an abnormal discharge from the breast, although a high percentage of false negative tests occur, as well as some false positive results. Absence of a mass is reassuring, but should not dissuade one from further diagnostic studies.

PAGET DISEASE

Paget disease of the breast is an uncommon type of cancer that occurs in only 1% to 4% of all women with breast cancer. Signs and symptoms include itching, burning, and redness or scaling of the surface of the nipple and areola. A bloody discharge may be present. The nipple may appear flattened against the breast. It has been mistaken for candidiasis during lactation, greatly delaying proper treatment. A biopsy of the areola is necessary. Mastectomy is usually recommended, although early lumpectomy may be adequate. Chemotherapy and radiation are recommended.

LUMPS IN THE BREAST

A lactating breast is lumpy to palpation, and the lumps shift day by day. The most common cause of a persistent lump is a plugged duct (see Chapter 8); the second most common cause is a mass associated with mastitis. Lumps that persist beyond a few days and do not respond to palliative treatment deserve investigation.[210,211] In young pregnant or lactating women, ultrasound is the ideal method for evaluation of the breast. It visualizes the breast architecture dynamically, facilitates differentiation between benign cysts and solid lesions, and further suggests if a solid mass is benign or malignant. It could be a benign shape with smooth edges. It also establishes a baseline for subsequent follow-up. The American College of Radiology standard for the performance of a breast ultrasound examination states that breast sonography is the initial imaging technique to evaluate

palpable masses in women younger than 30 years or in pregnant and lactating women.[10]

Ultrasound is also useful to diagnose and guide drainage of breast collections and check for abscess when mastitis presents. A small abscess, identified early, can be treated with percutaneous drainage before surgical drainage is necessary. When a mass is to be evaluated, a mother should nurse immediately before the procedure. If a mass is in a lactating breast that warrants biopsy, percutaneous core biopsy can be done. MRI is also useful because it can identify masses not detected by ultrasound and assist in the effort to do a needle biopsy.

Adenomas of the breast and ectopic breast under lactational influences were reviewed by O'Hara and Page.[203] They reported five ectopic lactating adenomas located in the axilla, chest wall, and vulva. Tubular adenomas have been associated with lactation and show lactational changes in a fibroadenoma, thus making diagnosis difficult by fine-needle aspiration. Fine-needle aspiration of the breast has been recommended as a safe, simple diagnostic tool to use in an ambulatory setting without interrupting lactation.[165]

Once a breast mass is palpated, prompt evaluation is indicated to rule out breast cancer. A palpable lump in pregnancy has been noted by investigators to delay the time to treatment as long as 8 months.[33]

Of women diagnosed with breast cancer, 3% are pregnant or lactating.[212] Data suggest that pregnant or lactating women with breast cancer, stage for stage, have similar survival rates as nonpregnant women. Average delay during the perinatal period is 2.2 months compared with 0.59 month in the total population of patients with breast cancer; thus a higher proportion of pregnant women are in advanced stages when first seen.[234] Lumpectomy can be performed safely during pregnancy and lactation.

FIBROCYSTIC DISEASE

Fibrocystic disease is a diffuse parenchymal process in the breasts that has many synonyms, none of which is satisfactory. The process involves hormonally produced benign proliferations of the alveolar system of varying degrees that occur in response to the normal menstrual cycle. A patient with full-blown disease has pain, tenderness, palpable thickenings, and nodules of varying sizes that are most symptomatic with menses. Fibrocystic disease is prominent in the childbearing years and regresses during pregnancy. It often disappears during menopause. It is not a contraindication to breastfeeding. Some women have achieved relief by totally eliminating caffeine and related products from their diet.

Diagnostic procedures include mammography and aspiration biopsy. When no fluid is obtained and a smooth, freely movable mass is present, lumpectomy can be performed. Microscopic examination will clarify the diagnosis and the need for further treatment.

A rare cause of hematemesis in the newborn was reported in which the mother had fibrocystic disease.[5] Spontaneous vomiting of blood began on day 3; the newborn had been breastfeeding without difficulty. Apt test demonstrated it was maternal blood. Pumping each breast revealed bloody milk only on the left. Ultrasound showed cystic disease only on the left with the bloody milk, which persisted for several months.

GALACTOGRAPHY

Galactography is radiography of the mammary ducts after the injection of radiopaque contrast material (see Figure 16-3). It is done to identify the cause of abnormal nipple discharge, especially when no lesion is palpable or radiologically detectable. Cytologic examination of the discharge material should always be done first. Positive cytologic examination is helpful, but false negative results do occur. The procedure involves cannulation of the duct with a blunt needle under sterile precautions with the slow injection of 2 mL of sterile, water-soluble contrast material. Preexisting mastitis or abscess is a contraindication to the procedure (see Figure 16-2). Galactographic findings in digital mammography can be helpful. The nipple discharge may be caused by ductal ectasia, fibrocystic changes, papilloma, papillomatosis, or intraductal carcinoma. Galactography is performed to localize the abnormality and not to make a histologic diagnosis, because the appearances of some benign and malignant lesions overlap significantly. In lactating women, fewer than 10% with abnormal discharge are malignant (Figure 16-12). IGM is a rare, inflammatory, chronic, and benign disease that mimicks malignant hyperplasia of the mammary gland, usually as a unilateral, distinct, painful mass. It is treated surgically by hemi-mastectomy or medically with azithromycin and prednisolone.

BREAST CYSTS

Benign cysts of the breast are being identified in younger and younger women, probably because of the more careful self-examination of the breast that is now recommended. They should be removed and biopsied but do not interfere with lactation. Fibroadenomas that result from a disturbance in the normal menstrual cycle usually proliferate and regress before age 30 years. Pregnancy and lactation stimulate their growth. They

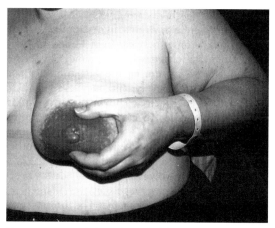

Figure 16-12. Bi-fed nipple or double nipple. Note milk at both orifices and third on face or surface of areola. With gentle pressure all three orifices have major spray.

are firm, smooth, lobulated masses and are freely movable without fixation. They can be diagnosed radiologically. They can be removed while the patient is under local anesthesia, if necessary, without causing cessation of breastfeeding.

LIPOMAS

Lipomas are common in the breasts, which have considerable fat in their stroma. They are usually solitary, asymptomatic, slowly growing, freely movable, soft, and well delineated. They can be easily identified radiologically or with ultrasound imagery in lactating breasts, which have less fat present.

FAT NECROSIS

Fat necrosis is usually associated with trauma and is caused by local destruction of fat cells with release of free lipid and variable hemorrhage. Organization with fibrosis may lead to fixation. Fat necrosis can be identified radiologically and appears as a fat density or oil cyst with a capsule.

HEMATOMAS

Hematomas of lactating breasts may occur from trauma or in women receiving anticoagulant therapy. They generally regress without treatment. When they occur with minimal trauma, the presence of a tumor should be considered.

GIGANTOMASTIA (BREAST HYPERTROPHY WITH PREGNANCY)

Massive hypertrophy of the breast with pregnancy is a rare condition of unknown etiology, referred to as gigantomastia of pregnancy.[190] It is reported in

were inappropriately low in depressed women who were breastfeeding. The authors suggest management should be different for breastfeeding and bottle-feeding women.[108]

Chlorpromazine or phenothiazine, used in psychotic disorders, appears in the milk in small amounts. Even at doses of 1200 mg, it does not appear to accumulate. Doses of 100 mg/day do not appear to cause symptoms in the infants. Fluoxetine (Prozac) appears in breast milk at one fourth to one fifth the levels in maternal plasma, and alternative therapies are recommended[122] (see Chapter 11).

Clinical experience with significantly depressed patients has shown that abrupt weaning from the breast may precipitate severe depression or even suicidal behavior. Whenever weaning is initiated in a woman with a psychiatric disorder, it should be initiated gradually and take place during 2 to 4 weeks or longer.

The impact of mental illness on the lactation process has been evaluated. Depressed mothers had more difficulties during breastfeeding than other women, and their attitudes were more negative. Depressed mothers complained more of too little milk or too much, of too much crying, of too little sleep, and of not getting enough support and help. It is difficult to determine cause and effect. Tamminen and Salmelin[257] noted frequent difficulties when they studied psychosomatic interaction between mother and infant during breastfeeding. They found that "depressed mothers in particular did not seem to understand that problems in nursing may be due to somatic rather than psychic reasons. Depressed mothers lacked satisfaction in the mother-infant relationship, failing to create reciprocity with their infant."

In assessing the relationship between infant-feeding method and maternal role adjustment at 1 month, studies find that women who breastfeed their infants have less anxiety and more mutuality; the adaptation of appropriate maternal behavior to the infant's state and behavioral cues, and the ability to adjust mothering activities to the infant's needs are improved.[257]

It is not possible with present knowledge to state definitely the impact of breastfeeding on the potential for mental illness in mothers, but breastfeeding clearly enhances mothering and mother-infant interaction and mutuality.[200] Under most circumstances, it is better to continue breastfeeding than to terminate it unnecessarily or prematurely.

POSTPARTUM DEPRESSION

Much has been written in the lay press about the "baby blues," and many mothers, predominantly primiparas, will admit to a few hours or a day of incredible emotional see-sawing in the first week after delivery (Table 16-12). Episodes in which a mother dissolves into tears when she has "so much to be thankful for" is the usual description. This is a transient state that has been attributed to the tremendous change in hormonal levels after the delivery of the placenta, although no studies confirm this belief. It is usually successfully treated with reassurance and rest. True postpartum depression does occur, however. Contrary to popular fantasy, it occurs in women who are breastfeeding, but usually only in women with a problem before pregnancy (Table 16-12).

Postpartum depression is not the baby blues, which have always been dismissed summarily as a transient reaction to hormonal change with a casual, "Buck up, girl, its just baby blues." Postpartum depression is a crippling mood disorder that leaves a mother in fear, confusion, and silence. "Joy is not an option" for some women, according to Beck[28,29] (Figure 16-21).

Theme #		Theme
1		Going to the movies: Please don't make me go!
2		A shadow of myself: Too numb to try and change
3		Seeking to have questions answered and wanting to talk, talk, talk
4		The dangerous trio of anger, anxiety, and depression: Spiraling downward
5		Isolation from the world of motherhood: Dreams shattered

Figure 16-21. Five essential themes of posttraumatic stress disorder due to childbirth. (Redrawn from Beck CT: Posttraumatic stress disorder due to childbirth: the aftermath, *Nurs Res* 53:216, 2004.)

Postpartum depression has been a catchall tag for many disorders. Misdiagnosis is common.

Postpartum panic disorder can occur for the first time after delivery. Panic attacks occur for brief intense periods, with extreme fear, palpitations, sweating, dypsnea, chest pain, dizziness, numbness, and even fear of death. Obsessive-compulsive disorder and bipolar disorder can occur postpartum and differ from the psychotic versions.

Postpartum depression is defined as five or more of the following symptoms for at least 2 weeks: insomnia or hypersomnia, psychomotor agitation or retardation, fatigue, changes in appetite, feelings of worthlessness or guilt, decreased concentration, and suicidality. Mothers who are depressed are less affectionate toward their infants and less responsive to their cries.[112]

Mothers with postpartum depression (Edinburgh Postnatal Depression score >12) at one week are more likely to wean by 4 to 8 weeks and be dissatisfied with their infant-feeding method, have breastfeeding problems, and report lower levels of breastfeeding self-efficacy. Findings were collected by questionnaires from over 500 postpartum mothers.[65]

A systematic review of the literature by Dennis and MacQueen[66] that identified 49 appropriate studies confirmed these findings. They concluded that postpartum depression results in poorer infant-feeding outcomes, including decreased breastfeeding initiation, duration, and exclusivity. There is need for early identification and treatment of postpartum women and breastfeeding mothers with depressive symptomatology to improve infant-feeding outcomes.

The incidence of psychiatric disorders during pregnancy is remarkably lower than age-adjusted rates in the general population. Rates in the postpartum period, however, increase dramatically to 1 to 2 per 1000, with 50% to 75% involving affective disorders, 10% to 20% schizophrenic illness, 2% to 12% organic psychiatric disorders, and 12% anxiety disorders.[45] Studies of clinically depressed postpartum women reveal that two of three have a major depression. With the introduction and use of antibiotics in the mid-1950s, many symptoms described as puerperal fever or milk fever, resulting in toxic-confusion or delirious behavior, no longer are reported.

A growing number of investigators have been unable to demonstrate significant evidence for a unique pattern of mental illness in puerperal compared with nonpuerperal psychiatric disorders. Although childbearing might make a woman more vulnerable to psychiatric stress, the patterns of illness symptomatology, course, and outcome are no different from those of nonpuerperal women or men. Prevailing views support a concept of multifactorial causes or the summation of stresses. Factors of ambivalence or negative attitude toward pregnancy, primary role conflict, lack of emotional and practical support, and increased numbers of life events are all part of the picture.

The relationship between breastfeeding and depression was studied in mothers who totally breastfed and in those who totally bottle fed. No relationship was found between depression and feeding method. A prospective study following 103 women postpartum recorded a 13% incidence of marked postnatal depressive illness and an additional 16% of minor depressive illness of at least 4 weeks' duration. No correlation was made with method of feeding until the mothers were asked about their feeding methods and oral contraceptive use in an attempt to determine the influence of hormones on depression. The authors speculated that the prolactin, estrogen, and progesterone levels would vary with the amount of breastfeeding, amount of other foods consumed by the baby, and amount of hormones taken in the form of contraceptives.[144] In this study the women who bottle fed received estrogen and progesterone as contraceptives, but women who breastfed received only progesterone. Women who were totally breastfeeding and were not taking contraceptives were somewhat more likely to report depressive symptoms. Feelings of fatigue may have influenced this. The mothers least likely to be depressed were those who were likely to have normal hormonal levels, that is, partial breastfeeders not taking contraceptives. Clearly, breastfeeding women are not immune to postpartum depression.[58]

The impact of a mother's depression on her breastfeeding and nursing attitudes was reported by Tamminen and Salmeun[257] in a study of 119 healthy primiparous women using the Beck Depression Inventory attitude scales and other questionnaires. Eight percent of the participants were clinically depressed, but 25% did not return the questionnaire, which is possibly more common in depressed subjects. Depressed mothers had more difficulty with breastfeeding.

In a continuing study as part of a larger study, qualitative analysis of mother-infant interactions during breastfeeding showed depressed mothers to be less able to sense the infant's needs, cues, and problems.[201] Furthermore, they saw the problems in psychologic terms; that is, the infant did not want their milk or did not like it.[257] They did not understand that difficulties in breastfeeding could be somatic in nature. Depressed mothers achieved less satisfaction and mutual pleasure in breastfeeding.

The impact of postpartum depression on the emotional and cognitive development of infants was found to be adverse in several studies, because depressed mothers are typically unresponsive to infant cues, which are manifest with flat affect or withdrawal.[192] Postnatally depressed mothers are likely to be socially isolated and emotionally unsupported. The relationship among family life events, maternal depression, and teacher and maternal ratings of child behavior up to age 6 years was reported. Both maternal depression and family life events made significant contributions to negative child behavior.[189]

The prevalence of postpartum depression varied between 7% and 14% during 34 weeks postpartum, based on the monitoring of a cohort of 293 women studied by Pop et al.[216] Peak incidence (14%) was at 10 weeks postpartum; in other studies the peak incidence has been as high as 40%. The symptoms of postpartum and other depressions are similar; however, the puerperium is a time of unique stress.[213] Table 16-12 lists major findings related to the "baby blues," postpartum depression, and psychosis.[139] The cause is uncertain, with hormonal change being a continuing theme. Other perinatal events have been noted to trigger true depression, especially negative birth experiences. At-risk infants, including premature infants, sick infants, and those with disabilities, are often triggers for maternal depressive episodes.[216]

Breastfeeding can be a source of distress for many new mothers who do not have a good support system at home, especially when no one knowledgeable about breastfeeding is available. The La Leche League International has made an enormous difference with their mother-to-mother program. Isolation often contributes to the depression, and having telephone contact with a League mother or resources such as a lactation consultant to assess the breastfeeding progress may be therapeutic.

The physician and other health care team members should be sensitive to the subtle signs and vague symptoms. When a woman says, "I am overwhelmed," "Nothing will ever be the same," or "I feel hopeless or out of control," the health care professional must listen to her. When she is anxious or nervous or has insomnia, especially waking in the early morning when she is exhausted, the professional must consider depression.[139] Use of a depression scale may be helpful when the mother answers general questions such as "How are things going?" with "Fine." A referral for professional psychiatric help or to a support program or hotline is the minimal response.

Studies support the recommendation that a primary care physician should identify the mother with depression using a simple inventory such as the 10-item Edinburgh Postnatal Depression Scale (EPDS) (Box 16-4). The EPDS has been validated and specifically designed for use by the primary

health care team during routine health care visits, and it relies on self-reporting.[192]

In a study conducted in the well baby clinic of a large teaching hospital, universal screening for postpartum depressive symptoms during the first year of an infant's life using the EPDS was administered at each well baby visit: 46% of visits had a filed completed form, 21% of completed forms had scores of 10 or greater, and 27% of all mothers who completed forms during the year had at least one score of 10 or greater (highly depressive symptoms). These clients were referred to social services. The authors concluded that pediatricians can play an active role in early detection and referral for postpartum depression.[51]

Appearing in the same journal was a report exploring maternal beliefs and perceptions about discussing the stress of parenting and symptoms of depression with their child's pediatricians. The population was from five community-based practices. The mothers were aware of the impact of their emotional health on their infants. Many were reluctant to discuss parenting stress and depressive symptoms with their child's pediatricians because of mistrust and fear of judgment. They liked open communication with their pediatrician and were receptive to written materials about parenting stresses and depression from their pediatrician, but did not want verbal counsel.[111]

The role of infant factors in postnatal depression and mother-infant interactions was evaluated in a large group of infants born to 188 primiparous women at risk for postnatal depression and a smaller group born to 43 mothers at low risk. By 8 weeks postpartum, poor motor scores and high irritability in the infants were strongly predictive of maternal depression. These factors also predicted less optimal infant behavior in face-to-face interactions with the mother at 8 weeks.[187]

When the crying behaviors of 3- and 6-month-old infants were compared, infants of depressed mothers cried significantly more per day than infants of nondepressed mothers at 3 months, but not at 6 months of age.[187]

A significant association exists with depressive disorder preceding the early cessation of breastfeeding, according to the results of two large, independent samples of puerperal women.[53] This was confirmed in a study in several large teaching centers, which examined the causes of early weaning, pointing out the effect of maternal depression and lack of clinical support.[258] Other factors associated with early weaning were low social class, low education, and young age of the mother. Depression is more common in winter in the Northern Hemisphere, when days are short and darkness is prolonged. The relationship of lower prolactin levels in the winter is not understood.[209]

BOX 16-4 Edinburgh Postnatal Depression Scale (EPDS)

The Edinburgh Postnatal Depression Scale (EPDS) has been developed to assist primary care health professionals to detect mothers suffering from postnatal depression, a distressing disorder more prolonged than the "blues" (which occur in the first week after delivery) but less severe than puerperal psychosis.

Previous studies have shown that postnatal depression affects at least 10% of women and that many depressed mothers remain untreated. These mothers may cope with their baby and with household tasks, but their enjoyment of life is seriously affected, and long-term effects on the family are possible.

The EPDS was developed at health centers in Livingston and Edinburgh. It consists of 10 short statements. The mother underlines which of the four possible responses is closest to how she has been feeling during the past week. Most mothers complete the scale without difficulty in less than 5 minutes.

The validation study showed that mothers who scored above a threshold of 12/13 were likely to be suffering from a depressive illness of varying severity. Nevertheless, the EPDS score should not override clinical judgment. A careful clinical assessment should be carried out to confirm the diagnosis. The scale indicates how the mother has felt during the previous week, and in doubtful cases it may be usefully repeated after 2 weeks. The scale will not detect mothers with anxiety neuroses, phobias, or personality disorders.

INSTRUCTIONS FOR USERS

1. The mother is asked to underline the response that is closest to how she has been feeling in the previous 7 days.
2. All 10 items must be completed.
3. Care should be taken to avoid the possibility of the mother discussing her answers with others.
4. The mother should complete the scale herself unless she has limited English or has difficulty with reading.
5. The EPDS may be used at 6 to 8 weeks to screen postnatal women. The child health clinic, postnatal check-up, or a home visit may provide suitable opportunities for its completion.

EDINBURGH POSTNATAL DEPRESSION SCALE (EPDS)

J. L. Cox, J. M. Holden, R. Sagovsky

Department of Psychiatry, University of Edinburgh
Name:
Address:
Baby's age:

As you have recently had a baby, we would like to know how you are feeling. Please UNDERLINE the answer which comes closest to how you have felt IN THE PAST 7 DAYS, not just how you feel today.
Here is an example, already completed.
  I have felt happy:
    Yes, all the time

Yes, most of the time
No, not very often
No, not at all
This would mean: "I have felt happy most of the time" during the past week. Please complete the other questions in the same way.

IN THE PAST 7 DAYS:

1. I have been able to laugh and see the funny side of things
   As much as I always could
   Not quite so much now
   Definitely not so much now
   Not at all
2. I have looked forward with enjoyment to things
   As much as I ever did
   Rather less than I used to
   Definitely less than I used to
   Hardly at all
*3. I have blamed myself unnecessarily when things went wrong
   Yes, most of the time
   Yes, some of the time
   Not very often
   No, never
4. I have been anxious or worried for no good reason
   No, not at all
   Hardly ever
   Yes, sometimes
   Yes, very often
*5. I have felt scared or panicky for no very good reason
   Yes, quite a lot
   Yes, sometimes
   No, not much
   No, not at all
*6. Things have been getting on top of me
   Yes, most of the time I haven't been able to cope at all
   Yes, sometimes I haven't been coping as well as usual
   No, most of the time I have coped quite well
   No, I have been coping as well as ever
*7. I have been so unhappy that I have had difficulty sleeping
   Yes, most of the time
   Yes, sometimes
   Not very often
   No, not at all
*8. I have felt sad or miserable
   Yes, most of the time
   Yes, quite often
   Not very often
   No, not at all
*9. I have been so unhappy that I have been crying
   Yes, most of the time
   Yes, quite often
   Only occasionally
   No, never

Continued

BOX 16-4 Edinburgh Postnatal Depression Scale (EPDS)—cont'd	
*10. The thought of harming myself has occurred to me Yes, quite often Sometimes	Hardly ever Never

J. L. Cox, MA, DM, FRCP(Edin), FRCPsych, Professor of Psychiatry, Department of Postgraduate Medicine, University of Keele. Consultant Psychiatrist. City General Hospital, Stoke-on-Trent, formerly Senior Lecturer. Department of Psychiatry, University of Edinburgh (Correspondence to: University of Keele, Thornburrow Drive, Hartshill, Stoke-on-Trent. Staffs S177QB). J. M. Holden, BSc., SRN, HVCert, Research Psychologist. R. Sagovsky, MB, ChB, MRCPsych, Research Psychiatrist, Department of Psychiatry, University of Edinburgh.

*Response categories are scored 0, 1, 2, and 3 according to increased severity of the symptom.

Items marked with an asterisk are reverse-scored (i.e., 3, 2, 1, and 0). The total score is calculated by adding together the scores for each of the 10 items.

Users may reproduce the scale without further permission, providing they respect copyright (which remains with the *British Journal of Psychiatry*) by quoting the names of the authors, the title, and the source of the paper in all reproduced copies (*Br J Psychiatry* 150:782, 1987).

Measurements of long-chain polyunsaturated fatty acids (LCPUFAs) in breast milk was done on the milk of 287 women enrolled in the Pregnancy, Infection, and Nutrition Study.[138] Levels were measured at <20 and 24 to 29 weeks in the mother and at 4 months postpartum in the breast milk. Multiple linear regression was used to examine association between depressive symptoms, as well as in the breast milk.[138] The authors express concern for early screening of LCPUFAs in the milk of depressed mothers and the nutritional value of their breast milk. Lower levels were found in pregnancy and associated with depressive symptoms, as well as in breast milk.

POSTTRAUMATIC STRESS DISORDER

Posttraumatic stress disorder has now been described with childbirth.[29] It was first listed in the *Diagnostic and Statistical Manual of Mental Disorders* in 1980 following the Vietnam War. It has been defined as "direct personal experience of an event that involves actual or threatened death or serious injury or a threat to the physical integrity of self or others." The individual's response is one of extreme fear, helplessness, or horror, according to the American Psychiatric Association. The reported prevalence of posttraumatic stress following childbirth ranges from 1.5% to 6% of births. Mothers experiencing stress disorder with childbirth struggle to survive each day, while battling nightmares and flashbacks of the birth, anger, anxiety, depression, and painful isolation from the world of motherhood.

As more is learned about this devastating state, more will be learned about feeding choice and breastfeeding success.

DYSPHORIC MILK EJECTION REFLEX

Dysphoric milk ejection reflex is described as a condition affecting lactating women that is "characterized by an abrupt dysphoria or negative emotions that occur just before milk release and continuing not more than a few minutes." It was first identified and described by Alia Macrina Heise, who is a mother of three children, Certified Lactation Counselor, Certified Postpartum Doula, and a trained birth doula (http://www.d-mer.org). Hundreds of women have come forward describing similar experiences. The current belief is that the condition is due to inappropriate dopamine activity at the time of milk ejection. They have distinguished it from a psychologic response to breastfeeding, from nausea and headache and other physical manifestation, from postpartum depression, and from breastfeeding aversion. The dysphoria, or negative emotion, has been described as a churning in the stomach, a hollow feeling, dread, anxiety, and anger. The problem is that it is real, and it is all about let-down. It has been ranked mild, moderate, and severe, the latter often resulting in weaning. No research has been published yet, but clinicians need to be aware of this phenomenon. Natural herbal remedies have been suggested. Antidepression therapy does not appear to help (http://www.d-mer.org).

REFERENCES

1. Adab P, Jiang CQ, Rankin E, et al: Breastfeeding practice, oral contraceptive use and risk of rheumatoid arthritis among Chinese women: the Guangzhou Biobank Cohort Study, *Rheumatology* 53:860–866, 2014.
2. Adamopoulos DA, Kapolla N: Prolactin concentration in milk and plasma of puerperal women and patients with galactorrhea, *J Endocrinol Invest* 7:273, 1984.
3. Akbari SAA, Alamolhoda SH, Baghban AA, et al: Effects of menthol essence and breastmilk on the improvement of nipple fissures in breastfeeding women, *J Res Med Sci* 19 (7):629–633, 2014.
4. Akbulut S, Yilmaz D, Bakir S: Methotrexate in the management of idiopathic granulomatous mastitis: review of 108 published cases and report of four cases, *Breast J* 17 (6):661–668, 2011.
5. Aksoy JT, Eras Z, Erdeve O, et al: A rare cause of hematemesis in newborn: fibrocystic breast disease of mother, *Breastfeed Med* 8(4):418–420, 2013.

6. Alipour S, Seifollahi A, Anbiaee R: Lactating breast abscess: a rare presentation of adenosquamous breast carcinoma, *Singapore Med J* 54(12):e247–e249, 2013.
7. Al-Khaffaf B, Knox F, Bundred NJ: Idiopathic granulomatous mastitis: a 25-year experience, *J Am Coll Surg* 206:269–273, 2008.
8. Alpert SE, Cormier AD: Normal electrolyte and protein content in milk from mothers with cystic fibrosis: an explanation for the initial report of elevated milk sodium concentration, *J Pediatr* 102:77, 1983.
9. Altintoprak F, Kivilcim T, Ozham OV: Aetiology of idiopathic granulomatous mastitis, *World J Clin Cases* 2(12): 852–858, 2014.
10. American College of Radiology Bulletin. Retrieved March 2002, from http://www.acr.org/.
11. Anbazhagan R, Bartek J, Monaghan P, et al: Growth and development of the human infant breast, *Am J Anat* 192:407, 1991.
12. Andersen LW, Qvist T, Hertz J, et al: Concentrations of thiopentone in mature breast milk and colostrum following an induction dose, *Acta Anaesthesiol Scand* 31:30, 1987.
13. Anderson JE, Held N, Wright K: Raynaud's phenomenon of the nipple: a treatable cause of painful breastfeeding, *Pediatrics* 113(4):e360–e364, 2004.
14. Angya JM, Gutierrez MA, Scopelitis E, et al: Hyperprolactinemia in primary Sjögren's syndrome, *Arthritis Rheum* 37:10, 1994.
15. Antevski BM, Smilevski DA, Stojovsky MZ: Extreme gigantomastia in pregnancy: case report and review of literature, *Arch Gynecol Obstet* 275:144–153, 2007.
16. Aono T, Aki T, Koike K, et al: Effect of sulpiride on poor puerperal lactation, *Am J Obstet Gynecol* 143:927, 1982.
17. Aoyama K, Koyama M, Matsuoka K-I, et al: Improved outcome of allogeneic bone marrow transplantation due to breastfeeding-induced tolerance to maternal antigens, *Blood* 113:1829–1833, 2009.
18. Applegate M: *Personal communication*, 2009, University of Albany School of Public Health.
19. Argyrion AA, Makris N: Review article: multiple sclerosis and reproductive risks in women, *Reprod Sci* 15:755–764, 2008.
20. Arroye R, Martin V, Maldonado A, et al: Treatment of infectious mastitis during lactation: antibiotics versus oral administration of lactobacilli isolated from breast milk, *Clin Infect Dis* 50:1551–1558, 2010.
21. Askmark H, Lundberg PO: Lactation headache—a new form of headache? *Cephalalgia* 9:119, 1989.
22. Asselin BL, Lawrence RA: Maternal disease as a consideration in lactation management, *Clin Perinatol* 14:71, 1987.
23. Baker PA, Schroeder D: Interpleural bupivacaine for postoperative pain during lactation, *Anesth Analg* 69:400, 1989.
24. Barbosa-Cesnik C, Schwartz K, Foxman B: Lactation mastitis, *JAMA* 289:1609–1612, 2003.
25. Barrett JH, Brennan P, Fiddler M, et al: Breast-feeding and postpartum relapse in women with rheumatoid and inflammatory arthritis, *Arthritis Rheum* 43:1010, 2000.
26. Barrett ME, Heller MM, Stone HF, et al: Raynaud phenomenon of the nipple in breastfeeding mothers, *JAMA Dermatol* 149(3):300–306, 2013.
27. Bartick MC, Stuebe AM, Schwarz EB, et al: Cost analysis of maternal disease associated with suboptimal breastfeeding, *Obstet Gynecol* 122(1):111–119, 2013.
28. Beck CT: Postpartum depression, *Am J Nurs* 106:40–50, 2006.
29. Beck CT: Post-traumatic stress disorder due to childbirth: the aftermath, *Nurs Res* 53(4):216–224, 2004.
30. Beischer NA, Hueston JH, Pepperell RJ: Massive hypertrophy of the breasts in pregnancy: report of 3 cases and reviewing of the literature, *Obstet Gynecol Surv* 44: 234–243, 1989.
31. Benjamin F: Normal lactation and galactorrhea, *Clin Obstet Gynecol* 37:887, 1994.
32. Bentley-Lewis R, Levkoff S, Stuebe A, et al: Gestational diabetes mellitus: postpartum opportunities for the diagnosis and prevention of type 2 diabetes mellitus, *Nat Clin Pract Endocrinol Metab* 4:552–558, 2008.
33. Berens P, Newton ER: Breast masses during lactation and the role of the obstetrician in breastfeeding, *ABM News Views* 3(2):4, 1997.
34. Bernstein J, Patel N, Moszczynski Z, et al: Colostrum morphine concentrations following epidural administration, *Anesth Analg* 68:S23, 1989.
35. Bitman J, Hamosh M, Hamosh P, et al: Milk composition and volume during the onset of lactation in a diabetic mother, *Am J Clin Nutr* 50:1364, 1989.
36. Bland KI, Romnell LJ: Congenital and acquired disturbances of breast development and growth. In Bland KI, Copeland EM III, editors: *The breast: comprehensive management of benign and malignant diseases*, Philadelphia, Pa., 1991, WB Saunders.
37. Borch-Johnsen K, Joner G, Mandrup-Poulsen T, et al: Relation between breastfeeding and incidence rates of insulin-dependent diabetes mellitus, *Lancet* 2:1083, 1984.
38. Brennan P, Silman A: Breast-feeding and the onset of rheumatoid arthritis, *Arthritis Rheum* 37:808, 1994.
39. Briggs GG, Freeman RK, Yaffe S: *Drugs in pregnancy and lactation*, ed 3, Baltimore, Md., 1990, Williams & Wilkins.
40. Briggs GG, Freeman RK, Yaffe SJ: *Drugs in pregnancy and lactation*, ed 10, Baltimore, 2014, Walters Kluwer/Lippincoll, Williams & Wilkens.
41. Brodie MJ: Management of epilepsy during pregnancy and lactation, *Lancet* 336:426, 1990.
42. Brun JG, Nilssen S, Kvale G: Breastfeeding, other reproductive factors and rheumatoid arthritis: a prospective study, *Br J Rheumatol* 34:542, 1995.
43. Brzozowski D, Niessen M, Evans BB, et al: Breast-feeding after inferior pedicle reduction mammaplasty, *Can J Public Health* 105:530, 2000.
44. Buddhadeb D, Perry MC: Bilateral non-Hodgkin's lymphoma of the breast mimicking mastitis, *South Med J* 90:328, 1997.
45. Burns PE: Absence of lactation in a previously radiated breast, *Int J Radiat Oncol Biol Phys* 13:1603, 1987 (letter).
46. Butte NF, Garza C, Burr R, et al: Milk composition of insulin-dependent diabetic women, *J Pediatr Gastroenterol Nutr* 6:936, 1987.
47. Bybee DE, Metzger BE, Freinkel N, et al: Amniotic fluid prolactin in the third trimester of pregnancies complicated by gestational or pregestational diabetes mellitus, *Metabolism* 39:714, 1990.
48. Campbell DA, Lorber MI, Sweeton JC, et al: Breastfeeding and maternal-donor renal allografts, *Transplantation* 37:340, 1984.
49. Cavallo MG, Fava D, Monetini L, et al: Cell-mediated immune response to b-casein in recent-onset insulin-dependent diabetes: implications for disease pathogenesis, *Lancet* 348:926, 1996.
50. Chan SC, Birdsell DC, Gradeen CY: Detection of toluenediamines in the urine of a patient with polyurethane-covered breast implants, *Clin Chem* 37:756, 1991.
51. Chaudron LH, Szilagyi PG, Kitzman HJ, et al: Detection of postpartum depressive symptoms by screening at well-child visits, *Pediatrics* 113:551, 2004.
52. Christensen AF, Al-Suliman N, Nielsen KR, et al: Ultrasound-guided drainage of breast abscesses: results in 151 patients, *Br J Radiol* 78:186–188, 2005.
53. Cooper PJ, Murray L, Stein A: Psychological factors associated with the early termination of breastfeeding, *J Psychosom Res* 37:171, 1993.
54. Cordero L, Treuer SH, Landon MB, et al: Management of infants of diabetic mothers, *Arch Pediatr Adolesc Med* 152:249, 1998.

55. Coulam CB, Moyer TP, Jiang NS, et al: Breastfeeding after renal transplantation, *Transplant Proc* 14:605, 1982.
56. Counsilman JJ, Mackay EV: Cigarette smoking by pregnant women with particular reference to their past and subsequent breastfeeding behaviour, *Aust N Z J Obstet Gynaecol* 25:101, 1985.
57. Courtiss EH, Goldwyn RM: Breast sensation before and after plastic surgery, *Plast Reconstr Surg* 58:1, 1976.
58. Cox JL, Connor Y, Kendall RE: Prospective study of the psychiatric disorders of childbirth, *Br J Psychiatry* 140:111, 1982.
59. Creasy RK, Resnik R, Iams JD, et al: *Creasy & Resnik's maternal-fetal medicine: principles and practice*, ed 7, Philadelphia, Pa., 2014, Elsevier/Saunders.
60. Crill E, Miracle D, Moore E: Lactation post-bariatric surgery: a qualitative study, *Breastfeed Med*, in press.
61. Dancey A, Khan M, Dawson J, et al: Gigantomasta-a classification and review of the literature, *J Plast Reconstr Aesthet Surg* 61:493–502, 2008.
62. Das UN: Breastfeeding prevents type 2 diabetes mellitus: but, how and why? *Am J Clin Nutr* 85:1436–1437, 2007.
63. David FC: Lactation following primary radiation therapy for carcinoma of the breast, *Int J Radiat Oncol Biol Phys* 11:1425, 1985.
64. Davis MK: Breastfeeding and chronic disease in childhood and adolescence, *Pediatr Clin North Am* 48:125, 2001.
65. Dennis CL, MacQueen K: Does maternal postpartum depressive symptomatology influence infant feeding outcomes? *Acta Paediatr* 96:590–594, 2007.
66. Dennis CL, MacQueen K: The relationship between infant-feeding outcomes and postpartum depression: a qualitative systematic review, *Pediatrics* 123:e736–e751, 2009.
67. Devereux WP: Acute puerperal mastitis, *Am J Obstet Gynecol* 108:78, 1970.
68. Diesing D, Axt-Fliedner R, Hornung D, et al: Granulomatous mastitis, *Arch Gynecol Obstet* 269:233, 2003.
69. Domino EF, Hornbach E, Demana T: The nicotine content of common vegetables, *N Engl J Med* 329:437, 1993.
70. Dosch HM, Becker DJ: Infant feeding and autoimmune diabetes, *Adv Exp Med Biol* 503:133, 2002.
71. Drinkwater BL, Chesnut CH: Bone density changes during pregnancy and lactation in active women: a longitudinal study, *Bone Miner* 14:153, 1991.
72. Dugh Pugh LC, Buchko BL, Bishop BA, et al: A comparison of topical agents to relieve nipple pain and enhance breastfeeding, *Birth* 23:88–93, 1996.
73. East CE, Dolan WJ, Forster DA: *Ante natal breast milk expression by women with diabetes for improving breast milk expression (Review)*. The Cochrane Collaboration, The Cochrane Library, 2014, issue 7: http://www.thecochranelibrary.com.
74. Edwards JE Jr: Should all patients with candidemia be treated with antifungal agents? *Clin Infect Dis* 15:422, 1992 (editorial).
75. Eglash A: Vasospasm of the nipples, *ABM News Views* 2 (1):1, 1996.
76. Eglash A: Treatment of maternal hypergalactia, *Breastfeed Med* 9(9):423–425, 2014.
77. Eidelman AI, Hoffmann NW, Kaitz M: Cognitive deficits in women after childbirth, *Obstet Gynecol* 81:764, 1993.
78. Esbjorner E, Jarnerot G, Wranne L: Sulphasalazine and sulphapyridine serum levels in children of mothers treated with sulphasalazine during pregnancy and lactation, *Acta Paediatr Scand* 76:137, 1987.
79. Feilberg VL, Rosenborg D, Christensen CB, et al: Excretion of morphine in human breast milk, *Acta Anaesthesiol Scand* 33:426, 1989.
80. Ferguson JH: Silicone breast implants and neurologic disorders, *Neurology* 48:1504, 1997.
81. Ferris AM, Dalidowitz CK, Ingardia CM, et al: Lactation outcome in insulin-dependent diabetic women, *J Am Diet Assoc* 88:317, 1988.
82. Fetherston CM, Lai CT, Hartmann PE: Relationships between symptoms and changes in breast physiology during lactation mastitis, *Breastfeed Med* 1:136–145, 2006.
83. Finkelstein SA, Keely E, Feig DS, et al: Breastfeeding in women with diabetes: lower rates despite greater rewards. A population based study, *Diabet Med* 30(9), 2013.
84. Flores HC, Cromwell JW, Leventhal JR, et al: Does previous breastfeeding affect maternal donor renal allograft outcome? A single-institution experience, *Transplant Proc* 25:212, 1993.
85. Forbes GB, Barton LD, Nicholas DL, et al: Composition of milk produced by a mother with galactosemia, *J Pediatr* 113:90, 1988.
86. Forester DA, McEgan K, Ford RF, et al: Diabetes and antenatal milk expressing: a pilot project to inform the development of a randomized trial, *Midwifery* 27:209–214, 2011.
87. Fort P, Lanes R, Dahlem S, et al: Breastfeeding and insulin-dependent diabetes mellitus in children, *J Am Coll Nutr* 5:439, 1986.
88. Foxman B, D'Arcy H, Gillespie B, et al: Lactation mastitis: occurrence and medical management among 946 breastfeeding women in the United States, *Am J Epidemiol* 155:103, 2002.
89. Gabbe SG, Niebyl JR, Simpson JL, editors: *Obstetrics: normal problem pregnancies*, ed 6, New York, 2012, Churchill Livingstone.
90. Gabby M, Kelly H: Use of metformin to increase breast milk production in women with insulin resistance: case series, *ABM News Views* 9:20, 2003.
91. Giampietro O, Ramacciotti C, Moggi G: Normoprolactinemic galactorrhea in a fertile woman with a copper intra-uterine device (copper IUD), *Acta Obstet Gynecol Scand* 63:23, 1984.
92. Giesecke AH Jr, Rice LJ, Lipton JM: Alfentanil in colostrum, *Anesthesiology* 63:A284, 1985.
93. Ginsberg JS, Hirsh J: Thromboembolic disorders of pregnancy. In Reese EA, Hobbins JC, Mahoney MJ, et al, editors: *Medicine of the fetus and mother*, Philadelphia, Pa., 1992, JB Lippincott.
94. Glatthaar D, Whittall DE, Welborn TA, et al: Diabetes in western Australian children: descriptive epidemiology, *Med J Aust* 148:117, 1988.
95. Glueck CJ, Salehi M, Sieve L, et al: Growth, motor, and social development in breast- and formula-fed infants of metformin-treated women with polycystic ovary syndrome, *J Pediatr* 148(5):628–632, 2006.
96. Gould BK, Randall RV, Kempers RD, et al: *Galactorrhea*, Springfield, Ill., 1974, Thomas.
97. Grange DK, Finlay JL: Nutritional vitamin B12 deficiency in a breast-fed infant following maternal gastric bypass, *Pediatr Hematol Oncol* 11:311–318, 1994.
98. Greenwald JH, Dubin A, Cardon L: Hypomagnesemic tetany due to excessive lactation, *Am J Med* 35:854, 1963.
99. Gruber HE, Gutteridge DH, Baylink DJ: Osteoporosis associated with pregnancy and lactation: bone biopsy and skeletal features in three patients, *Metab Bone Dis Rel Res* 5:159, 1984.
100. Gulick EE, Johnson S: Infant health of mothers with multiple sclerosis, *West J Nurs Res* 26:632–649, 2004.
101. Gupta R, Gupta AS, Duggal N: Tubercular mastitis, *Int Surg* 67:422, 1982.
102. Håkansson A, Cars H: Maternal cigarette smoking, breast feeding and respiratory tract infections in infancy, *Scand J Prim Health Care* 9:115, 1991.
103. Hale TW: *Medications and mother's milk*, ed 16, Amarillo, Tex., 2014, Hale Publishing LP.
104. Hale TW, Bateman TL, Finkelman MA, et al: The absence of *Candida albicans* in milk samples of women with clinical symptoms of ductal candidiasis, *Breastfeed Med* 4:57–61, 2009.
105. Hamosh M, Bitman J, Wood DL, et al: Human milk in cystic fibrosis: composition and enzyme content, *Pediatr Res* 16:164A, 1982.

106. Hanson LA: The mammary gland as an immunological organ, *Immunol Today* 3:168, 1982.

107. Hardwick-Smith S, Mastrobattista JM, Nader S: Breast engorgement and lactation associated with thyropin-releasing hormone administration, *Obstet Gynecol* 92:717, 1998.

108. Harris B, Johns S, Fung H, et al: The hormonal environment of postnatal depression, *Br J Psychol* 154:660, 1989.

109. Hattori N, Ishihara T, Ikekubo K, et al: Autoantibody to human prolactin in patients with idiopathic hyperprolactinemia, *J Clin Endocrinol Metab* 75:1226, 1992.

110. Heller MM, Fullerton-Stone H, Murase JE: Caring for new mothers: diagnosis, management and treatment of nipple dermatitis in breastfeeding mothers, *Int J Dermatol* 51:1149–1161, 2012.

111. Heneghan AM, Mercer MB, DeLeone NL: Will mothers discuss parenting stress and depressive symptoms with their child's pediatrician? *Pediatrics* 113:460, 2004.

112. Herrera E: Maternal touch and maternal child directed speech: effects of depressed mood in the postnatal period, *J Affect Disord* 81(1):29–39, 2004.

113. Higgins S, Haffty BG: Pregnancy and lactation after breast-conserving therapy for early stage breast cancer, *Cancer* 73:2175, 1994.

114. Hodnett DW, DeLuca HF, Jorgensen NA: Bone mineral loss during lactation occurs in absence of parathyroid tissue, *Am J Physiol* 262:E230–E233, 1992.

115. Holmquist DG, Papanicolaou GN: The exfoliative cytology of the mammary gland during pregnancy and lactation, *Ann N Y Acad Sci* 63:1422, 1956.

116. Hoover HC: Breast cancer during pregnancy and lactation, *Surg Clin North Am* 70:1151, 1990.

117. Hopkinson JM, Schanler RJ, Fraley JK, et al: Milk production by mothers of premature infants: influence of cigarette smoking, *Pediatrics* 90:934, 1992.

118. Hornstein E, Skornick Y, Rozin R: The management of breast carcinoma in pregnancy and lactation, *J Surg Oncol* 21:179, 1982.

119. Hoshiyama E, Tatsumoto M, Iwanami H, et al: Postpartum migraines: a long term prospective study, *Intern Med* 51:3119–3123, 2012.

120. Hummel S, Pflüger M, Kreichauf S, et al: Predictors of overweight during childhood in offspring of parents with type 1 diabetes, *Diabetes Care* 32:921–925, 2009.

121. Ingram AD, Mahoney MC: An overview of breast emergencies and guide to management by interventional radiologists, *Tech Vasc Interv Radiol* 17:55–63, 2014.

122. Isenberg KE: Excretion of fluoxetine in human breast milk, *J Clin Psychiatry* 51:169, 1990.

123. Isenberg DA, Black C: Raynaud's phenomenon, scleroderma, and overlap syndromes, *Br Med J* 310:795, 1995.

124. Jahanfar S, Ng CJ, Teng CL: *Antibiotics for mastitis in breastfeeding women (review).* Cochrane Review. Cochrane Library, Issue 2, 2009.

125. Jara LJ, Lavalle C, Espinoza LR: Does prolactin have a role in the pathogenesis of systemic lupus erythematosus? *J Rheumatol* 19:1333, 1992.

126. Jaques SC, Kingsbury A, Henshcke P, et al: Cannabis, the pregnant woman and her child: weeding out the myths, *J Perinatol* 34:1–8, 2014.

127. Jensen RG, Ferris AM, Lammi-Keefe CJ: Cholesterol levels and the breastfeeding mom, *JAMA* 262:2092, 1989.

128. Jorgensen C, Picot MC, Bologna C, et al: Oral contraception, parity, breastfeeding, and severity of rheumatoid arthritis, *Ann Rheum Dis* 55:94, 1996.

129. Joselin EP, Root HF, White P, et al: *The treatment of diabetes mellitus,* Philadelphia, Pa., 1959, Lea & Febiger.

130. Kalache A, Vessey MP, McPherson K: Lactation and breast cancer, *Br Med J* 280.223, 1980.

131. Kamble TK, Ookalka DS: Lactation hypomagnesemia, *Lancet* 2:155, 1989.

132. Kampmann J, Johansen K, Hansen JN, et al: Propylthiouracil in human milk, *Lancet* 1:736, 1980.

133. Kaneko S, Suzuki K, Sato T, et al: The problems of antiepileptic medication in the neonatal period: is breastfeeding advisable? In Janz D, Dam M, Richens A, et al, editors: *Epilepsy, pregnancy, and the child,* New York, 1982, Raven.

134. Kapcala LP: Galactorrhea and thyrotoxicosis, *Arch Intern Med* 144:2349, 1984.

135. Karjalainen J, Martin JM, Knip M, et al: A bovine albumin peptide as a possible trigger of insulin-dependent diabetes mellitus, *N Engl J Med* 327:302, 1992.

136. Karlson EW, Mandl LA, Hankinson SE, et al: Do breastfeeding and other reproductive factors influence future risk of rheumatoid arthritis? *Arthritis Rheum* 50:3458–3467, 2004.

137. Katz E, Adashi EY: Hyperprolactinemic disorders, *Clin Obstet Gynecol* 33:622, 1990.

138. Keim SA, Daniels JL, Siega-Riz AM, et al: Depressive symptoms during pregnancy and the concentration of fatty acids in breastmilk, *J Hum Lact* 28(2):189–195, 2012.

139. Kendall-Tackett KA, Kantor GK: *Postpartum depression. Sage series in clinical nursing research,* Newbury Park, Calif., 1993, Sage.

140. Kessler DA: The basis of the FDA's decision on breast implants, *N Engl J Med* 326:1713, 1992.

141. Key TC, Resnik R, Dittrich HC, et al: Successful pregnancy after cardiac transplantation, *Am J Obstet Gynecol* 160:367, 1989.

142. Kim SH, Cha ES, Kim HS, et al: Galactography acquired with digital mammography in patients with nipple discharge: a retrospective analysis, *Arch Gynecol Obstet* 280:217, 2009.

143. King EB, Goodson WH III: Discharges and secretions of the nipple. In Bland KI, Copeland EM III, editors: *The breast: comprehensive management of benign and malignant diseases,* Philadelphia, Pa., 1991, WB Saunders.

144. Kira J-I, Harada M, Yamaguchi Y, et al: Hyperprolactinemia in multiple sclerosis, *J Neurol Sci* 102:61, 1991.

145. Kiyak G, Dumlu EG, Kilinc I, et al: Management of idiopathic granulomatous mastitis: dilemmas in diagnosis and treatment, *BMC Surg* 14:66–70, 2014.

146. Klement E, Cohen RV, Boxman J, et al: Breastfeeding and risk of inflammatory bowel disease: a systemic review with meta-analysis, *Am J Clin Nutr* 80:1342–1352, 2004.

147. Kline TS, Kline IK: *Breast: guides to clinical aspiration biopsy,* New York/Tokyo, 1989, Igaku-Shoin Medical Publishers.

148. Kline TS, Lash SR: Nipple secretion in pregnancy: a cytologic and histologic study, *Am J Clin Pathol* 37:626, 1962.

149. Kline TS, Lash SR: The bleeding nipple of pregnancy and postpartum period: a cytologic and histologic study, *Acta Cytol* 8:336, 1964.

150. Kois WE, Campbell DA, Lorber MI, et al: Influence of breastfeeding on subsequent reactivity to a related renal allograft, *J Surg Res* 37:89, 1984.

151. Kossoy LR, Herbert CM, Wentz AC: Management of heart transplant recipients: guidelines for the obstetrician-gynecologist, *Am J Obstet Gynecol* 159:490, 1988.

152. Kostraba JN, Cruickshanks KJ, Lawler-Heavner J, et al: Early exposure to cow's milk and solid foods in infancy, genetic predisposition, and risk of IDDM, *Diabetes* 42:288, 1993.

153. Kostraba JN, Steenkiste AR, Dorman JS, et al: Early infant diet and risk of IDDM in blacks and whites, *Diabetes Care* 15:626, 1992.

154. Kreipe RE, Lewand AG, Dukarm CP, et al: Outcome for patients with bulimia and breast hypertrophy after reduction mammaplasty, *Arch Pediatr Adolesc Med* 151:176, 1997.

155. Kugyelka JG, Rasmussen KM, Frongillo EA: Maternal obesity and breastfeeding success among black and Hispanic women, *J Nutr* 134:1746–1750, 2004.

156. Kulski JK, Smith M, Hartmann PE: Normal and caesarean section delivery and the initiation of lactation in women, *Aust J Exp Biol Med Sci* 59:405, 1981.

157. Labrecque M, Marcoux S, Weber J-P, et al: Feeding and urine cotinine values in babies whose mothers smoke, *Pediatrics* 83:93, 1989.

158. Lafreniere R: Bloody nipple discharge during pregnancy: a rationale for conservative treatment, *J Surg Oncol* 43:228, 1990.

159. Lamberg BA, Ikonen E, Osterlund K, et al: Antithyroid treatment of maternal hyperthyroidism during lactation, *Clin Endocrinol (Oxf)* 21:81, 1984.

160. Langer-Gould A, Huang SM, Gupta R, et al: Exclusive breastfeeding and the risk of postpartum relapses in women with multiple sclerosis, *Arch Neurol* 66:958–963, 2009.

161. Law KL, Stroud L, LaGasse LL, et al: Smoking during pregnancy and newborn neurobehavior, *Pediatrics* 111: 1318–1323, 2003.

162. Lawlor-Smith LS, Lawlor-Smith CL: Raynaud's phenomenon of the nipple: a preventable cause of breastfeeding failure, *Med J Aust* 166:448, 1996.

163. Lawlor-Smith LS, Lawlor-Smith CL: Vasospasm of the nipple: a manifestation of Raynaud's phenomenon; case reports, *Br Med J* 314:644, 1997.

164. Lawrence R: Lactation, breastfeeding, infant care and mental illness. In Kuczmerczy AR, Reading AE, editors: *Handbook of behavioral obstetrics and gynecology*, New York, 1994, Plenum.

165. Lee GF: Fine-needle aspiration of the breast: the outpatient management of breast lesions, *Am J Obstet Gynecol* 156:1532, 1987.

166. Leis HP: Management of nipple discharge, *World J Surg* 13:736, 1989.

167. Leis HP, Urban JA: The other breast. In Gallager HS, editor: *The breast*, St Louis, Mo., 1978, Mosby.

168. Lindblad A, Mar Ahsál K: Influence of nicotine chewing gum on fetal blood flow, *J Perinat Med* 15:13, 1987.

169. Little RE, Lambert MD III, Worthington RB, et al: Maternal smoking during lactation: relation to infant size at one year of age, *Am J Epidemiol* 140:544, 1994.

170. Luck W, Nau H: Nicotine and cotinine concentrations in serum and urine of infants exposed via passive smoking or milk from smoking mothers, *J Pediatr* 107:816, 1985.

171. Luder E, Kaltan M, Tanzer-Torres G, et al: Current recommendations for breastfeeding in cystic fibrosis centers, *Am J Dis Child* 144:1153, 1990.

172. Lurie S, Rotmensch S, Feldman N, et al: Breast engorgement and galactorrhea during magnesium sulfate treatment of preterm labor, *Am J Perinatol* 19:239–240, 2002.

173. MacGregor EA: Migraine in pregnancy and lactation: a clinical review, *J Fam Plann Reprod Health Care* 33:83–93, 2007.

174. Magno R, Berlin A, Karlsson K, et al: Anesthesia for cesarean section. IV. Placental transfer and neonatal elimination of bupivacaine following epidural analgesia for elective cesarean section, *Acta Anaesthesiol Scand* 20:141, 1976.

175. Martin JN, Morrison JC, Files YC: Autoimmune thrombocytopenic purpura: current concepts and recommended practices, *Am J Obstet Gynecol* 150:86, 1984.

176. Matalon R, Michals K, Gleason L, et al: Strategies for dietary treatment and monitoring compliance, *Ann N Y Acad Sci* 477:223, 1986.

177. Matheson I, Rivrud GN: The effect of smoking on lactation and infantile colic, *JAMA* 261:42, 1989.

178. Matias SL, Dewey KG, Quesenberry CP, et al: Maternal prepregnancy obesity and insulin treatment during pregnancy are independently associated with delayed lactogenesis in women with recent gestational diabetes mellitus, *Am J Clin Nutr* 99(1):115–121, 2014.

179. Mayer EJ, Hamman RF, Gay EC, et al: Reduced risk of IDDM among breastfed children. The Colorado IDDM Registry, *Diabetes* 37:1625, 1988.

180. Meli MS, Rashidu MR, Delazar A, et al: Effect of peppermint water on prevention of nipple cracks in lactating primiparous women: a randomized controlled trial, *Int Breastfeed J* 2:7, 2007.

181. Mennella JA, Yourshaw LM, Morgan LK: Breastfeeding and smoking: short-term effects on infant feeding and sleep, *Pediatrics* 120:497–502, 2007.

182. Merland-Schultz K, Hill PD: Prevention of and therapies for nipple pain: a systematic review, *J Obstet Gynecol Neonatal Nurs* 34:428–437, 2005.

183. Meschengieser S, Lazzari MA: Breastfeeding in thrombocytopenic neonates secondary to maternal autoimmune thrombocytopenic purpura, *Am J Obstet Gynecol* 154:1166, 1986.

184. Metcalfe MA, Baum JD: Family characteristics and insulin dependent diabetes, *Arch Dis Child* 67:731, 1992.

185. Mezzacappa ES, Kelsey RM, Myers MM, et al: Breastfeeding and maternal cardiovascular function, *Psychophysiology* 38:988–997, 2001.

186. Michael SH, Mueller DH: Impact of lactation on women with cystic fibrosis and their infants: a review of five cases, *J Am Diet Assoc* 94:159, 1994.

187. Milgrom J, Westley DJ, McCloud PI: Do infants of depressed mothers cry more than other infants? *J Paediatr Child Health* 31:218, 1995.

188. Moazzez A, Kelsa RL, Towfigh S, et al: Breast abscess bacteriologic features in the era of community-acquired methicillin-resistant *Staphylococcus aureus* epidemics, *Arch Surg* 142:881–884, 2007.

189. Morrow-Tlucak M, Haude RH, Ernhart CB: Breastfeeding and cognitive development in the first two years of life, *Soc Sci Med* 26:635, 1988.

190. Moss TW: Gigantomastia with pregnancy, *Arch Surg* 96:27, 1968.

191. Mullins RJ, Russell A, McGrath GJ, et al: Breastfeeding anaphylaxis, *Lancet* 338:1279, 1991.

192. Murray L, Cooper PJ, Stein A: Postnatal depression and infant development: emotional and cognitive development of infants may be adversely affected, *Br Med J* 302:978, 1991.

193. Muscari A, Volta U, Bonazzi C, et al: Association of serum IgA antibodies to milk antigens with severe atherosclerosis, *Atherosclerosis* 77:251, 1989.

194. Nahas GG: Marijuana, *JAMA* 233:79, 1975.

195. Nahas GG, Suciu-Foca N, Armand J-P, et al: Inhibition of cellular mediated immunity in marijuana smokers, *Science* 183:419, 1974.

196. Neifert M, DeMarzo S, Seacat J, et al: The influence of breast surgery, breast appearance and pregnancy-induced breast changes on lactation sufficiency as measured by infant weight gain, *Birth* 17:31, 1990.

197. Neifert MR, McDonough SL, Neville MC: Failure of lactogenesis associated with placental retention, *Am J Obstet Gynecol* 140:477, 1981.

198. Newman J: *Serratia marcescens* and pink milk. Posting June 19, 2009 bfmed@eGroups.com.

199. Newton NR, Newton M: Relationship of ability to breastfeed and maternal attitudes toward breast feeding, *Pediatrics* 5:869, 1950.

200. Newton N, Newton M: Psychologic aspects of lactation, *N Engl J Med* 277:1179, 1967.

201. Nordstrom UL, Dallas JH, Morton HG, et al: Mothering problems and child mortality amongst "mothers with emotional disturbances," *Acta Obstet Gynecol Scand* 67:155, 1988.

202. O'Campo P, Brown H, Faden RR, et al: The impact of pregnancy on women's prenatal and postpartum smoking behavior, *Am J Prev Med* 8:8, 1992.

203. O'Hara MF, Page DL: Adenomas of the breast and ectopic breast under lactational influences, *Hum Pathol* 16:707, 1985.

204. Ohishl A, Nakashima T, Ogata T, et al: Early vitamin K deficiency bleeding in a neonate associated with maternal Crohn's disease, *J Perinatol* 34:636–639, 2014.

205. Olivares M, Albrecht S, Depalma G: Human milk composition differs in healthy mothers and mothers with celiac disease, *Eur J Nutr* 54(1):119–128, 2014. http://dx.doi.org/10.1007/s 00394-014-0692-1.

206. Omranipour R, Mohammadi S-F, Samimi P: Idiopathic granulomatous lobular mastitis—report of 43 cases from Iran, *Breast Care* 8(12):439–443, 2013.

207. Osborne MP: Breast development and anatomy. In Harris JR, Hellman S, Henderson IC, et al, editors: *Breast diseases*, Philadelphia, Pa., 1987, JB Lippincott.

208. Palmer JR, Viscidi E, Troester MA, et al: Parity, lactation, and breast cancer subtypes in African American women: results from the AMBER consortium, *J Natl Cancer Inst* 106(10): 2014.

209. Partonen T: Prolactin in winter depression, *Med Hypotheses* 43:163, 1994.

210. Paulus DD: Benign diseases of the breast, *Radiol Clin North Am* 21:27, 1983.

211. Pellegrini JR, Wagner RF Jr: Polythelia and associated conditions, *Am Fam Physician* 28:129, 1983.

212. Petrek JA: Abnormalities of the breast in pregnancy and lactation. In Harris JR, Lippman ME, Morrow M, editors: *Diseases of the breast*, Philadelphia, Pa., 1996, Lippincott-Raven.

213. Picazo O, Fernandez-Guasti A: Changes in experimental anxiety during pregnancy and lactation, *Physiol Behav* 54:295, 1993.

214. Pilnik S, Leis HP: Nipple discharge. In Gallager HS, editor: *The breast*, St. Louis, Mo., 1978, Mosby.

215. Pisacane A, Impagliazzo N, Russo M, et al: Breastfeeding and multiple sclerosis, *Br Med J* 308:1411, 1994.

216. Pop VJM, Essed GGM, deGeus CA, et al: Prevalence of postpartum depression, *Acta Obstet Gynecol Scand* 72:354, 1993.

217. Portaccio E, Ghezzia A, Hakiki B, et al: Breastfeeding is not related to postpartum relapses in multiple sclerosis, *Neurology* 77:145–150, 2011.

218. Qian X, Chen Y, Wan F: Granular cell tumor of the breast during lactation: a case report and review of the literature, *Oncol Lett* 8:2565–2568, 2014.

219. Ram KT, Bobby P, Hailpern S: Duration of lactation is associated with lower prevalence of the metabolic syndrome in midlife, *Am J Obstet Gynecol* 198:268.e1–268.e6, 2008.

220. Reddy P, Qi C, Zembower T, et al: Postpartum mastitis and community acquired methicillin-resistant *Staphylococcus aureus*, *Emerg Infect Dis* 13:298–301, 2007.

221. Rennie J: Formula for diabetes? *Sci Am* 267:24, 1992.

222. Rikwer M, Bergstrom U, Nisson JA, et al: Breastfeeding, but not the use of oral contraceptives, is associated with a reduced risk of rheumatoid arthrisitis, *Ann Rheum Dis* 68:526–530, 2009.

223. Russo IH, Russo J: Progestagens and mammary gland development: differentiation versus carcinogenesis, *Acta Endocrinol (Copenh)* 125:7, 1991.

224. Ruvalcaba RHA: Stress-induced cessation of lactation, *West J Med* 146:228, 1987.

225. Said G, Patois E, Lellouch J: Infantile colic and parenteral smoking, *Br Med J* 289:660, 1984.

226. Sakakura T: New aspects of stroma-parenchyma relations in mammary gland differentiation, *Int Rev Cytol* 125:165, 1991.

227. Salari P, Abdollahi M: The influence of pregnancy & lactation on maternal bone health: a systematic review, *J Fam Reprod Health* 8(12):135–148, 2014.

228. Sammaritana LR, Bermas BL: Rheumatoid arthritis medications and lactation, *Rheumatology* 26(3):354–360, 2014.

229. Scanlon JW, Ostheimer GW, Lurie AO, et al: Neurobehavioral responses and drug concentrations in newborns after maternal epidural anesthesia with bupivacaine, *Anesthesiology* 45:400, 1976.

230. Schiff M, Algert CS, Ampt A, et al: The impact of cosmetic breast implants on breastfeeding: a systematic review and meta-analysis, *Int Breastfeed J* 9:17–25, 2014.

231. Schnur PL, Weinzweig J, Harris JB, et al: Silicon analysis of breast and periprosthetic capsular tissue from patients with saline or silicone gel breast implants, *Plast Reconstr Surg* 98:798, 1996.

232. Schulte-Hobein B, Schwartz-Bickenbach D, Abt S, et al: Cigarette smoke exposure and development of infants throughout the first year of life: influence of passive smoking and nursing on nicotine levels in breastmilk and infant's urine, *Acta Paediatr Scand* 81:550, 1992.

233. Schwarz EB, Ray RM, Stuebe AM, et al: Duration of lactation and risk factors for maternal cardiovascular disease, *Obstet Gynecol* 113:974–982, 2009.

234. Scott-Conner CEH, Schorr SJ: The diagnosis and management of breast problems during pregnancy and lactation, *Am J Surg* 170:401, 1995.

235. Sert M, Tetiker T, Kirim S, et al: Clinical report of 28 patients with Sheehan's syndrome, *Endocr J* 50:297–301, 2003.

236. Shalev J, Frankel Y, Eshkol A, et al: Breast engorgement and galactorrhea after preventing premature contractions with ritodrine, *Gynecol Obstet Invest* 17:190–193, 1984.

237. Siemiatycki J, Colle E, Campbell S, et al: Case-control study of IDDM, *Diabetes Care* 12:209, 1989.

238. Silberstein SD: Headaches and women: treatment of the pregnant and lactating migraineur, *Headache* 33:533, 1993.

239. Sims CJ, Porter KB, Knuppel RA: Successful pregnancy after a liver transplant, *Am J Obstet Gynecol* 161:532, 1989.

240. Sirota L, Ferrera M, Lerer N, et al: Beta glucuronidase and hyperbilirubinemia in breastfed infants of diabetic mothers, *Arch Dis Child* 67:120, 1992.

241. Smith JL, Lear SR, Forte TM, et al: Effect of pregnancy and lactation on lipoprotein and cholesterol metabolism in the rat, *J Lipid Res* 39:2237–2249, 1998.

242. Smith PK, Tamlin N, Robertson E: Breastmilk and cystic fibrosis, *Med J Aust* 157:283, 1992.

243. Snell NJC, Coysh HL, Snell BJ: Carpal tunnel syndrome presenting in the puerperium, *Practitioner* 224:191, 1980.

244. Soltani H, Scott AMS: Antenatal breast expression in women with diabetes: outcomes from a retrospective cohort study, *Int Breastfeed J* 7:18, 2012.

245. Sorensen HJ, Mortensen EL, Reinisch JM, et al: Breastfeeding and risk of schizophrenia in Copenhagen perinatal cohort, *Acta Psychiatr Scand* 112:26–29, 2005.

246. Sowers MF, Corton G, Shapiro B, et al: Changes in bone density with lactation, *JAMA* 269:3130, 1993.

247. Stafford I, Hernandez J, Laibl V, et al: Community-acquired methicillin-resistant *Staphylococcus aureus* among patients with puerperal mastitis requiring hospitalization, *Obstet Gynecol* 112:533–537, 2008.

248. Steiner G, Myher JJ, Kuksis A: Milk and plasma lipid composition in a lactating patient with type I hyperlipoproteinemia, *Am J Clin Nutr* 41:121, 1985.

249. Steube AM, Schwarz EB, Grewen K, et al: Duration of lactation and incidence of maternal hypertension: a longitudinal cohort study, *Am J Epidemiol* 174(10):1147–1158, 2011.

250. Strom SS, Baldwin BJ, Sigurdson AJ, et al: Cosmetic saline breast implants: a survey of satisfaction, breastfeeding experience, cancer screening and health, *Plast Reconstr Surg* 100:1553–1557, 1997.

251. Stroud LR, Paster RL, Goodwin MS, et al: Maternal smoking during pregnancy and neonatal behavior: a large-scale community study, *Pediatrics* 123:e842–e848, 2009.

252. Stuebe AM, Rich-Edwards JW, Willett WC, et al: Duration of lactation and incidence of type 2 diabetes, *JAMA* 294:2601–2610, 2005.

253. Surian M, Imbasciati E, Cosci P, et al: Glomerular disease and pregnancy, *Nephron* 36:101, 1984.

254. Swelstad MR, Swelstad BB, Rao VK: Management of gestational gigantomastia, *Plast Reconstr Surg* 118:840–846, 2006.

255. Synderman RK: Augmentation mammoplasty. In Gallager HS, editor: *The breast*, St. Louis, Mo., 1978, Mosby.

256. Synderman RK: Reduction mammoplasty. In Gallager HS, editor: *The breast*, St. Louis, Mo., 1978, Mosby.

257. Tamminen TM, Salmelin RK: Psychosomatic interaction between mother and infant during breastfeeding, *Psychother Psychosom* 56:78, 1991.

258. Taveras EM, Capra AM, Braveman PA, et al: Clinician support and psychosocial risk factors associated with breastfeeding discontinuation, *Pediatrics* 112:108, 2003.

259. Terzi R, Terzi H, Ozert T, et al: A rare cause of postpartum low back pain: pregnancy and lactation—associated osteoporosis, *BioMed Res Int*, 2014. http://dx.doi.org/10.1155/2014/287832.

260. Thomsen AC: Infectious mastitis and occurrence of antibody-coated bacteria in milk, *Am J Obstet Gynecol* 144:350, 1982.

261. Thomsen AC, Espersen T, Maigaard S: Course and treatment of milk stasis, noninfectious inflammation of the breast, and infectious mastitis in nursing women, *Am J Obstet Gynecol* 149:492, 1984.

262. Vanky E, Isaksen H, Moen MH, et al: Breastfeeding in polycystic ovary syndrome, *Acta Obstet Gynecol Scand* 87:531–535, 2008.

263. Vidaeff AC, Ross PJ, Livingston CK, et al: Gigantomastia complicating mirror syndrome in pregnancy, *Obstet Gynecol* 101:1139–1142, 2003.

264. Voegeli DR: Galactography. In Peters ME, Voegeli DR, Scanlon KA, editors: *Breast imaging*, New York, 1989, Churchill Livingstone.

265. Wall VR: Breastfeeding and migraine headaches, *J Hum Lact* 8:209, 1992.

266. Wand JS: The natural history of carpal tunnel syndrome in lactation, *J R Soc Med* 82:349, 1989.

267. Wand JS: Carpal tunnel syndrome in pregnancy and lactation, *J Hand Surg (Br)* 15B:93, 1990.

268. Weiner CP, Buhimschi C: *Drugs for pregnant and lactating women*, Philadelphia, Pa., 2004, Churchill Livingstone.

269. Welch MJ, Phelps DL, Osher AB: Breastfeeding by a mother with cystic fibrosis, *Pediatrics* 67:664, 1981.

270. Whichelow MJ, Doddridge MC: Lactation in diabetic women, *Br Med J* 287:649, 1983.

271. Williams JM, Auerbach KG, Jacobi A: Lateral epicondylitis (tennis elbow) in breastfeeding mothers, *Clin Pediatr (Phila)* 28:42, 1989.

272. Woolridge MW: The "anatomy" of infant sucking, *Midwifery* 2:164, 1986.

273. Wu M, Chason R, Wong M: Raynaud's phenomenon of the nipple, *Obstet Gynecol* 119(2):447–449, 2012.

274. Wüst J: *Streptococcus pneumoniae* as an agent of mastitis, *Eur J Clin Microbiol Infect Dis* 14(156), 1995 (letter).

275. Yagnik PM: Carpal tunnel syndrome in nursing mothers, *South Med J* 80:1468, 1987.

276. Yoo H, Choi SH, Kim YJ, et al: Recurrent bilateral breast abscess due to nontuberculous mycobacterial infection, *J Breast Cancer* 17(3):295–298, 2014.

277. Zargar AH, Masoodi SR, Laway BA, et al: Familial puerperal alactogenesis: possibility of a genetically transmitted isolated prolactin deficiency, *Br J Obstet Gynaecol* 104:629, 1997.

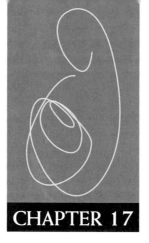

CHAPTER 17

Human Milk as a Prophylaxis

The Natural History of Atopic Disease

The association of allergy with cow milk has been documented in the literature for decades.[25,52,71] The incidence of this allergy in the general population has been noted to increase progressively since the original comments on the subject by Rowe[74] in 1931. The incidence has reportedly increased 10 times in 20 years. It has been attributed to increased recognition; increased incidence of exposure to known allergens; and a gradual decrease in infection as a source of morbidity, because the use of antibiotics and immunization revealed an underlying allergic component to chronic symptoms. Glaser[31] attributed this rapid increase in the development of allergic diseases to the abandonment of breastfeeding when safe, pasteurized milk became available. It was noted that 20% of all children were allergic by 20 years of age.

Studies of office pediatrics have shown that one-third of the visits are a result of allergy.[87] One third of all chronic conditions in patients younger than age 17 result from allergy and one third of lost school days from asthma. In the evaluation of 2000 consecutive, unselected newborns in pediatric practice, 50% had family histories of allergy. Grulee et al.[38] observed, as early as 1934, that eczema was seven times more common in infants fed cow milk than in breastfed infants. McCombs et al.[63] reported in 1979 that asthma caused more than 2000 deaths and the loss of 94 million days of activity. It initiated 183,000 hospital admissions and more than 1 million hospital days in 1 year in the United States alone.

Asthma is the most common chronic disease of childhood, affecting an estimated 6.3 million children, according to a Centers for Disease Control and Prevention (CDC) report in 2001.[66,92] These data indicate that, in the United States, people with asthma collectively have more than 100 million days of restricted activity and 470,000 hospitalizations annually, with more than 5000 deaths annually. Asthma hospitalization rates have been highest among black adults and children, with mortality rates consistently highest among black individuals ages 15 to 24 years. Asthma costs the American public billions of dollars every year. Decades of investigation have resulted in conflicting results. In a systematic review of the literature on how to prevent the development of food allergy,[18] there was one clear conclusion. Cow milk should be avoided for at least the first 4 months of life in children at risk for allergy. Maternal avoidance of allergens during pregnancy also produced conflicting results, except for the avoidance of cow milk during pregnancy when there was a family history. Maternal avoidance of cow milk resulted in lower levels of mucosal-specific IgA and a lower incidence of cow milk allergy in the infant.[43] The American Academy of Pediatrics (AAP) also agreed that cow milk and dairy products should be avoided in at-risk infants for the first year of life. The AAP and others have also declared that soy milk has no role in the prevention of allergy. The AAP is very supportive of breastfeeding for at least 6 months, as well as the delay in starting solids until 6 months.

Bone turnover is increased when mothers are on elimination diets that include cow milk, cow milk products, and eggs, even when they are on supplemental calcium. Mothers who were found to have some bone mobilization for 6 months recovered quickly when breastfeeding was discontinued.[2] Breastfeeding has increased in the new millennium. The incidence of allergy should diminish.

The Question of Heredity

Heredity undoubtedly plays a part in the development of allergic disease, an observation first recorded by Maimonides in his Treatise on Asthma in the twelfth century. Most studies in the past 60 years have concurred with the concept of a recessive mode of inheritance.[45]

Kern[51] has noted that the outstanding etiologic factor in human hypersensitivity is heredity. He states that few diseases exist in which heredity is so clearly identified and so common.

Hamburger reported that children with two atopic parents had a 47% chance of developing atopic disease. One atopic parent meant a 29% chance of developing atopy, and the risk dropped to 13% with no allergic parent.

In a study of asthmatic monozygotic twins, Falliers et al.[21] observed similar serum immunoglobulin E (IgE), blood eosinophil counts, and positive skin tests to allergens in both twins. However, they had dissimilar responses to infection and methacholine. This finding suggests an acquired component to bronchial hyperactivity. Apparently several mechanisms are involved in antigen processing.

To identify infants at high risk for developing atopy, several approaches have been suggested. Cord serum total IgE levels of greater than 100 U/mL are associated with a five to ten times greater risk than lower levels. Eosinophilia and lymphocytes may prove to be markers, but, at present, only the family allergy history and the cord blood IgE have been significantly reliable predictors.[9]

In the 1930s, Glaser[31] speculated that if a child was at a high risk for developing allergy, prophylaxis should be able to change the outcome. The original work on prophylaxis was done by Glaser and Johnstone[30] and reported in 1953. Only 15% of a group of children whose mothers controlled their own diet in pregnancy and the infants' diets and environments at birth did develop eczema. In contrast, 65% of the sibling controls and 52% of the nonrelated controls who received cow milk developed similar allergic illnesses. As a retrospective study, it was open to some criticism, although it did begin to look at a significant issue—reducing the incidence of allergic manifestations in high-risk individuals by a new type of preventive measure: avoidance of known antigens.

A second study was designed and carried out prospectively by Johnstone and Dutton,[46] in order to investigate dietary prophylaxis of allergic disease. They observed a difference of more than 10 years in the incidence of asthma and perennial allergic rhinitis in those fed soybean milk (18%) and those fed evaporated milk (50%). No infant in this study of 283 children was breastfed,

however. A study of 1753 children fed breast milk, soy milk, and cow milk from birth to 6 months of age, who were followed until they were 7 years or older, was published. The children included those with high-risk, low-risk, and no-risk family histories for allergy. No difference in outcome was related to early diet, but a relationship to the family history was seen.

In a prospective study to identify the development of reaginic allergy, infants of allergic parents were placed in a study or control group. The study group followed an allergen-avoidance regimen, including breastfeeding. At 6 months and 1 year, the study infants had less eczema than the control infants, as well as lower serum total IgE levels.[52]

Prophylaxis of Atopic Disease

Efforts to alter the incidence of atopic illness have continued to challenge investigators, who now have access to increased methodologic sophistication. Prevention of IgE-mediated disorders can be directed at the practice of interfering with any of the major forces responsible for the phenotypic expression of atopy. Practically, however, it is not yet possible to mask IgE genes or manipulate cellular components of the response organ. Clinicians are limited to manipulating the effect of the environment, by reducing the allergenic load.

Review of the plethora of studies directed at measuring the impact of dietary manipulations on the incidence of atopic disease demonstrates that retrospective studies show little or no difference in the incidence of asthma and eczema. Prospective studies, however, tend to demonstrate a significant reduction in atopic disease in the treated group (Table 17-1). In looking at these data, it is important to recognize that some studies did not consider the risk for the population developing atopic disease on a hereditary basis. In other studies, breastfeeding may have been carried out for only a few weeks or months.[22] The evidence is clear that exclusive breastfeeding for 6 months or longer makes a difference. None of these studies controlled for smoking in the household, and no data were reported on the incidence of respiratory syncytial virus. In addition, some studies did not control for the breastfeeding mother's diet, the weaning foods, or the use of cow milk beverages. However, when the long-term effects of breastfeeding, maternal smoking during pregnancy, and recurrent lower respiratory tract infections on asthma in children were examined, some discordance was observed. Breastfeeding for less than 3 months was not an effective deterrent. Breastfeeding reduced the effect of lower respiratory tract infections on asthma. Similarly, it reduced the effect of smoking.[55] The authors

TABLE 17-1	Prevention of Atopy: Prospective Studies				
Study	**Year Published**	**No. of Years Followed**	**No. of Subjects***	**Type of Milk/Feeding**	**Impact on Atopy[†]**
Johnstone and Dutton[12]	1966	10	235	Soy, cow	↓ Asthma, rhinitis
Matthew et al.[12]	1977	1	53 (26)	Breast, soy	↓ Eczema
Chandra[12]	1979	>2	134	Breast	↓ Eczema, asthma
Saarinen et al.[12]	1979	3	(256)	Breast	↓ Eczema, food allergy, asthma
Hamburger[12]	1981	1	(300)	Breast	↓ Eczema, asthma
Kaufman and Frick[12]	1976, 1981	2	(94)	Breast	↓ Asthma
Hide and Guyer[12]	1981	1	843 (266)	Breast <6 mo, soy, cow (maternal diet not controlled)	↓ Eczema slight, rhinitis
Gruskay[12]	1982	15	908 (328)	Breast 4 mo, soy, cow	↓ Breast symptoms; soy no effect
May et al.[12]	1982	1/2	67 normal	Soy, cow, modern formula	↑ Antibodies with no disease symptoms
Businco et al.[12]	1983	2	(101)	Breast <6 mo; soy, cow	↓ Asthma, eczema
Kajosaari and Saarinen[12]	1983	1	(135)	All breast milk <6 mo; half solid foods early	↑ Eczema/food intolerance in those fed solids
Moore et al.[12]	1985	1	525	Study—breastfed 3 mo; control—SMA	Not clear: 74% failed to breastfeed or gave cow milk in study group
Zeiger et al.[12]	1989	4	288	Maternal avoidance diet last trimester Controls unrestricted; mother's diet; infants given Nutramigen	↓ Atopy 16% in restricted infants ↑ Atopy in control infants (to 27%) ↓ Urticaria/GI symptoms in restricted group
Sigurs et al.[12]	1992	4	115	All breastfed; 65 mothers restricted diet for first 3 mo of lactation; 50 no restrictions	↓ Atopy/asthma among both groups ↓ Greater among restricted group

GI, Gastrointestinal. *SMA,* formula by Wyeth (no longer available).
*Number in study; parentheses indicate number at risk for atopy.
[†]Arrows indicate decrease or increase compared with control group.
Modified from Businco L, Marchetti F, Pellegrini G, et al: Prevention of atopic disease in "at-risk newborns" by prolonged breastfeeding, *Ann Allergy* 51:296, 1983.

concluded that asthma in childhood can be prevented by promoting breastfeeding, preventing smoking in pregnancy, and avoiding recurrent lower respiratory tract infections in early childhood. Recurrent wheezing episodes were evaluated for associated risk factors.[9] Cigarette smoking in the household, heating mode (open stove), and breastfeeding for less than 6 months were significant.

Hamburger et al.[41] carried out prospective prophylactic studies to include measuring IgE and skin radioallergosorbent tests (RASTs) on mothers, fathers, and infants. They found a significant correlation between maternal IgE and infant IgE and potential allergy in the infants (Tables 17-2

and 17-3). This study was done by controlling the environment and the diet. The process was initiated in pregnancy, in order to begin by protecting the fetus, and was then continued at birth. Therefore, considerable attention was directed toward breastfeeding in this and other studies.

Human milk consistently contains antibodies, especially secretory immunoglobulin A (IgA), to major food proteins. The levels are influenced by the mother's own external antigen exposure.

In a study of 500 babies born to families at a high risk for allergies, one group was deliberately not given cow milk and was fed soy milk by random assignment.[65] No benefit resulted from withholding

TABLE 17-2	Relationship of Maternal Total Serum IgE Level to Cord and 4-Month Serum IgE Levels in Infants in the Prophylaxis Group			
	Cord IgE (U/mL)		4-Month IgE (U/mL)	
Maternal IgE (U/mL)	<0.5, No. (%)	≥0.5, No. (%)	<5.0, No. (%)	≥5.0, No. (%)
≤100	35 (71)	14 (29)	41 (87)	6 (13)
>100	14 (42)	19 (58)	24 (73)	9 (27)
Total	49	33	65	15

$p < 0.01$ by chi-square test for maternal IgE <100 vs. >100 U/mL for cord IgE with a trend ($p < 0.08$) at 4-month IgE measurement.

From Hamburger RN, Heller S, Mellon MH, et al: Current status of the clinical and immunologic consequences of a prototype allergic disease prevention program, *Ann Allergy* 51:281, 1983.

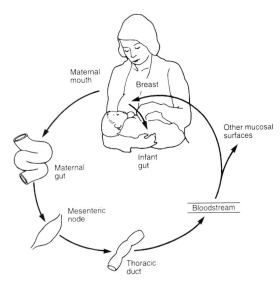

Figure 17-1. Maternal serum antibodies affect passage of foreign antigens into milk and processing of antigen in infant's intestine. (Redrawn from Kleinman RE: The role of developmental immune mechanisms in intestinal allergy, *Ann Allergy* 51:222, 1983.)

TABLE 17-3	Relationship of Paternal Total Serum IgE Level to Cord and 4-Month Serum IgE Levels in Infants in the Prophylaxis Group			
	Cord IgE (U/mL)		4-Month IgE (U/mL)	
Paternal IgE (U/mL)	<0.5, No. (%)	≥0.5, No. (%)	<5.0, No. (%)	≥5.0, No. (%)
≤100	29 (63)	17 (37)	40 (83)	8 (17)
>100	10 (56)	8 (44)	14 (82)	3 (18)
Total	39	25	54	11

From Hamburger RN, Heller S, Mellon MH, et al: Current status of the clinical and immunologic consequences of a prototype allergic disease prevention program, *Ann Allergy* 51:281, 1983.

cow milk, but breastfeeding, even for a short period, was clearly associated with a lower incidence of wheezing, prolonged colds, diarrhea, and vomiting. Smoking and environmental molds were also associated with wheezing. Merrett et al.[65] concluded from this that breastfeeding played a significant role in prophylaxis.

The effect of breastfeeding on allergic sensitization is both direct, through the elimination of nonhuman milk protein as an exposure to antigen, and indirect, by affecting the absorption of antigen through the intestinal tract.[52,53] Maternal antibodies are transferred to breastfed infants as part of what has been called the enteromammary immune system[48] (Figure 17-1). The secretory IgA antibody present in milk is the result of a mother's enteric immune response to antigens in her gut. Secretory IgA in a mother's milk provides protection against bacterial, viral, and toxic exposures. Prospective studies have shown that infants at a high risk for atopic illness,

from a hereditary standpoint, had significantly less disease when breastfed, especially if reared in a protected environment with delayed use of solid foods. This was compared with children of similar risk fed cow milk and regular solid foods. Serum IgE concentrations were also greatly reduced in infants younger than 6 months and 12 months of age in the breastfed group.[89]

Infants with a low incidence of T lymphocytes are at greater risk to develop allergies if fed cow milk rather than breast milk, according to Juto[47] and Juto and Bjorksten.[48] Infants with reduced T cells fed cow milk also demonstrated higher serum IgE levels and peripheral eosinophil counts. Juto[47] reported that with careful prophylaxis, more than 50% of infants who had both parents with IgE levels greater than 100 mg/mL showed elevated cord and 4-month IgE levels. More than 80% of those infants whose parents had IgE levels less than 100 mg/mL, however, had both low cord blood and low 4-month IgE levels. Such data confirm the genetic effect of both maternal and paternal genes.

Considerable work was reported from a laboratory in Newfoundland that promoted certain formulas as protective. This work has since been considered misleading.[14]

In a prospective study designed to examine asthma and atopy outcomes in male/female patients, Mandhane et al.[62] reported specific parental history of atopy and breastfeeding. The study members were born in New Zealand in 1972 to 1973 and followed to adulthood. Breastfeeding was considered positive if it lasted 4 weeks or more. There was no mention of exclusivity or when cow milk was introduced. Parental history was obtained.

Skin testing, spirometry, and bronchial challenge to methacholine was done from age 9 at intervals forward. They found that breastfeeding, in spite of its brevity, influenced development of atopy and asthma by sex and parental history. They found greater incidence of atopy in girls who were breastfed than boys who were breastfed and both who were bottle fed. They acknowledged the importance of a thorough breastfeeding history. The need to correlate the incidence of parental atopy, whose offspring were more likely to be breastfed, was also emphasized. Mai et al.[61] studied the relationship of breastfeeding, overweight, and asthma. They queried whether overweight and asthma shared common environmental influences, such as breastfeeding. They found that children who had been breastfed exclusively for less than 12 weeks had a risk for being overweight and of having asthma by 10 years of age. They also noted that they existed together but not separately. These mothers were obese in most cases, and the authors suggested that their obesity decreased their probability of successful breastfeeding. The long-term effects of maternal smoking during pregnancy and recurrent lower respiratory infections were associated with asthma in children. These effects were mitigated by breastfeeding in the long-term study of children in the Isle of Wight birth cohort.[50]

Long-Term Effects of Allergy Prophylaxis

In an 18-month study of atopic outcome, atopic mothers were randomly allocated to an intervention group or an unrestricted-diet group, and both were compared with nonatopic mothers on unrestricted diets. The intervention was a milk/dairy product-free diet during late pregnancy and lactation. After 7 weeks of the diet, serum β-lactoglobulin and immunoglobulin G (IgG) levels in the mothers were collated to the levels in cord blood. The infants were examined at 12 and 18 months, utilizing a single-blind allergy assessment by a pediatrician. Infants born to nonatopic parents had significantly less allergy than those born to atopic mothers with unrestricted diets.[58] The "restricted-diet group" of infants had comparable levels to the atopy-free group and had significantly less allergy than the unrestricted-diet group. The nature of the parents' disease also played a role in the type of illness in both groups.

Mothers who consumed a diet similar to the Mediterranean diet, rich in fruits, vegetables, and fish and ample in vitamin D, showed greater impact on suppression of atopic disorders than those who did not.[67] The role of vitamin D has just been recognized as being important in lactating women, especially those with restricted diets. All breastfeeding women should consume at least 1000 units of vitamin D while lactating.[55] A prospective longitudinal study of 988 healthy infants, from birth to 6 years of age, recorded feeding-history episodes of lower respiratory tract infection in the first 3 years of life and recurrent episodes of wheezing.[95] Being breastfed was associated with lower rates of recurrent wheeze (3.1% vs. 9.7%, $p < 0.01$) for nonatopic children. The authors concluded that recurrent wheeze at age 6 years is less common among nonatopic children who were breastfed as infants. This effect was independent of whether or not the child had a wheezing lower respiratory tract illness in the first 6 months of life (Table 17-4). These authors recorded smoking history, but it did not alter the compelling influence of breastfeeding on the outcome.[95]

Additional long-term studies have demonstrated that children who had ever been breastfed had a 50% lower incidence of wheezing than those who had not been breastfed. The effect persisted

---

TABLE 17-4   Odds Ratios and Confidence Intervals for Recurrent Wheeze at Age 6 Years by Logistic Regression

Factor	Odds Ratio (Confidence Interval)*		
	Total Group (n = 970)	Nonatopic Children (n = 420)	Atopic Children (n = 280)
Not breastfed	1.49 (0.80-2.77)	3.03† (1.05-8.69)	1.36 (0.49-3.73)
Maternal education ≤12 yr	1.48 (0.87-2.53)	1.58 (0.56-4.43)	0.92 (0.36-2.38)
Hispanic	2.48‡ (1.39-4.40)	2.45 (0.82-7.27)	2.50† (1.01-6.18)
Maternal hay fever	2.66§ (1.49-4.72)	2.64 (0.96-7.22)	2.35† (1.07-5.16)
Wheezing lower respiratory tract illness in first 6 mo	1.68 (0.88-3.19)	1.86 (0.55-6.25)	2.01 (0.74-5.48)

*Excludes children who were missing information for one or more of these factors.
†$p < 0.05$.
‡$p < 0.005$.
§$p < 0.0005$.
From Wright AL, Holberg CJ, Taussig LM, et al: Relationship of infant feeding to recurrent wheezing at age 6 years, *Arch Pediatr Adolesc Med* 49:762, 1995.

for the 7 years of the study in nonatopic children.[10] The authors attribute this, in part, to breastfeeding's protective effect against respiratory illness. They did not distinguish minimal from prolonged breastfeeding.

In a 17-year prospective study of 150 healthy children, researchers did consider length of breastfeeding.[75] The three groups had been breastfed: less than 1 month or not at all, 1 to 6 months, or more than 6 months. Prolonged breastfeeding was associated with the least eczema at 1 to 3 years, as well as fewer food and respiratory allergies. At age 17 years, the trends continued, leading the authors to conclude that breastfeeding is protective against atopic eczema, food allergy, and respiratory asthma throughout childhood and adolescence[75] (Figures 17-2 and 17-3).

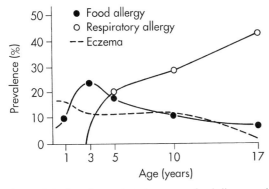

Figure 17-2. Prevalence of atopic eczema, food allergy, and respiratory allergy in full cohort of initial 236 children during follow-up for 17 years. (Modified from Saarinen UM, Kajossari M: Breastfeeding as prophylaxis against disease: prospective follow-up study until 17 years old, *Lancet* 346:1065, 1995.)

RECOMMENDATIONS OF COMMITTEE ON NUTRITION AND SECTION ON ALLERGY AND IMMUNOLOGY OF THE AMERICAN ACADEMY OF PEDIATRICS[16]

The incidence of atopic disease, including asthma, atopic dermatitis, and food allergies, has increased in the past decade. Asthma at age 4 years has increased 160% and atopic dermatitis 200% to 300%. The literature and the research have been abundant, but evidence is hindered by inadequate study design. Prevention of disease by dietary restrictions in pregnancy and lactation have had limited attention.[36] The following statements summarize the available evidence within the context of these limitations. It is accompanied by an extensive bibliography that supports these statements.

1. At the present time, evidence is lacking for the assertion that maternal dietary restrictions during pregnancy play a significant role in the prevention of atopic disease in infants. Similarly, antigen avoidance during lactation does not prevent atopic disease. Eczema is a possible exception, although more data are needed to substantiate this conclusion.

2. For infants at high risk for developing atopic disease, evidence shows that exclusive breastfeeding for at least 4 months decreases the cumulative incidence of atopic dermatitis and cow milk allergy in the first 2 years of life. This is compared with the feeding of intact cow milk protein formula.

3. Evidence supports that exclusive breastfeeding for at least 3 months protects against wheezing in early life. However, in infants at risk for

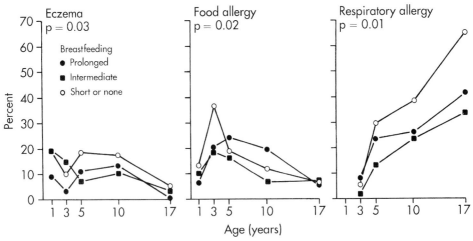

Figure 17-3. Prevalence of atopic eczema, food allergy, and respiratory allergy in infant feeding groups during follow-up for 17 years. Tests for differences during the appropriate age periods (eczema 1 to 3 years, food allergy 1 to 3 years, respiratory allergy at 5, 10, and 17 years) were done by analysis of variance and covariance with repeated measures. (Modified from Saarinen UM, Kajossari M: Breastfeeding as prophylaxis against disease: prospective follow-up study until 17 years old, *Lancet* 346:1065, 1995.)

developing atopic disease, the current evidence that exclusive breastfeeding protects against allergic asthma occurring beyond 6 years of age is not convincing.

4. Studies were done of infants who were not breastfed exclusively for 4 to 6 months or were formula fed and were at a high risk for developing atopic disease. Evidence from these studies is modest that atopic dermatitis may be delayed or prevented by the use of extensively or partially hydrolyzed formulas, compared with cow milk formula, in early childhood. Comparative studies of the various hydrolyzed formulas have also indicated that not all formulas have the same protective benefit. Extensively hydrolyzed formulas may be more effective than partially hydrolyzed in the prevention of atopic disease. In addition, more research is needed to determine whether these benefits extend into late childhood and adolescence. The higher cost of the hydrolyzed formulas must be considered in any decision-making process for their use. To date, the use of amino-acid-based formulas for atopy prevention has not been studied.

5. No evidence is convincing to support the use of soy-based infant formula for the purpose of allergy prevention.

6. Solid foods should not be introduced before 4 to 6 months of age. However, no current evidence is convincing that delaying their introduction beyond this period has a significant protective effect on the development of atopic disease. This is regardless of whether infants are fed cow milk protein formula or human milk. This includes delaying the introduction of foods that are considered to be highly allergic, such as fish, eggs, and foods containing peanut protein.

7. For infants older than 4 to 6 months of age, data are insufficient to support a protective effect of any dietary intervention for the development of atopic disease.

8. Additional studies are needed to document the long-term effect of dietary interventions in infancy to prevent atopic disease, especially in children older than 4 years and in adults.

9. This document describes means to prevent or delay atopic diseases through dietary changes. For a child who has developed an atopic disease that may be precipitated or exacerbated by ingested proteins (via human milk, infant formula, or specific complementary foods), treatment may require specific identification and restriction of causal food proteins. This topic was not reviewed in this document.

Analysis of infant and maternal variables in the 6 year follow-up study of a cohort of U.S. children revealed that socioeconomic and atopic factors were the most important predictors of probable food allergy at 6 years of age. Exclusive breastfeeding for 4 months or longer probably had a preventive effect on the development of food allergy after 1 year of age in non-risk children.

Immunologic Aspects of Allergy

Interest in identifying the immunologic aspects of clinical allergy led to a number of additional studies on infant feeding.[40,41] Kletter et al.[54] reported that hemagglutinating antibodies to cow milk were present in the sera of some newborns but usually at levels lower than those of the mother. The earliest rise in titer was detected at 1 month, and a peak was seen at 3 months in infants given cow milk from birth. Antibodies belonged mainly to the IgG group, with their rise and fall paralleling hemagglutinating antibodies. IgA antibodies were in low titer, and IgM antibodies were rarely detected.[60] The delayed exposure to cow milk in breastfed infants resulted in lower mean values of cow milk antibodies. Peak values were attained more slowly. An inverse relationship exists between duration of breastfeeding and levels of titers of humoral antibodies.

Freed and Green[23] investigated antibody-facilitated digestion and its implications for infant nutrition. They suggest a model of digestion in which oligopeptides in the small bowel are bound to secretory antibodies, which hold them in contact with proteases. This facilitates the breakdown and utilization of the oligopeptides. They consider immunity and digestion to be closely related. Breastfeeding with colostrum and then mature human milk provides the immature gut of the infant with both immunity and "digestivity."

The presence of periods of transient IgA deficiency in saliva in the first 12 months of life has been identified as a possible risk factor for the development of asthma, bronchial hyperactivity, and atopy.[33]

Savilahti et al.[77,79] studied 18 patients with documented malabsorption of cow milk. They were improved by feedings of human milk after having challenges with powdered milk. Eight patients had clinical reactions; the number of IgA- and IgM-containing cells increased by approximately 2.5 times in the intestinal mucosa. When breast milk feedings resumed, the findings returned to normal. Serum antibodies of both hemagglutination and IgA increased. No change was seen in IgE antibodies or serum complement. Many other findings, including villous atrophy and round cell infiltration, were noted. After age 2 years, all the infants became tolerant of milk, which may indicate that immunologic immaturity is part of the pathogenesis. Walker[94] presented similar arguments and conclusions in a symposium discussion.

When studying problems related to infant feeding, it is difficult to randomize groups to breastfeed or not. Many women with a strong family history of allergy are particularly adamant about breastfeeding. This was a factor in a study of 69 preterm infants and their subsequent allergic symptoms in childhood. A premature infant's intestine is also more permeable to proteins and their immune system more immature. The long-term incidence of atopy, however, was no different between the feeding groups at age 11 years, although those receiving breast milk had a strong family history of atopy.[79]

The low IgA content of milk, and the especially low colostral IgA, has been correlated with cow milk allergy in a group of 198 infants, seven of whom became allergic to cow milk.[78] All other measurements (immunoglobulins G, A, M; cow milk–specific antibodies; β-lactoglobulin) were similar among all 198 infants. The authors[58] suggest that an infant is more likely to develop cow milk allergy if the mother has insufficient protective factors, namely, IgA.

Some discrepancies among studies may be explained by measuring the concentration of bovine IgG in human milk using different methods. Levels were tested on the same milk samples using competition radioimmunoassay, competition enzyme-linked immunosorbent assay (ELISA), and sandwich ELISA. IgG levels were significantly higher using radioimmunoassay or ELISA.[63] Levels in the milk of mothers who went on a dairy product–free diet for a month still have measurable levels by radioimmunoassay and ELISA but not by sandwich ELISA.

Cantisani et al.[14] sought to resolve the question of the presence of specific secretory IgE for cow milk protein in the sera of breastfed infants who had never received cow milk. They measured secretory IgE in the sera of six breastfed infants with atopic dermatitis who were never in contact with cow milk. The secretory IgE to bovine β-lactoglobulin was not detected in any of the sera examined.

In the study of the role of heredity in allergy, unilateral family history was described as allergy in one parent and bilateral as involving both parents. Ninety-four infants were followed from birth for 24 months. Significantly more infants developed allergy if they were from a bilaterally allergic family. In the first 3 months, less atopic dermatitis occurred in the breastfed infants with unilateral history than with bilateral history. Businco et al.[12] presented similar relationships to family history in a study of breastfed infants.

These data are challenged by Murray's findings. Murray examined nasal-secretion eosinophilia in relationship to respiratory allergy, associated with a screening procedure for hearing loss. In a group

TABLE 17-5 Some Diseases Possibly Preventable by Protecting Relatively Immunodeficient Infants From Adverse Antigen Experience

Disease	Status
Eczema	Established
Asthma	Probable
Hay fever	Probable
Infantile gut and respiratory infection	Probable
Intestinal allergy	Probable
Septicemia and renal *Escherichia coli* infection	Probable
Sudden death	Probable
Ulcerative colitis	Possible

From Soothill JF: Some intrinsic and extrinsic factors predisposing to allergy, *Proc R Soc Med* 69:439, 1976.

of children with a history of allergy in the immediate family, an association between the early introduction of solid food and the presence of a nasal-secretion eosinophilia was significantly positive.

Although modern processing of cow milk has diminished the problem, it has not eliminated it. Given high-risk factors or strong family history of allergy, an effort to avoid unnecessary exposure to known allergens is an easy way to avoid some medical problems[96] (Table 17-5).

The Role of Intestinal Flora in Allergy

Microbes are important in the Earth's ecosystems. They are important in overall health and especially in infants' health. At birth, infants, usually sterile, are colonized with the mothers' bacteria coming through the birth canal. First feeds affect the colonization of the intestinal tract. Breast milk supports the growth of *Lactobacillus* and *Bifidobacterium*, which, in turn, enhance the maturity of the gut and promote digestion and absorption. *Bifidobacterium* constitute up to 90% of an infant's intestinal microbiota. A healthy intestinal microbiota, established through breastfeeding, has been confirmed to reduce the risk for atopic disease. The composition of the intestinal bacteria is one of the major contributors to the development of immune functions in newborn infants, thus affecting the problem of allergies.[37] Maternal allergic status can alter the number of bifidobacteria a woman can pass on to her breastfed infant. Grönlund et al.[37] have shown that allergic mothers have a reduced bifidobacteria count, as do their breastfed infants. At the same time, investigators are looking at the role of probiotics in health and disease and, more specifically, in formula-fed infants. This is in an effort to change the flora of the gut to the more physiologic bifido-bacteria of the breastfed infant. The committee on nutrition and the section on gastroenterology of the AAP have released a clinical report on Pro-biotics and Prebiotics in Pediatrics, accompanied by a 110-item bibliography.[16] They affirm that human milk is a natural prebiotic. Breastfed infants have a preponderance of naturally occurring probi-otic bacteria in their guts. They concede these bac-teria are probably associated with a reduction in atopic eczema. They also suggest it is related to humoral immunity (T-helper 2 type) in infancy. In pregnancy, the cytokine inflammatory response profile is diverted away from cell-mediated immu-nity (T-helper 1 type). The risk for allergic disease may well be related to a delay in humoral immunity and an ultimate imbalance in T-helper 1 and T-helper 2 inflammatory responses. A study of 4031 subjects in 20 cohorts in Europe, Asia, and Australia was reported in a meta-analysis of clinical trials. Studies included 25 double-blind, random-ized, and placebo-controlled trials. Probiotics were given prenatally and postnatally (10 studies), and directly to the child (9 studies). Atopic sensitiza-tion was measured by positive skin prick test or ele-vated serum-specific IgE level to any food or allergen. Asthma was diagnosed by physician or parent. Probiotics did not significantly reduce the prevalence of asthma or wheeze, although *lactobacil-lus* was associated with increased atopic sensitiza-tion, but not a reduction in the actual disease.[20]

A 7-year follow-up was done of a randomized controlled trial, where 184 Swedish children were given probiotic supplementation both prenatally and during infancy. All the children had a family history of allergic disease. At age 7 years, the chil-dren had a physical examination, a questionnaire, spirometry, and a measurement of fractional exhaled nitric oxide. An assessment of eczema, a skin prick, and IgE testing were also done. The out-comes of allergic diseases included symptomatic asthma, allergic rhinoconjunctivitis, allergic urti-caria, or eczema in the previous year.

The probiotic and placebo groups did not differ long term, even though there was a transient effect of reduced risk of sensitization in infancy.[1] Other studies also report lack of effect of probiotics on eczema and allergy.

Patterns of Clinical Disease Associated With Cow Milk Allergy in Childhood

Cow milk allergy affects 6% to 8% of infants youn-ger than 3 years old. Many poorly defined illnesses and pathologic lesions have been associated with the ingestion of milk, making clear diagnosis diffi-cult. Definitions have been proposed by the Amer-ican Academy of Allergy and Immunology and are described in a consensus paper,[38] as adapted by Anderson[5]:

- *Food intolerance* is an adverse reaction to the inges-tion of a food related to an enzyme deficiency or metabolic or pharmacologic reactions.
- *Food adverse reaction* with unknown mechanism is an idiosyncrasy; no immunologic mechanism is associated.
- *Food allergy* or *food hypersensitivity* is an adverse reaction to food caused by one or more immune hypersensitivity mechanisms and is not confined to IgE.
- *Food anaphylaxis* reactions are immediate hyper-sensitivity involving the immunologic activity of IgE homocytotropic antibody and the release of chemical mediators that may be life threatening.
- *Anaphylactoid reaction* to food is an anaphylaxis-like reaction to food as a result of a nonimmune release of chemical mediators.
- *Food toxicity* (poisoning) is toxin from the food itself and not an immune reaction (e.g., scom-broid fish poisoning, botulism).
- *Pharmacologic food reaction* is a naturally derived or added chemical that produces a pharmacologic reaction (caffeine in coffee or sodas).

Symptoms associated with food allergy include asthma, eczema, urticaria, and rhinitis, as well as colic and failure to thrive with chronic respira-tory and gastrointestinal disease.[15] Well-defined, but uncommon syndromes, including pulmonary hemosiderosis, bronchitis, protein- and iron-losing enteropathy, neonatal thrombocytopenia, and coli-tis, have been reported to result from cow milk allergy in both breastfed and formula-fed infants.[15] Sleep disturbances have been reported in a series of children evaluated with a prospective double-blind crossover design.[49] Another symptom, reported in two siblings, was insatiability despite adequate weight gain.[19] This was confirmed by history and reproducible reaction to dietary elimination and subsequent oral challenges.

The intestinal permeability test is a noninvasive but rigorous technique for detecting the deleteri-ous effect of food on the intestinal mucosa of aller-gic children. It requires overnight fasting of 6 hours, test feeding, and nothing but water for an additional 5 hours to collect urine samples for analysis. A 1-month-old breastfed infant with a history of regurgitation, diarrhea, difficult feed-ing, and malaise did not respond clinically to the elimination of dairy products from the mother's diet.[17] When the intestinal permeability test was performed with the mother's milk before and after dietary elimination of milk, no change occurred. When the mother eliminated pork and eggs, however, clinical and test results improved.

Acute Reactions to Cow Milk in Breastfed Infants

Hippocrates and Gojen described classic cases of milk allergy.[74] External reaction to cow milk was first described in the literature in the nineteenth century and then by Schloss[81] in 1920 and Tisdale and Erb[90] in 1925. At that time, the reaction was noted to occur during the first feeding of cow milk, which was provided in an effort to wean from the breast at several months of age. The event included sudden crying as if in pain; swelling of the lips, tongue, and throat; stridor; and even generalized urticaria and wheezing lasting for up to an hour.

This type of cow milk allergy is the first of two types described by Gerrard and Shenassa[27] and others. The second type is the well-known reaction to large amounts of cow milk in a cow milk–fed infant and is manifested by vomiting, diarrhea, or colic. This second type is not associated with cow milk–specific IgE antibodies. It usually subsides over time. The acute anaphylactic reactions, however, are associated with α-lactalbumin, β-lactoglobulin, and casein immunity.

Schwartz et al.[84] studied 29 breastfed or soy formula–fed infants who had experienced acute urticarial reactions while being fed cow milk for the first time. One infant had the reaction in the newborn nursery, suggesting in utero sensitization. When charts were carefully reviewed, 16 infants were identified as having been given formula, often without an order, in the newborn nursery. Twelve could have been sensitized in utero or through the breast milk. The authors identified elevated serum IgE levels; positive RASTs for α-lactalbumin, β-lactoglobulin, and casein; and recurrent wheezing in 55% of infants (16 of 29).

In a follow-up study challenging this group of children with whey and casein hydrolysate products, Schwartz et al.[84] found that 69% had positive prick tests to whey hydrolysate and 38% were positive to casein hydrolysate. Children with reactions to cow milk and both hydrolysates had severe reactions, including urticaria, angioedema, and wheezing. Hydrolysates of cow milk protein are not, therefore, hypoallergenic. Breastfeeding with occasional small amounts of cow milk can be a major risk factor in the development of IgE-mediated cow milk allergy in the rare, susceptible infant. Early exposures may occur in utero, through the breast milk, or with inadvertent feeds. Schwartz suggests

that isolated cow milk not be given to exclusively breastfed infants in the newborn period.[82,83]

The study confirms the importance of heredity in this acute reaction by its occurrence in twins and human leukocyte antigen-identical siblings, as well as in children of 28 parent pairs (89%) also sensitive to cow milk. Genetic homogeneity could not be demonstrated by human leukocyte antigen typing.

A case of anaphylactic shock from cow milk hypersensitivity in a breastfed infant was reported by Lifschitz et al.[57] They describe three episodes of shock from two separate feedings of formula and one while breastfeeding. After a prolonged course and the diagnosis of colitis, associated with numerous eosinophils, the infant was able to breastfeed at 21 days of age without difficulty. This was after his mother had been placed on a cow milk–free diet. When challenged, however, with breast milk that was pumped and stored while the mother was still consuming dairy products, the infant went into profound shock. The child was finally stabilized on breast milk and meat-based formula. At 6 months, cereal was added to the diet. At 12 months, soy and cow milk were well tolerated.

Intrauterine sensitization and allergy in the newborn breastfed infant were described by Matsumura in Japan. Glaser[32] also identified that under certain conditions, an infant with a predisposition for allergy may become actively sensitized in utero because of the mother's overindulgence in certain foods during pregnancy. For example, Shannon[86] demonstrated the presence of egg antigen in human breast milk in 1922. Infants then responded to re-exposure with allergic symptoms on first contact with that same food.[27,56] Kuroume et al.[56] showed that with intrauterine sensitization, hemagglutinating antibody titers against lactalbumin and soybean in the amniotic fluid are high. They suggest using measurement of amniotic fluid as an instrument to predict future allergy. Infant colic associated with maternal ingestion of cow milk is discussed in Chapter 18.

Multiple studies continue to confirm the value of elimination diets in pregnancy for women at a high risk for having an allergic infant.[13,24,42] These studies not only report a significantly reduced incidence of symptoms in the infants but also a significant reduction in β-lactoglobulin-specific IgA and α-casein-specific IgA levels in maternal serum and milk. Similar observations have been made with the elimination of egg. Consistently, breastfeeding was associated with reduced incidence of atopy in the infant with, and to a lesser degree without, dietary restrictions in mothers.[26]

Oral challenges must be physician-supervised for the diagnosis of food-allergic disease. In the case of an acute anaphylactic-type reaction that lacks evidence of food-specific IgE for a food highly suspected of provoking the reaction, a physician-supervised challenge is indicated to reintroduce the food. This is done in case a skin/RAST test was false-negative.[4] In a technical review, the American Gastroenterological Association comments that breastfeeding is cost effective, but maternally ingested protein can elicit allergic symptoms in infants. Thus maternal dietary manipulation is required, which should be done to avoid expensive alternative formulas.

When Giovannini et al.[28,29] studied growth and metabolic parameters of infants fed special formulas for atopy prevention, they noted differences compared with infants who were exclusively breastfed. Lower body mass index values and higher blood urea nitrogen levels were seen at 3 months.[28,29] Plasma aminoacidograms showed higher essential amino acids but lower branched-chain amino acids. Furthermore, the plasma taurine levels were lower in the formula-fed infants, even though the formulas had added taurine. These observations have been confirmed by other investigators, who are most concerned about the elevated threonine levels.[73]

The allergens of specific foods ingested by the mother have now been identified in the milk. Cant et al.[13] found 49 eczematous infants who were solely breastfed to be sensitized to cow milk and egg protein; these researchers also concluded that infants can be sensitized by foods eaten by the mother. They were able to demonstrate ovalbumin in the breast milk of 14 out of 19 mothers, who were tested 2 to 4 hours after eating raw egg. This was whether or not their infants had tested positive to egg albumin.

Troncone et al.[91] collected samples of breast milk at various times after the mothers were fed 20 g of gluten, after a period of deliberate gluten avoidance. Gliadin was found in 54 of 80 samples; levels peaked at 2 to 4 hours. Gliadin could not be detected in maternal serum. The transfer of gliadin to infants through the milk could be one of the factors producing a protective effect, because breastfeeding is known to decrease the risk for celiac disease.[34]

Allergies to Solid Foods

Foods ingested by a mother may present a problem for an allergic child. Well-known allergens have been discussed and include cow milk, bovine protein of any sort, eggs, and fish. In the hundreds of reports on children who develop atopy, eczema, and asthma in the first year of life, some authors claim restricting maternal diet prophylactically until a child is symptomatic is unnecessary.[59]

The increase in allergies to tree nuts is apparent even in breastfed infants. Peanuts (not tree nuts but legumes) belong to the same family as fenugreek, the ancient herb used a galactagogue. Mothers are taking large doses of fenugreek. Symptoms in the infants are usually colic, with and without diarrheal stools, fussiness, and crying. Stopping the fenugreek cures the symptoms. In a study of peanut allergies in children, 66% were boys, and 82% had a first-degree relative with atopy, including 68% with food allergy.[35] Median age of first exposure (known) was 14 months; median age of first reaction was 18 months. Children born before 2000 had the first reaction at 21 months; those born after 2000 had the first reaction at a mean of 14 months. It is recommended that children not be given peanuts in any form before the age of 3 years and that mothers of allergic children who are breastfeeding avoid peanuts. Allergy to tree nuts has been identified in breastfed infants whose mothers have ingested nuts on more than one occasion. Peanut allergy, in particular, can develop from skin contact and environmental exposure to the nut. Food protein–induced enterocolitis syndrome is commonly misdiagnosed as sepsis or a surgical abdominal energy. The most common triggers are cow milk and soy milk, given directly or consumed by the breastfeeding mother. Rice, a food commonly thought of as "hypoallergenic" and given to highly allergic children, has now been identified as a significant cause of hemorrhagic colitis. In one report,[64] 14 children had 26 episodes of colitis, which was likely to be misdiagnosed. Rice caused more severe reactions than cow's milk or soy in this report.[64]

Timing of solid food introduction in relation to atopic dermatitis and atopic sensitization is a controversial topic. No evidence to date shows that delaying the introduction of solids beyond 6 months is beneficial.[97] The controversy dwells on the 4- to 6-month period. Prescott et al.[70] state that the rising rates of food allergies in early childhood reflect increasing failure of early immune tolerance mechanisms. They are concerned that the practice of delaying complementary foods until 6 months of age may increase, rather than decrease, the risk for immune disorders. They feel a critical window exists in development, when exposure to these allergens is tolerated. The window may be 4 to 6 months. They concede that favorable colonization and breastfeeding may promote tolerance. It is agreed that this issue needs study. Breastfed infants are, of course, exposed via breast milk to many flavors and some foods.[3,70] The Australian Society of Clinical Immunology and Allergy[6] states that previous allergy prevention strategies have been ineffective. They admit that more research is needed but recommend starting solids at 4 to 6 months but not beyond 6 months. They do not

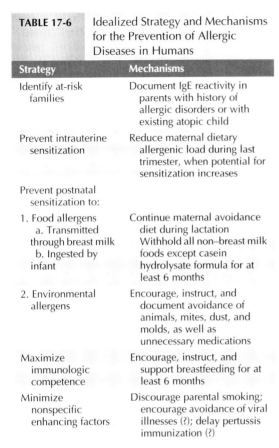

TABLE 17-6 Idealized Strategy and Mechanisms for the Prevention of Allergic Diseases in Humans

Strategy	Mechanisms
Identify at-risk families	Document IgE reactivity in parents with history of allergic disorders or with existing atopic child
Prevent intrauterine sensitization	Reduce maternal dietary allergenic load during last trimester, when potential for sensitization increases
Prevent postnatal sensitization to:	
1. Food allergens a. Transmitted through breast milk b. Ingested by infant	Continue maternal avoidance diet during lactation Withhold all non–breast milk foods except casein hydrolysate formula for at least 6 months
2. Environmental allergens	Encourage, instruct, and document avoidance of animals, mites, dust, and molds, as well as unnecessary medications
Maximize immunologic competence	Encourage, instruct, and support breastfeeding for at least 6 months
Minimize nonspecific enhancing factors	Discourage parental smoking; encourage avoidance of viral illnesses (?); delay pertussis immunization (?)

From Hamburger RN, Heller S, Mellon MH, et al: Current status of the clinical and immunologic consequences of a prototype allergic disease prevention program, *Ann Allergy* 51:281, 1983.

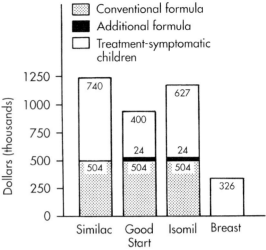

Figure 17-4. Estimated cost of management of symptomatic children with atopy in Newfoundland. Costs include physician fees, laboratory tests, hospitalization, and medication. For those fed Similac, cost of management until age 5 is $740,000 per annum. Standard cow milk formula (e.g., Similac) during first 6 months of life for all infants with parental history of allergy would cost $504,000. In those fed hydrolyzed formula (e.g., Good Start), cost is approximately the same as for standard formula but with savings of approximately 50% on management. An almost similar magnitude of reduction in allergic disease by feeding extensively hydrolyzed casein formula (e.g., Nutramigen) would cost three times more than in the cow milk group because of higher purchase value of such a formula. (Modified from Chandra RK: Five-year follow-up of high-risk infants with family history of allergy who were exclusively breast-fed or fed partial whey hydrolysate, soy, and conventional cow's milk formulas, *J Pediatr Gastroenterol Nutr* 24:388, 1997.)

this regimen will not prevent all the potential for allergy, it will help to minimize the insults by foreign protein. Another compelling reason to consider prophylaxis is the costly medical care required for the affected individual[13] (Figure 17-4).

The possible alleviation of atopic eczema in a breastfed infant by maternal supplementation with a fish oil concentrate has been reported by Jensen et al.[44] A 6-week-old infant who had eczema from the first week of life, despite treatment, cleared when the mother, who was part of a study of effects of fish oil supplementation, began the supplementation. The eczema returned when the fish oil was stopped, and cleared again when the mother added fish to her diet.

This clinical experience has been corroborated in the laboratory. Essential fatty acids are important in promoting the renewal of the protective hydrolipidic layer of the skin.[22] Altered essential fatty acid metabolism has been associated with atopic dermatitis.[37] Reduced levels of γ-linolenic acid and dihomo-α-linolenic acid appear in the plasma of patients with atopic dermatitis. The ratio of linoleic acid to the sum of its metabolites was found to

be the relevant feature related to atopy. Increased marine fat consumption by a breastfeeding mother appears to improve the ratio of polyunsaturated fatty acids,[11] although this treatment has not been incorporated into routine care.

Human milk is a carrier of biochemical messages through its hormones, growth factors, cytokines, and whole cells.[76] Nucleotides, glutamine, and lactoferrin have been shown to influence gastrointestinal development and host defenses. Basically, three separate processes are involved in the reaction of the immune system toward allergen challenge.[8] Deregulation in each of them may increase the susceptibility to developing gastrointestinal allergy. It is speculated that breast milk may help to shift the balance toward tolerance, rather than sensitization, when the infant is exposed to an allergen.[8]

Use of Pancreatic Enzymes

A novel treatment for allergic colitis, i.e., bloody diarrhea and colic in the breastfeeding infant, is the use of pancreatic enzymes by the mother.

The rationale for this treatment is that pancreatic enzymes will further break down the potential protein allergens in the maternal GI tract. Dosing is begun with the lowest dose of pancreatic enzyme (e.g., pancrelipase Creon® 6 in the United States or Kreon® in Europe, provided by Abbott Laboratories). There are 6000 USP units of lipase, 19,000 USP units of protease and 30,000 USP units of amylase.[72] Two capsules are taken with meals and one capsule with snacks. If necessary, doses can be doubled. No double-blind, controlled studies have been reported since Repucci first recommended this therapy. There are many reports of successful treatment. Schach and Haight have reported excellent results.[80]

Walker[94] summarizes his extensive research on the subject, by stating that antigens have been shown to cross the intestinal barrier in physiologic and pathologic states. He further states that it is most important to prevent excessive penetration of antigens, in patients who are susceptible to the disease, by implementing the following steps:

1. Identify the population at risk.
2. Encourage breastfeeding in infancy.
3. Decrease antigen load with elemental formulas.
4. Continue to conduct direct research at identification and prevention.

Summary

The role of prophylactic management in pregnancy and the initiation of breastfeeding at birth have a major impact on the long-term incidence of reactive airway disease. Beyond the medical risks, the high cost of medical management must be considered when an infant is not breastfed.

REFERENCES

1. Abrahamsson TR, Jakobsson T, Björksten B, et al: No effect of probiotics on respiratory allergies. A seven-year follow-up of a randomized controlled trial in infancy, Pediatr Allergy Immunol 24(6):556–561, 2013.
2. Adams J, Voutilainen H, Uillner PM, et al: The safety of maternal elimination diets in breastfeeding mothers with food allergic infants, Breastfeed Med 9(10):555–556, 2014.
3. Agostoni C, Decsi T, Fewtrell M, et al: Complementary feeding: a commentary by ESPGHAN (European Society for Pediatric Allergology and Clinical Immunology) committee on nutrition, J Pediatr Gastroenterol Nutr 46:99–110, 2008.
4. American Gastroenterological Association: AGA technical review on the evaluation of food allergy in gastrointestinal disorders, Gastroenterology 120:1304–1310, 2001.
5. Anderson JA: The establishment of common language concerning adverse reaction to foods and food additives, J Allergy Clin Immunol 78:140–144, 1986.
6. Australasian Society of Clinical Immunology and Allergy INC (ASCIA): Advice for Infant Feeding, 2008. www.allergy.org (Accessed September 2008).
7. Bergmann RL, Edenharter G, Bergmann KE, et al: Breast-feeding duration is a risk factor for atopic eczema, Clin Exp Allergy 32:205, 2002.
8. Bernt KM, Walker WA: Human milk as a carrier of biochemical messages, Acta Paediatr Suppl 88(430):27–41, 1999.
9. Bozaykut A, Paketoi A, Sezer RG, et al: Evaluation of risk factors for recurrent wheezing episodes, J Clin Med Res 5(5):395–400, 2013.
10. Burr M, Limb ES, Maguire MJ, et al: Infant feeding, wheezing, and allergy: a prospective study, Arch Dis Child 68:724, 1993.
11. Businco L, Ioppi M, Morse NL, et al: Breast milk from mothers of children with newly developed atopic eczema has low levels of long chain polyunsaturated fatty acids, J Allergy Clin Immunol 91:1134, 1993.
12. Businco L, Marchetti F, Pellegrini G, et al: Prevention of atopic disease in "at-risk newborns" by prolonged breast-feeding, Ann Allergy 51:296, 1983.
13. Cant AJ, Bailes JA, Marsden RA, et al: Effect of maternal dietary exclusion on breast fed infants with eczema: two controlled studies, Br Med J 293:231, 1986.
14. Cantisani A, Giuffrida MG, Fabris C, et al: Detection of specific IgE to human milk proteins in sera of atopic infants, FEBS Lett 412:515, 1997.
15. Committee on Nutrition American Academy of Pediatrics: Pediatric nutrition handbook, ed 7, Elkgrove, Ill., 2014, AAP, [#,63]? pp 845-862.
16. Committee on Nutrition (CON) and the Section on Gastroenterology, Hepatology and Nutrition (SOGHN) of the AAP. Clinical report: probiotics and prebiotics in pediatrics. Pediatrics 126, 2010.
17. de Boussieu D, Dupont C, Badoval J: Allergy to non-dairy proteins in mother's milk as assessed by intestinal permeability tests, Allergy 49:882, 1994.
18. de Silva D, Geromi M, Halken S, et al: Primary prevention of food allergy in children and adults: systematic review, Allergy (5):581–589, 2014.
19. Ducharme FM, Rousseau E, Seidman EG, et al: Apparent insatiability: an unrecognized manifestation of food intolerance in breast-fed infants, Pediatrics 93:1006, 1994.
20. Elazah N, Mendy A, Gasana J, et al: Probiotic administration in early life, atopy, and asthma: a meta-analysis of clinical trials, Pediatrics 132(3):e666–e676, 2013.
21. Falliers CJ, de Cardoso RR, Bane HN, et al: Discordant allergic manifestations in monozygotic twins: genetic identity vs. clinical, physiologic, and biochemical differences, J Allergy 47:207, 1971.
22. Fidler N, Koletzko B: The fatty acid composition of human colostrums, Eur J Nutr 39:31, 2000.
23. Freed DLJ, Green FHY: Hypothesis: antibody-facilitated digestion and its implications for infant nutrition, Early Hum Dev 1:107, 1977.
24. Fukushima Y, Kawata Y, Onda T, et al: Consumption of cow milk and egg by lactating women and the presence of beta-lactoglobulin and ovalbumin in breast milk, Am J Clin Nutr 65:30, 1997.
25. Gerrard JW: Allergy in infancy, Pediatr Ann 3:9, 1974.
26. Gerrard JW, Shenassa M: Food allergy: two common types as seen in breast and formula fed babies, Ann Allergy 50:375, 1983.
27. Gerrard JW, Shenassa M: Sensitization to substances in breast milk: recognition, management and significance, Ann Allergy 51:300, 1983.
28. Giovannini M, Agostoni C, Fiocchi A, et al: Antigen-reduced infant formulas versus human milk: growth and metabolic parameters in the first 6 months of life, J Am Coll Nutr 13:357, 1994.
29. Giovannini M, Fiocchi A, Agostoni C, et al: Nutrition in infancy and childhood. In Wüthrich B, Ortolani C, editors: Highlights in food allergy, Basel, 1996, Karger.

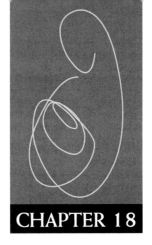

CHAPTER 18

Employment and Away from Home Activities while Breastfeeding

||||||||||||||||||||||||||||||||||||||||||||||||||||||||||||||||||||||||||||||||

Mothers are the fastest-growing segment of the labor force. Maternal employment has become more common in developed countries. Mothers who work and continue to breastfeed have also become more common. Part of the reason for this trend is the need for a second income in young households. Among professional women, the age of childbearing has been delayed to the 30s and early 40s, when a woman has established a career she wants to continue. Another reason for the increase of breastfeeding among employed mothers has been the exhaustive efforts by the United States Breastfeeding Committee, the Division of Nutrition Physical Activity and Obesity at the Centers for Disease Control and Prevention (CDC),[37] and the Center for Food Safety and Applied Nutrition of the Food and Drug Administration (FDA). The development of the Business Case for Breastfeeding campaign has been accomplished by their combined efforts. The Center for Economic and Policy Research reported on Parental Leave Policies in 21 countries, emphasizing their generosity, gender equality, the level of support provided to the parents, and the degree to which leave policies promote egalitarian distribution between mothers and fathers of the time devoted to child care. All 21 countries studied protect at least one parent's job for a period of weeks, months, or years at the birth of a child. Leaves vary from 14 weeks in Switzerland to over 300 weeks (about 6 years) in France and Spain. The United States is 20th out of 21, providing 24 weeks combined for both parents.

Switzerland also provides financial support of 80% of a mother's earnings.

In terms of money, most countries provide direct financial support between three months and one year at least for part of the protected leave time. The United States is one of two countries that provide a generous financial baby bonus but no paid leave; Australia is the other.

The Gender Equality Index is a single measure to examine the effect of parental leave policies on both the workplace and care giving. Sweden rated highest and the United States fell in the middle in terms of equality of gender in the workplace. Best practices require a generous, universal, gender-equalitarian, and flexible parental leave policy, financed through social insurance. There are states in the United States that provide some benefits but none provide generous benefits by international standards.

The issues of working women are no longer in the shadows. They are on the minds of federal legislators who are considering legislation to improve work environments, family leave, and accommodations for breastfeeding.[33] The Patient Protection and Affordable Care Act was signed into law in March of 2010; it includes an amendment to section 7 of the Fair Labor Standards Act (FLSA). This amendment requires employers to provide reasonable break time for an employee to express breast milk for her nursing child for a year after the child's birth.

Employers are required to provide a place, other than a bathroom, that is shielded from view and free

TABLE 18-1	Select Elements of the Reasonable Break Time for Nursing Mothers Legal Provisions
Elements	**Specifics**
Time and location of breaks	• Provide a reasonable amount of break time to express milk as frequently as needed by the nursing mother. • A bathroom, even if private, is not a permissible location. • The location must be functional as a space for expressing breast milk. • A temporarily created space is sufficient, provided it is shielded from view and free from any intrusion by coworkers and the public.
Coverage and compensation	• Employers with <50 employees are not subject to break time requirement if compliance with the provision would impose an undue hardship. • "Undue hardship" is determined by looking at the difficulty or expense of compliance for the employer. • Employers are not required to compensate nursing mothers for breaks taken for the purpose of expressing milk. • If employers already provide compensated breaks, and an employee uses such times to express milk, she must be compensated in the same way that other employees are compensated for break times. • The employee must be completely relieved from duty, or else the time must be compensated as work time.
Fair Labor Standards Act prohibitions on retaliation	• It is a violation to discriminate against any employee because such employee has filed any complaint under or related to this act. • Employees are protected regardless of whether the complaint is made orally or in writing.

Abridged from the Fact Sheet #73, Wages and Hours Division, U.S. Department of Labor.

from intrusion from coworkers and the public, which may be used by an employee to express breast milk. The break time requirement became effective when the Affordable Care Act was signed into law on March 23, 2010. The Wage and Hour Fact Sheet #73 is available from the U.S. Department of Labor Wage and Hour Division (Table 18-1).

Low income women who are predominantly minorities (black and Hispanic) return to work earlier and to jobs that do not accommodate breastfeeding. The barriers in the workplace include inflexible schedules and lack of support from employers and colleagues.

There were 127.1 million working age women (16 years of age or older) in the United States in 2013 and 72.7 million were in the labor force. Of that number, 99.5 million were white, 16.6 million were black, 7.1 million Asian, and 18.7 million Hispanic (Figure 18-1). By 2022 it is projected that women in the work force will increase by 5.4% compared to a 5.6% increase in the number of men. Women are expected to reach 46.8% of the labor force in 2022. The labor force participation rate of mothers with children under 18 years of age in 2013 was 69.9%, 74.7% for mothers with children 6 to 17 years of age, 63.9% for mothers with children under 6 years of age, 61.1% for mothers with children under 3, and 57.3% for mothers with infants (Figure 18-2). Of employed women, 74% worked full time (35 hours or more) and 24% worked part time compared to 86.9% and 13.1% of employed men. The largest percentage of employed women were in education and health services (36.2%), wholesale and retail trade industry (13.1%), professional and business services (10.5%), and leisure and hospitality (10.3%).

Education was a major factor with the over 64 million women 25 or older in the labor force; 6.7% had less than a high school diploma, 25.3% had no more than a diploma, 17.5% had some college, and 37.8% had a bachelor's degree or higher. The overall women-to-men ratio of earnings is 82.1%, with white women only 81.7% while black women are 91.3%, Hispanic women 91.1%, and Asian women only 77.3%.

Maternal employment, however, has been cited by many authors as the major reason for the decline in breastfeeding worldwide. International data do not actually support this conclusion. Year after year the Mothers Survey[34] in the United States confirmed that the highest percentage of women initiating breastfeeding in the hospital is among women who plan to return to full-time employment, the

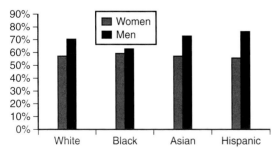

Figure 18-1. Labor force participation by sex, race, and Hispanic ethnicity, 2013 annual averages. (Data from U.S. Department of Labor, Women's Bureau, http://www.dol.gov./wb/stats/recentfacts.htm (Accessed 12.05.14.).)

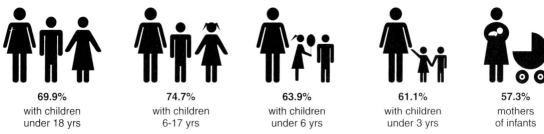

| **69.9%** | **74.7%** | **63.9%** | **61.1%** | **57.3%** |
| with children under 18 yrs | with children 6-17 yrs | with children under 6 yrs | with children under 3 yrs | mothers of infants |

Figure 18-2. Mothers' participation in the labor force. (Data from U.S. Department of Labor, Women's Bureau, http://www.dol.gov./wb/stats/recentfacts.htm (Accessed 12.05.14.).)

next highest among women who plan to return to part-time employment, and the lowest among those who plan to remain at home.[34] In 2002, initiation in the hospital was 69% among women fully employed, 72.9% among those employed part time, and 69% among those not employed. The duration, however, is affected by employment, with 36.8% of those employed part time still breastfeeding at 5 to 6 months, 35.2% of nonemployed women still breastfeeding at that point, and only 27.1% of those employed full time still breastfeeding at 5 to 6 months[34] (Figure 18-3). A mother who chooses to return to work and breastfeed is confronted by significant constraints, regardless of the statistical data. Although economic, cultural, and political pressures often confound decisions about infant feeding, the American Academy of Pediatrics (AAP) firmly adheres to the position that breastfeeding ensures the best possible health and the best developmental and psychosocial outcomes for infants.[4] Enthusiastic support and involvement of all physicians in the promotion and practice of breastfeeding are essential to the achievement of optimal infant and child health, growth, and development.[4]

The American College of Obstetricians and Gynecologists (ACOG) and the American Academy of Family Practice have made equally strong statements.[3,5]

Historical Perspective

In modern cultures, a stigma has been attached to a mother earning money while her children are young, but no such stigma is associated with leaving her children for social interaction, personal reasons, or a volunteer job. All women work when work is defined as expending energy for a purpose, but not all women are employed when it is defined as earning money for labor. Before industrialization, working mothers were the rule and not the exception. Home and work were separated by industrialization, making parenting a separate role for women.

Women's work has been described as domestic or productive, public or private, traditional or modern. Domestic work, when performed for the family, is unpaid, thus undervalued, and not considered

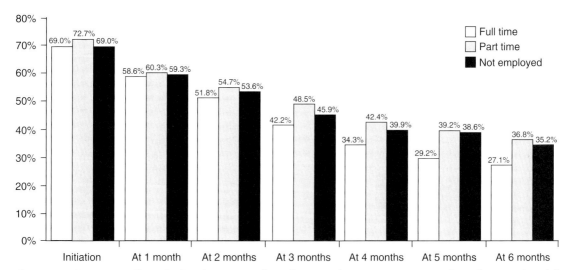

Figure 18-3. Comparison of breastfeeding duration rates during first 6 months postpartum among mothers who are working full time, working part time, and not employed. (From Ross Products Division, Abbott Laboratories: *Mothers survey: updated breastfeeding trends through 2002,* Columbus, Ohio, 2002, Abbott Laboratories.)

productive work. Domestic work is performed in the private domain, and "productive" work is associated with the public domain. Women had previously worked in agriculture and cottage industries as well as in small-scale marketing, whereas today they participate in formal work (i.e., they are employees), including clerical, factory, and professional jobs, predominantly in urban settings.

More women are employed outside the home today than previously. In 1900, 20% of the labor force were women; in 1950, 29%; in 1997, 56.6%; in 2003, 57.5%; and in 2008 (at the onset of a recession), 59.9%. Women with children younger than 6 years old are the fastest-growing segment of the female work force; their numbers reached 59% in 1992 and more than 65% in 1996 but dropped to 59.4% in 2002 and 63.6% in 2008. Even more important is that the number of employed mothers with infants younger than 1 year old rose to 48% of all women in 1985 and has continued to climb. Many more women facing the decision about infant feeding methods must include early return to work in their considerations. In 1998, at least 50% of women employed in the United States when they became pregnant returned to the labor force by the time their children were 3 months old. U.S. Department of Labor statistics show that 54.3% of mothers with children younger than 1 year old were in the work force in 1996 and 57.3% in 2008. This figure rises to 63.3% for women with children younger than 2 years of age. In Australia, 27% of women with infants younger than 1 year old return to work and 49% of women with children younger than 5 years old are part of the paid work force.

Generations ago, the woman who worked violated the Victorian norms of role definition. Even when forced to work by sheer necessity, she was accused of neglecting her primary responsibility to her children. The new ethic proclaims work a cardinal virtue for liberated women, so that now women who can and do stay home may begin to feel inadequate.

Knowing why women enter the work force is important to understanding the trend. Before 1970, the need to earn money motivated 3 million women either because the woman was a single parent or because husband-fathers were unable to earn an adequate income. For women whose husbands earned "enough," there was the desire to have a higher standard of living or to provide the father with greater freedom of career choice. Few women sought employment for the sake of having a career because the need for income was the only socially acceptable, defensible reason for a mother to work outside the home.

Since that time many women have found that the full-time care of a home leads only to higher standards of cleanliness with no greater sense of achievement or completion. Some believed that the exclusive investment of energy and emotion in the rearing of one to three children would involve a considerable hazard not only to a mother, but also to her children's ultimate achievement and ability to form a variety of responsive and satisfying personal relationships.[26] Women are responding to the pressures of a depressed economy, to the costs of higher education, to the opportunities for personal fulfillment, and to the growing market for service occupations.[8] Married women continue to carry at least 70% to 80% of the child care and household duties when both parents work.

Women have reached the point where marriage in itself has relatively little effect on the labor supply, according to Cohen and Bianchi. Educational differentials in the labor market have grown over time, widening the gap between more educated and less educated women, giving the former greater opportunities.[32,33]

Attitudes of Health Care Professionals Toward Working Mothers

Professional and lay[22] books alike on child rearing have viewed working negatively except for economic necessity, thus enhancing a working mother's guilt and providing little substantial advice about how to balance or how to continue breastfeeding.

The AAP strongly states that pediatricians should "encourage employers to provide appropriate facilities and adequate time in the workplace for breast-pumping."[4] The AAP provides extensive recommendations for a mother to prepare for returning to work and maintaining her milk supply when she does return.[36]

The ACOG[5] has acknowledged the current trend to work throughout pregnancy and to return to work promptly after delivery by preparing a physician's guide to patient assessment and counseling, which has not been updated since 1987. ACOG also provides a patient occupational questionnaire for the practitioner. This forms a basis of discussion with a patient and provides an opportunity to counsel the patient and her husband about plans to maintain a healthy environment and any special needs for child care. With few exceptions, "the normal woman with an uncomplicated pregnancy and a normal fetus, in a job that presents no greater potential hazards than those encountered in normal daily life in the community, may continue to work without interruption until the onset of labor and may resume working several weeks after an uncomplicated delivery."[5] An obstetrician has a role in facilitating continued breastfeeding after the return to work or school. This includes counseling regarding pumping and storing milk and avoiding exhaustion (Tables 18-2 and 18-3).

Physicians play an important role in guiding parents with information about quality and availability of child care facilities and with advice about coping strategies. Multiple studies have demonstrated the affect of clinician support and duration of breastfeeding.[40] As the family counselor, a physician can support mothers and fathers seeking to fulfill parental, occupational, and personal needs in a rapidly changing society. With the firm recommendation of the AAP to breastfeed throughout the first year and beyond, support from pediatricians will be critical.[4]

TABLE 18-2 Responses for Reasons to Recommend Work

Reason	Frequency No.	%
Economic	1709	25
Never recommend mother work	1566	22
Mother's emotional needs	1220	18
Mother's fulfillment	1059	15
Child is better off without mother	644	9
Reassure mother	270	4
Adequacy of child care	266	4
Child's age	170	2
Mother does important work	64	1
Total	6968	

From Heins M, Stillman P, Sabers D, et al: Attitudes of pediatricians toward maternal employment, *Pediatrics* 72:283, 1983; copyright© American Academy of Pediatrics, 1983.

TABLE 18-3 Responses for Reasons to Recommend Against Working

Reason	Frequency No.	%
Child's physical health	1724	24
Child's mental health	1445	20
Never recommend against work	1318	18
Inadequate child care	701	10
Child's age	591	8
Mother feels guilty	540	7
No economic need	459	6
Usually say, "Do not work"	72	1
Other	402	6
Total	7252	

From Heins M, Stillman P, Sabers D, et al: Attitudes of pediatricians toward maternal employment, *Pediatrics* 72:286, 1983; copyright© American Academy of Pediatrics, 1983.

Attitude of Employer and Employees Toward Working Women

Studies of employer attitudes toward working mothers, and specifically toward women who need accommodation to breastfeeding and to pump, reflected lack of knowledge. When employers understood the benefits of breastfeeding, attitudes changed.

Personal experience with breastfeeding had the greatest impact. Almost all at the managerial level were unaware of the existence of company policy. It appears that the greatest progress in supporting breastfeeding in the workplace has come when it has been mandated by state or federal policy.

Employers who accommodate lactating mothers can fear negative reactions from other workers. In a large U.S. corporation that provided a wide variety of accommodations for lactating mothers, 407 employees were studied by Suyes et al.[39] They observed that overall attitudes were favorable. Those who had previous exposure to a work colleague who was breastfeeding were associated with a positive attitude even after the investigators controlled for respondent's gender, length of employment, and personal exposure to breastfeeding. The authors concluded that lactation accommodations did not have a negative impact on the work environment or other employees.[39]

A program directed at the male employees has been functioning at the Los Angeles Department of Water and Power since 1990. There has been a full-time, on-site lactation program offered to the male employees. In addition to classes and individual instruction, information is available on the electronic pump and the pump kit and its use. Meetings with a lactation consultant and daily assistance for the mother when needed also are offered. It has grown by word of mouth, fathers' interest in the benefits of breastfeeding for the infant, and the female partners' interest in obtaining a free pump rental. It is a model that could well be implemented in any corporation.

Outcome for Children of Employed Mothers

Numerous studies since the early 1930s have looked at the effects of maternal employment. Assessment of infant behavior, school achievement and adjustment, children's attitudes, adolescence, and delinquency have all been used as outcome measures.[12] Annotated bibliographies covering the range of research in areas of medicine, psychology, sociology, and education are available.[11] The four major considerations are the variables that facilitate or impede maternal employment, the effect of maternal employment on children during the four developmental stages, the effects on the family, and the effects on society in general. Society is far more accepting of working mothers in the twenty-first century.

It has been emphasized that the presence of a mother in the home does not guarantee high-quality mothering. It has also been shown that well-educated (college) mothers, including those who are employed, spend time with their children at the expense of their own personal needs.[18] Because employed mothers encompass a large group of women with different educational levels, different reasons for working, and different opportunities for employment, it is difficult to generalize about effects. Literature reviews have emphasized critical factors that are more important than maternal employment, such as good substitute care, maternal role satisfaction, family stability, paternal attitude toward maternal employment, and the quality of the time spent with the children.[17] Despite the abundance of research on school-age children, there is still little reported about preschoolers because no school records or test results are available to use in large-population analysis.

To date, there is no direct effect of nonexclusive mothering per se. Studies of infants of adolescent mothers have shown that the children do better socially and academically if there are multiple caregivers instead of the adolescent mother alone.[23] No uniformly harmful effects on family life or on the growth and development of children have been demonstrated. Maternal employment may jeopardize family life when the conditions of the mother's employment are demeaning to self-esteem, when others are strongly disapproving of her work away from the home, or when arrangements for child care are not adequate.

Questions have been raised about the impact of separation of mother and infant and the timing of this separation.[8] Resumption of full-time employment when the child is younger than 1 year old has prompted studies. Using the Ainsworth "strange situation" validated techniques, no relationship between maternal work status and the quality of the infants' attachment to their mothers is reported.[1,2] Early resumption of employment may not impede development of a secure infant-mother attachment. A significantly higher proportion of insecure attachments to fathers in employed-mother families is reported for boys but not for girls. Boys are more insecurely attached than girls in most studies. It is believed that an infant's attachment relationship to mother emerges at approximately 7 months.[14] Other studies suggest that maternal employment can have a positive effect on girls but not boys. Whether breastfeeding accounts for some of the variability in these studies is not stated.[43] No study recorded feeding method or considered the impact breastfeeding has on the mother-infant relationship or the infant's development. One of the strategies suggested is to advocate for infant care centers that provide breastfeeding facilities in the workplace, schools, and other locations serving working women.

Breastfeeding and Employment

An important distinction must be made between work that separates mothers and infants for blocks of time and work that does not. In rural settings, women's work is usually compatible with all aspects of child care, including breastfeeding. Work in or around the home is usually flexible. If there are provisions for infants at the workplace, even formal urban work is compatible with child care and breastfeeding. The higher the education of the mother and the more advanced the job, the more opportunity exists for flexible arrangements that permit breastfeeding. Among the strategies available is pumping and saving milk while on the job to be fed to the baby by the babysitter the next day.

Overall, the breastfeeding rates for working women do not show that breastfeeding and employment are mutually exclusive. In Finland the incidence of mothers breastfeeding at 1 month is 78% among nonemployed and 80% among employed mothers. The duration is also unaffected: 29% of nonemployed and 32% of employed mothers are breastfeeding at 3 months, and 8% and 7%, respectively, at 6 months. Similar statistics are reported from Nigeria, the Philippines, and Chile.

An infant feeding practices study reported that those mothers at 6 months who were employed full time numbered 22,316 (26.6%), part time 12,186 (14.5%), and not employed 49,483 (58.9%). The same proportion (55%) of employed mothers as not employed mothers were breastfeeding when they left the hospital. Only 10% of full-time employed mothers were breastfeeding at 6 months compared with 24% of those who were not employed, however. The highest incidence of breastfeeding at birth and at 6 months was among mothers older than 30 years who are well educated and in a higher socioeconomic group. In 2002, the duration of breastfeeding at 6 months was as follows: of those mothers employed full time, 27.1% were breastfeeding, of those employed part time, 36.8% were breastfeeding, and of those not employed, 35.2% were breastfeeding—not a remarkable rate for those at home. At 6 months,

negative consequences of these requirements were studied by Haider et al.[15] They indicate that the national breastfeeding rate would have been 5.5% higher at 6 months in 2000 without this mandate. They further suggest that the negative consequences of this policy should be considered because the potential benefits of breastfeeding these at-risk infants are so great.[15]

A comparison of maternal absenteeism and infant illness rates among breastfeeding and formula-feeding women showed breastfeeding reduced absenteeism.[10] In two corporations with on-site lactation programs, one had 100 births among 2400, and the second had 30 births among 1200 female employees. Of the 101 mother-infant dyads studied, 59 were breastfed and 42 formula fed. The company provided lactation counseling as well as pumping and storing facilities. Of the 28% of the infants who had no illnesses, 86% were breastfed and 14% formula fed. Among mothers who were absent because of infant illness, 75% were formula feeding and only 25% were breastfeeding (Figure 18-5).

After a mail panel questionnaire study in which questionnaires were sent in late pregnancy and 10 times during the first year, mothers' work patterns were clarified. Working full time at 3 months decreased breastfeeding duration by 8.6 weeks relative to not working. Part-time work for 4 hours or less per day did not decrease duration of breastfeeding; part-time work more than 4 hours per day decreased breastfeeding duration only slightly. The authors concluded that part-time work is actually a good strategy to help mothers combine breastfeeding and work.

Planning to return to work before 6 weeks postpartum reduced the likelihood of initiating breastfeeding in a study of more than 10,000 mothers of singleton term infants.

Most of the studies concerning employment and breastfeeding were retrospective, relied on voluntary responses, and did not clearly define breastfeeding in terms of exclusivity or working in terms of part time or full time. A prospective study reported by Kurinij et al.[21] involving more than 1000 women confirmed the reports of others that women with professional occupations breastfeed longer than nonprofessionals and that part-time work is more conducive to longer duration than full-time jobs. Both groups of women found equal satisfaction from breastfeeding. The duration of breastfeeding was evaluated in a separate study in the same two corporations mentioned previously. Cohen et al.[9] reported that of the 187 participants, 75% who returned to work breastfed for 6 months or longer. The average duration for breastfeeding was 8.1 months. These rates were equal to the statistical norms for the region among women not employed outside the home.

The general consensus has been that returning to work diminishes breastfeeding. As the number of women who work outside the home increased and breastfeeding increased in the last decade, the trends have changed. A large study of U.S. mothers found that initiation rates among mothers who were not working after childbirth compared

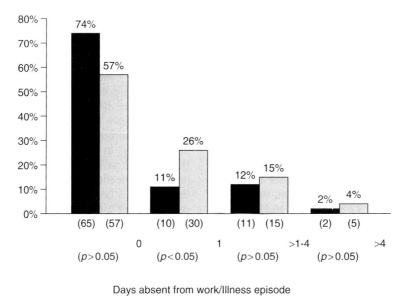

Days absent from work/Illness episode

■ Breastfed babies' illness episodes (*n* = 88)   ▨ Formula-fed babies' illness episodes (*n* = 117)

Figure 18-5. Distribution of illness episodes and maternal absenteeism by nutritional groups. (Modified from Cohen R, Mrtek MB, Mrtek RG: Comparison of maternal absenteeism and infant illness rates among breast-feeding and formula-feeding women in two corporations. *Am J Health Promot* 10:148, 1995.)

with mothers who were working part time were not different.[35] In 2001 to 2003 it was estimated that 67% of mothers of first children worked during the pregnancy, and most of them held full-time jobs.[19]

The Infant Feeding Practice Study II (IFPSII) was conducted by the FDA with the CDC from 2005 to 2007. It was a longitudinal study of women from late pregnancy through the infant's first year of life.[24] Similar to IFPSI conducted in 1992 to 1993, over 1400 mothers were involved. The expected number of hours she planned to work was used to categorize each dyad. The actual number of hours worked and baby's age at onset of work were categorized along with demographics, length of maternity leave, past breastfeeding experience, hospital experience, and degree of social support at home. This study showed that compared to not expecting to work, expecting to work less than 35 hours was not associated with breastfeeding initiation. Expecting to work full time, however, decreased breastfeeding initiation. Returning to work within 12 weeks, regardless of hours worked, was associated with less breastfeeding. Returning to work after 12 weeks but working more than 34 hours per week was also associated with shorter breastfeeding. The authors conclude that longer post partum leave and part-time work promote breastfeeding.[24]

The Early Childhood Longitudinal Study-Birth Cohort utilized a sample of singletons whose mothers had responded to a survey and had worked the 12 months before delivery. The study included 6150 women and classified them by the length of their maternity leave. Almost 70% initiated breastfeeding, which was not influenced by paid maternity leave. Those who returned to work within 1 to 6 weeks were less likely to initiate breastfeeding. Duration of breastfeeding was impacted by time of return to work. Those returning to work at or after 13 weeks were more apt to breastfeed for 3 months or longer.[30]

The dilemma every woman faces, whether breastfeeding or bottle-feeding, is leaving one's child. Mother's milk in a bottle given by any of several staff members at daycare is not equal to nursing at the breast. The decision to work or not work is a personal one and does not separate women into good and bad mothers. The role of the health professional is to discuss the mother's plans nonjudgmentally and assist her in adjusting her infant and herself to the process.

COUNSELING BREASTFEEDING MOTHERS WHO CHOOSE TO WORK

The AAP periodic survey of members that included questions about breastfeeding was conducted in 2004 and results were compared with a similar survey taken in 1995. Pediatricians in 2004 were less likely to believe that the benefits of breastfeeding outweigh the difficulties or inconveniences. Pediatricians with personal experience were much more likely to be supportive. Personal experience seemed to mitigate poor attitudes.

Part of a physician's counseling session before the birth of a baby should include inquiry about a mother's plan to work postpartum. Open discussion about work, breastfeeding, child care arrangements, and general stress will be helpful. Most well-educated women who plan to return to a career have thought out the entire process carefully but may want some reassurance or alternative suggestions. Physicians should know what services are available locally. It may be helpful to have a list of other working mothers who are willing to share experiences and knowledge of resources. It is often helpful for a woman to know another person who has experienced similar career choices. The physician, however, should not assume that personal experience should be the model recommended to the patient.

Some women have no experience with newborns and are totally unrealistic about the new responsibility and what it entails. Even pediatricians in training may be unrealistic. Pediatricians may have to recommend a more realistic view of parenting and urge the parents to plan carefully and practically for working and parenting. A new mother needs to appreciate that events occur that cannot be totally controlled. Even for a woman who has been an efficient career woman in total control of her destiny, an infant with normal needs may be overwhelming. Women who have jobs that are rigid from the standpoint of work hours and workplace will not find a few glib remarks in a pamphlet helpful when they want to maintain their milk supply.

Physicians may need to discuss specific issues of child care while a mother is working, as follows:

1. Child care arrangements should be sought that permit sufficient time for feeding an infant inexperienced with a bottle and sufficient time for extra cuddling of an infant who is used to a closer relationship with the "feeder." A child care specialist should be familiar with breastfeeding and sympathetic to the philosophy.
2. The advantages and disadvantages of child care in an infant's home, in a sitter's home, with or without a sitter's children, and with or without other children should be discussed. Is daycare a good arrangement for this family, and what centers take young infants and will work with breastfeeding mothers? Despite low costs, nursery "warehousing" should be avoided.

3. Are child care facilities available close to the workplace so that a mother could leave work on her breaks to breastfeed?

Plans for feeding an infant while the mother is working depend on the infant's age and feeding pattern. If an infant is totally breastfed and younger than 6 months of age, the mother can breastfeed if she can leave work and go to the infant or if the infant can be brought to the workplace. If a mother cannot leave work to nurse, she may choose to pump her milk at work and save it for the following day. This necessitates having a reasonably sanitary place to pump, such as a lounge or clean locker room, and a means of storing the milk until she gets home, either in a refrigerator at work or in a portable refrigerator system. Mothers have used insulated containers with ice, reusable cold packs, or dry ice. If no such arrangement for chilling can be made, the milk can be stored in a sterile container for 8 hours without refrigeration if collected under clean conditions.

A woman who is away from her breastfeeding infant past feeding time may need to pump to maintain her milk supply. A mother may also anticipate the infant's needs before she returns to work. She can practice pumping and storing a small amount of her milk daily for several weeks in her home freezer so that a stockpile is available while she is at work (see Chapter 21).

A mother should be instructed to introduce the baby to the bottle and an alternate caregiver before the first day of work. Developing a plan of organization and practicing it before the first day of work may avoid initial disaster. Also, returning to work part time at first may help minimize the adjustment. In addition, returning to work on a Wednesday or Thursday allows the first week to be a short one.

No evidence indicates that it is necessary to introduce a bottle sooner than 10 days before returning to work. Unless a mother is returning to work immediately after delivery, a bottle should not be introduced before lactation is well established (at least 4 weeks for most primiparas) because it interferes with a mother's milk-making rhythm. Furthermore, it may confuse the infant. Although some infants readily go back and forth between breast and bottle, no way exists to identify the infant who will develop sucking difficulties and "nipple confusion," ultimately resulting in preference for the bottle if it is introduced too early. Babies given a bottle well before 3 months may easily reject the breast after 3 months. For the infant who does not accept the bottle gracefully, the following techniques may facilitate the process:

1. Someone other than the mother should give the feeding.

2. The mother should be out of sight and hearing range, preferably out of the building, so the infant does not await her arrival.
3. The infant should be held by the "feeder" in the same position as for breastfeeding, that is, slightly elevated and close to the chest wall at about breast level. The bottle can be slipped down against the caregiver's chest wall.
4. Use a soft nipple and a small bottle at first for easy handling. A Volufeed, the clear plastic cylinder used for premature infants, allows a better view of the infant.
5. Create a soothing atmosphere; use a rocking chair, quiet music, and muted light.
6. The initial bottle-feedings, if not all of them, should contain warm mother's milk to reduce the elements of change being introduced.

If the bottle feedings do not go well and alternate feedings are needed, milk can be provided by medicine cup feeding (see Chapter 15).

If an infant is older than 6 months of age, a physician may consider introduction of other foods. The feeding given by the caregiver can be solids by spoon and liquids from a cup so that no breastfeeding is actually missed. A health professional can anticipate these issues and tailor feeding counseling accordingly. Some infants quickly learn the mother's schedule and may adjust their sleep pattern to allow a long stretch while mother is away. This may result in feedings during the night instead, but if the mother is informed of this phenomenon, she may be less anxious if it occurs.

Formula-fed infants have more infections and illnesses, which is another reason to encourage a mother to continue breastfeeding. This is especially important during the first weeks of adjustment to the transient, recurrent separation of mother and infant associated with the mother's return to work.

MATERNAL CONSIDERATIONS

Counseling a breastfeeding family when the mother returns to work should also include attention to mothering the mother. Fatigue is a significant problem for all postpartum women and many nursing mothers. It can easily become a major stress when the mother adds outside employment to her schedule. Several days or more of adjustment are necessary for a major change in one's schedule. If the mother can focus on a few essential concerns (infant, job, own well-being) as opposed to housework, fancy meals, or a social schedule, she will weather the transition without despair. The first casualty of fatigue may be breastfeeding unless some anticipatory action is taken.

Once the schedule has been adjusted and a routine established, breastfeeding may offer tremendous satisfaction for both mother and infant in terms of a sustained relationship as well as a reaffirmation for the mother of the quality of her parenting. One of the most difficult adjustments to motherhood is the need to set priorities and eliminate some chores of lesser urgency. Physicians need to reinforce this when a mother returns to work. Whether a mother continues to breastfeed, holding and cuddling her baby cannot become a lower priority. The mother's nourishment is also important and can be consumed during the time spent pumping. A mother should plan to have a beverage available every time she sits down to nurse or pump.

When mothers were asked what works for them when combining employment and breastfeeding, 43% pumped milk at work only, and 31% breastfed the baby while at work. Those mothers who neither fed nor pumped had the shortest duration of breastfeeding and working. Those who fed the baby either took the infant to work, went to the baby at daycare to feed the infant, or had the infant taken to the mother. These latter options require daycare that is nearby, a car, or a flexible caretaker who can take the baby to the mother.[13]

DAYCARE

Infants in daycare have created a special concern for parents, pediatricians, social scientists, and policymakers. Early published information did not discuss the impact of breastfeeding before or during an infant's involvement with daycare. Haskins and Kotch[16] first reviewed the literature (172 articles) and concluded, "Children in day care, especially those under three years old and sometimes their teachers and household contacts, have higher rates of diarrhea, hepatitis A, meningitis and possibly also otitis media than children not in day care." The data are less clear for respiratory illnesses and cytomegalovirus. Parents choosing daycare facilities for their children need to select them with consideration for health and safety. More than 60% of the children younger than 6 years of age of women who work are in out-of-home care, approximately 8 million children in the United States. In some situations, daycare may actually improve an infant's potential, especially when the mother is young, immature, depressed, overwhelmed, or without family support.

Concern about infant illness should result in the pediatricians' involvement in ensuring quality daycare in the local community. For an infant of an age appropriate for breastfeeding, one possible preventive measure would be to encourage a continuation of breastfeeding when possible. Furthermore, daycare policy and procedure should encourage and facilitate breastfeeding. Mothers should inquire

about daycare centers' policies toward breastfeeding. Physicians who consult for daycare centers should be well informed as well. Breast milk can safely stand at room temperature for 6 to 8 hours and need not be discarded if the first feeding attempt is incomplete. In contrast, formula must be refrigerated and discarded after the first feeding attempt because it contains no antibodies or infection protection factors. No infant feeding of any kind should be warmed in a microwave oven. Protective gloves are not necessary to feed breast milk. The accidental feeding of a different mother's milk is not cause for alarm, although it should be reported to the parents for public health reasons. One feeding of milk produced by a mother who is positive for human immunodeficiency virus (HIV) will probably not transmit the disease. Women who are HIV positive in developed countries, including the United States, are prevented from breastfeeding.

RESOURCES FOR PARENTS

The popular press has been inundated with books on child care and child rearing, with a significant number on breastfeeding, specifically breastfeeding and employment. These volumes can be extremely helpful to young parents, providing detailed information about how to manage. Many recognize that mothers, fathers, infants, jobs, child care arrangements, and support resources are all different. A disturbing number, however, are dogmatic and single-minded, giving the impression that the author's method is the only recipe for successful lactation. Pediatricians should become familiar with a few of these guidebooks and certainly not recommend any without reading them first. A few of these books have produced guilt in a working woman about leaving her infant.

The brochure *Working and Breastfeeding: Can You Do It?* was prepared by the National Healthy Mothers, Healthy Babies Coalition and is available free by calling the coalition in Alexandria, Virginia, at 703-837-4792. It is also available through local WIC nutritional programs. It is simple and direct, providing directions for managing a job and breastfeeding as well as collecting and storing breast milk.

Women in health care head the list of authors because many women physicians (especially residents), nurses, and hospital employees return to work while breastfeeding and then share their experiences in print. Even the worst setup in a hospital may surpass the resources available to the women working in another industry. Certainly hospitals and health care centers should provide models for other workplaces in supporting optimal daycare sources and making it possible for a mother-employee to return to work and maintain her milk supply.[20] Independent lactation practitioners provide an additional resource. Women should contact the International Lactation Consultants Association for consultants in their area (see Chapter 22). Some industries have hired certified lactation consultants to provide assistance to their employees in maintaining their milk supply. The company also usually provides "a pumping room" and equipment. As pointed out by Cohen et al.[9] this also reduces absenteeism because an infant who is provided the mother's milk has fewer illnesses.

In a survey conducted by the Women's Health Resource Center of 1000 working mothers in 2007, overall, 32% of new mothers gave up breastfeeding in less than 7 weeks after returning to work. When looked at by age, 51% of mothers younger than 24 years of age gave up and only 21% of older mothers gave up. They also noted that not meeting their breastfeeding goals and work was the reason more than 25% of the time. Mothers who were in retail jobs, were younger, and had lower paying jobs met the most significant barriers. Barriers at work were a lack of private space, a place to pump, a place to store milk, and an inflexible work schedule. Emotional barriers included discomfort about storing supplies in front of coworkers and anxiety about discussing this with supervisors.

Responding to parental needs, Brazelton[7] captured the quintessential challenge to parents in the title and the text of *Working and Caring*. It is possible for parents to both work and care! The two most powerful requirements for human existence are "love" and "work." Our culture had suggested that men work and women love in relation to family obligations. Today, it is possible not only for a mother to love her children and work, but also for a father to work and love his children.

SURGEON GENERAL'S WORKSHOP

The Report of the Surgeon General's Workshop on Breastfeeding and Human Lactation,[32] published in 1984, clearly enunciated that strategies need to be developed to reduce the barriers to breastfeeding while employed. All six categories of the report address the issue in some capacity. Twenty-five years later a summit on breastfeeding was convened to review the progress and reset the strategies.[33] The workgroups were the same: work, professional education, public education, health care systems, and support services. The issues were similar, as were the strategies. The urgency of legislative support, workplace support including daycare, paid maternity leave, child care, alternative work schedules (flextime), and job sharing were on the list for the workgroup on work. The workshop report also states that successful initiation and continuation of breastfeeding will require a broad spectrum of support services involving families, peers, care providers, employers, and community agencies and organizations.[32] Although little has been accomplished toward these specific goals, the U.S. Breastfeeding Committee has been formed in concert with the Innocenti Declaration recommendations.[41] The U.S. Breastfeeding Committee has undertaken as a major activity the improvement of the atmosphere for breastfeeding, working women. The Committee's policy paper on the subject states the following benefits for employers that adopt a breastfeeding support program[41]:

- Cost savings of $3 per $1 invested in breastfeeding support
- Less illness among the breastfed children of employees
- Reduced absenteeism to care for ill children
- Lower health care costs (an average of $400 per baby in the first year)
- Improved employee productivity
- Higher morale and greater loyalty
- Improved ability to attract and retain valuable employees
- Family-friendly image in the community

Each company or employer should tailor a program to its unique needs.

The Committee has suggested that several strategies are feasible, safe, and relatively easy to implement. They include developing a breastfeeding support program, distribution of support policy, consideration of a flexible scheduling option, sufficient break time to feed or pump, and providing useful information. The full statement is available at http://www.usbreastfeeding.org.

WORKPLACE KIT FOR AUSTRALIA

Women in Australia face the same challenges to working while breastfeeding as reported in many other countries. McIntrye et al.[25] report on a project that promoted balancing breastfeeding and paid work through the development, distribution, promotion, and evaluation of suitable materials to workplaces, employers, and employees. Materials for employees were translated into Arabic, Chinese, Turkish, Spanish, and Vietnamese.

In this project targeting employers, women, and workplaces in Australia, 500,000 information kits were distributed with preference for places that had women of childbearing age and women of diverse cultural backgrounds. The project was widely publicized in all media.

The kit contained a poster to display key points and a booklet to provide more detailed information in an easy-to-read format. The contents had been tested in focus groups and evaluated by other key

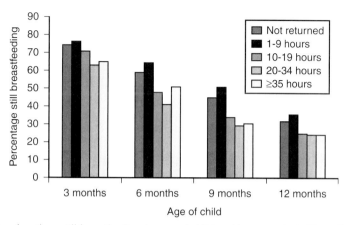

Figure 18-6. Percentage of mothers still breastfeeding, by age of child and hours worked. (From Cooklin AR, Donath SM, Amir LH: Maternal employment and breastfeeding: results from the longitudinal study of Australian children, *Acta Paediatr* 97:620–623, 2008.)

stakeholders, including a working mother and a lactation consultant.

The evaluation of the project included a simple survey sent via email or fax to 1571 organizations. Only 202 (12.8%) were returned. Those who responded thought it was excellent, more than half thought it would be useful, and two thirds thought the kit would provide suitable solutions to support balancing breastfeeding and work at their organization. The authors recognize the need for further work to implement the policies and procedures to support breastfeeding in the workplace. To investigate the effect of maternal postpartum employment on breastfeeding duration in Australia in the first 6 months after birth in 2008, Cooklin et al.[10] performed a secondary analysis of the Longitudinal Study of Australian Children. Data on 3697 children were completed. Multivariable logistic regression was used to measure the effect of the timing of a mother's return to work and the effect of employment on breastfeeding status. Maternal age, history of smoking during pregnancy, and socioeconomic status were adjusted for. Breastfeeding rates dropped to 39% at 6 months among employed mothers compared with unemployed mothers at 56%. Full-time employment before 6 months had a major impact; 44% of those who were employed part time were breastfeeding at 6 months. The authors concluded that in spite of controlling for risk factors, employment before 6 months had a negative impact on dedicated breastfeeding (Figure 18-6).

THE BUSINESS CASE FOR BREASTFEEDING

The *Business Case for Breastfeeding*[42] contains the steps for creating a breastfeeding-friendly worksite. This was developed by the U.S. Department of Health and Human Services (HHS), Health Resources and Services Administration's Maternal and Child Health Bureau (MCHB). It is a comprehensive resource kit that targets a broad spectrum of individuals and groups involved in supporting breastfeeding women. The kit provides a train-the-trainer approach that results in improving workplace lactation support for employed breastfeeding women. It is intended to provide training for reaching out to local businesses and is working with state breastfeeding coalitions and Healthy Start programs. Healthy Start is a HHS-funded program providing community-based initiatives to reduce infant mortality rates and to improve the health of women, infants, and children and their families. The training content is based on the MCHB workplace lactation resource kit in a community-based outreach program. Training is targeted at breastfeeding coalitions, Healthy Start Staff, International Board Certified Lactation Consultants, health care professionals, La Leche League Leaders, and WIC staff. It is a step-by-step program complete with script and slides. Format includes role play. Those who complete the course should be ready to approach employers with why and how to start a program that supports breastfeeding by their employees. The kit is well referenced. The bibliography is extensive. Materials are readily available.

The National Business Group on Health is a not-for-profit membership organization for large employers whose mission it is to identify and share best practices, link science and evidence to health benefit plan design, and be a national voice for large employers.[28] Membership includes half the Fortune 500 and 40% of the companies who made

Working Mother's Top 100 Best Companies to work for. Employers' budgets for health care benefits are limited, so that breastfeeding competes with smoking cessation, obesity prevention, and work-site wellness programs. The annual health care coverage costs will double in 10 years. Worksite breastfeeding programs have increased to cover more than 25% of large companies.[31] The number who offer breastfeeding programs is greatest among large employers. It has been shown that absenteeism is twice as high among mothers who bottlefed. Employee retention rates in companies who implemented breastfeeding support programs were 83% to 84% compared with the national average of 59%.[31] Other benefits of the programs beyond cost savings for health care are earlier return from maternity leave, higher productivity, morale, loyalty, and recognition as a "family-friendly" worksite. Employers decide what health benefits they will select based on medical evidence of effectiveness, impact on productivity indicators, cost savings, and good will. When making decisions about what health benefits to provide, employers often rely on a variety of sources of information, including the health plan itself and research they gather themselves. They do not consult government agencies or peer-reviewed academic journals.[28]

MATERNAL BENEFITS

In 1919 the International Labour Organization established the Maternity Protection Convention for working women. This document provided for two half-hour nursing breaks per day. It also recommended that employers provide crèches (day nurseries, especially European) or daycare when more than a given number of women are employed, but few countries hold to its tenets today. Maternity benefits vary from country to country and may include maternity leave with or without pay, nursing breaks, provision of daycare facilities, and prohibition of dismissal. Physicians who care for mothers and infants should take a leadership role in ensuring that mothers can continue breastfeeding even when the mother is employed.

The World Alliance of Breastfeeding Actions has stated that breastfeeding is a right of mothers and is a fundamental component in assuring a child's right to food, health, and good care. Recognition of the importance of maternity leave as a social function should be supported by public funds. The International Labour Organization in the document "Maternity Protection at Work" states, "Maternity protection is a precondition of genuine equality of opportunity and treatment for men and women." In the renewal of the Innocenti Declaration in 2005 one of the declarations was a charge to nations to "adopt maternity protection legislation and other measures that facilitate 6 months exclusive breastfeeding for women employed in all sectors."

Efforts in the United States, headed by the United States Breastfeeding Committee, include legislation for:

• Fully paid maternity leave with benefits and job security followed by paid breaks upon return to work (14 weeks' minimum paid leave recommended by the International Labour Organization)
• Cost sharing with state and federal funding tax incentives and legal mandates and protection of breastfeeding mothers (Civil Rights Act 1964)
• Provision of adequate facilities to feed one's infant or pump one's milk and store it safely

Many women, especially when faced with coping with a second or third child, reexamine the working issue in light of the needs of their children, even though they may have previously managed to breastfeed and work at one time. No one else can or should decide for a woman how she will handle parenting, especially in the early years of a child's life. No woman should be embarrassed to stay home or should apologize for working part time or not at all. Breast milk is not a substitute for good parenting, any more than "quantity parenting" is synonymous with quality parenting. It is possible to work and to care, however.

PHYSICIAN'S ROLE

The primary role of a pediatrician is as an advocate for children, but all physicians can help support fathers and mothers alike who are faced with fulfilling the roles of parent, employee, and citizen in a rapidly changing society. Physicians should be able to provide understandable information concerning a child's growth and development combined with a realistic view of the issues in parenting and family life. They should show an openness and willingness to discuss nonjudgmentally with the parents their specific situation, options, and choices for caring for their child.

If a physician is the medical consultant to the daycare program, the role can be to assure mothers who want to provide their milk that they will be supported by the staff. The physician should develop policies and procedures for the storage and use of the breast milk provided. In addition, space and facilities (at least a rocking chair and a screen) should be available for a mother to nurse the infant before leaving the child and on her return later before going home. If a physician is in the medical department of a large company or the pediatrician for a working breastfeeding mother, he or she can advocate for time and resources for pumping while at work as part of good preventive care.

The success of breastfeeding depends to a degree on ever-widening circles of support for the breastfeeding infant-mother dyad. Support should come first from the husband/father, then from other family members, other caregivers in the home, daycare facilities, employers and other employees, and community members to help the mother and family comfortably and safely breastfeed, work, and care for their child as they choose. Breastfeeding is not just a woman's issue. It is a family issue and a public health issue as well. Articles abound in the medical and lay literature describing how one can achieve success in breastfeeding and returning to work. Most authors list pumps and milk storage as important items. Each mother has to plan her own approach based on her job requirements, her own resources, and her support system, as well as her infant's needs. Although it is not easy to balance a job and breastfeed, it can be done, with adequate strategizing and planning, which is appropriate with or without breastfeeding and returning to work postpartum.

A physician's role in achieving a successful return to work for the breastfeeding mother includes the following steps:

1. Discuss the mother's plans for returning to work in advance.
2. Recommend appropriate local child care facilities that are "breastfeeding friendly."
3. Suggest that the mother discuss breastfeeding with her employer or supervisor.
4. Have a licensed, certified lactation consultant available in the practice or office, or if not, know where one can be contacted.
5. Provide recommendations for collecting and storing breast milk, which can be additionally covered in an office handout.
6. When medical problems arise, seek adequate information so that an appropriate solution can be recommended that supports continued breastfeeding.

Reading for Parents Regarding Breastfeeding and Working Outside the Home

Huggins K. *The nursing mother's companion*, ed 6, Cambridge, Mass., 2010, Harvard Common Press.

Meck JY, editor: *American Academy of Pediatrics new mother's guide to breastfeeding*, ed 2, New York, 2010, Bantam Books.

REFERENCES

1. Ainsworth MDS: The development of infant-mother attachment. In Caldwell BM, Ricciuti HN, editors: *Review of child development research*, Chicago, Ill., 1973, University of Chicago Press.
2. Ainsworth MDS, Blehar MC, Waters E, et al: *Patterns of attachment*, Hillsdale, N.J., 1978, Erlbaum.
3. American Academy of Family Physicians: *AAFP position paper on breastfeeding*, Leawood, Kan., 2001, KS American Academy of Family Physicians.
4. American Academy of Pediatrics: Section on breast-feeding: breastfeeding and the use of human milk, *Pediatrics* 115:496–506, 2005 (Revision 2010).
5. American College of Obstetricians and Gynecologists: *Breastfeeding: maternal and infant aspects. Educational bulletin 258*, July 2000, Washington, D.C., 1987, ACOG Publications.
6. Biagioli F: Returning to work while breastfeeding, *Am Fam Physician* 68:2199, 2003. Electronic article accessed at www.aafp.org/afp.
7. Brazelton TB: *Working and caring*, Reading, Mass., 1985, Addison-Wesley.
8. Bronfenbrenner U, Crouter AC: Work and family through time and space. In Kamerman SB, Hayes CD, editors: *Families that work: children in a changing world*, Washington, D.C., 1982, National Academy Press.
9. Cohen R, Mrtek MB, Mrtek RG: Comparison of maternal absenteeism and infant illness rates among breast-feeding and formula-feeding women in two corporations, *Am J Health Promot* 10:148, 1995.
10. Cooklin AR, Donath SM, Amir LH: Maternal employment and breastfeeding: results from the longitudinal study of Australian children, *Acta Paediatr* 97:620–623, 2008.
11. Easterbrooks MA, Goldberg WA: Effects of early maternal employment on toddlers, mothers and fathers, *Dev Psychol* 21:774, 1985.
12. Eiger MS, Olds SW: *The complete book of breastfeeding*, ed 3, New York, 2005, Workman.
13. Fein SB, Mandel B, Roc BE: Success of strategies for combining employment and breastfeeding. In *State breastfeeding coalition teleconference*, February 10. 2009.
14. Freud A, Dann S: An experiment in group upbringing, *Psychoanal Study Child* 6:127, 1961.
15. Haider SJ, Jacknowitz A, Schoeni RF: Welfare work requirements and child well-being: evidence from the effects on breastfeeding, *Demography* 40:479, 2003.
16. Haskins R, Kotch J: Day care and illness: evidence, costs, and public policy, *Pediatrics* 77(Suppl):951, 1986.
17. Hoffman LW: Effects of maternal employment on the child: a review of the research, *Dev Psychol* 10:204, 1974.
18. Hurst M, Zambrana RE: *Determinants and consequences of maternal employment*, Washington, D.C., 1981, Business and Professional Women's Foundation.
19. Johnson T: Maternity leave and employment patterns of first time mothers 1961-2003, *Curr Popul Rep* 1(19):70–113, 2008.
20. Katcher AL, Lanese MG: Breastfeeding by employed mothers: a reasonable accommodation in the work place, *Pediatrics* 75:644, 1985.
21. Kurinij N, Shiono PH, Ezrine SF, et al: Does maternal employment affect breastfeeding? *Am J Public Health* 79:1247, 1989.
22. La Leche League International: *The womanly art of breastfeeding*, ed 8, Schaumburg, Ill., 2014, La Leche League.
23. Lawrence RA: Early mothering by adolescents. In McAnarney ER, editor: *Premature adolescent pregnancy and parenthood*, New York, 1983, Grune & Stratton.
24. Mandel B, Roe BE, Fein SB: The differential effects of full-time and part-time work status on breastfeeding, *Health Policy* 97:79–86, 2010.
25. McIntrye E, Pisaniello D, Gun R, et al: Balancing breastfeeding and paid employment: a project targeting employers, women and workplaces, *Health Promot Int* 17:215, 2002.

26. Meyers D: Breastfeeding and returning to work in the physician's office, *Am Fam Physician* 68(11):2129, 2003.

27. Morse JM, Bottorff JL: Intending to breastfeed and work, *J Obstet Gynecol Neonatal Nurs* 18:493, 1989.

28. National Business Group on Health: *Survey: qualitative interviews NBGH members*, Washington, D.C., 2005, National Business Group on Health.

29. Noble S: ALSPAC Study Team: Maternal employment and the initiation of breastfeeding, *Acta Paediatr* 90:423, 2001.

30. Ogbuanu C, Glover S, Probst J, et al: The effect of maternity leave length and time of return to work on breastfeeding, *Pediatrics* 127:e1414–e1427, 2011.

31. Ortiz J, McGilligan K, Kelly P: Duration of breast milk expression among working mothers enrolled in an employer-sponsored lactation program, *Pediatr Nurs* 30 (2):111–119, 2004.

32. *Report of the Surgeon General's workshop on breastfeeding and human lactation, Lawrence RA (chair), DHHS Pub. No. HRS-D-MC 84-2*, Washington, D.C., 1984, Department of Health and Human Services.

33. Report 25th Anniversary of the Surgeon General's Workshop on Breastfeeding and Human Lactation: Summit #1 on Breastfeeding: Breastfeeding Medicine 4(Suppl 4), 2009.

34. Ryan AS, Wenjun Z, Acosta A: Breastfeeding continues to increase into the new millennium, *Pediatrics* 110:1103, 2002.

35. Ryan AS, Zhou WJ, Arensberg MB: The effect of employment status on breastfeeding in the United States, *Women Health Issues* 16(5):243–251, 2006.

36. Schanler RJ, editor: *Breastfeeding handbook for physicians*, Elk Grove Village, Ill., 2006, American Academy of Pediatrics.

37. Shealy KR, Li R, Benton-Davis S, et al: *The CDC guide to breastfeeding interventions*, Atlanta, 2005, US Department of Health and Human Services CDC.

38. Slusser WM, Lange L, Dickson V, et al: Breast milk expression in the workplace: a look at frequency and time, *J Hum Lact* 20:164–169, 2004.

39. Suyes K, Abrahams SW, Labbok MH: Breastfeeding in the workplace: other employees' attitudes towards services for lactating mothers, *Int Breastfeed J* 3:25–30, 2008.

40. Taveras EM, Capra AM, Braverman PA, et al: Clinician support and psychosocial risk factors associated with breastfeeding discontinuation, *Pediatrics* 112(1):108–115, 2003.

41. U.S. Breastfeeding Committee: *Workplace breastfeeding support*, http://usbfg.org (Accessed 07.07.10.).

42. U.S. Department of Health and Human Services, Health Resources and Services Administration's (HRSA), Maternal and Child Bureau (MCHB): *Implementing the business case for breastfeeding*, 2008. CD ROM available.

43. U.S. Department of Labor: *Office of the secretary: facts on women workers*, Washington, D.C., 2008, Women's Bureau.

44. United States Department of Labor, Wage and Hour Division. Break Time for Nursing Mothers Fact Sheet #73. http://www.dol.gov/whd/nursingmothers/.

45. United States Department of Labor. Women's bureau. http://dol.gov/wb/stats/recentfacts.htm, 2013.

46. Whaley SE, Meehan K, Lange L, et al: Predictors of breastfeeding duration for employees of the Special Supplemental Nutrition Program for Women, Infants, and Children (WIC), *Am J Obstet Gynecol* 102:1290, 2002.

47. Working Mother Magazine: *Working mother—the 100 best, 2003*. www.workingmother.com/oct03/100BestList.html 2003 (Accessed 07.07.10.).

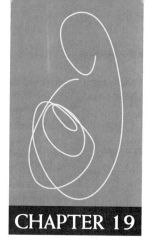

Induced Lactation and Relactation (Including Nursing an Adopted Baby) and Cross-Nursing

As breastfeeding has returned to being the preferred form of nourishment for the infant, there has been an increased interest in induced lactation. Induced lactation is the process by which a nonpuerperal woman is stimulated to lactate—in other words, breastfeeding without pregnancy. Relactation is the process by which a woman who has given birth but did not initially breastfeed is stimulated to lactate. This may also apply to a mother who may have initially breastfed her infant, weaned the infant, and then chooses to reinstitute lactation. Relactation can also involve a woman who previously breastfed a biologic child, even years before, and now is adopting a newborn. There are no blinded controlled research studies about either induced lactation or relactation. There are occasional observation reports about successes in a small series of dyads. The process has not been confirmed by clinical trials.[41] The literature is actually meager and predominantly in the animal research field.

Historical Perspective

Induced lactation and relactation are not new concepts but rather are well known to history and to other cultures. The motivation historically has been to provide nourishment for an infant whose mother has died in childbirth or is unable to nurse for some

reason. A friend or relative would take on the care of the child and with it the responsibility to nourish the infant at the breast because no other alternatives were available.

Relactation has been used in times of disaster or epidemics to provide safe nutrition to weaned or motherless infants. Numerous historical accounts of induced lactation are recorded in the medical literature and reviewed in the writings of Brown.[8] Mead[27] recorded the occurrence of relactation in her writings about New Guinea in 1935. Other anthropologists have made similar observations in other preindustrialized societies of women who have not borne children and, after a few weeks of placing the suckling infant to the breast, produce milk adequate to nourish the infant.[36] Until recently, Western world literature reported the phenomenon as an anecdotal report as part of the discussion of aberrant lactation. In 1971, Cohen[13] reported a patient who had been nursing an adopted child successfully for weeks when first seen in his pediatric office.

Today, the interest in induced lactation in the industrialized world stems from a desire on the part of adopting mothers to nurture an adopted child at the breast even though they were unable to carry the infant in utero. The interest in relactation comes from mothers of sick or premature infants who want to breastfeed their infants after the days

The following simple guidelines, developed as a result of experiences reported by several authors and many mothers, may be helpful to physicians in counseling mothers to induce lactation:

1. Before arrival of the baby, initiate frequent, brief manual stimulation of nipples and breasts, increasing time gradually to approximately 10 minutes per session. Initiate mechanical pumping stimulus after 2 weeks or so of manual stimulus, if time permits. Hand pumps usually cause more soreness. Modern electric pumps with milking action and pressure cycling are most effective. Pumps that can be controlled in cycle frequency and strength are best. Double-sided pumps maximize stimulus and save time.
2. On arrival of the baby, depending on the infant's age, limit sucking to breastfeeding, using a lactation supplementer if necessary.
3. Breastfeed before any other nourishment is provided for a given feeding.
4. Avoid stressing baby with hunger.
5. When supplementing, use donor human milk or prepared formula, not cow's milk, with its long stomach-emptying time and potential for allergic response.
6. Avoid rubber nipples and pacifiers to encourage appropriate suckling at breast.
7. Provide other supplements by dropper, spoon, cup, or supplementer.
8. Create a positive atmosphere; "mother the mother."

A trial of oxytocin nasal spray once the infant is established at the breast may facilitate let-down and even encourage prolactin release.

Rigid conformity to a system of feeding may be a symptom of a more serious problem. Women who are rigid and compulsive may have trouble lactating because of the inability to have a good ejection reflex, which can be inhibited by stress and emotional conflict. Mothers who demonstrate an inordinate attention to volume of production of milk more than the value of the relationship may feel as if they have failed.

WHEN ADOPTING MOTHERS ARE A SAME-SEX COUPLE

- As inducing lactation for an adopted infant by same-sex couples has become more common, so has the desire to breastfeed the infant by both women in a lesbian relationship.
- Physiologically inducing lactation is usually possible for both women although often one is more successful than the other. A case is reported by Wilson et al. in which both adopting women and the biologic mother breastfed the infant.

Milk induction was stimulated with hormones, domperidone, and scheduled breast pumping. Defining parental roles was complex and maintenance of milk production was difficult.

- Considerations are complex when the infant of a same-sex couple has been born to one member of the couple by artificial insemination, and both women plan to breastfeed the baby, one by lactation induction.
- A case is reported as an ethical issue when the physician refuses to assist the patient inducing lactation.[46] The conclusion of the ethics consults was that the physician's objections were unfounded. The value to the infant outweighed any objections. It was felt that the objection showed a troubling unfamiliarity with the clinical facts of lactation and a double standard for treating LGBTQ patients and heterosexual patients.[46]

NUTRITIONAL SUPPLEMENTATION

The need to supplement an infant's intake while the milk supply is being developed should be discussed. An older infant who has already been receiving solid foods can be continued on solids by spoon with careful attention to nutritional content so that the diet includes a balance of protein and other nutrients. Supplements with milk or formula should be appropriate to the age of the infant. The infant younger than 12 months should receive infant formula rather than whole milk if donor breast milk is not available. The milk supplements should be full strength, 20 kcal/oz, and provided during the feeding by dropper or supplementer or after the nursing by dropper, spoon, or cup in preference to artificial nipple, which may confuse the infant during adaptation to nursing at the breast.

POSTMENOPAUSAL LACTATION

Women have had infants after menopause thanks to modern fertility techniques and hormone therapy. The question, "Can they breastfeed?" arises. They will require maintenance hormone therapy paralleling levels in postpartum lactating women. The oxytocin and prolactin should respond with removal of the placenta and suckling of the infant at the breast. Three cases have been reported to the lactation center in which producing milk was successful. No long-term follow-up was available.

A postmenopausal woman may wish to induce lactation. Some of these women are young and had surgical menopause; however, most of them had emergency hysterectomies and still retain their ovaries. The situations are different; the treatment is different.

In natural menopause, the woman may be on hormone replacement therapy, which should be modified to match pregnancy levels of estrogen and progesterone. A program of regular systematic dual pumping should be initiated with the addition of galactagogues, such as domperidone, after the breast has responded with enlargement and turgescence and the first drops of milk. The woman who has retained her ovaries can be managed in the same manner as a premenopausal woman.

SUPPORT SYSTEMS

The process of induced lactation requires considerable commitment and determination.[48] It is far more arduous a task than initiating postpartum lactation, but it is possible and worth the effort, according to the many mothers who have attempted it. The situation is better managed if a doula is available. It is appropriate for a physician to suggest that, in addition to medical support, the mother seek counseling from a licensed, certified lactation consultant experienced in induced lactation. Day-by-day contact for verbal support may be helpful, and these needs may be beyond the scope of a busy office practice unless there is a lactation consultant on staff. A nurse practitioner may be invaluable in this situation, particularly if home visits are made.

Ensuring that the child grows appropriately is the responsibility of a pediatrician; however, this task is best carried out in a nonthreatening way so a mother can concentrate on nurturing and nourishing the infant.[17] Monitoring the usual growth parameters of weight and height as well as the patterns of voiding and stooling is essential.

PROTOCOLS FOR INDUCED LACTATION

The Newman-Goldfarb protocols were developed by Dr. Jack Newman and Ms. Lenore Goldfarb and are on the website Ask Lenore at http://www.asklenore.info/bfg/induced_lactation/regular. Also available are protocols for induced lactation with accelerated menopause. The protocols use hormonal stimulus using birth control pills and domperidone initially until the breasts have responded and enlarged; pumping is initiated within 1 month of the beginning of feeding. Various herbs recognized as galactagogues are also added.[31] Domperidone is not available in the United States by FDA mandate.[43] The authors point out that starting 9 months before the baby arrives is ideal preparation time. They also provide information for more rapid induction. They do not recommend pumping until the hormone treatment has been effective. They recommend stopping the

hormones as pumping is begun. Domperidone is maintained throughout. A woman should always consult her own physician before starting any protocol or trying any medication, hormones, or herbs.

Relactation

Relactation has assumed new significance as the plans for disaster preparedness are reviewed. World attention has been drawn to major disasters, hurricanes, earthquakes, tsunamis, tornadoes, and fires that leave infants without their mothers to nurse them. The drama has allowed people to recognize the value and safety of human milk and breastfeeding when simple things like clean water, sanitation, heat, and light are not available. Brown[8] recalls the 100,000 orphans in the city of Saigon, many of whom were newborns. In times of disaster surrogate mothers were housed in orphanages, fed well, and received a daily dose of chlorpromazine for a week. Many women were able to nourish two babies.

The need to relactate exists in a number of circumstances, including the following:

1. A sick or premature infant cannot be fed initially, or at all, until several weeks or months old (Figure 19-3).
2. An infant is weaned prematurely because of illness in the infant or in the mother.
3. An infant who was not previously breastfed develops an allergy or food intolerance.
4. A mother who has lactated weeks, months, or years earlier wants to nurse an adopted infant.
5. A mother who is nursing a biologic child wants to nurse an adopted child (without benefit of pregnancy).
6. A town or village is in a time of crisis in the area and infants need clean safe food.

Historical reviews provide many examples of infants suckled in times of crisis by women who have not lactated for years. The process of reestablishing lactation under these circumstances is generally easier than that of nonpuerperal lactation. Investigations have shown that a breast that has been previously primed by pregnancy to respond to prolactin will produce milk more readily (Table 19-4).

Relactation was reported in a series of 15 mothers being managed in a clinic in Davangere, Karnataka, India, who had stopped breastfeeding for 2 weeks or more.[6] The mothers had stopped because they thought they did not have enough milk and began supplementing. The management began immediately with putting the infant to the breast 10 to 12 times per day for at least 10 to 15 minutes on each breast. Key to success was the pouring of milk (formula or donor milk) by

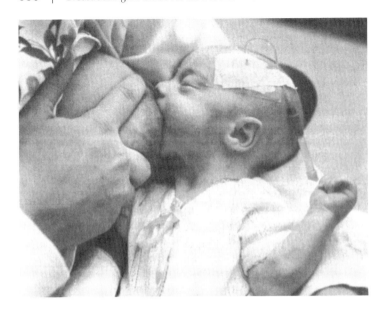

Figure 19-3. Premature infant at breast: infant weighed 1300 g at time of photograph.

TABLE 19-4	Historical and Clinical Data of Mothers in Relactation Study						
Case No.	Gestational Age	Time from Delivery to Entry into Study (days)	Time from Last Lactation to Entry into Study (days)	Postpartum Breast Involution*	Time to First Breast Milk (days)	Time to Half Breast Milk Supply† (days)	Time to Complete Relactation (days)
1	Term	10	10	None	1	4	8
2	Term	120	120	Incomplete	4	20	28
3‡	Twins, 31 wk	49	49	Complete	7	28	Never
4	32 wk	70	42	Complete	7	39	Never
5	28 wk	150	135	Complete	9	Never	Never
6	32 wk	30	16	None	4	17	58
7	Term (adopted)	5 yr	5 yr	Complete	21	Never	Never

*Mothers were asked if their brassiere size was different from that before this pregnancy.
†Estimated on the basis of a decrease in formula intake.
‡Ceased to suckle her infants after 28 days in the study to return to full-time employment.
From Bose CL, D'Ercole J, Lester AG, et al: Relactation by mothers of sick and premature infants, *Pediatrics* 67:565, 1981.

spoon or small cup by a helper (a nurse or relative). The amount of milk dripped over the breast was reduced as a mother's supply increased until the process could be stopped. The group of mothers included two with premature infants and two surrogate mothers who had not breastfed for 16 and for 6 years, respectively. Milk appeared at 7 and 8 days of pumping and exclusive breastfeeding was accomplished in 45 and 40 days. Follow-up and support was intense. Babies were seen and weighed weekly. Ten of the 15 were exclusively breastfed and five continued with some supplementation. The authors encourage clinicians to initiate relactation whenever a mother thinks her supply has dwindled.

These protocols have not been tested with placebo-controlled blinded studies but reflect the experience of a number of practitioners.

PSYCHOLOGIC FACTORS

Although the general process of nipple stimulation, having the infant suckle the breast, and setting the stage for lactation is similar, a woman who has experienced successful lactation previously may have not only the physiologic but also the psychologic edge. As Jelliffe[19] wrote, "Breastfeeding is a confidence game."

A prospective study of mothers whose infants were in the neonatal intensive care unit in Durham, North Carolina, was reported by Bose et al.[7] The profile of the mothers is listed in Table 19-4. Mother and baby were admitted to the clinical research unit, where they were assisted with relactating, including help using the Lact-Aid. The infant's nutritional intake was recorded. Mother and infant were discharged when the mother was comfortable with the Lact-Aid and feeding was established (approximately 3 days). Follow-up occurred every week or two. All but one infant were initially reluctant to suckle, but all received their entire nutritional intake at the breast, with or without Lact-Aid, within the first week of the study. Most of the mothers had trouble initiating suckling, with the most significant factor being the length of separation from their infants and not the degree of prematurity, postnatal age, weight, or feeding regimen. Nipple tenderness occurred in all mothers, but it was transient. All the mothers (except number seven, who was an adoptive mother) produced milk in 1 week, with maximum milk production occurring from 8 to 58 days, proportional to the time since delivery.

Although it was done with a small population, this study established some important information. Given appropriate techniques and support, many women appear to be able to relactate, and premature infants can learn to breastfeed after initial bottle feeding.

A retrospective study of relactation was reported by Auerbach and Avery[3] in which 366 women responded with a completed questionnaire of more than 500 contacted from a list of names obtained from manufacturers' lists, magazine ads, and requests to breastfeeding support groups. The bias was in favor of well-educated, affluent women who had probably obtained their lactation goals. The population included those who had untimely weaning ($n = 174$), after delivery of low-birth-weight infants ($n = 117$), and after hospitalization of mother or baby or both ($n = 75$).

An infant's willingness to nurse was related to previous suckling experience, but responses in the first week of effort were not directly correlated with ultimate successful suckling. After 1 month, 50% of mothers were able to discontinue supplementing; however, 24% were never able to eliminate supplements completely. Once established, the nursing patterns were similar to those of ordinary breastfeeding. The authors[3] point out that keeping the baby hungry in the mistaken notion that the infant will nurse more often and for longer periods does not help and may negatively influence outcome. It is of interest that fewer than 10% of respondents felt that they had received helpful advice from health care professionals.

Relactation in mothers of children older than 12 months of age was reported.[33,41] Six Australian children 12 to 18 months of age had been weaned by the mothers, with no further stimulus to the breast, and then were reinitiated to breastfeeding. The length of time without breastfeeding ranged from 1 week to 6 months (Table 19-5). All the

TABLE 19-5 Relactation in Mothers of Children Older Than 12 Months of Age

Case No.	Age of Child	Length of Time Off Breast	Methods	Evidence of Presence of Milk	How Long from Relactation to Weaning	Age at Final Weaning
1	48 mo	4 mo	Child suckled from breast Mother relaxed, not anxious over outcome	Child verbally reported presence of milk Mother saw whitish milk	After milk appeared	48 mo
2	12 mo	1 wk	Child took four feeds daily	Milk had not quite dried up	1 yr	2 yr
3	20½ mo	2½ mo	Mother gave in to demands of child and suckled her	Mother noticed child's swallowing while breastfeeding	>10 mo	Sometime after 2½ yr
4	2 yr	1 mo	Child suckled from both breasts avidly	Mother saw the milk flow was enough to soak the bed next morning Mother heard swallowing	Approx. 1 yr	>3 yr
5	>3 yr	6 wk	Child suckled from both breasts	Mother saw the milk Mother noticed swallowing	Approx. 2 yr	5 yr
6	Approx. 2 yr	Approx. 6 mo	Mother attached child to breast to demonstrate	Mother began to feel let-down of milk	12 mo	Almost 3 yr

From Phillips N: Relactation in mothers of children over 12 months, *J Trop Pediatr* 39:45, 1993.

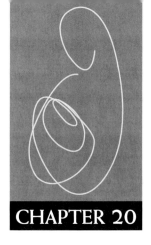

CHAPTER 20

Reproductive Function During Lactation

Complete and in-depth discussion of contraception during breastfeeding is provided in the Academy of Breastfeeding Medicine Protocol #13, recently revised by two of the Academy's most knowledgeable members on the subject.

Fertility

The understanding of the underlying mechanisms of infertility and fertility return during lactation has been increasing in the last 30 years, with studies of both animal and human models. Much has been learned from comparing the lactating and nonlactating hormonal physiology and from the study of the associated brain peptides. Although we understand more today, many significant questions remain.

LACTATIONAL INFERTILITY

The prolonged postpartum infertility associated with lactation has been attributed to changes in the hypothalamic-pituitary-ovarian axis mediated by gonadotropin secretion. Frequent suckling at the breast causes changes in gonadotropin-releasing hormone (GnRH), which impacts anterior pituitary hormone and disorganizes the pulsatility and levels of luteinizing hormone (LH) and follicle-stimulating hormone (FSH), disallowing the rhythmic patterns that result in ovulation. Frequent suckling also results in high prolactin levels; however, the role of prolactin in fertility suppression is less clear.[42]

Figure 20-1 illustrates the menstrual cycle and gonadotropic control. Key points include the following:

1. Follicular development is initiated by pituitary gonadotropin FSH.
2. Continued growth requires FSH and estradiol from the growing follicle in response to LH, which is released in a pulsatile fashion from the pituitary.
3. At midcycle, an increase in estradiol triggers the release of preovulatory surges of LH and FSH.
4. The follicle secretes predominantly progesterone (luteinization).
5. The oocyte is released 36 hours later.

The pulsatile release of GnRH from the hypothalamus stimulates the release of LH. In the cycling woman, estrogen increases GnRH secretion, and the combination of progesterone and estrogen decreases it.[42]

The postpartum period, however, is characterized hormonally by elevated levels of prolactin and low levels of gonadotropins, resulting in anovulation and amenorrhea. During breastfeeding, this state can persist for an extended period, even though prolactin levels decrease over time. As currently understood, the pulsatile secretion of GnRH is altered by the suckling stimulus, influencing ovarian activity.[42] Although the action of prolactin on multiple target organ sites has frequently been suggested as the cause of this ovarian quiescence, it appears that a suckling-induced alteration in hypothalamic GnRH production is the primary mechanism. Zinaman et al. found that when pulsatility is restored during lactation by administering exogenous pulsatile GnRH, LH values increase and FSH levels

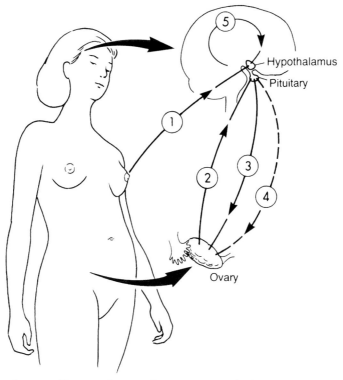

Figure 20-1. Possible mechanisms of lactational amenorrhea: nervous impulse from nipple produces not only a rise in prolactin (1) but also changes in hypothalamic sensitivity to ovarian steroid feedback (2) and changes in gonadotropin-releasing hormone (GnRH) (3), leading to changes in pituitary release of luteinizing hormone and follicle-stimulating hormone (4). Suckling may also stimulate release of β-endorphin (5), thus suppressing GnRH from hypothalamus. (Redrawn from Winikoff B, Semeraro P, Zimmerman M: *Contraception during breastfeeding: a clinician's source book*, New York, 1988, Population Council.)

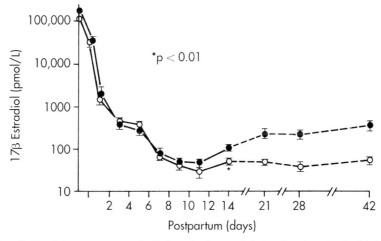

Figure 20-2. 17β-Estradiol levels in postpartum period in lactating (*open circles*) and nonlactating (*solid circles*) women. Levels in lactating women vary with intensity of suckling. (From Neville MC: Regulation of mammary development and lactation. In Neville MC, Neifert MR, editors: *Lactation: physiology, nutrition, and breastfeeding*, New York, 1983, Plenum.)

decrease while pulsatile organization of both increases, and the ovary responds accordingly.

The period of lactational amenorrhea depends on frequency and intensity of suckling (Figures 20-2 to 20-4). In these figures, open circles are lactating subjects, the solid circles are nonlactators postpartum.

Animal studies have shown that the release of FSH and LH is inhibited by intense suckling. In addition, when the nipple is stimulated while the milk ducts have been tied off there is still a suppression of estrous and menstrual cycles. Selye and McKeown[63] concluded that interruption of sexual cyclicity

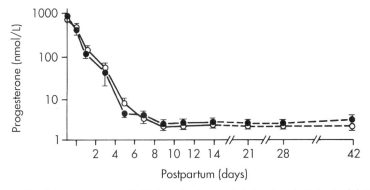

Figure 20-3. Progesterone levels in postpartum period in lactating (*open circles*) and nonlactating (*solid circles*) women. (From Neville MC: Regulation of mammary development and lactation. In Neville MC, Neifert MR, editors: *Lactation: physiology, nutrition, and breastfeeding,* New York, 1983, Plenum.)

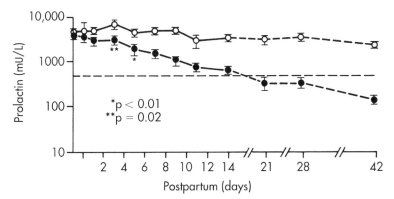

Figure 20-4. Prolactin levels in postpartum period in lactating (*open circles*) and nonlactating (*solid circles*) women. Levels in lactating women vary with intensity of suckling. (From Neville MC: Regulation of mammary development and lactation. In Neville MC, Neifert MR, editors: *Lactation: physiology, nutrition, and breastfeeding,* New York, 1983, Plenum.)

during lactation is a result of the suckling and not of the secretory activity of the mammary gland. This early animal work has stood the test of time. The more the suckling stimulus in frequency and duration, the more consistent is the suppression of ovulation.[42]

The levels of gonadotropin in all postpartum women for the first weeks of the postpartum period are decreased, which substantiates the theory of postpartum ovarian refractoriness. In the first 2 weeks postpartum, low levels of FSH are found in urine and plasma. Estrogen excretion is low with a linear increase during the first 5 to 8 weeks. In a longitudinal study of 48 women, endocrine profiles were assessed with morning blood samples from the first postpartum month until the recovery of ovulation.[13,14] Additional samples were drawn throughout 24 hours at the end of the third postpartum month in 10 exclusively nursing amenorrheic women. Prolactin, LH, FSH, estradiol (E_2), progesterone, cortisol, and dehydroepiandrosterone sulfate were measured. In response to suckling, there was a smaller increase in prolactin and higher levels of E_2 in women who

ovulated within 6 months postpartum compared with those who did not. Diaz et al.[16,17] suggest that this may explain some of the variability in duration of lactational amenorrhea. The greater prolactin response to suckling associated with longer amenorrhea may result from higher sensitivity to the breast-hypothalamus-pituitary system.[16]

PROLACTIN AND DOPAMINE

There is a relationship between lactational infertility and physiologic hyperprolactinemia; however, its role in fertility suppression is not as clear.[14] In an extensive study of prolactin levels in lactating women, Tay et al.[67] measured the pattern of prolactin secretion in relation to suckling and the return of ovarian activity. Blood samples were drawn at 10-minute intervals for 24 hours at 4 and 8 weeks, when weaning was initiated and suckling reduced, at first menses, and in the follicular phase of the first menstrual cycle after weaning. Mothers fed their infants on their usual pattern, with no restrictions or alterations, in an effort to replicate natural lactation.

These data confirmed that with frequent suckling, prolactin levels do not decline significantly between feeds. When suckling became less frequent, prolactin dropped to baseline levels between feeds but surged when suckling was initiated (see Chapter 3). The natural increase in prolactin at night was evident only after weaning. Prolactin also declined greatly in association with suckling after the return of menses. This occurred at 33.6 ± 3.5 weeks postpartum in this study. No relationship was seen between the duration of amenorrhea and plasma prolactin levels throughout a day, at night, or throughout lactation. The timing of the introduction of solids was strongly correlated with the duration of amenorrhea. The authors concluded that no exact link exists between release of prolactin during lactation and the duration of lactational infertility in breastfeeding women.[67]

However, at least one study has identified a differential response to different prolactins.

Another study explored the ability to predict duration of amenorrhea based on parameters during pregnancy. Campino et al.[7] followed 17 women at 34 and 38 weeks' gestation who fully breastfed for at least 6 months. During pregnancy, prolactin, estrogens (total estradiol, unconjugated estrone, unconjugated estriol), sex hormone binding globulin, dehydroepiandrosterone sulfate, progesterone, and placental lactogen, and during postpartum, prolactin, estrogens, and sex hormone binding globulin, were measured. Free estradiol in pregnancy and postpartum was calculated. They found that the 10 women who experienced long lactational amenorrhea (greater than 6 months) had a different hormonal profile during pregnancy than the seven who experienced a short duration (less than 6 months) of lactational amenorrhea. At 38 weeks' gestation, the women who experienced a long lactational amenorrhea had twice as much prolactin, approximately half the total estradiol, significantly lower sex hormone binding globulin concentration, but similar free estradiol concentration compared with those who experienced short lactational amenorrhea. They concluded that at 38 weeks' gestation, the higher ratio of prolactin/estradiol identified all women who would go on to experience a longer duration of their lactational amenorrhea, suggesting that duration of lactational amenorrhea is conditioned during pregnancy.[7]

The inhibition of dopamine secretion from the hypothalamus has been associated with the neural impulses from stimulation of the nipple during lactation. Normally dopamine inhibits the secretion of prolactin, and, conversely, when dopamine is inhibited, prolactin rises. Two pathways of ovulation inhibition are possible as a result of the rise in prolactin. One is a lack of responsiveness to ovarian steroids of the hypothalamic-pituitary axis of a lactating woman, leading to nonpulsatile release of pituitary gonadotropins, FSH, and LH, which in turn results in absent or reduced ovarian activity. FSH may actually be higher at some points; LH is nonpulsatile.

The fact that there are prolactin receptors on the ovary indicates that there may be a second mechanism contributing to the infertility through the impaired ovarian response to gonadotropins[5] (see Figure 20-1).

RETURN OF MENSES

The transition from amenorrhea to regular menstrual cycles is one of the most challenging times while breastfeeding and wishing to use natural family planning. The uncertainty of the onset of ovulation with the return of menses is especially difficult. The efficacy of a new postpartum transition protocol for avoiding pregnancy is reported by Bouchard et al. The use of an electronic hormonal fertility monitor (Clear Blue Easy Fertility Monitor, Swiss Precision Diagnostics, Geneva, Switzerland) identifies the fertile period. It measures changes in urinary estrone-3-glucuronide from baseline and urinary LH above a specific threshold. The device was developed to assist with conception; it has been shown to be equally effective when utilized to avoid pregnancy. The use of an online teaching and charting protocol has potential for avoiding pregnancy postpartum while lactating.

Clinically the proxy for the return of fertility is the onset of menstruation. Return of reproductive function varies depending on the length and degree of lactation. Most studies do not, in fact, report pattern of breastfeeding, that is, whether the infant is fully or exclusively breastfed or is also receiving solid foods or supplemental bottles.[20] By the end of the third month, only 33% of fully lactating women have had a menstrual period, whereas 91% of nonlactating women have had at least one period.[13]

Not all vaginal bleeds are menses; not all bleeds follow ovulation.[21] In 72 fully breastfeeding women studied prospectively from 42 days postpartum, vaginal bleeding was recorded daily if it occurred. Approximately half the women had some bleeding or spotting between 6 and 8 weeks postpartum. Those who experienced this bleeding eventually menstruated and ovulated earlier than those who did not, but differences were not significant. Seven women had ovarian follicular development before day 56, but neither bleeding nor follicular development was associated with ovulation in the first 8 weeks. The authors stated it was unlikely that vaginal bleeding before 8 weeks in a fully breastfeeding woman indicates a return to fertility and, therefore, is not the return of menses.[58]

Perez et al.[55] diagnosed the first postpartum ovulation by endometrial biopsy, basal body temperature, vaginal cytologic evaluation, and cervical mucus in a group of 200 women in a prospective study. The dates of first ovulation, first menses, and nursing status were analyzed. No woman demonstrated signs of ovulation before day 36, whether lactating or not. The intensity of nursing and time postpartum affected ovulation occurrence; 78% of the women ovulated before the first menses, but only 12 pregnancies occurred with first ovulation. Of the 170 women who breastfed, 24 ovulated while completely nursing, 49 while partially nursing, and 97 after weaning.

POSSIBILITY OF CONCEPTION

A nonlactating woman has a return of her period at 25 days at the earliest, a return of ovulation at 25 to 35 days, and a 5% chance of regaining fertility before 6 weeks postpartum.

Risk of ovulation during lactation was studied by Gray et al.[20] in Baltimore and in Manila.[18] During the first 6 months postpartum, amenorrheic women had a low risk of ovulation (less than 10%) with partial breastfeeding and a 1% to 5% risk with exclusive breastfeeding with either frequent short feeds or infrequent longer feeds. This would have resulted in a pregnancy rate of 2% and 1%, respectively.

In a detailed study of 130 women in Chile, Diaz et al.[17] found the cumulative probability of pregnancy at the end of 6 months postpartum in women who were exclusively nursing and amenorrheic to be 1.8%. For exclusively nursing women who had a return of menses it was 27.2%, and for those partially nursing it was 40.5%.

Although many investigators continue to evaluate the impact of lactation on ovulation and menstruation, the fundamental observations remain the same[68] (Table 20-1). Available data on return of ovulation and menstruation can be summarized as follows[60]:

I. Nursing mothers
   A. Ovulation generally occurs before menses return and varies 14% to 75%.
   B. The longer the first menses is delayed, the more likely the first cycle will be ovulatory.
   C. Continued suckling and elevated prolactin levels produce inadequate luteal function in first cycles.
   D. Exclusive breastfeeding: First bleed generally precedes ovulation return, and if an ovulation occurs it is generally inadequate for conception.
II. Nonnursing mothers
   A. Earliest possible menstruation is 4 weeks postpartum.

TABLE 20-1	Relative Risk for Ovulation in Relation to Breastfeeding Frequency*
Average Number of Feeds per Day	**Relative Risk**
0	1.0
1	0.62
2	0.43
3	0.28
4	0.19
5	0.12
6	0.08
7	0.05
8	0.04
9	0.02
10	0.01

*Breastfeeding episodes per day before ovulation: $p < 0.0001$.
From Gray RH, Campbell O, Eslamic S, et al: The return of ovarian function during lactation: results of studies from the United States and the Philippines. In Gray R, Leridon H, Spira A, editors: *Biomedical and demographic determinants of reproduction*, Oxford, 1993, Clarendon.

   B. Most women are menstruating by third month postpartum.
   C. Return of menstruation
      1. 6 weeks postpartum: 40%
      2. 12 weeks postpartum: 65%
      3. 24 weeks postpartum: 90%
   D. Earliest possible ovulation is 3½ to 5 weeks postpartum.
   E. Ovular cycles occur in 50% with first menstrual period postpartum.
   F. Early postpartum ovulation may occur late in menstrual cycle: Shortening of secretory phase and greater tendency toward irregular menses.
   G. Return of ovulation
      1. 6 weeks postpartum: 15%
      2. 12 weeks postpartum: 40%
      3. 24 weeks postpartum: 75%
III. Amenorrheic nonnursing mothers: Return of ovulation
   A. 12 weeks postpartum: 20%
   B. 16 weeks postpartum: 40%

MILK COMPOSITION DURING THE OVULATORY MENSTRUAL CYCLE

Acute changes in the composition of milk during the ovulatory menstrual cycle in lactating women were studied by Hartmann and Prosser[23] involving women during lactational amenorrhea, taking oral contraceptives, and during an ovulatory menstrual

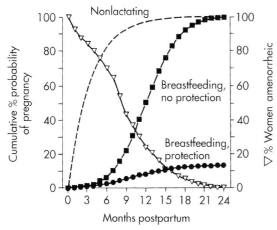

Figure 20-5. Cumulative probability of pregnancy during breastfeeding. —, Nonlactating women of normal fertility having unprotected intercourse; ■, breastfeeding women having unprotected intercourse throughout 24 months of lactation; ●, breastfeeding women having unprotected intercourse only during lactational amenorrhea and adopting effective contraceptive measures at resumption of menstruation. Percentage of women in lactational amenorrhea by month postpartum (∇) is also shown. (From Short RY, Lewis PR, Renfree MB, et al: Contraceptive effects of extended lactational amenorrhea: beyond the Bellagio consensus, *Lancet* 337:715, 1991.)

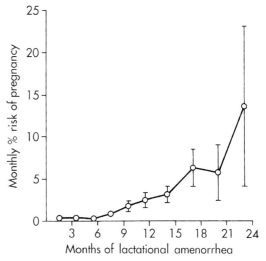

Figure 20-6. Monthly percentage probability of pregnancy during lactational amenorrhea with estimated standard errors. With cumulative percentage probability of pregnancy by months postpartum for these three groups of women, 50% of nonlactating women would be pregnant in less than 3 months, and 85% would be pregnant by 6 months. (From Short RY, Lewis PR, Renfree MB, et al: Contraceptive effects of extended lactational amenorrhea: beyond the Bellagio consensus, *Lancet* 337:715, 1991.)

cycle. Samples of milk were collected from each breast at each feed for each day for 28 days.

During the ovulatory menstrual cycle, two acute changes occurred. For the 5 to 6 days before ovulation and the 6 to 7 days after ovulation, the sodium and chloride values changed from 4.6 mM Na and 11.1 mM Cl to 10.1 and 22.0, respectively, and lactose and potassium decreased. The concentrations of lactose, Cl, K, and Na remained relatively constant during lactational amenorrhea, anovulatory menstrual cycles, and for those women taking oral contraceptives. The authors conclude that an increase in the permeability of the mammary epithelium was effected by changes related to ovulation. Perhaps the first acute change in composition is associated with the final stages of follicle maturation and the second with the regression of the corpus luteum during the ovulatory menstrual cycle (Figures 20-5 and 20-6).[66]

Nutritional status has virtually no effect on amenorrhea, except in the extremes. In a study of Guatemalan women, maternal energy supplements did not shorten length of lactational amenorrhea; however, supplementing their breastfed infants did shorten amenorrhea by reducing suckling. A difference exists between postpartum and nutritional amenorrhea: true nutritional amenorrhea is predictable on the basis of the height/weight ratio; lactational amenorrhea is hormonal, and when it occurs, nutrition has only a trivial role.[31]

BREASTFEEDING AND BIRTH INTERVAL

Among !Kung hunter-gatherers, long intervals pass between births, which has puzzled investigators because the tribes are well nourished, have low fetal wastage, and do not employ contraceptives or prolonged abstinence. The !Kung eat only what they hunt and gather. They have no agriculture. They are lean, spare people. They have late menarche (approximately 16 years of age), first pregnancy at age 18, and early menopause at approximately 40, leaving 24 reproductive years during which they produce 4.4 children, which, with some perinatal deaths, exactly replaces their society. This compares with industrial society, where productive years begin at 11 and end at 51. Konner and Worthman[35] report that the !Kung have unusual temporal patterns of nursing characterized by highly frequent nursing bouts with short space between nursings. The !Kung nurse several times an hour with only 15 minutes at most between bouts, which last only 15 to 120 seconds each. Serum estradiol and progesterone levels are correspondingly low. Infants are always in the immediate proximity of their mothers until they are weaned, at approximately 3½ years, during a new sibling's gestation.

In Nigeria, the effect of duration and frequency of breastfeeding on postpartum amenorrhea is comparable in that Nigerians breastfeed for 16.5 months with a frequency of 4.5 times a day. The mean length of amenorrhea is 12.5 months. Amenorrheic mothers who were lactating had lower levels of serum estradiol and lactic dehydrogenase. A significant association was seen between hyperprolactinemia with amenorrhea. The incidence of amenorrhea declined parallel to that of the hyperprolactinemia.

When fertility postpartum during lactation was studied in Edinburgh, suckling was the most important factor inhibiting the return to ovulation.[49] Suckling duration was the first factor to discriminate the mothers who experienced early ovulation. Those mothers who ovulated while breastfeeding had introduced two or more supplementary feeds per day and had reduced suckling to less than six times per day, with 60 minutes or less suckling time per day. The basal prolactin levels were less than 600 mU/L. The mothers who did not ovulate until after 40 weeks postpartum breastfed longest, suckled most intensely, maintained night feeds longest, and introduced supplementary feeds most slowly.[20] The prolactin levels remained substantially greater than 600 mU/L.

Another review of the effects of hormonal contraceptives on lactation by Hull[43] concludes that a significant number of reports indicate decrease in milk yield. The description of severe growth failure[16] in the nursling, even leading to "contraceptive marasmus," in Egypt and Tunisia is cause for concern.

Most large studies of birth interval and its relationship to method of feeding have been conducted in developing countries. However, Rosner and Schulman[60] reported on 112 Orthodox Jewish women from metropolitan New York with 266 birth experiences. The women strictly adhered to biblical and Rabbinic law that prohibits birth control. They were well-nourished, middle-class, educated women who breastfed on demand (210 infants) for a mean duration of 10.7 months, with 177 of the infants receiving formula less than once

a week. Significant positive correlations were found with duration of lactational amenorrhea, which increased as duration of breastfeeding increased. Delay in starting solids, continuation of night feedings, and postponement of other liquid feeds all were associated with prolongation of birth interval. The investigators found a longer mean duration of lactational amenorrhea (8.6 months) and mean birth interval (22 months) than other studies because of the more intensive feeding patterns[60] (Table 20-2).

Contraception During Lactation

MEDICAL ELIGIBILITY CRITERIA FOR CONTRACEPTIVE USE

WHO's Medical Eligibility Criteria for Contraceptive Use provides recommendations for policy makers to help rationalize the provision of various contraceptives in relation to the most up-to-date information available on the safety of the methods for people with certain health conditions. The document covers the following family planning methods: low-dose combined oral contraceptives (COCs), combined patch (P), combined vaginal ring (R), combined injectable contraceptives (CICs), progestin-only pills (POPs), depot medroxyprogesterone acetate (DMPA), norethindrone enanthate (NET-EN), levonorgestrel (LNG) and etonogestrel (ETG) implants, emergency contraceptive pills (ECPs), copper-bearing intrauterine devices (Cu-IUDs), levonorgestrel-releasing IUDs (LNG-IUDs), copper IUD for emergency contraception (E-IUD), barrier methods (BARR), fertility awareness-based methods (FAB), lactational amenorrhea method

| TABLE 20-2 | Comparison of Studies of Breastfeeding and Its Relationship to Birth Interval When Practiced in Absence of Birth Control |

Study	Mean Duration of Breastfeeding (mo)	Mean Lactational Amenorrhea (mo)	Mean Birth Interval (mo)
Bonte and van Balen[59]	N/A	15.2	25.2
Berman et al.[59]	7.0	7.1	21.6
Prema et al.[59]	19.8	11.1	23.8
Perez[59,*]	4.0	3.03[†]	N/A
Gioiosa[59]	10.27	N/A	21.92
Rosner and Schulman[59]	10.74	8.56	21.95
Adnan and Bakr[59]	36.0	12.0	N/A
Howie et al.[59]	10.0	8.1	N/A
Ojofeitimi[59]	16.5	12.5	N/A

N/A, Not available.

*Women did introduce family planning after menses return or after supplementation after 6 months.

†First postpartum ovulation.

Modified from Rosner AE, Schulman SK: Birth interval among breastfeeding women not using contraceptives, *Pediatrics* 86:747, 1990.

(LAM), coitus interruptus (CI), and female and male sterilization (STER).

The goal of this document is to provide policy- and decision-makers and the scientific community with a set of recommendations that can be used for developing or revising national guidelines on medical eligibility criteria for contraceptive use.[77,78]

LACTATIONAL AMENORRHEA METHOD

The Bellagio Consensus Conference[11] on breastfeeding as a family planning method established that a mother who is fully or nearly fully breastfeeding her infant and remains amenorrheic will have more than 98% protection from pregnancy in the first 6 months postpartum.[9,25,30] This was codified as a method of family planning the following year at a meeting at an international conference at Georgetown University.[13,37] The first study of the method per se found that only one woman in a study of 422 middle-class urban women in Chile became pregnant using the LAM as the only method of pregnancy avoidance in the first 6 months,[13,27] a protective rate of 99.5% (see Figures 20-5 and 20-6).

Menses as an indicator of ovulation has been studied with data collected not only on onset of menses but on urinary hormone assays. Among women who menstruated before 6 months postpartum, 67% of cycles were anovulatory, and the lag between anovular first menses and subsequent ovulation was 15.7 weeks.[16] On the other hand, after 6 months postpartum, the proportion of anovular first menses declined to 22%, and the lag to ovulation declined to 7.3 weeks. Comparing all menstrual episodes, the mean interval between first observed menses and ovulation was 8.4 weeks in the first 6 months and only 0.1 week after 6 months postpartum.

A significant distinction should be made between token breastfeeding with early solids and more rigid feeding schedules and the ad lib breastfeeding around the clock with no solids until the infant is 6 months old.[6] The amount and frequency of sucking are closely related to the continued amenorrhea in most women. When a totally breastfed infant sleeps through the night at an early age, requiring no suckling for 6 hours or so at night, the suppressive effect on menses diminishes. It has also been shown that if the infant uses a pacifier rather than receiving nonnutritive sucking at the breast, the suppression of ovulation is diminished.[37]

The degree of fertility inhibition associated with breastfeeding has decreased remarkably since the time of hunter-gatherers, cautions Diaz et al.[17] She points out that fertility rates vary; population and socioeconomic factors, urbanization, and nutrition influence not only breastfeeding patterns but associated ovarian quiescence. Lactational amenorrhea can provide protection against pregnancy for the first 6 months even in well-nourished women who are giving the infant some supplemental foods[32-34](Figure 20-7). For women who practice

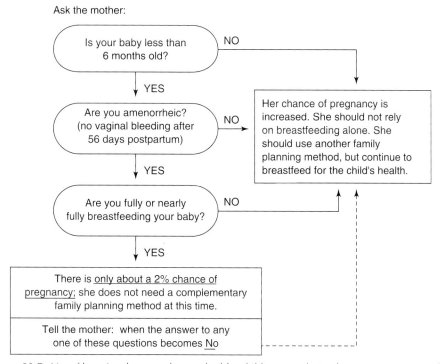

Ask the mother:

Is your baby less than 6 months old? — NO →

↓ YES

Are you amenorrheic? (no vaginal bleeding after 56 days postpartum) — NO →

↓ YES

Are you fully or nearly fully breastfeeding your baby? — NO →

↓ YES

Her chance of pregnancy is increased. She should not rely on breastfeeding alone. She should use another family planning method, but continue to breastfeed for the child's health.

There is only about a 2% chance of pregnancy; she does not need a complementary family planning method at this time.

Tell the mother: when the answer to any one of these questions becomes No

Figure 20-7. Use of lactational amenorrhea method for child spacing during first 6 postpartum months.

LAM, the efficacy is remarkably good (Table 20-3). Table 20-4 details the reestablishment of menses in breastfeeding women using LAM. *Bellagio and Beyond: Breastfeeding and LAM in Reproductive Health* was published as a final report in 1997 of the many years of work worldwide involving the use of LAM.[13] It was concluded that the efficacy of LAM is well established in prospective studies. Policy support is still needed to institute an additional method that increases the family planning choices of postpartum women.[10]

TABLE 20-3 Life Table Analysis of Lactational Amenorrhea Method Efficacy*

Month	No. of Pregnancies	WM	WMAC	R×100	P×100
1	0	384	384	0.00	0.00
2	0	327	711	0.00	0.00
3	0	272	983	0.00	0.00
4	0	243	1226	0.00	0.00
5	0	224	1450	0.00	0.00
6	1	221	1671	0.45	0.45

WM, Number of women using lactational amenorrhea method; *WMAC,* cumulative women-months of use; *R × 100,* monthly risk of conception; *P× 100,* cumulative risk of conception.

*Characteristics of women: Mean age (SEM; range) was 27.1 years (5.0; 18 to 39). Mean parity (SEM; range) was 2.0 (1.0; 1 to 5). 23.6% of the women had primary education, and only 5.4% had completed university studies.

From Perez A, Labbok MH, Queenan JT: Clinical study of the lactational amenorrhoea method for family planning, *Lancet* 339:968, 1992.

TABLE 20-4 Life Table of Reestablishment of Menses among Exclusively Breastfeeding Women Using Lactational Amenorrhea Method*

Month	Bleeding	WM	WMAC	R×100	P×100
1	0	384	384	0.00	0.00
2	8	327	711	2.45	2.42
3	18	272	983	6.62	8.67
4	11	243	1226	4.55	12.72
5	10	224	1450	4.46	16.53
6	6	221	1671	2.73	18.78

WM, Number of women using lactational amenorrhea method; *WMAC,* cumulative women-months of use; *R × 100,* monthly bleeding risk; *P× 100,* cumulative risk of bleeding.

*Characteristics of women: mean age (SEM; range) was 27.1 years (5.0; 18 to 39); mean parity (SEM; range) was 2.0 (1.0; 1 to 5); 23.6% of women had primary education, and only 5.4% had completed university studies.

From Perez A, Labbok MH, Queenan JT: Clinical study of the lactational amenorrhoea method for family planning, *Lancet* 339:968, 1992.

Gray et al.[21] studied a population of women in Baltimore in comparison to a group from Manila. Those in the Baltimore group were older, more educated, more frequently employed, and had fewer children. Women in Manila breastfed more frequently (at 10 weeks postpartum: 11.4 feeds in Manila versus 7.1 feeds in Baltimore). The mean duration of amenorrhea was 31.7 weeks versus 26.3 weeks, and mean delays before first ovulation were 38 versus 27 weeks (Manila and Baltimore, respectively). The frequency of suckling episodes was most strongly associated with ovulation in the Baltimore population, where small declines in breastfeeding were sufficient to permit the return of ovarian activity. Women in Manila, in contrast, maintained high suckling rates even when solids were introduced. More Baltimore women (49%) than Manila women (31%) ovulated before 6 months. There was no simple algorithm, however, to predict ovulation.[21,69]

The effects of age at introduction of complementary foods to breastfed infants on duration of lactational amenorrhea in Honduran women were reported by Dewey et al.[15] Introducing foods at 4 months significantly affected the likelihood of amenorrhea at 6 months but not thereafter. This effect was not seen, however, if breastfeeding frequency was maintained. The most significant determination of lactational amenorrhea was time spent breastfeeding (minutes per day), which was negatively associated with the infant's energy intake from complementary foods (Figure 20-8).

In a large prospective study of duration of lactational anovulation and amenorrhea in well-nourished Australian women—members of the Nursing Mothers' Association of Australia who

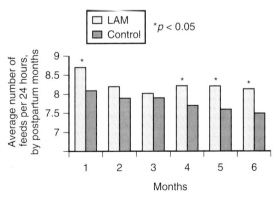

Figure 20-8. Average number of feeds per 24 hours by postpartum month. Lactational amenorrhea method may achieve higher efficacy than lactational amenorrhea as users of the lactational amenorrhea method would appear to practice a slightly more frequent pattern of feeding than fully lactating amenorrheic nonusers. Labbok M: Breastfeeding, birth spacing and family planning. In Hartmann PE, Hale TW, editors: *Hale and Hartmann's textbook of human lactation,* Amarillo, Tex., 2007, Hale Publishing.

breastfed for a long time—Short et al.[65] found that breastfeeding alone is not an effective form of contraception because all the women resumed ovulation while still breastfeeding. They compared breastfeeding women who had unprotected sex with breastfeeding women who had unprotected sex only during lactational amenorrhea and adopted other contraceptive measures after resumption of menstruation. Only 1.7% became pregnant during the first 6 months of amenorrhea, only 7% after 12 months, and 13% after 24 months.

Subsequent studies of the method show a range of high efficacies from studies in many countries. Comparisons of follicular development and hormonal profiles are important to understanding lactational amenorrhea. There is a profound dissociation between follicular growth and follicular endocrine activity, which suggests an alteration in the stimulus-response relationship at the follicular level according to Velasquez et al.[72,73] Serum FSH polymorphism during lactational amenorrhea was also studied by Velasquez et al. who concluded that FSH heterogeneity may be one of the critical factors contributing to incomplete follicular development and an ovulation during lactational amenorrhea.

The natural suppression of ovulation during early lactation and the concomitant amenorrhea induced by exclusive or nearly exclusive breastfeeding provide 98% or higher protection against pregnancy. Three conditions are necessary: amenorrhea, intensive breastfeeding day and night, and up to 6 months of exclusive breastfeeding postpartum. LAM can be used to time the introduction of any complementary method (barrier, etc.; Figure 20-9); it is not just for users of natural family planning.[37–40]

NATURAL FAMILY PLANNING

Although lactation provides protection early in the postpartum period, a woman who is not fully breastfeeding and who is interested in avoiding conception should be informed of her options. If she does not want to use contraceptives—medications or devices—she should be instructed in the external signs of ovulation, including ovulation method, LH-releasing hormone, and home tests.

Pregnancy rates and fertility-related behavior of users of the ovulation method were studied prospectively in Kenya and Chile in two groups of breastfeeding women.[38] The rate of unplanned pregnancy was less than 1% in the first 6 months. The rate of unplanned pregnancies increased after menses had begun and supplementary food was added to the infants' diets. The rates were compared with the rates among nonlactating women who were also using the ovulation method to avoid pregnancy. The breastfeeding women had followed the method closely, although clients who had not used the ovulation method before the pregnancy had an increased incidence of unplanned pregnancy.

One of the difficulties of studying the use/effectiveness and continuation of natural family planning methods is that terms have always been imprecise and markers have been different between studies.[48] The method is effective when properly used (failure rate 3.4%) but unforgiving when use is imperfect (failure rate 84.2% in the first year).[22]

Unplanned pregnancy rates rise among breastfeeders after menses return compared with the rates for those who use thermal or secretion surveillance methods when not lactating.[22] The increased pregnancy rate was related to poor compliance and understanding of the "rules" of the method.[19]

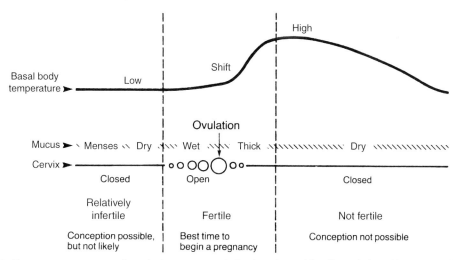

Figure 20-9. Temperature, mucus, and cervical assessments during lactation to identify ovulation. (Courtesy National Family Planning of Rochester, New York.)

The symptothermal method of fertility awareness during lactation was studied in Canada.[49] A special postpartum chart was designed to record morning temperature, cervical mucus, and other signs of fertility/infertility in relation to dates and postpartum days. The intensity of breastfeeding was also recorded. There were 54 breastfeeding experiences in 47 women whose ages ranged from 20 to 39. Parity ranged from 1 to 7, with an average of 3.3. The duration of full breastfeeding averaged 3.6 months (range 3 weeks to 8 months). The duration of partial breastfeeding ranged from 2 to 28 months, with an average of 8.8 months. These mothers found that in general they could predict their fertile times with accuracy while breastfeeding. During times of weaning or change in suckling pattern, special caution was suggested, during which the mothers watched for signs of first ovulation.[50]

The effectiveness of periodic abstinence for lactating women shows that long periods of lactational infertility can be identified by either lack of mucus or continuous unchanging mucus flow.

Cervical mucus accepts, filters, prepares, and releases sperm for successful transport to the egg for fertilization. The advancing sperm must penetrate the mucous structure or the small interstices between the mucous macromolecules. The interstices are largest in the periovular phase of the menstrual cycle.[54] As ovulation resumes, irregular mucous patterns that are difficult to interpret occur and, therefore, prolonged abstinence is required. A pregnancy rate with this method was 9.1 per 100 women-years. Because two thirds of the 82 women studied were totally breastfeeding, many of the ensuing postpartum cycles may have been anovulatory or had an inadequate luteal phase, thus helping to keep the pregnancy rate low.

Studies of cervical secretions alone (mucous patterns) during lactation have indicated that the same signs in mucus are reliable during lactation.[75] Charting is carried out in the usual manner, and feedings are also recorded. A woman who is following her pattern postpartum should be seen every 2 weeks for guidance until her pattern is well documented. The couple should make careful observations of when (1) the infant sleeps through the night, (2) the mother reduces the number of breastfeedings, (3) the infant begins solid foods, (4) the infant begins other liquids or a bottle, and (5) illness occurs in either mother or baby. Abstinence or LAM use is advised until the situation is clear. If there has been no previous ovulation or menstruation when weaning begins, ovulation may occur quite quickly.[5]

Figure 20-9 illustrates temperature, mucus, and cervical assessments during lactation.

Although contraceptive methods such as barrier methods and "the pill" have a statistically better record in avoiding pregnancy, that is a moot point for a woman for whom these methods are not an option for religious or medical reasons.[1] It is, therefore, important that a clinician be as well informed about natural child spacing as possible so the best advice can be provided. Ideally, the woman has used natural family planning before the pregnancy, so she is familiar with her own patterns, but it is more urgent that she knows how to check her mucus, her cervix, and her temperature, and is not trying to learn about her fertility signs during lactation. Natural family planning programs across the United States are gaining experience with lactating women using the ovulation method and are available to assist lactating women.[28] Further information can be obtained from the National Office of Natural Family Planning, 8514 Bradmoor Drive, Bethesda, MD 20817-3810, (301) 897-9323, if no local office is available; http://www.boma-usa.org and http://www.teenstar.org are the websites for the Billings Ovulation Method Association in the United States.

Natural Family Planning International can be reached at www.nfpandmore.org or at P.O. Box 11216, Cincinnati, OH 45211.

In a carefully designed study conducted in Chile by Perez et al.[55] at the Pontificia Universidad Católica de Chile Department of Obstetrics and Gynecology and by members of the faculty at Johns Hopkins University School of Hygiene and Public Health, 419 postpartum women were enrolled in the Natural Family Planning Program and were taught the method and how to record their observations. The purpose was to define cervical mucus patterns in relation to time since delivery, time of first bleed, frequency of feeding, introduction of supplements and solid foods, and time of weaning. The diaries of 110 women with detailed records were selected for critical evaluation; 49 have been reported and the preliminary observations evaluated by Barker.[1] Two characteristics of mucus (sensation and observation) were charted each day along with the women's breastfeeding patterns. Only seven women had used natural family planning previously. No woman menstruated before 4 months postpartum, when 10% did have first menses. By the fourth month, 50% of the women detected mucus, and not until the seventh month had 50% had first menses. Mucus was observed approximately 2 months before first menses. As women moved from total breastfeeding to partial and to complete weaning, the duration of episodes of mucus increased. Duration of mucus approached normal on weaning.

Rural women exposed to a breastfeeding education program prenatally and postpartum breastfed more and used fewer bottles than the comparison group, who had no training about lactational infertility.[55] However, no difference was seen in postpartum amenorrhea. No measures of ovulation or pregnancy were made. Rural women tend to breastfeed optimally naturally. Supplementary feeding affects the return of menses and ovulation as demonstrated in a study in rural China. There was a positive correlation with the start of solid food and the return of menses and the first ovulation.[76] A Cochran review of lactational amenorrhea for family planning was provided by Van der Wijden et al.[71] who found 459 relevant studies, of which only 159 investigated the risk of pregnancy during lactation and 14 were included. The length of lactational amenorrhea among women using LAM was very different between populations studied. They could not determine if LAM made a difference beyond amenorrhea while fully breastfeeding.

TOUCH SENSITIVITY AND OVULATION

In search of a simple method of identifying ovulation during lactation, urinary pregnanediol and estrogen and breast sensitivity were measured in six breastfeeding and six bottle feeding normal women. Two-point discrimination and touch sensitivity were measured. The mean duration of amenorrhea among breastfeeders was 24.3 weeks (range 14 to 35 weeks) and among bottle feeders 7.5 weeks (range 6 to 14 weeks). Findings, however, were not diagnostic of ovulation. Touch sensitivity tended to decrease as lactation progressed for months. The change is so gradual and difficult to detect that it has no practical value in determining ovulation.

ORAL CONTRACEPTIVES AND LACTATION

The significant issues related to lactation and the use of oral contraceptives are the potentially adverse effects of oral contraceptives on milk production, uterine involution, and growth and development of breastfed infants.[48] A single case of breast enlargement in a breastfed male infant whose mother began taking norethynodrel with ethinyl estradiol 3-methyl ether (Enovid) on the third day postpartum was reported. Breast enlargement began on the third week of life. The mother had noted her milk was not as "rich" and started supplements the second week. Nursing was discontinued at about 4 weeks of age, and the breasts of the infant returned to normal in 2 to 3 weeks. The additional risks to the mother of thromboembolism, hypertension, and cancer have also been discussed extensively in the literature. These occurred with the early high-dose products.

In a study of over 900 Latina women who had developed gestational diabetes during pregnancy, they were noted to develop diabetes postpartum

if they were given a progesterone-only oral contraceptive as compared with those who received a combinations oral contraceptive or nonhormonal contraception. This is an observation that requires follow-up. A Cochrane review of combined hormonal versus nonhormonal versus progestin-only contraception in lactation was inconclusive, and it was decided that existing trials were insufficient to establish any effect of hormone contraceptive therapy on milk quantity and quality.[70] The WHO recommendation regarding the use of progestin-only pills states delay of onset for 4 to 6 weeks postpartum is necessary. A depot medroxyprogesterone-only contraceptive providing highly effective, long acting, reversible contraception, usual dosing every 12 weeks, was studied by Rodriguez et al.,[58,59] who concluded that it was not a significant risk to breastfeeding or to the baby. It was further stated that risk of pregnancy outweighed all other considerations.

OTHER HORMONAL CONTRACEPTIVE USE

The impact of the distribution of oral contraceptives on breastfeeding and pregnancy status in rural Haiti indicated that it did not alter breastfeeding patterns in women who began the pills at 8 to 9 months postpartum. Pregnancy prevalence also decreased as a result.[64]

Studies of progestin-only pills beginning at 6 weeks postpartum showed that progestin-only pills do not suppress gonadotropins nor do they affect ovarian follicular development.[47] The contraceptive effect is believed to be mediated through local actions of the endometrium and cervix as in normally menstruating women.[50]

Birth control for women who are breastfeeding is still open for discussion. A Cochrane review surveyed the literature and found it grossly inadequate in spite of numerous articles published on hormonal and nonhormonal birth control utilized postpartum while breastfeeding. They found only five trials adequate for discussion but the dropout rate of participants was of concern. The authors found no major differences in infant growth or weight gain due to hormonal birth control use. They state that information is too limited to say whether women should use hormonal birth control or not. The impact on breastfeeding and the infant remains unclear.

IMPLANTS AND INJECTIONS

The recommendation for contraceptive use during lactation is the progestin-only products (Norplant System, Depo-Provera injections and minipills, progestin once-only pills). Use of these methods has not been associated with adverse effects on

TABLE 20-5 Effects of Contraceptive Agents on Milk Yield and Infant Development

Agent	Milk Yield	Effect on Infant
Combined estrogen/progestin	Moderate inhibitory effect Shorter breastfeeding Milk concentration unchanged Small amount of steroid in milk	Slower weight gain No long-term effects
Progestin only Minipill (Micronor, Nor-QD)	No effect on volume No effect on duration unless given before 6 weeks	No effect on weight gain No reported long-term effects
Other products: Injectable DMPA, Depo-Provera and norethindrone enanthate (NET-EN, Noristerat)	Breastfeeding lasts longer? Change in milk: protein increased, fat decreased Steroid present in milk	No long-term effects
Norplant System	No effect Small amount of steroid in milk	Normal growth No long-term effects
Vaginal rings containing natural hormone progesterone	No significant differences	No effect on growth Long-term effects under study

DMPA, Depot medroxyprogesterone acetate.
Modified from Winikoff B, Semeraro P, Zimmerman M: *Contraception during breastfeeding: a clinician's source book*, New York, 1987, Population Council.

infant growth or development and may even increase the volume of milk[39,62] (Table 20-5).

Injectable DMPA given as a contraceptive in the immediate postpartum period was reported to be a safe and effective alternative method with no deleterious effect on the mother's milk supply or the infant's growth for women in New Delhi, India. Because loss of milk supply after the injection has been documented to occur, this study, by Singhal et al., of 100 women is significant. It is important to note, however, that the injection was not given until the milk supply was well established. Some injections were not given for 10 days. Thus the establishment of a good milk supply before the injection was important to the outcome of this study. Practitioners in lactation medicine know well that depot injections and insertion of intrauterine devices can affect milk supply in spite of claims to the contrary. The mother must be warned and allowed to make an informed decision. DMPA should not be used for at least 6 weeks if there is a history of depression.

In a study of the effects of levonorgestrel (Norplant) in breast milk on thyroid activity, Bassol et al.[2] compared infants of mothers with the implant and those of women assigned to intrauterine device (IUD) use. The hormones (levonorgestrel) in the breast milk significantly decreased the infants' thyroid-stimulating hormone (TSH) levels at 3 months, and the TSH levels were even lower at 6 months of age.[2] The higher the levonorgestrel levels, the lower the TSH levels in the infants. It is recommended that the progestin-only method not be initiated until 6 weeks postpartum on the premise that the theoretic danger to the infants from exogenous steroids has passed by this time. The practice of injecting Depo-Provera immediately after delivery can interfere with the establishment of lactation, which is dependent upon the dramatic natural decline in progesterone postpartum.

Steroids are not bound well in plasma and not well conjugated by the liver or excreted by the immature kidneys of the neonate. Exogenous hormones may compete for receptor sites with natural ones in the liver, brain, or other tissues. As an infant's liver and kidneys mature, these issues disappear.[26] Medications that also contain estrogen suppress milk production.[63] With the many alternatives available, it should never be necessary to discontinue breastfeeding to initiate contraception.[24]

The growth and development of breastfed infants whose mothers received implants of Norplant containing levonorgestrel or injections of norethindrone enanthate were studied and compared with those whose mothers used IUDs.[10,24] The breastfeeding performance was similar. The infants were also similar in growth rate, development, and general health. Similarly, a group of mothers were given a vaginal ring that released 10 mg of "natural" progesterone every 24 hours, producing a maternal serum level of 4 ng/mL, which results in only a minimal amount in the milk and this is not absorbed by the infant gut. These infants also had normal growth and development and remained in good health.

LH-releasing hormone agonist for contraception has also been tested in nine fully breastfeeding women beginning 6 weeks postpartum. They received 300 mg LH-releasing hormone agonist (buserelin) intranasally once a day for the duration of their breastfeeding. Urinary excretion of LH, estrone, and pregnanediol was compared with that of nine control breastfeeding women. No ovulation occurred in the treated group, and seven of the nine untreated control subjects had one to six ovulations. LH-releasing hormone has potential as a safe, acceptable method of contraception while breastfeeding, according to Fraser et al.[19]

Home tests to monitor fertility are available; however, women must be tested during lactation and especially during the transition period when breastfeeding frequency and feeding duration are changing. Ovarian follicular dynamics can be accurately monitored through the noninstrumented analysis of daily estrone conjugates in urine samples at home.[36] Readings can be affected by urine osmolarity, either high or low, giving false positive or false negative results, respectively. Controlling intake of fluids would guard against this.

Two algorithms for initiating contraceptive treatment are shown in Figures 20-7 and 20-10.

INTRAUTERINE DEVICES AND OTHER CONTRACEPTIVE METHODS

Various alternatives to oral contraceptives exist and have different degrees of reliability (Table 20-6). The IUDs (95% to 98% effective), cervical caps and diaphragms (85% to 88% effective), condoms (80% to 85% effective), and vaginal suppositories, jellies, or creams (80% effective) have no known contraindication during breastfeeding because no chemicals are absorbed. The only contraceptive that is 100% effective is abstinence.

A study of 2271 postpartum women who had IUDs inserted between 1976 and 1981 and were followed for 6 to 12 months, was reported, with careful attention to details of lactation.[7] Data were analyzed separately for IUDs inserted immediately after birth (within 10 minutes of placental expulsion). The results of this analysis indicate that IUD insertion for breastfeeding women would be appropriate either immediately after delivery or much later (42 days or more postpartum). When inserted immediately postpartum, the delta loop and delta T were modified by adding projections of chromic sutures, which help the device remain in the uterus. The sutures biodegrade in 6 weeks, leaving a standard device in place. These authors report that breastfeeding is not a contraindication to IUD insertion, with no increased expulsion

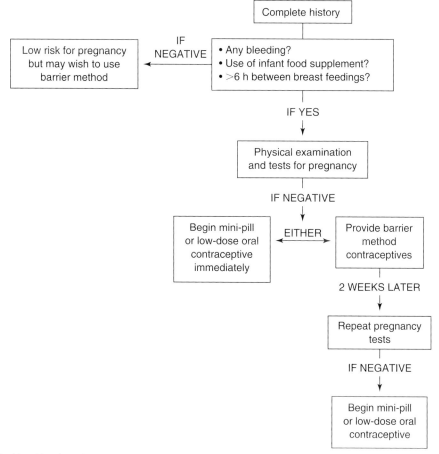

Figure 20-10. Algorithm for initiating contraceptive treatment in a breastfeeding woman. (Modified from Winikoff B, Semeraro P, Zimmerman M: *Contraception during breastfeeding: a clinician's source book*, New York, 1988, Population Council; Labbok M: Breastfeeding and contraception, *N Engl J Med* 308:51, 1983.)

TABLE 20-6 Family Planning Methods Presented by Relative Impact on Lactation

Method	Description	Efficacy	Risks to Lactation	Benefits for Lactation	Clinical/Counseling Suggestions and Special Considerations
No known impact on lactation					
LAM	Defined by three criteria that reflect reliable physiology for fertility delay	2/0.45	None	The required breastfeeding behaviors benefit maternal and child health and nutrition.	When any one of the criteria no longer applies, immediate transition to another method is recommended.
Abstinence/periodic abstinence/NFP methods • Complete abstinence • Calendar • Ovulation method • Symptothermal • Postovulation	Signs, symptoms, or timing of presumptive ovulation are used to identify periods of time when abstinence is necessary to avoid conception.	0 25 9 3 2	None; however, most methods may demand substantial periods of abstinence during lactation due to difficulty in assessing signs of ovulation.	None	Even experienced users of these methods will benefit from special counseling for their use during lactation because the signs and symptoms will vary and may be difficult to properly interpret during the hormonal changes that may occur during lactation.
Barrier methods: Condoms Male Female Diaphragms Cervical caps w/o spermicides alone/sponge	Condoms: Provides barrier to prevent ejaculum from coming in contact with cervical mucus. Diaphragms/caps: Generally used with spermicide, so provide elements of both physical and chemical barriers. Spermicides: Provide chemical barrier.	15/2 21/5 16/6 32/26 29/18 32/20	Some spermicides may provide lubrication; however, some varieties may cause additional sensitivity in some individuals.	Condoms: Lubricated varieties may be useful with lactational suppression of estrogenic vaginal lubricants.	Subject to user error; some individuals have allergies to ingredients; some couples may find methods inconvenient. Few side effects. Highly effective if used consistently and correctly. The condom can provide some protection against sexually transmitted diseases. If a patient has previously used a diaphragm or cervical cap, it should be refitted at the 6-week postpartum visit.
Little to no known impact on lactation					
IUD Noncopper/nonhormonal IUD Copper IUD: 7-10 yr	IUD functions as a foreign body in the uterus, provoking hormonal changes that reduce the possibility of fertilization of the egg and implantation of an embryo.	0.8/0.6 0.1/0.1	Some women may have excess lochia or contraction-associated uterine discharge.	Once inserted, no further action or intervention is needed during lactation.	An IUD should be inserted within the first 48 hours after delivery or delayed for at least 4 weeks as lactating women have strong uterine contractions. This also requires that IUD insertion be high in the uterus to decrease risk of expulsion.
Surgical sterilization Men: vasectomy Women: tubal ligation	Surgical blockage of path of gametes by bisecting, separating ends, and ligation of vas/fallopian tubes	0.15/0.10 0.5/0.5	Tubal ligation may necessitate temporary interruption in breastfeeding while surgery takes place. Milk should be expressed in advance for feeding during the procedure.	Once performed, no further intervention is needed. Both can be outpatient procedures.	Permanent decision. Reversal is expensive, requires surgical expertise, and may not be successful. Highly effective. Men: If coupled with postpartum infertility, simplifies contraception during the months necessary for healing. Male sterilization is easier and safer and may be performed in an office setting.

Some reports of negative impact on lactation

Method	Mechanism of action		Impact on milk supply		Common side effects
Progestin-only • Pills • Injectables (e.g., DMPA 3 months; norethisterone 2 months) • Implants (e.g., Number, size, and content of implanted rods offer different lengths of protection in years) • Levonorgestrel IUD: up to 5 yr	Mechanism of action includes some disruption of lactation and modification of intrauterine milieu and readiness for implantation. Progestin-only contraception during lactation does not suppress gonadotropins nor affect growth of ovarian follicles during breastfeeding. Thus the contraceptive effect of POP is likely mediated through local actions at the endometrium and cervix in a manner similar to that of menstruating women.[78]	5/0.5 3/0.3 0.05/0.05 0.1/0.1	May decrease milk supply if started before milk supply is well established. Anecdotal reports of immediate negative impact even when initiated after lactation is well established. Progestin IUD typically has minimal impact, but has the potential to have the same impact as other progestin-only methods.	Some studies report increased milk production with injectables.	Common side effects include irregular bleeding (less common in predominantly breastfeeding women), weight gain, and headaches. Return to fertility with injections may be delayed beyond expected duration—of potential concern for some women. Must develop routine for taking daily pills. Implants require procedure for placement and removal.

Expected to have negative impact on lactation

Method	Mechanism of action		Impact on milk supply		Common side effects
Combined pill • Contraceptive patch (e.g., ethinyl estradiol/norelgestromin) • Combined vaginal ring (e.g., ethinyl estradiol etonogestrel) • Combined injectables (e.g., estradiol/medroxyprogesterone)	Exogenous estrogen serves to suppress ovulation.	8/0.3 8/0.3 8/0.3 3/0.05	Significant risk of reducing milk supply. It is suggested that initiation be delayed until 6 months postpartum. Reduction of supply appears dose dependent. Injectables more difficult to stop if problems arise.	None	Several good noncontraceptive effects (e.g., reduced risk of ovarian and endometrial cancers, decreased anemia, regular menses). Not suitable for women with history of clotting problems, estrogen-dependent cancers, severe migraines, or women older than 35 who smoke.

From Labbok M: Breastfeeding, birth spacing and family planning. In Hartmann PE, Hale TW, editors: *Hale and Hartmann's textbook of human lactation*, Amarillo, Tex., 2007, Hale Publishing.

rate.[24] Conversely, the presence of an IUD has no adverse effect on lactation. The appropriate time for insertion should be selected to predate anticipated ovulation but guarantee patient compliance. A study showed that the use of the TCu-380A IUD in breastfeeding women resulted in fewer insertion-related complaints and lower removal rates for bleeding and pain in 12 months postpartum than in nonbreastfeeders. No intrauterine perforations were reported in either group. Copper IUDs are usually smaller, so there is little problem with the effects of let-down on the uterus.

A group of 32 women hospitalized for uterine perforation necessitating transperitoneal IUD removal and a matched control group of 497 women who had worn IUDs uneventfully were compared.[24] Of the women in the study, 97% were postpartum compared with 68% of the control subjects. Of the parous study group, 42% were lactating, and of the parous control subjects, 7% were lactating when the IUD was inserted. The risk of perforation was 10 times greater in the lactating than in the nonlactating women, unrelated to time of the insertion postpartum. In another group hospitalized for difficult transcervical IUD removal, the risk was 2.3 times greater for lactating women.[24] The authors recommend caution, not abandonment of the procedure, during lactation, because they believe the IUD is the best form of artificial contraception during lactation. The ideal candidate is a woman who wants reversible contraception to space births or limit size of the family, especially breastfeeding parous women in a monogamous relationship.[10]

The Technical Guidance/Competence Group of the United States Agency for International Development (USAID) and the WHO[77,78] recommends IUD insertion immediately postpartum as soon as the placenta is removed, whether by vaginal or cesarean delivery. They point out it must be done by a specially trained physician. From 10 minutes to 48 hours after delivery, however, the expulsion rate is high. If this window of opportunity is missed or no urgency exists, it is best to wait. Although immediate insertion is possible, a copper-T device may be safely inserted 4 or more weeks postpartum in breastfeeding women. Using the withdrawal technique minimizes the risk of perforation. Other IUDs should not be inserted until 6 weeks postpartum.

The IUD is a long acting, reversible method of contraception with expulsion rates of 5-15 per 100 woman-years of use when used as a postplacental method immediately after cesarean section. An IUD does not affect breastfeeding. These experiences are reported by Goldstuck and Steyn from South Africa.

Use of barrier and spermicidal products is an alternative contraceptive method during early lactation before hormonal methods or IUDs are introduced. These coital-dependent methods have no effect on lactation. The lubrication provided by the spermicidally treated condoms has the advantage of contributing lubrication when the hypoestrogenic vagina is exceptionally dry in association with lactation. A spermicide is more effective with a condom but is adequate early postpartum, when relative infertility is present. A diaphragm cannot be adequately fitted for 6 to 8 weeks postpartum, so it is not recommended during this period with or without lactation.

ABSTINENCE

Many cultures and societies place taboos on sexual intercourse for nursing mothers as an effective means of spacing children. Usually, there are no medical contraindications to sexual relationships during lactation. In a study on contraceptive use in the United States, among white women, 34% were not sexually active in the first month postpartum, 12.5% in the second month, and 4.3% during the third month. Among black women in the survey, 25% were not sexually active in the first month, 8.1% in the second, and 4.2% in the third. Contraceptive use among those sexually active was absent in 16%, 12.2%, and 13.8% in the first, second, and third postpartum months, respectively, among whites. Among blacks, no method was used by 27.3%, 22.7%, and 22.3%, in the first, second, and third postpartum months, respectively.

Sex and the Nursing Mother

SEXUAL AROUSAL ASSOCIATED WITH SUCKLING

If one examines normal adult women in regard to the menstrual cycle, sexual intercourse, pregnancy, childbirth, and lactation, one observes that these events are all influenced by the interaction of the same hormones—not only estrogen, progesterone, testosterone, FSH, and LH, but oxytocin and prolactin as well. The breast is known to respond during all these phases, enlarging before menstruation, during pregnancy, before orgasm, and during lactation. The nipples also respond during these phases. Furthermore, the uterus contracts during childbirth, orgasm, and lactation. Body temperature rises during ovulation, childbirth, orgasm, and lactation. As pointed out in Chapter 3, oxytocin is a critical element in the let-down reflex during lactation. Oxytocin levels also rise during orgasms and labor, and oxytocin causes the uterus to contract and the nipples to become erect. Newton and Newton[52,53] report other similarities in women, including sensory perception and emotional reactions, during these events.

The psychophysiologic similarities between lactation and coitus are as follows:

1. The uterus contracts.
2. The nipples become erect.
3. Breast stroking and nipple stimulation occur.
4. The emotions experienced involve skin changes (vascular dilatation and raised temperature).
5. Milk let-down (or ejection) reflex can be triggered.
6. The emotions experienced may be closely allied.
7. An accepting attitude toward sexuality may be related to an accepting attitude to breastfeeding (and vice versa).

Women also report hot flashes in association with some feeds, especially at night. This phenomenon has been studied by Marshall et al.,[45] who looked at oxytocin effect. Initiation of breastfeeding was accompanied by an increase in skin conductance resulting in increased skin temperature, especially of the breast. The pattern is similar to menopausal hot flashes.

Given the biologic and hormonal similarities of lactation to the other events in the sexual cycle of adult women, it is not surprising that some women experience some form of sexual gratification during suckling on certain occasions. In a study of 111 parturient women, only 24 of which breastfed, Masters and Johnson[46] reported that sexual arousal was experienced during suckling on some occasions. The exact incidence of this response is unknown, but it is thought to be uncommon. Nursing mothers may have an element of guilt surrounding these experiences and underreport. That guilt may lead to early weaning in some cases. For some women, the breasts are highly erogenous. The handling and manipulation of the breast necessary during lactation by both mother and infant can, in the right but unpremeditated circumstances, be stimulating. Clearly, the majority of women who enjoy breastfeeding have no feelings or responses to the stimulation of the breast that could be construed as sexual arousal, although they enjoy breastfeeding and the intimacy with their infant that it provides.

The erotic response to nursing the infant has no significance in terms of being normal or abnormal. The decline of breastfeeding because of feelings of shame, modesty, embarrassment, and distaste has been reported and interpreted as indicating that breastfeeding is viewed as a forbidden sexual activity. For such women, any sexual allusions and excitement accompanying breastfeeding are not permissible and cause shame. Such attitudes are more common in lower social groups and need to be considered in counseling mothers about breastfeeding prepartum or when premature weaning takes place. Major changes in the number of women who breastfeed may not be possible until society can accept the breast in its relationship to nurturing the infant and as an object of less sexual ambivalence.

The sensuousness of breastfeeding has been the topic of discussion in women's magazines as more has been written about women and their bodies. For the well-educated, well-read woman who breastfeeds her infant because she intellectually arrives at the decision, such discussions are an avenue of increased knowledge. Others may still be uncomfortable about breastfeeding if it is apt to be "pleasurable." The physician may sense this discomfort in a patient prenatally by her responses to bodily change during pregnancy. Cultural attitudes are an important part of this response and are deeply ingrained in an individual by the time she reaches the age of parenting. Professionals need to be sensitive to the patient and cautious about imposing cultural change on a patient while still being alert to needs for information and openness. A woman who experiences any erogenous reaction to breastfeeding, especially with an older child who may inadvertently roll the nipple while feeding, should not be criticized, but the phenomenon should be explained and discussed openly by the physician.

SEXUAL ACTIVITY OF NURSING MOTHERS

A review of the limited data available on lactating women in the study by Masters and Johnson[46] does indicate that in their group of 111 postpartum women, the nursing mothers were more eager than nonnursing mothers to resume sexual relations postpartum. The data were independent of the fear of pregnancy. They report that this interest was apparent 2 to 3 weeks postpartum. Individual reports through a questionnaire indicate that 30% of nursing mothers believed their sexual relationships were improved and only 2.5% believed they were worse postpartum. The individual testimonies of nursing mothers indicate they had a better feeling about themselves as well as their relationships with their husbands and family in general. In a study of sexual behavior during pregnancy and lactation, the desire returned by 4 weeks for most women, long before they thought it was safe. The longer they had been married and the more children, the sooner the interest returned and the sooner they felt it was safe. No change in interest or enjoyment occurred with weaning.

In studies of recovery after childbirth, the longer duration of breastfeeding (more than 5 months) has been associated with a longer duration of awareness of perineal damage (dyspareunia) during intercourse and a longer amenorrheic period in some women. High prolactin levels and decreased libido have also been observed in women with evidence of continued vaginal discomfort. In the clinical study of lactational amenorrhea in 422 women in Chile, however, Perez et al.[55] recorded the incidence of intercourse to be one to two times a week, beginning 4 weeks postpartum.

The frequency of coitus during breastfeeding was studied at four sites: Birmingham, United Kingdom; Montreal, Canada; Sydney, Australia; and Manila, the Philippines.[74] The frequency was lower than reported in other studies of married women, ranging from 4 to 30 episodes a month while averaging three to five times a month. Rates were not correlated with number of children but were related to maternal age, being slightly more frequent in younger women. The resumption of coital activity in these populations was more variable, with a median of 8 weeks postpartum, with 75% resuming activities by the end of the third postpartum month. Thus "normal" encompasses a broad range.

More general observations indicate that although some women may have increased interest in sexual relations while nursing, others may experience no interest at all for 6 months or so. Whether this results from the satiation of the mother's needs for intimate relationship and stimulus through nursing, general fatigue, or fear of pregnancy is debatable.[46] Sexual stimuli may trigger the ejection reflex, and milk ejection may have a negative effect on some men. A practical solution to spraying milk during lovemaking is feeding the infant or expressing some milk beforehand. The total knowledge of nursing and suckling as a biologic phenomenon will help couples understand such reactions and thus avoid inappropriate psychologic responses.

The conflict in some adult men over their role in regard to the nursing mother's breasts is usually a result of guilt or upbringing. There is no need to advise against fondling the lactating breast during lovemaking, although physicians have often imposed rigid restrictions on sexual activity in the lactating woman. No scientific basis for such restriction exists, and no difference in the incidence of infection and mastitis is associated with such activity. Unusually restrictive protocols are often imposed on patients without medical indication.

It is helpful to discuss with lactating women that the hormonal effect on the vagina may be excessive dryness with an increase in dyspareunia. With the abrupt withdrawal of gonadotropins and ovarian hormones and elevation of prolactin at the time of delivery of the infant and placenta, the vaginal epithelium becomes thin and atrophic.[57] Normally, the vagina and ectocervix are lined with stratified squamous epithelium, which is multilayered and protective. It is also responsive to ovarian hormones. The greatest maturation and thickness occur around ovulation in response to peak estrogen secretion. During pregnancy, progesterone inhibits the maturation of the epithelial cells. The vaginal lining retains its thickness, but cells do not fully mature because the effect of progesterone overtakes the effect of estrogen on the epithelium and cervical mucus; both hormones are abundant during pregnancy.

The lowered ovarian hormones that cause vaginal dryness and lack of cervical mucus during lactation lead to discomfort during intercourse. The dryness responds to locally applied lubricants and tends to improve over time. A sudden change may actually reflect ovulation. The breast that is being stimulated by feeding frequently may not be as sensitive during lovemaking. Usually this, too, is transient. Physicians should perhaps remind mothers that some adjustment to attend to fathers' needs may be necessary.

SEXUAL ABUSE AND BREASTFEEDING

In most cases, sexual abuse or any type of abuse during childhood takes its toll for a lifetime. Sexual abuse during adult life, especially during a relationship that results in pregnancy, impacts a mother's ability to accept the pregnancy, endure the labor, and mother the child. The role of abuse is being recognized as significant in all phases of women's pregnancies and postpartum periods. Anthropologists have identified abuse as a significant thread in the lives of low income women living in the most inhuman conditions in the world.[3,9,11,61] Those studying childbirth issues and breastfeeding have noted a relationship between alleged inadequate milk and abuse as well as an inability to breastfeed. Chin and Solomonik[9] have analyzed the term "inadequate," not just as a description by the woman for her milk supply but as a metaphor for the lives of low income women in the United States who have been identified in numerous statistical reports as the least likely to breastfeed.[9] Chin and Solomonik[9] note that everything about their lives is inadequate: education, income, health services, and life span. Their lives are saturated with violence, lack of safety, and fear even in their own homes. Chin and Solomonik[9] suggest an agenda to explore the relationship between these social inadequacies and the forces that compel these women to choose the less optimal infant feeding by bottle. Childhood sexual abuse is not limited to families in poverty but has been reported in as many as 20% of children.[56] Sexual abuse can have short- and long-term effects that manifest in various symptoms, including health problems, behavior problems, posttraumatic stress disorder, and interpersonal difficulties. Amnesia for the original abusive events can develop until the events of childbirth and subsequently putting the newborn to the breast triggers an anguished flashback. Kendall-Tackett[29] described the long-term effects of sexual abuse, which she divided into five domains: emotional distress, impaired sense of self, avoidance, interpersonal difficulties, and health problems. Avoidance is a major challenge to the physician. One mechanism of avoidance is the ability to numb one part of the body to avoid reliving the trauma inflicted. A mother may appear to be absent from her body when the baby is taken after breastfeeding. Physicians need to take careful and caring histories with any patients, but especially when a patient shows these signs and symptoms. It may be necessary to obtain a psychiatric referral if simple effort does not ameliorate the situation. As more information is brought forward, we learn of successful breastfeeding with mothers with a history of child abuse by a family member. Coles[11] interviewed eleven women and identified four key themes: "enhancement of the mother-baby relationship, validation of the maternal body, splitting of the breasts' dual role as maternal and sexual objects, and exposure and control when breastfeeding in public." A case report published by Beck[3] vividly described the original abuses, the victims' labors and deliveries, and breastfeeding that triggered panic attacks, disassociation, and flashbacks. After extensive interviewing of 18 women who were sexually abused by family members before the age of 16, Coles and Jones[12] reported two key themes: safety issues for survivors and their babies in clinical encounters and wishing for better and safer clinical experiences because of feelings of pain, fear, blame, helplessness, and guilt in the health care environment. The authors suggest important steps to make the health care experience more tolerable for these women who fear the intimacy of this care. Many of these suggestions are appropriate for all patients.

Severe physical violence between intimate partners during pregnancy is a major risk factor for early cessation of exclusive breastfeeding. This correlation has been made in many cultures around the world. Using a health services survey, the Conflict Tactics Scale, Moraes et al. investigated premature cessation of breastfeeding in Brazil. They concluded that severe physical violence during pregnancy was an important risk factor for early cessation of exclusive breastfeeding. They suggest that health care workers who deal with lactating women need to be trained beyond the biologic aspects of lactation to include the maternal, psychologic dimensions. Similar findings were reported from multiple African countries (Ghana, Kenya, Liberia, Malawi, Nigeria, Tanzania, Zambia, and Zimbabwe) by Misch and Yount. Partner violence was associated with early breastfeeding cessation. Screening for intimate partner violence victimization both prenatally and postpartum may mitigate the potential intergenerational effects of violence the authors recommend. Sexual assault has a pervasive negative effect on a new mother's sleep quality and risk of depression report

Kendall-Tackett et al., who studied over 6000 mothers with young infants using an online survey. Although assault history had negative effects, the effects were less severe for those mothers who breastfed than those who bottle fed or mixed fed. Abuse of any kind has long-term effects. Breastfeeding appears to trigger repressed memories of the events and becomes difficult for some women. Clearly, the process is not completely understood. A physician, initially during pregnancy and then postpartum, plays an essential role in helping a patient cope. The issue may go unidentified until a pediatrician enters the picture. As well as screening for depression, a pediatrician should be alert to a possible history of abuse, while carrying out care of the infant.

Nursing During Pregnancy and Tandem Nursing

Pregnancy can and does occur while a woman is lactating. When it does occur, it produces a number of questions. There is no need to wean the first infant from the breast, which is often ordered by a physician. It is possible to lactate throughout pregnancy and then to have two infants at the breast postpartum. This is now sufficiently common to be called *tandem nursing*.

The amount of nourishment provided the first infant at the breast depends on age and other supplements. When an infant at the breast is only a few months old when pregnancy occurs, there is some rationale to continue breastfeeding for the benefit of the infant until it is time to wean to solids and other liquids at 6 months of age or so. This child will be about a year old when the new infant arrives and, if still at the breast, may have demands in excess of the mother's ability to provide. Concern has been expressed that the older infant will take much of the nourishment needed by the new infant. In some societies, it is believed that a suckling infant will "take the spirit" from the newly conceived fetus; thus weaning is mandated once pregnancy is confirmed in these communities.

The milk produced immediately postpartum by the mother who never stopped nursing appears to be colostrum. The kangaroo has been observed to have a teat with mature milk for the older offspring and a teat for the new offspring who requires significantly different nourishment. Such a provision does not exist for humans. Mothers who want to maintain both infants at the breast have shown that it can be done without any apparent effect on the nourishment of the new infant. Counseling of such a mother should take into account the mother's resources to receive adequate rest, nourishment, and psychologic support to withstand the added demand, physically and mentally, on her.

If the first child will be older than 1 year of age when the new infant arrives, the need for physical nourishment is minimal, and continuation at the breast is more for the security and psychologic benefits. This is referred to as comfort nursing and may continue for several years (see Chapter 10). Abrupt weaning should be avoided, and consideration should be given to the impact of separation when the mother is confined during the birth of the new infant. This is an argument for 12-hour hospitalization for delivery for women who request it. The first few days of colostrum are most vital for the new infant, and the supply is not infinite; therefore, priorities need to be set concerning the older child. The new baby should be nursed first. Some older infants reject the colostrum.

The growth rate of children weaned during a subsequent pregnancy was compared with that of children weaned at the same age from nonpregnant mothers in a longitudinal study in Bhutan by Bohler and Bergstrom,[4] who followed 113 children closely for the first 3 years of life. The period of overlap for lactation and pregnancy was 5 months (median), increasing by 1 week for each month reduction in birth interval. When a child stopped breastfeeding during the mother's subsequent pregnancy, the growth rate was reduced during the last months before termination of breastfeeding compared with children weaned at the same age from nonpregnant mothers and with children who continued to breastfeed.

In a study of 503 La Leche League members, Newton and Theotokatos[53] reviewed breastfeeding during pregnancy practices and found that 69% of breastfeeding children weaned spontaneously when the mother became pregnant. Many of the children may have been at an age to wean even without an intercurrent pregnancy.

Moscone and Moore[51] conducted a questionnaire survey of 57 women who were concurrently pregnant and breastfeeding. The main reasons given for continuing breastfeeding after conception involved the emotional needs of the breastfeeding child; 43% of the children continued to breastfeed throughout pregnancy and after birth of the sibling. The main reason for mother-initiated weaning was breast and nipple pain. When the child weaned during the pregnancy, it occurred during the second trimester and seemed to be associated with diminished milk production. Three pregnancies terminated in spontaneous abortions (a rate higher than in the general population of 5%). The ages of the children at onset of pregnancy varied from 4 to 42 months. The feeding pattern was one to eight times a day for less than 5 minutes to more than

30 minutes. A descriptive study of 2617 women in a prenatal clinic in Egypt revealed that 95% had previously breastfed and 25.3% conceived while breastfeeding; 4.4% conceived in the first 6 months, 15.1% while still amenorrheic, and 28.1% while exclusively breastfeeding. Only 4 pregnancies (1.5%) occurred when all the prerequisites for the LAM method were present. In Egypt, especially in rural areas, infants are breastfed for at least 2 years. Pregnancy while breastfeeding is common in Egypt.[64]

Impact of Nursing During Pregnancy

Among rural Guatemalan women who were part of a nutrition supplementation trial, 253 of the 504 pregnant women had another pregnancy overlap while breastfeeding (50.2%); 41.4% of mothers with concurrent pregnancy and lactation continued to breastfeed into the second trimester and 3.2% into the third trimester. These "overlap" mothers received more supplements. The authors stated that overlap resulted in short recuperative periods (less than 6 months) requiring increased supplement intake and reduced maternal fat stores. The energetic stresses and short recovery time did not significantly affect fetal growth. It appeared the mother buffers the energy stress, protecting fetal growth.[44]

Significant decreases in bone mineral density do occur during breastfeeding when calcium demands are the greatest.[41] These changes are reversible and do not persist after a subsequent pregnancy according to Prentice et al.,[56] who studied calcium utilization and reproduction related osteoporosis extensively. They indicate that extended periods of breastfeeding and closely spaced pregnancies are unlikely to have a lasting effect on bone mineral status and osteoporosis when a mother is healthy and well nourished. Although short birth intervals and breastfeeding during pregnancy further deplete fat stores in a malnourished mother, healthy, well-nourished women fare well and replenish their stores during a subsequent pregnancy.[43,44]

INFANT HEALTH

Although pregnancy during lactation can cause flavor and volume changes that lead to early weaning, the milk still provides immunologic benefits. This is clearly demonstrated by Bohler and Bergstrom[4] among women in Bhutan in which abrupt weaning caused diarrhea, stunted growth, illness, and even death. Research in India showed that overlapping breastfeeding and pregnancy in a malnourished mother produced growth retardation in the older child. Healthy infants in the United States derive significant nutritional and immunologic benefit in the second year and beyond, however. The risk to a nursling depends on a child's age, other diet, and the amount of human milk available.

FETAL HEALTH

The nutritional status of a mother is key to adequate fetal growth. Varying results of fetal growth patterns are reported related to a mother's nutritional status before pregnancy. A significant issue is viability of the pregnancy. Breastfeeding stimulus triggers oxytocin release and concern focuses on the potential for initiating uterine contractions and fetal loss. Studies of oxytocin sensitivities in pregnancy and the state of oxytocin receptors during early pregnancy are graphically illustrated in Figure 3-19. The uterus is insensitive until close to 40 weeks in most women. It is well documented that nipple stimulation can be as effective as intravenous Pitocin for inducing labor at term.

Risk of Fetal Loss or Preterm Labor

Retrospective studies of fetal loss and preterm loss suggest that breast stimulus could be the source in some women. The Miscarriage Clinic in London states that once a pregnancy is clinically detectable, breastfeeding should pose no added risk of pregnancy loss, and there is no reason to link breastfeeding and miscarriage. Most obstetricians, however, caution against sex during pregnancy in a woman with a history of fetal loss or premature birth. Breast stimulus is equally proscribed in such circumstances. The stimulus is not exactly equal. In addition, the nursling will be nursing several times per day every day. Twin pregnancies and other multiples are considered high risk and weaning is usually recommended if the mother is nursing.

The decision to continue nursing when a new pregnancy is normal with no factors for a high-risk pregnancy should rest with the comfort level of the mother and child. The breast pain can be improved by wearing a supportive bra and repositioning during breastfeeding. The decrease in volume of milk is usually not remediable, but milk usually returns toward the end of pregnancy and is completely regenerated at delivery.[49]

In a study of 68 Peruvian women who breastfed during pregnancy and 65 who had not breastfed during the pregnancy, Marquis et al.[44] reported that on day 2 postpartum women who breastfed had higher concentrations of lactose and lysozyme but lower lactoferrin than women who did not breastfeed. At 1 month, immunoglobulin A was lower among women who breastfed. The infants of the women who breastfed were five times as likely to have respiratory symptoms ($p < 0.05$) in these early weeks.[44]

Women who were 2 months pregnant and weaning their infants showed a progressive loss of secretory activity by the mammary gland, seemingly due to an inhibition of milk secretion that overrides the stimulus provided by the infants. These results were compared to milk of women weaning without pregnancy.[52,53]

Many of the changes in child-rearing practices in recent years have increased the freedom and response to human needs. Carried to extremes, instant gratification becomes a right rather than a privilege. Sometimes a mother may need help in seeing that she need not feel guilty if she decides to wean the older child. If it is only an occasional feeding or suckling experience for added security, especially when security is threatened by the arrival of a new infant, it may be tolerable in terms of endurance for the mother, and she may agree willingly. When, however, continuing nursing becomes a strain or is painful or stressful, she should feel free to stop. When a mother feels real resentment toward the older child who is nursing, it is time to wean gently but firmly. If such a situation can be anticipated, it is probably easier for an older child to be weaned before delivery of the new infant.

Sore nipples are the most stressful symptom during pregnancy and may be the first sign of the new pregnancy as the hormonal milieu changes. There is no specific treatment, although having the toddler repositioned at the breast may ease the discomfort. If the toddler is old enough to understand, asking him or her to nurse more gently or "more softly" may help. The soreness may last for the first trimester or for the entire pregnancy until the new baby is born.

DECISION: SORTING OUT PERSONAL FEELINGS

Little is in the medical literature about nursing during pregnancy and tandem nursing. A mother must make up her own mind if there are no medical contraindications. Much depends on the age of a child, the nursing pattern, and the nutritional and emotional needs of the child. Medical indications to wean during pregnancy are uterine bleeding, signs of preterm labor, or failure to gain enough weight during pregnancy.

Tandem nursing for some women is too much "touching," especially when the infant and the toddler are a year or more apart in age. Nursing twins or triplets presents a similar situation for some mothers.

As with any such decisions to wean, it is best for a physician to work this out in frank discussion with a mother (and father, if available) so that any misgivings, resentment, or feeling of failure can be dealt with openly. Many patients automatically suspect the physician of being antagonistic to breastfeeding if the physician suggests weaning. Even when the reason is purely but urgently medical, discussion should be open and include options and alternatives and their risks. Weaning is part of a baby's growing up, but it is sometimes part of a mother's moving on as well.

While tandem nursing requires ordinary hygiene, it is usually not necessary to limit each child to one breast because any infections or colds have spread before the first symptom. There are a few precautions. If one child has thrush, assigning one breast may keep it under control. If the older child develops a herpetic lesion or cold sore, he or she must not nurse. The newborn could acquire a potentially fatal herpes infection.

The dilemma of tandem nursing and weaning an older child has been dealt with in other societies with various manipulations, such as painting the breast with pepper or bitter herbs to make it taste terrible. The mother may leave the child with other caregivers. The provision of love and affection during this difficult adaptation for the child is what makes the difference between a traumatic occasion and a step toward growing up. Equally important is the provision of some opportunity for a mother to express her concerns and doubts during the process to her physician, who should be neither judgmental nor unduly rigid in the medical care plan.

Reading for Parents

One book recommended for parents is *Adventures in Tandem Nursing (Breastfeeding During Pregnancy and Beyond)* by Hillary Flower, La Leche League International, Schaumburg, Ill., 2003.

REFERENCES

1. Barker DC: Use of natural family planning by breastfeeding women. In Shivanandan M, editor: *Breastfeeding and natural family planning. Fourth international symposium on natural family planning*, Chevy Chase, Md., 1985, KM Associate Publishers.
2. Bassol S, Nava-Hernandez MP, Hernandez-Morales C, et al: Effects of levonorgestrel implant upon TSH and LH levels in male infants during lactation, *Int J Gynaecol Obstet* 76:273, 2002.
3. Beck CT: An adult survivor of child sexual abuse and her breastfeeding experience: a case study, *MCN Am J Matern Child Nurs* 34:91–97, 2009.
4. Bohler E, Bergstrom S: Child growth during weaning depends on whether mother is pregnant again, *J Trop Pediatr* 42:104, 1996.
5. Brambilla F, Sirtori CM: Gonadotropin-inhibiting factor in pregnancy, lactation and menopause, *Am J Obstet Gynecol* 109:599, 1971.
6. Brown RE: Breast-feeding and family planning: a review of relationships between breast-feeding and family planning, *Am J Clin Nutr* 35:162, 1982.
7. Campino C, Torres C, Rioseco A, et al: Plasma prolactin/oestradiol ratio at 38 weeks gestation predicts the duration of lactational amenorrhea, *Hum Reprod* 16(12):2540–2545, 2001.
8. Chayen B, Tejani N, Verma U: Induction of labor with an electric breast pump, *J Reprod Med* 31:116, 1986.
9. Chin P, Solomonik A: Inadequate: a metaphor for the lives of low-income women? *Breastfeed Med* 4(Suppl 1):S-41–S-43, 2009.
10. Cole LP, McCann MF, Higgins JE, et al: Effects of breast-feeding on IUD performance, *Am J Public Health* 73:384, 1983.
11. Coles J: Qualitative study of breastfeeding after childhood sexual assault, *J Hum Lact* 25:317–324, 2009.
12. Coles J, Jones K: Universal precautions: perinatal touch and examination after childhood sexual abuse, *Birth* 36:230–236, 2009.
13. Cooney KA, Nahmias SR: *Bellagio and beyond: breast-feeding and LAM in reproductive health*, Washington, D.C., 1997, Institute for Reproductive Health, Georgetown University.
14. Delvoye P, Demaegd M, Nyampeta U, et al: Serum prolactin, gonadotropins, and estradiol in menstruating and amenorrheic mothers during two years' lactation, *Am J Obstet Gynecol* 130:635, 1978.
15. Dewey KG, Cohen RJ, Rivera LL, et al: Effects of age at introduction of complementary foods to breast-fed infants on duration of lactational amenorrhea in Honduran women, *Am J Clin Nutr* 65:1403, 1997.
16. Diaz S, Aravena R, Cardenas ME, et al: Contraceptive efficacy of lactational amenorrhea in urban Chilean women, *Contraception* 43:335, 1991.
17. Diaz S, Cardenas H, Brandeis A, et al: Early difference in the endocrine profile of long and short lactational amenorrhea, *J Clin Endocrinol Metab* 72:196, 1991.
18. Eslami SS, Gray RH, Apelo R, et al: The reliability of menses to indicate the return of ovulation in breastfeeding women in Manila, the Philippines, *Stud Fam Plann* 21:243, 1990.
19. Fraser HM, Dewart PJ, Smith SK, et al: Luteinizing hormone releasing hormone agonist for contraception in breastfeeding women, *J Clin Endocrinol Metab* 69:996, 1989.
20. Gray RH, Campbell OM, Apelo R, et al: Risk of ovulation during lactation, *Lancet* 335:25, 1990.
21. Gray RH, Campbell O, Eslamic S, et al: *The return of ovarian function during lactation: in results of studies from the United States and the Philippines, Biomedical demographic determinants*, Oxford, 1993, Clarendon.
22. Gross BA: Is the lactational amenorrhea method a part of natural family planning? Biology and policy, *Am J Obstet Gynecol* 165:2014, 1991.
23. Hartmann PE, Prosser CG: Acute changes in the composition of milk during the ovulatory menstrual cycle in lactating women, *J Physiol* 324:21, 1982.
24. Hartwell S, Schlesselman S: Risk of uterine perforation among users of IUD, *Obstet Gynecol* 61:31, 1983.
25. Heikkila M, Luukkainen T: Duration of breastfeeding and development of children after insertion of a levonorgestrel-releasing intrauterine contraceptive device, *Contraception* 25:279, 1982.
26. Howie P, McNeilly A, Houston M, et al: Fertility after childbirth: infant feeding patterns, basal PRL levels, and postpartum ovulation, *Clin Endocrinol (Oxf)* 17:315, 1982.
27. Howie P, McNeilly A, Houston M, et al: Fertility after childbirth: postpartum ovulation and menstruation in bottle and breastfeeding mothers, *Clin Endocrinol (Oxf)* 17:323, 1982.
28. Kambic RT: Natural family planning use—effectiveness and continuation, *Am J Obstet Gynecol* 165:2046, 1991.
29. Kendall-Tackett K: Breastfeeding and the sexual abuse survivor, *J Hum Lact* 14:125–130, 1995.
30. Kennedy KI, Labbok MH, Van Look PFA: Consensus statement: lactational amenorrhea method for family planning, *Int J Gynaecol Obstet* 54:55, 1996.
31. Kennedy KI, Rivera R, McNeilly AS: Consensus statement on the use of breastfeeding as a family planning method, *Contraception* 39:477, 1989.

32. Kennedy KI, Short RV, Tully MR: Premature introduction of progestin-only contraceptive methods during lactation, *Contraception* 55:347, 1997.

33. Kennedy KI, Visness CM: Contraceptive efficacy of lactational amenorrhea, *Lancet* 339:227, 1992.

34. Kent JC, Cox ML, Owens RA, et al: Breast volume and milk production during extended lactation in women, *Exp Physiol* 84:435, 1999.

35. Konner M, Worthman C: Nursing frequency, gonadal function, and birth spacing among !Kung hunter-gatherers, *Science* 207:788, 1980.

36. Kurz KM, Habicht J-P, Rasmussen KM: Influences of maternal nutrition and lactation on length of postpartum amenorrhea, *J Trop Pediatr* 37(Suppl):15, 1991.

37. Labbok M: Breastfeeding and contraception, *N Engl J Med* 308:51, 1983.

38. Labbok MH, Laukaran VH: Breastfeeding and family planning. In Sciarra JJ, editor: *Gynecology and obstetrics*, Philadelphia, 1994, Lippincott.

39. Labbok MH, Peréz A, Valdés F, et al: The lactational amenorrhea method (LAM): a postpartum introductory family planning method with policy and program implications, *Adv Contracept* 10:93, 1994.

40. Labbok MH, Stallings RY, Shah F, et al: Ovulation method use during breastfeeding: is there an increased risk of unplanned pregnancy? *Am J Obstet Gynecol* 165:2031, 1991.

41. Laskey MA, Prentice A: Bone mineral changes during and after lactation, *Obstet Gynecol* 94:608, 1999.

42. Lasley BL, Shideler SE, Munrol CJ: A prototype for ovulation detection: pros and cons, *Am J Obstet Gynecol* 165:1991, 2003.

43. Lewis PR, Brown JB, Renfree MB, et al: The resumption of ovulation and menstruation in a well-nourished population of women breastfeeding for an extended period of time, *Fertil Steril* 55:529, 1991.

44. Marquis GS, Penny ME, Zimmer JP, et al: An overlap of breastfeeding during late pregnancy is associated with subsequent changes in colostrum composition and morbidity rates among Peruvian infants and their mothers, *J Nutr* 133:2585, 2003.

45. Marshall WM, Cumming DC, Fitzsimmons GW: Hot flushes during breastfeeding? *Fertil Steril* 57:1349, 1992.

46. Masters WH, Johnson VE: *Human sexual response*, Boston, 1996, Brown.

47. McCann MF, Potter LS: Progestin-only oral contraception: a comprehensive review, *Contraception* 50:S1, 1994.

48. McNeilly AS: Lactation and fertility, *J Mammary Gland Biol Neoplasia* 2:291, 1997.

49. McNeilly AS: Lactational control of reproduction, *Reprod Fertil Dev* 13:583, 2001.

50. Merchant K, Martorell R, Haas J: Maternal and fetal responses to the stresses of lactation concurrent with pregnancy and of short recuperative intervals, *Am J Clin Nutr* 52:280, 1990.

51. Moscone SR, Moore MJ: Breastfeeding during pregnancy, *J Hum Lact* 9:83, 1993.

52. Newton N, Newton M: Psychologic aspects of lactation, *N Engl J Med* 277:1179, 1967.

53. Newton N, Theotokatos M: Breast-feeding during pregnancy in 503 women: does psychobiological weaning mechanism exist in humans?. In *Proc Fifth Int Congr Psychcosom Obstet Gymco*, 1979, p 845.

54. Nilsson S, Mellbin T, Hofvander Y, et al: Long-term follow-up of children breastfed by mothers using oral contraceptives, *Contraception* 34:443, 1986.

55. Perez A, Labbok MH, Queenan JT: Clinical study of the lactational amenorrhea method for family planning, *Lancet* 339:968, 1992.

56. Prentice JC, Lu MC, Lange L, et al: The association between childhood sexual abuse and breastfeeding initiation, *J Hum Lact* 18:212–226, 2009.

57. Prosser CG, Saint L, Hartmann PE: Mammary gland function during gradual weaning and early gestation in women, *Aust J Exp Biol Med Sci* 62:215, 1984.

58. Rodriguez MI, Kaunitz AM: An evidence-based approach to post partum use of depot medroxyprogesterone acetate in breastfeeding women, *Contraception* 80:4–6, 2009.

59. Rosner AE, Schulman SK: Birth interval among breastfeeding women not using contraceptives, *Pediatrics* 86:747, 1990.

60. Saadeh R, Benboozid D: Breastfeeding and child-spacing: importance of information collection for public health policy, *Bull World Health Organ* 68:625, 1990.

61. Sarkar NN: The impact of intimate partner violence on women's reproductive health and pregnancy outcome, *J Obstet Gynaecol* 28:266–271, 2008.

62. Sas M, Gellen JJ, Dusitsin N, et al: An investigation on the influence of steroidal contraceptives on milk lipid and fatty acids in Hungary and Thailand, *Contraception* 33:159, 1986.

63. Selye H, McKeown T: The effect of mechanical stimulation of the nipples on the ovary and the sexual cycle, *Surg Gynecol Obstet* 59:856, 1934.

64. Shaban OM, Glasier AF: Pregnancy during breastfeeding in rural Egypt, *Contraception* 77:350–354, 2008.

65. Short RV, Lewis PR, Renfree MB, et al: Contraceptive effects of extended lactational amenorrhea: beyond the Bellagio consensus, *Lancet* 337:715, 1991.

66. Tankeyoon M, Dusitsin N, Chalapati S, et al: Effects of hormonal contraceptives on milk volume and infant growth, *Contraception* 30:505, 1984.

67. Tay CCK, Glasier AF, McNeilly AS: Twenty-four-hour patterns of prolactin secretion during lactation and the relationship to suckling and the resumption of fertility in breastfeeding women, *Hum Reprod* 11:950, 1996.

68. Taylor RS: Physiology of the vagina and cervix in breastfeeding women. In Shivanandan M, editor: *Breastfeeding and natural family planning. Fourth international symposium on natural family planning*, Chevy Chase, Md., 1985, KM Associate Publishers.

69. Technical Guidance/Competence Group. USAID/WHO: Family Planning methods: New Guidance. Population Report XXIV, No. 2, Baltimore, Md., 1996, Johns Hopkins School of Public Health.

70. Truitt ST, Fraser AB, Gallop MF, et al: *Combined hormonal versus nonhormonal versus progestin-only contraception in lactation*, 2015, The Cochran Library, John Wiley & Sons Ltd., thecochranelibrary.com/view/0/index.htm.

71. Van der Wijden C, Brown J, Kleijnen J: *Lactational amenorrhea for family planning (Review)*, issue 3, 2009, The Cochran Library.

72. Velasquez EV, Creus S, Trigo RV, et al: Pituitary ovarian axis during lactational amenorrhea. II. Longitudinal assessment of serum FSH polymorphism before and after recovery of menstrual cycles, *Hum Reprod* 21:916–923, 2006.

73. Velasquez EV, Trigo RV, Creus S, et al: Pituitary ovarian axis during lactational amenorrhea. I. Longitudinal assessment of follicular growth, gonadotrophins, sex steroids and inhibin levels before and after recovery of menstrual cyclicity, *Hum Reprod* 21:909–915, 2006.

74. Visness CM, Kennedy KI, Gross BA, et al: Fertility of fully breast-feeding women in the early postpartum period, *Obstet Gynecol* 89:164, 1997.

75. Wade K, Sevilla F, Labbok M: Integrating the lactational amenorrhea method into a family planning program in Ecuador, *Stud Fam Plann* 25:162, 1994.

76. Wei LI, Yi Q: Relation of supplementary feeding to resumptions of menstruation and ovulation in lactating post partum women, *Chin Med J* 120:868–870, 2007.

77. WHO medical eligibility criteria for contraceptive use, Geneva, 2004, WHO.

78. World Health Organization Task Force for Epidemiological Research on Reproductive Health: Progestogen-only contraceptives during lactation. I and II. Infant development, *Contraception* 50:55, 1994.

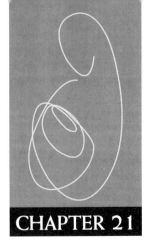

CHAPTER 21

The Collection and Storage of Human Milk and Human Milk Banking

Breast milk expression has become a very common practice. Although it is associated with maternal employment, it is also associated with the desire to make it possible for someone else to feed the infant. Pumping to donate the milk has been an uncommon reason, as has been pumping for a hospitalized infant. The prevalence of breast milk expression was determined by reviewing the data from the 2005 to 2007 Infant Feeding Practices Study II by the Center for Food Safety and Applied Nutrition, of the Food and Drug Administration (FDA), and the Centers for Disease Control and Prevention (CDC).[37] Of mothers whose infants were younger than 4½ months, 85% had expressed milk at some time since birth, 43% having done so occasionally and 25% on a regular schedule. The number was higher among first-time mothers and slowly declined as the infant became older (Figures 21-1 and 21-2).

The human milk bank has entered another era. The interest in providing human milk for infants with special needs, especially premature infants, has increased, but the concerns regarding donor milk have also escalated. Regulatory bodies have decreed that donor milk must be pasteurized. Milk banks have recognized the need for donors to be carefully screened and women at high risk for certain infections eliminated from the donor pool.

When there are risks associated with using even a mother's own milk for a given baby, the risk/benefit ratio is determined. Because of the effects of heating, cooling, freezing, and storing milk, some of the most valued and precious qualities are diminished or destroyed; feeding the milk fresh or at least fresh frozen and not heated preserves most of the constituents. The value of the milk produced by women who deliver prematurely has been discussed in Chapter 15.

Historical Perspective

When "wet nursing" was the immediate alternative feeding to replace a mother's own milk, and no safe ways were available to store milk of any species, no human milk banks existed.[7] As pasteurization became available and formulas based on milk from other species increased in popularity, the pool of human milk diminished. "Wet nurses" were increasingly difficult to locate, and often were not safe sources because of wet-nurse lifestyle, risk for infections, and poor nutrition. It had already been clearly demonstrated in the early twentieth century that infants who did not receive their mother's milk had six times the risk for dying in the first year of life (see Chapter 1).

The impetus behind milk banks at the turn of the twentieth century was actually the medical profession's desire to remove the control of infant feeding from wet nurses and separate the product (human milk) from the producer. Pediatricians, anxious to improve the prognosis for infants deprived of their own mother's milk for medical and social reasons, developed a means of storing human milk for general use for sick infants. The first milk bank was

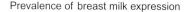

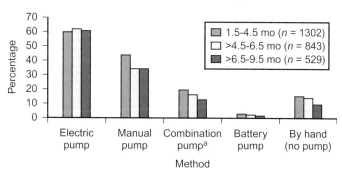

Figure 21-1. Percentage of breastfeeding mothers who had successfully expressed milk, according to method of milk expression and infant age group. The 1.5- to 4.5-month sample is based on breastfeeding mothers who responded about methods used to successfully express milk since their infant was born; the >4.5- to 6.5-month sample is based on mothers who responded in the previous 3 months; and the >6.5- to 9.5-month sample is based on mothers reporting about methods used in the previous 2 months. Samples are smaller than the total of those who had successfully expressed milk during a given period (1315, 845, and 653, respectively, for the successive age groups) as a result of question nonresponse. Respondents could mark all answers that applied; therefore percentages in each age group do not sum to 100%. [a]Combination pumps were defined as both electric and battery operated.

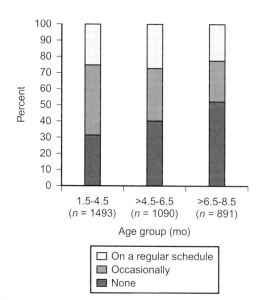

Figure 21-2. Breastfeeding mothers' prevalence of breast milk expression in the previous 2 weeks, according to infant age-group.

opened in Vienna in 1900. The first one in the United States was established 10 years later at the Massachusetts Infant Asylum, where wet nurses had been the only sources of human milk.[29] In 1919 the first human milk bank was founded in Germany in Magdeburg by Dr. Marie-Elise Kayser. In 1934, she wrote guidelines that were used throughout Europe for the creation and operation of milk banks.[67]

Early attempts at providing donor milk depended on casual screening of donors for tuberculosis, syphilis, and various acute contagious diseases.[47]

There was little research investigating human milk, but the dairy industry was rigorous in its attempt to store and market bovine and other mammalian milks. This technology was applied on a small scale, but other human milk banks appeared after Denny and Talbot created the one in Boston. The American Academy of Pediatrics (AAP) established its first formal guidelines for human milk banks in 1943.[10,11] Similar guidelines were provided in other countries. After World War II, milk banks were mandated on both sides of the Berlin Wall. In 1959 the Federal Republic of Germany (West Germany) had 24 milk banks, and the German Democratic Republic had 62.[66] The numbers gradually decreased.

As technology advanced in newborn care and in infant nutrition, science replaced nature. The interest in human milk faded, and with it the call for banked human milk, in the 1960s and into the 1970s. Experience in Rochester with short-gut syndrome and malabsorption syndromes, however, resulted in the development of a registry of lactating women, who donated fresh milk when needed. A milk bank was developed with donors providing frozen milk on a regular basis. By 1975, five large commercial milk banks were operating in Britain. Milk banks also sprang up across the United States. The system thrived with the establishment in 1985 of the Human Milk Banking Association of North America (HMBANA). The association not only facilitated communications among banks, but also began to investigate processes, develop uniform policies, and most importantly, provide professional and public education.[76]

The threat of human immunodeficiency virus (HIV) and hepatitis, the return of tuberculosis, and drug abuse have cast a long shadow on milk banks in the United States. This resulted in the closure of all but seven milk banks in North America and five in the United States in the nineties (see Appendix H). In Europe, milk banking has been key in the nourishment of premature and other high-risk infants. The Sorrento Maternity Hospital has supplied 50,000 L of milk from 10,000 donors in 40 years and provided 700 L a year both locally and across Britain in the nineties.[3] In 1994 the remaining 18 milk banks in unified Germany supplied about 15,000 L.

Many developing countries, especially in Central and South America, are establishing milk banks as part of national efforts to promote breastfeeding.[62] Studies done in nurseries in Guatemala have shown a marked decrease in mortality and morbidity rates by providing every infant with human milk, especially colostrum.[12] The United Nations Children's Fund (UNICEF) has encouraged and supported such efforts.[82]

The First International Congress on Human Milk Banking: A Vision of the Future was held in Brazil in 2000, sponsored by the Brazilian Association of Milk Banks. There are 154 milk banks in Brazil. Representatives from South America, France, United Kingdom, North America, and the Caribbean attended. All of the milk banks processed the milk. Some screened the serum of donors, but not all. None paid donors but some did provide pumps.[75] Regulations vary by locale. A resurgence of milk banks in the United States has occurred in the last 10 years, stimulated in part by the recognition of the value of human milk for premature and especially very-low-birth-weight infants by neonatologists. Another stimulus was the establishment of a for-profit milk bank in California, approved and licensed by the State of California. This milk bank, supported by venture capitalists, studied the safest ways to process milk. The milk bank was able to measure the caloric value of the milk and provide milk of 20, 22, 24, and 28 cal/oz. Its most important contribution has been the development of a supplement consisting only of human milk to be used to enhance the protein, calcium, and caloric content of a feeding of mother's milk for a premature or other compromised infant who requires extra calories, protein, and minerals.

Storing Human Milk

It is often necessary to store milk for infants, especially in the hospital. The storage of human milk involves two types of milk: mother's milk and donor milk. The distinction becomes important in how the milk is stored and prepared for an infant. It is also important because many states have developed codes for donor milk but fortunately have not regulated mother's milk as yet. Certain guidelines are appropriate for each milk. Indications for use of such milk were alluded to in other chapters but are briefly summarized here.

MOTHER'S MILK FOR A HEALTHY INFANT

The conditions under which a mother collects and stores milk while at work are not always ideal. At home, at work, or at school, milk should be collected with clean equipment, stored in sterile containers (dishwasher cleaned and dishwasher dried suffices), and handled with just-washed hands. The limits of temperature and time are an important consideration in the storage of milk.

To assess microbial growth and stability of milk protein and lipid at varying temperatures and for varying lengths of time, Hamosh et al.[30] collected samples from 16 healthy women with healthy babies who were exclusively breastfed. Sampling was done early in lactation (1 month postpartum) and late in lactation (5 to 6 months postpartum). The milk pH decreased from 7.02 ± 0.20 to 5.16 ± 0.26 after 24 hours of storage at $38°C$ ($100°F$), and significant differences in pH occurred at all temperatures at 24 hours or longer. Proteolysis was minimal at $15°C$ ($59°F$) and $25°C$ ($77°F$), but became apparent at $38°C$ ($100°F$) at 24 hours. Lipolysis was marked in the first 24 hours at all temperatures compared with freshly expressed milk. Bacterial growth or normal flora was minimal at $15°C$ at 24 hours, low at $25°C$ at 8 hours, and higher at $38°C$ by 4 hours.

The authors concluded that storage of human milk is safe at $15°C$ for 24 hours and $25°C$ (room temperature) for 4 hours and should not be stored at $38°C$. Proteins appear to maintain their structure and function in short-term storage. The marked lipolysis appears to slow bacterial growth at the same time.[30]

PASTEURIZING BREAST MILK AT HOME

Many women face the dilemma of discarding milk pumped when they had a *Candida* infection of the breast before it was diagnosed. Freezing does not destroy *Candida*. It has been suggested that milk could be "pasteurized" at home, for use at home by the mother's own infant. Below are the steps for home pasteurization for one's own infant, not a milk bank:

Pour all milk into a large saucepan, and place over medium heat on the stove.
Using a candy thermometer, gradually bring the milk to a temperature of 145°F (62.5°C).

Watch closely, and stir often, keeping milk at this temperature for 30 minutes.

Milk can then be poured into appropriate storage containers.

Label each container with the baby's name and the date and time of pasteurization.

Freeze the pasteurized milk in dishwasher-clean containers until ready for use.

Do not boil the milk (boiling occurs at 212°F or 100°C).

If performed correctly, this process will decrease nutritional and immunologic components by about 30%, but will destroy all microorganisms.

See Protocol 8 in Appendix P for more information. This milk should not be shared, but used only for the mother's baby.

MOTHER'S MILK FOR A SICK INFANT

The following situations are common scenarios for the use of mother's own milk.

1. A mother plans to breastfeed the infant ultimately but needs to provide pumped milk until the infant can be put to the breast.
2. An infant requires the special nutritional benefits of human milk (as with those infants who are recovering from intestinal surgery), but cannot nurse at the breast.
3. An infant weighs 1500 g or less and has difficulty digesting and absorbing other milks and is usually fed by nasogastric tube.

MILK SHARING

Milk sharing has become a popular source of human milk, and the various methods have generated much discussion in various media. Serious analysis of the activity has shown that it is not safe. A carefully executed study of milk samples purchased on the Internet showed high contamination with bacteria and, in some cases, pathogenic bacteria. The authors also reported poor collection, storage, and shipping practices. This study did not measure toxins, pharmaceuticals, or medications, which are also a risk in shared milk for the sick or premature infants. Caloric content and protein levels were not measured. Clearly, Internet sharing or selling milk by unscreened donors is not recommended. Small community-based nonprofit milk sharing systems where the donors are screened provide safety. They do not guarantee the caloric content, and it is known that the caloric content can be as low as 15 cal/oz. Neonatal intensive care units (NICUs) who need milk for high-risk infants should only accept milk from certified sources.

DONOR MILK FROM A MILK BANK

The following scenarios are common reasons for obtaining donor milk from a bank.

1. An infant is at risk for infection or necrotizing enterocolitis. Fresh colostrum is held to be especially protective and may be collected from low-risk, carefully screened mothers, who are not breastfeeding their own infants.
2. An infant has a gastrointestinal anomaly or other reasons for intestinal tract surgery, especially short-gut syndrome.
3. A physician thinks an infant would benefit from the nourishment in human milk because of prematurity, especially if the infant weighs less than 1500 g.
4. A mother is temporarily unable to nourish her own breastfed infant completely. It may be that the mother's supply is inadequate when she first puts the infant to the breast after weeks of pumping, or when the mother has been ill or hospitalized. Usually these infants are already at home.
5. Donor milk is an excellent transition from parenteral nutrition when mother's milk is not available. It allows earlier weaning from parenteral solution—earlier than when formula is known to be tolerated.
6. Metabolic disorders, especially amino acid disorders, respond well because of the physiologic profile of human milk (decreased casein, tyrosine, and phenylalanine). In addition, human milk is protective against infection, which may be a serious complication of these disorders.
7. An older infant or child has unique feeding difficulties, usually characterized by an inability to tolerate any oral nourishment except human milk (e.g., a child dying of HIV infection).

STRUCTURE OF A MILK BANK

Most informal and casual milk banks operating in conjunction with a NICU have disappeared.[61] NICUs may provide a deep freeze for storage of a mother's own milk for use by her infant. They store it for feeding of the infant and do not process it at all except to culture random samples for contamination. Most do not permit "donating" milk to other infants except by private arrangements between the two mothers with a physician's approval. No feeding is given to an infant in the hospital without a physician's order. Smaller public milk banks have phased out since state legislation or local medical practice standards have mandated strict surveillance of samples and pasteurization.

A few large, well-established banks operate in the United States and around the world (Figure 21-3). A network of these milk banks meets and shares information through the HMBANA in

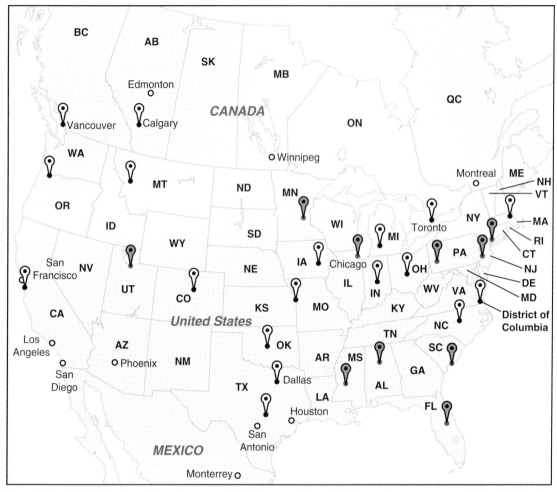

Figure 21-3. HMBANA milk bank locations in the United States and Canada. White markers represent established milk banks; gray markers represent banks in development. (Data from www.hmbana.org/locations (Accessed 26.05.15).)

North America.[2,76] Copies of the association's guidelines for milk storage are available for a fee. HMBANA works closely with the FDA concerning FDA regulations for human tissues and fluids. Appendix H provides the guidelines (Figure 21-4).

The Mother's Milk Bank of the Institute for Medical Research in San Jose, California, was established in 1974. It has a full-time coordinator and a medical director, provides milk for hundreds of infants, and contributes to the fund of knowledge on human milk. Because the milk is provided to patients only by physician's prescription, it is reimbursable by health insurance carriers of California. Mother's Milk Bank has developed procedures and policies regarding milk collection, storage, and processing. This was first described in detail by Asquith et al.[2] and documented with an extensive bibliography.

The State of New York passed an amendment to the public health law in 1980, in which it was declared policy that any and all infants requiring

human breast milk be assured access to sufficient quantities of wholesome human breast milk, donated by concerned lactating mothers on a continued and systematic basis. New York State has regulations, which have the force of law, governing human milk banks. They address construction, medical direction, donor qualifications, milk collection and storage, maintenance of records, and milk distribution. They are available on the Internet in Part 52, Subpart 52-9, of Title 10 (Health) of the New York Code of Rules and Regulations, which can be accessed from the New York State Department of Health's Public website at http://www.health.ny.gov/regulations/nycrr/title_10 (accessed 30 April 2015).

Neonatologists caution that the cavalier feeding of unsterile unsupplemented breast milk to premature infants may produce iatrogenic problems. Mothers who pump and save milk for their own infants should follow the instructions/guidelines for storing mother's own milk (see Appendix J, Protocol #8).

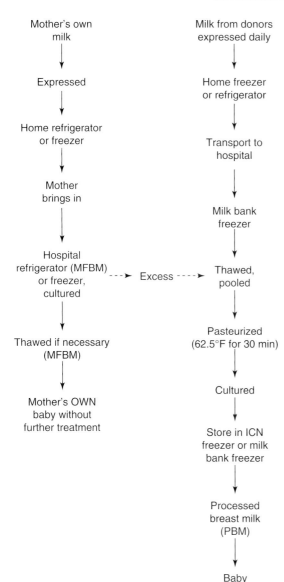

Figure 21-4. Flow chart of process for the mother at home pumping for her hospitalized infant *(left)*. The right column outlines the steps a donor takes when collecting milk for the bank. The mother described on the *left* can become a donor if she has an abundance of milk and is screened to be a donor. *MFBM,* Mother's frozen breast milk.

QUALIFICATIONS OF DONORS

A mother who is willing to donate milk should be healthy and fulfill the following qualifications (Box 21-1):

1. Normal pregnancy and delivery
2. Serologically negative for syphilis, hepatitis B surface antigen, cytomegalovirus (CMV), and HIV
3. No infection, acute or chronic (i.e., not at high risk)

BOX 21-1. Donor Screening Procedures

1. Donors answer questions on a verbal health history screening form. Primary health care providers for the prospective donor and her infant are asked for verification of health.
2. Donors are tested serologically for:
   a. HIV-1 and HIV-2
   b. HTLV-I and HTLV-II
   c. Hepatitis B
   d. Hepatitis C
   e. Syphilis
3. Repeat donors are treated as new donors with each pregnancy.
4. Milk banks will cover the cost of the serologic screening if the tests are done by the milk bank.

   Reasons for excluding a donor
- Receipt of a blood transfusion or blood products within last 12 months
- Receipt of an organ or tissue transplant within last 12 months
- Regular use of more than 2 oz of hard liquor or its equivalent in a 24-hour period
- Regular use of over-the-counter medications or systemic prescriptions (replacement hormones and some birth control hormones acceptable)
- Use of megadose vitamins or pharmacologically active herbal preparations
- Total vegetarians (vegans) who do not supplement their diet with vitamins
- Use of illegal drugs
- Use of tobacco products
- Silicone breast implants
- History of hepatitis, systemic disorders of any kind, or chronic infections (e.g., HIV, HTLV, TB)

---

4. Not taking medications, smoking, or using excessive alcohol
5. Capable of carrying out sterile technique
6. If donating for other infants, own child is healthy and without jaundice

When a directive from the Department of Health and Social Security in Great Britain mandated HIV testing for donors to milk banks, it was observed that the list of 19 established milk banks dwindled to six.[3] The Sorrento Maternity Hospital, however, in accordance with the directive of the Department of Health and Social Security, screened all donors for HIV antibodies. Only four mothers of 470 potential donors have refused to be tested, contrary to fears that the ruling would discourage donating.[3]

The donor should not be taking medications regularly, including certain oral contraceptives and any nonprescription medications, such as

TABLE 21-4 Comparison of Effects of Temperature on Vitamins, Fatty Acids, and Cultures

Microbial Analysis of Frozen and Thawed Breast Milk		Vitamin Analysis of Frozen and Thawed Breast Milk	
Conditions	CFU/mL	Vitamin A (IE/100 mL)	Vitamin C (mg/ 100 mL)
8°C for 4 hours	8.6×10^1	100	2.2
8°C for 24 hours	3.5×10^1	100	1.7
23°C for 4 hours	1.0×10^2	105	1.6
23°C for 8 hours	3.7×10^2	100	1.0
Repeated freeze-thaw	1.1×10^2	100	1.5
Control	1.1×10^2	100	2.2

CFU, Colony-forming units.

TABLE 21-5 Ranking of Samples

Fatty Acid	Highest Peaks					Lowest Peaks
C6	F	C	D	B	E	A
C8	F	C	D	B	E	A
C10	F	D	C	E	B	A
C12	C	D	F	B	E	A
C14	C	D	F	B	E	A
C16:1	C	F	B	D	A	E
C16	C	D	F	B	A	E
C18:2	C	B	F	D	A	E
C18:1	C	F	B	D	A	E

A = 8°C for 4 hours; B = 8°C for 24 hours; C = 23°C for 4 hours; D = 23°C for 8 hours; E = represented freeze-thaw; F = control.

Modified from Tables 2, 3, and 4 of Rechtman DJ, Lee ML, Berg H: Effect of environmental conditions on unpasteurized donor human milk, *Breastfeed Med* 1:24, 2006.

volumes in professional human milk banks. It requires establishing 72°C (87°F) for 15 seconds, which involves greater technical skill than the Holder method. The investigators report that HTST is effective in the elimination of bacteria as well as important pathogenic viruses. A time of 16 seconds is recommended rather than the original 15 seconds. Subsequently, they have demonstrated that HTST preserves the nutrients in human milk.

HTST treatment (72°F or 87°C up to 16 seconds) of human milk inoculated with endogenous bacteria and CMV rendered the milk bacteria free in 5 seconds and CMV-free in 15 seconds.[27] Folic acid and vitamins B_1, B_2, B_6, and C were

not affected. Bile salt-stimulated lipase was inactivated by these conditions. Lactoferrin and IgA and secretory IgA antibody activity were stable at 72°C (162°F) for 15 seconds. Lysozyme concentration and enzymatic activity were increased, suggesting that lysozyme may be sequestered in the milk.

The HTST technique was thoroughly studied by Terpstra et al.[73] to determine its effect on the bioburden of human milk. HTST was effective in eliminating all bacteria and lipid-enveloped viruses, as well as at least one nonlipid envelope virus from spiked samples. Furthermore, HTST preserved IgA and other proteins important to immune defences. The authors suggest HTST is the method of choice for milk banks[73] (Tables 21-6 and 21-7).

The effect of temperature on transforming growth factor (TGF)-α and TGF-$β_2$ of human milk concentrations during pasteurization (at temperatures commonly used by donor milk banks) slightly decreased TGF-α concentrations, but not milk TGF-$β_2$. There was little difference when temperature was increased to 71°C.[48]

PASTEURIZATION BY HOLDER METHOD

Recommended pasteurization of human milk for banks, according to HMBANA guidelines, follows these steps:[76,78]

1. All containers shall be tightly closed with new caps to prevent contamination of milk during heat treatment.
2. Heat processing.
   a. Aliquots of milk shall be processed by completely submerging the containers in a well-agitated or shaking water bath preheated to a minimum of 63°C.
   b. A control bottle, containing the same amount of milk or water as the most filled container of milk in the batch, shall be fitted with a calibrated thermometer to register milk temperature during heat processing. The control bottle should follow the same process as the rest of the batch at all times.
   c. The thermometer shall be positioned such that approximately 25% of the milk volume is below the measuring point of the thermometer.
   d. The monitored aliquot shall be placed into the water bath after all other aliquots and shall be positioned centrally among the treated aliquots.
   e. After the temperature of the monitored control bottle has reached a minimum of 62.5°C, the heat treatment shall continue for 30 minutes. Milk shall not reach a core temperature higher than 63°C.

TABLE 21-6 Effect of High-Temperature Short-Time (HTST) Pasteurization on Selected Vitamins in Human Milk

	Time (s)							
	0		**1**		**3**		**15**	
	P = V × I	n	P = V × I	n	P = V × I	n	P = V × I	n
Vitamin B₁ (mcg/mL)	0.104 ± 0.013	9						
72°C			0.098 ± 0.005	3	0.091 ± 0.008	3	0.088 ± 0.009	3
87°C	0.084 ± 0.011*	3			0.095 ± 0.027	3	ND	
Vitamin B₂ (mcg/mL)	0.724 ± 0.132	9						
72°C			0.75 ± 0.08	3	0.70 ± 0.09	3	0.56 ± 0.07	3
87°C			0.66 ± 0.13†	3	0.72 ± 0.22	3	ND	3
Vitamin B₆ (mcg/mL)	0.237 ± 0.081	9						
72°C			0.27 ± 0.05	3	0.26 ± 0.025	3	0.22 ± 0.012	3
87°C			0.25 ± 0.07	3	0.26 ± 0.02	3	ND	
Folic acid (mcg/mL)	0.106 ± 0.020	9						
72°C			0.089 ± 0.005‡	3*	0.065 ± 0.018	3	0.101 ± 0.012	3
87°C			0.088 ± 0.008	3	0.080 ± 0.023	3	ND	
Vitamin C (mcg/mL)	9.2 ± 2.4	9						
72°C			11.2 ± 1.2	3	21.5 ± 3.0*	3	8.7 ± 1.7	3
87°C			16.0 ± 4.9*	3	22.5 ± 13.3	3	ND	

*$p < 0.07$.
†$p < 0.001$.
‡$p < 0.04$.
From Goldblum RM, Dill CW, Albrecht TB, et al: Rapid high-temperature treatment of human milk, *J Pediatr* 104:380, 1984.

TABLE 21-7 Effect of High-Temperature Short-Time (HTST) Pasteurization on Immunologic Proteins in Human Milk

	Time (s)							
	0		**1**		**3**		**15**	
	P = V × I	n	P = V × I	n	P = V × I	n	P = V × I	n
Lactoferrin (mg/mL)	0.67 ± 0.10	8						
72°C			0.95 ± 0.21	2	0.58 ± 0.2	3	0.83 ± 0.05	3
87°C			0.50 ± 0.02	3	0.50 ± 0.2	3	0.47 ± 0.17	2
Lysozyme (mcg/mL)	15.0 ± 8.7	8						
72°C			86.0 ± 3.5*	2	78.0 ± 16.0	3†	59.0 ± 7.0*	3
87°C			86.0 ± 9.1*	3	59.0 ± 9.0	3†	36.0 ± 7.7	2
Total IgA (mg/mL)	0.37 ± 0.08	8						
72°C			0.37 ± 0.07	2	0.25 ± 0.06	3	0.3 ± 0.04	3
87°C			0.06 ± 0.04*	3	0.04 ± 0.02	3†	0.05 ± 0.03	2
sIgA Ab (reciprocal titer)	10.0 ± 4.8	7						
72°C			10.2 ± 12.4	2	10.6 ± 4.8	2	15.0 ± 3.5	3
87°C			<1	3	<1	2	<1	2

n, Number of experiments; *sIgA*, secretory immunoglobulin A.
*$p < 0.01$.
†$p < 0.05$.
From Goldblum RM, Dill CW, Albrecht TB, et al: Rapid high-temperature treatment of human milk, *J Pediatr* 104:380, 1984.

VIRUSES IN HUMAN MILK

The dilemma of CMV is a significant one because the virus does pass into the milk. In a study of postpartum women, CMV was recovered from the genital tract in 10%, from the urine in 7%, from the saliva in 2%, and from the breast milk in 30%. CMV does persist after storage at 4 and −20°C (39 and −4°F) in some specimens.[68] It is destroyed at 62.5°C after 30 minutes.[15] Donor milk should be accepted only from CMV-negative mothers. Mothers who are seropositive may be permitted

TABLE 21-10 Storage of Human Milk and Protein N Concentrations (mg N/dL)

Storage Time (h)	Storage Temperature		
	37°C	4°C	−72°C
4	187 ± 8*	181 ± 7*	
24	183 ± 7*,†	178 ± 5*,†	186 ± 8†
48	189 ± 8*	178 ± 5*	

Mean ± 1 SEM (n = 11).

*Effects from temperature significant when samples stored at 37°C and 4°C are compared (p < 0.05; F = 9.3).

†Comparison of storage temperature effects on samples stored only for 24 h not significant (p > 0.05; F = 1.4).

From Garza C, Johnson CA, Harrist R, et al: Effects of methods of collection and storage on nutrients in human milk, *Early Hum Dev* 6:295, 1982.

TABLE 21-11 Thermal Destruction of Milk Components (Follows First-Order Reaction Kinetics)

	D Value* at 60°C (s)	Z Value† (°C)
IgA	4.9×10^4	5.5
Lactoferrin	2.4×10^3	4.7
Thiamine	7.7×10^5	28.4
Folic acid	1.9×10^4	6.4

*90% degradation at 60°C in seconds.

†Temperature change to alter degradation rate by a factor of 10.

Modified from Morgan JN, Toledo RT, Eitenmiller RR, et al: Thermal destruction of immunoglobulin A, lactoferrin, thiamin, and folic acid in human milk, *J Food Sci* 51:348, 1986.

Freezing at −80°C significantly decreases the energy content of human milk both from fat and carbohydrate. Thus −80°C is not recommended for long-term storage.[42]

Because the nourishment of low-birth-weight (LBW) infants has been the purpose of many milk banks, the ability of preterm infants to utilize treated bank milk is relative. Pasteurization at 62.5°C for 30 minutes was reported not to influence nitrogen absorption or retention in LBW infants.[63] When raw, pasteurized, and boiled human milks were fed to very LBW (VLBW) (less than 1.3 kg) preterm infants in three separate consecutive weeks, fat absorption was reduced by one third in the heat-treated group. There was a reduction in the amount of nitrogen retained in the heat-treated group, as well, although the absorption was unaffected. The absorption and retention of calcium, phosphorus, and sodium were unaffected by heating or freezing. The mean weight gain was one third greater when the infants were fed raw human milk.[83]

Pasteurization decreased vitamin B_{12} by approximately 50% and folate-binding capacity by 10%[48] (see Table 21-11). Sterilization (100°C for 20 minutes), on the other hand, had similar effects on vitamin B_{12} binding and completely inactivated folate binding.[53] Vitamins A, D, E, B_2, and B_6, choline, niacin, and pantothenic acid were barely affected by pasteurization, whereas thiamine was reduced up to 25%, biotin up to 10%, and vitamin C up to 35%.[80]

Refrigeration at 4 to 6°C for 72 hours allows little bacterial growth and causes no change in nutrients or infection-protective properties. Freezing does have some effect on both, and the milk can be kept for months, whereas heating has significant effect, and the milk still requires freezing for storage. Quick freezing and frozen storage do not significantly affect levels of biotin, niacin, folic acid, vitamin E, and the fat-soluble vitamins. Photooxidation and absorption by the container or tubing are always a consideration. Vitamin C is reduced by both these processes.[23]

The effect of heating and freezing on the various constituents of human milk has been studied by a number of investigators. Their data should be considered before deciding how to store milk for special purposes, such as sick or premature infants.[64]

ANALYSIS

Routine analysis of the nutrient value of milk samples has been considered not practical, so gross screening by creamatocrit has been done by some banks and nurseries. A method of infrared analysis using a Milko-Scan 104 Infrared Analyzer (A/S Foss Electric, Hillerod, Denmark) has been described by Michaelsen et al.[50] It is simpler and more rapid than previous methods. These investigators in Denmark found a linear correlation between infrared results and the standard reference methods of Kjeldahl for nitrogen (protein), Roese Gottlieb for fat, and bomb calorimetry for energy. These techniques were used on all incoming milk, and on the outgoing pooled milk in banks in Denmark.

All the milk from the same mother was thawed, pooled, and stirred vigorously on arrival at the bank. A 10-mL sample was taken and stored at −5°C until analysis. Samples were collected every 2 weeks and were analyzed up to 2 to 3 weeks after expression. For the 2554 collections of milk contributed by 224 women, the mean protein content was 9 g/L and the fat was 39 g/L. The greater the body mass index of the mother, the greater was the protein and fat content.

The authors suggest that by selecting the milk with the highest protein content (12 g/L), a high-protein milk can be created with a higher energy content (725 kcal/L) for use in VLBW infants. Furthermore, they recommend pooling milk from up to five mothers to decrease the variability in nutrient levels.[50]

The product available from Prolacta Bioscience is labeled by both caloric content and protein content. Neo20 contains 20 cal/oz and 1.2 g of protein per 100 mL. Prolact20 also contains 20 cal/oz and 1.2 g protein/100 mL, as well as essential minerals. Prolacta Bioscience has also produced a human milk fortifier (Prolact + H^{2}MF) that contains only human milk. Nutritional constituents are provided on the label. This allows fortification of mother's milk or donor milk to meet the growth needs of VLBW infants using a human milk product. Ross Laboratory and Mead Johnson products called human milk fortifier (a misnomer) are made solely of bovine products.

At the Hvidovre Milk Bank in Copenhagen, monitoring of the macronutrients in donor milk is part of the bank's quality assurance standards. Donors are discontinued if their milk protein content becomes less than 8 g/L. Their milk was viewed as adequate for their own baby but not for high-risk infants, especially premature infants.

CREAMATOCRIT

Testing milk for protein, fat, and carbohydrate has not been done by most banks. However, Lucas et al.[44] have suggested a quick method of analysis. It involves standard hematocrit microtubes and a centrifuge. The percentage of cream, or "creamatocrit," is read from the capillary tube. Fat and energy content have a linear relationship, as follows:

$$Fat(g/L) = \frac{Creamatocrit[\%] - 0.59}{0.146}$$

$$kcal/L = 290 + (66.8 \times Creamatocrit[\%])$$

Accuracy is within 10%.

The Research Institute for Health Sciences provides the following formula for calculating the fat and energy content of milk, using the measurement of the creamatocrit (%)[59]:

$$Fat(g/L) = (6.24 \times Creamatocrit[\%]) - 3.08$$

$$[r = 0.98, 95\% \text{ confidence limit} = \pm 4.39 \, g/L]$$

$$kcal/dL = (5.57 \times Creamatocrit[\%]) + 45.13$$

$$[r = 0.92, 95\% \text{ confidence limit} = \pm 12.61 \, kcal/dL]$$

Studies done comparing energy value calculated by creamatocrit with energy value from percentage of carbon, as measured by Manchester bomb calorimeter using pooled pasteurized milk samples, were somewhat inaccurate compared with data obtained by creamatocrit on fresh or fresh-frozen samples.[65]

The methodology was validated with further analysis by Lemons et al.,[41] who repeated the studies and confirmed actual measurements of total fat and caloric content. Because the protein and lactose content remains relatively constant over time, the variation in fat content is the primary constituent affecting caloric value of the milk. Neither freezing for up to 2 months, nor pasteurization, affected the creamatocrit. There was no evidence of fat globule degradation during storage that affected the test.

Special cautions while performing this simple test should include the following:

- Use a representative, well-mixed sample.
- Complete a sample of pumping from at least one breast; do not take just a spot sample.
- Use a well-mixed 24-hour sample.
- Use a tube at least three fourths filled; seal one end.
- Centrifuge for 15 minutes in standard table-top centrifuge.

A new technology, the Creamatocrit Plus, has been reported by Meier et al.[49] The device is a special centrifuge that spins and calculates the creamatocrit. It automatically calculates the fat and calorie content. This device has been in use in research and in NICUs. Its accuracy was compared with the standard laboratory centrifuge with a hematocrit reader, and the standard laboratory centrifuge with digital calipers, utilizing 36 milk specimens from 12 women. The results varied less than 1% from each other. Laboratory measurements for lipids and calories were confirmatory.[49] NICUs that use mother's milk can easily check the content of a mother's milk with this device. Human milk fortifier derived solely from human milk (Prolact + H^{2}MF) and HM-derived cream (Prolact CR™) were combined with mother's milk and fed via feeding tube to premature infants in continuous enteral feedings. This mixture avoided the loss of fat and micronutrients and resulted in the benefits of bioactive elements from mother's milk and increased fat delivery. It improved infant weight gain.[72]

ULTRASONIC HOMOGENIZATION

Pooling specimens of human milk may not result in a milk of uniform fat content after storage. The separation of fat during processing, storage, and administration by continuous nasogastric infusion, whether by gravity flow or continuous mechanical pump, results in significant loss of fat and variation in the milk received (47.4% of fat with slow infusion and 16.8% with fast infusion).

Homogenization by ultrasonic treatment was studied by Martinez et al.,[45] who found that changes in fat concentration during infusion and loss of fat during administration, caused by the fat sticking to the container and tubes, were eliminated. Furthermore, the fat-soluble vitamins are preserved. Because 31% of iron, 15% of copper, 12% of zinc, 10% of calcium, and 2% of magnesium sulfate are in the fat fraction of both human and cow milk, preserving the fat is essential to maximizing nutrient intake from human milk, especially in compromised infants. Tube feedings have been noted to reduce vitamins B_2, B_6, A, and C in human milk.

Ultrasonic homogenization was accomplished in this study by subjecting the milk to treatment in a Tekmar Sonic Disruptor TSD-P 250 (Tekmar Co., Cincinnati, Ohio). The homogenization time (2, 4, or 8 minutes) is a function of the volume of milk and intensity of vibration. The procedure should be done with milk in an ice bath. It has not been tested to determine the amount of lipase, if any, that survives pasteurization and would be capable of digesting the fat after homogenizing.

MICROWAVE EFFECTS

Milk should be thawed in the refrigerator, and each bottle should be used completely within 24 hours. Defrosting in the microwave oven may lead to separation of layers, and microwaves decrease vitamin C content. The greatest danger of microwaving is that the milk heats and the container does not, so an infant could be burned or the milk significantly overheated.

The effects of microwave radiation on human milk have been much debated. The only nutritional effect identified has been the lowering of the vitamin C level. Lysozyme activity, total IgA, and specific IgA to *E. coli* serotypes 01, 04, and 06 were tested in 22 freshly frozen milk samples before and after heating for 30 seconds at low-power and high-power settings of the microwave oven.[59] Additional samples were tested at low (20 to 25°C), medium (60 to 70°C), and high (98°C or higher) microwave powers, before the addition of *E. coli*

suspension. Microwaving at high temperatures (72 to 98°C) greatly decreased all the tested antiinfective factors (Table 21-12). *E. coli* growth at 98°C or higher was 18 times that of untreated thawed human milk. Low temperatures did not affect total IgA or specific IgA to *E. coli* serotypes 01 and 04 or specific IgA to *E. coli* serotype 06. At only 20 to 25°C, the growth of *E. coli* was five times that of the untreated thawed milk.[59]

In the experimental laboratories, the microwaves are carefully controlled. In the home, they vary tremendously. Ovesen et al.[56] admitted that the temperature had to stay under 60°C (140°F). Above that, antibodies were decreased and at 77°C (170°F), they were totally destroyed. Vitamins B_1 and E were apparently stable, but they did not test for vitamin C. It is very clear that IgA, secretory IgA, and lysozyme were affected by microwaving at 14 to 25°C (i.e., lower temperatures). Time is important because even at 30% power the temperature will increase over time.

Microwaving clearly interferes with the antiinfective properties of human milk—the higher the temperature, the greater the effect (Table 21-13)—and is not appropriate for heating human milk.

SPECIALTY MILKS

New technologies offer the potential for providing specialty milks. Simple homogenization would preserve the fat, as noted. However, because of the presence of active enzymes, once the fat membrane is ruptured by homogenization, the milk should be used promptly to prevent excessive fat breakdown. Lyophilization, or freeze drying, is an opportunity to concentrate the nutrients without increasing the volume. Adding a freeze-dried aliquot to liquid human milk is preferable to using the commercial

TABLE 21-12	Impact of Microwaving on Antiinfective Factors in Human Milk*			
	No.	Control	Low Microwave	High Microwave
Lysozyme activity (mcg/mL)	22	23.7 ± 4.0	19.2 ± 3.4	0.9 ± 0.72
			$p < 0.005$	$p < 0.0005$
Total IgA (mg/dL)	22	73.3 ± 16.1	48.9 ± 15.8	1.55 ± 1.54
			$NS^\dagger$	$p < 0.0005$
Antigen-specific antigen to **E. coli** *serotype*				
01	22	100%	$91 \pm 9.2^\ddagger$	$24.9 \pm 10.0^\ddagger$
04	22	100%	$90.3 \pm 6.5^\ddagger$	$12.3 \pm 3.7^\ddagger$
06	22	100%	$79.8 \pm 5.7^\ddagger$	$17.1 \pm 3.6^\ddagger$
			$p < 0.005$	$p < 0.0005$

IgA, Immunoglobulin A.

*Results are mean ± SEM. All significant differences were also confirmed by the Fisher protected least significant difference test.

[†]Not significant.

[‡]Percentage of control.

From Quan R, Yang C, Rubinstein S, et al: Effects of microwave radiation on anti-infective factors in human milk, *Pediatrics* 89:667, 1992.

TABLE 21-13 Impact of Microwaving on *Escherichia coli* Growth in Human Milk at 3½ Hours*

	No.	Colony Count
Control	10	$8.4 \pm 2.7 \times 10^7$
Low microwave	10	$43.9 \pm 11.4 \times 10^{7\dagger}$
Medium microwave	10	$90.1 \pm 24.1 \times 10^{7\ddagger}$
High microwave	10	$152 \pm 43 \times 10^{7\ddagger}$

*Results are mean $\pm$ SEM. All significant differences were also confirmed by the Fisher protected least significant difference test.
$\dagger p = 0.005$ compared with control.
$\ddagger p = 0.001$ compared with control.
From Quan R, Yang C, Rubinstein S, et al: Effects of microwave radiation on anti-infective factors in human milk, *Pediatrics* 89:667, 1992.

bovine-based products. Such a human milk product is available from Prolacta. In Denmark, infrared analysis of milk donations is used to provide high-protein or high-fat pools of milk. In Canada and the United States, some banks identify donors with dairy-free diets for specific infants with bovine protein allergies.[1-3] Gluten free milk from mothers on gluten free diets is available. Fat free milk can be prepared from a mother's own milk by NICU staff for an infant with chylothorax that does not need pasteurization. It is described in Chapter 14.

CONTAMINATION WITH COW MILK

Donor milk is at risk for being contaminated with cow milk by the donor. The California Mother's Milk Bank checks its contributions with a simple test directed at precipitating the casein. It mixes 1 mL of donor milk with 1 mL of 8 N sulfuric acid and 8 mL of water, and lets it sit at room temperature for 5 hours. If cow milk is present, it will precipitate.[54] Human milk makes a floccular curd. A quicker, more accurate method is to check the DNA of the sample to match the donor. This is done by both Medolac and Prolacta.

SOUR MILK FOLLOWING STORAGE

For decades, women have reported to the Lactation Study Center that their fresh-frozen breast milk smells sour, and even rancid. When thawed, it is rejected by their infant. Although a slightly soapy odor had sometimes been noted, it had never been reported to be harmful or to be rejected by the infant. This soapy smell has been attributed to a change in the lipid structure associated with the freeze-thaw effects of the self-defrost cycle in the freezer-refrigerator.

The cases reported to the Center, however, have suggested true lipid breakdown is associated with the rancid smell. The speculation first suggested in

the first edition in 1979 was that some women have more lipase activity than others, as noted in the study of lipase and hyperbilirubinemia. Some mothers reported that their milk began to smell as soon as it cooled, whether refrigerated or frozen. Others have noted that their stockpile of milk, meticulously stored in anticipation of returning to work, was rancid and rejected by their infants when thawed months later. When these mothers heated their milk to a scald (not boiling) immediately after collection and then quickly cooled and froze it, the effect was not apparent, and their infants accepted the heat-treated milk. That process, it was speculated, inactivated the lipase and halted the process of fat digestion. On the other hand, scalding rancid milk will not improve the flavor or smell. Scalding does not work for all mothers. A few mothers have noted improvement when they lowered the pressure and speed of the pump. This is also noted in the bovine literature.

In the over 4 decades since the first thoughts about sour milk were published, many women have experienced the devastation of discovering they had stored quarts and quarts of sour milk. Some women found scalding helped prevent souring. But no studies were done predominately because no investigator could accumulate enough samples to study lipase levels. This problem was solved thanks to the wise thinking of the Medolac Bank leadership. Medolac had received thousands of donor milk samples and, in the screening process, identified some that were sour. They separated the sour milk samples out, kept them frozen, and shared them with the Lactation Study Center at the University of Rochester. Analysis of lipase activity, fatty acids, and pH were done. The samples had already been cultured at Medolac, and no samples had excessive growth, or any species except skin flora. Cultures were unremarkable.

Lipase levels were compared with levels in known normal milk samples. Lipase in the sour milk was half that of the normal samples, not increased. Lactic acid was increased and lactate was low or unmeasurable, similar to the normal samples. This was reported by the Academy of Breastfeeding Medicine meetings in Los Angeles, California, in October, 2015. Further studies are underway at the Lactation Study Center. The cause of the souring or human milk is still unconfirmed.

FINANCIAL ASPECTS OF BANKING

Established milk banks have various financial structures.[3] Charges can include fees for equipment rental and for processing milk. Certainly a hospital should recover costs of collecting and processing. Precedent for this has been set in the United States. Because some states have passed legislation mandating the availability of human milk for all babies who need it, reimbursement and funds must be available for its proper handling.

All banks have a minimal charge that partially covers the costs of processing, such as labor, equipment, and supplies. The largest cost is shipping it frozen overnight. As with blood banks, the recipient is not charged for the milk itself. Third-party payers do reimburse for this, and Women, Infants, and Children (WIC) programs also provide this reimbursement in more and more states.

The recommendations from the State of New York suggest that the monitoring of standards of a hospital-based bank be absorbed into existing hospital surveillance. New York State has not approved a bank in the state, however one should be approved by the end of 2015. Freestanding banks would be monitored by the state and local health departments. Economic analysis indicates that the primary costs would be administrative overhead costs. Also acknowledged are staff costs, minimal equipment costs, and laboratory costs, as well as costs to the state health department to administer the system. Much consideration is being given to limiting banks to hospital settings, where health professionals and equipment are readily available, and quality control is part of the system.

The average processing fee charged by milk banks in the United States begins over $4.00 per ounce, although it does not totally cover costs.[3] No infant is refused access for lack of funds, and milk banks cover their costs by various methods, including donations, subsidies, and grants. With proper physician orders and paperwork, most third-party payers cover the cost of banked human milk. The cost of milk from Prolacta Bioscience is higher, but it only covers costs of operation and preparation. They provide information about the milk (calories, protein, fat, etc.). Prolacta makes a supplement to add to mother's milk that contains additional protein and fat from human milk. The supplement made by formula companies is made form bovine milk. The bovine-based supplement made by formula companies carries a significant charge.

Costs of necrotizing enterocolitis (NEC) and the cost-effectiveness of exclusively human milk-based products in feeding extremely premature infants were determined by Ganapathy et al.[24] NEC is costly in terms of medical needs and increased length of stay in the hospital. When costs were calculated for infants receiving bovine supplement, compared to the cost of caring for infants who do not get NEC, there was a huge saving. The cost of patients without NEC averaged $74,000, and with NEC $236,000. The cost of bovine supplement was $1.30 per packet. The cost of human milk supplement was $6.25 per mL. The calculated saving per infant given human milk was over $8000. Cost ignores the benefit of avoiding the lifelong burden of NEC.

While banks in North America, HMBANA, and parts of Europe have been not-for-profit and do not pay the donors for their milk, historically that has not always been true. For hundreds of years, when the need for human milk was a life-or-death matter, donors (called wet nurses) were given room and board for themselves and their infant, or some other "pay." British royalty always hired women to take care of the offspring. When the child was young enough to be breastfed, one attendant would be labeled the dry nurse; the breastfeeding nurse was the wet nurse. They were employees. Recently, the Mother's Milk Cooperative was organized in Michigan, the state best known for cooperatives organized for various purposes by official legal documentaries and co-op lawyers. Co-ops are owned by the members. The Mother's Milk Co-op is owned by the donors, and the donors make the decisions. Donors receive pay for their milk, which they can keep or turn into the co-op pool. Most mothers are able to earn enough money so they can stay home with their infants instead of going back to work.

The science of milk banking has been advanced in recent years. Prolacta was designed in California and funded by venture capitalists who wanted to improve the science behind this priceless commodity, human milk. Prolacta has developed the best pasteurization program that preserves the most nutrients and antiinfective properties. They have designed a human milk supplement made entirely of human milk. The calories and nutrients of all their products are on the label. The milk costs more than HMBANA, but it is sterile and quality controlled.

Medolac, a newer company, has developed a product of human milk that is made entirely of human milk, is sterile, shelf stable for over a year, and does not need to be frozen or refrigerated. The constituents are on the label. It is cheaper than frozen products and has been approved by the FDA. Medolac pays the Mother's Milk Co-op for the milk it purchases.

Minimum requirements for human milk prepared for fragile premature infants include that it must be sterile and have standard calories and nutrients.

Breast-Pumping Equipment

Breast pumps have assumed an undeserved prominence in breastfeeding management in the last decade. Stimulated by the need to return to work for some women, but also by promotion by lactation professionals, the rise has persisted. Sadly, lactation professionals may also sell or rent this equipment that they recommend as necessary, thus setting up an egregious conflict of interest. Not all women need a pump. For thousands of years, women breastfed successfully without a pump. For everyday problems like engorgement or a plugged duct, a mother can use her hands. Every mother should be trained in how to manually express her breasts before she leaves the hospital. Even before a pump is applied, the breast should be massaged and milk gently expressed. This approach reduces trauma and enhances the let-down reflex. Breast pumps are medical devices. They have multiple roles, including relieving engorgement, stimulating and increasing milk production, collecting milk for a sick infant who cannot nurse, or providing donor milk to a milk bank. The FDA regulates breast pumps. It monitors the performance of medical devices by several pathways, including mandatory reporting programs and a passive surveillance system that receives reports on adverse events and product problems. FDA databases list FDA-cleared breast pumps, characterize adverse breast pump events, and identify any FDA-initiated or manufacturer pump recalls. The medical device reporting regulation requires reporting of significant medical device-related adverse events by manufacturers, importers, and users. Examples of a significant event are device-related deaths, serious injury, and malfunction. All reports are entered into the Manufacturer and User Facility Device Experience database, which dates back to 1991. Two medical device epidemiologists at the FDA have reported on the events listed in FDA databases, along with an independent epidemiologist from the University of Michigan and a nurse consultant at the FDA, who reviews postmarked adverse events. The FDA recorded 37 reports between 1992 and 2003; 81% were for electric or battery-powered pumps. Tables 21-14 and 21-15 record the pump type and adverse events. Most reports were for device malfunction, which means failure of the device to meet specifications. Table 21-16 is a brief summary of five incidents reported to the FDA. The patient problems were predominantly pain, soreness, discomfort, and tissue damage from the electric pump. The most common problems for the manual pump were tissue damage and infection. The authors point out the importance of reporting such events to the FDA so that the problems can be corrected. The FDA toll free number is 1-888-463-6332. The website for Med-Watch is http://www.fda.gov/Safety/MedWatch (Accessed 30 April 2015).

As noted earlier, several types of breast-pumping devices have provoked questions concerning the sterility of milk collected. Additional issues need to be considered, including efficiency, ease of use, potential for breast trauma, availability, and cost. A good pump should be capable of completely emptying the breast and of stimulating production. It should be clean and easy to keep clean, contamination free, easy to use, and atraumatic.

TABLE 21-14	Patient and Device Problems Reported to the Food and Drug Administration for Electric and Manual Breast Pumps	
	Pump Type, No. (%)	
Problem*	Electric/ Battery ($n = 30$)	Manual ($n = 7$)
Patient problem[†]		
Report had at least one patient problem code	20 (66.7)	4 (57.1)
Pain, soreness, discomfort	17 (56.7)	1 (14.3)
Medical care or intervention	6 (20.0)	1 (14.3)
Tissue damage	4 (13.4)	2 (28.6)
Erythema, fever, swelling	2 (6.7)	0 (0.0)
Not able to continue breastfeeding	2 (6.7)	0 (0.0)
Bruise, thrombus	1 (3.4)	1 (14.3)
Healing impaired	0 (0.0)	1 (14.3)
Infection	0 (0.0)	2 (28.6)
Device problem[‡]		
Report had at least 1 device problem code	23 (76.7)	5 (71.4)
Suction high	4 (13.4)	1 (14.3)
Suction inadequate	4 (13.4)	0 (0.0)
Device design or structure problem	2 (6.7)	2 (28.6)
Device motor or pump failure	2 (6.7)	–
Milk bled back into motor	1 (3.4)	–
Device fluid leak	0 (0.0)	1 (14.3)
Device instructions inadequate	1 (3.4)	0 (0.0)
Device not sterile	1 (3.4)	0 (0.0)
Device misassembled	1 (3.4)	1 (14.3)
Tear, rip, or hole in device	1 (3.4)	0 (0.0)
Device out of box failure	1 (3.4)	0 (0.0)

*Multiple problems may be coded in each report. Each report does not necessarily have a coded patient or device problem.
[†]Patient problem when specified. For 6 reports, a patient problem was coded as "unknown" or "other."
[‡]Device problem when specified. For 14 reports, a device problem was coded with such nonspecific information as "performance," "malfunction," "unknown," or "other."
From Brown L, Bright R, Dwyer D, et al: Breast pump adverse events: reports to the Food and Drug Administration, *J Hum Lact* 21:169, 2005.

HAND PUMPS

The "bicycle horn" pump has been marketed in drugstores for years without instructions for use or cleaning. At the museum at the Corning Glass Works in Corning, New York, a glass and rubber hand pump made by Davol (circa 1830) is on display next to glass baby bottles and pewter nipples. The current model is the same, except the glass has

TABLE 21-15 Characteristics of Adverse Events Reported to the Food and Drug Administration for Electric and Manual Breast Pumps

Characteristic	Electric/Battery Pump No. (%)	Manual Pump No. (%)
Adverse event type		
Malfunction	11 (36.7)	4 (57.1)
Injury	7 (23.3)	1 (14.3)
Other or not specified	12 (40.0)	2 (28.6)
Reporter		
Health care professional*	13 (43.4)	1 (14.3)
Patient or consumer	9 (30.0)	2 (28.6)
Other†	2 (6.7)	3 (42.8)
Not specified	6 (20.0)	1 (14.3)
Event location		
Home	14 (46.7)	1 (14.3)
Hospital	4 (13.3)	4 (57.2)
Outpatient facility	1 (3.4)	0 (0.0)
Not specified	11 (36.7)	2 (28.6)
Patient age (yr)		
15-20	2 (6.7)	0 (0.0)
21-30	9 (30.0)	1 (14.3)
31-40	3 (10.0)	1 (14.3)
Not specified	16 (53.3)	5 (71.4)

*Includes one physician, six nurses, three lactation consultants, and four health care professionals not otherwise specified.
†*Other* includes risk manager, biomedical engineer, and caregiver.

TABLE 21-16 Examples of Medical Device Reports Submitted to the United States Food and Drug Administration and Retrieved from the Manufacturer and User Facility Device Experience Database

Case	Event Reported
1	This was reported for a manual breast pump by a consumer in January 2003. The pump was applied to the engorged breast to relieve pain and pressure. The suction created on the nipple tissue was so great that it pulled a clot to the surface. The action tore approximately one fourth of the nipple off, resulting in bleeding and leaving the breast susceptible to infection. The infection was treated with antibiotics; however, the nipple did not heal for 7 weeks and made successful breastfeeding nearly impossible.
2	This was reported for a manual breast pump by a health professional in January 1999. In late September 1998, in the NICU, a set of premature twins became ill. The organism, *Pseudomonas aeruginosa*, was isolated as the cause of their illness. Because this organism is easily spread and is life threatening to infants in a NICU, swift action was taken. These infants were placed in isolation, and more than 50 items in the NICU were cultured as the possible source of this organism. All these cultures were negative. The mother of the twins was aware of the seriousness of the situation and the actions we were taking to find the source. She reported that the tubing from her breast pump system always seemed to have liquid in it. She wondered if this could be the source. Immediately, the company (breast pump manufacturer) gave her another kit and sent her complete kit to the laboratory to be tested. The tubing, breast shield, and valve from the kit, in addition to her pumped breast milk, all grew *P. aeruginosa*. After another course of antibiotics and discontinuation of the previously pumped breast milk, the infection abated. In response to this incident, a committee composed of a neonatologist, infection control director, lactation consultant, and manager met to develop a strategy to prevent any further incidents. This group recommended that the manufacturer make changes to their breast pump system.
3	This was reported by a consumer for an electric breast pump in December 2000. The unit got stuck on the breast, and the suction release did not work.
4	This was reported for an electric breast pump in April 1999. When using this single-breast electric pump, the reporter experienced extreme pain. The suction was so much that even on the lowest setting, it hurt badly. The pump did not get enough milk, resulting in engorgement.
5	This was reported by a lactation consultant for an electric pump in October 1997. The mother had been using the breast pump for 24 to 48 hours when she began experiencing skin breakdown on her nipples. The breakdown resulted in wounds with bleeding, pain, two cracks on her right nipple, and four cracks on her left nipple. The wounds had since scabbed over. The mother sought medical advice from the lactation consultant who advised her to switch to a different barrier on her nipples. The lactation consultant claims this particular breast pump has a history of causing tissue damage. The device squeezes and pulls on the nipples, which leads to tissue damage.

NICU, Neonatal intensive care unit.

been replaced by plastic. The dangers of this pump are many. They can be summarized by saying the milk is contaminated, a spray of milk can go directly into the bulb, the pump requires constant emptying, and it can be quite traumatic to the nipple, areola, and breast and predispose women to mastitis.[21]

Modifications of the bicycle horn pump insert a removable collecting bottle in place of the well. The modification permits feeding the infant directly from the collecting vessel by placing a nipple on it. Milk does not wash back over the breast, and pumping is not interrupted for emptying. The bulb still may harbor bacteria because it is difficult to clean. The limitations of the effect of creating a simple vacuum and applying a simple, rigid, sharp-edged flange against the breast are still present. This pump is satisfactory for temporary use, but it takes time to become proficient in its use, and it may never create enough pressure to be effective. Another model (Nurture) with a special flexible silicone funnel overcomes some of these problems. The cylindrical pump is comprised of two all-plastic cylindrical tubes that fit inside one another to create a vacuum. A rigid flange at the top of the inner tube accommodates the nipple and areola. The flange also has a gasket for tight fit at the other end. The outer tube collects the milk and is adapted for use as a feeding unit when an artificial nipple is attached on top. The mother creates the vacuum by pulling the outer tube, and creates rhythm by alternately pushing the outer tube in and out (Figure 21-7). It is simple, easy to clean, and the milk is usable directly from the collecting cylinder with a nipple attached. This pump is excellent in the hands of an experienced, dexterous mother. The product

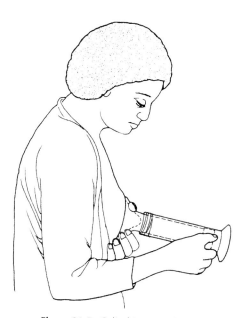

Figure 21-7. Cylindric pump in use.

has several manufacturers, and models differ slightly. Some have a choice of flanges. The only precaution is that 220 mm Hg of negative pressure can be produced if the cylinder is drawn at least three quarters of the way out when empty or when there is fluid (pumped milk) in the cylinder. The pressure desired can be achieved by pulling out the cylinder only a fraction. Most cylinder pumps are marked by the manufacturer to indicate degree of a cycle.

ELECTRIC MECHANICAL PUMPS

Battery-operated pumps are available, but they have all the disadvantages of most battery-operated devices. In most cases, they are not sufficiently powerful to stimulate the breast adequately. They are ineffective for women whose infants are not feeding at the breast, such as premature infants or those hospitalized in NICUs. These small hand pumps work for some fully lactating women and for those who have no trouble with volume but need a pump that fits in their purse for use while at work or school.

Small, purse-size electric pumps may be effective for the fully lactating woman (see Figure 21-5). They have an advantage over a manually powered hand pump, in that the electric power frees one hand for the mother to stroke the breast and encourage let-down. If flow is going well, the hand is free to perform other tasks, such as read, hold a telephone, or write, not an insignificant advantage for a busy, working, breastfeeding woman. Most small electric models have a small hole in the flange base that must be closed with a finger to develop the suction, as in many hospital suctioning devices. This also gives the mother control over the pressure. By rhythmically opening and closing the hole with the finger, the operator can simulate a milking action that is effective in extracting milk. The manufacturers, unfortunately, do not always point this out.

Hand-held mechanical devices may not be enough for a woman trying to build up a supply when the infant cannot stimulate the breast directly. A new mother may become discouraged at the low volume of her production and discontinue the process. Part of the management of a sick infant is to be sure that the mother's milk production is also progressing. Most hospitals provide a lactation consultant for lactating women with babies in the NICU, or have trained the unit's nursing staff to provide assistance. NICUs in the United States should provide a room with electric pumps for the mothers of infants in the NICU to learn how to pump their milk and breastfeed their infants. This is a key resource for any NICU because appropriate nourishment is key for the survival of infants in NICUs. Newly designed NICU's should have pumping resources beside the infant's isolette or warmer.

Full-size electric pumps are the most efficient, because the motor applies the mechanical effort. The mother can concentrate on applying the cup to her breast, massaging the breast, and relaxing so that adequate let-down can take place. All electric pumps are not equal, and some guidance is needed to be sure that the mother understands the principles involved. Nursery staff should be familiar with the equipment. The pumps are no challenge to skilled nurses in the NICU, who are adept at handling much more complicated electronic equipment.

A pump that cycles pressure instead of maintaining constant negative pressure will be less likely to cause petechiae or internal trauma to the breast.

The ultimate effect of pressure also depends on the length of time the pressure is applied. Tissue cannot withstand sustained high pressure. Pressure sustained for 2 seconds or at a rate of 30 pumps per minute is considered maximum time or minimum rate.[18] Negative pressures should have a governing mechanism to avoid excessive pressures. Mean sucking pressures of most normal full-term infants range from -50 to -155 mm Hg/in^2, with a maximum of -220 mm Hg/in^2. Manufacturers recommend about 200 mm Hg/in^2 to initiate flow in most women.

A careful study by Johnson[35] of more than 1000 patients at the University of Texas, using a variety of pumps, has confirmed some facts about pumps. The amount of negative pressure possible and the control mechanisms were recorded (Tables 21-17 to 21-19).

TABLE 21-17 Electric Pumping Devices

Mechanical Pump	Advantages	Disadvantages
Medela	Comfortable Automatic cycling Adjustable vacuum Double or single pump	
Classic electric breast pump Heavy duty for hospital use (available to rent)		

Lactina Select electric breast pump Light, portable, economical		

TABLE 21-18	Hand Pumping Devices	
Hand Pump	**Advantages**	**Disadvantages**
Bicycle horn	Inexpensive Portable	Difficult to clean Bulb retains bacteria Works as vacuum No instructions Can cause trauma Not appropriate for donor milk Milk washes back over nipple Requires constant emptying Not recommended
Evenflo	Inexpensive	Difficult to clean Bulb harbors bacteria even when boiled
White River	Pliable flange Can feed baby from collecting container Works well for less experienced mother with good let-down No milk contacts mechanism	

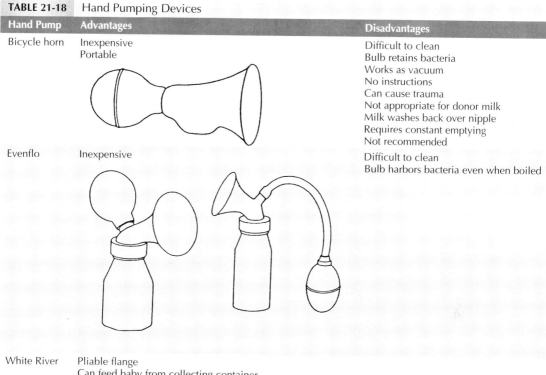

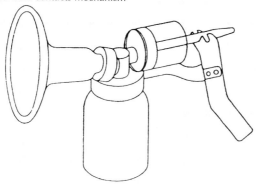

An increasing number of pumps on the market have similar designs, but each has its special nuances. A standard electric pump capable of cycling pressures to 220 mm Hg (2.5 to 8.5 psi/Hg) is usually required to stimulate production de novo (that is, when an infant is unavailable to suckle directly, such as a small premature infant on a ventilator in the NICU). Breast pumps have been identified repeatedly for years as the source of infection.[52] Improvement in design, with a safety trap between the collecting vessel and the machine to prevent milk getting into the mechanism, is important. In addition, all equipment that comes in contact with milk or the breast should be sterilizable or disposable. The well-designed electric pump properly used is the best system for stimulating lactation and increasing volume for hospitalized infants.

In the hospital, as with all special equipment, it is advisable to select the best equipment to fill the needs of that hospital, and then purchase more of the same model so that staff can learn how to use one model properly and can instruct the patient.

Similarly, the equipment should be checked on a routine basis, cleaned, and bacteriologically tested.

TABLE 21-19 Hand Pumping Devices

Hand Pump	Advantages	Disadvantages
Cylindric		
Two all-plastic cylindric tubes fit inside one another to create vacuum; inner tube has flange at top and rubber or nylon gasket	Less expensive than electric Portable Can feed baby from collecting container Easily cleaned and sterilized	Requires some dexterity Works as vacuum with some rhythm Rigid flange Can achieve >220 mm Hg of pressure Must follow instructions

Lloyd		
Glass flange attached to collecting jar; trigger handle mechanism creates vacuum; has vacuum relief switch	Less expensive than electric Portable Can be cleaned No milk contacts mechanism	Handle difficult to squeeze Hand becomes cramped Awkward Large breast and nipple may hit flange Transfer of milk to feeding unit necessary

Accessory equipment (disposable) can be resterilized for the same patient but not for a second patient.

Although attention is usually given to the pressure mechanisms, the cup or flange that is applied to the breast is equally important. The diameter and depth of the flare are fixed for the hand pumps, but a choice is offered for the standard electric pumps (Figure 21-8). The nipple should have room to be drawn out, and the flange should be adequate to transmit pressure or milking action to the collecting ampullae under the areola. The hand pumps are too small; however, bigger is not always better. A mother may find that the smaller model of the two offered may be more physiologically suited to her anatomy. This feature does not correlate directly with overall size of the breast. The ideal range is 68- to 82-mm outer diameter and 35- to 40-mm depth of flare (see Figure 21-8).[33] Silicone funnels adapt well to all sizes and shapes because of their flexibility. Study of type of pump, hand and electric, shows the difference in effect on prolactin production and milk volumes obtained. See Figures 21-9, 21-10, and 21-11 and Table 21-20.

The WIC branch of the Hawaii Department of Health studied whether an electric or a manual pump would increase breastfeeding duration for those women returning to work or school.[32] Of 246 women, 76.8% of women who used the manual pump (76 of 107) and 72.3% of those using the electric pump (94 of 139) breastfed for 6 months. The manual pump only pumped one breast at a time, so pumping took longer. The groups were matched for age, parity, ethnicity, and socioeconomic status. Contrary to most studies, the women with some college education breastfed for a shorter

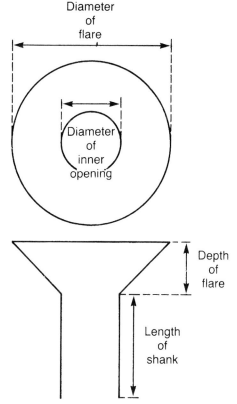

Figure 21-8. Measurement of nipple cups. (From Johnson CA: An evaluation of breast pumps currently available on the American market, *Clin Pediatr (Phila)* 22:40, 1983.)

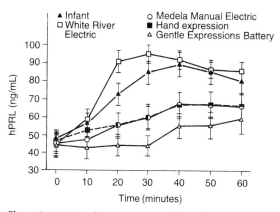

Figure 21-9. Mean human serum prolactin (hPRL) levels for each of five expression methods. Data given as mean ±SEM. (Modified from Zinaman MJ, Hughes V, Queenan JT, et al: Acute prolactin, oxytocin responses and milk yield to infant suckling and artificial methods of expression in lactating women, *Pediatrics* 89:437, 1992.)

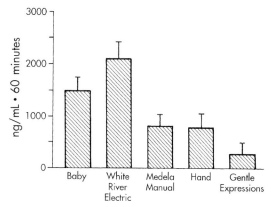

Figure 21-10. Serum prolactin results, with breast stimulation calculated as mean net area under curves for each of five methods. Data given as mean ±SEM. (Modified from Zinaman MJ, Hughes V, Queenan JT, et al: Acute prolactin, oxytocin responses and milk yield to infant suckling and artificial methods of expression in lactating women, *Pediatrics* 89:437, 1992.)

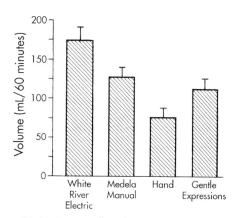

Figure 21-11. Mean milk volumes obtained with breast stimulation for four of the five expression methods (infant not included). Data given as mean ±SEM. (Modified from Zinaman MJ, Hughes V, Queenan JT, et al: Acute prolactin, oxytocin responses and milk yield to infant suckling and artificial methods of expression in lactating women, *Pediatrics* 89:437, 1992.)

TABLE 21-20	Oxytocin Results*	
Method	**Mean Net AUC**	**SEM**
Infant	224.7	75.4
White River Electric	174.1	41.3
Medela Manual	218.5	157.5
Hand expression	140.5	66.5
Gentle Expressions Battery	186.7	67.6

*Levels of plasma oxytocin with breast stimulation calculated as mean net area under the curves (AUC) for each of the five methods for the 60-minute sampling session. No significant differences were noted.

From Zinaman M, Hughes V, Queenan JT, et al: Acute prolactin, oxytocin responses and milk yield to infant suckling and artificial methods of expression in lactating women, *Pediatrics* 89:437, 1992.

period of time. This study suggests manual pumps work well when one is also breastfeeding an infant, in contrast to pumping for a hospitalized child.[32] In a study of two electric pumps, healthy women with healthy babies intending to return to work or school were randomly assigned to use a novel (Embrace, Playtex, Westport, Conn) or a standard (pump-in-style, Medela, Baar, Switzerland) electric pump. Milk extraction was greater with the standard pump; 24-hour production did not differ. However, women were equally likely to select either of the two pumps.[34]

The universal availability of a double collecting system, so both breasts are "pumped" simultaneously, greatly enhances production and saves time.

Tables 21-21 and 21-22 provide data on expression and pump methods and logistic model factors.

To test the effect on milk ejection, an electric pump was programmed to cycle 45 to 125 times per minute with vacuums between 45 and 273 mm

Hg by the research laboratories of Hartman. The time it took for milk to be ejected was determined by ultrasound of the opposite breast measuring the dilation of lactiferous ducts. Ejection occurred between 136 ± 12 and 104 ± 10 seconds. This compares with ejection time when the infant suckles at 56 ± 4 seconds. The vacuum affected the volume of milk, but not the time of ejection.[38]

When this same research group investigated means of assessing milk injection and breast milk flow, they measured milk flow rates while the mother pumped milk with an electric pump at different settings. They determined the milk duct diameter by ultrasound in the other breast simultaneously. They reported a direct relationship

TABLE 21-21 Expression and Pumping Methods

Type	Action	Equipment	Availability
Hand expression	Hand action stimulates milk ejection reflex and compresses milk ducts	None	Universal
Hot jar (base cooled with cold cloth)	Cooling creates a vacuum so that the milk flows from breast (higher pressure) to the jar (lower pressure); suction pressure may be difficult to control	Suitable glass jar, hot water, cold water, cloth	Widespread
Manual pump: Compressing a bulb, pulling on two connected cylinders, or squeezing and releasing a handle	Negative pressure created by hand; arm action of the pump causes milk to flow from breast to pump; suction pressure may be difficult to control; some brands designed to reduce arm/hand fatigue; some work on a "draw and hold" principle rather than an even in-out action	Pump Cleaning supplies Most pumps have at least 3 parts One-handed pumps available and 2 pumps can be used for double pumping	Depends on market demand/distribution
Battery pump: Power provided by battery, manner of creating pressure may vary	Negative pressure at pump causes milk to flow from breast to pump; adjustable suction pressure and cycling time in some brands; some work on a "draw and hold" principle rather than even in-out action	Pump Batteries: New batteries may be needed after 2-4 hours use; some have AC adapters available Cleaning supplies Most pumps have at least 4 parts Most are hand-held so weight of pump plus milk may be a concern	Depends on market demand/distribution
Small pump: Electric, diaphragm	Negative pressure created by pump action of the pump causes milk to flow from breast to pump; adjustable suction pressure and cycling time in some brands	Pump Electricity supply Cleaning supplies Most pumps have many parts Two collection sets can be used for double pumping for most brands	Depends on market demand/distribution

Continued

TABLE 21-21   Expression and Pumping Methods—cont'd

Type	Action	Equipment	Availability
Large electric: Piston pump, rotary vane pump, diaphragm pump; power may be provided by car battery or by foot treadle	Negative pressure created by action of the pump causes milk to flow from breast to pump; suction pressure may be difficult to control; some brands designed to reduce arm/hand fatigue; some work on a "draw and hold" principle rather than an even in-out action	Electricity supply or other power source Cleaning supplies Most pumps have 10 or more parts Two collection sets can be used	Depends on market demand/distribution; larger pumps generally purchased by hospitals or rental companies for loan to mothers

Note: Some brands of pump have a flexible breast cup that compresses the breast, and some have a choice of sizes of breast cup. Multiuser pumps require high-quality cleaning procedures and frequent servicing.

There is no one type of pump that is suitable for all mothers and all circumstances. To obtain quantities of milk by any method requires an effective milk ejection reflex.

From Becker GE, McCormick FM, Renfrew MJ: Methods of milk expression for lactating women, *Cochrane Database Syst Rev* 8(4):CD006170, 2008.

TABLE 21-22   Logistic Model Factors and Adjusted Odds Ratios (95% Confidence Intervals) Associated With Regular Milk Expression Compared With Occasional Milk Expression Among Breastfeeding Mothers Who Expressed Milk in the Previous 2 Weeks According to Infant Age Group

Characteristic	1.5 to 4.5 mo (N = 853)	>4.5 to 6.5 mo (N = 558)	>6.5 to 9.5 mo (N = 362)
Mother's education			
Some college vs. high school or less	0.53 (0.30-0.92)*	1.43 (0.64-3.21)	0.95 (0.32-2.78)
College graduate vs. high school or less	0.76 (0.44-1.32)	2.07(0.93-4.57)*	1.37 (0.48-3.09)
Household income			
185%-350% vs. <185% poverty level	1.23 (0.82-1.84)	1.52 (0.91- 2.52)	2.10 (1.04-4.22)*
>350% vs. <185% poverty level	1.82 (1.15-2.87)*	1.50 (0.84- 2.67)	2.48 (1.16-5.27)
Region			
Northwest vs. West	1.24 (0.75-2.09)	1.30 (0.70-2.41)	0.78 (0.35-1.70)
Midwest vs. West	1.36 (0.88-2.11)	1.22 (0.72-2.06)	0.64 (0.32-1.25)
South vs. West	1.73 (1.12-2.66)*	1.49 (0.87-2.55)	1.05 (0.53-2.10)
Infant delivery			
Vaginal birth with pain medication vs. without pain medication	0.95 (0.60-1.50)	0.97 (0.56-1.69)	0. 69(0.35-1.35)
Cesarean delivery vs. vaginal birth without pain medication	1.10 (0.67-1.82)	0.72 (0.39-1.32)	0.52 (0.25-1.11)
Infant gestation, ≥37 vs. 35 to <37 wk	0.37 (0.16-0.81)*	1.58 (0.56-4.52)	0.55 (0.14-2.17)
Breastfed other infant, yes vs. no[†]	0.64 (0.45-0.90)*	0.49 (0.31-0.76)*	0.71 (0.40-1.27)
Prenatal intent to breastfeed, ≥12 vs. <12 mo	0.72 (0.45-1.14)	0.49 (0.30-0.81)*	0.58 (0.32-1.06)*
Employed in previous 4 wk, yes vs. no	3.99 (2.86-5.56)*	4.02 (2.68- 6.04)*	5.94 (3.47-10.17)*
Embarrassed to breastfeed in public, yes vs. no	1.34 (0.97-1.85)*	0.87 (0.59-1.09)	1.11 (0.66-1.87)
Type of breast pump device used most often[‡]			
Combination of electric/battery vs. electric pump	0.66 (0.43-1.02)	0.55 (0.33-0.92)*	0.87 (0.42-1.82)
Manual pump vs. electric pump	0.51 (0.35-0.75)*	0.39 (0.23-0.65)*	0.31 (0.16-0.59)*
Age of first breast pump use (wk)	0.91 (0.84-0.98)*	1.02 (0.96-1.09)	1.02 (0.96-1.09)

Analysis was limited to those with complete data on the relevant questions.

*Indicates statistical significance at the $p < 0.05$ level.

[†]Includes mothers with no other children and mothers with other children whom they did not breastfeed.

[‡]Hand expression was not a response option on the question that asked about the type of pump device used most often.

From Labiner-Wolfe J, Fein SB, Shealy KR, et al: Prevalence of breast milk expression and associated factors, *Pediatrics* 122: S63–S68, 2008.

between increases in duct diameter and increases in milk flow rates.[59]

Breast pump efficiency was studied by Hartmann et al.,[31] utilizing a procedure for objective determination of breast pump efficiency by measuring milk removal from one breast in a 5-minute period in 30 women using an electric breast pump (vacuum pattern of Medela Classic). They compared these data with breastfeeding characteristics. They determined each woman's breastfeeding characteristics by collecting milk samples before and after each feed from each breast, by either manual breast pump (Medela AG) or hand expression, by test weighing the infant, measuring degree of fullness, and direct measurement of breast volume, techniques standardized in their laboratory. The authors concluded that pump efficiency can be measured if maternal characteristics, and the amount of milk in the breast available to be expressed, are known. The proportion of available milk expressed varied greatly between mothers.

Investigators in this same laboratory looked at the impact of vacuum on volume of milk expressed. They looked at 23 mothers (two were expressing milk only and not feeding the infant), who expressed their milk for 15 minutes. The pumps were set at their own maximum comfort levels and then at lesser vacuum levels. The mother's maximum comfort level produced more milk than at lesser pressures. Milk flow was greatest at the onset, and cream level was highest at the end of the 15 minutes at maximum comfort level.[36] Milk output from the right and left breasts was compared in mothers who were exclusively pumping and had not fed their infants at the breast.[18] It was reported that differences between right and left breasts are common, with the right often more productive. The difference was not related to handedness, but was consistent through the day and over time.

Methods of milk expression for lactating women were reviewed for the Cochrane Collaboration by Becker et al.[4] They found 12 studies that met criteria, of which six could be utilized, involving 397 mothers. Compared with hand expression, a study found that a greater volume of milk could be collected utilizing an electric pump. Providing a relaxing tape to be played while pumping resulted in a greater volume of milk. Pumping both breasts simultaneously took less time, but no difference in total volume was found in this study. There was no difference in milk contamination, breastfeeding at hospital discharge, fat content of milk, or serum prolactin by method of pumping. No data were reported on maternal satisfaction, adverse effects, or economic advantages.[4]

A complete assessment of all the pumps readily available on the market and details about other equipment for breastfeeding are provided by the U.S. Food and Drug Administration website: http://www.fda.gov/MedicalDevices/Productsand MedicalProcedures (Accessed 30 April 2015). The information is extensive, including renting or buying, where to get, how to assemble, how to use and how to clean various pumps.

Information can also be found at company websites. In order to obtain unbiased information, one should seek online sources that are familiar with all the brands and are not also marketing a particular brand.

REFERENCES

1. Arnold LDW: The statistical state of human milk banking and what's in the future, *J Hum Lact* 7:25, 1991.
2. Asquith MT, Pedrotti PW, Stevenson DK, et al: Clinical uses, collection, and banking of human milk, *Clin Perinatol* 14:173, 1987.
3. Balmer SE, Wharton BA: Human milk banking at Sorrento Maternity Hospital, Birmingham, England, *Arch Dis Child* 67:556, 1992.
4. Becker GE, Mc Cormick FM, Renfrew MJ: Methods of milk expression for lactating women (Review), The Cochrane Collaboration, *The Cochrane Library* 3:1–40, 2009.
5. Beerens H, Romond C, Neut C: Influence of breastfeeding on the bifid flora of the newborn intestine, *Am J Clin Nutr* 33:2434, 1980.
6. Berkow SE, Freed LM, Hamosh M, et al: Lipases and lipids in human milk: effects of freeze-thawing and storage, *Pediatr Res* 18:1257, 1984.
7. Brown RE: Relactation: an overview, *Pediatrics* 60:116–120, 1977.
8. Carroll L, Osman M, Davies DP: Does discarding the first few milliliters of breast milk improve the bacteriological quality of bank breast milk? *Arch Dis Child* 55:898, 1980.
9. Carroll L, Osman M, Davies DP, et al: Bacteriological criteria for feeding raw breast-milk to babies on neonatal units, *Lancet* 2:732, 1979.
10. Committee on Mother's Milk: American Academy of Pediatrics: operation of mother's milk bureaus, *J Pediatr* 23:112, 1943.
11. Committee on Nutrition: American Academy of Pediatrics: human milk banking, *Pediatrics* 68:854, 1980.
12. Cruz JR, Gil L, Cano F, et al: Protection by breastfeeding against gastrointestinal infection and disease in infancy. In Atkinson SA, Hanson LA, Chandra RK, editors: *Nutrition, infection and infant growth in developed and emerging countries*, Saint John's, Newfoundland, Canada, 1990, Arts Biomedical Publishers.
13. Davidson DC, Poll RA, Roberts G: Bacteriological monitoring of unheated human milk, *Arch Dis Child* 54:760, 1979.
14. Donowitz LG, Marsik FJ, Fisher KA, et al: Contaminated breast milk: a source of Klebsiella bacteremia in a newborn intensive care unit, *Rev Infect Dis* 3:716, 1981.
15. Dworsky M, Stagno S, Pass RF, et al: Persistence of cytomegalovirus in human milk after storage, *J Pediatr* 101:440, 1982.
16. Eglin RP, Wilkinson AR: HIV infection and pasteurization of breast milk, *Lancet* 1:1093, 1987.
17. Eidelman AI, Szilagyi G: Patterns of bacterial colonization of human milk, *Obstet Gynecol* 53:550, 1979.
18. Enstrom JL, Meier PP, Jegier B, et al: Comparison of milk output from right and left breasts during simultaneous pumping in mothers of very low birthweight infants, *Breastfeed Med* 2(2):83–91, 2007.
19. Evans TJ, Ryley HC, Neale LM, et al: Effect of storage and heat on antimicrobial proteins in human milk, *Arch Dis Child* 53:239, 1978.

20. Ford JE, Law BA, Marshall VM, et al: Influence of heat treatment of human milk on some of its protective constituents, *J Pediatr* 90:29, 1977.

21. Foxman B, D'Arcy H, Gillespie B: Lactation mastitis: occurrence and medical management among 946 breastfeeding women in the United States, *Am J Epidemiol* 155:115, 2002.

22. Freier S, Faber J: Loss of immune components during the processing of human milk. In Williams AF, Baum J, editors: *Human milk banking. Nestle nutrition*, New York, 1984, Vevey/Raven.

23. Friend BA, Shahani KM, Long CA, et al: The effect of processing and storage on key enzymes, B vitamins, and lipids of mature human milk. I. Evaluation of fresh samples and effects of freezing and frozen storage, *Pediatr Res* 17:61, 1983.

24. Ganapathy V, Hay JW, Kim JH: Costs of necrotizing enterocolitis and cost-effectiveness of exclusively human milk-based products in feeding extremely premature infants, *Breastfeed Med* 6(2):1–8, 2011.

25. Garza C, Johnson CA, Harrist R, et al: Effects of methods of collection and storage on nutrients in human milk, *Early Hum Dev* 6:295, 1982.

26. Gibbs JH, Fisher C, Bhattacharya S, et al: Drip breast milk: its composition, collection and pasteurization, *Early Hum Dev* 1:227, 1977.

27. Goldblum RM, Dill CW, Albrecht TB, et al: Rapid high-temperature treatment of human milk, *J Pediatr* 104:380, 1984.

28. Goldblum RM, Goldblum AS, Garza C, et al: Human milk banking. II. Relative stability of immunologic factors in stored colostrum, *Acta Paediatr Scand* 71:143, 1982.

29. Golden J: From wet nurse directory to milk bank: the delivery of human milk in Boston, 1909-1927, *Bull Hist Med* 62:589, 1988.

30. Hamosh M, Ellis LA, Pollock DR, et al: Breastfeeding and the working mother: effect of time and temperature of short-term storage on proteolysis, lipolysis, and bacterial growth in milk, *Pediatrics* 97:492, 1996.

31. Hartmann PE, Mitoulas LR, Gurrin LC: Physiology of breastmilk expression using an electric breast pump, *J Nutr* 131:3016S, 2001.

32. Hayes DK, Prince CB, Espinueva V, et al: Comparison of manual and electric breast pumps among WIC women returning to work or school in Hawaii, *Breastfeed Med* 3 (1):3–10, 2008.

33. Hernandez J, Lemons P, Lemons J, et al: Effect of storage processes on the bacterial growth-inhibiting activity of human breast milk, *Pediatrics* 63:597, 1979.

34. Hopkinson J, Heird W: Maternal response to two electric breast pumps, *Breastfeed Med* 4:17–23, 2009.

35. Johnson CA: An evaluation of breast pumps currently available on the American market, *Clin Pediatr (Phila)* 22:40, 1983.

36. Kent JC, Mitoulas LR, Cregan MD, et al: Importance of vacuum for breastmilk expression, *Breastfeed Med* 3:11–19, 2008.

37. Labiner-Wolfe J, Fein SB, Shealy KR, et al: Prevalence of breast milk expression and associated factors, *Pediatrics* 122:S63–S68, 2008.

38. Landers S, Updegrove K: Bacteriological screening of donor human milk before and after Holder pasteurization, *Breastfeed Med* 5(3):117–121, 2010.

39. Lavine M, Clark RM: Changing patterns of free fatty acids in breast milk during storage, *J Pediatr Gastroenterol Nutr* 6:769, 1987.

40. Lawrence RA: *Breastfeeding: a guide for the medical profession*, ed 1, St Louis, Mo., 1979, CV Mosby.

41. Lemons JA, Schreiner RL, Gresham EL: Simple method for determining the caloric and fat content of human milk, *Pediatrics* 66:626, 1980.

42. Lev HM, Ovental A, Mandel D, et al: Major losses of fat, carbohydrates and energy content of preterm human milk frozen at −80°C, *J Perinatol* 34:396–398, 2014.

43. Lucas A: Human milk banks, *Lancet* 1:103, 1982.

44. Lucas A, Gibbs JA, Lyster RL, et al: Creamatocrit: simple clinical technique for estimating fat concentration and energy value of human milk, *Br Med J* 1:1018, 1978.

45. Martinez FE, Desai ID, Davidson AG, et al: Ultrasonic homogenization of expressed human milk to prevent fat loss during tube feeding, *J Pediatr Gastroenterol Nutr* 6:593, 1987.

46. McDougal JS, Martin LS, Cort SP, et al: Thermal inactivation of the acquired immunodeficiency syndrome virus, human T lymphotropic virus-III/lymphadenopathy-associated virus, with special reference to antihemophilic factor, *J Clin Invest* 76:875, 1985.

47. McEnery G, Chattopadhyay B: Human milk bank in a district general hospital, *Br Med J* 2:794, 1978.

48. McPherson RJ, Wagner CL: The effect of pasteurization on TGFa and TGFb2 concentrations in human milk, *Adv Exp Med Biol* 501:359, 2001.

49. Meier PP, Enstrom JL, Zuleger JL, et al: Accuracy of a user-friendly centrifuge for measuring creamatocrits on mother's milk in the clinical setting, *Breastfeed Med* 1(2):79–87, 2006.

50. Michaelsen KF, Skafte L, Badsberg JH, et al: Variation in macronutrients in human bank milk: influencing factors and implications for human milk banking, *J Pediatr Gastroenterol Nutr* 11:229, 1990.

51. Moffatt PA, Lammi-Keefe CJ, Ferris AM, et al: Alpha and gamma tocopherols in pooled mature human milk after storage, *J Pediatr Gastroenterol Nutr* 6:225, 1987.

52. Moloney AC, Quoraishi AH, Parry P, et al: A bacteriological examination of breast pumps, *J Hosp Infect* 9:169, 1987.

53. Morgan JN, Toledo RT, Eitenmiller RR, et al: Thermal destruction of immunoglobulin A, lactoferrin, thiamin, and folic acid in human milk, *J Food Sci* 51:348, 1986.

54. Mother's Milk Unit: *California Transplant Bank: procedures and protocols*, San Jose, Calif., 1988, The Mother's Milk Bank, The Institute for Medical Research.

55. Orloff SL, Wallingford JC, McDougal JS: Inactivation of human immunodeficiency virus type I in human milk: effects of intrinsic factors in human milk and of pasteurization, *J Hum Lact* 9:300, 1993.

56. Ovesen L, Jakobsen J, Leth T, et al: The effect of microwave heating on vitamins B1 and E, and linoleic and linolenic acids, and immunoglobulins in human milk, *Int J Food Sci Nutr* 47:427, 1996.

57. Paxson CI, Cress CC: Survival of human milk leukocytes, *J Pediatr* 94:61, 1979.

58. Pittard WB, Bill K: Human milk banking: effect of refrigeration on cellular components, *Clin Pediatr (Phila)* 20:31, 1981.

59. Quan R, Yang C, Rubinstein S, et al: Effects of microwave radiation on anti-infective factors in human milk, *Pediatrics* 89:667, 1992.

60. Rechtman DJ, Lee ML, Berg H: Effect of environmental conditions on unpasteurized donor human milk, *Breastfeed Med* 1(1):24–26, 2006.

61. Reynolds GJ, Lewis-Jones DI, Isherwood DM, et al: A simplified system of human milk banking, *Early Hum Dev* 7:281, 1982.

62. Rogers IS: Relation, *Early Hum Dev* 49(Suppl):S75, 1997.

63. Schmidt E: Effects of varying degrees of heat treatment on milk protein and its nutritional consequences, *Acta Paediatr Scand Suppl* 296:41, 1982.

64. Silprasert A, Dejsarai W, Keawvichit R, et al: Effect of storage on the creamatocrit and total energy content of human milk, *Hum Nutr Clin Nutr* 40C:31, 1986.

65. Smith L, Bickerton J, Pilcher G, et al: Creamatocrit, carbon content, and energy value of pooled banked human milk: implications for feeding preterm infants, *Early Hum Dev* 11:75, 1985.

66. Sosa R, Barness L: Bacterial growth in refrigerated human milk, *Am J Dis Child* 141:111, 1987.

67. Springer S: Human milk banking in Germany, *J Hum Lact* 13:65, 1997.

68. Stagno S, Reynolds DW, Pass RF: Breast milk and the risk of cytomegalovirus infection, *N Engl J Med* 302:1073, 1980.

69. Steele C, Bixby C: Centralized breastmilk handling and bar-code scanning improve safety and reduce breastmilk administration errors, *Breastfeed Med* 9(9):426–429, 2014.

70. Stocks RJ, Davies DP, Carroll LP, et al: A simple method to improve the energy value of bank human milk, *Early Hum Dev* 8:175, 1983.

71. Sunshine P, Asquith MT, Liebhaber M: The effects of collection and processing on various components of human milk. In Frier S, Eidelman AI, editors: *Human milk: its biological and social value*, Amsterdam, 1980, Excerpta Medica.

72. Tabata M, Abdelrahman K, Hair AB, et al: Fortifier and cream improve fat delivery in continuous enteral infant feeding of breast milk, *Nutrients* 7(2):1174–1183, 2015.

73. Terpstra FG, Rechtman DJ, Lee ML, et al: Antimicrobial and antiviral effect of high-temperature short-time (HTST) pasteurization applied to human milk, *Breastfeed Med* 2(1):27–33, 2007.

74. Thiry L, Sprecher-Goldberger S, Jonckheer T, et al: Isolation of AIDS virus from cell-free breast milk of three healthy virus carriers, *Lancet* 2:891, 1985.

75. Tully MR: Excelencia em bancos de leite humano: Uma visao do futuro—the First International Congress on Human Milk Banking, *J Hum Lact* 17:51, 2001.

76. Tully MR, Jones F: *Guidelines for the establishment and operation of a donor human milk bank*, Raleigh, N.C., 2003, Human Milk Banking Association of North America.

77. Tyson JE, Edwards WH, Rosenfeld AM, et al: Collection methods and contamination of bank milk, *Arch Dis Child* 57:396, 1982.

78. Undergrove KH: Donor human milk banking: growth, challenges, and the role of HMBANA, *Breastfeed Med* 8(5):435–437, 2013.

79. US Food and Drug Administration. Breast Pumps. 2015. http://www.fda.gov/MedicalDevices/ProductsandMedical Procedures (Accessed 30.04.15.).

80. Van Zoeren-Grobben D, Schrijver J, Van Den Berg H, et al: Human milk vitamin content after pasteurisation, storage or tube feeding, *Arch Dis Child* 62:161, 1987.

81. Welsh JK, May JT: Anti-infective properties of breast milk, *J Pediatr* 93:1, 1979.

82. WHO/UNICEF joint statement: Meeting on infant and young child feedings, *J Nurse Midwifery* 25:31, 1980.

83. Williamson S, Finucane E, Ellis H, et al: Effect of heat treatment of human milk on absorption of nitrogen, fat, sodium, calcium, and phosphorus by preterm infants, *Arch Dis Child* 53:555, 1978.

84. Wills ME, Han VE, Harris DA, et al: Short-time low-temperature pasteurisation of human milk, *Early Hum Dev* 7:71, 1980.

85. Ziegler JB, Cooper DA, Johnson RO, et al: Post-natal transmission of AIDS-associated retrovirus from mother to infant, *Lancet* 1:896, 1985.

86. Zinaman MJ, Hughes V, Queenan JT, et al: Acute prolactin, oxytocin responses and milk yield to infant suckling and artificial methods of expression in lactating women, *Pediatrics* 89:437, 1992.

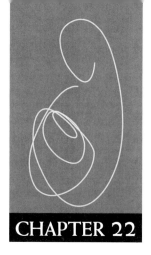

CHAPTER 22

Breastfeeding Support Groups and Community Resources

Certain changes in cultural aspects of Western civilization have contributed to the widespread use of artificial feedings for human infants as well as to the changing structure of the family. Urbanization has been associated not only with industrialization but also with the separation of generations. This has produced the nuclear family. Nuclear families are smaller, mobile, isolated families often stranded in a large urban population. In a nuclear family, a young couple and their new infant are totally without personal human resources. That is, no one cares enough to give individual support to the family. They have no one to turn to and from whom to receive advice, encouragement, and support.

Historical Perspective

Rites of passage were described by the French author Van Gennep[28] as the ceremonies and rituals that mark special changes in people's lives. The list includes marriage, motherhood, birth, death, circumcision, graduation, ordination, and retirement. In our present culture, support exists for most of these events except birth and motherhood. The most critical rite of passage in a woman's life, Raphael[22] points out, is when she becomes a mother. Raphael further distinguishes this period of transition with the term *matrescence*, "to emphasize the mother and to focus on her new life-style." Traditional cultures herald a mother giving birth, whereas our culture announces the birth of an infant. The former highlights the mother, the latter the infant. Matrescence is a time of coddling. In preindustrial societies, a mother is coddled for some time after birth, having only the responsibility of the infant's

care while the mother's needs are met by doulas. Mothering the mother should be part of the postpartum support for a new mother.

A number of other forces added momentum to the bottle feeding trend that began in the 1920s, when manufacturers finally were able to mass produce an inexpensive container and rubber nipple with which to feed infants inexpensively. Pediatrics was a new specialty to guard the health of children. The focus was on measuring and calculating. Physicians seemed more secure when they could prescribe a measure of nutrition. The rise in the female labor force has also been credited with having an impact on the method of feeding infants, who were no longer taken everywhere with the mothers to be nursed but instead were left behind to be bottle fed. The technology of the infant food industry was a continuing influence on the nutritional thinking of both medical and lay groups.

Breastfeeding was never totally abandoned. Always groups of women prepared themselves for childbirth and read and researched feeding and nutrition and chose to breastfeed. In the mid-1940s, Dr. Edith Jackson began the Rooming-In Project at Yale University in New Haven, Connecticut. Families in New Haven who sought "childbirth without fear" and an opportunity to room-in with their infants usually chose to breastfeed. In the rooming-in unit, breastfeeding was often "contagious" because one mother successfully nursing would encourage others to try. Hospital stays averaged 5 to 7 days, during which time a mother-infant couple was cared for as a pair. More than 70% of the patients left this hospital breastfeeding. The national average at that time (1945 to 1955) was less than 25%.

Students and staff who were exposed to the philosophy of this unit went to many parts of the country, taking with them tremendous commitment to prepared childbirth and nurturing through breastfeeding. The classic article on the management of breastfeeding by Barnes et al.[2] was published as a result of counseling hundreds of nursing mothers. The students of Jackson inoculated many hundreds of hospitals and communities with a zeal for breastfeeding.

Development of Mother Support Groups

The need remained for nuclear families to have access to support and conversation about healthy infants, mothering, and breastfeeding. The La Leche League, developed by a group of seven mothers to meet these needs, was established in Franklin Park, Illinois, in 1957. The original intent was to provide other nursing mothers with information, encouragement, and moral support. Thousands of local chapters and a network of 32,000 state and regional coordinators synchronized their activities with the headquarters in Schaumburg, Illinois. La Leche League International's (LLLI) 4000 groups were in 66 countries, including the United States, Canada, parts of Europe, New Zealand, Africa, and other parts of the world.[14]

An excellent publication, *The Womanly Art of Breastfeeding*,[14] was prepared by the original group of mothers involved in the La Leche League. The League celebrated its fiftieth anniversary in Chicago in 2007 and published the eighth edition of this publication. La Leche League continues to provide information and updated publications about common questions that arise during lactation. Local groups offer classes to prepare mothers to breastfeed. They help with suggestions about the nitty-gritty details of preparation, nutrition, clothing, and mothering in general. They also provide every mother with a telephone counselor. To be qualified to serve as a counselor to another mother, a member must demonstrate knowledge and expertise in breastfeeding as well as an understanding of how to counsel and render support. "Telephone mothers" do not give medical advice and are instructed to tell a troubled mother to call her own physician for such advice. Interested local physicians provide medical expertise for the group when a medical opinion is appropriate. The league provides support for mothers to reduce the time the physician needs to spend counseling on the non-medical aspects of lactation. Most information needed by new mothers is not medical.

In the decades that this support system has been in place, no good substitute for this mother-to-mother program has evolved because a woman needs a true doula.

Similar programs have been developed in more than 70 other countries. A well-established and respected program in Norway is Ammehjelpen International Group; in Australia, the Nursing Mothers' Association of Australia; and in the United Kingdom, the National Childbirth Trust.

The group dynamics are important and feelings of normalcy are reinforced. The information and experience were shown to be important, but the support from the group had far greater influence on success in breastfeeding. Meara reports similar observations on league activities in a nonsupportive culture.

The Breastfeeding Association of South Africa is a nongovernmental, nonprofit, voluntary organization founded in 1978 by South Africans for the express needs of South African women. Their special problems and solutions are well described by Bergh.[4] Support groups for all life's events, especially those covering health, have become a common feature (more than 150 parent support groups exist). In the field of perinatal care, groups are available for infertile couples; couples who are expecting; those who have experienced pregnancy loss, loss of a premature infant, or loss of a term baby; those who had a cesarean delivery; and so on. Physicians should be aware of the groups that function in their communities and the policies and philosophies they embrace.

The International Childbirth Education Association also provides resources for a new family in many countries. Its program makes preparation and training available for couples during pregnancy and afterward as parents. Its scope embraces the entire childbirth concept, of which breastfeeding is part.

Adolescents need special support to improve the outcome of their pregnancies, to encourage them to breastfeed, and to establish the special relationship with, and commitment to, their infants. A study done in the Breastfeeding Educated and Supported Teen Club in Melbourne, Florida, looked at the impact of specific breastfeeding education provided by a lactation consultant in group classes. Teens were randomly assigned to the program or as a control; ethnicity and age were not significant factors. Of the 43 adolescents in the education group, 28 (65%) initiated breastfeeding, but of the 48 control subjects without education, only 7 (14.6%) initiated breastfeeding ($p < 0.001$). The authors concluded that targeted education makes a difference in adolescents.[29]

When a similar study was performed involving low-income women, a community-based program studied a hospital, home visit, and telephone support system provided by a community health nurse and a peer counselor for 6 months. After random assignment, those receiving intervention breastfed longer. The infants had fewer sick visits and use of medicines than the group with "standard care." The cost of the program per mother was $301, which was offset by the savings on the cost of formula and health care.[21]

In another study, adult women without a personal breastfeeding support system at home were randomized to receive support or not. The support group received support in the hospital and at home from a practicing midwife in the community. She visited in the hospital daily and was available by pager continually. After discharge, she telephoned within 72 hours and then weekly for 4 weeks. At home, the participants had access to the midwife by phone and pager. One home visit was made the first week and then as necessary. In the supported group, 26 of 26 were still breastfeeding at 1 month, but only 17 of 25 (68%) in the unsupported group were breastfeeding, proving that intensive professional support works. The costs of the program were not provided.[19]

Active support outreach clearly affects the duration of breastfeeding and ultimately saves health care dollars. Such programs can be included in private practice.

Community Resources

Most hospitals provide training in preparation for childbirth. Part of the program is about the new infant and how to plan for neonatal care. These programs often serve as the initial stimulus to consider breastfeeding. Many such programs are given by hospital-based lactation consultants.

When a large health maintenance organization looked at 5213 new mothers enrolled in a commercial managed care plan by telephone survey at 4 to 6 months postpartum, 75% had breastfed for some time. Of these, 75% breastfed for more than 6 weeks. Breastfeeding for more than 6 weeks was associated with level of education, employment status (part-time, 84%), and adequacy of postpartum information. Health plans and employers should consider promoting breastfeeding, concluded the authors.[8]

Because hospitals have become competitive and are marketing their services, many are developing birthing centers and are trying to capture the attention of the childbearing public with special services. These services often include classes on child rearing, including breastfeeding. Physicians should investigate the programs and printed materials distributed by the hospitals where their patients deliver. Many pediatricians are coping with the flood of patient information from conflicting sources by printing up an office manual (desktop printers make this quite feasible). This is especially helpful if the patients give birth at more than one hospital or more than one lay advocacy group is active in the community. Hospital procedures and policies can influence the success or failure of breastfeeding mothers.[26] Pediatricians should be aware of the policies at the hospital(s) with which they are associated.

In a few short decades, we have gone from a paucity of support groups and resource literature to an overwhelming flood. Health care books and childbearing and family-rearing advice books are cascading off the presses, written by everyone from qualified experts to poorly informed freelance writers. Some are written by health care professionals who have personal experience in childbearing. Pediatricians should be familiar with a few good references for parents and provide a list for patients in the practice.

The Young Women's Christian Association (YWCA) in most communities may also provide preparation for childbirth. Its classes usually provide programming that appeals to young and unwed women, a group in need of services rarely provided by other sources.

The Visiting Nurses Association and the public health nurses on the staff of the local county health department are special resources particularly skilled at counseling new mothers with their infants. They can provide valuable information to the physician who is working with an infant who fails to thrive at the breast by witnessing the breastfeeding scene at home. As discharge from the hospital occurs earlier and earlier, pediatricians should consider employing nurse practitioners who are prepared to make house calls immediately after birth.

Many other organizations, local and national in scope, have the perinatal period and the family as their focus. Many of these are also interested in promoting breastfeeding as part of their overall goals.

The World Health Organization (WHO) and United Nations International Children's Education Fund (UNICEF) have joined an international effort to create a supportive atmosphere in hospitals around the world by developing the Baby Friendly Hospital Initiative (BFHI) (see Chapter 1). Both WHO and UNICEF provide international support for breastfeeding, especially in developing countries. The ten steps toward becoming a Baby Friendly Hospital are listed in Box 1-2 in Chapter 1.

The BFHI was designed originally to rid hospitals of their dependence on artificial infant formulas and to encourage the support of breastfeeding in these facilities. It is designed to create a supportive atmosphere with trained and knowledgeable staff.

The ten steps describe the essentials of the program. In 2009, the BFHI materials were revised by WHO. The program was expanded to integrate BFHI with the Global Strategy for Infant and Young Child Feeding. This revision included the expectation that staff be trained to provide support and education for mothers who were not breastfeeding. The 2009 update also included a review of labor and delivery practices. Step 4 has been extensively revised to promote skin-to-skin and the process of the infant finding the breast and latching on, immediately after delivery. BFHI expects that every infant will spend up to an hour accomplishing the first feeding while skin-to-skin with the mother.

Worldwide achievement of Baby Friendly Hospitals accreditation has been extensive. In the United States progress has been slow. The provision of millions of dollars in grant money has allowed many hospitals to train their staff and rebuild their programs to meet the 10 steps and achieve accreditation.

GOVERNMENT ORGANIZATIONS

The United States government has taken an active interest in the promotion of breastfeeding as well. In the goals for national health prepared by a multidisciplinary task force in 1978, it is stated that by 1990, 75% of infants leaving the hospital shall be breastfed and at 6 months of age at least 35% will still be breastfeeding.[20] The rates in 1990 fell well short of the goals, and they were thus restated to be achieved by the year 2000, extending to 50% the number to still be breastfeeding at 5 to 6 months. The goals for 2010 included 75% breastfeeding at hospital discharge, 50% at 6 months, and at least 25% breastfeeding at 1 year. A midcourse correction indicated that 60% exclusive breastfeeding should continue for at least 3 months and exclusivity should continue for 6 months for 25%.[20] National statistics continue to fall short of predictions although the gap is shrinking.

The U.S. Office of the Surgeon General conducted a national workshop on breastfeeding and human lactation in Rochester, New York, in June 1984 to develop recommendations for national policy. A publication from the workshop was available from the U.S. Government Printing Office in Washington, District of Columbia. A follow-up workshop was held in Washington, District of Columbia in 1985, gathering the representatives of the major official national organizations for obstetrics, pediatrics, and family physicians, including the credentialing organizations for physicians, nurses, nurse midwives, and dietitians. The organizations responded to a request for each to approve a model statement in support of breastfeeding. This was accomplished by January 1987.

The organizations prepared a review of curriculum within their disciplines to ensure adequate education, training, and accreditation regarding human lactation and breastfeeding for their members. Although improvements have been made and certifying examinations have incorporated questions about breastfeeding and human lactation, curriculum development in most institutions has lagged behind. Available curricula to solve this problem have been developed by the AAP/ACOG and Wellstart.

Although C. Everett Koop, U.S. Surgeon General in the 1980s, maintained his commitment to breastfeeding, later Surgeons General did not. Twenty-five years to the day later, June 9, 2009, the Academy of Breastfeeding Medicine convened the first summit on breastfeeding in Washington, District of Columbia. Dr. Koop opened the meeting with a televised message, the same message he concluded with in 1984. The summit was directed at a different audience, not at breastfeeding zealots and supporters but the United States government and its many agencies and the health care and insurance industries. The purpose was to educate the participants on the value of breastfeeding and the necessity to support breastfeeding, including reimbursement for services provided to patients in hospitals and at home. Progress has been made. The Centers for Disease Control and Prevention (CDC), the Office of Women's Health, and the Surgeon General took action and have participated in collecting data, and changing programs. The sitting Surgeon General issued the first "call to action" charge.

The Office of Women's Health and others invested time, talent, and resources in the issues of maternal employment. Annual summits were convened, continuing to involve the government agencies, the health care industry, and insurance providers.

Six summits have been convened and the seventh will have been held in June 2015, sponsored and executed by the Academy of Breastfeeding Medicine. Most significant has been the generous grant support from the WW Kellogg Foundation from the very first summit. Not only did Kellogg fund the summits but the foundation has dedicated its grant resources to breastfeeding issues across the country. Kellogg now supports over 100 programs large and small. Nothing has done more to facilitate the progress of breastfeeding than the commitment of the Kellogg Foundation. The credit for this contact goes to the brilliant grant writing by ABM and the overwhelming support of Mary Ann Liebert Publishers, Inc.

During these 6 years of summits, much progress has occurred among minority groups who have formed their own organizations such as Mocha

Mothers and Black Mother's Breastfeeding Association. The Women, Infants, and Children (WIC) program has changed its policy to encourage breastfeeding and support breastfeeding mothers. Employers are supporting their lactating employees one company at a time.

Issues of rural health have begun to include those surrounding birth and the infant's welfare. Programs are being developed to increase breastfeeding among rural women. Although the incidence of breastfeeding has increased among well-educated, self-motivated, middle-class Americans, the number of impoverished, less well-educated women who breastfeed remains small. Progress is being made, community by community, by dedicated health care workers, dietitians, and WIC staff. Health professionals often serve as a catalyst in developing such programs but should always be ready to serve as knowledgeable, supportive consultants to the efforts of others.[11]

The U.S. Department of Agriculture's Supplemental Nutrition Program for Women, Infants, and Children (WIC) nutrition services provides supplemental nutrition and counseling to more than 50% of U.S. families with young children. There are large differences in rates of breastfeeding among the different racial groups in WIC. A study of services in North Carolina confirmed the racial/ethnic disparities in breastfeeding rates.[9]

The differences in availability of support services were also associated with racial/ethnic composition of the catchment area. These observations of disparity among services at WIC were also reported in an analysis of data from the Early Childhood Longitudinal Study-Birth Cohort. Breastfeeding duration was a result of cultural trends, not WIC programming. Multiple studies have done analysis outcomes at WIC sites. When the barriers to reaching the national goals for breastfeeding among the WIC population were counted, they were (1) lack of support in and outside the hospital; (2) returning to work; (3) practical issues; (4) WIC related issues; and (5) social, cultural barriers.[12] Issues included young age, non-Hispanic ethnicity, obesity, and depression.

Solutions that worked for local WIC programs have been peer counselors, breast pump programs, and discontinuing free formula at the hospital and by the WIC program. The major obstacle to WIC program success is budgetary. Nationally, WIC spends 25 times more money on formula than on breastfeeding initiatives.[3] The new food packages, however, implemented in the fall of 2009, have improved breastfeeding outcomes in Los Angeles County where exclusive breastfeeding rates at 3 and 6 months have doubled.[15]

The U.S. Department of Agriculture's breastfeeding program, through the WIC's Nutrition Program, has launched a major effort to increase breastfeeding initiation and duration throughout the 50 states. The program, Best Start, included social marketing research, a media campaign, a staff support kit, a breastfeeding resource guide, a training conference, and continuing education and technical assistance. WIC has been made a permanent national health and nutrition program, and breastfeeding has been written into the legislation (see Chapter 1). The program even mandates that every WIC agency must have accommodations for employees who are breastfeeding their infants to pump and store their milk.[25]

BEST START: THE CONCEPT OF SOCIAL MARKETING

Using the concept of social marketing, Bryant et al.[5] designed an approach to promoting breastfeeding that utilized the counseling strategies, educational materials, policies, and community-based activities that formed the Best Start Program. Social marketing "combines the principles of commercial marketing with health education to promote a socially beneficial idea, practice or product."[4] Typically a well-articulated program involves a combination of mass media, print materials, personal counseling, and community-based activities and services.

From these findings, a multifaceted breastfeeding promotion campaign was designed for new mothers, family members, health professionals, and the community at large. The Best Start Program proved to be extremely successful and has been replicated by others successfully.

Utilizing strategies developed in social marketing and segmentation modeling for health communication,[17] Best Start developed a multimedia program, Loving Support Makes Breastfeeding Work. This program was the substance of the WIC National Breastfeeding Promotion Project launched in April 1997.[1,5] Best Start has turned the program over to WIC for its continuation.

THE UNITED STATES BREASTFEEDING COMMITTEE

In order to fulfill a mandate of the Innocenti Declaration signed in 1990 in Italy by representatives of 90 countries, including Audrey Nora, MD, Assistant Surgeon General of the United States, a group of interested breastfeeding supporters and advocates met in Florida in January 1996. The declaration states that each member country should have a national breastfeeding committee, and many countries have complied.

This small group of breastfeeding advocates met to discuss the need for coordination of breastfeeding activities in the United States. After conducting an intensive needs assessment, the National Alliance for Breastfeeding Advocacy (NABA) was formed to address needs not being met by organizations, government agencies, or individuals, and convened the first National Breastfeeding Leadership Roundtable to determine if another organization was needed to move breastfeeding forward in this country.[30] Working on the international model, the formation of this committee, if successful, would satisfy one of the four operational targets set forth by the 1990 Innocenti Declaration. This was to establish a multisectoral, national breastfeeding committee composed of representatives from relevant government departments, nongovernmental organizations, and health professional associations in every country.

It was agreed at that meeting of 19 breastfeeding leaders to do four things: (1) to support ongoing breastfeeding projects in the United States; (2) to develop a strategic plan for breastfeeding in the United States; (3) to reorganize the National Breastfeeding Leadership Roundtable into the U.S. Breastfeeding Committee (USBC); and finally, (4) to incorporate the organization of the USBC and its leadership. The organization continued to meet twice a year and in January 1998 voted to declare itself, with the encouragement of Assistant Surgeon General Audrey Nora, MD, the USBC.

The USBC is a collaborative partnership of organizations. The mission of the committee is to protect, promote, and support breastfeeding in the United States. The USBC exists to assure the rightful place of breastfeeding in society. Major organizations that are members include but are not limited to the American College of Obstetricians and Gynecologists (ACOG), the American Academy of Pediatrics (AAP), the American Academy of Family Practice (AAFP), the LLLI, the International Lactation Consultant Association (ILCA), and Wellstart and the NABA. The National Institutes of Health (NIH), Maternal and Child Health Bureau of the Health Resources Division of the U.S. Department of Health and Human Services, Women's Health, the Food and Drug Administration (FDA), and the CDC also participated. After more than 10 years of developing its organizational skill and attracting more than 30 organizational members, it has assumed a vital role in national breastfeeding activity. It has organized coalitions in all states, has hosted coalition meetings to train state representatives, and provided a forum for sharing strategies among the members. USBC is an organization of organizations, not individuals. An important effort has been to create federal legislation to support breastfeeding women. The problems of employment for working mothers have been a major thrust that has resulted in cooperation of the summits in the development of the national program, the

Business Case for Breastfeeding. Because of the interdisciplinary nature of its membership as a forceful network, USBC has been developed to promote, protect, and support breastfeeding. The USBC's website is http://www.usbreastfeeding.org.

WELLSTART INTERNATIONAL

A program to extend the scope of global breastfeeding promotion was launched by Wellstart International in a cooperative agreement with the U.S. Agency for International Development (AID). Wellstart International, a private, nonprofit organization headquartered in San Diego, grew out of clinical and teaching experiences at the University of California, San Diego Medical Center in the late 1970s.[18] In 1983, in response to a clear need to improve the breastfeeding knowledge of health professionals, a Lactation Management Education program was initiated with funding from AID. Almost 400 participants of the Lactation Management Education program now form a network of Wellstart Associates in 28 countries.

In late 1991, Wellstart joined in a cooperative agreement with AID to expand and diversify its global breastfeeding promotion activities.[18] The Expanded Promotion of Breastfeeding can work in any country at the request of the local AID mission. Wellstart continues to provide educational information for the training of physicians, nurses, and dietitians. Wellstart was active in global events as well.[31] These activities include the development of the "ten steps" for hospital care of the mother-baby dyad and the Innocenti Declarations of 1990 and 2005, the formation of the World Alliance for Breastfeeding Advocates, and the initiation of World Breastfeeding Week and the BFHI; Wellstart also and they served as one of the initial organizers of the USBC.

Other lactation centers were created in health care facilities. The purpose of these programs was to provide consultation services for mothers as well as education, training, and information for health care workers. Efforts have been made to change hospital policy regarding breastfeeding to increase the success rate. An impressive program was initiated in the Philippines. It has not only increased the incidence of breastfeeding but also lowered the morbidity rate from sepsis, diarrhea, and malnutrition. Breastfeeding programs now exist in many large cities in the United States and around the world.

BREASTFEEDING AND HUMAN LACTATION STUDY CENTER

The Lactation Study Center of the University of Rochester School of Medicine and Dentistry in New York encourages and promotes human lactation and breastfeeding through physician education and support. The goal is to provide information that will help practitioners encourage and support breastfeeding for all patients. Information is available to the health care professional by telephone. Originally federally funded and established at the request of the Office of the Surgeon General in 1984, the center now depends on private grants and donations from users. The drug information line operates Monday through Friday from 9 AM to 4 PM EST. Physician consultation is available by call back.

Lactation Consultants

For years, many medical and nursing professionals have served as lactation consultants ready to respond to any colleague's request for knowledge and expertise. With the great national movement to embrace breastfeeding, however, a new type of lactation consultant has evolved from the vast pool of women who have served in local mother-to-mother programs to help others breastfeed. The health care professional needs to ensure that the lactation resources available in the community are truly of professional quality and background and that the individuals have obtained proper certification and licensure. Counseling on any topic is a special skill requiring more than personal experience with the situation.

The International Board of Lactation Consultant Examiners (IBLCE) was developed as a separate organization by the LLLI to credential individuals who want to counsel about breastfeeding.[13] Those who successfully complete the IBLCE certification process, which includes a written examination, are entitled to use the designation IBCLC (International Board Certified Lactation Consultant) after their names. The IBLCE has defined lactation consultants as "allied health care providers who possess the necessary skills, knowledge, and attitudes to facilitate breastfeeding." These lactation consultants perform as employees in some situations and as independent contractors in states where the medical practice act allows such activity. A lactation consultant should have professional liability insurance coverage and a license to practice in the health field in the state. Nurses, midwives, nurse practitioners, and dietitians are usual candidates. Some physicians have taken the examination.

The International Lactation Consultants Association stated, "A lactation consultant is a health care professional whose scope of practice is focused upon providing education and management to prevent and solve breastfeeding problems and to encourage a social environment that effectively supports the breastfeeding mother/infant dyad." The International Lactation Consultants Association has published Standards of Practice for Lactation Consultants, which are available in print and at the website ILCA.com.

LACTATION SPECIALIST AS MEMBER OF HEALTH CARE TEAM

Modern medicine has developed a team approach to the management of many patient populations, such as elderly or handicapped persons.[16] A team approach also is used in the management of many categories of diseases, such as cancer and diabetes. A health care team provides medical service for the family during the perinatal period. This team includes an obstetrician and a pediatrician or a family physician; nurse midwives; nurses working in prenatal care, obstetrics, neonatal care, and public health; social workers; dietitians; and when a problem develops, perinatologists, neonatologists, and the skilled team from the perinatal center. These team members are well-educated and extensively trained professionals. Together they have lowered the morbidity and mortality rates of childbirth. The long-range prognosis for the intact survival of infants has been significantly improved.

Thus medical progress has occurred concomitantly with the isolation of the nuclear family. The result is a medically successful birth to a family poorly prepared emotionally and socially to cope. The family is inadequately prepared to take over when the mother and infant are discharged from the hospital and instantly placed on their own without a transitional period of adjustment with close support and supervision.

Lactation specialists become an important addition to the health care team, replacing the traditional family support system. Specialists not only must know their role as counselors interacting with the family, but also must understand how they interact with other members of the health care team. The professional team members are beginning to understand the importance of lactation specialists and how to work most effectively with them. Some physicians, however, provide a nurse practitioner, whose role is to fill that gap between medical care and family support. The nurse practitioner is usually skilled in well-baby care, especially breastfeeding, and in the era of early postpartum discharge home, may make house calls within 48 hours of arrival home.[24]

Lactation consultants quickly earn the respect of health care teams when they communicate openly with them, support mothers in a positive manner, and encourage a relationship of mutual trust and respect between the mothers and the teams.[16]

Peer Counseling

Peer counseling is part of a system developed by health care providers and health educators to change personal health behavior.[27] It is an adaptation of a cultural technique that has been used for generations wherein the family provided a personal advocate or ombudsman to help the individual carry out good health practices. In lay midwifery, for example, members of the group attend women throughout pregnancy, delivery, and the postpartum period. The important point is that the peer counselor is a member of the same sociocultural group as the recipient, is selected for leadership qualities and experience, and is trained in special issues.

Public health programs have used peer counselors to encourage women to seek prenatal care or well-child care for their children. Other programs have provided peer counselors for individuals with hypertension, diabetes, or other chronic diseases to help the patient access health care and carry out instructions for treatment. This concept has been applied to the WIC program.[27] A model program was developed in south Georgia in the mid-1980s by Wanda Grogan, PhD, and was effective in encouraging women to carry out health care advice, to keep appointments for health care, and appropriately to breastfeed their infants.[23] This system has been expanded to many parts of the country.

The most successful programs involve the peer counselor in all health issues so that the relationship between counselor and client continues. These peer programs are integrated with efforts to improve health habits in general and especially those associated with childbearing. The best programs train community counselors to support women through pregnancy, delivery, and early child rearing, of which breastfeeding is a part. This type of program encourages the development of a relationship that lasts several years.

Because the lowest incidence and duration of breastfeeding are among low-income women and among black mothers, a peer-support program among these clients has the highest probability of success.[23] Using the same model for training candidates that has been developed for other health projects has facilitated initiating the program. The local WIC program or health department is ideal for undertaking a peer-support program because the permanent, full-time staff are knowledgeable about nutrition and lactation and can provide continuity when peer counselors leave the program and new ones need training. This stability is essential to developing some consistency and permanency for the system. The WIC program supports women from early pregnancy through postpartum and early infancy periods.

Because a peer counselor is an individual from the social or cultural community who is selected because of good health behaviors and an innate ability to help others and gain respect, a peer counselor for breastfeeding is a respected member

of the community or neighborhood, is of the same or similar ethnic background and of similar educational and economic level, and has breastfed one or more children. The tremendous success of the La Leche League was based on peer counseling among well-educated, white, middle-class American women.

Some physician practices have employed (yes, peer counselors should be trained and paid) peer counselors successfully to take some of the roles of health care professionals who lack the time to relate on an even plane with a client of different educational or socioeconomic status. Well-established peer-counseling programs have even inspired the counselors to obtain further training as nurses' aides, licensed practical nurses, or registered nurses.

Peer-support programs have been developed in Britain and Canada.[7] In a randomized controlled trial of a telephone-based peer-support intervention, increased duration of breastfeeding and increased satisfaction with the experience were observed. Women valued the support of a counselor in another study in London and South Essex, but the impact on duration was not as dramatic, probably because mothers had to ask for help after discharge and were not routinely contacted.[10]

A peer counselor will complement the work of the health professionals but should never replace the role of the health care provider (Table 22-1).

A woman was more likely to initiate breastfeeding if she had a WIC peer counselor contact her before delivery and was more likely to continue breastfeeding with peer counselor support postpartum in a study of at-risk women enrolled in WIC in Texas.[6] A review of peer counseling publications to evaluate the effectiveness of breastfeeding peer counseling showed overwhelmingly improved rates of breastfeeding initiation, duration, and exclusivity. Secondary gains included a decreased incidence of infant diarrhea and a significant increase in the duration of lactational amenorrhea. These results were reported from both developed and underdeveloped countries. From these findings, a multifaceted breastfeeding promotion campaign was designed for new mothers, family members, health professionals, and the community at large. The Best Start Program proved to be extremely successful and has been replicated by others successfully.

The effectiveness of breastfeeding peer counseling has been shown by secondary gains including a decreased incidence of infant diarrhea and a significant increase in the duration of lactational amenorrhea. These results were reported from both developed and underdeveloped countries.

TABLE 22-1	Child Care Providers' Perceived Advantages and Disadvantages of Breast Milk Versus Formula	
	Breast Milk % (N)	Formula % (N)
Advantages		
Better bonding with mother	86 (171)	3 (5)
Better nutritionally	83 (166)	5 (10)
Diapers not as "smelly"	29 (58)	15 (30)
Helps make infants smarter	34 (68)	2 (4)
Infant is easier to care for	22 (43)	31 (61)
It is easier (in general)	40 (79)	45 (89)
Less illness	77 (153)	3 (5)
Less risk for diseases in adult life	59 (118)	1 (1)
Less risk for obesity	36 (72)	1 (2)
Less trash	53 (105)	4 (8)
More convenient	41 (81)	45 (89)
No advantage	2 (4)	28 (56)
Not embarrassing	11 (22)	28 (55)
Saves family money	85 (170)	2 (3)
Other	2 (4)	7 (14)
Disadvantages		
Do not have a regular feeding schedule	29 (57)	3 (6)
Eat more frequently	42 (83)	3 (6)
Embarrassing	9 (17)	1 (2)
Harder for infants to leave mothers	55 (110)	1 (2)
More diaper changes	18 (35)	6 (4)
No disadvantage	25 (50)	38 (76)
Not as healthy	1 (I)	47 (94)
Uncomfortable for staff	13 (26)	1 (1)
Other	3 (6)	8 (3)

From Clark A, Anderson J, Adams E, et al: Assessing the knowledge, attitudes, behaviors and training needs related to infant feeding, specifically breastfeeding, of child care providers, *Matern Child Health J* 12:128, 2008.
I = individual.

WHO SHALL COUNSEL?

Among those working closely with people in critical life situations, some people make good counselors and some equally good people are not appropriate as counselors and should have other jobs in the organization.[16]

Counseling is a profession, and professional counselors are carefully screened, educated, and trained. Therefore, individuals who help mothers breastfeed should be screened, educated, and trained as well. They should have the following special abilities:

- To listen
- To avoid judgment

- To understand other lifestyles
- To admit it when they do not know
- To seek appropriate help from professionals
- To recognize incompatibility in a given relationship

In the past few decades, peer counseling has become widespread and has been successful, not only with breastfeeding and childbirth, but also with chronic diseases such as cystic fibrosis and with devastating illnesses such as cancer. The first fact that all these groups had to acknowledge is that just because one has experienced a life event, one is not automatically qualified to counsel others experiencing similar situations.

A candidate must first put personal experiences into perspective and understand the motivation for seeking this counseling role. Counseling is an opportunity to help by listening, and being a sympathetic listener is the most important quality. This is not a time to talk about the counselor's pregnancies. The counselor cannot have a personal agenda and press personal views or lifestyle choices on a mother being counseled, nor should counseling be used as a personal platform to promote organizational biases.

A counselor must understand that assuming a place on a health care team demands time and effort. One must be available at the convenience and need of a client, even when this is inconvenient to the counselor.

LEARNING TO HELP MOTHERS

The suggestions to guide a counselor in training must be general guidelines about attitude. The emphasis is on listening, encouraging a mother to talk, and ultimately helping her to solve her own problem by understanding it. Professional counselors are trained using didactic sessions, role play, and supervisory sessions until skills are developed. Continued reinforcement of philosophy and techniques forms the basis of growth and improvement. A lay counselor should attend counselor-training sessions provided by the parent organization and work closely with the supervisor. Sharing counseling situations with others with more experience will give further insight. Returning to reference materials again and again will bring to light new thoughts that have been read before but not truly assimilated initially because of lack of experience.[24]

A peer counselor does not provide medical advice. A counselor can encourage a mother to contact her physician. When an infant is doing poorly or is sick, the pediatrician should be consulted promptly. The rare condition of failure to thrive while breastfeeding is increasing in frequency, paralleling the increased incidence of breastfeeding. It has serious implications for infants and for the continuation of breastfeeding unless treatment is initiated promptly by the physician. A counselor must be able to recognize when a situation is beyond her skills. A physician is powerless to help if not consulted. When an infant's problem is identified and it is prudent to continue breastfeeding, a counselor can be an invaluable asset in supporting and reassuring the mother.

Maternal problems such as mastitis should respond well if treated early, but recurrent mastitis may develop when home remedies are substituted for proper treatment. The role of a counselor in such situations is significant. Encouraging a mother to seek medical care promptly is most important. Reinforcing medical advice will further enhance its effectiveness. For example, if rest is prescribed, a counselor can help a mother to understand how critical rest is to recovery and then help her determine how she is going to cope at home with family responsibilities and a newborn and still rest.

The role of a counselor is support of a mother. A counselor should work in concert with the medical health care team as a team player, not as a competitor or as an adversary, but as a facilitator. The mission of the team is successful lactation, a satisfying mothering experience, and a healthy infant. The health care team will continue to be responsible for a family long after lactation has been discontinued. The confidence and trust developed between the health team and family will be critical to lasting success. The counselor should be remembered as a gentle facilitator and a caring support person who was present and supportive through the rite of passage of matrescence.

A physician working with a lactation counselor or consultant needs to recognize this specialist's skills and limitations. As in other, similar situations, the physician is the leader of the health care team and carries the ultimate responsibility.

REFERENCES

1. Albreht TL, Bryant C: Advances in segmentation modeling for health communication and social marketing campaigns, *J Health Commun* 1:65, 1996.
2. Barnes GR, Lethin AN, Jackson EB, et al: Management of breastfeeding, *JAMA* 151:192, 1953.
3. Baumgartel KL, Spatz DL: WIC (The Special Supplemental Nutrition Program for Women, Infants, Children): policy versus practice regarding breastfeeding, *Nurs Outlook* 61(6):466–470, 2013.
4. Bergh A-M: The role of a nongovernmental organization in breast feeding education, *J Nutr Educ* 19:117, 1987.
5. Bryant CA, Coreil J, D'Angelo SL, et al: A strategy for promoting breastfeeding among economically disadvantaged women and adolescents, *NAACOGS Clin Issu Perinat Womens Health Nurs* 3:723, 1992.
6. Campbell LA, Wan J, Speck PM, et al: Women, infant and children (WIC) peer counselor contact with first time breastfeeding mothers, *Public Health Nurs* 31(1):3–9, 2013.
7. Dennis CL, Hodnett E, Gallop R, et al: The effect of peer support on breast-feeding duration among primiparous women: a randomized controlled trial, *Can Med Assoc J* 166:21, 2002.
8. Deshpande AD, Gazmararian JA: Breast-feeding education and support: association with the decision to breast-feed, *Eff Clin Pract* 3:116, 2000.
9. Evans K, Labbok M, Abrahams SW: WIC and breastfeeding support services: does the mix of services offered vary with race and ethnicity? *Breastfeed Med* 6(6):401–406, 2011.
10. Graffy J, Taylor J, Williams A, et al: Randomised controlled trial of support from volunteer counselors for mothers considering breast feeding, *BMJ* 328:26, 2004. Accessed at www.bmj.com.
11. Gussler J, Bryant C: *Helping mothers breastfeed: program strategies for minority communities*, Health Action Papers (vol. I), Lexington, Ky., 1984, Lexington Fayette County Health Department, University of Kentucky Medical Behavioral Sciences Department.
12. Hedberg IC: Barriers to breastfeeding in the WIC population, *MCN Am J Matern Child Nurs* 38(4):244–249, 2013.
13. International Board of Lactation Consultant Examiners, 7309 Arlington Blvd., Suite 300, Falls Church, Va. 22042.
14. La Leche League International: *The womanly art of breastfeeding*, ed 9, Shomberg, Ill., 2005, La Leche League.
15. Langellier BA, Chaparro MP, Wang ML, et al: The new food package and breastfeeding outcomes among women, infants, and children participants in Los Angeles County, *Am J Public Health* 104:5112–5118, 2014.
16. Lawrence RA: Introduction. In Lauwers J, Woessner C, editors: *Counseling the nursing mother: a reference handbook for health care providers and lay counselors*, Wayne, N.J., 1983, Avery.
17. Mitra AK, Khoury AJ, Carothers C, et al: The loving support breastfeeding campaign: awareness and practices of health care providers in Mississippi, *J Obstet Gynecol Neonatal Nurs* 32:753, 2003.
18. Naylor A, Wester R: Providing professional lactation management consultation, *Clin Perinatol* 14:33, 1987.
19. Porteous R, Kaufman K, Rush J: The effect of individualized professional support on duration of breastfeeding: a randomized controlled trial, *J Hum Lact* 16:303, 2000.
20. Public Health Service: Implementation plans for attaining the objectives for the nation. In *Healthy people 2010: national health promotion and disease prevention objectives midcourse review*, Washington, D.C., 2006, U.S. Government Printing Office. DHHS Pub. No. (PHS) 91-50213.
21. Pugh LC, Milligan RA, Frick KD, et al: Breastfeeding duration, costs, and benefits of a support program for low-income breastfeeding women, *Birth* 29:95, 2002.
22. Raphael D: *The tender gift: breast feeding*, New York, 1976, Schocken.
23. Report of the Surgeon General's Workshop on Breastfeeding and Human Lactation, Washington, D.C., 1984, U.S. Government Printing Office. DHHS Pub. No. HRS-DMC 84-2.
24. Riordan J: *Breastfeeding and human lactation*, ed 9, Boston, 2005, Jones and Bartlett Publishers Inc.
25. Schwartz JB, Popkins BA, Tognetti J, et al: Does WIC participation improve breastfeeding practices? *Am J Public Health* 85:729, 1995.
26. Scrimshaw SCM: The cultural context of breastfeeding in the United States, In *Report of the Surgeon General's Workshop on Breastfeeding and Human Lactation*, Washington, D.C.,

1984, U.S. Government Printing Office. DHHS Pub. No. HRS-D-MC 84-2.

27. Spisak S, Gross SS: *Second follow-up report: the Surgeon General's Workshop on Breastfeeding and Human Lactation,* Washington, D.C., 1991, National Center for Education in Maternal and Child Health.

28. Van Gennep A: *Rites of passage,* London, 1960, Routledge & Kegan Paul (translated by Vizedom MB and Caffee GL).

29. Volpe EM, Bear M: Enhancing breastfeeding initiation in adolescent mothers through the Breastfeeding Educated and Supported Teen (BEST) club, *J Hum Lact* 16:196, 2000.

30. Walker M: *Breastfeeding management for the clinician: using the evidence,* Boston, 2006, Jones and Bartlett Publishers Inc.

31. Wellstart International: *Lactation management self-study modules,* ed 3, Shelbourne, Vt., 2009, Wellstart International.

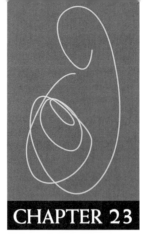

CHAPTER 23

Educating and Training the Medical Professional

The 1984 Surgeon General's Workshop on Breast-feeding and Human Lactation[19] was the first national meeting to focus exclusively on breastfeeding. The breastfeeding strategies developed at that workshop are still being used as the United States and the world move toward the breastfeeding objectives set in *Healthy People 2010: National Health Promotion and Disease Prevention Objective*.[10]

Although many of the objectives have been addressed, the education of the health care professional remains a challenge.[13] A second meeting of the National Planning Committee of the Surgeon General's Workshop convened in Washington, District of Columbia in 1985 to address the issue of that education. The leaders of major professional organizations attended, including the American College of Obstetricians and Gynecologists, American Academy of Pediatrics (AAP), American Academy of Family Physicians, National Association of Pediatric Nurse Practitioners, American Dietetic Association, Nurses of American College of Obstetricians and Gynecologists, National Association of Nurse-Midwives, and National Board of Medical Examiners. These organizations developed and ratified a policy in support of educating and certifying its membership in human lactation and breastfeeding. Discussion was initiated about developing a curriculum appropriate to each professional level of training and specialization.

In June 2009, 25 years later, an anniversary meeting commemorating the first Surgeon General's Workshop was held in Washington, District of Columbia to review the progress that had been made and look at the gaps. Professional education was once again a workshop. The challenges were similar but the strategies more aggressive. It was suggested that federal funds be allocated specifically for professional education. Consistency of curriculum and a system of accreditation were urged. Accountability for professional training on the part of the educational institutions was deemed essential through all professional levels.

Continuing Efforts

Most physicians who are supportive of breastfeeding have breastfed their own children but acknowledge their training was insufficient.[1] Work continues in scattered ad hoc special presentations that may or may not have some affiliation with a medical school or hospital. However, no central unified program has been developed to change the curriculum at the seat of learning: United States medical schools and nursing schools.

Lack of support or encouragement from physicians and nurses was a continuing barrier, and no substantive progress had been made in developing curricula or credentialing. Excellent programs have been provided by Wellstart International[25,27] for teams consisting of a physician, a nurse, a nutritionist, and a hospital administrator from the same institution. Wellstart's programs have been international, and they provide resources around the world. Many other universities have served as cosponsors for a program, seminar, or workshop in their own geographic area. However, the programs have not been integrated into the total medical school curriculum or the training in a residency program, and they are not taught by medical school faculty at all levels of training.

The failure of medical schools to address the issue of education about the breast and training in the clinical issues of breastfeeding was addressed at the University of Texas at San Antonio by Newton.[15] He initiated a program on the obstetric service for medical students and residents. He also reported the results of his national survey of medical schools' curricula: 55% of the 127 United States obstetric and pediatric departments had no didactic lectures for medical students. Of obstetric and pediatric residencies, 30% provided no didactic lectures to their students. Most programs relied on clinical opportunities for learning.

When Freed et al.[9] investigated the attitudes and education of pediatric house staff concerning breastfeeding, they found that third-year residents did not know any more than interns about the subject. Furthermore, only personal experience seemed to provide any in-depth knowledge about simple problems, such as sore nipples.

The Problem

That breastfeeding is important to infants and their mothers for nutritional, immunologic, psychologic, and other health reasons is an established fact. Since the first Surgeon General's Workshop, United States health goals have been to increase the incidence and duration of breastfeeding. Little formal education is provided on the topic in medical schools and residency training programs. No planned curricula or testing mechanisms have been available.

Breastfeeding has another unique problem of interest to the lay persons who have become involved. Many nonphysicians have become involved in training. Some attempts at educating physicians have been made by nonphysicians and sometimes by people who are not health care professionals.[3,5] The message to medical students is that understanding and encouraging breastfeeding are not in a physician's job description. When other care providers give presentations to medical students or residents, it is assumed the provider is describing the work for information only and not for its role in a physician's work. Childbirth is of great interest to the lay public and to consumer advocacy groups as well, but they do not provide physicians' training in childbirth. This training is provided by skilled specialists who have doctoral degrees, residency training, board certification, and, in many cases, additional fellowship training and subspecialty certification, which are minimal qualifications for medical school faculty.

How much do residents and physicians know about managing breastfeeding? The data suggest the answer is "very little." In a study of obstetric

residents, Freed et al.[6] mailed a survey to more than 600 residents, and 64% responded. Only 38% had any education from the faculty about breastfeeding and indicated what little they knew came from other residents and nurses. All participants agreed, however, that they should have a role in the management of breastfeeding for their patients. A survey of 87 of a possible 108 pediatric residents (81%) evenly distributed among levels I, II, and III in a large hospital reported that level III residents were no more competent than their PL-1 counterparts.[8] If they or their spouse breastfed, they were more confident in their knowledge base. No differences were found between men and women or between those breastfed or not breastfed as an infant.[8,9]

The knowledge, training, and attitudes of obstetricians concerning the management of breastfeeding were evaluated by the American College of Obstetricians and Gynecologists.[17] A survey was sent to 1200 fellows of the college, and only 397 (33%) practitioners responded. Obstetricians considered counseling their patients and managing breastfeeding care an important part of their clinical responsibilities. They thought that they were very qualified to treat mastitis, prescribe maternal medications, and advise their lactating patients about contraception. They were less confident about educating their patients about breastfeeding and solving any problems. Personal breastfeeding experience for the women was a predictor of confidence. Four of ten physicians thought their training was inadequate in lactation.[17]

A subsequent study confirmed that residents' knowledge was low and their misinformation disturbingly high.[8] The authors concluded that residency training programs must provide comprehensive education on breastfeeding to prepare residents to meet the needs of patients and other parents. Another study of pediatricians in training given a 15-minute, self-administered, and anonymous questionnaire resulted in 53% participation (29 respondents).[26] On a six-point scale of support of breastfeeding, the group averaged 2.6 (1 being most supportive), revealing an attitude barely above neutral. They averaged only 53% on the management questions, and their confidence in their skills was low, confirming the need for didactic and clinical training in breastfeeding.

The effect of an educational intervention about breastfeeding on the knowledge, confidence, and behaviors of pediatric resident physicians was evaluated using before and after questionnaires. Their behaviors in the clinical setting were also measured before and after an interactive multimedia curricular intervention to increase their knowledge about common lactation issues. The investigators also telephoned the mothers after the clinic visit.

Acceptable management of breastfeeding adequacy and the correct management went from 22% to 65% after the training. The resident physicians especially improved in assessing of problems[11] (Figures 23-1 and 23-2).

A national survey of 1099 family medicine residents, 71% of whom responded, indicated that they thought they should be involved in breastfeeding promotion and support.[7] They demonstrated significant deficits, however, in knowledge about benefits

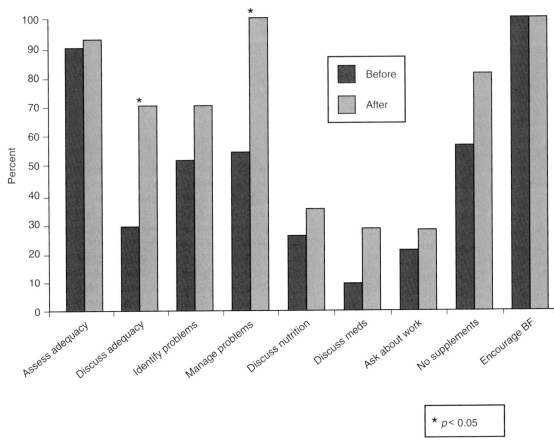

Figure 23-1. Change in resident behaviors: Percentage of residents demonstrating each behavior before and after the educational intervention. *BF*, Breastfeeding. (From Hillenbrand KM, Larsen PG: Effect of educational intervention about breastfeeding on the knowledge, confidence, and behaviors of pediatric resident physicians, *Pediatrics* 110:e59, 2002.)

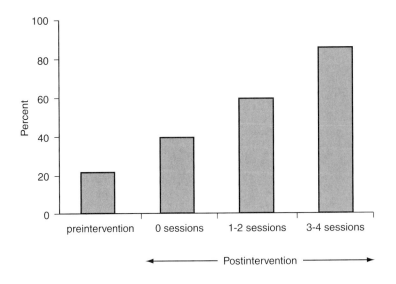

Figure 23-2. Percentage of residents with "acceptable performance" of desired behaviors (at least 6 of 9) compared with number of sessions attended. (From Hillenbrand KM, Larsen PG: Effect of educational intervention about breastfeeding on the knowledge, confidence, and behaviors of pediatric resident physicians, *Pediatrics* 110:e59, 2002.)

and clinical management. These same investigators also polled practitioners regarding their beliefs and knowledge base.[8] The results indicated a similar level of support and lack of knowledge.

Others have investigated the level of knowledge of physicians in training in other countries. A self-administered questionnaire was returned by 76 obstetric residents (84%) in metropolitan areas of South Korea.[12] Korean breastfeeding rates have decreased, especially among well-educated women; the rate was only 17% in 1994. The questionnaire responses indicated that the residents were neutral about breastfeeding. They considered themselves competent to handle breastfeeding situations, but they scored only 38% on the management quiz.

Improved breastfeeding education clearly is needed in obstetrics, pediatrics, and family medicine, the physicians who should be most involved in supporting and promoting breastfeeding.

The Solution

To begin to solve this educational problem, a curriculum should be developed. It should span all 4 years of medical school, being carefully woven into the fabric of medical school for all students, as well as into the residency years for those specializing in obstetrics, pediatrics, and family medicine.

The program should be taught by physicians who are qualified faculty members recognized by their peer group and certified by specialty examining boards. The classes should be part of the total curriculum and not something a student can elect to do only in the fourth year, when most of the assignments are by electives. Graduate physicians in practice rarely will go to a teaching day exclusively on breastfeeding, and they rarely attend programs directed at a broad-based audience of nonphysicians. It does not serve their educational needs when they are also responsible for keeping up to date on the constant flow of advancements in every branch of medicine.

Breastfeeding topics should become part of a well-rounded continuing education program that includes a number of other important issues, such as infectious diseases, endocrine problems, growth, development, and perinatology. When breastfeeding is included in programs on infant nutrition and presented by a physician, it will gain the status it needs.

Suggested Curriculum for Medical Students

If first-year students have a program in human nutrition, breastfeeding can be presented in the section on child nutrition, and the discussion should provide information about the reasons breastfeeding and human milk are superior to formula feeding.

When second-year students have a program on women's health issues, including hormonal maturation, menarche, sex, contraception, childbearing, menopause, and the breast, the additional curriculum can be dedicated to the use of the breast, that is, the anatomy and physiology of lactation. The pathology, including augmentation mammoplasty, reduction mammoplasty, and benign and malignant tumors, is an additional topic.

The third year begins with the general clerkship, wherein skills in history taking and physical examination are sharpened. Obstetrics and gynecology concentrates on breast and pelvic examinations. It is expected that all students, residents, and practitioners will always make these physical examinations part of the physical examination of women.

Third-year medical students spend time on obstetrics, treating patients prenatally, intrapartum, at delivery, and postpartum. Breastfeeding should be part of that continuum, from the discussion of infant feeding prenatally through the postpartum checks for physiologic engorgement and the mother's questions about her afterpains, for example.

The third-year students also spend time on the pediatric service, including the ward, the outpatient, and emergency service. Each student spends a short time in the newborn nursery going crib to crib, checking the newborn's adaptation to extrauterine life. The student also examines infants and talks to mothers. Observing a feeding is part of all discharge examinations on the nursery service and mandatory if the infant is breastfed. The student learns about the breastfed infants' feeding and weight patterns and early lactation. The student learns to identify problems and treat them.

The weeks in the clinic provide additional experience when seeing well babies. The students are exposed to the early weeks and months of breastfeeding and learn about infant weight gain and any problems that arise. The preceptors are experienced, board-certified pediatricians. The daily lecture series, which starts the day for all the residents and students assigned to the outpatient service, is directed at reviewing routine clinical issues. At least one of ten lectures should be about breastfeeding. Students are encouraged to visit their patients while they breastfeed and to accompany the mother-baby nurse when assisting the nursing dyad. They also attend the breastfeeding classes for mothers given by the lactation consultants, who are college-prepared nurses and board-certified lactation consultants (IBCLC).

Fourth-year medical students have a few required courses but the rest of the year is given to electives. A student may elect extra time in the

---

BOX 23-1. Wellstart International Model Hospital Breastfeeding Policies for Full-Term Normal Newborn Infants

Definition and purpose: To promote a philosophy of maternal and infant care that advocates breastfeeding and supports the normal physiologic functions involved in this maternal-infant process. The goal is to ensure that all families who elect to breastfeed their infants will have a successful and satisfying experience.

1. Hospital administrative, medical, nursing, and nutrition staff should establish a strategy that promotes and supports breastfeeding through the formation of an interdisciplinary team responsible for the implementation of hospital policies and provision of ongoing educational activities.
2. All pregnant women should receive information before delivery regarding the benefits and management of breastfeeding.
3. Every mother should be allowed to have a close companion stay with her continuously throughout labor.
4. Infants are to be put to breast as soon after birth as feasible for both mother and infant. This is to be initiated in either the delivery room or the recovery room, and every mother is to be instructed in proper breastfeeding technique and reevaluated before discharge.
5. Breastfeeding mother-infant couples are to room-in together on a 24-hour basis.
6. The infant is to be encouraged to nurse at least 8 to 12 times or more in 24 hours, for a minimum of 8 feedings per 24 hours.
7. Specific timing at the breast is not necessary. Infants usually fall asleep or release the nipple spontaneously when satiated.
8. Infants should spontaneously finish at the first breast, then should be encouraged to try the second breast at each feed.
9. If a feeding at the breast is incomplete or ineffective, the mother should be instructed to begin regular expression of her breasts in conjunction with continued assistance by an experienced staff member. The colostrum or milk obtained by expression should be given to the baby.
10. No supplementary water or milk is to be given unless specifically ordered by a physician or nurse practitioner.
11. Pacifiers are not to be given to any breastfeeding infant unless specifically ordered by a physician or nurse practitioner. The use of bottle nipples and nipple shields should be discouraged.
12. Breastfeeding mothers are to have breasts examined for evidence of lactation or breastfeeding problems at least once every nursing staff shift.
13. Discharge gift packs offered to breastfeeding mothers should contain only noncommercial materials that provide educational information and promote breastfeeding.
14. All breastfeeding mothers are to be advised to arrange for an appointment for their baby's first checkup within 1 week after discharge.
15. At discharge, each mother is to be given a phone number to call for breastfeeding assistance.
16. Mothers who are separated from their babies are to be instructed on how to maintain lactation.

From Naylor AJ, Creer AE, Woodward-Lopez G, et al: Lactation management education for physicians, *Semin Perinatol* 18:525, 1994.

Pan American Health Organization of the World Health Organization, provides an excellent description of such a program. This text is directed at nursing school faculties. The target audience is undergraduate nursing students, although the text could serve as a guide for postgraduate and continuing education programs. A well-trained student will be able to teach mothers optimal breastfeeding and weaning techniques. Students will also be able, within the scope of the total health team, to promote, maintain, and protect breastfeeding.[18]

The learning objectives for nurses include being able to do the following:

- Apply acquired knowledge and skills
- Assist mothers in initiating and continuing breastfeeding
- Promote breastfeeding
- Organize and conduct breastfeeding education seminars for other members of the nursing staff
- Plan and implement breastfeeding services in clinical sites

A training guide for experienced health care professionals was prepared by Best Start and Bryant and Roy.[2] The work is culturally sensitive and is based on a thorough study of social marketing.

Other resources for education and training are listed in Appendix K. Nursing schools should seek the same quality in their lactation resources as they have in all other phases of nursing. When the professional nursing certifying organizations develop appropriate certification for lactation throughout perinatal nursing to accompany the certification already established for labor and delivery, normal newborn, postpartum care, and other areas, the curriculum will come into place quickly.

The Ontario Public Health Association, Toronto, Canada, has developed a series of modules covering the basic essential information regarding breastfeeding, which it recommends be incorporated into the undergraduate curricula of all health care professionals who work with childbearing families. Breastfeeding resource material can be accessed on its website at http://www.hc-sc.gc.ca.

BOX 23-2. Lactation Management Self-Study Modules

MODULE ONE

Breastfeeding: A Basic Health Promotion Strategy in Primary Care
Objectives
After completing this module, you will be able to:

1. Describe the reasons why breastfeeding is important as well as evidence-based risks of not breastfeeding for the infant, mother, family, and community at large.
2. Identify factors that contribute to the breastfeeding decision.
3. Counsel a woman about breastfeeding.

Introduction
All mothers want to provide what's best for their babies and often turn to their health care provider for advice. This module will help prepare you for this discussion by reviewing human milk composition and some of the major benefits of breastfeeding for infant, mother, family, and the community. Some of the factors that influence how women make their infant feeding choice will also be described.

MODULE TWO

Basics of Breastfeeding: Getting Started
Objectives
After completing this module, you will be able to:

1. Describe the process of milk production and removal.
2. Recognize correct attachment and effective suckling at the breast.
3. Identify components of anticipatory guidance for all women.
4. Recognize the impact of perinatal hospital practices on breastfeeding.

Introduction
Although the mother's body produces milk as a normal part of the reproductive cycle, the technique of breastfeeding is a learned skill enhanced by practice and support. While parents need helpful information prenatally to know what to expect, the opportunity postpartum to practice attaching the baby to the breast and assessing the baby's breastfeeding effectiveness can provide the family with confidence as they embark on this particular experience of parenthood.

The key to helping new breastfeeding families is an understanding of the basic anatomy of the breast and physiology of the milk production and removal process. This module will focus on the science of lactation and practical clinical skills to help mothers get started. The module is applicable to both the obstetric and pediatric sides of the equation, as the management of the peripartum course and newborn care can profoundly affect the early breastfeeding experience and later infant feeding outcomes. As far as breastfeeding is concerned, the mother and baby are a biologic unit; whatever influences one affects the other.

MODULE THREE

Common Breastfeeding Problems
Objectives
After completing this module, you will be able to:

1. Discuss causes and prevention of common breastfeeding problems.
2. Recognize that infants and mothers with special health care needs can breastfeed.
3. Recommend treatment options compatible with breastfeeding.
4. Recognize when and how lactation can be sustained during mother-infant separation.

Introduction
From time to time, mothers encounter problems with breastfeeding. Most problems are preventable with good breastfeeding practices: correct positioning and attachment, frequent unlimited feeds, and attention to the effectiveness of the infant's suckling. When problems do occur, early recognition and treatment enable a mother to begin or continue to enjoy breastfeeding and help reach the recommended goals of exclusive breastfeeding for six months and continued breastfeeding for a year and beyond.

From Wellstart International: Home page. Available at www.wellstart.org (Accessed 28.01.15.).

POSTGRADUATE LEARNING OPPORTUNITIES FOR NURSES AND LACTATION CONSULTANTS

Numerous programs across the United States are geared toward nurses and often are provided by nurses. Many of these focus on curricula designed to assist the participant in passing the certifying examination provided by the International Board of Lactation Consultant Examiners. Postgraduate teaching for lactation consultants is provided by the International Lactation Consultants Association and by independent professional groups.

POSTGRADUATE LEARNING OPPORTUNITIES BY MEDICAL GROUPS FOR PHYSICIANS

Postgraduate educational opportunities are one of the major goals of the ABM, an international organization founded in 1994 and limited to physicians from all disciplines and physician trainees. The ABM holds an annual meeting with plenary sessions, workshops, and submitted papers and posters on the wide range of topics involving breastfeeding and human lactation. ABM's mission is to encourage and support breastfeeding, especially through physician education. ABM has developed a program—*What Every Physician Needs to Know About Breastfeeding (WEPNKAB)*—which is presented by a team of experts every year preceding the annual meeting. It has been recorded on video and is available from the ABM on its website as well.

The Milk Club is a group that meets in conjunction with the American Pediatric Society, Society for Pediatric Research, and Academic Pediatric Association. Their mission is to bring new science in the field to the attention of all investigators. The format is usually a symposium with discussion and a poster session at the Pediatric Academic Society (PAS) annual meeting.

The International Society for Research in Human Milk and Lactation is an organization of investigators who meet annually in conjunction with the Federation of American Societies for Experimental Biology and meet biannually and independently at international sites to discuss current knowledge of laboratory and clinical research. Membership is limited to qualified investigators in the field. Appendix K provides the addresses for these organizations.

The AAP, American College of Obstetricians and Gynecologists, and American Academy of Family Practice have increased their programming about human lactation at their annual and regional meetings. The AAP established a Work Group on Breastfeeding that became the section on Breastfeeding of the AAP. The section has prepared a position paper on breastfeeding every five years that was most recently published in *Pediatrics*. It is available at http://www.AAP.org/breastfeeding.

The statement has been updated and published in 2010.[23] It includes the additional AAP recommendation for vitamin D to be given to breastfed infants by 2 months of age because of a deficiency of sunlight exposure in present lifestyles. The dose is 400 IU of vitamin D daily starting shortly after birth. Members of the AAP are welcome to join the section. The section is the sponsor of the Program on Breastfeeding in Pediatric Offices, which is now offered to the American College of Obstetricians and Gynecologists and all obstetricians as well as to the American Academy of Family Practice and its members. The section has also prepared a speaker's kit on breastfeeding with presentation slides for a physician to present his or her own lecture in the practice area. The section has authored a book for parents edited by Joan Meek, MD now in its second edition, and a handbook for physicians edited by Richard Schanler, MD, also in its second edition.

Physicians Who Breastfeed

Pregnancy is becoming more common in residency and over 50% are female in new millennium. A study

of Obstetric Residency reported 80% of the residents are female whereas in pediatrics 63% are female and in family medicine 53% are female. In a study by Orth et al.[16] 404 responded, and of those, 22% had personal experience with breastfeeding, all of whom felt support from faculty and fellow residents. Resident mothers felt it placed extra burden on their colleagues. Two thirds of the breastfeeding residents struggled with low milk supply and stopped breastfeeding before they planned to, in spite of the supportive atmosphere. Sustaining breastfeeding was also reported by Riggins et al.[21] in a Pediatric Residency Program. The rate of initiation was high (98%) above state averages and national goals. At 6 months 68% were breastfeeding, also higher than state averages (38%) and national goals (61%), but at one year it was 12% below averages and goals. Three quarters of the women had difficulties and 73% were able to continue. Twenty-seven percent were unsuccessful and did not meet their breastfeeding goals, and most felt they had failed. Suggestions they made to improve outcome were: on-site daycare, need for pumping facilities, or better facilities with a phone. They tended to seek help from books, lactation consultants, or friends but not other physicians.

Summary

To establish breastfeeding and human lactation as an integral part of medical student education, the topic should be inserted into the present curriculum at the appropriate natural points, whether it is a class on anatomy, physiology, nutrition, endocrinology, women's health, or infant care. The class should be taught by recognized faculty who also teach the other parts of the subject material. Finally, the material should be included in the examination for the subject. When it is not on the examination it is ignored. Much remains to be learned in modern medicine, and lactation should be part of it. The residency training programs in obstetrics, pediatrics, and family medicine can access the residency curriculum from the AAP website and introduce it into their residency programs. It is available at http://aap.org/breastfeeding/curriculum/ (Tables 23-2 and 23-3).

As more and more education is available electronically, breastfeeding resources need to be available. An Internet-based program called "Breastfeeding Basics" is available free of charge. This source was evaluated. Of the 3456 who accessed the program, 2237 (65%) completed one or more pretests. The mean pretest/posttest scores showed improvement. The lowest scores were on vitamin D, breastfeeding physiology, infant growth, and infant problems. Pre- and posttests are an important factor in the value of learning over the Internet.

TABLE 23-2   Comparison of Intervention Differences (I) to Control Site Differences (C) by Specialty: Mean Difference (p)

		Pediatrics	OB/GYN	Family Practice
Knowledge	I	14	18	18
		(0.057)	(0.007)	(0.009)
	C	9.0	5.0	2.0
Practice patterns	I	0.48	0.35	0.59
		(0.277)	(0.063)	(0.302)
	C	0.35	−0.05	0.31
Confidence	I	1.0	0.94	1.21
		(0.0015)	(0.052)	(0.072)
	C	0.58	0.13	0.50

TABLE 23-3   Comparison of Scores for All Maternal-Child Health Care Providers Who Completed Both the Pretest and the Posttest of the Modules

Module	Number (%) Completing	Mean Score ± 1 SD Pretest	Posttest	Statistical Significance*
Benefits/barriers	1629 (47%)	91 ± 8.2%	96 ± 6.4%	$p < 0.001$
Anatomy/physiology	1280 (37%)	79 ± 14.1%	93 ± 9.1%	$p < 0.001$
Growth/development	1072 (31%)	72 ± 15.1%	91 ± 11.0%	$p < 0.001$
Breastfeeding around the world	962 (28%)	84 ± 12.1%	93 ± 8.5%	$p < 0.001$
Mother-infant couple	1021 (30%)	82 ± 13.6%	92 ± 8.7%	$p < 0.001$
Breastfed infant with problems	918 (27%)	77 ± 15.7%	91 ± 10.4%	$p < 0.001$
Breast milk and drugs	928 (27%)	81 ± 11.8%	89 ± 11.3%	$p < 0.001$

*By paired Student's t test.

REFERENCES

1. Anchondo I, Berkeley L, Mulla ZD, et al: Pediatricians', obstetricians', gynecologists', and family medicine physicians' experiences with and attitudes about breastfeeding, South Med J 105(5):243–248, 2012.
2. Bryant CA, Roy M: Best start training manual: breastfeeding for healthy mothers, healthy babies, Tampa, Fla., 1990, Best Start.
3. Department of Human Services: WIC State Agency: District of Columbia breastfeeding peer counselor program: training manual, Washington, D.C., 1990, Department of Health and Human Services.
4. Feldman-Winter L, Barone L, Milcareck KB, et al: Residency curriculum improves breastfeeding care, Pediatrics 126:289–297, 2009, http://dx.doi.org/10.1542/peds.2009-3250.
5. Food and Nutrition Service: U.S. Department of Agriculture: promoting breastfeeding in WIC: a compendium of practical approaches, Alexandria, Va., 1988, Nutrition and Technical Services Division, USDA.
6. Freed GL, Clark SJ, Cefalo RC, et al: Breast-feeding education of obstetrics-gynecology residents and practitioners, Am J Obstet Gynecol 173:1607, 1995.
7. Freed GL, Clark SJ, Curtis P, et al: Breast-feeding education and practice in family medicine, J Fam Pract 40:263, 1995.
8. Freed GL, Clark SJ, Lohr JA, et al: Pediatrician involvement in breast-feeding promotion: a national study of residents and practitioners, Pediatrics 96:490, 1995.
9. Freed GL, Jones MTM, Fraley JK: Attitudes and education of pediatric house staff concerning breastfeeding, South Med J 85:484, 1992.
10. Healthy People 2010: National health promotion and disease prevention objectives, Washington, D.C., 2000, U.S. Government Printing Office. DHHS Pub. No. (PHS) 91-50213.
11. Hillenbrand KM, Larsen PG: Effect of an educational intervention about breastfeeding on the knowledge, confidence, and behaviors of pediatric resident physicians, Pediatrics 110: e59, 2002.
12. Kim HS: Attitudes and knowledge regarding breast-feeding: a survey of obstetric residents in metropolitan areas of South Korea, South Med J 89:684, 1996.
13. Lawrence RA: Review of the Surgeon General's Workshop on Breastfeeding and Human Lactation. In Presented at American Public Health Association meetings, San Diego, November. 1984.
14. Naylor AJ, Creer AE, Woodward-Lopez G, et al: Lactation management education for physicians, Semin Perinatol 18:525, 1994.
15. Newton E: Breastfeeding/lactation and the medical school curriculum, J Hum Lact 8:122, 1992.
16. Orth TA, Drachmen D, Habak P: Breastfeeding in obstetrics residency: exploring maternal and colleague resident perspectives, Breastfeed Med 8(4):394–400, 2013.
17. Power ML, Locke E, Chapin J, et al: The effort to increase breast-feeding: do obstetricians, in the forefront, need help? J Reprod Med 48:72, 2003.
18. Powers NG, Naylor AJ, Wester RA: Hospital policies: crucial to breastfeeding success, Semin Perinatol 18:517, 1994.
19. Report of the Surgeon General's Workshop on Breastfeeding and Human Lactation, Washington, D.C., 1984, U.S. Government Printing Office. DHHS Pub. No. HRS-D-MC 84-2.

20. Ricciotti HA, Hacker MR, De Flesco LD, et al: Randomized, controlled trial of a normal pregnancy virtual patient to teach medical students counseling skills, *J Reprod Med* 55 (11&12):498–502, 2010.

21. Riggins C, Rosenman MB, Szucs KA: Breastfeeding experiences among physicians, *Breastfeed Med* 7(3):151–154, 2012.

22. Rodriguez-Garcia R, Schaefer LA, Yunes J: *Lactation education for health professionals*, Washington, D.C., 1990, Pan American Health Organization.

23. Section on Breastfeeding AAP: Policy statement: breastfeeding and the use of human milk, *Pediatrics* 129:e827–e841, 2012.

24. Tully MR, Overfield ML: *Educating health professionals for breastfeeding support, SPRANS Grant*, Athens, Ga., 1986, University of Georgia.

25. Wellstart International: *Model hospital breastfeeding policies for full-term normal newborn infants*, San Diego, Calif., 1990, Wellstart.

26. Williams EL, Hammer LD: Breastfeeding attitudes and knowledge of pediatricians-in-training, *Am J Prev Med* 11:26, 1995.

27. Woodward-Lopez G, Creer AE, editors: *Lactation management curriculum: a faculty guide for schools of medicine, nursing and nutrition*, ed 4, San Diego, Calif., 1994, Wellstart International and University of California at San Diego.

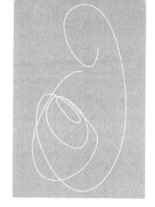

Appendices

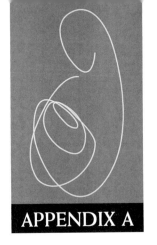

APPENDIX A

Composition of Human Milk

TABLE A-1	Composition of Human Colostrum and Mature Breast Milk	
Constituent (per 100 mL)	**Colostrum 1-5 Days**	**Mature Milk >30 Days**
Energy (kcal)	58	70
Total solids (g)	12.8	12.0
Lactose (g)	5.3	7.3
Total nitrogen (mg)	360	171
Protein nitrogen (mg)	313	129
Nonprotein nitrogen (mg)	47	42
Total protein (g)	2.3	0.9
Casein (mg)	140	187
α-Lactalbumin (mg)	218	161
Lactoferrin (mg)	330	167
IgA (mg)	364	142
Amino acids (total)		
Alanine (mg)	—	52
Arginine (mg)	126	49
Aspartate (mg)	—	110
Cystine (mg)	—	25
Glutamate (mg)	—	196
Glycine (mg)	—	27
Histidine (mg)	57	31
Isoleucine (mg)	121	67
Leucine (mg)	221	110
Lysine (mg)	163	79
Methionine (mg)	33	19
Phenylalanine (mg)	105	44
Proline (mg)	—	89
Serine (mg)	—	54
Threonine (mg)	148	58
Tryptophan (mg)	52	25
Tyrosine (mg)	—	38
Valine (mg)	169	90
Taurine (free) (mg)	—	8

Continued

TABLE A-1	Composition of Human Colostrum and Mature Breast Milk—cont'd	
Constituent (per 100 mL)	**Colostrum 1-5 Days**	**Mature Milk >30 Days**
Urea (mg)	10	30
Creatine (mg)	—	3.3
Total fat (g)	2.9	4.2
Fatty acids (% total fat)		
12:0 tauric	1.8	5.8
14:0 myristic	3.8	8.6
16:0 palmitic	26.2	21.0
18:0 stearic	8.8	8.0
18:1 oleic	36.6	35.5
18:2, n-6 linoleic	6.8	7.2
18:3, n-3 linolenic	—	1.0
C_{20} and C_{22} polyunsaturated	10.2	2.9
Cholesterol (mg)	27	16
Vitamins		
Fat soluble		
Vitamin A (retinol equivalents) (mcg)	89	67
β-Carotene (mcg)	112	23
Vitamin D (mcg)	—	0.05
Vitamin E (total tocopherols) (mcg)	1280	315
Vitamin K (mcg)	0.23	0.21
Water soluble		
Thiamin (mcg)	15	21
Riboflavin (mcg)	25	35
Niacin (mcg)	75	150
Folic acid (mcg)	—	8.5
Vitamin B_6 (mcg)	12	93
Biotin (mcg)	0.1	0.6
Pantothenic acid (mcg)	183	180
Vitamin B_{12} (ng)	200	26
Ascorbic acid (mg)	4.4	4.0
Minerals		
Calcium (mg)	23	28
Magnesium (mg)	3.4	3.0
Sodium (mg)	48	18
Potassium (mg)	74	58
Chlorine (mg)	91	42
Phosphorus (mg)	14	15
Sulfur (mg)	22	14
Trace elements		
Chromium (ng)	—	50
Cobalt (mcg)	—	1
Copper (mcg)	46	25
Fluorine (mcg)	—	16
Iodine (mcg)	12	11
Iron (mcg)	45	40
Manganese (mcg)	—	0.6±
Nickel (mcg)	—	2
Selenium (mcg)	—	2.0
Zinc (mcg)	540	120

Data from multiple references (see Chapter 4). Figures have been averaged.

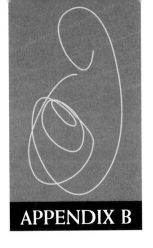

APPENDIX B

Normal Serum Values for Breastfed Infants

TABLE B-1	Serum Chemical Values of Normal Breastfed Infants*											
Concentration/100 mL of Serum	Age 28 Days			Age 56 Days			Age 84 Days			Age 112 Days		
	N	Mean	SD	N	Mean	SD	N	Mean	SD	N	Mean	SD
Males												
Total protein (g)	22	5.87	0.50	36	5.96	0.42	29	6.16	0.57	51	6.29	0.51
Albumin (g)	22	4.02	0.35	36	4.14	0.34	29	4.27	0.39	51	4.38	0.40
Globulins (g)												
α_1	22	0.14	0.03	36	0.17	0.03	29	0.18	0.03	51	0.17	0.04
α_2	22	0.53	0.10	36	0.60	0.11	29	0.74	0.14	51	0.81	0.19
β	22	0.61	0.11	36	0.67	0.13	29	0.69	0.20	51	0.67	0.11
γ	22	0.57	0.14	36	0.38	0.09	29	0.28	0.08	51	0.26	0.10
Cholesterol (mg)	21	139	31	32	153	34	25	133	32	47	145	26
Triglycerides (mg)	18	122	36	32	106	57	25	170	76	46	148	57
Urea nitrogen (mg)	43	8.5	3.2	49	6.6	2.1	47	7.0	2.7	51	7.3	4.2
Calcium (mg)	41	10.2	0.8	47	10.3	1.0	42	10.4	0.8	48	10.3	0.8
Phosphorus (mg)	43	6.6	0.7	49	6.4	0.7	47	6.2	0.5	49	6.2	0.7
Alkaline phosphatase[†]	31	**22**	6	40	**21**	7	35	21	8	44	18	7
Magnesium (mg)	40	2.0	0.2	47	2.1	0.2	45		0.2	50	2.2	0.2
Females												
Total protein (g)	18	6.04	0.40	27	5.86	0.44	21	6.21	0.57	42	6.31	0.62
Albumin (g)	18	4.07	0.27	27	4.03	0.35	21	4.29	0.37	42	4.36	0.42
Globulins (g)												
α_1	18	0.15	0.02	27	0.17	0.04	21	0.17	0.03	42	**0.19**	0.04
α_2	18	0.55	0.07	27	0.65	0.12	21	0.74	0.18	42	0.78	0.17
β	18	0.70	0.18	27	0.63	0.11	21	0.71	0.13	42	0.67	0.16
γ	18	0.57	0.10	27	0.38	0.10	21	0.30	0.06	42	**0.31**	0.10
Cholesterol (mg)	13	**180**	35	25	157	37	20	**155**	29	40	**165**	36
Triglycerides (mg)	9	**157**	43	24	112	53	18	195	56	38	**170**	52
Urea nitrogen (mg)	37	8.3	2.3	33	6.4	2.2	40	6.4	2.2	42	6.6	3.5
Calcium (mg)	37	10.3	0.8	33	10.3	0.8	40	10.3	0.8	42	10.7	0.7

Continued

TABLE B-1   Serum Chemical Values of Normal Breastfed Infants—cont'd

Concentration/100 mL of Serum	Age 28 Days			Age 56 Days			Age 84 Days			Age 112 Days		
	N	Mean	SD	N	Mean	SD	N	Mean	SD	N	Mean	SD
Phosphorus (mg)	39	6.9	0.8	33	6.4	0.8	40	6.1	0.7	42	6.1	0.7
Alkaline phosphatase	31	19	5	28	17	5	32	17	5	36	17	5
Magnesium (mg)	39	2.0	0.4	32	2.0	0.2	40	2.1	0.2	41	2.1	0.3

*Bold figures indicate that value is greater than the corresponding value for infants of the opposite sex and that the difference is statistically significant at the 95% level of confidence.

†King-Armstrong units.

From Fomon SJ, Filer LJ, Thomas LN, et al: Growth and serum chemical values of normal breastfed infants, *Acta Paediatr Scand Suppl* 202:1, 1970.

TABLE B-2   Leptin Levels in Infants

	Leptin (ng mL^{-1})	In (Leptin) (ng mL^{-1})	In (Leptin)/Weight (ng mL^{-1} per kg)	In (Leptin)/BMI (ng m^2 mL^{-1} per kg)
Total ($n=35$)	7.35±6.87	1.19±0.89	0.21±0.20	0.08±0.06
M ($n=18$)	6.92±5.72	0.96±1.01	0.13±0.22	0.05±0.07
F ($n=17$)	7.79±8.02	1.43±0.73	0.29±0.17	0.1±0.05
BF ($n=13$) (7M, 6F)	8.04±5.01	1.62±0.73*	0.30±0.13*	0.11±0.05*
FF ($n=22$) (llM, 1lF)	6.93±7.91	0.94±0.95*	0.16±0.20*	0.06±0.07*

Data are mean±SD.

BF, Breastfed; *BMI*, body mass index; *F*, female; *M*, male.

*$p<0.05$.

From Savino F, Costamagna M, Prino A, et al: Leptin levels in term breastfed (BF) and formula-fed (FF) infants, *Acta Paediatr* 91:897, 2002.

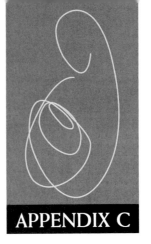

APPENDIX C

Herbals and Natural Products

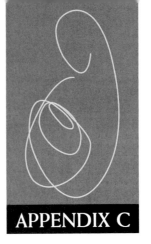

Herb Common Name/Rating*	Synonyms	Active Ingredient	Uses	Present in Milk	Safety/Efficacy
Aloe vera AAP – H L3 W –	Aloe barbadensis, A. capensis, vera	Polysaccharide, glucomannan	Wound healing and small burns	Unknown, probably none when applied to skin	Orally is a strong purgative; oral dosing not recommended during lactation. Dermal use ok.[11,12]
Asparagus	Wild asparagus root	Asparagus racemosus			Nourishing herb; used in those debilitated or conv galactagogue (1 g powdered root per day in milk or juice).[17]
Blessed thistle AAP – H L3 W –		Many chemicals and volatile oils	Gastrointestinal symptoms	Unknown	This is not a galactagogue. It is a different plant from milk thistle. No known toxicity.[11] Many uses.
Borage AAP – H L5 W –	Borage officinalis Toxin	Pyrrolizidine alkaloid	Pain therapy		Contraindicated in pregnancy and lactation.[30]
Botulism AAP – H L3 W –					In natural cases of botulism toxin does not get into the milk. Pharmaceutical product Botox treatment unlikely to reach milk.[23]
Cannabis AAP 2 H L5 W –	Marijuana Capsicum	Δ9-Tetrahydro-cannabinol (THC)	Sedative, hallucinogen	Yes	Remains in infant's system for weeks, especially in fat.[2,11,13,32]
Capsaicin AAP – H L3 W –		Topical anesthesia		Unknown	Available as a cream, lotion, or oral tablets. Used where vasodilation or warmth is needed. Can cause burning, stinging. Do not use on breasts.[12,28]
Chamomile AAP – H L3 W –	Matricaria recutita, Aster Aceae family	Terpenoids (coumarins), flower heads	Antiinflammatory, carminative, antiseptic, sedative (all unproved)	Unknown	Potential for allergic reaction. Animal studies question safety in pregnancy and lactation.[2,6]
Cohosh (black) AAP – H L4 W –	Cimicifuga racemosa, black cohosh, black snakeroot, found in Lydia Pinkham's compound	Estrogenic compounds, tannins, terpenoids, use roots and rhizome	Dysmenorrheal, dyspepsia, rheumatism, menopause	Unknown	May cause hypotension; could decrease milk production? Efficacy and safety in lactation.[31]
Cohosh (blue) AAP – H L5 W –	Caulophyllum, blue cohosh, squaw root	Roots and rhizome, methylcytosine, caulosaponin	Uterine stimulant, emmenagogue, increased blood pressure, like nicotine, induces labor		Safety of concern, can constrict coronary vessels; leaves and seeds are known to be toxic. Can induce labor.[30]
Comfrey FDA banned AAP – H L5 W –	Symphytum officinale	Roots and rhizome and leaves, allantoin, hepatotoxic, pyrrolizidine alkaloids	"Wonder drug," heals wounds, used as poultice, used as tea	Yes	Venoocclusive disease causing hepatic failure. Banned in many countries; unsafe.[1,5,4,11,15,24,26]

Continued

Herb Common Name/Rating*	Synonyms	Active Ingredient	Uses	Present in Milk	Safety/Efficacy
Echinacea AAP – H L3 W –	Echinacea angustifolia, coneflower	Whole plant, flowers, dried roots	Immunostimulant, antiinfective, tested for upper respiratory infections	Unknown	Has been studied; effective in short courses, not continual use. No known toxicity; probably safe during lactation.[8,11,12,21]
Evening primrose AAP – H L3 W –	Oenothera biennis	Biennis, oil from seeds, cis-gamma-linoleic acid (GLA), a precursor of prostaglandin E_1, essential fatty acids (EFA)	Lower cholesterol, lower blood pressure, lower dysmenorrhea, mastalgia, eczema	Yes	Efficacy: conflicting reports. Safety: +/− probably in small amounts. Supplements increase EFA in milk[9]; increase bleeding time.[27] Do not use with phenol thiazines.
Fennel AAP – H L4 W –	Foeniculum vulgare	Dried ripe fruit, volatile oil, transanethole estrogenic effect	Carminative, loosen phlegm, galactagogue, increase libido	Probable	Volatile oil can be toxic; use only fruits (seeds). Because of estrogenic effect, its reputation as a galactagogue is questioned.[11]
Fenugreek AAP – H L3 W –	Trigonella foenum-graecum, Greek hayseed	Dried ripe seeds, diosgenin, and alkaloids smell like maple syrup	Hypoglycemia, galactagogue, anticoagulant, see text	Probable	Risk: cross allergy to chrysanthemum family. Probably in milk; infants smell of maple syrup. No studies of efficacy.[13,14,17,22,25,29]
Feverfew Not rated	Chrysanthemum partenium Bachelor's button	Leaves extract tincture	Associated with migraines. Menstrual irregularity antiinflammatory	Unknown	Enhances effect of warfarin contraindicated during pregnancy. Value as galactagogue undocumented; decreases platelet aggregation.[30]
Garlic (Supplement form) AAP – H L3 W –	Lily family: Allium sativum, pocr man's treacle, clove garlic, common garlic, allium, stinking rose	Alliin, ajoens	Has 125 different uses, some contradictory, both high and low blood pressure, antibacterial, antithrombotic, lower cholesterol	Yes	Can cause colic in breastfed infants. Can enhance warfarin. Not tolerated by some infants.[7]

Antigalactagogues: decrease milk supply. Fennel and estrogenic effects; oil is toxic. Peppermint, sage, parsley (tabbouleh salad) agnus castus (monk's pepper) Jasmine flowers applied to breast

Galactagogues: increase milk supply

Fenugreek (Greek hayseed)

Goats rue (Galega officinalis)

Alfalfa (member pea family) seeds can be toxic

Borage contains amabilene/ relieves pain can cause venoocclusive disease

Ginkgo AAP – H L3 W –	Ginkgo biloba	Flavones and glycosides, seeds, ginkgotoxin, ginkgo biloba extract (GBE), leaves for tea	Herbal antioxidant	Unknown	Placebo-controlled studies suggest no efficacy in young adults. Use in elderly more effective. Conflicting reports of safety. Not recommended in lactation.[7,31] Enhances the effect of warfarin. Can cause bleeding even alone.
Ginseng AAP – H L3 W –	Panax ginseng (P. quinquefolius), Asian ginseng	Root and extracts	Panacea, cure-all, adaptogen, strengthening, increasing mental capacity	Unknown	Too much has been written, with considerable conflict of opinion. Ginseng abuse syndrome; research done mostly by manufacturers. Safety: not long-term use; efficacy questionable.[3,16,20] Not recommended in lactation.[7] Reduces effect of warfarin.
Grapefruit seed extract AAP – H – W – Grape seed AAP – H – W –		Flavonols Capsules, tablets (50-100 mg daily supplementation/ 150-300 mg daily therapeutic	Antimicrobial inhibits intestinal cytochrome 450		Noted to have autoinfection, antiviral, antibacterial, and antifungal effects. Grapefruit is known to contain quinine, especially in the bitter skin and section fibers. Recommended as an extract for use by direct application on sore nipples. If it has antiinfectious properties, it should be effective when traumatized nipples have become infected.[26] Antioxidant, anticancer agent for varicose veins, circulatory problems. May increase risk for bleeding.
Herbal teas	Tablets, powders, tea leaves	May include Gerry mander, comfrey, mistletoe, skull cap, pennyroyal, all of which are toxic. Always check constituents.			Many cause hepatotoxicity and/or venous occlusive disease. Many associated with hemorrhagic disease.[9,31]
Kava AAP – H L5 W –	Piper methysticum, Kew, tonga	Roots/rhizomes, dihydropyrones with central nervous system activity, kavapyrones	Inebriation, muscle relaxants, alternative to penzodiapams	Unknown	Unsafe in pregnancy and lactation. Numbs the mouth; nauseating. Causes yellow discoloration of the skin, hair, nails.[11,12]
Licorice root	Glycyrrhiza glabra family	Glycyrrhizin acid rhizomes and roots	Laxative and cure for gastritis	Laxative, gastritis, hypokalemia	Known for 4000 years; large doses: weakness, edema, weight loss, hypertension, hypokalemia, and confusion. Consumption should be avoided in pregnancy and lactation.[7,33]

Continued

Herb Common Name/Rating*	Synonyms	Active Ingredient	Uses	Present in Milk	Safety/Efficacy
Milk thistle (holy thistle) (not blessed thistle) AAP – H L3 W –; Raspberry root AAP – H – W –	Silybum marianum, St. Mary's thistle, Rubis idaeus leaves	Fruits, flavolignans, inhibits oxidative damage to cells Promote diverse urinary tract infections, morning sickness, ease labor	Protective effect, concentrates in the liver	Unknown	Galactagogue. Problem: can cause allergy; low oral bioavailability. Probably safe.[11] Poor oral bioavailability. Safe in pregnancy and lactation.[28]
Sage AAP – H L4 W –	Salvia officinalis	Fresh leaves and fresh flowering aerial parts, dried leaves, and oils prepared as extracts and teas	Loss of appetite, inflammation of mouth and pharynx, excessive perspiration	Unknown	Contraindicated in pregnancy. Suppresses lactation. Okay as a flavoring.[23]
St. John's wort AAP – H L2 W –	Hypericum perforatum Hyperforin	Naphthodianthrones, phloroglucinols Antioxidant	Depression	Not detected Galactagogue	Can cause photosensitivity. Risk for self-medication for a serious psychiatric problem. Can reduce the effect of warfarin, induce cytochrome P-450 enzyme system.[18,19,31] Dose variable in different products. Poorly soluble in water micronized for oral use as galactagogue.[9,10,28]
Silymarin (micronized) AAP – H L3 W –	Flavonolignans seeds Silybum marianum, Milk thistle, BIO-C	Liver protectant possibly			
Valerian root AAP – H L3 W –	Valeriana officinalis, all-heal, Amantilla, setwell, setewale, capon's tail, heliotrope, vandal root	Liquid, tablets, tea, volatile oil	Nervousness and insomnia	Unknown	Not recommended in lactation. Used as a sedative, hypnotic.[12]

*Ratings for each drug represent three classification systems. American Academy of Pediatrics (AAP), Hale (H), and Weiner (W). See text for a complete listing of categories in each system. A dash indicates that the drug is not listed in that system.

REFERENCES

1. Abbot PJ: Comfrey: assessing the low-dose health risk, *Med J Aust* 149:678, 1988.
2. American Academy of Pediatrics: Committee on drugs: the transfer of drugs and other chemicals into human milk, *Pediatrics* 108:776, 2001.
3. Awang DV: Maternal use of ginseng and neonatal androgenization, *JAMA* 265:1828, 1991.
4. Bach N, Thung SN, Schaffner F: Comfrey herb tea-induced hepatic veno-occlusive disease, *Am J Med* 87:97, 1989.
5. Bach N, Thung SN, Schaffner F: Comfrey herb tea-induced hepatic veno-occlusive disease, *Am J Med* 87:97, 1998.
6. Barr RG: Herbal teas for infantile colic, *J Pediatr* 123:669, 1993.
7. Briggs GC, Freeman RK, Yaffe SJ: *Drugs in pregnancy and lactation, A reference guide to fetal and neonatal risk*, ed 6, Philadelphia, Pa., 2002, Lippincott, Williams & Wilkins.
8. Burger RA, Torres AR, Warren RP, et al: Echinacea induced cytokine production by human macrophages, *Int J Immunopharmacol* 19:371, 1997.
9. Cant A, Shay J, Horrobin DF: The effect of maternal supplementation with linoleic and gamma-linoleic acids on the fat composition and content of human milk: a placebo-controlled trial, *J Nutr Sci Vitaminol (Tokyo)* 37:573, 1991.
10. Di Pierro F, Callegari A, Carotenuto D, et al: Clinical efficacy, safety and tolerability of BIO-C$_k$ (micronized Silymarin) as a galactogogue, *Acta Biomed* 79:205–210, 2008.
11. Doughty C, Walker A, Brenchley J: Herbal mind altering substances: an unknown quantity? *Emerg Med J* 21:253, 2004.
12. Foster S, Tyler VE: *Tyler's honest herbal: a sensible guide to the use of herbs and related remedies*, New York, 1999, The Haworth Herbal Press.
13. Hale TW: *Medications and mother's milk*, ed 13, Amarillo, Tex., 2008, Pharmasoft Publishing.
14. Huggins KE: Fenugreek: one remedy for low milk production, *Medela Messenger Winter* 15:16, 1998.
15. Huxtable RJ, Luthy J, Zweifel U: Toxicity of comfrey pepsin preparations, *N Engl J Med* 315:1095, 1986.
16. Koren G, Randor S, Martin S, et al: Maternal ginseng use associated with neonatal androgenization, *JAMA* 264:2866, 1990.
17. Koupparis LS: Harmless herbs: a cause for concern, *Anaesthesia* 55:101, 2000 (correspondence).
18. Linde K, Ramirez G, Mulrow CD, et al: St. John's wort for depression—an overview and meta-analysis of randomized clinical trials, *BMJ* 313:253, 1996.
19. Low Dog T: The use of botanicals during pregnancy and lactation, *Altern Ther Health Med* 15:54–58, 2009.
20. McRae S: Elevated serum digoxin levels in a patient taking digoxin and Siberian ginseng, *Can Med Assoc J* 155:293, 1996.
21. Mullins RJ: Echinacea-associated anaphylaxis, *Med J Aust* 168:170, 1998.
22. Patil SP, Niphadkap PV, Bapat MM: Allergy to fenugreek (*Trigonella foenum graecum*), *Ann Allergy Asthma Immunol* 78:297, 1997.
23. *Physicians desk reference for herbal medicines*, ed 2, Montvale, N.J., 2000, Medical Economics Co.
24. Ramsay HM, Goddard W, Gill S, et al: Herbal creams used for atopic eczema in Birmingham, UK illegally contain potent corticosteroids, *BMJ* 88:2056, 2003.
25. Rengers B, Foote J: Fenugreek: an aid to lactation? *Breastfeed Update* 5:3, 1997.
26. Ridker PM, McDermott WV: Hepatotoxicity due to comfrey herb tea, *Am J Med* 87:701, 1989.
27. Rotblatt M, Ziment I: *Evidence-based herbal medicine*, Philadelphia, Pa., 2002, Hanley and Belfus.
28. Roulet M, Laurini R, Rivier L, et al: Hepatic venoocclusive disease in newborn infant of a woman drinking herbal tea, *J Pediatr* 112:433, 1988.
29. Sewell AC, Mosandl A, Bohles H: False diagnosis of maple syrup urine disease owing to ingestion of herbal tea, *N Engl J Med* 341:769, 1999.
30. Skidmore-Roth L: Mosby's handbook of herbs and natural supplements. In Schaefer C, Peters P, Miller RK, editors: *Drugs during pregnancy and lactation*, ed 2, San Diego, Calif., 2007, Academic Press.
31. Stickel F, Poschl G, Seitz HK, et al: Acute hepatitis induced by greater celandine (*Chelidonium majus*), *Scand J Gastroenterol* 38:565, 2003.
32. U.S. Food and Drug Administration: *FDA advises dietary supplement manufacturers to remove comfrey products from the market*, Rockville, Md., 2001, U.S. Food and Drug Administration.
33. Weiner CP, Buhimschi C: *Drugs for pregnant and lactating women*, New York, 2004, Churchill Livingstone.

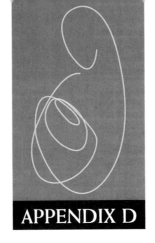

APPENDIX D

Precautions and Breastfeeding Recommendations for Selected Maternal Infections

TABLE D-1	Precautions and Breastfeeding Recommendations for Selected Maternal Infections*		
Organism, Syndrome, or Condition[+,‡]	**Empiric Precautions[§]**	**Breastfeeding Acceptable[¶]**	**Compatibility of Medications with Breastfeeding[‖]**
Adenoviruses			
Conjunctivitis	Contact		
Upper/lower respiratory infections	Droplet	Yes[#]	
Gastroenteritis	Standard		
Amebiasis			
Entamoeha histolytica			
Intestinal	Standard	Yes	Iodoquinol, paromomycin, metronidazole, tinidazole
Extraintestinal	Standard	Yes	
Anthrax			
Bacillus anthracis (cutaneous, inhalation, gastrointestinal)	Standard, add contact precautions for draining cutaneous lesions	Yes, if cutaneous lesion is not on the breast and can be covered	Ciprofloxacin
Arboviruses			
Arthropod-borne infections, meningoencephalitis, hemorrhagic fevers, hepatitis	Standard	Yes**	
California encephalitis	Standard	Yes	
Colorado tick fever	Standard	Yes	
Dengue fever	Standard	Yes	

TABLE D-1	Precautions and Breastfeeding Recommendations for Selected Maternal Infections—cont'd		
Organism, Syndrome, or Condition'	**Empiric Precautions**	**Breastfeeding Acceptable**	**Compatibility of Medications with Breastfeeding**
Eastern equine encephalitis	Standard	Yes	
Japanese encephalitis	Standard	Yes	
St. Louis encephalitis	Standard	Yes	
West Nile virus	Standard	Yes**	
Yellow fever	Standard	Yes	
Yellow fever vaccine virus	Standard	No**	
Arcanobacterium haemolyticus			
Pharyngitis, skin infections	Standard	Yes	Erythromycin, azithromycin clindamycin, cefuroxime, tetracycline
Ascaris lumbricoides			
Gastrointestinal infections, pneumonitis	Standard	Yes	Pyrantel pamoate, mebendazole, albendazole, piperazine
Aspergillosis			
Bronchopulmonary, sinus, or invasive infections	Standard	Yes	Amphotericin B, flucytosine, rifampin
Astroviruses			
Gastroenteritis	Standard, but contact for incontinent individuals	Yes	
Babesiosis			
Babesia microti			
Subacute/chronic febrile illness	Standard	Yes	Clindamycin+quinine, atovaquone +azithromycin
Blastocystis hominis			
Gastrointestinal infection	Standard	Yes	Metronidazole, nitazoxanide, trimethoprim-sulfamethoxazole (TMP-SMX)
Blastomycosis			
Blastomyces dermatitidis			
Pulmonary, cutaneous, or invasive infection	Standard	Yes	Amphotericin B, fluconazole, itraconazole
Borrelia			
Relapsing fever			
Borrelia hermsii	Standard (tick-borne)	Yes	Penicillin, erythromycin, tetracycline
Borrelia recurrentis	Contact (louse-borne)	Yes	
Borrelia turicatae	Standard (tick-borne)	Yes	Doxycycline
Botulism			
Clostridium botulinum			
Hypotonia, progressive weakness, toxin-mediated paralysis	Standard	Yes	

Continued

TABLE D-1   Precautions and Breastfeeding Recommendations for Selected Maternal Infections—cont'd

Organism, Syndrome, or Condition'	Empiric Precautions	Breastfeeding Acceptable	Compatibility of Medications with Breastfeeding
Breast abscess (see Mastitis)			
Staphylococcus aureus *Enterobacteriaceae* *Streptococcus pyogenes*	Contact (24 h)	Yes (after 24 h if no drainage into breast milk; discard breast milk for first 24 h after surgery)	First-generation cephalosporin, amoxicillin/ clavulanate, ampicillin/ sulbactam
Brucellosis			
Febrile illness with variable manifestations	Standard	Yes (after 48 h of therapy in mother; discard breast milk for 48 h)	Doxycycline, TMP-SMX, rifampin, gentamicin, streptomycin, tetracycline
Brucella abortus *Brucella melitensis* *Brucella suis*	Contact (for draining wounds)	Yes	
Calciviruses			
Gastroenteritis	Standard, but contact for incontinent individuals	Yes	
Campylobacter			
Gastrointestinal infection *Campylobacter fetus* *Campylobacter jejuni*	Standard, but contact for incontinent individuals	Yes	Erythromycin, azithromycin, ciprofloxacin
Candidiasis			
Mucocutaneous infection, vulvovaginitis, invasive infections *Candida albicans* *Candida krusei* *Candida tropicalis*	Standard	Yes (therapy for the infant simultaneous with mother's therapy)**	Topical agents, fluconazole, ketoconazole, itraconazole, amphotericin B, flucytosine
Cat-scratch disease			
Skin infection, regional lymphadenitis, and rarely, invasive infection *Bartonella henselae*	Standard	Yes	Azithromycin, TMP-SMX, rifampin, ciprofloxacin, gentamicin, doxycycline, erythromycin
Chlamydia			
Chlamydophila pneumonia	Standard	Yes	Tetracycline, doxycycline, erythromycin, azithromycin
Pharyngitis, pneumonia			
Chlamydophila psittaci Psittacosis, pneumonia, rarely invasive infection	Standard	Yes	Tetracycline, doxycycline, erythromycin, azithromycin,
Chlamydia trachomatis Urethritis, vaginitis, endometritis, salpingitis, lymphogranuloma venereum, conjunctivitis, pneumonia	Standard	Yes (consider treating the infant simultaneously)	Erythromycin, azithromycin, doxycycline, sulfonamide, levofloxacin, ofloxacin
Clostridia			
Clostridium botulinum			
Toxin-mediated paralysis	Standard	Yes	Antibiotic therapy not indicated

TABLE D-1 Precautions and Breastfeeding Recommendations for Selected Maternal Infections—cont'd

Organism, Syndrome, or Condition·	Empiric Precautions	Breastfeeding Acceptable	Compatibility of Medications with Breastfeeding
Clostridium difficile			
Antimicrobial-associated diarrhea, pseudomembranous colitis	Contact	Yes	Metronidazole, vancomycin, fidaxomicin
Clostridium perfringens			
Food poisoning, wound infection, gas gangrene, myonecrosis	Standard	Yes	
Coccidioides immitis			
Pulmonary, invasive infections rarely, extrapulmonary	Standard, but contact for draining lesions	Yes	Amphotericin B, fluconazole, itraconazole
Conjunctivitis			
Adenovirus	Contact	Yes	
Chlamydia trachomatis	Standard	Yes	Tetracycline, doxycycline, erythromycin
Neisseria gonorrhoeae	Standard	Yes[††]	Penicillin, ceftriaxone
Cryptococcus neoformans			
Meningitis, pneumonia	Standard	Yes	Amphotericin B, flucytosine, fluconazole
Cryptosporidiosis			
Cryptosporidium parvum			
Diarrhea	Contact	Yes	Nitazoxanide, paromomycin, azithromycin
Cytomegalovirus (CMV)			
Asymptomatic infection	Standard	Yes (for full-term infants)	
Infectious mononucleosis	Standard	No (for premature or immunodeficient infants, do not give expressed breast milk)**	
Dengue fever			
Acute febrile illness, hemorrhagic fever	Standard	Yes	
Diphtheria			
Corynebacterium diphtheriae			
Membranous nasopharyngitis	Droplet (DI)	Yes (with infant receiving chemoprophylaxis-P)	Erythromycin, penicillin
Obstructive laryngotracheitis	Droplet (DI)		
Cutaneous infection, toxin-mediated myocarditis, or neurologic disease	Contact (cover lesions)	No (only if skin lesion involves breast)	
Diarrhea			
Campylobacter fetus	Standard	Yes	Azithromycin
Campylobacter jejuni	Standard + Contact for infants	Yes	Erythromycin, ciprofloxacin
Escherichia coli (O157:H7)	Contact	Yes	None indicated
Giardia lamblia	Standard	Yes	Metronidazole, tinidazole, nitazoxanide
Rotavirus	Contact	Yes	
Salmonella enteritidis	Standard	Yes	

Continued

TABLE D-1   Precautions and Breastfeeding Recommendations for Selected Maternal Infections—cont'd

Organism, Syndrome, or Condition'	Empiric Precautions	Breastfeeding Acceptable	Compatibility of Medications with Breastfeeding
Shigella boydii	Contact	Yes	Ciprofloxacin, ceftriaxone, TMP-SMX
Shigella dysenteriae	Contact	Yes	Ciprofloxacin, ceftriaxone, TMP-SMX
Shigella flexneri	Contact	Yes	Ciprofloxacin, ceftriaxone, TMP-SMX
Shigella sonnei	Contact	Yes	Ciprofloxacin, ceftriaxone, TMP-SMX
Vibrio cholerae	Standard	Yes	Doxycycline, azithromycin, tetracycline, ciprofloxacin, furazolidone
Vibrio parahaemolyticus	Standard	Yes	None
Yersinia enterocolitica	Standard + Contact for incontinent persons	Yes	For sepsis or invasive disease— ciprofloxacin, norfloxacin, ceftriaxone, TMP-SMX, doxycycline
Yersinia pseudotuberculosis	Standard	Yes	
Ebola virus	Contact, droplet, and airborne	No (do not give expressed breast milk)	
Encephalitis			
Enteroviruses	Standard	Yes	
Lyme disease (*Borrelia burgdorferi*)	Standard	Yes	Ceftriaxone, doxycycline, amoxicillin
Rabies	Standard	No (BM+)	Rabies immune globulin, rabies vaccine
Endometritis, pelvic inflammatory disease			
Anaerobic organisms	Standard	Yes	Clindamycin, metronidazole, cefoxitin, cefmetazole
Chlamydia trachomatis	Standard	Yes	Erythromycin, azithromycin, tetracycline, levofloxacin
Enterobacteriaceae	Standard	Yes	Ampicillin, aminoglycosides, cephalosporins
Group B streptococci	Standard	Yes** (after 24 h of therapy for mother, breast milk is permissible with observation of infant) No** (if infant is sick with suspected or proven group B streptococcal infection and the breast milk is being cultured to identify a source of infection; permissible if breast milk is culture negative)	Penicillin, cephalosporin, macrolides

TABLE D-1	Precautions and Breastfeeding Recommendations for Selected Maternal Infections—cont'd		
Organism, Syndrome, or Condition	**Empiric Precautions**	**Breastfeeding Acceptable**	**Compatibility of Medications with Breastfeeding**
Mycoplasma hominis	Standard	Yes	Clindamycin, tetracycline
Neisseria gonorrhoeae	Standard	Yes[++]	Ceftriaxone, spectinomycin, doxycycline, azithromycin
Ureaplasma urealyticum	Standard	Yes	Erythromycin, azithromycin, clarithromycin, tetracycline
Enteroviruses			
Myocarditis: respiratory, gastrointestinal, skin, central nervous system, and eye infections	Adults: standard Children: contact		
Coxsackievirus		Yes	
Echovirus		Yes	
Polioviruses		Yes	
Epstein-Barr virus			
Infectious mononucleosis, broad range of infections	Standard	Yes	
Erythema infectiosum			
Parvovirus B19	Standard	Yes (no infectious risk after the appearance of the rash in immune-competent individuals)	
Food poisoning			
Bacillus cereus			
Toxin mediated	Standard	Yes	
Clostridium perfringens			
Toxin mediated	Standard	Yes	
Escherichia coli (O157:H7) Enterohemorrhagic	Contact	Yes	
Hepatitis A	Standard	Yes (immune serum globulin and hepatitis A vaccine for the infant)	
Norwalk virus	Standard	Yes	
Salmonella enteritidis	Standard	Yes	
Shigella	Contact	Yes	Ciprofloxacin, TMP-SMX
Staphylococcus aureus			
Enterotoxin	Standard	Yes	
Gastroenteritis (see Diarrhea or Food Poisoning)			
Giardiasis			
Giardia lamblia	Standard, no contact with incontinent individuals	Yes	Metronidazole, tinidazole, nitazoxanide
Gonorrhea			
Genital, pharyngeal, conjunctival, or disseminated infection			
Neisseria gonorrhoeae	Standard	Yes[++]	Ceftriaxone, azithromycin, erythromycin, doxycycline

Continued

TABLE D-1   Precautions and Breastfeeding Recommendations for Selected Maternal Infections—cont'd

Organism, Syndrome, or Condition'	Empiric Precautions	Breastfeeding Acceptable	Compatibility of Medications with Breastfeeding
Haemophilus influenzae			
Meningitis, epiglottitis, pneumonia, cellulitis, sinusitis, bacteremia	Droplet	Yes (24 h after initiating therapy in mother; breast milk[†]; *P*** if infant has not been fully immunized, observation)	Cefotaxime, ceftriaxone, ampicillin
Hantavirus			
Pulmonary syndrome, hemorrhagic fever with renal syndrome	Standard	Yes	Intravenous ribavirin is investigational
Hemorrhagic fevers			
African hemorrhagic fever			
Ebola virus	Contact	No (no expressed breast milk)	
Marburg virus	Contact	No (no expressed breast milk)	
Dengue virus (1–4)	Standard	Yes (breast milk +)	
Hantavirus	Standard	Yes (breast milk +)	
Lassa fever	Contact	No (no expressed breast milk)	Intravenous ribavirin?
Yellow fever	Standard	Yes** (breast milk +)	Vaccine
Yellow fever vaccine virus immunization in mother**	Standard	No**	
Hepatitis**			
A Acute only	Standard, but contact for incontinent individuals	Yes (after immune serum globulin [ISG] and vaccine)	
B Chronic hepatitis, cirrhosis, hepatocellular carcinoma	Standard	Yes (after hepatitis B immunoglobulin [HBIG] and vaccine)	
C Chronic hepatitis, cirrhosis, hepatocellular carcinoma	Standard	Yes	
D Associated with hepatitis B	Standard	Yes (after HBIG and vaccine)	
E Severe disease in pregnant women	Standard	Yes	
G	Standard	Inadequate data	
Herpesviruses			
Cytomegalovirus (CMV)	Standard	Yes for full-term infants	Ganciclovir, valganciclovir, foscarnet
Asymptomatic, infectious mononucleosis-like syndrome: severe disease in the immunodeficient person		No for premature or immunodeficient infants (infant of CMV-negative mother should not receive milk from CMV-positive mothers)	
Epstein-Barr virus			
Asymptomatic, infectious mononucleosis, associated with chronic fatigue syndrome, African Burkitt lymphoma, and nasopharyngeal carcinoma	Standard	Yes	
Herpes simplex			
Types 1, 2 (HSV$_{1,2}$)			
Mucocutaneous	Contact	Yes (in the absence of breast lesions)	Acyclovir, valacyclovir, famciclovir
Neonatal	Contact		
Encephalitis	Standard		

TABLE D-1	Precautions and Breastfeeding Recommendations for Selected Maternal Infections—cont'd		
Organism, Syndrome, or Condition'	**Empiric Precautions**	**Breastfeeding Acceptable**	**Compatibility of Medications with Breastfeeding**
Varicella-zoster virus**			
Varicella	Airborne	No (Breast milk+is permissible in absence of lesions on the breast). Give VariZIG for the exposed infant.	Acyclovir, valacyclovir, famciclovir
Zoster	Standard in normal patient		
	Airborne/contact in immunocom-promised individuals	No, VariZIG for the exposed infant, especially less than 1 month of age**	
Human herpesvirus 6 (HHV-6)			
Roseola (exanthema subitum, sixth disease), acute febrile illness	Standard	Yes	
Histoplasmosis			
Acute pulmonary disease, disseminated	Standard	Yes	Amphotericin B, itraconazole, fluconazole
Human immunodeficiency viruses (HIV)**			
HIV-1	Standard	Yes/no**	Limited information on antiretrovirals in breast milk** Antiretroviral medications for the mother and/or infant through period of lactation
HIV-2	Standard	Yes/no**	
Human T-cell leukemia viruses (HTLV)			
HTLV-1			
T-cell leukemia/lymphoma, myelopathy, dermatitis, adenitis, Sjögren's syndrome	Standard	No**	
HTLV-II			
Myelopathy, arthritis, glomerulonephritis	Standard	No**	
Impetigo	Contact	Yes	Oxacillin, dicloxacillin, erythromycin, first-generation cephalosporins
Infectious mononucleosis (see CMV, EBV)			
Influenza	Droplet	Yes	Osetamavir, zanamivire, amantadine, rimantadine
Junin virus			
Argentine hemorrhagic fever	Contact	No (do not give expressed breast milk)	
Lassa fever	Contact	No (do not give expressed breast milk)	Intravenous ribavirin
Legionnaires' disease			
Legionella pneumophila	Standard	Yes	Azithromycin, erythromycin, levofloxacin

Continued

| TABLE D-1 | Precautions and Breastfeeding Recommendations for Selected Maternal Infections—cont'd |

Organism, Syndrome, or Condition'	Empiric Precautions	Breastfeeding Acceptable	Compatibility of Medications with Breastfeeding
Pneumonia ± gastrointestinal, central nervous system, or renal involvement			
Leprosy			
Mycobacterium leprae	Standard	Yes	Dapsone, rifampin, clofazimine
Chronic disease of skin, peripheral nerves, and respiratory mucosa			
Leptospirosis			
Abrupt febrile illness, often biphasic, with multiple organ involvement			
Leptospira interrogans	Standard	Yes (no mother-infant contact except for breastfeeding)	Penicillin, cefotaxime, ceftriaxone
Leptospira icterohaemorrhagiae			
Leptospira canicola			
Listeria monocytogenes			
In adults: Nonspecific febrile illness; in neonates: meningitis, pneumonia, sepsis, granulomatosis infantisepticum	Standard	Yes	Ampicillin, penicillin, TMP-SMX
Lyme disease			
Borrelia burgdorferi			
Multistaged illness of skin, joint, and peripheral or central nervous system	Standard	Yes, with informed discussion**	Ceftriaxone, ampicillin, doxycycline
Lymphocytic choriomeningitis			
Aseptic meningitis to severe encephalitis, with variable presentation of other symptoms	Standard	Yes	
Malaria	Standard	Yes	Pyrimethamine-sulfadoxine, chloroquine, quinidine, quinine, tetracycline, mefloquine
Marburg virus			
Hemorrhagic fever	Contact	No (no expressed breast milk)	
Mastitis			
Candida albicans	Standard	Yes, with simultaneous treatment of the infant**	Nystatin, ketoconazole, fluconazole
Enterobacteriaceae	Standard	Yes	First-generation cephalosporin,
Staphylococcus aureus	Contact	Yes** (after 24 h of therapy, during which milk must be discarded) (If infant becomes ill during evaluation and treatment of mother, infant should be treated for presumed staphylococcal infection, and breast milk should be withheld until proven to be culture negative.)	Dicloxacillin, oxacillin, erythromycin

TABLE D-1   Precautions and Breastfeeding Recommendations for Selected Maternal Infections—cont'd

Organism, Syndrome, or Condition	Empiric Precautions	Breastfeeding Acceptable	Compatibility of Medications with Breastfeeding
Group A streptococcus	Contact	Yes** (after 24 h of therapy, during which milk must be discarded) (If infant becomes ill during evaluation and treatment of mother, infant should be treated for presumed streptococcal infection, and breast milk should be withheld until proven to be culturally negative.)	Ampicillin, third-generation cephalosporin
Mycobacterium tuberculosis	Standard (if mother has pulmonary involvement, then airborne precautions as well)	No** (breastfeeding for 2 weeks of maternal therapy, consider prophylactic INH for infant [see Figures 16-1 and 16-2], breast milk permissible with INH)	Isoniazid, rifampin, ethambutol, pyrazinamide ethionamide
Measles			
Febrile illness with coryza, conjunctivitis, cough, and an erythematous maculopapular rash	Airborne	Yes (after 72 h of rash in mother and after infant receives ISG, expressed breast milk is permissible)	Ribavirin is experimental
Meningitis			
Aseptic meningitis (nonbacterial, viral meningitis)	Standard	Yes	
Fungal meningitis	Standard	Yes	Amphotericin, itraconazole, flucytosine
Haemophilus influenzae	Droplet (for first 24 h of appropriate therapy and carrier eradication with ceftriaxone or rifampin)	Yes (after 24 h of maternal therapy, with the infant receiving prophylaxis, P; begin infant vaccination; expressed breast milk is permissible)	Ceftriaxone, ampicillin, chloramphenicol, rifampin
Neisseria meningitidis	Droplet (24 h of appropriate therapy and carrier eradication with ceftriaxone or rifampin)	Yes (after 24 h of maternal therapy, with the infant receiving prophylaxis, P; expressed breast milk is permissible)	Ceftriaxone, penicillin, chloramphenicol
Streptococcal pneumoniae	Standard	Yes	Ceftriaxone, penicillin, vancomycin
Mumps	Droplet	Yes	
*Mycobacterium tuberculosis***	Standard and airborne	Yes	Antituberculosis medications are acceptable during breastfeeding (see Chapter 13, section on Tuberculosis and ** *Red Book*, 30th Edition)
Mycoplasma pneumoniae			
Bronchitis, pneumonia, pharyngitis, otitis media, and a broad range of unusual manifestations, including central nervous system, cardiac, skin, muscle, and joint involvement	Droplet	Yes	Erythromycin, clarithromycin, azithromycin, tetracycline

Continued

TABLE D-1 Precautions and Breastfeeding Recommendations for Selected Maternal Infections—cont'd

Organism, Syndrome, or Condition	Empiric Precautions	Breastfeeding Acceptable	Compatibility of Medications with Breastfeeding
Neisseria meningitidis			
Meningitis, meningococcemia	Droplet (for 24 h of appropriate therapy and carrier eradication with ceftriaxone or rifampin)	Yes (after 24 h of appropriate therapy, and with prophylaxis for the infant)	Penicillin, ceftriaxone, chloramphenicol, rifampin
Norwalk agent			
Gastroenteritis	Standard	Yes	
Papillomaviruses			
Skin or mucous membrane warts, laryngeal papillomas	Standard	Yes (in the absence of breast involvement)	
Parainfluenza viruses			
Laryngotracheobronchitis, upper and lower respiratory infections	Standard (contact for infants and children)	Yes	
Parvovirus B19			
Erythema infectiosum, fifth disease, aplastic crisis, arthritis	Standard Droplet for mothers with aplastic crisis or immunodeficient and prolonged illness	Yes (no infectious risk after the appearance of the rash in immune-competent individuals) No (for aplastic crisis or infection in individuals with hemoglobinopathy or immune deficiency infection for the duration of the illness [DI])§	
Pelvic inflammatory disease (see Endometritis)			
Pertussis			
Whooping cough, pneumonia, bronchitis, encephalitis			
Bordetella parapertussis and *Bordetella pertussis*	Droplet (for 5 days of appropriate therapy)	Yes (after 5 days of appropriate therapy and chemoprophylaxis for the infant, expressed breast milk is permissible) If no appropriate Rx is given then 3 weeks of droplet precautions	Erythromycin, clarithromycin, TMP-SMX
Pneumocystis jiroveci pneumonia (previously *Pneumocystis carinii* pneumonitis)	Standard	Yes, but suspect HIV infection if mother develops symptoms and reassess breastfeeding with HIV infection in mind	Pentamidine, TMP-SMX, atovaquone, prednisone
Pneumonia (see specific causative agents)			
Poliomyelitis	Standard	Yes	
Rabies			
Severe, progressive central nervous system infection, generally fatal	Standard	No** (when mother is clinically sick) Yes** (BM+) (during postexposure immunization of mother without symptoms; yes if both mother and infant are receiving postexposure immunization)	Rabies immune globulin, rabies vaccine
Rat-bite fever			
Spirillum minus	Standard	Yes	Tetracycline, chloramphenicol, streptomycin
Streptobacillus moniliformis	Standard	Yes	Penicillin

TABLE D-1	Precautions and Breastfeeding Recommendations for Selected Maternal Infections—cont'd		
Organism, Syndrome, or Condition	**Empiric Precautions**	**Breastfeeding Acceptable**	**Compatibility of Medications with Breastfeeding**
Relapsing fever			
Borrelia recurrentis	Standard (tick-borne)	Yes	Tetracycline, doxycycline, TMP-SMX, streptomycin, rifampin
	Contact if louse infested	Yes with simultaneous treatment of mother and infant for lice	
Respiratory syncytial virus			
Upper respiratory infection, pneumonia, bronchiolitis	Contact	Yes	Ribavirin
Retroviruses			
(see Human immunodeficiency viruses 1, 2 and Human T-cell leukemia viruses I, II)			
Rickettsial diseases			
Fever, rash, vasculitis; arthropod, louse-borne			
Ehrlichiosis, leukopenia	Standard	Yes	Doxycycline, tetracycline
Ehrlichia chaffeensis			
Q fever			
Coxiella burnetii			
Pneumonia, hepatosplenomegaly, endocarditis	Standard	Yes	Doxycycline, tetracycline, TMP-SMX
Rickettsial pox			
Rickettsia akari			
Scab or eschar, rash, regional lymphadenopathy, self-limited	Standard	Yes	Doxycycline, tetracycline, fluoroquinolones
Rocky Mountain spotted fever			
Rickettsia rickettsii	Standard	Yes	Doxycycline
Typhus (flea-borne)			
Rickettsia typhi	Standard	Yes	Doxycycline, fluoroquinolones
Typhus (louse-borne)			
Rickettsia prowazekii	Standard	Yes	Doxycycline (in epidemic situations a single dose may be adequate), chloramphenicol
Rotavirus			
Diarrhea, vomiting, "winter vomiting disease"	Contact	Yes	
Rubella virus			
Self-limited, mild exanthem with fever: congenital rubella syndrome	Contact	Yes	
Salmonella (see Diarrhea/gastroenteritis)			
SARS-associated coronavirus, severe acute respiratory syndrome	Droplet	Yes	

Continued

TABLE D-1   Precautions and Breastfeeding Recommendations for Selected Maternal Infections—cont'd

Organism, Syndrome, or Condition[*]	Empiric Precautions	Breastfeeding Acceptable	Compatibility of Medications with Breastfeeding
Shigella (see Diarrhea)			
Smallpox			
Variola virus (variola major)	Contact, airborne	No (no expressed breast milk)	
Vaccinia virus (smallpox vaccine) secondary contact infection	Contact	Yes, except if breast involved with lesions	
Staphylococcus aureus			
Cellulitis, abscess	Contact	Yes	Oxacillin, dicloxacillin, first-generation cephalosporins, erythromycin, vancomycin
Enterocolitis, diarrhea	Standard	Yes	
Scalded-skin syndrome	Contact	Yes (after 24 h of effective therapy; discard breast milk for 24 h)	
Toxic shock syndrome	Standard	Yes**	
Methicillin-resistant *S. aureus* (MRSA)	Contact	Yes** (after 24 h of therapy, during which milk must be discarded) (If infant becomes ill during evaluation and treatment of mother, infant should be treated for presumed MRSA infection, and breast milk should be withheld until proven to be culture negative.)	Vancomycin, TMP-SMX, clindamycin, linezolid
Staphylococcus epidermidis			
Opportunistic infections	Standard	Yes	Oxacillin, dicloxacillin, vancomycin
Streptococcus			
Group A: Cellulitis, pharyngitis, pneumonia, myositis/fasciitis, scarlet fever	Standard	Yes (24 h after beginning appropriate therapy; discard breast milk for 24 h)	Penicillin, erythromycin, cephalosporin
	Contact (for extensive skin infection unable to be covered until after 24 h of therapy)	Yes (24 h after beginning appropriate therapy; discard breast milk for 24 h)	
Group B: Urinary tract infection, endometritis, mastitis; infants: sepsis, pneumonia, meningitis, osteomyelitis, arthritis	Standard	Yes** (after 24 h of therapy, during which milk must be discarded) (If infant becomes ill during evaluation and treatment of mother, infant should be treated for presumed Streptococcal infection, and breast milk should be withheld until proven to be culture negative.)	Penicillin, ampicillin, third-generation cephalosporin
Streptococcus pneumoniae			
Pneumonia, occult bacteremia, otitis media, sinusitis	Standard	Yes	Penicillin, ceftriaxone, vancomycin, cefotaxime, rifampin

TABLE D-1 Precautions and Breastfeeding Recommendations for Selected Maternal Infections—cont'd

Organism, Syndrome, or Condition	Empiric Precautions	Breastfeeding Acceptable	Compatibility of Medications with Breastfeeding
Syphilis			
Treponema pallidum			
Multisystem, multistage infection with widely varying presentations, congenital infection	Standard	Yes (after 24 h of effective therapy; discard breast milk for 24 h)	Penicillin, doxycycline, tetracycline
Open skin lesions of breast or nipples	Contact	No, until 24 h of effective therapy in mother if open skin lesions involve breasts	Penicillin, doxycycline, tetracycline
Tetanus			
Exotoxin-mediated severe muscular spasms *Clostridium tetani*	Standard	Yes (age-appropriate vaccination of the child, no tetanus immunoglobulin [TIG] necessary for infant)	Penicillin, metronidazole
Tinea capitis			
Microsporum audouinii	Standard	Yes	Griseofulvin, terbinafine, selenium sulfide shampoo, prednisone
Microsporum canis			
Trichophyton tonsurans			
Tinea corporis, cruris, pedis			
Epidermophyton floccosum	Standard	Yes	Topical agents
Trichophyton canis			
Trichophyton rubrum			
Tinea versicolor			
Malassezia furfur	Standard	Yes	Topical agents, ketoconazole, itraconazole
Toxoplasmosis			
Toxoplasma gondii	Standard	Yes	Pyrimethamine, sulfadiazine, TMP-SMX, dapsone, atovaquone, clindamycin
Asymptomatic or mononucleosis-like illness with lymphadenopathy, ocular symptoms; congenital infection			
Toxic shock			
(see *S. aureus, Streptococcus* [group A])			
Toxin-mediated illness (see specific agents)			
Bacillus cereus			
Botulism			
Food poisoning			
Staphylococcal scalded-skin syndrome (SSSS)			
Trichinosis			
Trichinella spiralis			
Asymptomatic, or may cause myalgia, periorbital edema, myocardial failure, CNS involvement, or pneumonitis	Standard	Yes	Albendazole, mebendazole, thiabendazole, prednisone

Continued

TABLE D-1   Precautions and Breastfeeding Recommendations for Selected Maternal Infections—cont'd

Organism, Syndrome, or Condition¹	Empiric Precautions	Breastfeeding Acceptable	Compatibility of Medications with Breastfeeding
Trichomonas vaginalis			
Vaginitis, urethritis, or asymptomatic infections	Standard	Yes	Metronidazole, tinidazole
Trypanosomiasis			
Trypanosoma brucei			
"Sleeping sickness"; tsetse fly vector (African)	Standard	No	Suramin, pentamidine, eflornithine, melarsoprol
Trypanosoma cruzi			
Chagas disease (American)	Standard	Yes	Nifurtimox, benznidazole
TT virus			
Hepatitis	Standard	Yes	
Tuberculosis (see *mycobacterium* in this Appendix; see Chapter 13, Figures 13-2 and 13-3 and Table 13-1; see ** *Red Book*, 30th Edition)			
Tularemia			
Francisella tularensis			
Acute febrile illness with various syndromes; oculoglandular, ulceroglandular, glandular, oropharyngeal, typhoidal, pneumoniae	Standard	Yes	Streptomycin, gentamicin doxycycline, ciprofloxacin
Ureaplasma urealyticum			
Nongonococcal urethritis (NGU), endometritis, pelvic inflammatory disease	Standard	Yes	Doxycycline, erythromycin, azithromycin, clarithromycin, ciprofloxacin
Urinary tract infection			
Group B streptococcus (see *Streptococcus* [group B])	Standard	Yes	Ampicillin, aminoglycosides, cephalosporin
Enterobacteriaceal	Standard	Yes	Ampicillin, cephalosporins, fluoroquinolones
Staphylococcus saprophyticus	Standard	Yes	Vancomycin, clindamycin +rifampin
Vaginitis			
Bacterial	Standard	Yes	Metronidazole, clindamycin
Candida albicans (see Candidiasis)			
Varicella-zoster virus (see Herpesviruses)			
West Nile virus	Standard	Yes**	
Asymptomatic, fever, meningoencephalitis			
Whooping cough			
Bordetella parapertussis and *Bordetella pertussis*: see also Adenovirus, *Chlamydia* (*Chlamydia pneumoniae*, *Chlamydia trachomatis*), *Mycoplasma pneumoniae* as other agents may mimic the clinical picture of whooping cough	Droplet (for 5 days of appropriate therapy and chemoprophylaxis for infant)	Yes, after 5 days of appropriate therapy, breast milk+, P**	Erythromycin, clarithromycin, TMP-SMX

TABLE D-1	Precautions and Breastfeeding Recommendations for Selected Maternal Infections—cont'd		
Organism, Syndrome, or Condition·	Empiric Precautions	Breastfeeding Acceptable·	Compatibility of Medications with Breastfeeding
Yellow fever			
Yellow fever virus	Standard	Yes**	
Yellow fever vaccine virus	Standard	No**	Avoid yellow fever vaccine virus immunization during lactation if possible**
Yersinia enterocolitica			
Diarrhea, pseudoappendicitis, focal infections, and bacteremia	Contact precautions for incontinent individuals	Yes	Cefotaxime, aminoglycosides, TMP-SMX, fluoroquinolones
Yersinia pseudotuberculosis			
Fever, rash, abdominal symptoms	Standard	Yes	TMP-SMX

*To ensure that appropriate empiric precautions are always implemented, hospitals must have systems in place to routinely evaluate patients according to these criteria as part of their preadmission and admission care.

†Patients with the syndromes or conditions listed may present with atypical signs and symptoms (e.g., pertussis in neonates and adults may not have paroxysmal or severe cough). A clinician's index of suspicion should be guided by the prevalence of specific conditions in the community as well as clinical judgment.

‡The organisms listed are not intended to represent the complete, or even most likely diagnoses, but rather possible etiologic agents that may require additional precautions, beyond *standard precautions*, until they can be excluded.

§These are the usual precautions (Standard. Airborne, Contact, and Droplet) outlined in the text, as proposed by the Centers for Disease Control and Prevention. Symbols for duration of precautions: *24 hours,* 24 hours of antibiotic therapy; *CN,* until off antibiotics and culture negative; *DI,* duration of the illness; *PI,* period of infectivity.

◆*Yes* means that if, in a hospitalized mother and infant, the proposed precautions are followed, breastfeeding is acceptable and may be beneficial to the infant. Any infant breastfeeding during a maternal infection should be observed closely for signs or symptoms of illness.

‖See Chapter 12 on medications in breast milk, in this book, and refer to LactMed at http://toxnet.nlm.nih.gov/newtoxnet/lactmed.htm.

#Adenovirus types 4 and 7 have been known to cause severe respiratory disease in premature infants or individuals with immunodeficiency or underlying respiratory disease. In certain situations, feeding of expressed breast milk to an infant may not be advisable.

**See text for more complete explanation. *P,* Prophylactic antibiotics for the infant. See the 2015 Report of the Committee on Infectious Diseases, *Red Book,* 30th edition, for current recommendations on the specific antibiotics for the specific condition.

††Breastfeed immediately if mother receives ceftriaxone intramuscularly or intravenously. Breastfeed after 24-hour antibiotic therapy for other treatment regiments, with feeding expressed breast milk for the first 24 hours.

Modified from Garner JS: Hospital Infection Control Practices Advisory Committee guidelines for isolation precautions in hospitals, *Infect Control Hosp Epidemiol* 17:53, 1996.

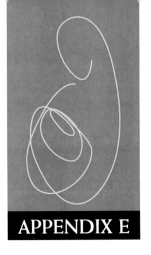

Manual Expression of Breast Milk

A health care professional should be familiar with the technique of manual expression and be able to diagnose improper technique.

Technique

All breastfeeding women should be familiar with the basic technique of manual expression of milk from the breast, and ideally this technique is acquired before discharge from the hospital and with the assistance of the nursery or postpartum nursing staff.

Reasons to express breast milk include the following:

1. To initiate flow and assist an infant to grasp the breast properly
2. To encourage production of milk early in lactation when an infant is premature or ill
3. To relieve engorgement
4. To remove milk when it is not possible to nurse an infant at a given feeding
5. To maintain lactation when an infant cannot be fed
6. To pump and save milk for feeding an infant at another time
7. To contribute to a milk bank
8. To pump and discard milk while temporarily on a specific medication

Manual expression is appropriate to initiate flow before applying a hand pump or an electric pump. Not many women can manually pump large volumes over time without mechanical assistance.

The breast should always be massaged, and flow initiated, before applying any pump.

Procedure

Step 1. Always wash hands before handling a breast.

Step 2. Breast massage: Whether planning to manually express or mechanically pump, preparing the breast for ejecting the milk facilitates the process. The release of oxytocin and the ejection reflex are stimulated by external stimuli: a baby's cry, a picture of the baby, or gentle handling of the breast. Prolactin release and milk production are stimulated by "sucking" stimulation.

After the mother finds a comfortable sitting position and is relaxed, the breast is exposed and gently stroked with the fingertips from periphery to areola (Figure E-1). As this stroking is intensified, one should avoid slipping the hand across skin and irritating tissues. Gently massage. A warm washcloth soak is also helpful in initiating flow through the ducts. Gentle fingertip massage around all quadrants should follow and be repeated several times during extended mechanical pumping. It should not leave red marks or hurt.

Step 3. Position hands on the breast: Usually placing the fingers below and thumb on top is natural for most women. One hand placed above and one hand placed below the areola may be easier when the hand is small compared with breast size. The target area is beyond the ampullae, which are the collecting areas of the main ducts that radiate out from the nipple to the areola.

The ampullae are approximately 3 cm from the nipple base, which may not be at the edge of the areola. Press toward the chest wall, and then compress the thumb and fingers together (Figure E-2). Continue to compress the breast while moving the hand away from the chest wall in a "milking" action toward the nipple (Figure E-3). (Avoid pulling, squeezing, or rubbing motions.) Perform this motion in a repeated rhythmic manner at a comfortable, but not abrasive, rate. Infant suckling does not involve movement (stroking) of the tongue along the elongated areola and nipple, but an undulating motion of the tongue itself. Simulating that motion is the goal of manual expression. This action is similar to a peristaltic motion. The hand should be rotated around the breast to massage and stroke all quadrants, including the periphery and the axillae.

Use one or both hands to find the most productive grasp. Preventing trauma is essential; thus, avoid squeezing, rubbing, or pulling the breast tissue. Every mother develops her own natural pattern, so rigid adherence to methods may be counterproductive. Effectiveness is measured by the comfortable release of milk.

Total emptying of the breast will require 20 to 30 minutes of manual stimulation. Warm compresses, hot showers, or suspending the breast in a bowl of warm water may help, especially if engorgement or mastitis is present. Leaning over and gently shaking the breast may help stimulate flow. Manual expression while leaning over may help empty the lower quadrants.

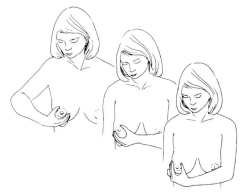

Figure E-1

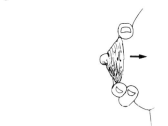

Figure E-2

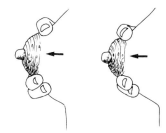

Figure E-3

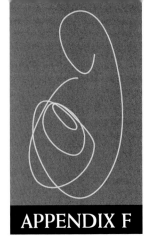

The Storage of Human Milk

Academy of Breastfeeding Medicine's Human Milk Storage Information for Home Use for Healthy Full-Term Infants

Please see Appendix J-8, Table F-1, and Box F-1 for guidelines on milk storage and thawing.

Human Milk Banking and the HMBANA

The Human Milk Banking Association of North America (HMBANA) was established in 1985, drawing together representatives of donor milk banks and members of the medical community. The goals of HMBANA are as follows:

1. Provide a forum for networking among experts in the field on issues relating to human milk banking;
2. Provide information to the medical community on the benefits and appropriate uses of banked human milk;
3. Develop and annually review guidelines for milk banking practices in North America;
4. Communicate among member milk banks to ensure adequate supplies for all patients;
5. Encourage research into the unique properties of human milk and its uses;
6. Act as a liaison between member institutions and governmental regulatory agencies;
7. Ensure quality control of donor human milk banking among member banks through adherence to the mandatory guidelines and periodic inspection of member banks.

WHAT IS A HUMAN MILK BANK?

A donor human milk bank is a service established for the purpose of collecting, screening, processing, storing, and distributing donated human milk to meet the specific medical needs of individuals for whom human milk is prescribed by physicians. A small processing fee is charged by each milk bank on a per-ounce basis.

HOW DOES A HUMAN MILK BANK OPERATE?

Donor human milk banks solicit lactating mothers to donate milk. Donors are carefully screened for health behaviors and tested for communicable diseases before they are accepted as donors.

Donors are taught how to express their milk using sanitary collecting methods.

Donated milk is heat treated to destroy any bacteria or viruses that may be present.

Frozen, heat-treated milk is dispensed to recipients with a medical need for donor milk. A physician's prescription is required.

Frequent Reasons for Prescribing Donor Milk

NUTRITIONAL USES

Prematurity
Failure to thrive
Malabsorption syndromes
Short-gut syndrome
Renal failure
Feeding intolerance
Inborn errors of metabolism
Postsurgical nutrition

TABLE F-1	Storage of Human Milk for Home Use		
Breast Milk	**Room Temperature**	**Refrigerator**	**Freezer**
Freshly expressed into closed container	6-8 h (78°F or lower)	3-5 days (39°F or lower)	2 weeks in freezer compartment inside refrigerator 3 to 6 months in freezer section of refrigerator with separate door; 6-12 months in deep freeze (0°F or lower)
Previously frozen Thawed in refrigerator but not warmed or used	4 h or less (i.e., next feeding)	Store in refrigerator 24 h	Do not refreeze
Thawed outside refrigerator in warm water	For completion of feeding	Hold for 4 h or until next feeding	Do not refreeze
Infant has begun feeding	Only for completion of feeding; then discard	Discard	Discard

Developed from recommendations of the Human Milk Banking Association of North America and current literature. See References, Chapter 21.

BOX F-1. Suggestions for Milk Storage for Infant at Home

- Wash hands thoroughly.
- Polyethylene bags are acceptable for home use.
- Refrigerate or freeze milk after expressing.
- Use fresh milk whenever possible.
- Freeze milk that will not be used within 2 days.
- Use milk stored in a self-defrosting freezer within 3 months (top of refrigerator).
- Use milk stored in a deep freezer within 12 months.
- Use the oldest milk first. Date container at time of collection.

Cardiac problems
Bronchopulmonary dysplasia
Pediatric burn cases

MEDICINAL/THERAPEUTIC USES

Treatment for infectious diseases, such as intractable diarrhea, gastroenteritis, infantile botulism, sepsis, pneumonia, and hemorrhagic conjunctivitis
Postsurgical healing (omphalocele, gastroschisis, intestinal obstruction/bowel fistula, colostomy repair)
Immunodeficiency diseases (severe allergies, IgA deficiencies)
Inborn errors of metabolism
Solid-organ transplants (including use for adults)
Noninfectious intestinal disorders (ulcerative colitis, irritable bowel syndrome)

PREVENTIVE USES

Necrotizing enterocolitis
Crohn disease
Colitis

Allergies to bovine and soy milks/feeding intolerance
During immune suppression therapy

Donor Milk Banks in the United States, Canada, and Mexico

Human Milk Banking Association of North America
1500 Sunday Drive, Suite 102
Raleigh, NC 27607
Phone: 919-787-5181
Website: http://www.hmbana.org

Mothers' Milk Bank
751 South Bascom
P.O. Box 5730
San Jose, CA 95150
Phone: 408-998-4550
E-mail: mothersmilkbank@hhs.co.santaclara.ca.us

Triangle Mothers' Milk Bank
Wake Medical Center
3000 New Bern Avenue
Raleigh, NC 27610
Phone: 919-350-8599
E-mail: mmould@wakemed.org or abuckley@wakemed.org

Mothers' Milk Bank at P/SL Medical Center
1719 East 19th Avenue
Denver, CO 80218
Phone: 303-869-1888
E-mail: mmilkbank@health1.org

Mothers' Milk Bank at Austin
900 E. 30th Street, Suite. 214
Austin, TX 78705
Phone: 512-494-0800
E-mail: info@mmbaustin.org

Mother's Milk Bank of Iowa
Division of Nutrition
Department of Pediatrics
Children's Hospital of Iowa
University of Iowa Hospitals and Clinics
Iowa City, Iowa 52242
Phone: 877-891-5347 (toll-free)
Website: http://www.uihealthcare.com/milkbank

Mothers' Milk Bank
Special Care Nursery
Christiana Hospital
Christiana Care Health Systems
4755 Ogletown-Stanton Road
Newark, DE 19718
Phone: 302-733-2340 or 800-NICU, ext. 101
  (toll-free)

Lactation Support Service
BC Childrens' Hospital
4480 Oak Street
Vancouver, BC V6H 3V4, Canada
Phone: 604-875-2282
E-mail: francesjones@shaw.ca

Banco de Leche Humana
Av. Adalfo Ruiz Cortines #2903
CP 91020
Xalapa, Veracruz, Mexico
Phone: 52-55-14-4500

DEFINITIONS

Donor human milk bank: A donor human milk bank is a service established for the purpose of collecting, screening, processing, storing, and distributing donated human milk to meet the specific needs of individuals for whom human milk is prescribed by health care providers who are licensed to prescribe.

Donor milk: Donor milk is voluntarily given by women other than the biologic mother of the recipient. Donors are not paid.

Fresh-raw milk: Milk stored continuously at approximately 4°C for use not longer than 72 hours after expression.

Fresh-frozen milk: Fresh-raw milk that has been frozen and held at approximately −20°C for not longer than 12 months from the date of collection.

Heat-processed milk: Fresh-raw or fresh-frozen milk that has been heated to a minimum of 62.5°C, but no more than 63°C, for 30 minutes, to minimize loss of the unique beneficial properties of the milk.

Pooled milk: Milk received from more than one donor.

Preterm milk: Milk pumped within the first month postpartum by a mother who delivered at or before 36 weeks' gestation.

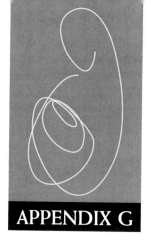

Measurements of Growth in Breastfed Infants

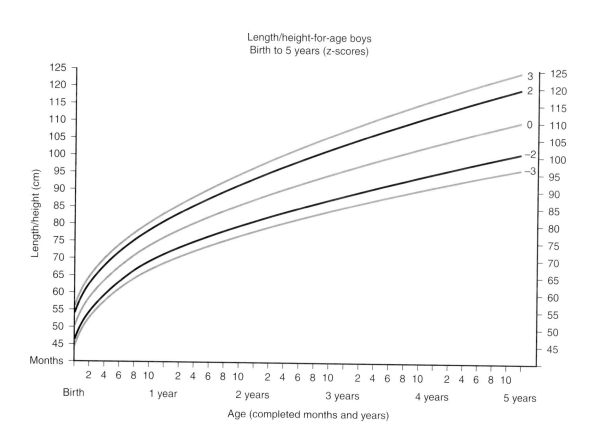

Length/height-for-age boys
Birth to 5 years (z-scores)

Length/height-for-age girls
Birth to 5 years (z-scores)

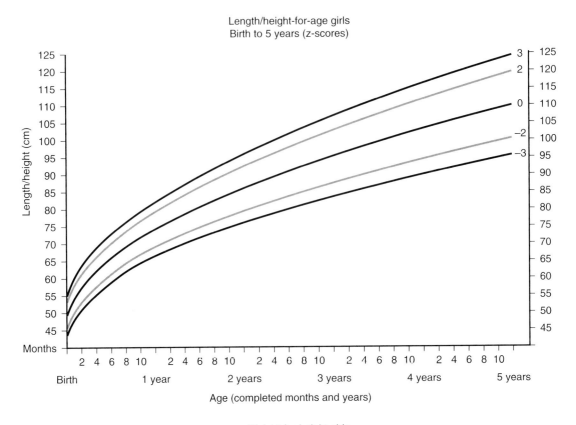

Age (completed months and years)

Weight-for-height girls
2 to 5 years (z-scores)

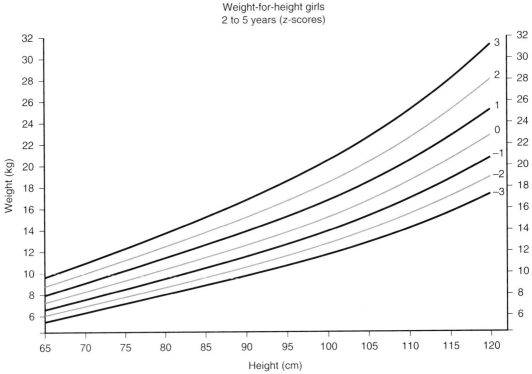

Height (cm)

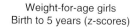

Weight-for-age girls
Birth to 5 years (z-scores)

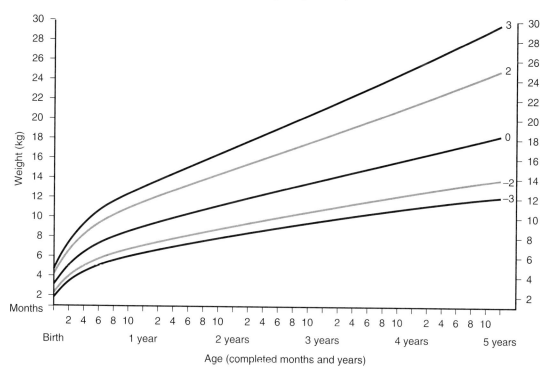

Head circumference-for-age girls
Birth to 13 weeks (z-scores)

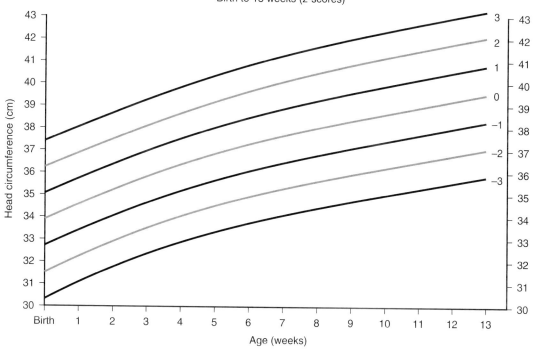

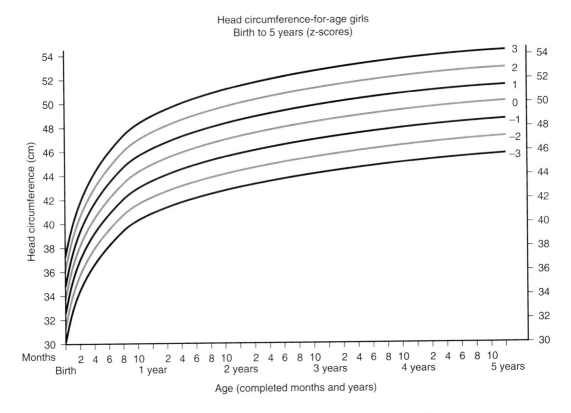

Head circumference-for-age girls
Birth to 5 years (z-scores)

Body mass index-for-age percentiles:

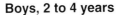

Boys, 2 to 4 years

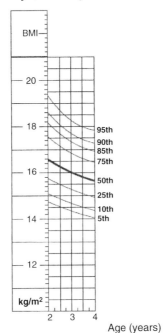

Girls, 2 to 4 years

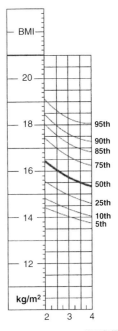

Published May 30, 2000.
Source: Developed by the National Center for Heath Statistics in collaboration with
the National Center for Chronic Disease Prevention and Health Promotion (2000).

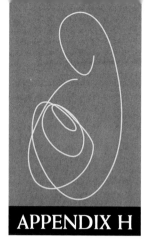

APPENDIX H

Organizations Interested in Supporting and Providing Materials for Breastfeeding

Government Agencies

Food and Nutrition Information Center
Nutrient Data Laboratory
USA-ARS
10300 Baltimore Avenue
Beltsville, MD 20705-2350
Phone: 301-504-5414
Fax: 301-504-6409
E-mail: ndlinfo@ars.usda.gov
Website: http://ndb.nal.usda.gov

The center serves the informational needs of people interested in human nutrition, nutrition education, food service management, consumer education, and food technology. It acquires and lends books, journal articles, and audiovisual materials dealing with these areas of concern, including breastfeeding research and education.

International Nutrition Communication Service
Education Development Center
43 Foundry Avenue
Waltham, MA 02453-8313
Phone: 617-969-7100
Fax: 617-969-5979
TTY: 617-964-5448
Website: http://www.edc.org

Funded by the U.S. Agency for International Development, the service provides support and assistance in designing, implementing, and evaluating nutrition training projects in Third World countries. It has also published the *Nutrition Training Manual Catalogue*, which contains reviews of 116 training manuals. The manuals focus on nutrition in developing countries. Breastfeeding training manuals are included.

National Health Information Center
Office of the Assistant Secretary for Health, Office of the Secretary
U.S. Department of Health and Human Services
1101 Wootton Parkway, Suite LL100
Rockville, MD 20852
Phone: 240-453-8280
Fax: 240-453-8282
E-mail: info@nhic.org
Website: http://www.health.gov/NHIC/

The Clearinghouse helps the public locate health information by identifying health information resources. Health questions are referred to appropriate health agencies that, in turn, respond directly to inquirers.

World Health Organization
Publications Center, USA
5 Sand Creek Rd.
Albany, NY 12205-1400
Phone: 518-436-9686
Fax: 518-436-7433
E-mail: QCORP@compuserve.com

Publications available include a statement on infant and young child feeding, a breastfeeding guide for use by community health workers, and a study on patterns of breastfeeding.

Private Educational and Support Organizations

Clearinghouse on Infant Feeding and Maternal Nutrition

American Public Health Association
1015 Fifteenth Street, NW
Washington, DC 20005
Phone: 202-789-5712

The clearinghouse serves as a resource primarily for health professionals who work in Third World countries. It also responds to domestic requests as time and staffing permit. It has a large collection of materials of all types on breastfeeding. It makes available bibliographies and lists of resources on a variety of topics, and refers inquiries to appropriate sources for information.

Health Education Associates

327 Quaker Meeting House Road
East Sandwich, MA 02537-1300
Phone: 888-888-8077 (toll-free); 508-888-8044
Fax: 508-888-8050
E-mail: info@healthed.cc

Health Education Associates make inexpensive pamphlets and other materials available as teaching aids on breastfeeding. They sponsor training programs for breastfeeding counseling and promotion techniques.

International Childbirth Education Association

1500 Sunday Drive, Suite 102
Raleigh, NC 27607
Phone: 919-863-9487
Fax: 919-787-4916
E-mail: info@icea.org
Website: http://www.icea.org/info.htm

The association's *Bookmarks* catalog has a large selection of books and inexpensive pamphlets on breastfeeding, childbirth, and parenting. It publishes *ICEA News*, with news about childbirth, prenatal, and parenting issues, and *ICEA Review*, which provides in-depth reviews of current perinatal issues. It also has a resource committee on breastfeeding.

International Lactation Consultant Association

2501 Aerial Center Parkway, Suite 103
Morrisville, NC 27560
Phone: 919-861-5577
Fax: 919-459-2075
E-mail: info@ilca.org

The International Lactation Consultant Association (ILCA) provides many member services, including newsletters and annual conferences.

Lact-Aid International, Inc.

P.O. Box 1066
Athens, TN 37371-1066
Phone: 423-744-9090 (orders outside U.S., information, and consulting); 866-866-1239 (toll-free ordering in the U.S.)
Fax: 1-423-744-9116
E-mail: orders@lact-aid.com
Website: http://www.lact-aid.com

Lact-Aid International, Inc. formerly published a quarterly journal, *Keeping Abreast, Journal of Human Nurturing*. It makes available back issues of the journal and reprints of selected articles. It also produces and markets the Lact-Aid Nursing Trainer and specializes in giving information and consultation on specific breastfeeding situations, including prematurity, relactation, adoptive nursing, and failure to thrive.

Also available is a special counseling service, LAMBS (Lact-Aid Mom's Buddies), which consists of peer counselors ready to assist a mother with the same special problem. Resource LAMBS who have personal experience nursing infants with a variety of problems (e.g., cleft palate, Down syndrome) can be reached by calling the Lact-Aid "Warmline."

La Leche League International, Inc.

35 E. Wacker Drive, Suite 850
Chicago, IL 60601
Phone: 312-646-6260; 1-800-LaLeche
Fax: 312-644-8557
E-mail: info@llli.org
Website: http://www.llli.org

La Leche's publications catalog includes a large variety and broad scope of materials for mothers and health professionals to use in promoting and supporting breastfeeding. There is also a directory of league area coordinators by state and foreign country. The coordinators can give information about local support groups.

Nursing Mothers Counsel, Inc.

P.O. Box 5024
San Mateo, CA 94402-0024
Phone: 650-327-6455
Website: http://www.nursingmothers.org

The counsel makes available a variety of publications on breastfeeding for mothers and health professionals.

Wellstart International
Corporate Headquarters
P.O. Box 602
Blue Jay, CA 92317-0602
Phone: 714-724-1675
Fax: 802-985-8794
E-mail: info@wellstart.org
Website: http://www.wellstart.org

Wellstart International is a private, nonprofit organization dedicated to the global promotion of healthy families through breastfeeding. Its purpose is to promote breastfeeding for future generations, to expand and share knowledge and understanding of breastfeeding and its benefits to families throughout the world, and to provide leadership for global change.

Wellstart International uses the following methodologies to build on existing resources and ensure quality and sustainability:

- Knowledge and skill transfer
- Development of health professional faculty as core resources of in-country expertise
- Short- and long-term technical assistance, follow-up, and field support
- Assessment of infant feeding practices
- Program evaluation, impact appraisal, and trends monitoring
- Network development and utilization
- Policy and economic analyses
- Information dissemination, including publications and meetings
- Funding support for national program activities

These methodologies are used to spread knowledge, skills, and information in the following subject areas:

- Clinical lactation management
- Scientific fundamentals of lactation and breastfeeding
- Communication and social marketing
- Community outreach and mother-to-mother support
- Evaluation and research methodologies
- Education and training methodologies

Wellstart International has been designated as a WHO Collaborating Center on Breastfeeding Promotion and Protection, with particular emphasis on lactation management education. The organization has also been involved in a variety of global breastfeeding initiatives, including preparation for the Innocenti Declaration, the World Summit for Children, and the Baby-Friendly Hospital Initiative.

Other National and International Breastfeeding Support Programs

For information about Baby-Friendly Hospital Initiative, contact:

Baby Friendly, USA
Corporate Headquarters
125 Wolf Rd, Suite 402
Albany, NY 12205
Phone: 518-621-7982
Fax: 518-621-7983
E-mail: info@babyfriendlyusa.org
Website: http://www.babyfriendlyusa.org

The World Alliance for Breastfeeding Action (WABA) is a network of organizations and individuals dedicated to protecting, promoting, and supporting breastfeeding as a right of all children and women. For information, contact:

WABA Secretariat: World Alliance for Breastfeeding Action
P.O. Box 1200
10850 Penang
Malaysia
Fax: 60-4-657 2655
E-mail: waba@waba.org.my
Website: http://www.waba.org.my

Other international support organizations are:

Australian Breastfeeding Association (ABA)
P.O. Box 4000
Glen Iris, Victoria 3146
Australia
Phone: 03-9885-0855, or from outside Australia +61-3-98850855
Fax: 03-9885-0866, or from outside Australia +61-3-98850866
E-mail: info@breastfeeding.asn.au
Website: http://www.breastfeeding.asn.au

Baby Milk Action Group
34 Trumpington St.
Cambridge CB2 1QY, United Kingdom
Phone: 01223-464420 (UK); +44-1223-464420 (Int'l)
Website: http://www.babymilkaction.org

Center for Science in the Public Interest
1220 L St. N.W. Suite 300
Washington, DC 20005
Phone: 202-332-9110
Fax: 202-265-4954
E-mail: cspi@cspinet.org
Website: http://www.cspinet.org

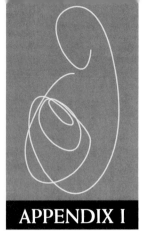

Breastfeeding Health Supervision

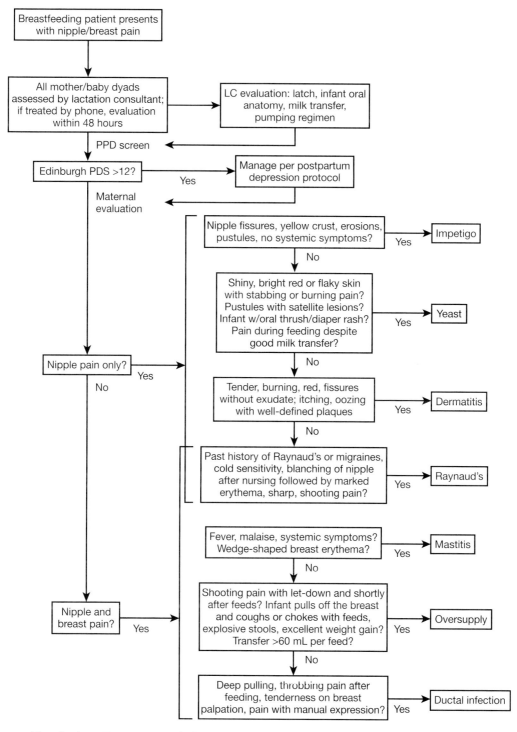

Courtesy Alison Stuebe, MD, Department of Obstetrics and Gynecology, University of North Carolina School of Medicine, Chapel Hill, North Carolina.

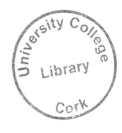

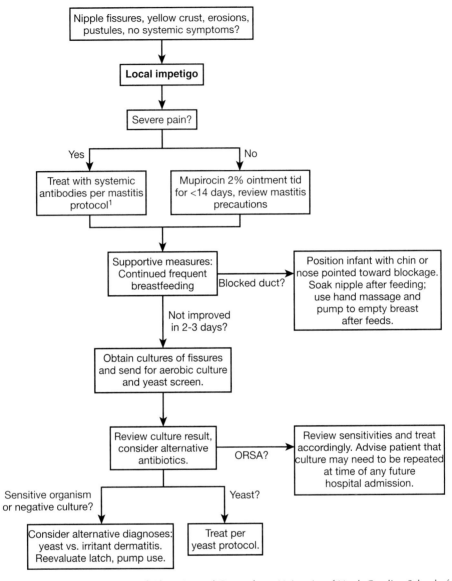

Courtesy Alison Stuebe, MD, Department of Obstetrics and Gynecology, University of North Carolina School of Medicine, Chapel Hill, North Carolina.

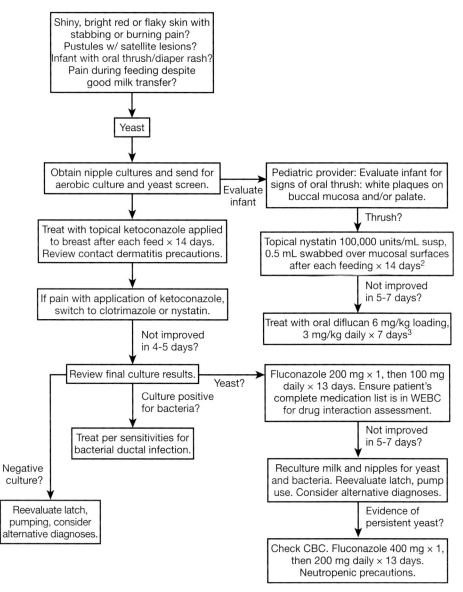

Courtesy Alison Stuebe, MD, Department of Obstetrics and Gynecology, University of North Carolina School of Medicine, Chapel Hill, North Carolina.

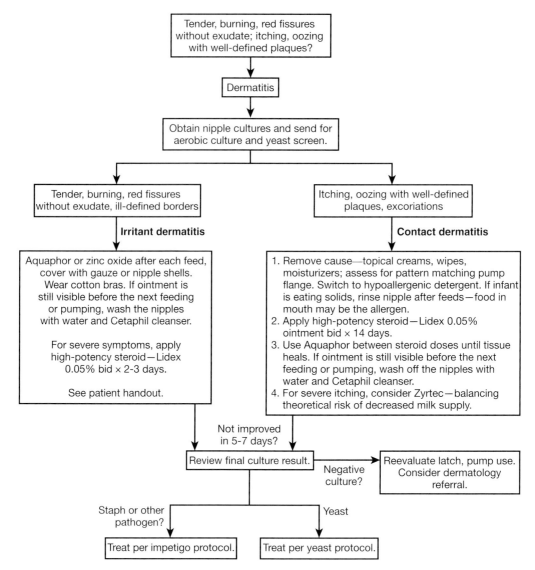

Courtesy Alison Stuebe, MD, Department of Obstetrics and Gynecology, University of North Carolina School of Medicine, Chapel Hill, North Carolina.

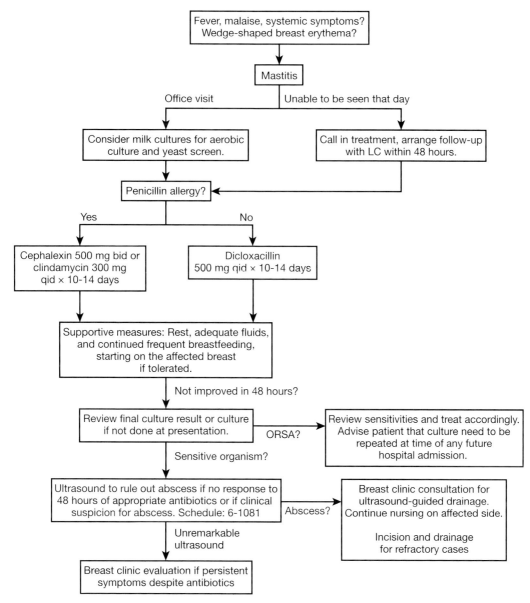

Fever, malaise, systemic symptoms?
Wedge-shaped breast erythema?

↓

Mastitis

Office visit ← → Unable to be seen that day

Consider milk cultures for aerobic culture and yeast screen.

Call in treatment, arrange follow-up with LC within 48 hours.

Penicillin allergy?

Yes / No

Cephalexin 500 mg bid or clindamycin 300 mg qid × 10-14 days

Dicloxacillin 500 mg qid × 10-14 days

Supportive measures: Rest, adequate fluids, and continued frequent breastfeeding, starting on the affected breast if tolerated.

Not improved in 48 hours?

Review final culture result or culture if not done at presentation.

ORSA?

Review sensitivities and treat accordingly. Advise patient that culture need to be repeated at time of any future hospital admission.

Sensitive organism?

Ultrasound to rule out abscess if no response to 48 hours of appropriate antibiotics or if clinical suspicion for abscess. Schedule: 6-1081

Abscess?

Breast clinic consultation for ultrasound-guided drainage. Continue nursing on affected side.

Incision and drainage for refractory cases

Unremarkable ultrasound

Breast clinic evaluation if persistent symptoms despite antibiotics

Courtesy Alison Stuebe, MD, Department of Obstetrics and Gynecology, University of North Carolina School of Medicine, Chapel Hill, North Carolina.

RAYNAUD PHENOMENON

Anderson JE, Held N, Wright K: Raynaud's phenomenon of the nipple: a treatable cause of painful breastfeeding, *Pediatrics* 113:e360–e364, 2004.

Delgado S, Collado MC, Fernandez L, et al: Bacterial analysis of breast milk: a tool to differentiate Raynaud's phenomenon from infectious mastitis during lactation, *Curr Microbiol* 59:59–64, 2009.

OVERSUPPLY

Woolridge MW, Fisher C: Colic, "overfeeding," and symptoms of lactose malabsorption in the breast-fed baby: a possible artifact of feed management? *Lancet* 2:382–384, 1988.

DUCTAL INFECTION

Eglash A, Plane MB, Mundt M: History, physical and laboratory findings, and clinical outcomes of lactating women treated with antibiotics for chronic breast and/or nipple pain, *J Hum Lact* 22:429–433, 2006.

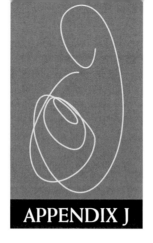

APPENDIX J

Protocol 1: Academy of Breastfeeding Medicine Protocols Guidelines for Blood Glucose Monitoring and Treatment of Hypoglycemia in Term and Late-Preterm Neonates

Nancy Wight, Kathleen A. Marinelli, and the Academy of Breastfeeding
Medicine Protocol Committee

A central goal of the Academy of Breastfeeding Medicine is the development of clinical protocols for managing common medical problems that may impact breastfeeding success. These protocols serve only as guidelines for the care of breastfeeding mothers and infants and do not delineate an exclusive course of treatment or serve as standards of medical care. Variations in treatment may be appropriate according to the needs of an individual patient.

Purpose

To provide guidance in the first hours/days of life to:

- Prevent clinically significant hypoglycemia in infants
- Appropriately monitor blood glucose levels in at-risk term and late-preterm infants
- Manage documented hypoglycemia in infants

- Establish and preserve maternal milk supply during medically necessary supplementation for hypoglycemia or during separation of mother and baby

Background

PHYSIOLOGY

The term "hypoglycemia" refers to a low blood glucose concentration. Clinically significant neonatal hypoglycemia reflects an imbalance between the supply and utilization of glucose and alternative fuels and may result from several disturbed regulatory mechanisms.[1] Transient hypoglycemia in the first hours after birth is common, occurring in almost all mammalian newborns. In healthy term human infants, even if early enteral feeding is withheld, this phenomenon is self-limited, without clinical signs, and considered to be part of adaptation to postnatal life, as glucose levels spontaneously rise within the first 24 hours after birth (for some, it is even longer but still physiological).[60,33,15,37,40] Most neonates compensate for this "physiological" low blood glucose with endogenous fuel production through gluconeogenesis, glycogenolysis, and ketogenesis, collectively called "counter-regulation." Even in those situations where low blood glucose concentrations do develop secondary to prolonged intervals (>8 hours) between breastfeeding, a marked ketogenic response occurs. The enhanced capability of the neonatal brain to utilize ketone bodies provides glucose-sparing fuel to the brain, protecting neurological function.[33,47,23,68] The compensatory provision of alternate fuels constitutes a normal adaptive response to transiently low nutrient intake during the establishment of breastfeeding,[33,13] resulting in most breastfed infants tolerating lower plasma glucose levels without any significant clinical manifestations or sequelae.[13]

No studies have shown that treating transiently low blood glucose levels results in better short-term or long-term outcomes compared with no treatment, and in fact there is no evidence at all that hypoglycemic infants with no clinical signs benefit from treatment.[8,46] Increases in neurodevelopmental abnormalities have been found in infants who have hypoglycemia associated with abnormal clinical signs, especially those with severe, persistent hyperinsulinemic hypoglycemia.[8,46,45,20,9,49] Rozance and Hay[52] have delineated the conditions that should be present before considering that long-term neurologic impairment might be related to neonatal hypoglycemia. Transient, single, brief periods of hypoglycemia are unlikely to cause permanent neurologic damage.[64,24,35,65] Therefore, the monitoring of blood glucose concentrations in healthy, term, appropriately grown neonates is unnecessary and potentially harmful to parental well-being and the successful establishment of breastfeeding.[64,24,35,65,34,31]

DEFINITION OF HYPOGLYCEMIA

The definition of hypoglycemia in the newborn infant has remained controversial because of a lack of significant correlation among plasma glucose concentration, clinical signs, and long-term sequelae.[13,44,58] An expert panel convened in 2008 by the U.S. National Institutes of Health concluded that there has been no substantial evidence-based progress in defining what constitutes clinically important neonatal hypoglycemia, particularly regarding how it relates to brain injury.[36] Multiple reviews have concluded that there is no specific plasma or blood glucose concentration or duration of low blood glucose level that can be linked to either clinical signs

or permanent neurologic injury.[52,58,51] In addition, blood glucose test results vary enormously with the source of the blood sample, the assay method, and whether whole blood, plasma, or serum glucose concentration is determined. Plasma or serum glucose concentrations are 10% to 15% higher than in whole blood.[7,16]

Breastfed, formula-fed, and mixed-fed infants follow the same pattern of glucose values, with an initial fall in glucose level over the first 2 hours of life, followed by a gradual rise in glucose level over the next 96 hours, whether fed or not.[60,37,40] Artificially fed infants tend to have slightly higher levels of glucose and lower levels of ketone bodies than breastfed infants.[33,37,64,63,22,14]

The incidence of "hypoglycemia" varies with the definition.[56,28] Many authors have suggested numeric definitions of hypoglycemia, usually between 30 and 50 mg/dL (1.7 to 2.8 mmol/L) and varying by postnatal age.* There is no scientific justification for the value of <47 mg/dL (2.6 mmol/L) that has been adopted by some clinicians.[13,58,36,51,48] Cornblath et al.[13] summarized the problem as follows:

Significant hypoglycemia is not and cannot be defined as a single number that can be applied universally to every individual patient. Rather, it is characterized by a value(s) that is unique to each individual and varies with both their state of physiologic maturity and the influence of pathology.

A meta-analysis of studies published from 1986 to 1994 looked at low plasma glucose thresholds in term healthy newborns who were mostly mixed-fed (breastfed and formula-fed) or formula-fed. It presented statistical ranges of low thresholds for plasma glucose level based on hours after birth in healthy term infants (Table J-1).[3] The authors specifically noted that given the known lower plasma glucose levels in healthy term breastfed infants as compared with formula-fed infants, the low thresholds for exclusively breastfed infants might even be lower. Table J-1 gives recommendations for this timed threshold approach.

This information is translated into guidelines for clinical intervention by the operational treatment

TABLE J-1	Population Low Thresholds: Plasma Glucose Level[3]	
Hour(s) After Birth	**≤5th Percentile Plasma Glucose Level**
1-2 (nadir)	28 mg/dL (1.6 mmol/L)
3-47	40 mg/dL (2.2 mmol/L)
48-72	48 mg/dL (2.7 mmol/L)

*Refs. 60,37,64,44,36,56,12,61,54,2.

TABLE J-2	Operational Thresholds for Treatment of Plasma Glucose Levels[13]	
Infant	**Plan/PGL**	**Treatment**
Infant with clinical signs	If <45 mg/dL (2.5 mmol/L)	Clinical interventions to increase blood glucose concentration
Infants with risk factors*	Initiate glucose monitoring as soon as possible after birth, within 2-3 hours after birth and before feeding, or at any time there are abnormal signs. If plasma glucose concentration is <36 mg/dL (2.0 mmol/L), close surveillance should be maintained. Intervention is recommended if plasma glucose remains below this level, does not increase after a feed, or if abnormal clinical signs develop.	Clinical interventions to increase blood glucose concentration: at very low glucose concentration (20-25 mg/dL, 1.1-1.4 mmol/L), intravenous glucose infusion to raise plasma glucose levels to >45 mg/dL (2.5 mmol/L) is indicated.

PGL, Plasma glucose level.
  *See Table J-3.

guidance of Cornblath et al.[13] As they stated, an operational threshold is that concentration of plasma or whole blood glucose at which clinicians should consider intervention, based on the evidence currently available in the literature (Table J-2). It needs to be underscored that the therapeutic objective (45 mg/dL [2.5 mmol/L]) is different from the operational threshold for intervention (36 mg/dL [2.0 mmol/L]), which is different from the population low thresholds in normal babies with no clinical signs or risk factors who do not need to be treated (Table J-1). The higher therapeutic goal was chosen to include a significant margin of safety in the absence of data evaluating the correlation between glucose levels in this range and long-term outcome in full-term infants.[13]

Given this information, it is clear that routine monitoring of blood glucose in healthy term infants is not only unnecessary, but is instead potentially harmful to the establishment of a healthy mother-infant relationship and successful breast-feeding patterns.[1,35,34,31,55,30] This recommendation has been supported by the World Health Organization,[64] the American Academy of Pediatrics,[1,55] the U.S. National Institutes of Health,[36] and the National Childbirth Trust of the United Kingdom.[50] These organizations all conclude that (1) early and exclusive breastfeeding is safe to meet the nutritional needs of healthy term infants and that (2) healthy term infants do not develop clinically significant hypoglycemia simply as a result of a time-limited duration of underfeeding.

TESTING METHODS

Bedside glucose reagent test strips are inexpensive and practical but are not reliable, with significant variance from true blood glucose levels, especially at low glucose concentrations.[34,2,4,39,41] Bedside glucose tests may be used for screening, but laboratory levels sent STAT (immediate determination, without delay) (e.g., glucose oxidase, hexokinase,

or dehydrogenase method) must confirm results before a diagnosis of hypoglycemia can be made, especially in infants with no clinical signs.[1,64,34] Other bedside rapid measurement methods such as reflectance colorimetry and electrode methods may be more accurate.[25,19,57,53] Continuous subcutaneous glucose monitoring, as is used in diabetic patients, has been used experimentally in neonates with good correlation with laboratory glucose values but is not currently recommended for screening.[29,27]

RISK FACTORS FOR HYPOGLYCEMIA

Neonates at increased risk for developing neonatal hypoglycemia should be routinely monitored for blood glucose levels irrespective of the mode of feeding. At-risk neonates fall into two main categories:

1. Excess utilization of glucose, which includes the hyperinsulinemic states
2. Inadequate production or substrate delivery[14,21,17]

Infant risk factors for hypoglycemia are listed in Table J-3.[†]

CLINICAL MANIFESTATIONS OF HYPOGLYCEMIA

The clinical manifestations of hypoglycemia are nonspecific, occurring with various other neonatal problems. Even in the presence of an arbitrary low glucose level, the physician must assess the general status of the infant by observation and physical examination to rule out other disease entities and processes that may need additional laboratory evaluation and treatment. Some common clinical signs are listed in Table J-4.

[†]Refs. 33,13,64,24,65,63,14,28,21,17,62,43.

TABLE J-3	At-Risk Infants for Whom Routine Monitoring of Blood Glucose Is Indicated: Small for Gestational Age: <10th Percentile for Weight Commonly Cited in the United States; <2nd Percentile Cited in the United Kingdom as Above This Considered Small Normal*

Babies with clinically evident wasting of fat and muscle bulk

LGA: >90th percentile for weight and macrosomic appearance[†]

Discordant twin: weight 10% < larger twin

All infants of diabetic mothers, especially if poorly controlled

Low birth weight (<2500 g)

Prematurity (<35 weeks, or late-preterm infants with clinical signs or extremely poor feeding)

Perinatal stress: severe acidosis or hypoxia-ischemia

Cold stress

Polycythemia (venous Hct > 70%)/hyperviscosity

Erythroblastosis fetalis

Beckwith-Wiedemann's syndrome

Microphallus or midline defect

Suspected infection

Respiratory distress

Known or suspected inborn errors of metabolism or endocrine disorders

Maternal drug treatment (e.g., terbutaline, beta-blockers, oral hypoglycemics)

Infants displaying signs associated with hypoglycemia (see Table J-4)

Hct, hematocrit.
*As per Dr. Jane Hawdon (personal communication).
[†]Unnecessary to screen all large for gestational age (LGA) babies. Glucose monitoring is recommended for infants from maternal populations who were unscreened for diabetes during the pregnancy where LGA may represent undiagnosed and untreated maternal diabetes.

TABLE J-4	Clinical Manifestations of Possible Hypoglycemia

Irritability, tremors, jitteriness
Exaggerated Moro reflex
High-pitched cry
Seizures or myoclonic jerks
Lethargy, listlessness, limpness, hypotonia
Coma
Cyanosis
Apnea or irregular breathing
Tachypnea
Hypothermia; temperature instability
Vasomotor instability
Poor suck or refusal to feed

A recent study found that of the 23 maternal/infant risk factors and infant signs/symptoms studied, only jitteriness and tachypnea were statistically significant at predicting low blood glucose—not even maternal diabetes![38] A diagnosis of hypoglycemia also requires that signs abate after normoglycemia is restored (the exception being if brain injury has already been sustained).

General Management Recommendations (Table J-5)

Any approach to management needs to account for the overall metabolic and physiologic status of the infant and should not unnecessarily disrupt the mother-infant relationship and breastfeeding.[1,65] Because severe, prolonged hypoglycemia with clinical signs may result in neurologic injury,[8,20,9,67] immediate intervention is needed for infants with clinical signs. Several authors have suggested algorithms for screening and treatment.[1,52,36,51,42] (Quality of evidence [levels of evidence I, II-1, II-2, II-3, and III] is based on the U.S. Preventive Services Task Force Appendix A Task Force Ratings[6] and is noted in parentheses.)

A. **Initial management**

Early and exclusive breastfeeding meets the nutritional and metabolic needs of healthy term newborn infants. Healthy term infants do not develop clinically significant hypoglycemia simply as a result of time-limited underfeeding.[64,24,65] (III)

TABLE J-5	General Management Recommendations for All Term Infants

A. Early and exclusive breastfeeding meets the nutritional and metabolic needs of healthy term newborn infants.

1. Routine supplementation is unnecessary.

2. Initiate breastfeeding within 30-60 minutes of life and continue on demand.

3. Facilitate skin-to-skin contact of mother and infant.

4. Feedings should be frequent, 10-12 times per 24 hours in the first few days after birth.

B. Glucose screening is performed only on at-risk infants or infants with clinical signs.

1. Routine monitoring of blood glucose in all term newborns is unnecessary and may be harmful.

2. At-risk infants should be screened for hypoglycemia with a frequency and duration related to the specific risk factors of the individual infant.

3. Monitoring continues until normal, prefeed levels are consistently obtained.

4. Bedside glucose screening tests must be confirmed by formal laboratory testing.

1. Healthy, appropriate weight for gestational age, term infants should initiate breastfeeding within 30 to 60 minutes of life and continue breastfeeding on cue, with the recognition that crying is a very late sign of hunger.[55,5,66] (III)

2. Initiation and establishment of breastfeeding, and reduction of hypoglycemia risk, are facilitated by skin-to-skin contact between the mother and her infant immediately after birth for at least the first hour of life and continuing as much as possible. Such practices will maintain normal infant body temperature and reduce energy expenditure (thus enabling maintenance of normal blood glucose) while stimulating suckling and milk production.[22,55] (II-2, III)

3. Feedings should be frequent, at least 10 to 12 times per 24 hours in the first few days after birth.[55] (III) However, it is not unusual for term infants to feed immediately after birth and then sleep quite a long time (up to 8 to 12 hours) before they become more active and begin to suckle with increasing frequently. They mount protective metabolic responses throughout this time so it is not necessary to try to force-feed them. However, an unusually, excessively drowsy baby must undergo clinical evaluation.

4. Routine supplementation of healthy term infants with water, glucose water, or formula is unnecessary and may interfere with the establishment of normal breastfeeding and normal metabolic compensatory mechanisms.[33,63,55,50] (II-2, III)

B. **Blood glucose screening**

Glucose screening should be performed only on at-risk infants and those with clinical signs compatible with hypoglycemia. Early breastfeeding is not precluded just because the infant meets the criteria for glucose monitoring.

1. At-risk infants should be screened for hypoglycemia with a frequency and duration related to the specific risk factors of the individual infant.[1,24] (III) Monitoring should begin no later than 2 hours of age for infants in risk categories.[1] Hawdon[32] recommended blood glucose monitoring should commence before the second feeding (i.e., not so soon after birth that the physiologic fall in blood glucose level causes confusion and overtreatment). (III)

2. Monitoring should continue until acceptable, prefeed levels are consistently obtained, meaning until the infant has had at least two consecutive satisfactory measurements.[32] A reasonable (although arbitrary) goal is to maintain plasma glucose concentrations between 40 and 50 mg/dL (between 2.2 and 2.8 mmol/L)[1] or >45 mg/dL (2.5 mmol/L).[13] (III)

3. Bedside glucose screening tests must be confirmed by formal laboratory testing, although treatment should begin immediately in infants with clinical signs.

Table J-5 summarizes these recommendations.

Management of Documented Hypoglycemia (Table J-6)

A. **Infant with no clinical signs (absence of clinical signs can only be determined by careful clinical review)**

1. Continue breastfeeding (approximately every 1 to 2 hours) or feed 1 to 3 mL/kg (up to 5 mL/kg)[64] of expressed breastmilk or substitute nutrition (pasteurized donor human milk, elemental formulas, partially hydrolyzed formulas, or routine formulas). Glucose water is not suitable because of insufficient energy and lack of protein. Recent reports of mothers

TABLE J-6	Management of Documented Hypoglycemia

A. Infant with no clinical signs

1. Continue breastfeeding (approximately every 1-2 hours) or feed 1-5 mL/kg of expressed breastmilk or substitute nutrition.

2. Recheck blood glucose concentration before subsequent feedings until the value is acceptable and stable.

3. Avoid forced feedings (see above).

4. If the glucose level remains low despite feedings, begin intravenous glucose therapy.

5. Breastfeeding may continue during intravenous glucose therapy.

6. Carefully document response to treatment.

B. Infant with clinical signs or plasma glucose levels <20-25 mg/dL (<1.1-1.4 mmol/L)

1. Initiate intravenous 10% glucose solution with a mini-bolus.

2. Do not rely on oral or intragastric feeding to correct extreme or clinically significant hypoglycemia.

3. The glucose concentration in infants who have had clinical signs should be maintained at >45 mg/dL (>2.5 mmol/L).

4. Adjust intravenous rate by blood glucose concentration.

5. Encourage frequent breastfeeding.

6. Monitor glucose concentrations before feedings while weaning off the intravenous treatment until values stabilize off intravenous fluids.

7. Carefully document response to treatment.

with diabetes expressing and freezing colostrum prenatally (beginning at 34 to 36 weeks of gestation) to have it available after birth to avoid artificial feedings should their infant become hypoglycemic are mixed in terms of association with earlier births, and currently this procedure is not widely recommended.[18,26,59,10,11] (III)

2. Recheck blood glucose concentration before subsequent feedings until the value is acceptable and stable (usually >40 mg/dL [2.2 mmol/L]). If staff is unavailable to check blood glucose and an infant has no clinical signs, breastfeeding should *never* be unnecessarily delayed while waiting for the blood glucose level to be checked.

3. If the infant is simply worn out and not otherwise ill, nasogastric feeds of human milk can be initiated, watching carefully for signs of intolerance or evidence of significant underlying illness. If the neonate is too ill to suck or enteral feedings are not tolerated, avoid forced oral feedings (e.g., nasogastric tube) and instead begin intravenous (IV) therapy (see below). Such an infant is not normal and requires a careful examination and evaluation in addition to more intensive therapy. Term babies should not be given nasogastric feedings. They are much more likely to fight and aspirate.

4. If the glucose level remains low despite feedings, begin IV glucose therapy and adjust the IV rate by blood glucose concentration. Avoid bolus doses of glucose unless blood glucose is unrecordable or there are severe clinical signs (e.g., seizures or coma). If a bolus dose is given, use 5 mg/kg of glucose in 10% dextrose preparation.

5. Breastfeeding should continue during IV glucose therapy when the infant is interested and will suckle. Gradually wean from the IV glucose as the serum glucose level normalizes and feedings increase.

6. Carefully document physical examination, screening values, laboratory confirmation, treatment, and changes in clinical condition (i.e., response to treatment).

7. The infant should not be discharged until reasonable levels of blood glucose are maintained through a fast of 3 to 4 hours. Monitoring must be recommenced if there are adverse changes in feeding.

B. **Infants with clinical signs or with plasma glucose levels <20 to 25 mg/dL (<1.1 to 1.4 mol/L)**
   1. Initiate IV 10% glucose solution with a bolus of 3 mL/kg and continuous IV treatment at 5 to 8 mg/kg/minute.
   2. Do not rely on oral or intragastric feeding to correct extreme or symptomatic hypoglycemia.

Such an infant most likely has an underlying condition and, in addition to IV glucose therapy, requires an immediate and careful examination and evaluation.

3. The glucose concentration in infants with clinical signs should be maintained at >45 mg/dL (>2.5 mmol/L).

4. Adjust the IV rate by blood glucose concentration.

5. Encourage frequent breastfeeding after initiation of IV therapy.

6. Monitor glucose concentrations before feedings while gradually weaning from the IV solution, until values are stabilized off IV fluids.

7. Carefully document physical examination, screening values, laboratory confirmation, treatment, and changes in clinical condition (i.e., response to treatment).

Supporting the Mother

Giving birth to an infant who develops hypoglycemia is of concern to both the mother and family and thus may jeopardize the establishment of breastfeeding. Mothers should be explicitly reassured that there is nothing wrong with their milk and that supplementation is usually temporary. Having the mother hand-express or pump milk that is then fed to her infant can overcome feelings of maternal inadequacy as well as help establish a full milk supply. It is important for the mother to provide stimulation to the breasts by manual or mechanical expression with appropriate frequency (at least eight times in 24 hours) until her baby is latching and suckling well to protect her milk supply. Keeping the infant at breast or returning the infant to the breast as soon as possible is important. Skin-to-skin care is easily accomplished with an IV line in place and may lessen the trauma of intervention, while also providing physiologic thermoregulation, thus contributing to metabolic homeostasis.

Recommendations for Future Research

1. Well-planned, well-controlled studies are needed that look at plasma glucose concentrations, clinical signs, and long-term sequelae to determine what levels of blood glucose are the minimum safe levels.

2. The development and implementation of more reliable bedside testing methods would increase the efficiency of diagnosis and treatment of significant glucose abnormalities.

3. Studies to determine a clearer understanding of the role of other glucose-sparing fuels and the methods to measure them in a clinically meaningful way and time frame are required to aid in understanding which babies are truly at risk of neurologic sequelae and thus must be treated.
4. For those infants who do become hypoglycemic, research into how much enteral glucose, and in what form, is necessary to raise blood glucose to acceptable levels is important for clinical management.
5. Randomized controlled studies of prenatal colostrum expression and storage for mothers with infants at risk of hypoglycemia are important to determine if this is a practical and safe treatment modality.

Summary

Healthy term infants are programmed to make the transition from their intrauterine constant flow of nutrients to their extrauterine intermittent nutrient intake without the need for metabolic monitoring or interference with the natural breastfeeding process. Homeostatic mechanisms ensure adequate energy substrate is provided to the brain and other organs, even when feedings are delayed. The normal pattern of early, frequent, and exclusive breastfeeding meets the needs of healthy term infants.

Routine screening and supplementation are not necessary and may harm the normal establishment of breastfeeding. Current evidence does not support a specific blood concentration of glucose that correlates with signs or that can predict permanent neurologic damage in any given infant. At-risk infants should be screened, followed up as needed, and treated with supplementation or IV glucose if there are clinical signs or suggested thresholds are reached. Bedside screening is helpful, but not always accurate, and should be confirmed with laboratory glucose measurement. A single low glucose value is not associated with long-term neurologic abnormalities, provided the treating clinician can be assured that the baby was entirely well up until the time of the low value. Hypoglycemic encephalopathy and poor long-term outcome are extremely unlikely in infants with no clinical signs and are more likely in infants who manifest clinical signs and/or with persistent or repeated episodes of severe hypoglycemia.

Acknowledgments

This work was supported in part by a grant from the Maternal and Child Health Bureau, U.S. Department of Health and Human Services.

REFERENCES

1. Adamkin DH: Committee on Fetus and Newborn: Postnatal glucose homeostasis in late-preterm and term infants, *Pediatrics* 127:575–579, 2011.
2. Alkalay A, Klein A, Nagel R, et al: Neonatal nonpersistent hypoglycemia, *Neonatal Intensive Care* 14:25–34, 2001.
3. Alkalay AL, Sarnat HB, Flores-Sarnat L, et al: Population meta-analysis of low plasma glucose thresholds in full-term normal newborns, *Am J Perinatol* 23:115–119, 2006.
4. Altimier L, Roberts W: One Touch II hospital system for neonates: correlation with serum glucose values, *Neonatal Netw* 15(2):15–18, 1996.
5. American Academy of Pediatrics, American College of Obstetricians and Gynecologists: *Guidelines for perinatal care*, ed 6, Elk Grove Village, Ill., 2008, American Academy of Pediatrics.
6. Appendix A. Task Force Ratings Guide to Clinical Preventive Services: Report of the U.S. Preventive Services Task Force, ed 2. www.ncbi.nlm.nih.gov/books/NBK15430. Accessed March 28, 2014.
7. Aynsley-Green A: Glucose: a fuel for thought!, *J Paediatr Child Health* 27:21–30, 1991.
8. Boluyt N, van Kempen A, Offringa M: Neurodevelopment after neonatal hypoglycemia: a systematic review and design of an optimal future study, *Pediatrics* 117:2231–2243, 2006.
9. Burns C, Rutherford M, Boardman J, et al: Patterns of cerebral injury and neurodevelopmental outcomes after symptomatic neonatal hypoglycemia, *Pediatrics* 122:65–74, 2008.
10. Chapman T, Pincombe J, Harris M: Antenatal breast expression: a critical review of the literature, *Midwifery* 29:203–210, 2013.
11. Chapman T, Pincombe J, Harris M, et al: Antenatal breast expression: exploration and extent of teaching practices amongst International Board Certified Lactation Consultant midwives across Australia, *Women Birth* 26:41–48, 2013.
12. Cole MD, Peevy K: Hypoglycemia in normal neonates appropriate for gestational age, *J Perinatol* 14:118–120, 1994.
13. Cornblath M, Hawdon JM, Williams AF, et al: Controversies regarding definition of neonatal hypoglycemia: suggested operational thresholds, *Pediatrics* 105:1141–1145, 2000.
14. Cornblath M, Ichord R: Hypoglycemia in the neonate, *Semin Perinatol* 24:136–149, 2000.
15. Cornblath M, Reisner SH: Blood glucose in the neonate and its clinical significance, *N Engl J Med* 273:378–381, 1965.
16. Cornblath M, Schwartz R: Hypoglycemia in the neonate, *J Pediatr Endocrinol* 6:113–129, 1993.
17. Cowett RM, Loughead JL: Neonatal glucose metabolism: differential diagnoses, evaluation, and treatment of hypoglycemia, *Neonatal Netw* 21:9–19, 2002.
18. Cox SG: Expressing and storing colostrum antenatally for use in the newborn period, *Breastfeed Rev* 14:11–16, 2006.
19. Dahlberg M, Whitelaw A: Evaluation of HemoCue blood glucose analyzer for the instant diagnosis of hypoglycaemia in newborns, *Scand J Clin Lab Invest* 57:719–724, 1997.
20. Dalgic N, Ergenekon E, Soysal S, et al: Transient neonatal hypoglycemia—long-term effects on neurodevelopmental outcome, *J Pediatr Endocrinol Metab* 15:319–324, 2002.
21. de Lonlay P, Giurgea I, Touati G, et al: Neonatal hypoglycaemia: aetiologies, *Semin Neonatol* 9:49–58, 2004.
22. Durand R, Hodges S, LaRock S, et al: The effect of skin-to-skin breast-feeding in the immediate recovery period on newborn thermoregulation and blood glucose values, *Neonatal Intensive Care* 10:23–29, 1997.
23. Edmond J, Auestad N, Robbins RA, et al: Ketone body metabolism in the neonate: development and the effect of diet, *Fed Proc* 44:2359–2364, 1985.
24. Eidelman AI: Hypoglycemia and the breastfed neonate, *Pediatr Clin North Am* 48:377–387, 2001.

25. Ellis M, Manandhar DS, Manandhar N, et al: Comparison of two cotside methods for the detection of hypoglycaemia among neonates in Nepal, *Arch Dis Child Fetal Neonatal Ed* 75:F122–F125, 1996.

26. Forster DA, McEgan K, Ford R, et al: Diabetes and antenatal milk expressing: a pilot project to inform the development of a randomised controlled trial, *Midwifery* 27:209–214, 2011.

27. Harris D, Battin M, Weston P, et al: Continuous glucose monitoring in newborn babies at risk of hypoglycemia, *J Pediatr* 157:198–202, 2010.

28. Harris DL, Weston PJ, Harding JE: Incidence of neonatal hypoglycemia in babies identified as at risk, *J Pediatr* 161:787–791, 2012.

29. Harris D, Weston P, Williams C, et al: Cot-side electroencephalography monitoring is not clinically useful in the detection of mild neonatal hypoglycemia, *J Pediatr* 159:755–760, 2011.

30. Haninger NC, Farley CL: Screening for hypoglycemia in healthy term neonates: effects on breastfeeding, *J Midwifery Womens Health* 46:292–301, 2001.

31. Hawdon JM: Neonatal hypoglycemia: the consequences of admission to the special care nursery, *Child Health* 48–51, 1993.

32. Hawdon JM: Neonatal hypoglycemia: are evidence-based clinical guidelines achievable? *NeoReviews* 15:e91–e98, 2014.

33. Hawdon JM, Ward Platt MP, Aynsley-Green A: Patterns of metabolic adaptation for preterm and term infants in the first neonatal week, *Arch Dis Child* 67(4 Spec No.):357–365, 1992.

34. Hawdon JM, Platt MP, Aynsley-Green A: Neonatal hypoglycaemia—blood glucose monitoring and baby feeding, *Midwifery* 9:3–6, 1993.

35. Hawdon JM, Ward Platt MP, Aynsley-Green A: Prevention and management of neonatal hypoglycaemia, *Arch Dis Child Fetal Neonatal Ed* 70:F60–F64, 1994 (discussion F65).

36. Hay WW, Raju T, Higgens R, et al: Knowledge gaps and research needs for understanding and treating neonatal hypoglycemia: workshop report from Eunice Kennedy Shriver National Institute of Child Health and Human Development, *J Pediatr* 155:612–617, 2009.

37. Heck LJ, Erenberg A: Serum glucose levels in term neonates during the first 48 hours of life, *J Pediatr* 110:119–122, 1987.

38. Hoops D, Roberts P, VanWinkle E, et al: Should routine peripheral blood glucose testing be done for all newborns at birth? *MCN Am J Matern Child Nurs* 35:264–270, 2010.

39. Ho HT, Yeung WK, Young BW: Evaluation of "point of care" devices in the measurement of low blood glucose in neonatal practice, *Arch Dis Child Fetal Neonatal Ed* 89:F356–F359, 2004.

40. Hoseth E, Joergensen A, Ebbesen F, et al: Blood glucose levels in a population of healthy, breast fed, term infants of appropriate size for gestational age, *Arch Dis Child Fetal Neonatal Ed* 83:F117–F119, 2000.

41. Hussain K, Sharief N: The inaccuracy of venous and capillary blood glucose measurement using reagent strips in the newborn period and the effect of haematocrit, *Early Hum Dev* 57:111–121, 2000.

42. Jain A, Aggarwal R, Jeeva Sankar M, et al: Hypoglycemia in the newborn, *Indian J Pediatr* 77:1137–1142, 2010.

43. Kalhan S, Parmimi P: Gluconeogenesis in the fetus and neonate, *Semin Perinatol* 24:94–106, 2000.

44. Kalhan S, Peter-Wohl S: Hypoglycemia: what is it for the neonate? *Am J Perinatol* 17:11–18, 2000.

45. Kinnala A, Rikalainen H, Lapinleimu H, et al: Cerebral magnetic resonance imaging and ultrasonography findings after neonatal hypoglycemia, *Pediatrics* 103:724–729, 1999.

46. Koivisto M, Blanco-Sequeiros M, Krause U: Neonatal symptomatic and asymptomatic hypoglycaemia: a follow-up study of 151 children, *Dev Med Child Neurol* 14:603–614, 1972.

47. Lucas A, Boyes S, Bloom SR, et al: Metabolic and endocrine responses to a milk feed in six-day-old term infants: differences between breast and cow's milk formula feeding, *Acta Paediatr Scand* 70:195–200, 1981.

48. McGowan JE: Commentary: neonatal hypoglycemia—fifty years later, the questions remain the same, *NeoReviews* 5:e363–e364, 2004.

49. Menni F, deLonlay P, Sevin C, et al: Neurologic outcomes of 90 neonates and infants with persistent hyperinsulinemic hypoglycemia, *Pediatrics* 107:476–479, 2001.

50. National Childbirth Trust, Kingdom: Hypoglycemia of the newborn: guidelines for the appropriate blood glucose screening of breast-fed and bottle-fed babies in the UK, *Midwives* 110:248–249, 1997.

51. Rozance PJ, Hay WW: Hypoglycemia in newborn infants: features associated with adverse outcomes, *Biol Neonate* 90:74–86, 2006.

52. Rozance PJ, Hay WW Jr.: Describing hypoglycemia—definition or operational threshold? *Early Hum Dev* 86:275–280, 2010.

53. Schlebusch H, Niesen M, Sorger M, et al: Blood glucose determinations in newborns: four instruments compared, *Pediatr Pathol Lab Med* 18:41–48, 1998.

54. Schwartz RP: Neonatal hypoglycemia: how low is too low? *J Pediatr* 131:171–173, 1997.

55. Section on Breastfeeding: Breastfeeding and the use of human milk, *Pediatrics* 129:e827–e841, 2012.

56. Sexson WR: Incidence of neonatal hypoglycemia: a matter of definition, *J Pediatr* 105:149–150, 1984.

57. Sharief N, Hussein K: Comparison of two methods of measurement of whole blood glucose in the neonatal period, *Acta Paediatr* 86:1246–1252, 1997.

58. Sinclair JC: Approaches to the definition of neonatal hypoglycemia, *Acta Paediatr Jpn* 39(Suppl 1):S17–S20, 1997.

59. Soltani H, Scott AM: Antenatal breast expression in women with diabetes: outcomes from a retrospective cohort study, *Int Breastfeed J* 7:18, 2012.

60. Srinivasan G, Pildes RS, Cattamanchi G, et al: Plasma glucose values in normal neonates: a new look, *J Pediatr* 109:114–117, 1986.

61. Stanley CA, Baker L: The causes of neonatal hypoglycemia, *N Engl J Med* 340:1200–1201, 1999.

62. Sunehag AL, Haymond MW: Glucose extremes in newborn infants, *Clin Perinatol* 29:245–260, 2002.

63. Swenne I, Ewald U, Gustafsson J, et al: Inter-relationship between serum concentrations of glucose, glucagon and insulin during the first two days of life in healthy newborns, *Acta Paediatr* 83:915–919, 1994.

64. Williams AF: *Hypoglycemia of the newborn: review of the literature*, Geneva, 1997, World Health Organization.

65. Wight N: Hypoglycemia in breastfed neonates, *Breastfeed Med* 1:253–262, 2006.

66. World Health Organization UNICEF: *Protecting, promoting and supporting breast-feeding: the special role of maternity services, a joint WHO/UNICEF statement*, Geneva, 1989, World Health Organization.

67. Yager J: Hypoglycemic injury to the immature brain, *Clin Perinatol* 29:651–674, 2002.

68. Yager JY, Heitjan DF, Towfighi J, Vannucci RC: Effect of insulin-induced and fasting hypoglycemia on perinatal hypoxic-ischemic brain damage, *Pediatr Res* 31:138–142, 1992.

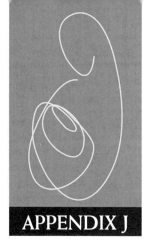

APPENDIX J

Protocol 2: Guidelines for Hospital Discharge of the Breastfeeding Term Newborn and Mother: "The Going Home Protocol"

Amy Evans, Kathleen A. Marinelli, Julie Scott Taylor, and
the Academy of Breastfeeding Medicine

A central goal of the Academy of Breastfeeding Medicine is the development of clinical protocols for managing common medical problems that may impact breastfeeding success. These protocols serve only as guidelines for the care of breastfeeding mothers and infants and do not delineate an exclusive course of treatment or serve as standards of medical care. Variations in treatment may be appropriate according to the needs of an individual patient.

Background

The ultimate success of breastfeeding is measured in part by both the duration of and the exclusivity of breastfeeding. Anticipatory attention to the needs of the mother and infant at the time of discharge from the hospital is crucial to ensure successful, long-term breastfeeding. The following principles and practices are recommended for consideration prior to sending a mother and her full-term infant home.

Clinical Guidelines

1. A health professional trained in formal assessment of breastfeeding should perform and document an assessment of breastfeeding effectiveness at least once during the last 8 hours preceding discharge of the mother and infant. Similar assessments should have been performed during the hospitalization, preferably at least once every 8 to 12 hours. In countries such as Japan, where the hospital stay may last up to a week, assessment should continue until breastfeeding is successfully established and then may decrease in frequency. These should include evaluation of positioning, latch, milk transfer, clinical jaundice, stool color and transition, stool and urine output, and notation of uric acid crystals if present. Infant's weight and percentage weight loss should be assessed but do not need to be checked frequently. For example, in Australia, infants are weighed at birth and at discharge or

825

on day 3 of life, whichever comes first. All concerns raised by the mother such as nipple pain, inability to hand express, perception of inadequate supply, and any perceived need to supplement must also be addressed.[35,43,5,24,7,1,36] (I; II-3; III) (Quality of evidence [levels of evidence I, II-1, II-2, II-3, and III] for each recommendation as defined in the U.S. Preventive Services Task Force Appendix A Task Force Ratings[9] is noted in parentheses.) It is important to ask detailed questions—many mothers may not bring up these concerns if not directly questioned.

2. Prior to discharge, anticipation of breastfeeding problems should be assessed based on maternal and/or infant risk factors (Tables J-7 and J-8). (III)

   All problems with breastfeeding, whether observed by hospital staff or raised by the mother, should be attended to and documented in the medical record prior to discharge of the mother and infant. This includes prompt recognition and treatment plans for possible ankyloglossia, which can affect latch, lactogenesis, and future breastfeeding.[17,10] (An updated clinical protocol is in development.) (I) A plan of action that includes follow-up of the problem after discharge must be in place.[51,3,12,20] (II-3) If the mother's and infant's caregivers are not the same person, there needs to be coordinated communication of any issues between the obstetric and pediatric providers for optimal follow-up care (see Guideline #10).

3. Physicians, midwives, nurses, and all other staff should encourage the mother to breastfeed exclusively for the first 6 months of the infant's life and to continue breastfeeding through at least the first year and preferably to 2 years of life and beyond.[5,4,30] (III) This is the recommendation of the World Health Organization, as well as organizations from many individual countries such as the National Health and Medical Research Council in Australia.[39] The Joint Commission, an organization that accredits hospitals and health care institutions in the United States and globally, is now mandating documentation of exclusive breastfeeding rates as part of its accreditation process for hospitals and birthing centers in the United States. The U.S. Centers for Disease Control and Prevention has similar recommendations.[20,49,48,31,50] (III) The addition of appropriate complementary food should occur at 6 months of life.[34] (I) Mothers benefit from education about the rationale for and practical advice on exclusive breastfeeding. The medical, psychosocial, and societal benefits for both mother and infant and why artificial milk supplementation is

TABLE J-7 Maternal Risk Factors for Lactation Problems

Factors

History/social
- Primiparity
- Intention to both breastfeed and bottle or formula feed at less than 6 weeks
- Intention to use pacifiers/dummies and/or artificial nipples/teats at less than 6 weeks
- Early intention/necessity to return to school or work
- History of previous breastfeeding problems or breastfed infant with slow weight gain
- History of infertility
- Conception by assisted reproductive technology
- Significant medical problems (e.g., untreated hypothyroidism, diabetes, cystic fibrosis, polycystic ovaries)
- Extremes of maternal age (e.g., adolescent mother or older than 40 years)
- Psychosocial problems (e.g., depression, anxiety, lack of social support for breastfeeding)
- Prolonged labor
- Long induction or augmentation of labor
- Use of medications during labor (benzodiazepines, morphine, or others that can cause drowsiness in the newborn)
- Peripartum complications (e.g., postpartum hemorrhage, hypertension, infection)
- Intended use of hormonal contraceptives before breastfeeding is well established (6 weeks)
- Perceived inadequate milk supply
- Maternal medication use (inappropriate advice about compatibility with breastfeeding is common)

Anatomic/physiologic
- Lack of noticeable breast enlargement during puberty or pregnancy
- Flat, inverted, or very large nipples
- Variation in breast appearance (marked asymmetry, hypoplastic, tubular)
- Any previous breast surgery, including cosmetic procedures (important to ask—not always obvious on exam)
- Previous breast abscess
- Maternal obesity (body mass index ≥ 30 kg/m^2)
- Extremely or persistently sore nipples
- Failure of "secretory activation" lactogenesis II. (Milk did not noticeably "come in" by 72 hours postpartum. This may be difficult to evaluate if mother and infant are discharged from the hospital in the first 24-48 hours postpartum.)
- Mother unable to hand-express colostrum
- Need for breastfeeding aids or appliances (such as nipple shields, breast pumps, or supplemental nursing systems) at the time of hospital discharge

Adapted with permission from Neifert[40,p.285] and the *Breastfeeding Handbook for Physicians.*[43,p.90] (III)

TABLE J-8	Infant Risk Factors for Lactation Problems

Factors

Medical/anatomic/physiologic

- Low birth weight or premature (<37 weeks)
- Multiples
- Difficulty in latching on to one or both breasts
- Ineffective or unsustained suckling
- Oral anatomic abnormalities (e.g., cleft lip/palate, macroglossia, micrognathia, tight frenulum/ankyloglossia with trained medical assessment)
- Medical problems (e.g., hypoglycemia, infection, jaundice, respiratory distress)
- Neurologic problems (e.g., genetic syndromes, hypertonia, hypotonia)
- Persistently sleepy infant
- Excessive infant weight loss (>7-10% of birth weight in the first 48 hours)

Environmental

- Mother-infant separation
- Breast pump dependency
- Formula supplementation
- Effective breastfeeding not established by hospital discharge
- Discharge from the hospital at <48 hours of age[16]
- Early pacifier use

Adapted with permission from Neifert[40,p.285] and the *Breastfeeding Handbook for Physicians*.[43,p.91] (III)

discouraged should be emphasized. Such education is a standard component of anticipatory guidance that addresses individual beliefs and practices in a culturally sensitive manner.[45,19,44] Special counseling is needed for those mothers planning to return to outside employment or school (see Guideline #7).[27] (II-2)

4. Families will benefit from appropriate, noncommercial educational materials on breastfeeding (as well as on other aspects of child health care).[42] (I) Discharge packs containing infant formula, pacifiers, commercial advertising materials specifically referring to infant formula and foods, and any materials not appropriate for a breastfeeding mother and infant should not be distributed. These products may encourage poor breastfeeding practices, which may lead to premature weaning.[42]

5. Breastfeeding mothers and appropriate others (fathers, partners, grandmothers, support persons, etc.) will benefit from simplified anticipatory guidance prior to discharge regarding key issues in the immediate future. (I) Care must be given not to overload mothers. Specific information should be provided in written form to all parents regarding:

a. prevention and management of engorgement
b. interpretation of infant cues and feeding "on cue"
c. indicators of adequate intake (evacuation of all meconium stools, three to four stools per day by day 4, transitioning to yellow bowel movements by day 5, at least five to six urinations per day by day 5, and regaining birth weight by day 10 to 14 at the latest)
d. signs of excessive jaundice[24,6] (III)
e. sleep patterns of newborns, including safe co-sleeping practices[2] (III)
f. maternal medication, cigarette, and alcohol use
g. individual feeding patterns, including normality of evening cluster feedings
h. regarding the use of pacifiers (in communities where the use of sanitary pacifiers is commonly recommended to prevent sudden infant death syndrome [SIDS]), discouraging their use until breastfeeding is well established, at least 3 to 4 weeks. (These recommendations are in accordance with the U.S.-based American Academy of Pediatrics recommendations for the use of pacifiers as a possible prevention of SIDS. Breastfeeding, in itself, is thought to be preventative for SIDS. The Japanese Ministry of Health, Labour and Welfare supports breastfeeding, no smoking, and back sleeping but does not encourage pacifier use.)[33,46,47,11,28] (I)
i follow-up and contact information

6. Every breastfeeding mother should receive instruction on the technique of expressing milk by hand (whether or not she uses a pump) so she is able to alleviate engorgement, increase her milk supply, maintain her milk supply, and obtain milk for feeding to the infant should she and the infant be separated or if the infant is unable to feed directly from the breast.[22,23,29] (II-1)

7. Every breastfeeding mother should be provided with the names and phone numbers of individuals and medical services that can provide advice, counseling, and health assessments related to breastfeeding, ideally on a 24-hour-a-day basis.[35,5] (I)

8. Every breastfeeding mother should be provided with lists of various local peer support groups and services (e.g., mother-to-mother support groups such as La Leche League, Australian Breastfeeding Association, hospital/clinic-based support groups, governmental supported groups [e.g., Special Supplemental Nutrition Program for Women, Infants, and Children (WIC) in the United States]

with phone numbers, contact names, and addresses). (II-1; III) Mothers should be encouraged to contact and consider joining one of these groups.[41,8,25,14,13,37,26] (II-3; III)

9. If a mother is planning on returning to school or outside employment soon after delivery, she may benefit from additional information.[23,29] (II-1) This should include the need for ongoing social support, possible milk supply issues, expressing and storing milk away from home, the possibility of direct nursing breaks with the infant, and information about any relevant regional and/or national laws regarding accommodations for breastfeeding and milk expression in the workplace. It is prudent to provide her with this information in written form, so that she has resources when the time comes for her to prepare for return to school or work.

10. In countries where hospital discharge is common within 72 hours after birth, appointments for the infant and mother where breastfeeding can be viewed should be made prior to discharge for an office or home visit within 3 to 5 days of age by a physician, midwife, or a physician-supervised breastfeeding-trained health care provider. All infants should be seen within 48 to 72 hours after discharge; infants discharged before 48 hours of age should be seen within 24 to 48 hours after discharge.[35,5] (III) In countries where discharge is 5 to 7 days after birth, the infant can be seen several times by the physician prior to discharge. In Japan, where this is the case, the next routine visit is recommended at 2 weeks unless there is a problem. Based on the mother's choice, her postpartum visit can be scheduled before discharge, or she can be given the information to make the appointment herself once she is settled at home. In many countries this appointment will be with the obstetrician, family physician, or midwife who participated in the birth of her infant. In other countries such as Australia, if she gave birth in a public hospital, it will be with her general practitioner or family practitioner, who did not attend her birth.

11. Additional visits for the mother and the infant are recommended even if discharge occurs at later than 5 days of age, until all clinical issues such as adequate stool and urine output, jaundice, and the infant attaining birth weight by 10 to 14 days of age are resolved.

An infant who is not back to birth weight by the first 10 days of life, but who has demonstrated a steady, appropriate weight gain for several days, is likely fine. This baby needs continued close follow-up but may not need intervention.

Any baby exhibiting a weight loss approaching 7% of birth weight by 5 to 6 days of life needs to be closely monitored until weight gain is well established. Should 7% or more weight loss be noted after 5 to 6 days of life, even more concern and careful follow-up must be pursued. These infants require careful assessment. By 4 to 6 days infants should be gaining weight daily, which makes their percentage weight loss actually more significant when that lack of daily weight gain is taken into account. In addition to attention to these issues, infants with any of these concerns must be specifically evaluated for problems with breastfeeding and milk transfer.[35,43,5,24,7,1,36] (III)

12. If the mother is medically ready for hospital discharge but the infant is not, every effort should be made to allow the mother to remain in the hospital either as a patient or as a "mother-in-residence" with access to the infant to support exclusive breastfeeding. Maintenance of a 24-hour rooming-in relationship with the infant is optimal during the infant's extended stay.[48,31,37] (II-1)

13. If the mother is discharged from the hospital before the infant is discharged (as in the case of a sick infant), the mother should be encouraged to spend as much time as possible with the infant, to practice skin-to-skin technique and kangaroo care with her infant whenever possible, and to continue regular breastfeeding.[21,15,18,32,38] (I; II-2) During periods when the mother is not in the hospital, she should be taught to express and store her milk and to bring it to the hospital for the infant. At the least she should demonstrate successful expression of her milk before hospital discharge. If she has problems with her milk supply, early referral to a lactation consultant and/or a physician skilled in breastfeeding management and medicine is indicated. (III) Milk may be expressed at home and brought in to the hospital for use by the baby. Some countries discourage this practice, but there is no evidence to contradict this recommendation and much evidence to support the use of mother's milk for these fragile infants.[5]

Suggestions for Future Research

Although the majority of the clinical recommendations in this policy are firmly evidence-based, areas for future study remain. We know that in some areas of the world, initiation rates are high in the hospital but fall precipitously after hospital discharge. Once mothers and infants receive the best evidence-based information and assistance possible in the hospital, what best practices need to be established to ensure that the process of "going home" is a smooth one? What culturally appropriate safety nets of support, help, and advice need to be readily and easily available to them, regardless of where they live and their socioeconomic or educational level? There is much work that can be done in this area to develop and test model policies and plans of action that could then be replicated in similar areas to determine best practices to support exclusive breastfeeding.

A Cochrane Review was done in 2002[16] looking at the effect of "early discharge" (less than 48 to 72 hours) on maternal/infant outcomes, including breastfeeding out to 6 months. The results were equivocal, with no differences in sample and control groups, but there was no standardization of definitions or any attempt to quantify teaching in hospital and follow-up on "going home." This is an area ripe for examination as we try to discern when a dyad is ready for discharge home.[7] Finally, if future research deliberately uses the same primary and secondary outcome measures currently described in the literature, then meta-analysis of these data will become possible.[38]

Acknowledgments

This work was supported in part by a grant from the Maternal and Child Health Bureau, U.S. Department of Health and Human Services.

REFERENCES[1]

1. Academy of Breastfeeding Medicine Board of Directors: Position on breastfeeding, *Breastfeed Med* 3:269–270, 2008.
2. Academy of Breastfeeding Medicine Protocol Committee: ABM clinical protocol #6: Guideline on co-sleeping and breastfeeding. Revision, March, 2008, *Breastfeed Med* 3:38–43, 2008.
3. Ahluwalia IB, Morrow B, Hsia J: Why do women stop breastfeeding? Findings from the pregnancy risk assessment and monitoring system, *Pediatrics* 116:1408–1412, 2005.
4. American Academy of Family Physicians. Breastfeeding Policy Statement, 2013. www.aafp.org/about/policies/all/breastfeeding.html. Accessed December 13, 2013.
5. American Academy of Pediatrics, Section on Breastfeeding: Policy statement: breastfeeding and the use of human milk, *Pediatrics* 129:e327–e341, 2012.
6. American Academy of Pediatrics Subcommittee on Hyperbilirubinemia: Management of hyperbilirubinemia in the newborn infant 35 or more weeks of gestation, *Pediatrics* 114:297–316, 2004.
7. American College Obstetricians Gynecologists: Committee Opinion No. 570: breastfeeding in underserved women:

increasing initiation and continuation of breastfeeding, *Obstet Gynecol* 122:323–428, 2013.
8. Anderson AK, Damio G, Young S, et al: A randomized trial assessing the efficacy of peer counseling on exclusive breastfeeding in a predominantly Latina low-income community, *Arch Pediatr Adolesc Med* 159:836–841, 2005.
9. Appendix A Task Force Ratings Guide to Clinical Preventive Services: Report of the U.S. Preventive Services Task Force, ed 2, www.ncbi.nlm.nih.gov/books/NBK15430. Accessed December 15, 2013.
10. Ballard J: Academy of Breastfeeding Medicine Protocol Committee. Clinical protocol #11: Guidelines for the evaluation and management of neonatal ankyloglossia and its complications in the breastfeeding dyad, 2004 [Members Only page]. http://www.bfmed.org/Media/Files/Protocols/ankyloglossia.pdf. Accessed December 19, 2013.
11. Blair PS, Sidebotham P, Evason-Coombe C, et al: Hazardous cosleeping environments and risk factors amenable to change: case control study of SIDS in South West England, *BMJ* 339:b3666, 2009.
12. Britton JR, Baker A, Spino C, et al: Postpartum discharge preferences of pediatricians: results from a national survey, *Pediatrics* 110:53–60, 2002.
13. Bronner Y, Barber T, Davis S: Breastfeeding peer counseling: policy implications, *J Hum Lact* 17:105–109, 2001.
14. Bronner Y, Barber T, Vogelhut J, et al: Breastfeeding peer counseling: results from the national WIC survey, *J Hum Lact* 17:119–168, 2001.
15. Browne JV: Early relationship environments: physiology of skin-to-skin contact for parents and their preterm infants, *Clin Perinatol* 31:287–298, 2004.
16. Brown S, Small R, Argus B, et al: Early postnatal discharge from hospital for healthy mothers and term infants, *Cochrane Database Syst Rev* 3:CD002958, 2002.
17. Buryk M, Bloom D, Shope T: Efficacy of neonatal release of ankyloglossia: a randomized trial, *Pediatrics* 128:280–288, 2011.
18. Carfoot S, Williamson PR, Dickson R: A systematic review of randomized controlled trials evaluating the effect of mother/baby skin-to-skin care on successful breastfeeding, *Midwifery* 19:148–155, 2003.
19. Centers for Disease Control and Prevention: Racial and ethnic differences in breastfeeding initiation and duration, by state—national immunization survey, United States, 2004-2008, *MMWR Morb Mortal Wkly Rep* 59:327–334, 2010.
20. Centers for Disease Control and Prevention (CDC): Vital signs: hospital practices to support breastfeeding, United States, 2007 and 2009, *MMWR Morb Mortal Wkly Rep* 60:1020–1025, 2011.
21. DiGirolamo AM, Grummer-Strawn LM, Fein SB: Effect of maternity-care practices on breastfeeding, *Pediatrics* 122 (Suppl 2):S43–S49, 2008.
22. Eglash A: Academy of Breastfeeding Medicine Protocol Committee: ABM clinical protocol #8: human milk storage information for home use for full-term infants (original protocol March 2004; revision #1 March 2010), *Breastfeed Med* 5:127–130, 2010.
23. Eldridge S, Croker A: Breastfeeding friendly workplace accreditation. Creating supportive workplaces for breastfeeding women, *Breastfeed Rev* 13:17–22, 2005.
24. Gartner L: ABM Clinical Protocol #22: guidelines for management of jaundice in the breastfeeding infant equal or greater than 35 weeks gestation, *Breastfeed Med* 5:87–93, 2010.
25. Graffy J, Taylor J: What information, advice, and support do women want with breastfeeding? *Birth* 32:179–186, 2005.
26. Gross SM, Resnik AK, Nanda JP, et al: Early postpartum: a critical period in setting the path for breastfeeding success, *Breastfeed Med* 6:407–412, 2011.
27. Guendelman S, Kosa JL, Pearl M, et al: Juggling work and breastfeeding: effect of maternity leave and occupational characteristics, *Pediatrics* 123:e38–e46, 2009.

[1]ABM protocols expire 5 years from the date of publication. Evidence-based revisions are made within 5 years or sooner if there are significant changes in the evidence.

28. Hauck FR, Thompson JM, Tanabe KO, et al: Breastfeeding and reduced risk of sudden infant death syndrome: a meta-analysis, *Pediatrics* 128:1–8, 2011.

29. Health Resources and Services Administration. The Business Case for Breastfeeding. Steps for Creating a Breastfeeding Friendly Worksite: Bottom Line Benefits, 2008. http://mchb.hrsa.gov/pregnancyandbeyond/breastfeeding/. Accessed December 13, 2013.

30. James DC, Dobson B: American Dietetic Association: Position of the American Dietetic Association: promoting and supporting breastfeeding, *J Am Diet Assoc* 105:810–818, 2005.

31. Joint Commission Perinatal Core Measures. http://manual.jointcommission.org/releases/TJC2013A/PerinatalCare.html. Accessed December 13, 2013.

32. Kirsten GF, Bergman NJ, Hann FM: Kangaroo mother care in the nursery, *Pediatr Clin North Am* 48:443–452, 2001.

33. Kramer MS, Barr RG, Dagenais S, et al: Pacifier use, early weaning, and cry/fuss behavior, *JAMA* 286:322–326, 2001.

34. Kramer MS, Kakuma R: Optimal duration of exclusive breastfeeding, *Cochrane Database Syst Rev* 1:CD003517, 2002.

35. Langan RC: Discharge procedures for healthy newborns, *Am Fam Physician* 73:849–852, 2006.

36. Lawrence RA, Lawrence RM: *Breastfeeding: a guide for the medical professional*, ed 7, Philadelphia, Pa., 2010, Saunders.

37. Mickens AD, Modeste N, Montgomery S, et al: Peer support and breastfeeding intentions: among black WIC participants, *J Hum Lact* 25:157–162, 2009.

38. Moore ER, Anderson GC, Bergman NJ: Early skin-to-skin contact for mothers and their healthy newborn infants, *Cochrane Database Syst Rev* 3:CD003519, 2011.

39. National Health and Medical Research Council: *Infant feeding guidelines*, Canberra, 2012, National Health and Medical Research Council.

40. Neifert MR: Prevention of breastfeeding tragedies, *Pediatr Clin North Am* 48:273–297, 2001.

41. Phillip BL: Every call is an opportunity. Supporting breastfeeding mothers over the telephone, *Pediatr Clin North Am* 48:525–532, 2001.

42. Sadacharan R, Grossman X, Matlak S, et al: Hospital discharge bags and breastfeeding at 6 months: data from the Infant Feeding Practices Study II, *J Hum Lact*, 2013. http://dx.doi.org/10.1177/0890334413513653. http://jhl.sagepub.com/content/early/2013/11/25/0890334413513653.full.pdf+html. Accessed December 19, 2013 [Epub ahead of print].

43. Schanler RJ, Krebs N, Mass S, editors: *Breastfeeding handbook for physicians*, ed 2, Elk Grove Village, Ill., 2014, American Academy of Pediatrics and American College of Obstetrics and Gynecologists.

44. Segawe M: Buddhism and breastfeeding, *Breastfeed Med* 3:124–128, 2008.

45. Setrakian HU, Rosenman MB, Szucs K: Breastfeeding and the Bahá'í faith, *Breastfeed Med* 6:221–225, 2011.

46. Task Force on Sudden Infant Death Syndrome: SIDS and other sleep related infant deaths: expansion of recommendations for a safe infant sleeping environment, *Pediatrics* 128:1030–1039, 2011.

47. Task Force on Sudden Infant Death Syndrome: Technical report: SIDS and other sleep related infant deaths: expansion of recommendations for a safe infant sleep environment, *Pediatrics* 128:e1341–e1367, 2011.

48. U.S. Department of Health and Human Services: *The surgeon general's call to action to support breastfeeding*, Washington, D.C., 2011, Office of the Surgeon General, U.S. Department of Health and Human Services.

49. World Health Organization, United Nations Children's Fund: Protecting, promoting and supporting breastfeeding: the special role of maternity services (a joint WHO/UNICEF statement), *Int J Gynaecol Obstet* 31:171–183, 1990.

50. World Health Organization. The Optimal Duration of Exclusive Breastfeeding: Report of an Expert Consultation. March 2001. www.who.int/nutrition/publications/optimal_duration_of_exc_bfeeding_report_eng.pdf. Accessed December 13, 2013.

51. Yanicki S, Hasselback P, Sandilands M, et al: The safety of Canadian early discharge guidelines, *Can J Public Health* 93:26–30, 2002.

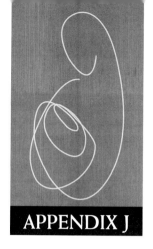

APPENDIX J

Protocol 3: Hospital Guidelines for the Use of Supplementary Feedings in the Healthy Term Breastfed Neonate

The Academy of Breastfeeding Medicine Protocol Committee

A central goal of the Academy of Breastfeeding Medicine is the development of clinical protocols for managing common medical problems that may impact breastfeeding success. These protocols serve only as guidelines for the care of breastfeeding mothers and infants and do not delineate an exclusive course of treatment or serve as standards of medical care. Variations in treatment may be appropriate according to the needs of an individual patient.

Definitions

- *Supplementary feedings:* Feedings provided in place of breastfeeding. This may include expressed or banked breastmilk and/or breastmilk substitutes/formula. Any foods given prior to 6 months, the recommended duration of exclusive breastfeeding, are thus defined as supplementary.
- *Complementary feedings:* Feedings provided in addition to breastfeeding when breastmilk alone is no longer sufficient. This term is used to describe foods or liquids given in addition to breastfeeding after 6 months, a "complement" to breastfeeding needed for adequate nutrition.

Background

Given early opportunities to breastfeed, breastfeeding assistance, and instruction, the vast majority of mothers and babies will successfully establish breastfeeding. Although some infants may not successfully latch and feed during the first day (24 hours) of life, they will successfully establish breastfeeding with time, appropriate evaluation, and minimal intervention. Unfortunately, formula supplementation of healthy newborn infants in the hospital is commonplace, despite widespread recommendations to the contrary.[13,28] The most recent scientific evidence indicates that *exclusive breastfeeding* (only breastmilk, no food or water except vitamins and medications) for the first 6 months is associated with the greatest protection against major health problems for both mothers and infants.[34,43,54]

NEWBORN PHYSIOLOGY

Small colostrum feedings are appropriate for the size of the newborn's stomach;[58,75,94] are sufficient to prevent hypoglycemia in the healthy, term, appropriate for gestational age infant;[88–90] and easy to manage as the infant learns to coordinate sucking, swallowing, and breathing. Healthy term infants also have sufficient body water to meet their metabolic needs, even in hot climates.[19,31,50,67,73,72,77] Fluid necessary to replace insensible fluid loss is adequately provided by breastmilk alone.[72,5,76] Newborns lose weight because of a physiologic diuresis of extracellular fluid following transition to extrauterine life.[94] The normal maximal weight loss is 5.5% to 6.6% of birth weight in optimally exclusively breastfed infants[50,67,48,52] and occurs between days 2 and 3 of life (48-72 hours after birth).[50,67,48] Optimally, breastfed infants regain birth weight at an average (95% confidence interval) of 8.3 days (7.7 to 8.9) with 97.5% having regained their birth weight by 21 days.[48] Percentage weight loss should be followed closely for outliers in this regard, but the majority of breastfed infants will not require supplementation.

EARLY MANAGEMENT OF THE NEW BREASTFEEDING MOTHER

Because some breastfeeding mothers question the adequacy of colostrum feedings and may receive conflicting advice, they may benefit from reassurance, assistance with breastfeeding technique, and education about the normal physiology of breastfeeding. Inappropriate supplementation may undermine a mother's confidence about her ability to meet her infant's nutritional needs[8] and give inappropriate messages that may result in continued supplementation of the breastfed infant at home.[66]

Postpartum mothers with low confidence levels are very vulnerable to external influences, such as advice to offer breastfeeding infants supplemention such as glucose water or artificial baby milk.[8] Well-meaning health care professionals often offer supplementation as a means of protecting mothers from tiredness or distress, although this at times conflicts with their role in promoting breastfeeding.[17,46] Inappropriate reasons for supplementation and associated risks are multiple (see Appendix for quick reference).

There are common clinical situations where evaluation and breastfeeding management may be necessary, but supplementation is not indicated, including:

1. The sleepy infant with fewer than 8 to 12 feedings in the first 24 to 48 hours with less than 7% weight loss and no signs of illness
   - Newborns are normally sleepy after an initial approximately 2-hour alert period after birth.[25,80] They then have variable sleep-wake cycles, with an additional one or two wakeful periods in the next 10 hours whether fed or not.[25]
   - Careful attention to an infant's early feeding cues and gently rousing the infant to attempt breastfeeding every 2 to 3 hours is more appropriate than automatic supplementation after 6, 8, 12, or even 24 hours.
   - The general rule in the first week is: "an awake baby is a hungry baby!"
   - Increased skin-on-skin time can encourage more frequent feeding.
2. The healthy, term, appropriate for gestational age infant with bilirubin levels less than 18 mg/dL (mol/L) after 72 hours of age when the baby is feeding well and stooling adequately and weight loss is less than 7%[4]
3. The infant who is fussy at night or constantly feeding for several hours
4. The tired or sleeping mother

For both points 3 and 4 above, breastfeeding management that optimizes infant feeding at the breast may make for a more satisfied infant and allow the mother to get more rest.

Before any supplementary feedings are begun, it is important that a formal evaluation of each mother-baby dyad, including a direct observation of breastfeeding, is completed. The following guidelines address indications for and methods of supplementation for the healthy, term (37- to 42-week), breastfed infant. Indications for supplementation in term, healthy infants are few[65,23] (Table J-9).

TABLE J-9	Indications for Supplemental Feeding in Term, Healthy Infants (Situations Where Breastfeeding Is Not Possible)

1. Separation
   - Maternal illness resulting in separation of infant and mother (e.g., shock or psychosis)
   - Mother not at the same hospital
2. Infant with inborn error of metabolism (e.g., galactosemia)
3. Infant who is unable to feed at the breast (e.g., congenital malformation, illness)
4. Maternal medications (those contraindicated in breastfeeding)[20]

TABLE J-10	Possible Indications for Supplementation in Term, Healthy Infants

1. Infant indications

   a. Asymptomatic hypoglycemia documented by laboratory blood glucose measurement (not bedside screening methods) that is unresponsive to appropriate frequent breastfeeding. Symptomatic infants should be treated with intravenous glucose. (Please see ABM Hypoglycemia Protocol for more details.[88,89])

   b. Clinical and laboratory evidence of significant dehydration (e.g., >10% weight loss, high sodium, poor feeding, lethargy, etc.) that is not improved after skilled assessment and proper management of breastfeeding[92,59]

   c. Weight loss of 8-10% accompanied by delayed lactogenesis II (day 5 [120 hours] or later)

   d. Delayed bowel movements or continued meconium stools on day 5 (120 hours)[59,40]

   e. Insufficient intake despite an adequate milk supply (poor milk transfer)[59]

   f. Hyperbilirubinemia

     i. "Neonatal" jaundice associated with starvation where breastmilk intake is poor despite appropriate intervention (please see ABM Jaundice in the Breastfed Infant Protocol)

     ii. Breastmilk jaundice when levels reach >20-25 mg/dL (mol/L) in an otherwise thriving infant and where a diagnostic and/or therapeutic interruption of breastfeeding may be helpful

   g. When macronutrient supplementation is indicated

2. Maternal indications

   a. Delayed lactogenesis II (day 3-5 or later [72-120 hours]) and inadequate intake by the infant[59]

     i. Retained placenta (lactogenesis probably will occur after placental fragments are removed)

     ii. Sheehan's syndrome (postpartum hemorrhage followed by absence of lactogenesis)

     iii. Primary glandular insufficiency, occurs in less than 5% of women (primary lactation failure), as evidenced by poor breast growth during pregnancy and minimal indications of lactogenesis

   b. Breast pathology or prior breast surgery resulting in poor milk production[60]

   c. Intolerable pain during feedings unrelieved by interventions

Adapted with permission from Powers and Slusser.[65]

   Table J-10 lists possible indications for the administration of such feedings. The physician must decide if the clinical benefits outweigh the potential negative consequences of such feedings.

Recommendations

1. Healthy infants should be put skin-to-skin with the mother immediately after birth to facilitate breastfeeding,[4,23,69] because the delay in time between birth and initiation of the first breastfeed is a strong predictor of formula use.[46,79]

2. Antenatal education and in-hospital support can significantly improve rates of exclusive breastfeeding.[82] Both mothers and health care providers should be aware of the risks of unnecessary supplementation.

3. Healthy newborns do not need supplemental feedings for poor feeding for the first 24 to 48 hours, but babies who are too sick to breastfeed or whose mothers are too sick to allow breastfeeding are likely to require supplemental feedings.[65]

4. Hospitals should strongly consider instituting a policy regarding supplemental feedings to require a physician's order when supplements are medically indicated and informed consent of the mother when supplements are not medically indicated. It is the responsibility of the health professional to provide information, document parental decisions, and support the mother after she has made the decision.[35] When the decision is not medically indicated, efforts to educate the mother ought to be documented by the nursing and/or medical staff.

5. All supplemental feedings should be documented, including the content, volume, method, and medical indication or reason.

6. If mother-baby separation is unavoidable, established milk supply is poor or questionable, or milk transfer is inadequate, the mother needs instruction and encouragement to pump or manually express her milk to stimulate production and provide expressed breastmilk as necessary for the infant.[5,65,23,40]

7. When supplementary feeding is necessary, the primary goals are to feed the baby and also to optimize the maternal milk supply while determining the cause of poor feeding or inadequate milk transfer.

8. Whenever possible, it is ideal to have the mother and infant room-in 24 hours per day to enhance opportunities for breastfeeding and hence lactogenesis.[5,65,23,40]

9. Optimally, mothers need to express milk each time the baby receives a supplemental feeding, or about every 2 to 3 hours. Mothers should be encouraged to start expressing on the first day (within the first 24 hours) or as soon as possible. Maternal breast engorgement should be

avoided as it will further compromise the milk supply and may lead to other complications.[65,23]

10. All infants must be formally evaluated for position, latch, and milk transfer prior to the provision of supplemental feedings.[5,40] Most babies who remain with their mothers and breastfeed adequately lose less than 7% of their birth weight. Weight loss in excess of 7% may be an indication of inadequate milk transfer or low milk production.[59] Although weight loss in the range of 8% to 10% may be within normal limits, if all else is going well and the physical exam is normal, it is an indication for careful assessment and possible breastfeeding assistance.

11. The infant's physician should be notified if:
   a. The infant exhibits other signs of illness in addition to poor feeding.
   b. The mother-infant dyad meets the clinical criteria in Table J-9.
   c. The infant's weight loss is greater than 7%.

Choice of Supplemental Feeding

1. Expressed human milk is the first choice for supplemental feeding,[5,29] but sufficient colostrum in the first few days (0 to 72 hours) may not be available. The mother may need reassurance and education if such difficulties occur. Hand expression may elicit larger volumes than a pump in the first few days and may increase overall milk supply.[55] Breast massage along with expressing with a mechanical pump may also increase available milk.[56]

2. If the volume of the mother's own colostrum does not meet her infant's feeding requirements, pasteurized donor human milk is preferable to other supplements.[29]

3. Protein hydrolysate formulas are preferable to standard artificial milks as they avoid exposure to cow milk proteins, reduce bilirubin levels more rapidly,[32] and may convey the psychological message that the supplement is a temporary therapy, not a permanent inclusion of artificial feedings. Supplementation with glucose water is not appropriate.

4. The physician must weigh the potential risks and benefits of other supplemental fluids, such as standard formulas, soy formulas, or protein hydrolysate formula, with consideration given to available resources, the family's history for risk factors such as atopy, the infant's age, the amounts needed, and the potential impact on the establishment of breastfeeding.

Volume of Supplemental Feeding

Several studies give us an idea of intakes at the breast over time. In one study the mean yield of colostrum (using infant test-weighing) for over the first 24 hours after birth was 37.1 g (range, 7 to 122.5 g) with an average intake of 6 g per feed and six feedings in the first 24 hours.[74] A similar study also using test-weighing revealed a mean intake of 13 g/kg/24 hours (range, 3 to 32 g/kg/24 hours) for the first 24 hours, increasing to a mean of 98 g/kg/24 hours (range, 50 to 163 g/kg/24 hours) on day 3 (by 72 hours).[14] Yet another study[26] noted breastmilk transfer of 6 mL/kg/24 hours for day 1 (24 hours), 25 mL/kg/24 hours for day 2 (48 hours), 66 mL/kg/24 hours for day 3 (72 hours), and 106 mL/kg/24 hours for day 4 (96 hours) in healthy, vaginally delivered infants allowed on-demand breastfeeding. Interestingly, the intake of infants delivered by cesarean section was significantly less during days 2 to 4 (within 48 to 96 hours).[26] In a study where there was no rooming in and infants were fed every 4 hours, the average intake was 9.6 mL/kg/24 hours on day 1 and 13 mL/kg/24 hours on day 2 (48 hours).[24] In most studies, the range of intake is wide, with formula-fed infants usually taking in larger volumes than breastfed infants.

1. Infants fed artificial milks ad libitum commonly have higher intakes than breastfed infants.[24] Acknowledging that ad libitum breastfeeding recapitulates evolutionary feeding and considering recent data on obesity in artificially fed infants, it can be concluded that such artificially fed infants may well be overfed.

2. As there is no definitive research available, the amount of supplement given should reflect the normal amounts of colostrum available, the size of the infant's stomach (which changes over time), and the age and size of the infant.

3. Based on the limited research available, suggested intakes for term healthy infants are given in Table J-11, although feeding should be by infant cue to satiation.

TABLE J-11	Average Reported Intakes of Colostrum by Healthy Breastfed Infants[74,14,26,24]
Time	Intake (mL/feed)
1st 24 hours	2-10
24-48 hours	5-15
48-72 hours	15-30
72-96 hours	30-60

Methods of Providing Supplementary Feedings

1. When supplementary feedings are needed there are many methods from which to choose: a supplemental nursing device at the breast, cup feeding, spoon or dropper feeding, finger feeding, syringe feeding, or bottle feeding.[87]
2. There is little evidence about the safety or efficacy of most alternative feeding methods and their effect on breastfeeding; however, when cleanliness is suboptimal, cup feeding is the recommended choice.[29] Cup feeding has been shown safe for both term and preterm infants and may help preserve breastfeeding duration among those who require multiple supplemental feedings.[37,38,42,51,49,47]
3. Supplemental nursing systems have the advantage of supplying appropriate supplement while simultaneously stimulating the breast to produce more milk and reinforcing the infant's feeding at the breast. Unfortunately, most systems are awkward to use, difficult to clean, expensive, and require moderately complex learning.[87] A simpler version, supplementing with a dropper or syringe while the infant is at breast, may be effective.
4. Bottle feeding is the most commonly used method of supplementation in more affluent regions of the world but is of concern because of distinct differences in tongue and jaw movements, differences in flow, and long-term developmental concerns.[87] Some experts have recommended a nipple with a wide base and slow flow to try to mimic breastfeeding, but no research has been done evaluating outcomes with different nipples.
5. An optimal supplemental feeding device has not yet been identified, and they may vary from one infant to another. No method is without potential risk or benefit.[87,18]
6. When selecting an alternative feeding method, clinicians should consider several criteria:
   a. Cost and availability
   b. Ease of use and cleaning
   c. Stress to the infant
   d. Whether adequate milk volume can be fed in 20 to 30 minutes
   e. Whether anticipated use is short- or long-term
   f. Maternal preference
   g. Whether the method enhances development of breastfeeding skills.

Research Needs

1. Research is necessary to establish evidence-based guidelines on appropriate supplementation volumes for specific conditions and whether this varies for colostrum versus artificial milk. Other specific questions include: Should the volume be independent of infant weight or a per kg volume? Should supplementation make up for cumulative losses? Should feeding intervals be different for different supplements?
2. Research is also lacking on what is the optimal method of supplementation. Are some methods best for infants with certain conditions, ages, and available resources? Which methods interfere least with establishing direct breastfeeding?

Notes

This protocol addresses the term healthy newborn. For information regarding appropriate feeding and supplementation for the late preterm infant (35 to 37 weeks), see "ABM Protocol #10: Breastfeeding the Near-Term Infant"[1] and "Care and Management of the Late Preterm Infant Toolkit."[12]

The World Health Organization is currently updating its annex to the Global Criteria for the Baby Friendly Hospital Initiative: "Acceptable Medical Reasons for Supplementation."[6] The annex has been broadened to acceptable reasons for use of breastmilk substitutes in all infants. The handout (#4.5) is available at: http://www.who.int/nutrition/publications/infantfeeding/WHO_NMH_NHD_09.01/en/.

Acknowledgments

This work was supported in part by a grant to the Academy of Breastfeeding Medicine from the Maternal and Child Health Bureau, U.S. Department of Health and Human Services.

Contributors

*Nancy E. Wight, MD, FABM, FAAP
*Robert Cordes, MD, FAAP
Protocol Committee
Caroline J. Chantry, MD, FABM, Co-Chairperson
Cynthia R. Howard, MD, MPH, FABM, Co-Chairperson
Ruth A. Lawrence, MD, FABM
Kathleen A. Marinelli, MD, FABM, Co-Chairperson
Nancy G. Powers, MD, FABM
Maya Bunik, MD, MSPH, FABM

APPENDIX	Inappropriate Reasons for Supplementation, Responses, and Risks	
Concerns	**Responses**	**Risks of Supplementation**
There is no milk, or colostrum is insufficient, until the milk "comes in"	• Mother and family should be educated about the benefits of colostrum (e.g., liquid gold) including dispelling myths about the yellow substance. Small amounts of colostrum are normal, physiologic, and appropriate for the term healthy newborn.	• Can alter infant bowel flora.[9,68] • Potentially sensitizes the infant to foreign proteins.[70,71,83,36] • Increases the risk of diarrhea and other infections,[16,39,41,63] especially where hygiene is poor.[23,81] • Potentially disrupts the "supply-demand" cycle, leading to inadequate milk supply and long-term supplementation.
Concern about weight loss and dehydration in the postpartum period	• A certain amount of weight loss is normal in the first week of life and is due to both a diuresis of extracellular fluid received from the placenta and passage of meconium. • There is now evidence that too *little* weight loss in the newborn period is associated with an increased risk of obesity later in life.[81]	• Supplementation in the first few days interferes with the normal frequency of breastfeedings.[23,86] • If the supplement is water or glucose water, the infant is at risk for increased bilirubin,[44,21,61,62,85] excess weight loss,[30] and potential water intoxication.[76]
Concern about infant becoming hypoglycemic	• Healthy, full-term infants do not develop symptomatic hypoglycemia simply as a result of suboptimal breastfeeding.[90]	• Risk for weight loss/dehydration.
Concern about jaundice	• The more frequent the breastfeeding, the lower the bilirubin level.[4,93,22] • Bilirubin is a potent antioxidant.[45] The appropriately breastfed infant has *normal* levels of bilirubin unless affected by another pathologic process such as hemolysis (e.g., ABO or Rh incompatibility). • Colostrum acts as a natural laxative, helping to eliminate the retained pool of bilirubin contained in meconium.	• Risk for weight loss/dehydration.
Not enough time to counsel mother about exclusive breastfeeding, mothers may request supplement	• Training all staff in how to assist mothers with breastfeeding is important. • Mothers may also benefit from education about artificial feeds and/or how supplements may adversely affect subsequent breastfeeding.[17,79] • Help health care professionals understand that time spent on passive activities and interactions such as listening to and talking with mothers is of critical importance as opposed to other more active interventions (which may be viewed more as "real work" to them).[17,79]	• If the supplement is artificial milk, which is slow to empty from the stomach[15,84] and often fed in larger amounts,[24] the infant will breastfeed less frequently.[24] • Depending on the method of supplementation[87,53] or the number of supplements,[38,87] an infant may have difficulty returning to the breast. • Prelacteal feeds (as opposed to supplementation) are associated with delayed initiation of breastfeeding and negatively associated with exclusivity and duration of breastfeeding.[38,27,10,64]
Medications that may be contraindicated with breastfeeding	• Accurate references are easily available to providers (e.g., Lactmed on Toxnet website,[57] AAP policy,[3] *Medications and Mothers' Milk*[33]).	• Risk of decreasing breastfeeding duration or exclusivity.
Mother too malnourished or sick to breastfeed	• Even malnourished mothers can breastfeed. • Reasons for supplementation with maternal illness that are listed in text.	• Risk of decreasing breastfeeding duration or exclusivity.
Need to quiet a fussy or unsettled baby	• Infants can be unsettled for many reasons. They may wish to "cluster feed" (several short feeds in a short period of time) or simply need additional skin-to-skin time or holding.[87] • Filling (and often *overfilling*) the stomach with artificial milk may make the infant sleep longer,[84] missing important opportunities to breastfeed, and demonstrating to the mother a short-term solution that may generate long-term health risks. • Teaching other soothing techniques to new mothers such as breastfeeding, swaddling, swaying, side lying techniques, encouraging father or other relatives to assist. Again, caution should be taken to not ignore early feeding cues.[11]	• Risk of decreasing breastfeeding duration or exclusivity.[42,61,53,91,2,8,17,46] • Studies have noted delayed lactogenesis II (also known as "secretory activation" or "milk coming in").[79] Maternal engorgement due to decreased frequency of breastfeeding in the immediate postpartum period.[66,7]

Continued

APPENDIX	Inappropriate Reasons for Supplementation, Responses, and Risks—cont'd	
Concerns	**Responses**	**Risks of Supplementation**
Accommodate growth or appetite spurts or periods of cluster feeds	• Periods when infants demand to nurse more and/or excrete less stool are sometimes interpreted by mothers as insufficient milk. This may happen in later weeks but also in the second or third night (48-72 hours) at home, in the immediate postpartum period. • Anticipatory guidance may be helpful.	• Risk of decreasing breastfeeding duration or exclusivity.
Mother needs to rest or sleep	• Postpartum mother has been shown to be restless when separated from her infant and actually gets less rest.[17] • Mothers lose the opportunity to learn their infant's normal behavior and early feeding cues.[40] • The highest risk time of day for an infant to receive a supplement is between 7 PM and 9 AM.[2]	• Risk of decreasing breastfeeding duration or exclusivity.
Taking a break will help with sore nipples	• Sore nipples are a function of latch, positioning, and sometimes individual anatomic variation, like ankyloglossia, not length of time nursing.[78] • There is no evidence that limiting time at the breast will prevent sore nipples.	• Problem with latch not addressed. • Risk of shortening breastfeeding duration or cessation of breastfeeding.

Compiled by Maya Bunik, MD, MSPH.
AAP, American Academy of Pediatrics.

REFERENCES[1]

1. ABM Protocol #10: Breastfeeding the Near-Term Infant. http://www.bfmed.org. Accessed July 30, 2009.
2. Akuse R, Obinya E: Why healthcare workers give prelacteal feeds, *Eur J Clin Nutr* 56:729–734, 2002.
3. American Academy of Pediatrics Committee on Drugs: Transfer of drugs and other chemicals into human milk, *Pediatrics* 108:776–789, 2001.
4. American Academy of Pediatrics: Management of hyperbilirubinemia in the newborn infant 35 or more weeks of gestation, *Pediatrics* 114:297–316, 2004.
5. American Academy of Pediatrics, Section on Breastfeeding: Policy statement: breastfeeding and the use of human milk, *Pediatrics* 115:496–506, 2005.
6. Annex to the Global Criteria for the Baby Friendly Hospital Initiative (A39/8 Add.1). World Health Organization, Geneva, 1992, pp. 122–135.
7. Blomquist HK, Jonsbo F, Serenius F, et al: Supplementary feeding in the maternity ward shortens the duration of breast feeding, *Acta Paediatr* 83:1122–1126, 1994.
8. Blyth R, Creedy D, Dennis C, et al: Effect of maternal confidence on breastfeeding duration: an application of breastfeeding self-efficacy theory, *Birth* 29:278–284, 2002.
9. Bullen C, Tearle P, Stewart M: The effect of "humanized" milks and supplemented breast feeding on the faecal flora of infants, *J Med Microbiol* 10:403–413, 1977.
10. Bunik M, Beaty B, Dickinson M, et al: Early formula supplementation in breastfeeding mothers: how much is too much for breastfeeding success? [abstract 18], *Breastfeed Med* 1:184, 2007.
11. Bystrova K, Matthiesen AS, Widström AM, et al: The effect of Russian Maternity Home routines on breastfeeding and neonatal weight loss with special reference to swaddling, *Early Hum Dev* 83:29–39, 2007.
12. California Perinatal Care Collaborative. Care and Management of the Late Preterm Infant Toolkit. http://www.cpqcc.org. Accessed July 30, 2009.
13. California WIC Association, UC Davis Human Lactation Center. A fair start for better health: California hospitals must close the gap in exclusive breastfeeding rates. http://www.calwic.org. Accessed November 2007.
14. Casey CE, Neifert MR, Seacat JM, et al: Nutrient intake by breast-fed infants during the first five days after birth, *Am J Dis Child* 140:933–936, 1986.
15. Cavell B: Gastric emptying in infants fed human milk or infant formula, *Acta Paediatr Scand* 70:639–641, 1981.
16. Chen A, Rogan WJ: Breastfeeding and the risk of postneonatal death in the United States, *Pediatrics* 113:e435–e439, 2004.
17. Cloherty M, Alexander J, Holloway I: Supplementing breast-fed babies in the UK to protect their mothers from tiredness or distress, *Midwifery* 20:194–204, 2004.
18. Cloherty M, Alexander J, Holloway I, et al: The cup-versus-bottle debate: a theme from an ethnographic study of the supplementation of breastfed infants in hospital in the United Kingdom, *J Hum Lact* 21:151–162, 2005; quiz 63-66.
19. Cohen RJ, Brown K, Rivera L, et al: Exclusively breastfed, low birth weight term infants do not need supplemental water, *Acta Paediatr* 89:550–552, 2000.
20. Committee on Drugs, The American Academy of Pediatrics: The transfer of drugs and other chemicals into human milk, *Pediatrics* 108:776–789, 2001.
21. de Carvalho M, Hall M, Harvey D: Effects of water supplementation on physiological jaundice in breast-fed babies, *Arch Dis Child* 56:568–569, 1981.
22. De Carvalho M, Klaus MH, Merkatz RB: Frequency of breast-feeding and serum bilirubin concentration, *Am J Dis Child* 136:737–738, 1982.
23. Division of Child Health and Development, World Health Organization: *Evidence for the Ten Steps to Successful Breastfeeding*,

---

[1]ABM protocols expire 5 years from the date of publication. Evidence-based revisions are made within 5 years or sooner if there are significant changes in the evidence.

Geneva, 1998, World Health Organization. Publication WHO/CHD/98.9.

24. Dollberg S, Lahav S, Mimouni FB: A comparison of intakes of breast-fed and bottle-fed infants during the first two days of life, *J Am Coll Nutr* 20:209–211, 2001.

25. Emde R, Swedberg J, Suzuki B: Human wakefulness and biological rhythms after birth, *Arch Gen Psychiatry* 32:780–783, 1975.

26. Evans KC, Evans RG, Royal R, et al: Effect of caesarean section on breast milk transfer to the normal term newborn over the first week of life, *Arch Dis Child Fetal Neonatal Ed* 88:F380–F382, 2003.

27. Feinstein JM, Berkelhamer JE, Gruszka ME, et al: Factors related to early termination of breast-feeding in an urban population, *Pediatrics* 78:210–215, 1986.

28. Gagnon AJ, Leduc G, Waghorn K, et al: In-hospital formula supplementation of healthy breastfeeding newborns, *J Hum Lact* 21:397–405, 2005.

29. World Health Organization/UNICEF: *Global strategy for infant and young child feeding*, Geneva, 2003, World Health Organization/UNICEF.

30. Glover J, Sandilands M: Supplementation of breastfeeding infants and weight loss in hospital, *J Hum Lact* 6:163–166, 1990.

31. Goldberg N, Adams E: Supplementary water for breast-fed babies in a hot and dry climate—not really a necessity, *Arch Dis Child* 58:73–74, 1983.

32. Gourley GR, Kreamer B, Cohnen M, et al: Neonatal jaundice and diet, *Arch Pediatr Adolesc Med* 153:184–188, 1999.

33. Hale TW: *Medications and mothers' milk*, Amarillo, Tex., 2008, Hale Publishing.

34. Heinig M: Host defense benefits of breastfeeding for the infant. Effect of breastfeeding duration and exclusivity, *Pediatr Clin North Am* 48:105–123, 2001.

35. Henrikson M: A policy for supplementary/complementary feedings for breastfed newborn infants, *J Hum Lact* 6:11–14, 1990.

36. Host A: Importance of the first meal on the development of cow's milk allergy and intolerance, *Allergy Proc* 12:227–232, 1991.

37. Howard CR, de Blieck EA, ten Hoopen CB, et al: Physiologic stability of newborns during cup- and bottle-feeding, *Pediatrics* 104:1204–1207, 1999.

38. Howard CR, Howard FM, Lanphear B, et al: Randomized clinical trial of pacifier use and bottle-feeding or cupfeeding and their effect on breastfeeding, *Pediatrics* 111:511–518, 2003.

39. Howie PW, Forsyth JS, Ogston SA, et al: Protective effect of breast feeding against infection, *BMJ* 300:11–16, 1990.

40. International Lactation Consultant Association: *Clinical guidelines for the establishment of exclusive breastfeeding*, 2005: http://www.ilca.org/files/resources/ClinicalGuidelines2005.pdf. Accessed July 30, 2009.

41. Ip S, Chung M, Raman G, et al: *Breastfeeding and maternal and infant health outcomes in developed countries. Evidence Report/Technology Assessment No. 153*, Rockville, Md., 2007, Agency for Healthcare Research and Quality. AHRQ Publication 07-E007.

42. Kramer MS, Chalmers B, Hodnett ED, et al: Promotion of Breastfeeding Intervention Trial (PROBIT): a randomized trial in the Republic of Belarus, *JAMA* 285:413–420, 2001.

43. Kramer MS, Kakuma R: The optimal duration of exclusive breastfeeding: a systematic review, *Adv Exp Med Biol* 554:63–77, 2004.

44. Kuhr M, Paneth N: Feeding practices and early neonatal jaundice, *J Pediatr Gastroenterol Nutr* 1:485–488, 1982.

45. Kumar A, Pant P, Basu S, et al: Oxidative stress in neonatal hyperbilirubinemia, *J Trop Pediatr* 53:69–71, 2007.

46. Kurinij N, Shiono P: Early formula supplementation of breastfeeding, *Pediatrics* 88:745–750, 1991.

47. Lang S, Lawrence CJ, Orme RL: Cup feeding: an alternative method of infant feeding, *Arch Dis Child* 71:365–369, 1994.

48. MacDonald P, Ross S, Grant L, et al: Neonatal weight loss in breast and formula fed infants, *Arch Dis Child Fetal Neonatal Ed* 88:F472–F476, 2003.

49. Malhotra N, Vishwambaran L, Sundaram KR, et al: A controlled trial of alternative methods of oral feeding in neonates, *Early Hum Dev* 54:29–38, 1999.

50. Marchini G, Stock S: Thirst and vasopressin secretion counteract dehydration in newborn infants, *J Pediatr* 130:736–739, 1997.

51. Marinelli KA, Burke GS, Dodd VL: A comparison of the safety of cupfeedings and bottlefeedings in premature infants whose mothers intend to breastfeed, *J Perinatol* 21:350–355, 2001.

52. Martens PJ, Phillips SJ, Cheang MS, et al: How babyfriendly are Manitoba hospitals? The Provincial Infant Feeding Study. Breastfeeding Promotion Steering Committee of Manitoba, *Can J Public Health* 91:51–57, 2000.

53. Matheny RJ, Birch LL, Picciano MF: Control of intake by human-milk-fed infants: relationships between feeding size and interval, *Dev Psychobiol* 23:511–518, 1990.

54. Mihrshahi S, Ichikawa N, Shuaib M, et al: Prevalence of exclusive breastfeeding in Bangladesh and its association with diarrhoea and acute respiratory infection: results of the multiple indicator cluster survey 2003, *J Health Popul Nutr* 25:195–204, 2007.

55. Morton J: Early hand expression affects breastmilk production in pump-dependent mothers of preterm infants [abstract 7720.9]. In Pediatric Academic Societies Scientific Program. Pediatric Academic Societies, Toronto, 2007.

56. Morton J: Breast massage maximizes milk volumes of pump-dependent mothers [abstract 444]. In Pediatric Academic Societies Scientific Program. Pediatric Academic Societies, Toronto; 2007.

57. National Library of Medicine. TOXNET, LactMed. http://toxnet.nlm.nih.gov/cgi-bin/sis/htmlgen?LACT. Accessed July 30, 2009.

58. Naveed M, Manjunath C, Sreenivas V: An autopsy study of relationship between perinatal stomach capacity and birth weight, *Indian J Gastroenterol* 11:156–158, 1992.

59. Neifert MR: Prevention of breastfeeding tragedies, *Pediatr Clin North Am* 48:273–297, 2001.

60. Neifert MR, Seacat JM, Jobe WE: Lactation failure due to insufficient glandular development of the breast, *Pediatrics* 76:823–828, 1985.

61. Nicoll A, Ginsburg R, Tripp JH: Supplementary feeding and jaundice in newborns, *Acta Paediatr Scand* 71:759–761, 1982.

62. Nylander G, Lindemann R, Helsing E, et al: Unsupplemented breastfeeding in the maternity ward. Positive long-term effects, *Acta Obstet Gynecol Scand* 70:205–209, 1991.

63. Paricio Talayero JM, Lizan-Garcia M, Otero Puime A, et al: Full breastfeeding and hospitalization as a result of infections in the first year of life, *Pediatrics* 118:e92–e99, 2006.

64. Perez-Escamilla R, Segura-Millan S, Canahuati J, et al: Prelacteal feeds are negatively associated with breast-feeding outcomes in Honduras, *J Nutr* 126:2765–2773, 1996.

65. Powers NG, Slusser W: Breastfeeding update. 2: Clinical lactation management, *Pediatr Rev* 18:147–161, 1997.

66. Reiff MI, Essock-Vitale SM: Hospital influences on early infant-feeding practices, *Pediatrics* 76:872–879, 1985.

67. Rodriquez G, Ventura P, Samper M, et al: Changes in body composition during the initial hours of life in breast-fed healthy term newborns, *Biol Neonate* 77:12–16, 2000.

68. Rubaltelli F, Biadaioli R, Pecile P, et al: Intestinal flora in breast- and bottle-fed infants, *J Perinat Med* 26:186–191, 1998.

69. Saadeh R, Akre J: Ten steps to successful breastfeeding: a summary of the rationale and scientific evidence, *Birth* 23:154–160, 1996.

70. Saarinen K, Juntunen-Backman K, Jarvenpaa A, et al: Supplementary feeding in maternity hospitals and the risk of cow's milk allergy: a prospective study of 6209 infants, *J Allergy Clin Immunol* 104:457–461, 1999.
71. Saarinen U, Kajosaari M: Breastfeeding as prophylaxis against atopic disease: prospective follow-up study until 17 years old, *Lancet* 346:1065–1069, 1995.
72. Sachdev H, Krishna J, Puri R, et al: Water supplementation in exclusively breastfed infants during summer in the tropics, *Lancet* 337:929–933, 1991.
73. Sachdev H, Krishna J, Puri R: Do exclusively breast fed infants need fluid supplementation? *Indian Pediatr* 29:535–540, 1992.
74. Saint L, Smith M, Hartmann PE: The yield and nutrient content of colostrum and milk of women from giving birth to 1 month post-partum, *Br J Nutr* 52:87–95, 1984.
75. Scammon R, Doyle L: Observations on the capacity of the stomach in the first ten days of postnatal life, *Am J Dis Child* 20:516–538, 1920.
76. Scariati P, Grummer-Strawn L, Fein S: Water supplementation of infants in the first month of life, *Arch Pediatr Adolesc Med* 151:830–832, 1997.
77. Shrago L: Glucose water supplementation of the breastfed infant during the first three days of life, *J Hum Lact* 3:82–86, 1987.
78. Slaven S, Harvey D: Unlimited suckling time improves breastfeeding, *Lancet* 1:392–393, 1981.
79. Smale M: Working with breastfeeding mothers: the psychosocial context. In Clement S, editor: *Psychological perspectives on pregnancy and childbirth*, Edinburgh, 1998, Churchill Livingstone, pp 183–204.
80. Stern E, Parmalee A, Akiyama Y, et al: Sleep cycle characteristics in infants, *Pediatrics* 43:67–70, 1969.
81. Stettler N, Stallings VA, Troxel AB, et al: Weight gain in the first week of life and overweight in adulthood: a cohort study of European American subjects fed infant formula, *Circulation* 111:1897–1903, 2005.
82. Su LL, Chong YS, Chan YH, et al: Antenatal education and postnatal support strategies for improving rates of exclusive breast feeding: randomised controlled trial, *BMJ* 335:596, 2007.
83. Vaarala O, Knip M, Paronen J, et al: Cow's milk formula feeding induces primary immunization to insulin in infants at genetic risk for Type 1 diabetes, *Diabetes* 48:1389–1394, 1999.
84. Van Den Driessche M, Peeters K, Marien P, et al: Gastric emptying in formula-fed and breast-fed infants measured with the 13C-octanoic acid breath test, *J Pediatr Gastroenterol Nutr* 29:46–51, 1999.
85. Verronen P, Visakorpi JK, Lammi A, et al: Promotion of breast feeding: effect on neonates of change of feeding routine at a maternity unit, *Acta Paediatr Scand* 69:279–282, 1980.
86. Victora CG, Smith PG, Vaughan JP, et al: Evidence for protection by breast-feeding against infant deaths from infectious diseases in Brazil, *Lancet* 2:319–322, 1987.
87. Wight NE: Management of common breastfeeding issues, *Pediatr Clin North Am* 48:321–344, 2001.
88. Wight N: Hypoglycemia in breastfed neonates, *Breastfeed Med* 1:253–262, 2006.
89. Wight N, Marinelli K: ABM Protocol Committee: ABM Clinical Protocol #1: guidelines for glucose monitoring and treatment of hypoglycemia in breastfed neonates, *Breastfeed Med* 1:178–184, 2006.
90. Williams A: *Hypoglycemia of the newborn: review of the literature*, Geneva, 1997, World Health Organization.
91. Williams HG: 'And not a drop to drink'—why water is harmful for newborns, *Breastfeed Rev* 14:5–9, 2006.
92. Yaseen H, Salem M, Darwich M: Clinical presentation of hypernatremic dehydration in exclusively breast-fed neonates, *Indian J Pediatr* 71:1059–1062, 2004.
93. Yamauchi Y, Yamanouchi I: Breast-feeding frequency during the first 24 hours after birth in full-term neonates, *Pediatrics* 86:171–175, 1990.
94. Zangen S, DiLorenzo C, Zangen T, et al: Rapid maturation of gastric relaxation in newborn infants, *Pediatr Res* 50:629–632, 2001.

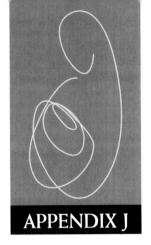

Protocol 4: Mastitis

Lisa H. Amir and the Academy of Breastfeeding Medicine Protocol Committee

Introduction

Mastitis is a common condition in lactating women; estimates from prospective studies range from 3% to 20%, depending on the definition and length of postpartum follow-up.[31,10,15] The majority of cases occur in the first 6 weeks, but mastitis can occur at any time during lactation. There have been few research trials in this area.

Quality of evidence (levels of evidence I, II-1, II-2, II-3, and III) for each recommendation as defined in the U.S. Preventive Services Task Force Appendix A Task Force Ratings[16] is noted in parentheses in this document.

Definition and Diagnosis

The usual clinical definition of mastitis is a tender, hot, swollen, wedge-shaped area of breast associated with temperature of 38.5°C (101.3°F) or greater, chills, flu-like aching, and systemic illness.[13] However, mastitis literally means, and is defined herein, as an inflammation of the breast; this inflammation may or may not involve a bacterial infection.[33,32] Redness, pain, and heat may all be present when an area of the breast is engorged or "blocked"/"plugged," but an infection is not necessarily present. There appears to be a continuum from engorgement to noninfective mastitis to infective mastitis to breast abscess.[32] (II-2)

Predisposing Factors

The following factors may predispose a lactating woman to the development of mastitis.[32,1] Other than the fact that these are factors that result in milk stasis, the evidence for these associations is generally inconclusive (II-2):

- Damaged nipple, especially if colonized with *Staphylococcus aureus*
- Infrequent feedings or scheduled frequency or duration of feedings
- Missed feedings
- Poor attachment or weak or uncoordinated suckling leading to inefficient removal of milk
- Illness in mother or baby
- Oversupply of milk
- Rapid weaning
- Pressure on the breast (e.g., tight bra, car seatbelt)
- White spot on the nipple or a blocked nipple pore or duct: milk blister or "bleb" (a localized inflammatory response)[28]
- Maternal stress and fatigue

Investigations

Laboratory investigations and other diagnostic procedures are not routinely needed or performed for mastitis. The World Health Organization publication on mastitis suggests that breastmilk culture and sensitivity testing "should be undertaken if

- there is no response to antibiotics within 2 days
- the mastitis recurs
- it is hospital-acquired mastitis
- the patient is allergic to usual therapeutic antibiotics or
- in severe or unusual cases."[32] (II-2)

Breastmilk culture may be obtained by collecting a hand-expressed midstream clean-catch sample into a sterile urine container (i.e., a small quantity of the initially expressed milk is discarded to avoid contamination of the sample with skin flora, and subsequent milk is expressed into the sterile container, taking care not to touch the inside of the container). Cleansing the nipple prior to collection may further reduce skin contamination and minimize false-positive culture results. Greater symptomatology has been associated with higher bacterial counts and/or pathogenic bacteria.[11] (III)

Management

EFFECTIVE MILK REMOVAL

Because milk stasis is often the initiating factor in mastitis, the most important management step is frequent and effective milk removal:

- Mothers should be encouraged to breastfeed more frequently, starting on the affected breast.
- If pain interferes with the letdown, feeding may begin on the unaffected breast, switching to the affected breast as soon as letdown is achieved.
- Positioning the infant at the breast with the chin or nose pointing to the blockage will help drain the affected area.
- Massaging the breast during the feed with an edible oil or nontoxic lubricant on the fingers may also be helpful to facilitate milk removal. Massage, by the mother or a helper, should be directed from the blocked area moving toward the nipple.
- After the feeding, expressing milk by hand or pump may augment milk drainage and hasten resolution of the problem.[20] (III)

An alternate approach for a swollen breast is fluid mobilization, which aims to promote fluid drainage toward the axillary lymph nodes.[29] The mother reclines, and with gentle hand motions starts stroking the skin surface from the areola to the axilla.[29] (III)

There is no evidence of risk to the healthy term infant of continuing breastfeeding from a mother with mastitis.[32] Women who are unable to continue breastfeeding should express the milk from breast by hand or pump, as sudden cessation of breastfeeding leads to a greater risk of abscess development than continuing to feed.[20] (III)

SUPPORTIVE MEASURES

Rest, adequate fluids, and nutrition are important measures. Practical help at home may be necessary for the mother to obtain adequate rest. Application of heat—for example, a shower or a hot pack—to the breast just prior to feeding may help with the letdown and milk flow. After a feeding or after milk is expressed from the breasts, cold packs can be applied to the breast in order to reduce pain and edema.

Although most women with mastitis can be managed as outpatients, hospital admission should be considered for women who are ill, require intravenous antibiotics, and/or do not have supportive care at home. Rooming-in of the infant with the mother is mandatory so that breastfeeding can continue. In some hospitals, rooming-in may require hospital admission of the infant.

PHARMACOLOGIC MANAGEMENT

Although lactating women are often reluctant to take medications, women with mastitis should be encouraged to take appropriate medications as indicated.

Analgesia

Analgesia may help with the letdown reflex and should be encouraged. An anti-inflammatory agent such as ibuprofen may be more effective in reducing the inflammatory symptoms than a simple analgesic like paracetamol/acetaminophen. Ibuprofen is not detected in breastmilk following doses up to 1.6 g/day and is regarded as compatible with breastfeeding.[21] (III)

Antibiotics

If symptoms of mastitis are mild and have been present for less than 24 hours, conservative management (effective milk removal and supportive measures) may be sufficient. If symptoms are not improving within 12 to 24 hours or if the woman is acutely ill, antibiotics should be started.[32] Worldwide, the most common pathogen in infective mastitis is penicillin-resistant S. aureus.[17,19] Less commonly, the organism is a Streptococcus or Escherichia coli.[20] The preferred antibiotics are usually penicillinase-resistant penicillins,[13] such as dicloxacillin or flucloxacillin 500 mg by mouth four times per day,[27] or as recommended by local antibiotic sensitivities. (III) First-generation cephalosporins are also generally acceptable as first-line treatment, but may be less preferred because of their broader spectrum of coverage. (III)

Cephalexin is usually safe in women with suspected penicillin allergy, but clindamycin is suggested for cases of severe penicillin hypersensitivity.[27] (III) Dicloxacillin appears to have a lower rate of adverse hepatic events than flucloxacillin.[25] Many authorities recommend a 10- to 14-day course of antibiotics[14,8]; however, this recommendation has not been subjected to controlled trials. (III)

S. aureus resistant to penicillinase-resistant penicillins (methicillin-resistant *S. aureus* [MRSA], also referred to as oxacillin-resistant *S. aureus*) has been increasingly isolated in cases of mastitis and breast abscesses.[24,2,9,30] (II-2) Clinicians should be aware of the likelihood of this occurring in their community and should order a breastmilk culture and assay of antibiotic sensitivities when mastitis is not improving 48 hours after starting first-line treatment. Local resistance patterns for MRSA should be considered when choosing an antibiotic for such unresponsive cases while culture results are pending. MRSA may be a community-acquired organism and has been reported to be a frequent pathogen in cases of breast abscess in some communities, particularly in the United States and Taiwan.[2,6,30] (I, II-2) At this time, MRSA occurrence is low in other countries, such as the United Kingdom.[23] (I) Most strains of methicillin-resistant staphylococci are susceptible to vancomycin or trimethoprim/sulfamethoxazole but may not be susceptible to rifampin.[18] Of note is that MRSA should be presumed to be resistant to treatment with macrolides and quinolones, regardless of susceptibility testing results.[3] (III)

As with other uses of antibiotics, repeated courses place women at increased risk for breast and vaginal *Candida* infections.[26,12]

Follow-up

Clinical response to the above management is typically rapid and dramatic. If the symptoms of mastitis fail to resolve within several days of appropriate management, including antibiotics, a wider differential diagnosis should be considered. Further investigations may be required to confirm resistant bacteria, abscess formation, an underlying mass, or inflammatory or ductal carcinoma. More than two or three recurrences in the same location also warrant evaluation to rule out an underlying mass or other abnormality.

Complications

EARLY CESSATION OF BREASTFEEDING

Mastitis may produce overwhelming acute symptoms that prompt women to consider cessation of breastfeeding. Effective milk removal, however, is the most important part of treatment.[32] Acute cessation of breastfeeding may actually exacerbate the mastitis and increase the risk of abscess formation; therefore, effective treatment and support from health care providers and family are important at this time. Mothers may need reassurance that the antibiotics they are taking are safe to use during breastfeeding.

ABSCESS

If a well-defined area of the breast remains hard, red, and tender despite appropriate management, then an abscess should be suspected. This occurs in about 3% of women with mastitis.[5] (II-2) The initial systemic symptoms and fever may have resolved. A diagnostic breast ultrasound will identify a collection of fluid. The collection can often be drained by needle aspiration, which itself can be diagnostic as well as therapeutic. Serial needle aspirations may be required.[4,7,22] (III) Ultrasound guidance for needle aspiration may be necessary in some cases. Fluid or pus aspirated should be sent for culture. Consideration of resistant organisms should also be given depending on the incidence of resistant organisms in that particular environment. Surgical drainage may be necessary if the abscess is very large or if there are multiple abscesses. After surgical drainage, breastfeeding on the affected breast should continue, even if a drain is present, with the proviso that the infant's mouth does not come into direct contact with purulent drainage or infected tissue. A course of antibiotics should follow drainage of the abscess. (III)

Photographs of breast abscesses and percutaneous aspiration can be found in a 2013 review by Kataria et al.[34]

CANDIDA INFECTION

Candida infection has been associated with burning nipple pain or radiating breast pain symptoms.[14] Diagnosis is difficult, as the nipples and breasts may look normal on examination, and milk culture may not be reliable. Careful evaluation for other etiologies of breast pain should be undertaken with particular attention to proper latch and ruling out Raynaud's/vasospasm and local nipple trauma. When wound cultures are obtained from nipple fissures, they most commonly grow *S. aureus*. (I)

A recent investigation of women with these typical symptoms, using breastmilk cultures after cleansing the nipples, found that none of the 35 cultures from the control group of women grew *Candida*, whereas only 1 of 29 in the symptomatic group grew the organism. (I) There was also no significant difference in the measurement of a by-product of *Candida* growth $[(1,3)\beta\text{-D-glucan}]$ between groups. Yet, evidence is conflicting as another recent study on milk culture found that 30% of symptomatic mothers were positive for *Candida*, whereas 8% of women in the asymptomatic group grew the organism. (I)

Women with burning nipple and breast pain may also be more likely to test positive for *Candida* on nipple swab by polymerase chain reaction.

Using molecular techniques as well as standard culture, a large cohort study of women followed up for 8 weeks postpartum found that burning nipple pain with breast pain was associated with *Candida* species but not with *S. aureus*. (II-2)

Further research in this area is required. Until then, a trial of antifungal medications, either with or without culture, is the current expert consensus recommendation. (III)

Prevention (III)[1]

EFFECTIVE MANAGEMENT OF BREAST FULLNESS AND ENGORGEMENT

- Mothers should be helped to improve infants' attachment to the breast.
- Feeds should not be restricted.
- Mothers should be taught to hand-express when the breasts are too full for the infant to attach or the infant does not relieve breast fullness. A breast pump may also be used, if available, for these purposes, but all mothers should be able to manually express as the need for its use may arise unexpectedly.

PROMPT ATTENTION TO ANY SIGNS OF MILK STASIS

- Mothers should be taught to check their breasts for lumps, pain, or redness.
- If the mother notices any signs of milk stasis, she needs to rest, increase the frequency of breastfeeding, apply heat to the breast prior to feedings, and massage any lumpy areas as described in the section "Effective milk removal."
- Mothers should contact their health care provider if symptoms are not improving within 24 hours.

PROMPT ATTENTION TO OTHER DIFFICULTIES WITH BREASTFEEDING

Skilled help is needed for mothers with damaged nipples or an unsettled discontented infant or those who believe that they have an insufficient milk supply.

REST

As fatigue is often a precursor to mastitis, health care providers should encourage breastfeeding mothers to obtain adequate rest. It may also be helpful for health care providers to remind family members that breastfeeding mothers may need more help and encourage mothers to ask for help as necessary.

GOOD HYGIENE

Because *S. aureus* is a common commensal organism often present in hospitals and communities, the importance of good hand hygiene should not be overlooked.[17] It is important for hospital staff, new mothers, and their families to practice good hand hygiene. Breast pump equipment may also be a source of contamination and should be washed thoroughly with soap and hot water after use.

Recommendations for Further Research

There are several aspects of prevention, diagnosis, and treatment of mastitis that require research. First, a consensus on a definition of mastitis is vital. We need to know when antibiotics are needed, which are the most appropriate antibiotics, and the optimal duration of treatment. The role of probiotics in prevention and treatment needs to be determined. Finally, the role of massage to prevent and treat breast engorgement and infection needs to be clarified.

Acknowledgments

This work was supported in part by a grant from the Maternal and Child Health Bureau, U.S. Department of Health and Human Services.

REFERENCES[1]

1. Aabo O, Matheson I, Aursnes I, et al: Mastitis in general practice. Is bacteriologic examination useful? *Tidsskr Nor Laegeforen* 110:2075–2077, 1990.
2. Amir LH, Forster D, McLachlan H, et al: Incidence of breast abscess in lactating women: report from an Australian cohort, *BJOG* 111:1378–1381, 2004.
3. Amir LH, Garland SM, Dennerstein L, et al: *Candida albicans*: is it associated with nipple pain in lactating women? *Gynecol Obstet Invest* 41:30–34, 1996.
4. Amir LH, Garland SM, Lumley J: A case-control study of mastitis: nasal carriage of *Staphylococcus aureus*, *BMC Fam Pract* 7:57, 2006.
5. Andrews JI, Fleener DK, Messer SA, et al: The yeast connection: is *Candida* linked to breastfeeding associated pain? *Am J Obstet Gynecol* 197, 2007. 424.e1–424.e4.
6. Christensen AF, Al-Suliman N, Nielson KR, et al: Ultrasound-guided drainage of breast abscesses: results in 151 patients, *Br J Radiol* 78:186–188, 2005.
7. Collignon PJ, Grayson ML, Johnson PDR: Methicillin-resistant *Staphylococcus aureus* in hospitals: time for a culture change [editorial], *Med J Aust* 187:4–5, 2007.

[1]ABM protocols expire 5 years from the date of publication. Evidence-based revisions are made within 5 years or sooner if there are significant changes in the evidence.

8. Dinsmoor MJ, Viloria R, Lief L, et al: Use of intrapartum antibiotics and the incidence of postnatal maternal and neonatal yeast infections, *Obstet Gynecol* 106:19–22, 2005.
9. Dixon JM: Repeated aspiration of breast abscesses in lactating women, *BMJ* 297:1517–1518, 1988.
10. Foxman B, D'Arcy H, Gillespie B, et al: Lactation mastitis: occurrence and medical management among 946 breastfeeding women in the United States, *Am J Epidemiol* 155:103–114, 2002.
11. Hale T: *Medication and mother's milk*, ed 11, Amarillo, Tex, 2004, Pharmasoft Medical Publishing.
12. Hale TW, Bateman T, Finkelman M, et al: Detection of *Candida albicans* in control and symptomatic breastfeeding women using new methodology [abstract 26], *Breastfeed Med* 2:187–188, 2007.
13. Inch S, Renfrew MJ: Common breastfeeding problems. In Chalmers I, Enkin M, Keirse M, editors: *Effective care in pregnancy and childbirth*, Oxford, UK, 1989, Oxford University Press, pp 1375–1389.
14. Kader AA, Kumar A, Krishna A: Induction of clindamycin resistance in erythromycin-resistant, clindamycin susceptible and methicillin-resistant clinical staphylococcal isolates, *Saudi Med J* 26:1914–1917, 2005.
15. Kinlay JR, O'Connell DL, Kinlay S: Incidence of mastitis in breastfeeding women during the six months after delivery: a prospective cohort study, *Med J Aust* 169:310–312, 1998.
16. Lawrence RA: The puerperium, breastfeeding, and breast milk, *Curr Opin Obstet Gynecol* 2:23–30, 1990.
17. Lawrence RA, Lawrence RM: *Breastfeeding: a guide for the medical profession*, ed 6, Philadelphia, Pa., 2005, Elsevier Mosby.
18. Livingstone VH, Willis CE, Berkowitz J: *Staphylococcus aureus* and sore nipples, *Can Fam Physician* 42:654–659, 1996.
19. Neifert MR: Clinical aspects of lactation: promoting breastfeeding success, *Clin Perinatol* 26:281–306, 1999.
20. Niebyl JR, Spence MR, Parmley TH: Sporadic (nonepidemic) puerperal mastitis, *J Reprod Med* 20:97–100, 1978.
21. Olsson R, Wiholm BE, Sand C, et al: Liver damage from flucloxacillin, cloxacillin and dicloxacillin, *J Hepatol* 15:154–161, 1992.
22. Panjaitan M, Amir LH, Costa A-M, et al: Polymerase chain reaction in detection of *Candida albicans* for confirmation of clinical diagnosis of nipple thrush [letter], *Breastfeed Med* 3:185–187, 2008.
23. Peterson B, Berens P, Swaim L: Incidence of MRSA in postpartum breast abscess [abstract 33], *Breastfeed Med* 2:190, 2007.
24. Pirotta MV, Gunn JM, Chondros P: "Not thrush again!" Women's experience of post-antibiotic vulvovaginitis, *Med J Aust* 179:43–46, 2003.
25. Reddy P, Qi C, Zembower T, et al: Postpartum mastitis and community-acquired methicillin-resistant. *Staphylococcus aureus*, *Emerg Infect Dis* 13:298–301, 2007.
26. Saenz RB: Bacterial pathogens isolated from nipple wounds: a four-year prospective study [abstract 34], *Breastfeed Med* 2:190, 2007.
27. Saiman L, O'Keefe M, Graham PL, et al: Hospital transmission of community-acquired methicillin-resistant *Staphylococcus aureus* among postpartum women, *Clin Infect Dis* 37:1313–1319, 2003.
28. Thomsen AC, Espersen T, Maigaard S: Course and treatment of milk stasis, noninfectious inflammation of the breast, and infectious mastitis in nursing women, *Am J Obstet Gynecol* 149:492–495, 1984.
29. Therapeutic guidelines: antibiotic. North Melbourne, Australia, 2006, Therapeutic Guidelines Ltd.
30. Ulitzsch D, Nyman MKG, Carlson RA: Breast abscess in lactating women: US-guided treatment, *Radiology* 232:904–909, 2004.
31. Waldenstrom U, Aarts C: Duration of breastfeeding and breastfeeding problems in relation to length of postpartum stay: a longitudinal cohort study of a national Swedish sample, *Acta Paediatr* 93:669–676, 2004.
32. Walker M: Mastitis in lactating women, *Lactation consultant series two*, Schaumburg, Ill., 1999, La Leche League International. Unit 2.8.
33. World Health Organization: *Mastitis: causes and management*, Geneva, 2000, World Health Organization. Publication Number WHO/FCH/CAH/00.13.
34. Kataria K, Srivastava A, Dhar A: Management of lactational mastitis and breast abscesses: review of current knowledge and practice, *Indian J Surg* I 75(6):430–435, 2013.

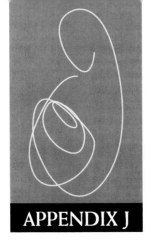

Protocol 5: Peripartum Breastfeeding Management for the Healthy Mother and Infant at Term

〜〜〜〜〜〜〜〜〜〜〜〜〜〜〜〜〜〜〜〜〜〜〜

Background

Hospital policies and routines greatly influence breastfeeding success.[28,65,38,44,68,6,59,16,3,61] The Baby-Friendly Hospital Initiative (BFHI) has defined the Ten Steps to Successful Breastfeeding, and 20 years of research has now verified that "the achievement of BFHI certification leads to substantially improved breastfeeding outcomes, especially increases in breastfeeding initiation and exclusivity."[28]

The peripartum hospital experience should include adequate support, instruction, and care to ensure the successful initiation of breastfeeding. Such management is part of a continuum of care and education that begins during the prenatal period, promotes breastfeeding as the optimal method of infant feeding, and includes information about maternal and infant benefits. The following principles and practices are recommended for care in the peripartum hospital setting.

Recommendations

Quality of evidence (levels of evidence I, II-1, II-2, II-3, and III) for each recommendation as defined in the U.S. Preventive Services Task Force Appendix A Task Force Ratings[8] is noted in parentheses.

Prenatal

1. All pregnant women must receive education about the benefits and management of breastfeeding to allow an informed decision about infant feeding.[68,6,59,16,3,61] An evidence-based review of practices that improve the duration or initiation of breastfeeding found that "prenatal combined with postnatal interventions are more effective than usual care in prolonging the duration of breastfeeding...."[20] Information and advice from a health professional early in pregnancy are also supported by the American College of Obstetricians and Gynecologists and the American Academy of Family Physicians in their policy statements, which read "Advice and encouragement of the obstetrician-gynecologist are critical in making the decision to breastfeed"[6] and "Family-centered care (the belief that health care staff and the family are partners, working together to best meet the needs of the patient) allows support of breastfeeding practices throughout the lifecycle to all family members."[3] (I, II-1, II-2, II-3, III)

2. Prenatal education should include information about the benefits to mother and baby of exclusive breastfeeding initiated in the first hour after birth.[68] Educational materials produced by formula manufacturers are inappropriate sources of information about infant feeding.[30,2] (I, III)

for the breastfeeding mother, revised 2012, *Breastfeed Med* 7:547–553, 2012.

47. Moore ER, Anderson GC, Bergman N, et al: Early skin-to-skin contact for mothers and their healthy newborn infants, *Cochrane Database Syst Rev* 5, 2012. CD003519.

48. Morton J, Hall JY, Wong RJ, et al: Combining hand techniques with electric pumping increases milk production in mothers of preterm infants, *J Perinatol* 29:757–764, 2009.

49. Mottl-Santiago J, Walker C, Ewan J, et al: A hospital-based doula program and childbirth outcomes in an urban, multicultural setting, *Matern Child Health J* 12:372–377, 2008.

50. Murray EK, Ricketts S, Dellaport J: Hospital practices that increase breastfeeding duration: results from a population-based study, *Birth* 34:202–211, 2007.

51. Nommsen-Rivers LA, Mastergeorge AM, Hansen RL, et al: Doula care, early breastfeeding outcomes, and breastfeeding status at 6 weeks postpartum among low-income primiparae, *J Obstet Gynecol Neonatal Nurs* 38:157–173, 2009.

52. O'Connor NR, Tanabe KO, Siadaty MS, et al: Pacifiers and breastfeeding: a systematic review, *Arch Pediatr Adolesc Med* 163:378–382, 2009.

53. Perez-Escamilla R, Pollitt E, Lonnerdal B, et al: Infant feeding policies in maternity wards and their effect on breastfeeding success: an analytical overview, *Am J Public Health* 84:89–97, 1994.

54. Perrine CG, Scanlon KS, Li R, et al: Baby-Friendly Hospital practices and meeting exclusive breastfeeding intention, *Pediatrics* 130:54–60, 2012.

55. Preer G, Pisegna JM, Cook JT, et al: Delaying the bath and in-hospital breastfeeding rates, *Breastfeed Med* 8:485–490, 2013.

56. Renfrew MJ, McCormick FM, Quinn WA, et al: Support for healthy breastfeeding mothers with healthy term babies, *Cochrane Database Syst Rev* 5, 2012. CD001141.

57. Righard L, Alade MO: Effect of delivery room routines on success of first breast-feed, *Lancet* 336:1105–1107, 1990.

58. Righard L, Alade MO: Sucking technique and its effect on success of breastfeeding, *Birth* 19:185–189, 1992.

59. Rotundo G: Centering pregnancy: the benefits of group prenatal care, *Nurs Womens Health* 15:508–517, 2011.

60. Sachs HC, Committee on Drugs: The transfer of drugs and therapeutics into human breast milk: an update on selected topics, *Pediatrics* 132:e796–e809, 2013.

61. Section on Breastfeeding: Breastfeeding and the use of human milk, *Pediatrics* 129:e827–e841, 2012.

62. Sudfeld CR, Fawzi WW, Lahariya C: Peer support and exclusive breastfeeding duration in low and middle-income countries: a systematic review and meta-analysis, *PLoS One* 7, 2012. e45143.

63. Thukral A, Sankar MJ, Agarwal R, et al: Early skin-to-skin contact and breast-feeding behavior in term neonates: a randomized controlled trial, *Neonatology* 102:114–119, 2012.

64. Toxnet: Toxicology Data Network. Drugs and Lactation Database (LactMed). http://toxnet.nlm.nih.gov/cgi-bin/sis/htmlgen?LACT. Accessed October 31, 2013.

65. UNICEF Breastfeeding Initiatives Exchange. The Baby Friendly Hospital Initiative. www.unicef.org/programme/breastfeeding/baby.htm. Accessed October 31, 2013.

66. Waldenstrom U, Swenson A: Rooming-in at night in the postpartum ward, *Midwifery* 7:82–89, 1991.

67. Webb JA, Thomsen HS, Morcos SK, et al: The use of iodinated and gadolinium contrast media during pregnancy and lactation, *Eur Radiol* 15:1234–1240, 2005.

68. World Health Organization, UNICEF, Wellstart International: *Baby-Friendly Hospital Initiative. Revised, Updated and Expanded for Integrated Care,* 2009: www.unicef.org/nutrition/files/BFHI_2009_s1.pdf. Accessed October 31, 2013.

69. www.who.int/maternal_child_adolescent/documents/9789241599535/en/. Accessed October 30, 2013.

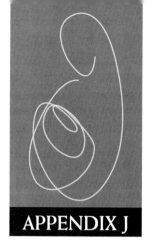

Protocol 6: Guideline on Co-Sleeping and Breastfeeding

Introduction

The Academy of Breastfeeding Medicine is a worldwide organization of physicians dedicated to the promotion, protection, and support of breastfeeding and human lactation. One of the goals of the Academy of Breastfeeding Medicine is the facilitation of optimal breastfeeding practices. This clinical guideline addresses an aspect of parenting that has a significant impact on breastfeeding: infant sleep locations.

Background

The terms *co-sleeping* and *bed sharing* are often used interchangeably. However, bed sharing is only one form of co-sleeping. Co-sleeping, in reality, refers to the diverse ways in which infants sleep in close social and/or physical contact with a caregiver (usually the mother).[19] This operational definition includes an infant sleeping alongside a parent on a different piece of furniture/object as well as clearly unsafe practices such as sharing a sofa or recliner. Around the world the practice of co-sleeping can be quite variable, and, as such, all forms of co-sleeping do not carry the same risks or benefits.[3] Some forms of parent-child co-sleeping provide physical protection for the infant against cold and extend the duration of breastfeeding, thus improving the chances of survival of the slowly developing human infant.[19,14–16] The human infant, relative to other mammals, develops more slowly, requires frequent feedings, and is born neurologically less mature.[19,14–16] In malaria

settings, co-sleeping is recommended as the most efficient use of available bed nets, and co-sleeping may be necessary in other geographic areas where available bedding or housing is inadequate. Bed sharing and co-sleeping have also long been promoted as a method to enhance parenting behavior or "attachment parenting" and also to facilitate breastfeeding.[19,3,14–16,4,6,7,11,26,34,33,28]

Bed sharing and some forms of co-sleeping have been rather controversial in the medical literature in recent years and have received considerable negative comment.[4,6,7,11,26] Some public health authorities have discouraged all parents from bed sharing.[34,33]

Bed Sharing and Infant Mortality

The concerns regarding bed sharing and increased infant mortality have been centered around mechanical suffocation (asphyxiation) and sudden infant death syndrome (SIDS) risks.

ASPHYXIATION RISK

Several studies using *unverified death certificate* diagnoses concluded that a significant number of infants were asphyxiated as they slept in unsafe sleep environments caused by either accidental entrapment in the sleep surface or overlying by a sleeping adult or older child.[4,6,7,11,26] The U.S. Consumer Product Safety Commission (USCPSC), using data from some of these studies, has made recommendations against the use of all types and forms of co-sleeping and advised parents against sleeping with their infants under any circumstances. The USCPSC is concerned about the absence of infant safety standards for adult beds and the hazards that may result from an infant sleeping in an unsafe environment.[34] All of these studies lack data on the state of intoxication of the co-sleeping adult (drugs or alcohol) and fail to consider the sleep position of the baby at time of death, even though a prone sleep position appears to be one of the most significant risk factors for SIDS. The USCPSC also groups all bed sharing into one category, not separating known unsafe sleep environments such as sofas and couches, waterbeds, and upholstered chairs from other, safer sleep surfaces. In these studies, there is no assurance of the quality of the data collection, no consistency in the criteria employed in using the term "overlay," and no validation of the conclusions. Bias by medical examiners and coroners may lead them to classify infant deaths that occur in an adult bed, couch, or chair in the presence of an adult as a rollover death even where there is no evidence that an actual overlay occurred. This is especially a problem in the absence of a death scene examination and detailed interviews of those present at the time of death. There is no autopsy method to differentiate between death caused by SIDS versus death from accidental or intentional causes such as infant homicide by pillow smothering. Thus infant deaths that occur in a crib are usually designated as SIDS, whereas deaths in a couch or adult bed are usually labeled as smothering. Further complicating analyses of infant deaths is the diversity of bed-sharing behaviors among different populations and even within the same families (i.e., bed sharing during the day vs. at night or when a baby is ill vs. when a baby is well), suggesting different levels of risk. A home visit study of families considered to be at high risk for SIDS because of socioeconomic status found that those who practiced bed sharing were more likely to place infants in the prone position and to use softer bed surfaces.[8] Similarly, a population-based retrospective review found that "Bed-sharing subjects who breastfed had a risk profile distinct from those who were not breastfed cases. Risk and situational profiles can be used to identify families in greater need of early guidance and to prepare educational content to promote safe sleep."[27]

SIDS PREVENTION AND RISK

Several epidemiological studies and a meta-analysis have found a significant association between breastfeeding and a lowered SIDS risk, especially when breastfeeding was the exclusive form of feeding during the first 4 months of life.[9,20]

However, there is insufficient evidence at this time to show a causal link between breastfeeding and the prevention of SIDS. Several studies have consistently demonstrated an increased risk of SIDS when infants bed share with mothers who smoke cigarettes.[3,23,21,24,30,31,29,22] Exposure to cigarette smoke as a fetus and in infancy appears to contribute to this risk and is independent of other known risk factors, including social class. This has led to the recommendation, which is well supported in the medical literature, that infants not bed share with parents who smoke. A large meta-analysis, after review of over 40 studies, concluded that, "Evidence consistently suggests that there may be an association between bed sharing and sudden infant death syndrome (SIDS) among smokers (however defined), but the evidence is not as consistent among nonsmokers. This does not mean that no association between bed sharing and SIDS exists among nonsmokers, but that existing data do not convincingly establish such an association."[10]

Ethnic Diversity

The rates of SIDS deaths are low in Asian cultures in which co-sleeping is common. However, some argue that co-sleeping in these cultures is different from the bed sharing that occurs in the United States. As Blair and colleagues note in their study, "A baby sleeping at arm's length from the mother on a firm surface, as is often the case in Hong Kong, or a Pacific Island baby sleeping *on* the bed rather than *in* the bed is in a different environment from a baby sleeping in direct contact with the mother on a soft mattress and covered by a thick duvet."[3] Similarly, even within the United States there seems to be variation in bed-sharing practices based on ethnicity and race. A large, prospective study using multivariate analysis of bed sharing found that race or ethnicity appears to have the strongest association with bed sharing at all follow-up periods, with black, Asian, and Hispanic mothers four to six times more likely to bed share than white mothers.[13]

In a study in Alaska, where there is a high rate of co-sleeping among Alaska Native people, researchers found that almost all SIDS deaths associated with parental bed sharing occurred in conjunction with a history of parental drug use and occasionally in association with prone sleep position or sleeping on surfaces such as couches or waterbeds.[12] A study using the PRAMS (Pregnancy Risk Assessment Monitoring System) data set in Oregon found that "The women most likely to bed share are non-white, single, breastfeeding, and low-income. Non-economic factors are also important, particularly among blacks and Hispanics. Campaigns to decrease bed sharing by providing cribs may have limited effectiveness if mothers are bed sharing because of cultural norms."[12]

Controlled Laboratory Studies

McKenna and colleagues have studied bed sharing in the greatest scientific detail in a laboratory setting and have found that infants who shared a bed with the mother had more sleep arousals and spent less time in Stage 3 and 4 sleep. This may be protective against SIDS as deep sleep and infrequent arousals have been considered as possible risk factors for SIDS.[14,17,25]

A similar study that was conducted in the natural physical environment of home instead of a sleep lab "compared the two different sleep practices of bed sharing and cot sleeping quantifying factors that have been identified as potential risks or benefits. Overnight video and physiologic data of bed-share infants and cot-sleep infants were recorded in the infants' own homes."[1] This study concluded that "Bed-share infants without known risk factors for sudden infant death syndrome (SIDS) experience increased maternal touching and looking, increased breastfeeding, and faster and more frequent maternal responses."[1] This increased interaction between mothers and babies may be protective.

Parental Factors

The contribution of other parental factors to the risk of bed sharing is unclear. Blair and colleagues found in a multivariate analysis that maternal alcohol consumption of more than two drinks (one drink = 12 oz beer, 5 oz wine, or 1.5 oz distilled alcohol) and parental tiredness were associated with sudden infant death.[3] A study in New Zealand, however, did not show a clear link with alcohol consumption.[30] The role of obesity was examined in one study of SIDS cases. They found the mean pre-gravid weights of bed-sharing mothers to be greater than those of nonbed-sharing mothers.[6]

If overlying is thought to be the mechanism of infant suffocation, it would seem plausible that the psychological and physical states of those sharing the bed with an infant could be of importance.

Room sharing with parents (infants sharing the same room as their parents as opposed to being in a separate room) appears to be protective against SIDS.[3,32,5]

Infant Factors

There is some evidence that bed sharing with younger babies <8 to 14 weeks may increase the risk of SIDS.[3,32,5]

Breastfeeding and Bed Sharing

Research continues to show the strong relationship between breastfeeding and bed sharing/co-sleeping. A study of bed sharing and breastfeeding in the United States found that infants who routinely shared a bed with their mothers breastfed approximately three times longer during the night than infants who routinely slept separately. There was a twofold increase in the number of breastfeeding episodes, and the episodes were 39% longer.[18] Proximity to and sensory contact with the mother during sleep facilitates prompt responses to signs of the infant's readiness to breastfeed and provides psychological comfort and reassurance to the dependent infant as well as the parents. A large prospective study of more than 10,000 infants in the United State found that up to 22% of 1-month-old infants were bed sharing and that breastfeeding mothers were three times more likely to bed share than mothers who did not breastfeed. Ninety-five percent of infants who shared a bed did so with a parent.[13] Similarly, a study of parent-infant bed sharing in England found that "Breast feeding was strongly associated with bed-sharing, both at birth and at 3 months."[2]

Based on the above information and literature, the Academy of Breastfeeding Medicine has the following recommendations for health care providers.

Recommendations

A. Because breastfeeding is the best form of nutrition for infants, any recommendations for infant care that impede its initiation or duration need to be carefully weighed against the many known benefits to infants, their mothers, and society.

B. It should not be assumed that all families are practicing only one sleeping arrangement all night every night and during the daytime as well. Health care providers should consider ethnic, socioeconomic, feeding, and other family circumstances when obtaining a history on infant sleep practices.[3,8,27]

C. Parents need to be encouraged to express their views and to seek information and support from their health care providers. Sensitivity to cultural differences is necessary when obtaining sleep histories.

D. There is currently not enough evidence to support routine recommendations against co-sleeping. Parents should be educated about risks and benefits of co-sleeping and unsafe co-sleeping practices and should be allowed to make their own informed decision.

Bed sharing/co-sleeping is a complex practice. Parental counseling about infant sleep environments should include the following information:

1. Some potentially unsafe practices related to bed sharing/co-sleeping have been identified either in the peer-reviewed literature or as a consensus of expert opinion:
   - Environmental smoke exposure and maternal smoking[3,23,21,24,30,31,29,22,10]
   - Sharing sofas, couches, or daybeds with infants[3,7,11,26,34,33]
   - Sharing waterbeds or the use of soft bedding materials[4,7,11,26,34,33]
   - Sharing beds with adjacent spaces that could trap an infant[4,7,11,26,34,33]
   - Placement of the infant in the adult bed in the prone or side position[4,7,11,26,34,33]
   - The use of alcohol or mind-altering drugs by the adult(s) who is bed sharing[3]
   - Infants bed sharing with other children[10]
   - Bed sharing with younger babies <8 to 14 weeks of age may be more strongly associated with SIDS.[3,6,10,32,5]
2. Families also should be given all the information that is known about safe sleep environments for their infants, including:
   - Place babies in the supine position for sleep.[10]
   - Use a firm, flat surface and avoid waterbeds, couches, sofas, pillows, soft materials, or loose bedding.[4,7,11,26,34,33]
   - If blankets are to be used, they should be tucked in around the mattress so that the infant's head is less likely to be covered.[10]
   - Ensure that the head will not be covered. In a cold room the infant could be kept in an infant sleeper to maintain warmth.[4,7,11,26,34,33]
   - Avoid the use of quilts, duvets, comforters, pillows, and stuffed animals in the infant's sleep environment.[4,7,11,26,34,33]
   - Never put an infant down to sleep on a pillow or adjacent to a pillow.[4,7,11,26,34,33]
   - Never leave an infant alone on an adult bed.[4,7,11,26,34,33]
   - Inform families that adult beds have potential risks and are not designed to meet federal safety standards for infants.[4,7,11,26,34,33]
   - Ensure that there are no spaces between the mattress and headboard, walls, and other surfaces, which may entrap the infant and lead to suffocation.[4,7,11,26,34,33]
   - Placement of a firm mattress directly on the floor away from walls may be a safe alternative. Another alternative to sharing an adult bed or sharing a mattress is the use of an infant bed that attaches to the side of the adult bed and provides proximity and access to the infant but a separate sleep surface. There are

currently no peer-reviewed studies on the safety or efficacy of such devices.
   - Room sharing with parents appears to be protective against SIDS.[3,10,32,5]

Recommendations for Future Research

A. The Academy of Breastfeeding Medicine urges that more research be undertaken so that the benefits and risks of co-sleeping and bed sharing and their association with breastfeeding can be better understood.
B. Researchers should employ well-designed, impartial, prospective protocols with standardized, well-defined data collection methods. Control data for comparison are an essential part of such research. Studies should be population-based, so that actual risk of sudden infant death and overlying smothering due to bed sharing or co-sleeping can be computed. A denominator is needed for calculation of risk and for comparison with a population not practicing co-sleeping or bed sharing. In the final analysis, it is critical that dangerous, modifiable "factors" associated with bed sharing not be considered the same as bed sharing itself.
C. The diversity of bed sharing/co-sleeping practices among the different ethnic groups in the United States and throughout the world needs to be carefully considered and documented as part of research protocols.
D. Continuing study of the impact of co-sleeping on infant behavior, SIDS, and breastfeeding is essential.

REFERENCES

1. Baddock SA, Galland BC, Bolton DP, et al: Differences in infant and parent behaviors during routine bed sharing compared with cot sleeping in the home setting, *Pediatrics* 117:1599–1607, 2006.
2. Blair PS, Ball HL: The prevalence and characteristics associated with parent-infant bed-sharing in England, *Arch Dis Child* 89:1106–1110, 2004.
3. Blair PS, Fleming PJ, Smith IJ, et al: Babies sleeping with parents: case-control study of factors influencing the risk of the sudden infant death syndrome. CESDI SUDI research group, *BMJ* 319:1457–1461, 1999.
4. Byard RW, Beal S, Bourne AJ: Potentially dangerous sleeping environments and accidental asphyxia in infancy and early childhood, *Arch Dis Child* 71:497–500, 1994.
5. Carpenter RG, Irgens LM, Blair PS, et al: Sudden unexplained infant death in 20 regions in Europe: case control study, *Lancet* 363:185–191, 2004.
6. Carroll-Pankhurst C, Mortimer EA Jr., : Sudden infant death syndrome, bedsharing, parental weight, and age at death, *Pediatrics* 107:530–536, 2001.
7. Drago DA, Dannenberg AL: Infant mechanical suffocation deaths in the United States, 1980-1997, *Pediatrics* 103:1999. e59.

8. Flick L, White DK, Vemulapalli C, et al: Sleep position and the use of soft bedding during bed sharing among African American infants at increased risk for sudden infant death syndrome, *J Pediatr* 138:338–343, 2001.

9. Ford RP, Taylor BJ, Mitchell EA, et al: Breastfeeding and the risk of sudden infant death syndrome, *Int J Epidemiol* 22:885–890, 1993.

10. Horsley T, Clifford T, Barrowman N, et al: Benefits and harms associated with the practice of bed sharing: a systematic review, *Arch Pediatr Adolesc Med* 161:237–245, 2007.

11. Kemp JS, Unger B, Wilkins D, et al: Unsafe sleep practices and an analysis of bedsharing among infants dying suddenly and unexpectedly: results of a four-year, population-based, death-scene investigation study of sudden infant death syndrome and related deaths, *Pediatrics* 106:2000. e41.

12. Lahr MB, Rosenberg KD, Lapidus JA: Maternal-infant bed-sharing: risk factors for bedsharing in a population-based survey of new mothers and implications for SIDS risk reduction, *Matern Child Health J* 11:277–286, 2007.

13. McCoy RC, Hunt CE, Lesko SM, et al: Frequency of bed sharing and its relationship to breastfeeding, *J Dev Behav Pediatr* 25:141–149, 2004.

14. McKenna JJ: An anthropological perspective on the sudden infant death syndrome (SIDS): the role of parental breathing cues and speech breathing adaptations, *Med Anthropol* 10:9–92, 1986.

15. McKenna JJ, Mosko S: Evolution and infant sleep: an experimental study of infant-parent co-sleeping and its implications for SIDS, *Acta Paediatr Suppl* 82(Suppl 389):31–36, 1993.

16. McKenna JJ, Mosko SS: Sleep and arousal, synchrony and independence, among mothers and infants sleeping apart and together (same bed): an experiment in evolutionary medicine, *Acta Paediatr Suppl* 397:94–102, 1994.

17. McKenna JJ, Mosko S, Dungy C, et al: Sleep and arousal patterns of co-sleeping human mother/infant pairs: a preliminary physiological study with implications for the study of sudden infant death syndrome (SIDS), *Am J Phys Anthropol* 83:331–347, 1990.

18. McKenna JJ, Mosko SS, Richard CA: Bedsharing promotes breastfeeding, *Pediatrics* 100:214–219, 1997.

19. McKenna JJ, Thoman EB, Anders TF, et al: Infant-parent co-sleeping in an evolutionary perspective: implications for understanding infant sleep development and the sudden infant death syndrome, *Sleep* 16:263–282, 1993.

20. McVea KL, Turner PD, Peppler DK: The role of breastfeeding in sudden infant death syndrome, *J Hum Lact* 16:13–20, 2000.

21. Mitchell EA, Esmail A, Jones DR, et al: Do differences in the prevalence of risk factors explain the higher mortality from sudden infant death syndrome in New Zealand compared with the UK? *N Z Med J* 109:352–355, 1996.

22. Mitchell EA, Scragg L, Clements M: Factors related to infants bed sharing, *N Z Med J* 107:466–467, 1994.

23. Mitchell EA, Taylor BJ, Ford RP, et al: Four modifiable and other major risk factors for cot death: the New Zealand study, *J Paediatr Child Health* 28(Suppl 1):S3–S8, 1992.

24. Mitchell EA, Tuohy PG, Brunt JM, et al: Risk factors for sudden infant death syndrome following the prevention campaign in New Zealand: a prospective study, *Pediatrics* 100:835–840, 1997.

25. Mosko S, Richard C, McKenna J: Infant arousals during mother-infant bed sharing: implications for infant sleep and sudden infant death syndrome research, *Pediatrics* 100:841–849, 1997.

26. Nakamura S, Wind M, Danello MA: Review of hazards associated with children placed in adult beds, *Arch Pediatr Adolesc Med* 153:1019–1023, 1999.

27. Ostfeld BM, Perl H, Esposito L, et al: Sleep environment, positional, lifestyle, and demographic characteristics associated with bed sharing in sudden infant death syndrome cases: a population-based study, *Pediatrics* 118:2051–2059, 2006.

28. Rosenberg KD: Sudden infant death syndrome and co-sleeping, *Arch Pediatr Adolesc Med* 154:529–530, 2000.

29. Scragg RK, Mitchell EA: Side sleeping position and bed sharing in the sudden infant death syndrome, *Ann Med* 30:345–349, 1998.

30. Scragg R, Mitchell EA, Taylor BJ, et al: Bed sharing, smoking, and alcohol in the sudden infant death syndrome. New Zealand Cot Death Study Group, *BMJ* 307:1312–1318, 1993.

31. Scragg R, Stewart AW, Mitchell EA, et al: Public health policy on bed sharing and smoking in the sudden infant death syndrome, *N Z Med J* 108:218–222, 1995.

32. Tappin D, Ecob R, Brooke H: Bedsharing, roomsharing, and sudden infant death syndrome in Scotland: a case-control study, *J Pediatr* 147:32–37, 2005.

33. The changing concept of sudden infant death syndrome. Diagnostic coding shifts, controversies regarding the sleeping environment, and new variables to consider in reducing risk, *Pediatrics* 116:1245–1255, 2005.

34. U.S. Consumer Products Safety Commission. CPSC Warns Against Placing Babies in Adult Beds. Report Number SPSC Document #5091. Washington, D.C., 1999, U.S. Consumer Products Safety Commission.

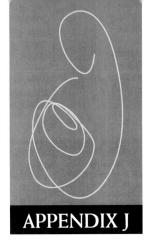

APPENDIX J

Protocol 7: Model Breastfeeding Policy

Purpose

The purpose of this protocol is to promote a philosophy of maternal infant care that advocates breastfeeding and supports the normal physiologic functions involved in the establishment of this maternal-infant process and to assist families choosing to breastfeed with initiating and developing a successful and satisfying experience.

This policy is based on recommendations from the most recent breastfeeding policy statements published by the Office on Women's Health of the U.S. Department of Health and Human Services,[19] the American Academy of Pediatrics,[17] the American College of Obstetricians and Gynecologists,[3] the American Academy of Family Physicians,[18] the World Health Organization,[21] the American Dietetic Association,[11] the Academy of Breastfeeding Medicine,[1] and the UNICEF/WHO evidence-based *Ten Steps to Successful Breastfeeding.*[21,20,22]

Policy Statements

1. The *"name of institution"* staff will actively support breastfeeding as the preferred method of providing nutrition to infants. A multidisciplinary, culturally appropriate team comprising hospital administrators, physician and nursing staff, lactation consultants and specialists, nutrition staff, parents, and other appropriate staff shall be established and maintained to identify and eliminate institutional barriers to breastfeeding. On a yearly basis, this group will compile and evaluate data relevant to breastfeeding support services and formulate a plan of action to implement needed changes.

2. A written breastfeeding policy will be developed and communicated to all health care staff. The *"name of institution"* breastfeeding policy will be reviewed and updated routinely (biannually) using current research as an evidence-based guide.

3. All pregnant women and their support people as appropriate will be provided with information on breastfeeding and counseled on the benefits of breastfeeding, contraindications to breastfeeding, and risk of formula feeding.

4. The woman's desire to breastfeed will be documented in her medical record.

5. Mothers will be encouraged to exclusively breastfeed unless medically contraindicated. The method of feeding will be documented in the medical record of every infant.
   - Exclusive breastfeeding is defined as providing breast milk as the sole source of nutrition. Exclusively breastfed babies receive no other liquids or solids.

6. At birth or soon thereafter all newborns, if baby and mother are stable, will be placed skin-to-skin with the mother. Skin-to-skin contact involves placing the naked baby prone on the mother's bare chest. Mother-infant couples will be given the opportunity to initiate breastfeeding within 1 hour of birth. Post-cesarean-birth babies will be encouraged to breastfeed as soon as possible. The administration of vitamin K and prophylactic antibiotics to prevent ophthalmia neonatorum should be delayed for

the first hour after birth to allow uninterrupted mother-infant contact and breastfeeding.[13]

7. Breastfeeding mother-infant couples will be encouraged to remain together throughout their hospital stay, including at night (rooming-in). Skin-to-skin contact will be encouraged as much as possible.

8. Breastfeeding assessment, teaching, and documentation will be done on each shift and whenever possible with each staff contact with the mother. After each feeding, staff will document information about the feeding in the infant's medical record. This documentation may include the latch, position, and any problems encountered. For feedings not directly observed, a maternal report may be used. Every shift, a direct observation of the baby's position and latch-on during feeding will be performed and documented.

9. Mothers will be encouraged to utilize available breastfeeding resources, including classes, written materials, and video presentations, as appropriate. If clinically indicated, the clinician or nurse will make a referral to a lactation consultant or specialist.

10. Breastfeeding mothers will be instructed about
    a. proper positioning and latch-on;
    b. nutritive suckling and swallowing;
    c. milk production and release;
    d. frequency of feeding/feeding cues;
    e. expression of breastmilk and use of a pump if indicated;
    f. how to assess if infant is adequately nourished; and
    g. reasons for contacting the clinician.
    These skills will be taught to primiparous and multiparous women and reviewed before the mother goes home.

11. Parents will be taught that breastfeeding infants, including cesarean-birth babies, should be put to breast at least 8 to 12 times each 24 hours. Infant feeding cues (e.g., increased alertness or activity, mouthing, or rooting) will be used as indicators of the baby's readiness for feeding. Breastfeeding babies will be breastfed at night.

12. Time limits for breastfeeding on each side will be avoided. Infants can be offered both breasts at each feeding but may be interested in feeding only on one side at a feeding during the early days.

13. No supplemental water, glucose water, or formula will be given unless specifically ordered by a physician or nurse practitioner or by the mother's documented and informed request. Prior to nonmedically indicated supplementation, mothers will be informed of the risks of supplementing. The supplement should be fed to the baby by cup if possible and will be no more than 10 to 15 mL in a term baby.[7,6,9] Alternative feeding methods such as syringe or spoon-feeding may also be used; however, these methods have not be shown to be effective in preserving breastfeeding. Bottles will not be placed in a breastfeeding infant's bassinet.

14. This institution does not give group instruction in the use of formula. Those parents who, after appropriate counseling, choose to formula feed their infants will be provided individual instruction.

15. Pacifiers will not be given to normal full-term breastfeeding infants. The pacifier guidelines at *"name of institution"* state that preterm infants in the Neonatal Intensive Care or Special Care Unit or infants with specific medical conditions may be given pacifiers for nonnutritive sucking. Newborns undergoing painful procedures (e.g., circumcision) may be given a pacifier as a method of pain management during the procedure. The infant will not return to the mother with the pacifier. *"Name of institution"* encourages "pain-free newborn care," which may include breastfeeding during the heel stick procedure for the newborn metabolic screening tests.

16. Routine blood glucose monitoring of full-term, healthy, appropriate for gestational age (AGA) infants is not indicated. Assessment for clinical signs of hypoglycemia and dehydration will be ongoing.[14]

17. Antilactation drugs will not be given to any postpartum mother.

18. Routine use of nipple creams, ointments, or other topical preparations will be avoided unless such therapy has been indicated for a dermatologic problem. Mothers with sore nipples will be observed for latch-on techniques and will be instructed to apply expressed colostrum or breast milk to the areola after each feeding.

19. Nipple shields or bottle nipples will not be routinely used to cover a mother's nipple to treat latch-on problems or prevent or manage sore or cracked nipples or when a mother has flat or inverted nipples. Nipple shields will be used only in conjunction with a lactation consultation.

20. After 24 hours of life, if the infant has not latched on or fed effectively, the mother will be instructed to begin breast massage and hand expression of colostrum into the baby's mouth during feeding attempts. Skin-to-skin contact will be encouraged. (Parents will be instructed to watch closely for feeding cues and whenever these are observed to awaken and feed the infant.) If the baby continues to feed poorly,

pumping with skilled hand expression or a double set-up electric breast pump will be initiated and maintained approximately every 3 hours or a minimum of eight times per day. Any expressed colostrum or mother's milk will be fed to the baby by an alternative method. The mother will be reminded that she may not obtain much milk or even any milk the first few times she pumps her breasts. Until the mother's milk is available, a collaborative decision should be made among the mother, nurse, and clinician regarding the need to supplement the baby. Each day clinicians will be consulted regarding the volume and type of the supplement. Pacifiers will be avoided. In cases of problem feeding, the lactation consultant or specialist will be consulted.[13]

21. If the baby is still not latching on well or feeding well when going home, the feeding/pumping/supplementing plan will be reviewed in addition to routine breastfeeding instructions. A follow-up visit or contact will be scheduled within 24 hours. Depending on the clinical situation it may be appropriate to delay discharge of the couplet to provide further breastfeeding intervention, support, and education.

22. All babies should be seen for follow-up within the first few days postpartum. This visit should be with a pediatrician or other qualified health care practitioner for a formal evaluation of breastfeeding performance, a weight check, assessment of jaundice, and age-appropriate elimination:
    - For infants discharged at less than 2 days of age (<48 hours): Follow-up at 2 to 4 days of age.
    - For infants discharged at more than 2 days of age (>48 hours): Follow-up at 4 to 5 days of age.
    - All newborns should be seen by 1 month of age.

23. Mothers who are separated from their sick or premature infants will be
    a. instructed on how to use skilled hand expression or the double set-up electric breast pump—instructions will include expression at least eight times per day or approximately every 3 hours for 15 minutes (or until milk flow stops, whichever is greater) around the clock and the importance of not missing a pumping session during the night;
    b. encouraged to breastfeed on demand as soon as the infant's condition permits;
    c. taught proper storage and labeling of human milk; and

d. assisted in learning skilled hand expression or obtaining a double set-up electric breast pump prior to going home.

24. Before leaving the hospital,[15] breastfeeding mothers should be able to
    a. position the baby correctly at the breast with no pain during the feeding;
    b. latch the baby to breast properly;
    c. state when the baby is swallowing milk;
    d. state that the baby should be nursed approximately 8 to 12 times every 24 hours until satiety;
    e. state age-appropriate elimination patterns (at least six urinations per day and three to four stools per day by the fourth day of life);
    f. list indications for calling a clinician; and
    g. manually express milk from their breasts.

THE TEN STEPS TO SUCCESSFUL BREASTFEEDING

1. Have a written breastfeeding policy that is routinely communicated to all health care staff.
2. Train all health care staff in skills necessary to implement this policy.
3. Inform all pregnant women about the benefits and management of breastfeeding.
4. Help mothers initiate breastfeeding within 1 hour of birth.
5. Show mothers how to breastfeed and how to maintain lactation, even if they are separated from their infants.
6. Give newborn infants no food or drink other than breast milk, unless medically indicated.[1]
7. Practice rooming-in—allow mothers and infants to remain together—24 hours a day.
8. Encourage breastfeeding on demand.
9. Give no artificial teats or pacifiers to breastfeeding infants.
10. Foster the establishment of breastfeeding support groups and refer mothers to them on discharge from the hospital or clinic.

25. Prior to going home, mothers will be given the names and telephone numbers of community resources to contact for help with breastfeeding, including (the support group or resource recommended by "name of institution").

26. "Name of institution" does not accept free formula or free breastmilk substitutes. Nursery or NICU discharge bags offered to all mothers

---

[1]A hospital must pay fair market price for all formula and infant feeding supplies that it uses and cannot accept free or heavily discounted formula and supplies.

will not contain infant formula, coupons for formula, logos of formula companies, or literature with formula company logos.

27. *"Name of institution"* health professionals will attend educational sessions on lactation management and breastfeeding promotion to ensure that correct, current, and consistent information is provided to all mothers wishing to breastfeed.

APPLICATION

All breastfeeding patients.

EXCEPTIONS

Breastfeeding is contraindicated in the following situations:

- HIV-positive mother in developed countries (e.g., United States, Europe)
- Mother using illicit drugs (e.g., cocaine, heroin) unless specifically approved by the infant's health care provider on a case-by-case basis
- A mother taking certain medications. Although most prescribed and over-the-counter drugs are safe for the breastfeeding infant, some medications may make it necessary to interrupt breastfeeding. These include radioactive isotopes, antimetabolites, cancer chemotherapy, and a small number of other medications. The references used at *"name of institution"* are *Medications and Mothers' Milk* by Thomas Hale,[5] *Breastfeeding: A Guide for the Medical Profession* by R.A. Lawrence and R.M. Lawrence,[8] and the American Academy of Pediatrics Statement on the Transfer of Drugs into Human Milk.[4]
- Mother has active, untreated tuberculosis
- Infant has galactosemia
- Mother has active herpetic lesions on her breast(s)—breastfeeding can be recommended on the unaffected breast (The Infectious Disease Service will be consulted for problematic infectious disease issues.)
- Mother has varicella that is determined to be infectious to the infant
- Mother has HTLV1 (human T-cell leukemia virus type 1)

RESPONSIBILITY

- RN
- LPN
- LC
- PNP
- MD
- CNM

FORMS

- Newborn Flow Sheet
- Maternal Flow Sheet

OTHER RELATED POLICIES

- Policy #
- Other references/resources[8,12,16,2,10]

Initiated by

Contributing Departments

Acknowledgment

The development of this protocol was supported in part by a grant from the Maternal and Child Health Bureau, U.S. Department of Health and Human Services.

Copyright © 2003 by the Academy of Breastfeeding Medicine, Inc.

Protocol Committee

Caroline J. Chantry, MD

Co-Chairperson

Cynthia R. Howard, MD, MPH, FABM

Co-Chairperson

Barbara L. Philipp, MD

This article has been cited by:

1. Xena Grossman, Jana Chaudhuri, Lori Feldman-Winter, Jessica Abrams, Kimberly Niles Newton, Barbara L. Philipp, Anne Merewood. 2009. Hospital Education in Lactation Practices (Project HELP): does clinician education affect breastfeeding initiation and exclusivity in the hospital? *Birth* 36:1, 54–59. [CrossRef].
2. Philip O. Anderson, Verónica Valdés. 2007. A critical review of pharmaceutical galactagogues. *Breastfeed Med* 2:4, 229–242. [Abstract] [PDF] [PDF Plus].

REFERENCES

1. Academy of Breastfeeding Medicine Board of Directors. ABM Mission Statement, 2003. Available at www.bfmed .org.
2. American Academy of Pediatrics: *Redbook: 2003 Report of the Committee on Infectious Diseases*, ed 26, Elk Grove, Ill., 2003, American Academy of Pediatrics.
3. American College of Obstetricians and Gynecologists and Committees on Health Care for Underserved Women and Obstetric Practice. In: Queenan JT, editor: Breastfeeding: maternal and infant aspects, 2000, The American College of Obstetricians and Gynecologists: Washington, D.C. ACOG Educational Bulletin.
4. Committee on Drugs. The American Academy of Pediatrics: The transfer of drugs and other chemicals into human milk, *Pediatrics* 108:776–789, 2001.
5. Hale TW: *Medications and mother's milk*, ed 10, Amarillo, Tex., 2002, Pharmasoft Medical Publishing.

6. Howard CR, de Blieck EA, ten Hoopen CB, et al: Physiologic stability of newborns during cup- and bottlefeeding, *Pediatrics* 104:1–7, 1999.

7. Howard CR, Howard FM, Lanphear B, et al: Randomized clinical trial of pacifier use and bottle-feeding or cup-feeding and their effect on breastfeeding, *Pediatrics* 111:511–518, 2003.

8. Lawrence RA, Lawrence RM: *Breastfeeding: a guide for the medical profession*, ed 5, St. Louis, Mo., 1999, Mosby.

9. Marinelli KA, Burke GS, Dodd VL: A comparison of the safety of cup feedings and bottle feedings in premature infants whose mothers intend to breastfeed, *J Perinatol* 21:350–355, 2001.

10. Merewood A, Philipp BL: *Breastfeeding: conditions and diseases*, Amarillo, Tex., 2001, Pharmasoft Publishers.

11. Position of the American Dietetic Association: Breaking the barriers to breastfeeding, *J Am Diet Assoc* 01:1213–1220, 2001.

12. Protocol Committee Academy of Breastfeeding Medicine. In: Chantry C, Howard CR, McCoy RC, editors: *Clinical Protocol #5: peripartum breastfeeding management for the healthy mother and infant at term*. Academy of Breastfeeding Medicine, 2002, New Rochelle, N.Y. Available at: www.bfmed.org.

13. Protocol Committee Academy of Breastfeeding Medicine. In: Cordes R, Howard CR, editors: *Clinical Protocol #3: hospital guidelines for the use of supplementary feedings in the healthy term breastfed newborn*. Academy of Breastfeeding Medicine, 2002, New Rochelle, N.Y. Available at: www.bfmed.org.

14. Protocol Committee Academy of Breastfeeding Medicine. Eidelman AI, Howard CR, Schanler RJ, Wight NE: *Clinical protocol number 1: guidelines for glucose monitoring and treatment of hypoglycemia in breastfed neonates*. ABM News and Views 5 (1999) (insert).

15. Protocol Committee Academy of Breastfeeding Medicine. In: Gartner L, Howard CR, editors: *Clinical protocol #2: guidelines for hospital discharge of the breastfeeding term infant and mother, "The Going Home Protocol."* Academy of Breastfeeding Medicine, 2002, New Rochelle, N.Y. Available at: www.bfmed.org.

16. Riordan JM, Auerbach KG: *Breastfeeding and human lactation*, Boston, Mass., 1993, Jones & Bartlett Publishers.

17. The American Academy of Pediatrics: Work Group on Breastfeeding. Breastfeeding and the use of human milk, *Pediatrics* 100:1035–1039, 1997.

18. The American Academy of Family Physicians. Family Physicians Supporting Breastfeeding: Breastfeeding Position Paper 2002. The American Academy of Family Physicians. In: *Compendium of AAFP positions on selected health issues*, 2002, The American Academy of Family Physicians, Kansas City, Mo. Available at: http://www.aafp.org/policy/x1641.xml.

19. U.S. Department of Health and Human Services. HHS Blueprint for Action on Breastfeeding. In: U.S. Department of Health and Human Services, 2000, Office on Women's Health: Washington, D.C.

20. WHO/UNICEF Joint Statement: Meeting on Infant and Young Child Feeding, *J Nurse Midwifery* 25:31–38, 1980.

21. World Health Organization: United Nations Children's Fund. Protecting, promoting and supporting breastfeeding: the special role of maternity services (a joint WHO/UNICEF statement), *Int J Gynecol Obstet* 31:171–183, 1990.

22. World Health Organization and United Nations Children's Fund: *Innocenti declaration on the protection, promotion and support of breastfeeding*, New York, 1990, UNICEF.

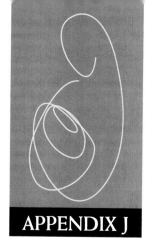

Protocol 8: Human Milk Storage Information for Home Use for Healthy Full-Term Infants

‖‖‖

Storage Containers

1. Hard-sided containers, such as hard plastic or glass, are the preferred containers for long-term human milk storage. These containers should have an airtight seal.[3]
2. Plastic bags specifically designed for human milk storage can be used for short-term (less than 72 hours) milk storage.[3,11] Use of plastic bags is not recommended for long-term storage as they may spill, leak, or become contaminated more easily than hard-sided containers, and some important milk components may adhere to the soft plastic and be lost.

General Guidelines

1. Hands must be washed prior to expressing or pumping milk.
2. Use containers and pumping equipment that have been washed in hot, soapy water and rinsed. If available, cleaning in a dishwasher is acceptable; dishwashers that additionally heat the water may improve cleanliness. If a dishwasher is not available, boiling the containers after washing is recommended. Boiling is particularly important where the water supply may not be clean.
3. Store in small portions to minimize waste. Most breastfed babies take between 2 and 4 ounces (60 to 120 mL) of milk when beginning with an alternative feeding method. Storing in 2-ounce (60-mL) amounts and offering additional amounts if the baby is still hungry will prevent having to throw away unfinished milk.
4. Consider storing smaller size portions [1 to 2 ounces (30 to 60 mL) each] for unexpected situations. A small amount of milk can keep a baby happy until mom comes to nurse the baby.
5. Several expressions throughout a day may be combined to get the desired volume in a container. Chill the newly expressed milk for at least 1 hour in the main body of the refrigerator or in a cooler with ice or ice packs, and then add it to previously chilled milk expressed on the same day.
6. Do not add warm breast milk to frozen milk because it will partially thaw the frozen milk.
7. Keep milk from one day separate from other days.
8. Do not fill the container; leave some room at the top because breast milk expands as it freezes.
9. Label containers clearly with waterproof labels and ink, if possible.
10. Indicate the date that the milk was expressed and the child's name (for day care).
11. Expect that the milk will separate during storage because it is not homogenized. The cream will rise to the top of the milk and look thicker and whiter. Before feeding, gently swirling the container of milk will mix the cream

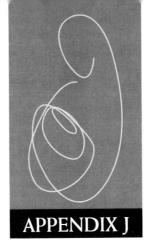

Protocol 9: Use of Galactogogues in Initiating or Augmenting Maternal Milk Supply

Background

Galactogogues (or lactogogues) are medications or other substances believed to assist initiation, maintenance, or augmentation of maternal milk production. Because low milk supply is one of the most common reasons given for discontinuing breast-feeding,[30] both mothers and physicians have sought medicine to address this concern. Breast milk production is a complex physiologic process involving physical and emotional factors and the interaction of multiple hormones, the most important of which is believed to be prolactin. With parturition and expulsion of the placenta, progesterone falls and a full milk supply is initiated (Lactogenesis II).[27] Through interaction with the hypothalamus and anterior pituitary, dopamine agonists inhibit, and dopamine antagonists increase, prolactin secretion and thereby milk production (endocrine control). Thereafter, prolactin levels gradually decrease but milk supply is maintained or increased by local feedback mechanisms (autocrine control).[20] Therefore, an increase in prolactin levels is needed to increase, but not maintain, milk supply. If the breasts are not emptied regularly and thoroughly, milk production declines. Likewise, more frequent and thorough emptying of the breasts typically results in increased milk production. Use of galactogogues for faltering milk supply should generally be reserved for situations after both a thorough evaluation for treatable causes (e.g., maternal hypothyroidism or medication) and increased frequency of breastfeeding or pumping or expression has not been successful.

Indications for Galactogogues

Common indications for galactogogues are adoptive nursing (induction of lactation in a woman who was not pregnant with the current child), relactation (reestablishing milk supply after weaning), and increasing a faltering milk supply because of maternal or infant illness or separation. Mothers who are not directly breastfeeding but are expressing milk by hand or with a pump often experience a decline in milk production after several weeks. One of the most common indications for galactogogues is to augment a declining milk supply in mothers of preterm or ill infants in the neonatal intensive care unit.

Procedure

1. Before using any substance to try to increase milk supply, a full evaluation of current maternal milk supply and effectiveness of milk transfer is imperative. Attention must be directed to the evaluation and augmentation of frequency and thoroughness of milk removal. This can be accomplished through increased frequency and duration of breastfeeding (if the infant has been shown to be effective at emptying the breasts) or

pumping. A full-size, automatic cycling breast pump, capable of draining both breasts ("hospital grade") at the same time is recommended, if available. Problems such as inappropriate timing and duration of feedings, inappropriate supplementation, mother-infant separation, ineffective latch, and inadequate milk transfer should be corrected.

2. Women should be informed of any data (or lack thereof) regarding the efficacy, safety, and timing of use of galactogogues. With the exception of adoptive nursing, where galactogogues are started *before* the birth of the baby, there is no research to suggest that starting galactogogues within the first week postpartum is efficacious.

3. Mothers should be screened for contraindications to the chosen medication or substance and informed as to possible side effects. Although a lactation consultant may recommend the medication or herb, it is the physician's responsibility to prescribe medications and follow the mother and infant.

4. The physician who prescribes the medication is obligated to follow, or to ensure appropriate follow-up, of both mother and infant regarding milk supply and any side effects. In practice, many times it is the nurse practitioner, pediatrician, or neonatologist who is asked to prescribe a galactogogue and not the obstetrician-gynecologist. As is commonly found when dealing with lactation, family physicians are ideally situated to manage this issue.

5. Although short-term use (1 to 3 weeks) has been evaluated for some of these substances, long-term use has not been studied. Anecdotal reports suggest no increase in side effects with the most commonly used medications (metoclopramide, domperidone, and fenugreek), but long-term effects on both mother and infant are unknown.

Specific Galactogogues

Many medications, foods, and herbal therapies have been recommended as galactogogues. The medications used often exert their effects through antagonism of dopamine receptors, resulting in increased prolactin. In many cases, the mechanism(s) of action are unknown.

METOCLOPRAMIDE

Metoclopramide (Reglan) is the most well studied and most commonly used medication for inducing or augmenting lactation in the United States. It promotes lactation by antagonizing the release of dopamine in the central nervous system, thereby

increasing prolactin levels.[26] It is an antiemetic and also commonly used for gastroesophageal reflux in infants. Although levels found in breastmilk have been measured higher than maternal serum levels, levels in infants have been undetectable or well below infant therapeutic levels with no reported side effects.[17] Metoclopramide does not appear to alter milk composition significantly.[9,8] Many studies have shown its efficacy in the induction and augmentation of milk production.[31,12,21,33,18,19,8,16,11,10,23,2] However, there is one controlled trial that failed to show efficacy.[22]

Maternal restlessness, drowsiness, fatigue, and diarrhea may occur but usually do not require stopping the medication.[26,16] The drug should be discontinued if any of the rare extrapyramidal side effects of sleeplessness, headache, confusion, dizziness, mental depression, or feelings of anxiety or agitation occur. Acute dystonic reactions are very rare (<0.05%) and may require diphenhydramine (Benadryl) treatment. Metoclopramide should not be used if patients have epilepsy or are on antiseizure medications, have a history of significant depression or are on antidepressant drugs, have a pheochromocytoma or uncontrolled hypertension, have intestinal bleeding or obstruction, or have a known allergy or prior reaction to metoclopramide.[26] Metoclopramide does transfer into the milk, but research has demonstrated no side effects in the infants of mothers taking metoclopramide.[31,12,21,33,18,19,8,16,11,10,23,2,13]

The usual dose is 30 to 45 mg/day in three or four divided doses, with a dose-response effect up to 45 mg daily.[18] It is usually given for 7 to 14 days at full dose with a taper off over 5 to 7 days. Longer periods of use may be associated with an increased incidence of depression. Occasionally a mother's milk supply will falter as the dose is reduced, and the lowest effective dose has been continued for longer periods successfully. Some experts also advise a gradual increase when beginning the dosage.

DOMPERIDONE (MOTILIUM)

Domperidone is also a dopamine antagonist that is available outside the United States for the treatment of gastroesophageal reflux and emesis.[15] Because of its drug characteristics it is less likely to cross the maternal blood-brain barrier, resulting in fewer extrapyramidal side effects than metoclopramide. Domperidone is also less likely than metoclopramide to cross into the breastmilk.[33] Administration of domperidone results in significant increases in mean serum prolactin levels in normal women.[7,28] Domperidone is the only galactogogue evaluated in a randomized controlled trial and shown to be safe and effective in increasing breastmilk production.[7]

Side effects are very uncommon and include dry mouth, headache (resolved with decreased dosage), and abdominal cramps.[15] Chronic high-dose treatment with domperidone in rodents has been associated with increased numbers of breast tumors. This has not been reported in humans. Domperidone is contraindicated in patients with known sensitivity to the drug and in situations in which gastrointestinal stimulation might be dangerous (e.g., gastrointestinal hemorrhage, mechanical obstruction, or perforation). Despite the fact that domperidone is approved for use in most of the developed world and has been used for many years with an excellent safety record, the U.S. Food and Drug Administration (FDA) issued a warning against its use in the United States based on safety concerns with IV use and risks associated with drug importation.[34a] There is no evidence that oral administration is associated with toxicity in either mother or infant.[34a] The usual dosage is 10 to 20 mg three to four times per day taken for 3 to 8 weeks. Most women respond within 3 to 4 days, but some women respond in 24 hours, and some require 2 to 3 weeks to get maximum effect.[28]

SULPIRIDE (EGONYL) AND CHLORPROMAZINE (THORAZINE)

Sulpiride is an antipsychotic (neuroleptic) medication not available in the United States that acts as a galactogogue by increasing prolactin-releasing hormone from the hypothalamus. Two studies have shown an increase in milk supply over placebo. Maternal side effects may include the extrapyramidal effects listed above for metoclopramide and possibly weight gain. The suggested dosage is 50 mg two or three times daily.[1,35,36]

Psychiatric practitioners have long noted galactorrhea in both males and females taking chlorpromazine (also a neuroleptic). A dose of 25 mg orally three times daily for 1 week has been shown in case reports to increase milk supply.

As both sulpiride and chlorpromazine increases prolactin levels by blocking dopamine receptors (and therefore the prolactin-inhibiting action of dopamine), extrapyramidal side effects are again possible.[1]

HUMAN GROWTH HORMONE

One randomized, double-blind, placebo-controlled trial of human growth hormone in a dose of 0.1 international unit/kg/day subcutaneously noted a significant increase in milk volume by day 7 in 16 healthy lactating women. There were no documented changes in milk composition or side effects reported in the mothers. The usefulness of this expensive, injectable galactogogue appears limited.[13,4]

THYROTROPIN-RELEASING HORMONE

Thyrotropin-releasing hormone (TRH) is used in the United States to assess thyroid function. It causes the release of both thyroid-stimulating hormone and prolactin from the pituitary. The most recent study suggests short-term use is both safe and effective, but long-term use has not been evaluated. Dosage was one spray (1 mg TRH) four times daily.[5] Other studies used IV (200 mcg) or oral (5 mg) forms.[34] TRH is not commonly used.

HERBAL/NATURAL GALACTOGOGUES

Throughout world history women have used certain herbs or foods to enhance their milk supply. Most of these substances have not been scientifically evaluated, but traditional use suggests safety and some efficacy. The mechanisms of action for all are unknown. Herbs commonly mentioned as galactogogues include fenugreek, goat's rue, milk thistle, anise, basil, blessed thistle, fennel seeds, marshmallow, and others. Beer is commonly used in some cultures, but alcohol may actually reduce milk production, and there is no evidence to support that the yeasts in beer are effective galactogogues.

It is of note that herbs and dietary supplements were removed by the Federal 1994 Dietary Supplement Act from undergoing the rigorous evaluation by the U.S. Food and Drug Administration that is required for drugs. The composition of herbal and dietary supplements is unknown, and they have been known to contain toxic substances. This is especially true for herbs from mainland China. There is no standard dosing, preparation, or composition, and fraudulent preparations may be a risk.

Fenugreek (*Trigonella foenum-graecum*) is the most commonly recommended herbal galactogogue, treasured as a spice and medicine throughout India and the Middle East for thousands of years. It is a member of the pea family listed as GRAS (generally regarded as safe) by the U.S. Food and Drug Administration. Usual dose is one to four capsules (580 to 610 mg) three to four times per day, although as with most herbal remedies there is no standard dosing. The higher of these doses may be required in relactating or adoptive mothers. Alternatively, it can be taken as one cup of strained tea three times per day (1/4 tsp seeds steeped in 8 oz water for 10 minutes).[24] Huggins[14] reported the anecdotal use of fenugreek in at least 1200 women with increased milk supply within 24 to 72 hours. Reported side effects are rare: maple-like odor to sweat, milk, and urine; diarrhea; and increased asthmatic symptoms. Use during pregnancy is not recommended because of its uterine stimulant effects. Fenugreek is known to lower blood glucose, so caution is advised. Two recent preliminary reports suggest effectiveness.[32,6]

Goat's rue (*Galega officinalis*) is a traditional galactogogue, widely recommended in Europe, based on observations of increased milk supply when fed to cows in the 1900s. No controlled human trials have been done, and no adverse effects have been reported with the following possible exception: Maternal ingestion of a lactation tea containing extracts of licorice (*Glycyrrhiza glabra*), fennel, anise, and goat's rue was linked to drowsiness, hypotonia, lethargy, emesis, and poor suckling in two breastfed neonates. An infection work-up was negative, and symptoms and signs resolved on discontinuation of the tea and a 2-day break from breastfeeding.[29] The tea was not tested for contaminants or adulterants, and there have been no other adverse events reported in Europe or South America, where the herb is also used as a hypoglycemic agent. It is usually used as a tea (1 tsp dried leaves steeped in 8 oz water for 10 minutes) with 1 cup taken three times a day.[24]

Milk thistle (*Silybum marianum*) has been used historically throughout Europe, but there are no randomized controlled trials to validate its use. The plant is still commonly known as St. Mary's thistle in honor of the Virgin Mary. Early Christians believed that the white colored veins in the leaves were symbolic of her breast milk. The American Herbal Products Association gives it a rating of 1, meaning that the herb may be safely consumed when used appropriately and does not contraindicate its use during lactation.[25] It is used as a strained tea (simmer 1 tsp crushed seeds in 8 oz water for 10 minutes) taking two to three cups per day.[24]

Conclusions

Of the substances used to induce, maintain, or augment milk production, domperidone and metoclopramide appear to be the most clinically useful. Prior to the use of any galactogogue, evaluation and correction of any modifiable factors such as frequency and thoroughness of breast emptying should be addressed. Medication should never replace evaluation and counseling on modifiable factors or reassurance when appropriate. As with any medication given to lactating women, close follow-up of both mother and baby is essential.

Acknowledgment

Supported in part by a grant from the Maternal and Child Health Bureau, U.S. Department of Health and Human Services.

The Academy of Breastfeeding Medicine Protocol Committee
Caroline J. Chantry, MD, FABM, Co-Chairperson
Cynthia R. Howard, MD, MPH, FABM, Co-Chairperson
*Anne Montgomery, MD, FABM
*Nancy Wight, MD, FABM
*Lead Author(s)

REFERENCES

1. Aono T, Ari T, Koike K, et al: Effect of sulpiride on poor puerperal lactation, *Am J Obstet Gynecol* 143:927, 1982.
2. Bose CL, D'Ercole J, Lester AG, et al: Relactation by mothers of sick or premature infants, *Pediatrics* 67:565, 1981.
3. Brown RE: Relactation: an overview, *Pediatrics* 60:116, 1977.
4. Budd SS, Erdman SH, Long DM, et al: Improved lactation with metoclopramide. A case report, *Clin Pediatr* 32:53, 1993.
5. Caron RW, Janh GA, Deis RP: Lactogenic actions of different growth hormone preparations in pregnant and lactating rats, *J Endocrinol* 142:535, 1994.
6. Co MM, Hernandez EA, Co BG: A comparative study on the efficacy of the different galactogogues among mothers with lactational insufficiency. In Abstract, AAP Section on Breastfeeding (2002 NCE), 2002.
7. daSilva OP, Knoppert DC, Angelini MM, et al: Effect of domperidone on milk production in mothers of premature newborns: a randomized, double-blind, placebo-controlled trial, *Can Med Assoc J* 164:17–21, 2001.
8. deGezelle H, Ooghe W, Thiery M, et al: Metoclopramide and breast milk, *Eur J Obstet Gynecol Reprod Biol* 15:31–36, 1983.
9. Ehrenkrantz RA, Ackerman BA: Metoclopramide effect on faltering milk production by mothers of premature infants, *Pediatrics* 78:614, 1986.
10. Ertl T, Sulyok E, Ezer E, et al: The influence of metoclopramide on the composition of human breast milk, *Acta Paediatr Hung* 31:415–422, 1991.
11. Gabay MP: Galactogogues: medications that induce lactation, *J Hum Lact* 18:274–279, 2002.
12. Gupta AP, Gupta PK: Metoclopramide as a lactogogue, *Clin Pediatr* 24:269–272, 1985.
13. Guzman V, Toscano G, Canales ES, et al: Improvement of defective lactation by using oral metoclopramide, *Acta Obstet Gynecol Scand* 58:53–55, 1979.
14. Huggins KE: *Fenugreek: one remedy for low milk production*, http://www.breastfeedingonline.com/fenuhugg.shtml. Retrieved July 16, 2004.
15. Hutchinson TA, Shahan DR, Anderson ML, editors: *DRUG-DEX®system*, Englewood, Colo., 2004, MICROMEDEX: Healthcare Series 121 (Edition expires).
16. Kauppila A, Anunti P, Kivinen S, et al: Metoclopramide and breast feeding: efficacy and anterior pituitary responses of the mother and child, *Eur J Obstet Gynecol Reprod Biol* 19:19–22, 1985.

17. Kauppila A, Arvel P, Koivisto M, et al: Metoclopramide and breastfeeding: transfer into milk and the newborn, *Eur J Clin Pharm* 25:619–623, 1983.

18. Kauppila A, Kivinen S, Ylikorkala O: A dose response relation between improved lactation and metoclopramide, *Lancet* 1(8231):175–1177, 1981.

19. Kauppila A, Kivinen S, Ylikorkala O: Metoclopramide increases prolactin release and milk secretion in puerperium without stimulating the secretion of thyrotropin and thyroid hormones, *J Clin Endocrinol Metab* 52:436–439, 1981.

20. Lawrence RA, Lawrence RM: *Breastfeeding: a guide for the medical profession*, ed 5, St. Louis, 1999, Mosby.

21. Lewis PJ, Devenish C, Kahn C: Controlled trial of metoclopramide in the initiation of breast feeding, *Br J Clin Pharmacol* 9:217–219, 1980.

22. Lewis PA, Devenish C, Kahn C: Controlled trial of metoclopramide in the initiation of breast feeding, *Brit J Clin Pharmacol* 9:217–219, 1980.

23. Liu JH, Lee DW, Markoff E: Differential release of prolactin variants in postpartum and early follicular phase women, *J Clin Endocrinol Metab* 71:605–610, 1990.

24. Low Dog T: Lactogogues. In Presentation at International Lactation Consultants Association (ILCA) Annual Meeting, 2001.

25. McGuffin M, Hobbs C, Upton R, et al, editors: *American Herbal Products Association's botanical safety handbook*, Boca Raton, Fla., 1997, CRC Press, p 107.

26. Murray L, editor: *Physicians' desk reference*, ed 56, Montvale, N.J., 2002, Medical Economics.

27. Neville MC, Morton J, Unemura S: Lactogenesis: transition from pregnancy to lactation, *Ped Clin North Am* 48:45–52, 2001.

28. Newman J. Handout #19: Domperidone, January 1998. Retrieved 7 1.04 from http://bflrc.com/newman/lbreast feeding/domperid.htm.

29. Rosti L, Nardini A, Bettinelli ME, et al: Toxic effects of an herbal tea mixture in two newborns, *Acta Pediatr* 83:683, 1994.

30. Sjolin S, Hofvander Y, Hillervik C: Factors related to early termination of breastfeeding: a retrospective study in Sweden, *Acta Paediatr Scand* 66:505–511, 1977.

31. Sousa PLR, Barros FC, Pinheiro GNM, et al: Reestablishment of lactation with metoclopramide, *J Trop Pediatr Environ Child Health* 21:214, 1975.

32. Swafford S, Berens P: Effect of fenugreek on breast milk volume. In Abstract, 5th International Meeting of the Academy of Breastfeeding Medicine, Tucson, Ariz, 2000.

33. Tolino A, Tedeschi A, Farace R, et al: The relationship between metoclopramide and milk secretion in puerperium, *Clin Exp Obstet Gynecol* 8:93–95, 1981.

34. Tyson JE, Perez A, Zanartu J: Human lactational response to oral thyrotropin releasing hormone, *J Clin Endocrinol Metab* 43:760–776, 1976.

34a. U.S. Food and Drug Administration: FDA talk paper. June 7, 2004. www.fda.gov/bbs/topics/answers.

35. Ylikorkali O, Kauppila A, Kivinen S, et al: Sulpiride improves inadequate lactation, *Br Med J* 285:299, 1982.

36. Ylikorkali O, Kauppila A, Kivinen S, et al: Treatment of inadequate lactation with oral sulpiride and buccal oxytocin, *Obstet Gynecol* 63:57, 1984.

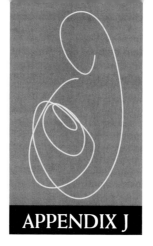

APPENDIX J

Protocol 10: Breastfeeding the Near-Term Infant (35 to 37 Weeks' Gestation)

Goals

1. Promote, support, and sustain breastfeeding in the near-term infant.
2. Maintain optimal health of infant and mother.

Purpose

1. Allow infants born at 35 to 37 weeks of gestation to breastfeed and/or breastmilk feed to the greatest extent possible.
2. Heighten awareness of difficulties near-term infants and their mothers may experience with breastfeeding.
3. Offer strategies to anticipate, identify promptly, and manage breastfeeding problems that the near-term infant and mother may experience in the inpatient and outpatient setting.
4. Prevent medical problems such as dehydration, hypoglycemia, hyperbilirubinemia, and failure to thrive in the near-term infant.
5. Maintain awareness of mothers' needs.

Definition

"Near-term infant" refers to infants born between 35 0/7 and 36 6/7 weeks of gestation. Many problems of the near-term infant are also found in the larger 34- to 35-week preterm infant and the borderline term infant of 37 0/7 to 37 6/7 weeks'

gestation, and, therefore, the following guidelines may be applicable to these infants as well.

Background

The advantages of breastmilk feeding for premature infants appear to be even greater than those for term infants. Establishing breastfeeding in the near-term infant, however, is frequently more problematic than in the full-term infant. Because of their immaturity, near-term infants may be sleepier and have less stamina; more difficulty with latch, suck, and swallow; more difficulty maintaining body temperature; increased vulnerability to infection; greater delays in bilirubin excretion; and more respiratory instability than the full-term infant. The sleepiness and inability to suck vigorously is often misinterpreted as sepsis, leading to unnecessary separation and treatment. Alternatively, the near-term infant may appear deceptively vigorous at first glance. Physically large newborns are often mistaken for being more developmentally mature than their actual gestational age. (Remember the 3.84-kg baby born at 40 weeks was 3.0 kg at 36 weeks of gestation.) Near-term infants are more likely to be separated from their mother as a result of the infant being ill or requiring a screening procedure such as evaluation for sepsis, IV placement for antibiotics, and phototherapy.

Mothers who deliver near, but not at, term are more likely to deliver multiples or have a medical condition such as diabetes, pregnancy-induced hypertension, prolonged rupture of membranes, chorioamnionitis, Pitocin induction, or a C-section delivery that may affect the success of breastfeeding. Any one or a combination of these conditions places these mothers and infants at risk for difficulty in establishing successful lactation or for breastfeeding failure.

The potential maternal and infant problems listed above place the near-term breastfeeding infant at increased risk for hypothermia, hypoglycemia, excessive weight loss, dehydration, slow weight gain, failure to thrive, prolonged artificial milk supplementation, exaggerated jaundice, kernicterus, dehydration, fever secondary to dehydration, rehospitalization, and breastfeeding failure. In places where early discharge is the norm, these infants will be sent home soon after delivery. Discussion and parental education become crucial in the proper management of breastfeeding.

Near-term infants have a greater chance of exclusive breastfeeding in hospitals that adhere to the Ten Steps to Successful Breastfeeding. To this end, practitioners should become knowledgeable in the Ten Steps and work with the administration in their maternity hospitals to endorse the guidelines set forth in the Ten Steps (see Protocol #7).

Most of the acute problems encountered in the newborn are managed on the postpartum floor in the first few hours and days after parturition; however, there are times that an infant's condition deteriorates in the interval between discharge and the first office visit. Therefore, timely evaluation of the near-term infant after discharge is critical. Just as many hospitals are becoming breastfeeding friendly, the outpatient office or clinic needs to be not only supportive of the breastfeeding mother, but also able to assist mothers with uncomplicated problems or questions related to breastfeeding. In addition, it is essential to be able to refer mothers and infants in a timely manner to a trained lactation professional for more complicated breastfeeding problems. A lactation referral should be viewed with the same medical urgency as any other acute medical referral.

Principles of Care

1. Optimal communication
   a. Pathway and order set for breastfeeding the near-term infant.
   b. Written feeding plan to follow on hospital discharge.
   c. Facilitate communication among physician, nurses, and lactation consultants in the inpatient and outpatient settings.

   d. Avoid conflicting advice to mother and family of the near-term infant.
2. Assessment/reassessment
   a. Objective assessment of gestational age and associated risk factors.
   b. Daily assessment of breastfeeding on the postpartum floor or special care nursery.
   c. Careful assessment of breastfeeding issues in the outpatient setting.
3. Timely lactation support in the inpatient and outpatient setting
4. Avoid separation of mother and infant
   a. Immediate postpartum period.
   b. In cases in which either mother or infant is hospitalized for medical reasons.
5. Prevent frequently encountered problems in breastfed near-term infant
   a. Hypoglycemia.
   b. Hypothermia.
   c. Hyperbilirubinemia.
   d. Dehydration or excessive weight loss.
6. Education
   a. Ongoing education of staff and care providers of issues specific to breastfeeding the near-term infant in the inpatient and outpatient settings.
   b. Have one (or two) outpatient office support person (RN or lactation educator) trained in breastfeeding support, assessment, basic breastfeeding problem solving, and near-term breastfeeding issues.
   c. Educate parents about breastfeeding the near-term infant.
7. Discharge/follow-up
   a. Develop criteria for discharge readiness.
   b. Establish a feeding plan to follow after discharge.
   c. Facilitate timely and frequent outpatient follow-up to assure effective breastfeeding after discharge.
   d. Careful outpatient monitoring of mother and near-term infant.

INPATIENT: IMPLEMENTATION OF PRINCIPLES OF CARE

1. Initial steps
   a. Communicate the feeding plan through a prewritten order set that can be easily modified.
   b. Encourage immediate and extended skin-to-skin contact to improve postpartum stabilization of heart rate, respiratory effort, temperature control, metabolic stability, and early breastfeeding.

c. Assessment of gestational age by obstetrical estimate and Dubowitz scoring. Observe infant closely for 12 to 24 hours to assure physiologic stability (e.g., temperature, apnea, tachypnea, hypoglycemia).

d. Encourage rooming-in 24 hours a day. If the infant is physiologically stable and healthy, allow the infant to remain with the mother while receiving IV antibiotics or phototherapy. Depending on the individual situation, use of the biliblanket during breastfeeds, as well as limiting time outside more intense phototherapy, may be necessary.

e. Allow free access to the breast, encouraging initiation of breastfeeding within 1 hour after birth. Encourage continuous skin-to-skin contact as much as possible.

f. Breastfeeding ad libitum (on demand) should be encouraged. It is very important that the infant be breastfed (or breastmilk fed) *at least* eight times per 24-hour period. Sometimes it may be necessary to wake the baby if he or she does not indicate hunger. A mother may need to express her milk and give it to the baby using a cup or other alternative feeding method. Mothers should be warned that use of bottles at this stage might prevent breastfeeding in some babies.

2. Ongoing care

a. Communicate daily changes in feeding plan either directly or with use of a written bedside tool such as a crib card.

b. Formal evaluation from a lactation consultant or other certified health professional with expertise in lactation management should be completed within 24 hours of delivery.

c. Assess and document breastfeeding at least three times per day by at least two different providers with use of a standardized tool (e.g., LATCH Score,[5] IBFAT,[7] Mother/Baby Assessment Tool[10]).

d. Educate the mother about breastfeeding her infant (e.g., position, latch, duration, early feeding cues, etc.).

e. Monitor vital signs, weight change, stool and urine output, and milk transfer. Pre/post feeding weights where available, may be helpful, especially once lactogenesis II has occurred. Monitor for frequently occurring problems (e.g., obtain bilirubin if jaundiced before discharge, glucose screen before feeds for the first three feeds or until stable if hypoglycemia has occurred [see Protocol #1]). It is recommended to routinely screen for hyperbilirubinemia in near-term infants and to use standardized nomograms to assess risk of hyperbilirubinemia as well as plan for follow-up testing.

f. Avoid excessive weight loss or dehydration. Losses greater than 3% of birth weight by day 1 or greater than 7% by day 3, ineffective milk transfer, or exaggerated jaundice are considered excessive and merit further evaluation and monitoring.

i. The infant may need to be supplemented after breastfeeding with small quantities (5 to 10 mL per feeding on day 1, 10 to 30 mL per feeding thereafter) of expressed breast milk or formula. Mothers may supplement using a supplemental nursing device at the breast, cup feeds, finger feeds, syringe feeds, or bottle depending on clinical situation and mother's preference. Cup feedings have demonstrated safety in both preterm[6] and term infants.[3] Cup feeding may also preserve breastfeeding duration among both preterm[2] and term[4] infants who require multiple supplemental feeds. However, there is little evidence about the safety or efficacy of other alternative feeding methods or their effect on breastfeeding. When cleanliness is suboptimal, cup feeding may be the best choice.[12]

ii. If supplementing, the mother should pump or express milk regularly (use of a hospital-grade electric pump is recommended when feasible) during the day (e.g., every 3 hours) until the baby is breastfeeding well or if the mother and infant are separated and unable to breastfeed.

iii. Consider use of an ultrathin silicone nipple shield if there is difficulty with latch or evidence of ineffective milk transfer.[8] The use of nipple shields is controversial and generally requires close supervision of a trained lactation consultant or knowledgeable health care professional. Inappropriate or prolonged nipple shield use can decrease milk supply, and in some situations, nipple shields decrease, rather than increase, milk transfer.

g. Avoid thermal stress by using skin-to-skin (e.g., kangaroo) care or by double wrapping if necessary and by dressing the baby in a shirt and hat. Consider intermittent use of an incubator to maintain temperature. Where it is culturally acceptable, mothers can sleep with their babies to provide warmth.

3. Discharge planning.
   a. Assess readiness for discharge, including physiologic stability and adequate intake exclusively at breast or with supplements. May use 24-hour test weights, with a scale designed with adequate precision for such weights, for infants with >7% weight loss.[9]
   b. Develop discharge-feeding plan. Consider diet, milk intake (mL/kg/day), and method of feeding (breast, bottle, supplemental device, etc.). If supplementing, determine method most acceptable to mother for use after discharge.
   c. Make an appointment for follow-up within 48 hours of discharge to recheck weight, feeding adequacy, jaundice.
   d. Communicate discharge-feeding plan to pediatric outpatient provider. Written communication is preferred.

OUTPATIENT: IMPLEMENTATION OF PRINCIPLES OF CARE

1. Initial visit.
   a. The first outpatient office or home health visit should be when the infant is 3 to 5 days of life or 1 or 2 days after discharge.
   b. Review the inpatient maternal and infant records including prenatal, perinatal, infant, and feeding history (e.g., need for supplement in the hospital, problems with latch, need for phototherapy, etc.). Gestational age, birth weight, and weight at discharge should be recorded in the outpatient chart.
   c. Physician review of breastfeeding since discharge needs to be very specific regarding frequency, approximate duration of feedings, and how baby is being fed (e.g., at breast, expressed breast milk with supplemental device such as supplemental nursing system, finger feeds, or bottle with artificial nipple). Information about stool and urine output, color of stools, baby's state (e.g., crying, not satisfied after a feed, sleepy and difficult to keep awake at the breast during a feed, etc.) should be obtained. If parents have a written feeding record, it should be reviewed.
   d. Examination of the infant must include an accurate weight without clothes and calculation of change in weight from birth and discharge, state of alertness, and hydration. Assess for jaundice with cutaneous bilirubin screen and/or serum bilirubin determination if indicated.
   e. Assess the mother's breast for nipple shape, pain and trauma, engorgement, and mastitis.

The mother's emotional status and degree of fatigue should be considered, especially when considering supplemental feeding routines. Observe the baby feeding at the breast, looking at the latch, suck, and swallow.

2. Problem solving.
   a. Poor weight gain (<20 g/day) is most likely the result of inadequate intake. Median daily weight gain of a healthy newborn is 26 to 31 grams per day.[11] The care provider must determine whether the problem is insufficient breastmilk production, inability of the infant to transfer enough milk, or a combination of both. The infant who is getting enough breastmilk should have six to eight voids and yellow seedy stools daily by day 4, have lost no more than 8% of birth weight, and be satisfied after 20 to 30 minutes of nursing. Consider feeding more frequently or supplementing (preferably with expressed breast milk) after suckling if the mother is not already doing so or increasing the amount of supplement. Consider instituting or increasing frequency of pumping or manual expression. Consider referral to a lactation specialist.
   b. For infants with latch difficulties, the baby's mouth should be examined for anatomical abnormalities [e.g., ankyloglossia (tongue-tied),[1] cleft palate], and a digital suck exam performed. A referral to a trained professional lactation specialist or in the case of ankyloglossia a referral to someone trained in frenotomy may be indicated.
   c. The jaundiced near-term infant poses more of a problem when considering management of hyperbilirubinemia. Keep in mind all risk factors should be determined, and if the principal factor is lack of milk the primary treatment is to provide milk (preferably through improved breastfeeding or expressed breastmilk) to the baby. Institution of phototherapy for breastfeeding jaundice either in the home or in the hospital may actually interfere with the primary treatment of getting increased quantities of milk to the baby.
   d. Consider the use of a galactogogue (a medicine or herb that increases breast milk supply) in mothers who have a documented low breastmilk supply (see Protocol #9).
   e. The mother's ability to cope and manage the feeding plan needs to be evaluated. If the mother is not coping well, work with her to find help, and/or modify the feeding plan to something that is more manageable.

3. Follow-up: The near-term infant should have weekly weight checks until 40 weeks' postconceptual age or until it is demonstrated that he or she is thriving with no supplements.

   a. Babies who are not gaining well and for whom adjustments are being made to the feeding plan may need a visit 2 to 4 days after each adjustment. A home health provider, preferably trained in medical evaluation of the newborn and in lactation support, who reports the weight to the primary care provider could make this visit.

   b. Near-term infants have less vitamin D stored at birth, increasing their risk for later deficiency. Depending on sunlight exposure and skin color, vitamin D supplements (200 IU/day) may be indicated if the infant is exclusively breastfed. Strong consideration should be given to starting these supplements earlier than the 2 months of age recommended for term infants in the United States. Consideration should also be given to supplementing the near-term exclusively breastfed infant with iron, as iron stores in these infants are not those of the full-term infant. The American Academy of Pediatrics Committee on Nutrition recommends 2 mg/kg/day of elemental iron for preterm breastfed infants in the form of iron drops from 1 to 12 months of age.

   c. After the first week, infants should be monitored for adequate growth and evidence of normal biochemical indices (see Table P-4 from Protocol #12). Weight gain should average more than 20 g/day, and length and head circumference should each increase by an average of more than 0.5 cm/week.

Acknowledgment

Supported in part by a grant from the Maternal and Child Health Bureau, U.S. Department of Health and Human Services.

Protocol Committee
Eyla Boies, main author,
Co-Chairperson
Caroline J. Chantry, MD, FABM,
Co-Chairperson
Cynthia R. Howard, MD, MPH, FABM,
Co-Chairperson
Yvonne Vaucher, MD

APPENDIX Baby Friendly Hospital Initiative Steps for Successful Breastfeeding

1. Have a written breastfeeding policy.
2. Train all health care staff in the skills necessary to implement the policy.
3. Inform all mothers of the benefits of breastfeeding.
4. Help mothers initiate breastfeeding within 1 hour of birth.
5. Show mothers how to breastfeed and how to maintain lactation, even if they are to be separated from their infant.
6. Give newborn infants no food or drink other than breast milk, unless medically indicated.
7. Practice rooming-in—allow mothers and infants to remain together—24 hours a day if medically stable.
8. Encourage breastfeeding on demand.
9. Give no artificial teats or pacifiers to breastfeeding infants.
10. Foster the establishment of breastfeeding support groups and refer mothers to them, on discharge from the hospital or clinic.

REFERENCES

1. Ballard MD, Auer CE, Khoury JC: Ankyloglossia: assessment, incidence, and effect of frenuloplasty on the breast-feeding dyad, Pediatrics 110:e63, 2002.
2. Collins CT, Ryan P, Crowther CA, et al: Effect of bottles, cups, and dummies on breast feeding in preterm infants: a randomised controlled trial, Br Med J 329:193–198, 2004.
3. Howard CR, de Blieck EA, ten Hoopen CB, et al: Physiologic stability of newborns during cup- and bottlefeeding, Pediatrics 104(5 Pt 2):1204–1207, 1999.
4. Howard CR, Howard FM, Lanphear B, et al: Randomized clinical trial of pacifier use and bottle-feeding or cupfeeding and their effect on breastfeeding, Pediatrics 111:511–518, 2003.
5. Jensen D, Wallace S, Kelsay P: LATCH: a breastfeeding charting system and documentation tool, J Obstet Gynecol Neonatal Nurs 23:27–32, 1994.
6. Marinelli K, Burke G, Dodd V: A comparison of the safety of cup feedings and bottle feedings in premature infants whose mothers intend to breastfeed, J Perinatol 21:350–355, 2001.
7. Matthews MK: Developing an instrument to assess infant breastfeeding behaviour in the early neonatal period, Midwifery 4:154–165, 1988.
8. Meier PP, Brown LP, Hurst NM, et al: Nipple shields for preterm infants: effect on milk transfer and duration of breastfeeding, J Hum Lact 16:106, 2000.
9. Meier PP, Engstrom JL, Crichton C, et al: A new scale for in-home test-weighing for mothers of preterm and high-risk infants, J Hum Lact 10:63–68, 1994.
10. Mulford C: The mother-baby assessment (MBA): an Apgar "score" for breastfeeding, J Hum Lact 8:79–82, 1992.
11. National Research Council: Food and Nutrition Board, National Academy of Science: recommended daily allowances, ed 10, Washington, DC, 1989, U.S. Government Printing Office.
12. United Nations Children's Fund: Feeding low birth weight babies, 1996, UNICEF Division of Information and Public Affairs.

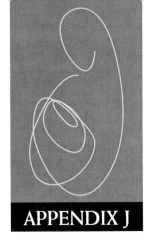

APPENDIX J

Protocol 11: Guidelines for the Evaluation and Management of Neonatal Ankyloglossia and Its Complications in the Breastfeeding Dyad

Definition

Ankyloglossia, partial: The presence of a sublingual frenulum that changes the appearance or function of the infant's tongue because of its decreased length, lack of elasticity, or attachment too distal beneath the tongue or too close to or onto the gingival ridge. In this document we will refer to partial ankyloglossia as simply "ankyloglossia." "True" or "complete ankyloglossia," extensive fusion of the tongue to the floor of the mouth, is extremely rare and is not within the scope of this discussion.

Background

At birth, the infant's tongue is normally able to extend over and past the mandibular gum pad. Significant ankyloglossia prevents an infant from anteriorly extending and elevating the tongue, and many breastfeeding experts believe that these limitations alter the normal peristaltic motion of the tongue during feeding, resulting in the potential for nipple trauma and problems with effective milk transfer and infant weight gain.

Ankyloglossia, commonly known as tongue-tie, occurs in approximately 3.2% to 4.8% of consecutive term infants at birth[14,1] and in 12.8% of infants with breastfeeding problems.[1] The condition has been associated with an increased incidence of breastfeeding difficulties: 25% in affected versus 3% in unaffected infants.[14]

Various methods have been suggested to diagnose and evaluate the severity of ankyloglossia[7,11] and to determine the criteria for intervention.[13,21] Short- and long-term consequences of ankyloglossia may include feeding and speech difficulties,[5,15] as well as orthodontic and mandibular abnormalities[23,22,24,6] and psychological problems.[10]

In the 1990s a number of case reports and observational studies were published that documented an association between ankyloglossia and breastfeeding problems.[8,18,2,12,17] There is considerable controversy regarding the significance of ankyloglossia and its management, both within and among medical specialty groups.[3,16] Both the diagnosis of ankyloglossia and the use of frenotomy, an incision or "snipping" of the frenulum, to treat ankyloglossia vary widely. The frenotomy procedure, carefully performed, has recently been shown to decrease maternal nipple pain to improve infant latch[1] and to improve milk transfer (personal communication, J. Ballard, July 27, 2004). There is a growing tendency among breastfeeding medicine specialists to favor releasing the tongue of the infant to facilitate breastfeeding and to protect the breastfeeding experience. To date, no randomized trials exist to demonstrate frenotomy for ankyloglossia is effective in treating infant or maternal breastfeeding problems.

Assessment of Ankyloglossia

All newborn infants, whether healthy or ill, should have a thorough examination of the oral cavity that assesses function as well as anatomy. This examination should include palpation of the hard and soft palate, gingivae, and sublingual areas in addition to the movements of the tongue, and the length, elasticity, and points of insertion of the sublingual frenulum.

When breastfeeding difficulties are encountered and a short or tight sublingual frenulum is noted, the appearance and function of the tongue may be semi-quantified using a scoring system such as the Hazelbaker[7] (Table J-12). The Hazelbaker scale has been tested for interrater reliability (personal communication, J. Ballard, July 27, 2004) and validated in a sample of term neonates.[1] Hazelbaker scores consistent with significant ankyloglossia have been shown to be highly correlated with difficulty with latching the infant onto the breast and maternal complaints of sore nipples.[1] Alternatively, ankyloglossia may be qualified as mild, moderate, or severe by the appearance of the tongue and of the frenulum.

Assessment of the Breastfeeding Dyad

Breastfeeding complications caused by ankyloglossia can generally be placed into broad categories of those caused by maternal nipple trauma or failure of the infant to breastfeed effectively. Specific complaints include difficulty latching or sustaining a latch, infant becoming frustrated or falling asleep at breast, prolonged feedings, a dissatisfied baby, gumming or chewing at the breast, poor weight gain, or failure to thrive. Maternal complaints include traumatized nipples, severe unrelenting pain with feeding, inability to let down because of pain, incomplete breast drainage, breast infections, and plugged ducts.

The physician should interview the mother to ascertain her degree of confidence and comfort while breastfeeding. This can be done semiquantitatively by using a scoring system such as the

TABLE J-12	Hazelbaker Assessment Tool for Lingual Frenulum Function*
Appearance Items	**Function Items**
Appearance of tongue when lifted	Lateralization
2: Round or square	2: Complete
1: Slight cleft in tip apparent	1: Body of tongue but not tongue tip
0: Heart- or V-shaped	0: None
Elasticity of frenulum	Lift of tongue
2: Very elastic	2: Tip to mid-mouth
1: Moderately elastic	1: Only edges to mid-mouth
0: Little or no elasticity	0: Tip stays at lower alveolar ridge or rises mid-mouth only with jaw closure
Length of lingual frenulum when tongue lifted	Extension of tongue
2: >1 cm	2: Tip over lower lip
1: 1 cm	1: Tip over lower gum only
0: <1 cm	0: Neither of the above, or anterior or mid-tongue humps
Attachment of lingual frenulum to tongue	Spread of anterior tongue
2: Posterior to tip	2: Complete
1: At tip	1: Moderate or partial
0: Notched tip	0: Little or none
Attachment of lingual frenulum to inferior	Cupping alveolar ridge
2: Entire edge, firm cup	2: Attached to floor of mouth or well below ridge
1: Side edges only, moderate cup	1: Attached just below ridge
0: Poor or no cup	0: Attached at ridge
	Peristalsis
	2: Complete, anterior to posterior
	1: Partial, originating posterior to tip
	0: None or reverse motion
	Snapback
	2: None
	1: Periodic
	0: Frequent or with each suck

*The infant's tongue is assessed using the five appearance items and the seven function items. Significant ankyloglossia is diagnosed when the appearance score total is 8 or less and/or the function score total is 11 or less.[1,7]
Modified with permission from Hazelbaker AK: *The assessment tool for lingual frenulum function (ATLFF): use in a lactation consultant private practice.* Master's Thesis, 1993, Pacific Oaks College.

LATCH score or a similar tool.[9] The LATCH score has been shown to correlate with breastfeeding duration, but only due to subscores for breast comfort.[20]

If the mother describes nipple pain, the physician may wish to use a pain scale in order to semi-quantify her perception of the degree of her pain. This serves to follow trends in the severity of pain, which may help in determining the effectiveness of an intervention.

The infant should be weighed, and the rate of weight gain since birth should be assessed. The physician should observe the mother and infant while breastfeeding to assess the effectiveness of the feeding and provide assistance as appropriate. Problems including an inadequate or nonsustained latch, and ineffective feedings should be noted. Test weights may be useful in assessing milk transfer. The infant should be weighed prior to and after breastfeeding without a change in clothing or diaper; the difference between the weights in grams indicates the amount of breastmilk consumed in milliliters.

The mother's nipples should be examined carefully for creases, bruises, blisters, cracks, or bleeding. Areolar edema and erythema should be noted as possible signs of nipple infection. A family history of bleeding diatheses should be elicited.

Recommendations

Conservative management of tongue-tie may be sufficient, requiring no intervention beyond breastfeeding assistance, parental education, and reassurance.[3] For partial ankyloglossia, if a tongue-tie release is deemed appropriate, the procedure should be performed by a physician or pedodontist experienced with the procedure; otherwise a referral should be made to an ear, nose, and throat specialist or oral surgeon. Release of the tongue-tie appears to be a minor procedure, but it may be ineffective in solving the immediate clinical problem and may cause complications such as infant pain and distress and postoperative bleeding, infection, or injury to the Wharton duct.[3] Complications are rare, however.[14,1,13,23]

Frenotomy, or simple incision or "snipping," of a tongue-tie is the most common procedure performed for partial ankyloglossia. It should be recognized that postoperative scarring may further limit tongue movement.[3] Excision with lengthening of the ventral surface of the tongue or a z-plasty release is a procedure with less postoperative scarring, but it carries the additional risks of general anesthesia.[3]

The Frenotomy Procedure

Instruments: Iris scissors and grooved retractor.
 Supplies: Clean gloves and gauze; gelatin foam.

Method: Parents should be counseled about risks, benefits, and alternatives of the procedure, and informed consent should be obtained. This counseling should include a discussion of the possibility that the clinical breastfeeding problem will not improve.

The frenulum may be transilluminated to check for translucency and lack of vasculature. The frenulum is usually a thin, translucent hypovascular membrane, where a simple frenotomy results in an almost bloodless procedure. Rarely, it may be thick and fibrous or muscular and relatively vascular. Thicker frenula are best incised by an otolaryngologist or oral surgeon under controlled conditions.

The frenulum is almost devoid of sensory innervation. Infants under 4 months of age can usually tolerate the frenotomy very well without any local anesthesia. Alternatively, topical anesthetic (e.g., benzocaine gel or paste) may be applied with cotton applicators to both sides of the frenulum in the area to be incised. This, however, may have the undesirable effect of numbing the mouth, such that the baby may not be able to suck effectively after the frenotomy is completed.

The infant is placed supine on the examining table or mother's lap. An assistant holds the baby's elbows firmly against the ears and stabilizes the chin with one index finger. Alternatively, the infant may be swaddled with a receiving blanket to immobilize the arms while the assistant stabilizes the head. Slight extension of the infant's neck allows better visualization of the tongue and frenulum. Using the grooved retractor or physician's fingers, the physician lifts the tongue to expose the frenulum. With the tips of the iris scissors an incision is made in the thinnest portion of the frenulum, close to the retractor and parallel to the tongue. Care is taken not to incise the tongue, the genioglossus muscle, or the gingival tissue. The incision should extend into the sulcus between the tongue and the genioglossus muscle, just beyond the level of the muscle, carefully avoiding the floor of the mouth. This ensures complete detachment of the tongue from the gingiva, without causing damage to the sublingual mucosa or to the salivary duct (Figure J-1).

The site beneath the tongue is blotted with gauze until little or no blood is seen. In the event of unexpected bleeding beyond 2 to 3 minutes, a strip of gelatin foam may be used to achieve rapid hemostasis. The infant may be returned to the mother immediately to be breastfed. Infant latch and maternal nipple pain should be reassessed at this time. There is no specific aftercare required except for breastfeeding. A small white patch or eschar is seen in some infants for 1 or 2 weeks during the healing process. Infection of the site is exceedingly rare if clean technique is used as described.

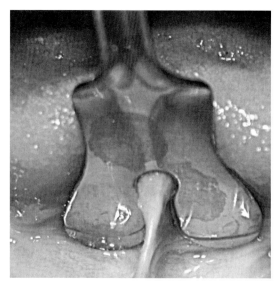

Figure J-1. Using a Lorenz tongue elevator, the lingual frenum is exposed. Pulling upward on the tongue stretches and allows visualization of the frenum and the floor of the mouth. In this infant an 8-mm incision was needed to allow sufficient movement of the tongue for effective breastfeeding to occur. Courtesy Dr. Larry Kotlow.

Medical equipment used in this procedure should be sterilized or disinfected in accordance with the guidelines of the Centers for Disease Control and Prevention.[4]

Management of Maternal and Infant Complications of Ankyloglossia

If nipple damage or infection is present, a problem-specific treatment program should be instituted. Mastitis and yeast infections should be treated according to established guidelines.[19]

Some mothers may need nipple rest for one to several days to allow healing to occur before reinstituting feedings at the breast. These mothers should be encouraged to express their breastmilk to maintain their milk supply and to feed their milk to the baby by an alternate method.

Suppressed lactation should be addressed and every attempt made to reestablish the mother's milk supply. Infants who have been gaining weight slowly or failing to thrive may need to receive supplements of expressed breastmilk or formula temporarily.

Follow-up for resolution of maternal and infant complications of ankyloglossia should take place by the mother's or infant's primary health care provider within 3 or 4 days of the frenotomy.

Further Research

This protocol was developed by the Academy of Breastfeeding Medicine to provide clinicians with guidance about the assessment and treatment of ankyloglossia and associated breastfeeding problems. More definitive recommendations await future research in this area. The Academy of Breastfeeding Medicine urges that more research be undertaken so that the benefits and risks of frenotomy for ankyloglossia and its effectiveness in treating breastfeeding concerns can be better understood. We specifically recognize that the Hazelbaker and LATCH instruments cited in this document require further interrater and intrarater reliability and validity testing. We recognize that a critical need exists for clinical tools to assess breastfeeding performance as well as the degree of ankyloglossia and function of the tongue. In addition, a randomized investigator-blinded clinical trial is needed to assess the effectiveness of frenotomy in treating infant and maternal breastfeeding problems associated with ankyloglossia.

REFERENCES

1. Ballard JL, Auer CE, Khoury JC: Ankyloglossia: assessment, incidence, and effect of frenuloplasty on the breastfeeding dyad, *Pediatrics* 110:e63, 2002.
2. Berg KL: Tongue-tie (ankyloglossia) and breastfeeding: a review, *J Hum Lact* 6:109–112, 1990.
3. Canadian Paediatric Society: Community Paediatrics Committee: Canadian Paediatric Society Statement: ankyloglossia and breastfeeding, *Paediatr Child Health* 7:269–270, 2002.
4. Centers for Disease Control: *Sterilization or disinfection of medical devices: general principles*, 2002, www.cdc.gov/ncidod/hip/Sterile/Sterilgp.htm.
5. Garcia Pola MJ, Gonzalez Garcia M, Garcia Martin JM, et al: A study of pathology associated with short lingual frenum, *ASDC J Dent Child* 69:59–62, 2002.
6. Hasan N: Tongue tie as a cause of deformity of lower central incisor, *J Pediatr Surg* 8:985, 1973.
7. Hazelbaker AK: *The assessment tool for lingual frenulum function (ATLFF): use in a lactation consultant private practice.* Master's Thesis, 1993, Pacific Oaks College.
8. Jain E: Tongue-tie: its impact on breastfeeding, *AARN News Lett* 51:18, 1995.
9. Jensen D, Wallace S, Kelsay P: LATCH: a breastfeeding charting system and documentation tool, *J Obstet Gynecol Neonatal Nurs* 23:27–32, 1994.
10. Ketty N, Sciullo PA: Ankyloglossia with psychological implications, *ASDC J Dent Child* 41:43–46, 1974.
11. Kotlow LA: Ankyloglossia (tongue-tie): a diagnostic and treatment quandary, *Quintessence Int* 30:259–262, 1999.
12. Marmet C, Shell E, Marmet R: Neonatal frenotomy may be necessary to correct breastfeeding problems, *J Hum Lact* 6:117–121, 1990 (review).
13. Masaitis NS, Kaempf JW: Developing a frenotomy policy at one medical center: a case study approach, *J Hum Lact* 12:229–232, 1996.
14. Messner AH, Lalakea ML: Ankyloglossia: controversies in management, *Int J Pediatr Otorhinolaryngol* 54:123–131, 2000.
15. Messner AH, Lalakea ML: The effect of ankyloglossia on speech in children, *Otolaryngol Head Neck Surg* 127:539–545, 2002.

16. Messner AH, Lalakea ML, Aby J, et al: Ankyloglossia: incidence and associated feeding difficulties, *Arch Otolaryngol Head Neck Surg* 126:36–39, 2000.

17. Nicholson WL: Tongue-tie (ankyloglossia) associated with breastfeeding problems, *J Hum Lact* 7:82–84, 1991.

18. Notestine GE: The importance of the identification of ankyloglossia (short lingual frenulum) as a cause of breastfeeding problems, *J Hum Lact* 6:113–115, 1990.

19. Protocol Committee Academy of Breastfeeding Medicine, Amir LH, Chantry C, Howard CR: *Clinical Protocol Number 4: Mastitis.* www.bfmed.org, 2002, Academy of Breastfeeding Medicine.

20. Riordan J, Bibb D, Miller M, et al: Predicting breastfeeding duration using the LATCH breastfeeding assessment tool, *J Hum Lact* 17:20–23, 2001.

21. Sanchez-Ruiz I, Gonzalez LG, Perez GV, et al: Section of the sublingual frenulum. Are the indications correct? *Cir Pediatr* 12:161–164, 1999 (Spanish).

22. Williams WN, Waldron CM: Assessment of lingual function when ankyloglossia (tongue-tie) is suspected, *J Am Dent Assoc* 110:353–356, 1985.

23. Wright JE: Tongue-tie, *J Paediatr Child Health* 31:276–278, 1995.

24. Yoel J: Tongue tie and speech disorders, *Trib Odontol (B Aires)* 60:195–196, 1976.

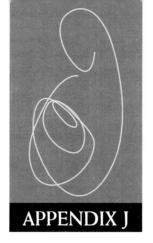

APPENDIX J

Protocol 12: Transitioning the Breastfeeding/Breast-Milk-Fed Premature Infant from the Neonatal Intensive Care Unit to Home

Introduction and Background

The practice of breastfeeding or providing expressed mother's milk to premature infants is promoted because of the considerable benefits to their health and well-being.[15,1] Exclusive breastfeeding has been shown to result in adequate postdischarge weight gain even in very-low-birth-weight infants.[18] The following guidelines include recommendations for monitoring and optimizing nutritional support of premature infants after they are discharged from the hospital. These guidelines represent expert opinions and have not been validated experimentally.

This protocol addresses the care of premature infants less than 37 weeks' gestation and less than 2500 g at birth, who are being transitioned from the hospital to home. Depending on the unit, these infants often weigh 1750 to 2000 g at discharge or less if a kangaroo mother care (also known as skin-to-skin) program is practiced, which may allow for more rapid development of feeding skills. Many of the infants weighing 2000 to 2500 g are not admitted to NICU; they may be either in a transitional nursery or in the postnatal ward with their mothers. (Please also refer to Protocol #10.) The plan does not

distinguish in utero appropriately grown (AGA) from growth-restricted (SGA) infants but bases decisions on current nutritional status and body weight.

For infants less than 1500 g at birth, it is recommended that they be fed their mothers' milk fortified with nutrients and calories. Infants 1500 g or more may breastfeed ad libitum as they are able, provided they are supplemented with multivitamins and iron. Near the time of discharge, a decision must be made as to the feeding in the postdischarge period (to 1 year corrected age). Many of these infants do well after discharge with full or partial breastfeeding, or receiving mother's milk by bottle, cup,[10,4] syringe, nasogastric tube, or supplemental nursing (feeding tube) device. Growth faltering, however, has been observed in some premature infants in the postdischarge period if they receive exclusive human milk feedings without nutrient and caloric fortification.[8,2,16,3,5,9]

Most slow growth in these babies, with the exception of the extremely low-birth-weight infant (ELBW is defined as less than 1000 g at birth), is a function of absolute intake rather than milk composition such that every effort to ensure optimal milk volume should be exhausted prior to switching feedings to formula.

Predischarge: Discharge Planning

A. The clinician should work with the mother to devise a feeding plan well before the actual date of discharge. Rooming-in by the mother for a few days prior to discharge during this transition period is strongly recommended. The baby will preferably be on exclusive breastmilk, either suckling straight from the breast or by use of expressed breastmilk. Less often, the plan may include a combination of breastmilk (directly from the breast or expressed) and formula.

B. The following aspects of the current feeding plan should be assessed when making post-discharge plans.

1. "Type" of feeding: Unfortified human milk, fortified human milk, formula, or a combination.
2. "Amount" of feeding: Milk intake (mL/kg/day): This includes either measuring the mothers' pumped milk volume or performing daily test weights[13] for infants who feed at the breast. If the baby is already growing adequately, it is not typically necessary to perform test weights.
3. "Method" of feeding: Oral (breast, bottle, cup, supplemental nursing device, other, or a combination of methods) versus, or in combination with, tube-feeding (nasal or orogastric) or use of a feeding device (e.g., gastrostomy tube).
4. "Adequacy of growth": In-hospital growth noted as daily rate of weight gain and weekly rate of length gain calculated or plotted on appropriate growth charts (Table J-13).

5. "Adequacy of nutrition": In-hospital biochemical nutritional status, when feasible (Table J-13).
   (NOTE: It is recognized that biochemical monitoring is not feasible in all settings. In such situations, dietary adequacy is based on optimal growth and absence of clinical rickets.)
6. Summary of current nutritional assessment: optimal versus suboptimal.
   a. Optimal status (includes *all* of the following).
      i. Infant can achieve entire intake orally, by breastfeeding or alternate methods.
      ii. Volume of intake is approximately 180 mL/kg/day or more. (Rarely, lower volumes will be adequate if both of the following criteria are met.)
      iii. Growth (weight and length) is within normal limits or improving.
      iv. Biochemical indices (phosphorus, alkaline phosphatase, blood urea nitrogen) are within normal limits (Table J-5) or improving.
   b. Suboptimal (includes *any* one or more of the following).
      i. Infant's intake is less than 160 mL/kg/day (with rare exceptions).
      ii. Infant cannot consume all feedings orally.
      iii. Growth is less than adequate (weight gain less than 20 g/day and/or length gain less than 0.5 cm/week).
      iv. Biochemical indices are abnormal and are not improving.

C. Transition to postdischarge nutrition for infants with "optimal assessment":
1. If the infant has been receiving fortified human milk with or without preterm formula, the diet may be changed to unfortified human milk ad libitum, by breastfeeding or alternative feeding methods, at least 1 week before anticipated discharge.
   a. Prior to this transition it is necessary to assure that mother's milk supply is appropriate for a trial of breastmilk without fortification. This can be done by reviewing the mother's pumping record. Ideally, the mother has been pumping or expressing breastmilk regularly. It is recommended that the mother continue pumping or expressing milk at least three times per day to have an "oversupply" to facilitate adequate volume consumption by the premature infant at the breast. For some mothers, pumping after each feeding ensures optimal drainage of the breast, optimal milk production, and expression of the highest fat content (hindmilk) for

TABLE J-13	Biochemical* and Growth Monitoring for Premature Infants in the Postdischarge Period
Parameter	**Action Values**
Growth	
Weight gain	<20 g/day
Length increase	<0.5 cm/wk
Head circumference increase	<0.5 cm/wk
Biochemical markers	
Phosphorus	<4.5 mg/dL
Alkaline phosphatase	>450 international units/L
Blood urea nitrogen	<5 mg/dL

*It is recognized that biochemical monitoring is not feasible in all settings; presence or absence of clinical rickets then becomes a substitute parameter.
Modified from Hall RA: Nutritional follow-up of the breastfeeding premature infant after hospital discharge, *Pediatr Clin North Am* 48:453, 2001; Schanler RJ: Nutrition support of the low birth weight infant. In Walker WA, Watkins JB, Duggan CP, editors: *Nutrition in pediatrics*, ed 3, Hamilton, ON, Canada, 2003, BC Decker Inc., pp. 392-412.

supplemental feedings. This technique of breastfeeding, then feeding previously pumped breastmilk, and then pumping any residual volume from the breast is termed "triple feeding."

(NOTE: In many areas manual expression is the norm or only available method for milk expression. Preliminary evidence suggests that greater volumes may be obtained with electric, hospital-grade pumps.[14] Therefore, whenever possible, use of the latter is recommended.)

b. For infants receiving formula supplements, a trial without formula is appropriate while increasing human milk intake to approximately 180 mL/kg/day, if possible. Use of hindmilk to increase caloric intake for some feedings may be appropriate.

c. Add iron, 2 mg/kg/day. If enriched post-discharge formula is used, a decrease in the quantity of iron and multivitamin supplementation is indicated. Generally, if formula constitutes about 50% of the diet, the dose for iron is 1 mg/kg/day and multivitamin preparation is half the doses listed below.

d. Add a complete multivitamin preparation. (Dosed to receive at least the following amounts of vitamin A [1500 IU/day], C [20 to 70 mg/day], and D [400 IU/day]; vitamin C requirements of preterm infants are poorly studied. B vitamins are also necessary for the former preemie receiving unfortified human milk. Typically, appropriate amounts of all vitamins will be provided by infant multivitamin [MVI] preparations at 1 mL/day.) See note under iron above C1 (c) if providing enriched post-discharge formula supplements.

e. Monitor milk intake and growth (weight and length) during this week. Volumes of pumped or expressed milk and daily test weights (for infants fed at the breast) should be recorded during this period.[13]

f. If intake and growth are adequate, continue this diet after discharge.

g. If intake and growth are suboptimal, follow D (d) below.

2. If the infant has been receiving unfortified human milk:

a. Continue iron (2 mg/kg/day).

b. Continue multivitamin preparation [see dosing above, C,1 (c)].

c. Continue this diet after discharge.

D. Transition to postdischarge nutrition for infants with "suboptimal assessment":

1. If the infant has been receiving fortified human milk:

a. Change the diet to unfortified human milk, with or without preterm formula, ad libitum (by breastfeeding and/or alternative feeding methods) plus a minimum of two to three feedings of enriched post-discharge formula prepared per manufacturer instructions (≈ 22 kcal/oz) at least 1 week before anticipated discharge.

(NOTE: Many neonatologists and institutions add powdered discharge premature formula to expressed breastmilk to provide enriched feeds while still providing the advantages of breastmilk. There is no evidence to recommend for or against this practice. This use of powdered premature formula is off-label and the potential for error is great, so be advised to be extremely cautious if using this approach.)

b. Recommend that the mother continue pumping or expressing milk at least three times/per day [see C,1 (a) above].

c. Monitor milk intake and growth during this week.

d. Assess adequacy of breastfeeding and address problems or potential problems.

i. Latch.

ii. Milk transfer/milk volume. If lactation has been suppressed or the baby is not adequately draining the breast, it may be necessary to intervene to increase volume (i.e., increased pumping after feeds or pumping at some feeds and feeding the expressed milk in lieu of or in addition to feeding at the breast.) (Please also see Protocol #9.)

iii. Maternal milk content. Consider the use of hindmilk for some feedings to increase caloric content. This must be considered in conjunction with milk transfer and volume as it may be particularly important if the baby is getting only foremilk and leaving hindmilk.

iv. Frequency of feeds at breast (please note that with "sleepy preemies" subtle feeding cues may be missed).

v. Optimize milk transfer. Suggested techniques may include pumping or expressing to let down before putting baby to breast or using breast compression during feedings.

vi. Maternal satisfaction. Mothers may have preferences regarding timing of feeds, feeding devices, and so on that fit best with the family's needs and can be accommodated without compromising the infant's nutrition.

vii. Consider use of a feeding device.

    (A) Nipple shield to improve milk transfer.[6]

      (NOTE: Any mother who is discharged using a nipple shield must be closely monitored by a competent lactation professional to watch for potential associated complications.)

    (B) Supplemental nursing (feeding tube) device while at breast.

    (C) May be able to use nipple shield and supplemental nursing device together effectively (e.g., by placing tube inside nipple shield so when baby suckles, the volume of milk available for transfer is increased).

    (D) Test weighing.[13]

      (I) Monitor milk intake and growth (weight and length) during this week. Record volumes of pumped or expressed milk and daily test weights (for infants fed at the breast) during this period.[13]

      (II) If intake and growth are adequate during this week after switching:

        (a) Add iron (1 to 2 mg/kg/day), depending on how much formula is fed.

        (b) Add multivitamin preparation (half to full dose described above C,1 [c]), depending upon how much formula is fed.

      (III) Continue this diet after discharge.

2. If the infant has been receiving unfortified human milk, assess the adequacy of breastfeeding and address problems or potential problems as above, D,1 (d).

  a. If addressing any existing breastfeeding problems does not result in "optimal assessment," add two to three feedings of enriched postdischarge formula prepared per manufacturer instructions ($\approx$ 22 kcal/oz) [see note under D,1 (a) above]. Ensure that the mother is expressing milk to maintain and optimize her milk production. Anticipate at least 1 more week of continued hospitalization before discharge.

    i. Monitor milk intake and growth during this week.

ii. Continue iron and multivitamin supplement.

iii. If the feeding assessment continues to be suboptimal after 1 week, increase the number of feedings of enriched postdischarge formula or increase the concentration of enriched formula to 24 to 30 kcal/oz.

Postdischarge Assessment

A. Nutrition monitoring 1 week after discharge.

  1. Assess intake.

    a. History.

    b. Observation of feeding.

    c. Consider test weighing if concerns persist.[13]

  2. Growth—weight and length (Table J-13).

  3. Biochemical indices of nutritional status (Table J-13).

  4. Reassess nutritional status as "Optimal" versus "Suboptimal."

    a. Infants with an "Optimal" assessment may be reevaluated at 1 month after discharge (see III,B, below).

    b. For infants with a "Suboptimal assessment":

      i. Assess adequacy of breastfeeding.

        (A) Latch.

        (B) Milk transfer/volume.

        (C) Maternal satisfaction.

        (D) Milk content—consider hindmilk.

        (E) Consider use of feeding devices.

          (I) Nipple shield to improve milk transfer.[12]

          (II) Test weighing[13] to evaluate milk volume.

      ii. If addressing any existing breastfeeding problems does not result in an "optimal assessment," add additional feedings of enriched postdischarge formula, prepared as below, per clinical judgment according to the individual infant's assessment.

        (A) Prepared per manufacturer instructions ($\approx$ 22 kcal/oz).

        (B) Concentrated to 24 to 30 kcal/oz.

        (C) Ensure that the mother is expressing milk to maintain and optimize her milk production.

      iii. Frequent follow-up visits for ongoing nutritional monitoring.

B. Nutrition monitoring 1 month after discharge.
1. Assess intake.
   a. History.
   b. Observation of feeding.
   c. Consider test weighing if concerns persist.[13]
2. Growth—weight and length (Table J-13).
3. Biochemical indices of nutritional status (Table J-13).
4. Reassess nutritional status as "Optimal" versus "Suboptimal."
   a. Infants with an "Optimal" assessment may be reevaluated at every 2 months to 1 year corrected age.
   b. For infants with a "Suboptimal assessment":
      i. Ensure optimal milk production, breastfeeding.
      ii. Add additional feedings of enriched postdischarge formula, individualizing preparation either prepared per manufacturer instructions ($\approx$ 22 kcal/oz) or concentrated to 24 to 30 kcal/oz.
      iii. Frequent follow-up visits for ongoing nutritional monitoring.
C. Once nutrition has been optimized, nutritional monitoring can occur every 2 months until 1 year corrected age.
D. With regard to enriched formula, a few studies have demonstrated a positive effect on growth using enriched formulas for 6 to 9 months. Until more definitive data are available for breastfed former preemies, we recommend continuing an enriched postdischarge formula for a minimum of 6 months.
   See Figure J-2 for an algorithm for care of premature infants postdischarge.

General Strategies

A. Enriched postdischarge formula is used because it provides greater nutrient intake than term infant formula. Human milk fortifier usually is not recommended postdischarge because its nutrient content is too great for the infant at the time of discharge and it is expensive and very difficult to prepare according to specifications.
B. Hindmilk, if used, provides extra calories (estimated at 22 to 24 cal/oz) but no increase in the intake of minerals or protein. (Hindmilk is the fat-rich milk that occurs at the end of the feeding.)
C. It is imperative that the hospital physician communicate with the physician who will provide follow-up care to ensure that the desired plan is carried out and to convey any unique concerns about growth, diet, feeding patterns, and biochemical monitoring.

Support for Breastfeeding Mothers of Premature Infants

A. Support mothers to initiate kangaroo (skin-to-skin) care as early as possible in-hospital.[15,6]
B. Encourage mothers to express their milk soon after delivery and approximately every 3 hours on an ongoing basis. Aim for at least eight pumping sessions in 24 hours, so that if pumping does not occur exactly every 3 hours, sessions will not be missed. Instruct mothers on the use of effective breast pumping methods, either electric rental-grade or effective manual pumps or manual expression. Whenever possible, electric rental-grade pumps should be used for maximal stimulation, particularly for the establishment of milk supply. Skin-to-skin contact, simultaneous milk expression, and nonnutritive suckling at the breast may facilitate the establishment of the milk supply.
C. Educate mothers that early feeding behaviors emerge during skin-to-skin holding and that mothers can follow the infant's cues for early feeding attempts. Mothers should understand that early feeding attempts are gradual and not expected to result in a full feeding for the infant.
D. Sustained suckling with swallowing for 5 minutes is one indicator that the infant may be ready to transition from nasogastric tube to breastfeeding.[7,19] Other studies suggest that early introduction of oral feeding hastens the development of oral motor skills.[17] Nursing supplementers may provide additional volume.[11]
E. Have trained personnel evaluate breastfeeding (position and latch) on a regular basis. A correct latch is critical for efficient milk removal.
F. Monitor mothers for nipple soreness. If present, this may be an indication of shallow latch. Temporary use of silicone nipple shields is a helpful adjunct for milk transfer and more efficient latch-on for premature infants with shallow latch.[6]
G. If the infant is achieving partial intake directly at the breast, consider "triple feeding"—put the baby to breast, supplement with expressed breastmilk or formula (at breast with the supplemental nursing [tube feeding] device or after the breastfeeding), and then pump or express milk afterward to maintain the milk supply.

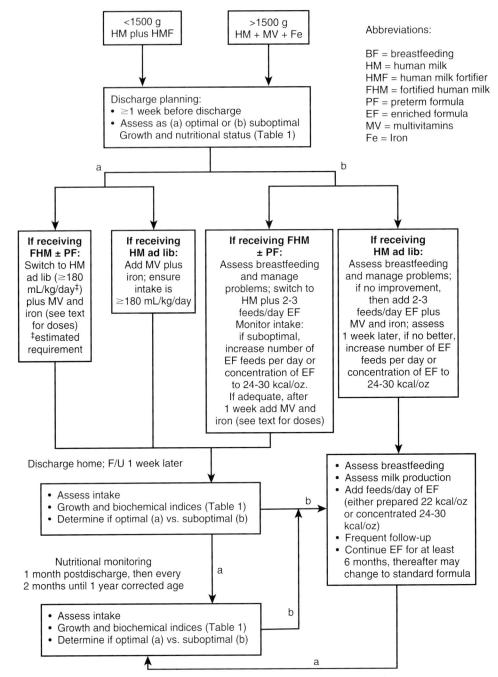

Figure J-2. Algorithm for care of prematures postdischarge by weight (<1500 g or >1500 g).

H. If the baby is discharged with partial feedings at the breast, consider a scale sensitive enough to distinguish milk intake for home use to help with the transition to total feedings at the breast.

I. Refer and coordinate supportive care services such as community support, visiting nurse, lactation consultant visits, social services, and WIC.

Acknowledgment

Supported in part by a grant from the Maternal and Child Health Bureau, U.S. Department of Health and Human Services.

Protocol Committee
Caroline J. Chantry, MD, FABM, Co-Chairperson

*Lori Feldman-Winter, MD,
Co-Chairperson
Cynthia R. Howard, MD, MPH, FABM
*Richard J. Schanler, MD

REFERENCES

1. Bier JAB, Ferguson AE, Morales Y, et al: Breastfeeding infants who were extremely low birth weight, *Pediatrics* 100:e3, 1997.
2. Carver JD, Wu PJK, Hall RT, et al: Growth of preterm infants fed nutrient-enriched or term formula after hospital discharge, *Pediatrics* 107:683–689, 2001.
3. Chan GM: Growth and bone status of discharged very low birth weight infants fed different formulas or human milk, *J Pediatr* 123:439–443, 1993.
4. Collins CT, Ryan P, Crowther CA, et al: Effect of bottles, cups, and dummies on breast feeding in preterm infants: a randomised controlled trial, *Br Med J* 329:193–198, 2004.
5. Greer FR: Feeding the preterm infant after hospital discharge, *Pediatr Ann* 30:658–665, 2001.
6. Kirsten GF, Bergman NJ, Hann FM: Kangaroo mother care in the nursery, *Pediatr Clin North Am* 48:443–452, 2001.
7. Kliethermes PA, Cross ML, Lanese MG, et al: Transitioning preterm infants with nasogastric tube supplementation: increased likelihood of breastfeeding, *J Obstet Gynecol Neonatal Nurs* 28:264–273, 1999.
8. Lucas A, Bishop NJ, King FJ, et al: Randomized trial of nutrition for preterm infants after discharge, *Arch Dis Child* 67:324–327, 1992.
9. Lucas A, Fewtrell MS, Morley R, et al: Randomized trial of nutrient-enriched formulas versus standard formula for post-discharge preterm infants, *Pediatrics* 108:703–711, 2001.
10. Marinelli K, Burke G, Dodd V: A comparison of the safety of cup feedings and bottle feedings in premature infants whose mothers intend to breastfeed, *J Perinatol* 21:350–355, 2001.
11. Meier PP: Breastfeeding in the special care nursery: prematures and infants with medical problems, *Pediatr Clin North Am* 48:425–442, 2001.
12. Meier PP, Brown LP, Hurst NM, et al: Nipple shields for preterm infants: effect on milk transfer and duration of breastfeeding, *J Hum Lact* 16:106–113, 2000.
13. Meier PP, Engstrom JL, Crichton C, et al: A new scale for in-home test-weighing for mothers of preterm and high-risk infants, *J Hum Lact* 10:63–68, 1994.
14. Ramsethu J, Jeyaseelan L, Kirubakaran C: Weight gain in exclusively breastfed preterm infants, *J Trop Pediatr* 39:152–159, 1993.
15. Schanler RJ: Human milk for premature infants, *Pediatr Clin North Am* 48:207–219, 2001.
16. Schanler RJ, Burns PA, Abrams SA, et al: Bone mineralization outcomes in human milk-fed preterm infants, *Pediatr Res* 31:583–586, 1992.
17. Simpson C, Schanler R, Lau C: Early introduction of oral feeding in preterm infants, *Pediatrics* 110:517–522, 2002.
18. Slusher T, Slusher I, Biomdo M, et al: Electric breast pump use increases maternal milk volume and decreases time to onset of adequate maternal milk volume in African nurseries, *Pediatr Res* 55(4, Part 2):445A, 2004.
19. Valentine CJ, Hurst NM: A six step feeding strategy for preterm infants, *J Hum Lact* 11:7–8, 1995.

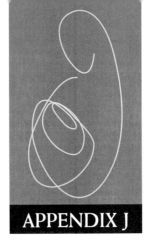

APPENDIX J

Protocol 13: Contraception During Breastfeeding

Pamela Berens, Miriam Labbok, and the Academy of Breastfeeding Medicine

Purpose

The purpose of this protocol is to outline considerations in assisting breastfeeding families to achieve optimal birth spacing by selecting a contraceptive method that is effective, unlikely to disrupt lactation, and satisfactory for the mother and her partner. The protocol covers the use of contraceptive methods during breastfeeding and provides guidance on the lactational amenorrhea method (LAM).

This protocol assumes that the practitioner is well versed in the risks and benefits of different types of contraception, including all pharmaceutical, permanent, and periodic abstinence/natural family planning methods.

Issues in Counseling and Selection of Contraceptives During Breastfeeding

CONSIDERATIONS FOR CLINICIAN COUNSELING AND METHOD USE

Postpartum contraception, like breastfeeding, should be discussed with women during their own obstetric prenatal and postpartum visits and the infant's pediatric well-baby visits. A woman's contraceptive choice depends on many factors such as previous experience with contraceptives, future childbearing plans, husband or partner's attitude, level of user attention required for use, medical considerations, return of menses, and the woman's lactation status. If a woman is not comfortable with a method, she may not use it effectively.

ADVANTAGES AND DISADVANTAGES OF AVAILABLE OPTIONS

Contraceptive counseling during breastfeeding extends beyond issues of efficacy, because the selected method must be appropriate for a woman's breastfeeding expectations. Table J-14 provides useful information for counseling the breastfeeding mother. Considerations include the potential for hormonal methods to either disrupt milk synthesis or expose the infant to synthetic hormones. Because a falling progesterone level after birth is necessary for onset of milk production, initiation of hormonal contraception before lactation is established is of particular concern. Published evidence is insufficient to exclude these risks. At the same time, long-acting reversible hormonal methods have high contraceptive efficacy. Health care providers should discuss the limitations of the available data within the context of a mother's desire to breastfeed, her risk of low milk production, and her risk of unplanned pregnancy, so that she can make an autonomous and informed decision.

TABLE J-14	General Principles for Counseling Breastfeeding Women Concerning Contraceptive Selection and Birth Spacing	
Issues	**Considerations**
1. Breastfeeding patterns, status, and plans	• Consider both short- and long-term breastfeeding intent as well as well birth spacing plans. There is the potential for hormonal methods to have an impact depending on when they are started • Mothers may plan to exclusively breastfeed; some may do so to use LAM, others may use LAM because they are already fully breastfeeding. LAM users should be counseled to have another method in hand for when menses return or breastfeeding patterns change. Effectiveness of LAM in exclusively breastmilk pumping mothers may not be equivalent to direct breastfeeding • Many women who intend to breastfeed exclusively are not able to achieve their goals
2. Child's age/time postpartum	• Many methods should not be introduced until breastfeeding is well established (i.e., at 4-6 weeks), as there may be potential for hormonal methods to directly impact lactogenesis and/or to impact the infant
3. Maternal age and future childbearing plans	• Choices depend on desire to space births or desire to limit family size. Globally recommended interpregnancy intervals are at least 18 months to 2+ years for maternal health, depending on the setting, and about 3-5 years for child health outcomes
4. Previous contraceptive experience	• Discussion of previous contraceptive experience, including compliance, satisfaction, side effects, and social issues, is essential. These issues can influence compliance and satisfaction, particularly as they pertain to prior lactation experiences
5. Partners/interactions	• Partner's experiences and opinions may impact compliance, particularly for barrier methods, LAM, and natural family planning • The woman's social and behavioral considerations, such as number of partners and sexual activity, should be explored. A woman's history of unplanned pregnancy and short interpregnancy interval should be reviewed and discussed
6. Previous lactation experience/medical conditions	• Prior insufficient milk supply or inadequate infant growth • Prior breastfeeding experience did NOT meet goals (either exclusivity or duration), AND supply was a potential reason • Physical examination suggestive of insufficient glandular tissue • Prior breast surgery • Medical conditions potentially adversely affecting supply (polycystic ovary syndrome, infertility, obesity) • Multiple gestation • Preterm infant(s)

LAM, Lactational amenorrhea method.

LAM for Contraception in the Early Postpartum Period and for the Introduction of Other Methods

BACKGROUND

Data published in the 1970s showed that women who breastfed were less likely to ovulate early postpartum and that if breastfeeding were more intensive, they were less likely than partial or non-breastfeeders to experience a normal ovulation prior to the first menstrual-like bleed.[33] In 1988, at a Bellagio Conference, a group of expert scientists proposed three criteria as sufficient to predict fertility return. This three-criteria approach described in further detail below as the "Lactational Amenorrhea Method" was subsequently tested.[32,27] Studies of the acceptability and contraceptive efficacy of active LAM use continue to confirm the original findings, demonstrating that LAM is acceptable, learnable, user-friendly, and as effective as many other alternatives.[43,42,25,34,17,22] (II-2) (Quality of evidence [levels of evidence I, II-1, II-

2, II-3, and III] is based on the U.S. Preventive Services Task Force Appendix A Task Force Ratings[1] and is noted throughout this protocol in parentheses.)

METHOD: WHAT IS LAM?

LAM is presented as an algorithm (Figure J-3) and includes three criteria for defining the period of lowest pregnancy risk. If one of these criteria is not met, women should immediately initiate another method. Clinically, the mother is asked these three questions:

• "Are you amenorrheic?" meaning that you have not had a menstrual bleed or any bleed of >2 days in duration (discounting any bleed in the first 2 months).
• "Are you fully or nearly fully breastfeeding?" This includes not giving your baby any supplementary foods or fluids in addition to breastfeeding (greater than once or twice a week)?
• "Is your infant less than 6 months of age?"

Ask the mother, or advise her to ask herself, these three questions:

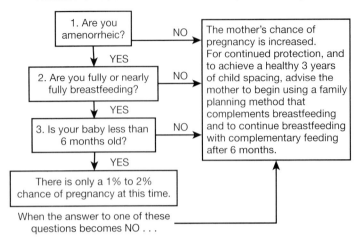

Figure J-3. The lactational amenor-rhea method (LAM).

If she answers "yes" to all three questions, she meets the requirements for LAM. If any of the above three questions is answered "no," then her chance of pregnancy is increased, and she should be advised to initiate another form of contraception to prevent pregnancy. If the mother is interested in and qualifies for LAM, she should review these three questions regularly. Clinicians should ensure that she has chosen her next method of contraception and either has it on hand or knows how to obtain it if it is an implant or intrauterine device (IUD).

DEFINITIONS FOR LAM USE

To use LAM correctly, it is important that the patient understand each of the three criteria, which can be remembered using the letters "LAM" to indicate Lactation, Amenorrhea, and the number of Months:

1. Lactation. Full or nearly full breastfeeding includes exclusive, nearly exclusive, and some irregularly provided supplements, as long as they do not disrupt the frequency of feeds.[26]
2. Amenorrhea. For the purposes of LAM use, menses return is defined as any bleeding that occurs after 56 days postpartum that is perceived by the patient as a menses or any two consecutive days of bleeding.
3. Months. The "6 months" criterion is added primarily because this is the time that complementary feeding should begin. If breastfeeding continues at the same frequency and complementary foods are offered after the breastfeed, efficacy apparently remains high as long as amenorrhea continues. In Rwanda, the method was used up to 9 months, by maintaining the breastfeeding frequency experienced during

month 6.[9] This was achieved by feeding before each complementary feeding. Another study in Pakistan found a continued high efficacy under these conditions for up to 12 months.[21] (II-2)

EFFICACY

A Cochrane Review[47] (and assessed as up-to-date in 2008) concluded that fertility rates are low among fully breastfeeding, amenorrheic women. In controlled studies of LAM, pregnancy rates for 6 months ranged from 0.45% to 2.45%. In six uncontrolled studies of LAM users, pregnancy ranged from 0% to 7.5%. The World Health Organization (WHO) carried out a prospective trial on lactational amenorrhea and fertility return; although this was not a study of women selecting and using LAM, the findings confirmed the physiological potential for high efficacy as seen in the LAM trials.[43,42] Subsequently, studies of method use have consistently found a 6-month pregnancy rate averaging 2%[15] (I, II-2)

LAM MANAGEMENT ISSUES

Suggested behaviors contributing to method success and duration include:

1. Number of feedings. One controlled study found exclusively breastfeeding women using LAM are more likely to be amenorrheic at 6 months than exclusively breastfeeding controls (84% vs. 69.7%, respectively).[28] Women using LAM had a higher feeding frequency and a shorter interfeeding interval than other exclusively breastfeeding women.
2. LAM can be used beyond the sixth month. The two studies mentioned above in Rwanda[9] and

Pakistan[21] have indicated that the efficacy of LAM can be maintained during the 6- to 12-month period, provided the mother continues to breastfeed before giving complementary foods at less than 4-hour intervals during the day and 6-hour intervals at night while remaining amenorrheic. (II-2)

3. LAM effectiveness has not as yet been adequately tested to offer the method with confidence to women who are giving supplemental feedings daily or expressing milk by hand or pump instead of breastfeeding.[46] (II-2) Women who are expressing milk more than a few times per week should be counseled to initiate an additional contraceptive method. (III)

TRANSITION TO OTHER METHODS

LAM may also be used as an introductory method to inform the user when it is time to initiate use of another method. Of note is that fully breastfeeding women are very unlikely to conceive in the first 56 days postpartum so secondary methods can be delayed until at least 8 weeks postpartum. When LAM criteria no longer apply or whenever a breastfeeding woman wishes to use an alternate family planning method, she should have an alternative method readily available. Alternative methods are discussed in terms of advantages and disadvantages and special issues related to breastfeeding.

Additional Comments on Individual Methods

Table J-15 provides additional specific information for many individual methods, including advantages, disadvantages, and potential issues related to breastfeeding for each.

TABLE J-15	Use of Contraceptive Methods During Lactation: Advantages, Disadvantages, and Impact on Lactation		
Method	**Advantages**	**Disadvantages**	**Effects Related to Breastfeeding**
Lactational amenorrheic method			
Natural family planning			
• Billings ovulation • Creighton model • Marquette • Symptothermal	• No side effects • Effectiveness rates comparable with other user-directed methods of birth control (i.e., pills or barriers) • Low cost for most methods	• Requires special instruction for use during breastfeeding • ClearBlue fertility monitor expense with Marquette • May require long periods of abstinence	• None
Barrier methods			
• Diaphragm/cap • Spermicide • Condoms	• Few side effects • Effective with diligent and appropriate use • Easily accessible as "back-up" • Low cost • Also provide protection from sexually transmitted infection	• Potential for user error • Allergy possible • May be inconvenient and limit spontaneity • Cervical cap and diaphragm require fitting	• None • Use of lubricant may be beneficial with condoms in setting of vaginal atrophy
Other contraceptive options			
IUDs			
• Copper IUD (ParaGard T380A), 10 years • Levonorgestrel IUD (Mirena), 5 years • Levonorgestrel IUD (Skyla), 3 years	• Highly effective • Reversible • Long-term contraceptives • Little user attention required (typical use and perfect use are similar)	• Small risk of infection, perforation, expulsion • Requires provider insertion and removal • Copper contraindicated with Wilson's disease and copper allergy • Short-term use costly; long-term use cost-effective	• Copper IUD: no known impact on lactation • Possible risk of perforation at insertion requiring surgical removal, which may necessitate short interruption in breastfeeding • Levonorgestrel IUD (Mirena) placed immediately postpartum may be associated with shorter duration of breastfeeding. No adverse effect on breastfeeding reported when placed 6 weeks postpartum or later

Continued

TABLE J-15   Use of Contraceptive Methods During Lactation: Advantages, Disadvantages, and Impact on Lactation—cont'd

Method	Advantages	Disadvantages	Effects Related to Breastfeeding
Sterilization			
• Male (vasectomy) • Female: postpartum; laparoscopic; hysteroscopic	• Highly effective • Male vasectomy and female hysteroscopic occlusion may be performed on an outpatient basis	• Permanent; risk of regret • Surgical procedural risks • Cost related to surgery • Requires surgeon • Risk of ectopic pregnancy with female procedures	• Male sterilization: none • Female sterilization: postpartum procedure separates mother and infant and may require use of maternal narcotics (ideally avoid procedures in first 1-2 hours to allow skin-to-skin, initial breastfeeding, etc.)
Progestin-only hormonal options[a]			
• Injectible (DMPA) every 3 months • Oral daily pills (norethindrone) • Progestin-releasing IUD (see above): LNG IUD (Mirena), 5 years; LNG IUD (Skyla), 3 years • Progestin vaginal rings • Implants: etonogestrel (Implanon/Nexplanon), 3 years (Jadelle), 5 years	• Long-term options highly reliable	• Common side effect of irregular bleeding may be less problematic in breastfeeding mothers • Potential for user failure with daily pills • Other progestin side effects: headache, acne, weight gain, bloating, depressed mood • DMPA may have delayed return to fertility • Implant and IUDs require provider insertion and removal	• Theoretical potential to adversely impact milk supply when started in the early postpartum period prior to establishing a milk supply. Insufficient data to determine risk at this time • If milk supply decreases with DMPA, cannot be discontinued or removed • LNG IUD (Mirena) placed immediately postpartum may be associated with shorter duration of breastfeeding (single study). No adverse effect on breastfeeding reported when placed 6 weeks postpartum or later
Estrogen-containing combined hormonal options			
• COC pills, daily • Estrogen-containing vaginal ring (NuvaRing), monthly • Estrogen-containing transdermal patch (Ortho-Evra), weekly	• Options can be self-administered • Regular menstrual cycles (extended cycle options have more breakthrough bleeding) • Noncontraceptive benefits: decreased bleeding, less anemia, improved acne, improved dysmenorrhea	• Potential for user failure (especially with COCs) • Increased risk of blood clots • Potential for drug interactions • Multiple medical contraindications	• Ideally avoid until lactation/milk supply well established • Potential for adverse effect on milk supply. Risk appears more pronounced with higher estrogen levels than used in contemporary products • If used by a breastfeeding mother, begin lowest possible dose as late as possible into well-established breastfeeding
Emergency contraceptives			
• Combined estrogen/progestin pills (Preven, Yuzpe method) • Progestin-only pills—LNG (Plan B) • Mifepristone • Ulipristal • Copper IUD	• Most effective within 72 hours of exposure • LNG options appear to have superior efficacy to COC with fewer side effects • Copper IUD most effective and provides continued contraception • Mifepristone similar or superior to LNG in efficacy	• Estrogen-containing options cause nausea/vomiting and often require use of antiemetics • No data for ulipristal in lactation currently available • Limited data on mifepristone in lactation	• LNG preferred over estrogen-containing options in breastfeeding mothers owing to previously described concerns related to estrogen and milk supply

COC, Combined oral contraceptive; *DMPA*, depo-medroxyprogesterone acetate; *IUD*, intrauterine device; *LNG*, levonorgestrel.

[a]Conclusive research regarding the clinical implications of progestin contraceptive administration in the early postpartum period is contradictory and insufficient.

Natural Family Planning

Four methods of "fertility awareness" natural family planning include the Billings ovulation method (OM), the Creighton model system, the sympto-thermal method, and the Marquette method. Each of these methods can be used even when a woman's menses has not yet returned because of breastfeeding. These methods rely on observation of various combinations of cervical mucus, temperature, and/or hormonal monitoring, and then couples abstain during fertile periods. All of these methods have specific protocols for women to use during the postpartum period so they may plan accordingly if they wish to delay another pregnancy. The Marquette model has a recent peer-reviewed study to show the efficacy of its postpartum protocol.[3]

These methods may require significant periods of abstinence. Research on the use of the Billings OM during the postpartum period found that those who were using OM and were breastfeeding had a lower pregnancy rate than those using OM but not breastfeeding. The rate of unplanned pregnancy was less than 1% during the first 6 months of lactational amenorrhea. However, OM-associated pregnancy rates were elevated among breastfeeders after menses returned (36% vs. 13% for nonlactating women) and when infant feeding supplementation was started. This increase in unplanned pregnancies was not directly attributable to OM nonadherence. Special emphasis on both the need for improved breastfeeding support to delay menses return and the increased potential for method failure among new users during this period of time should be incorporated into OM training and support programs.[29]

HORMONAL CONTRACEPTIVE METHOD: GENERAL COMMENTS

Controversy exists in the literature regarding hormonal contraceptive effects on milk supply. Although Koetsawang[24] reported an increase, Tankeyoon et al.[40] noted a 12% decline in milk supply with progestin-only contraception compared with placebo. Other studies have not found an effect. A recent study quantified the effect of hormonal contraception on infant's milk ingestion between days 42 and 63 using deuterium as a marker.[2] Forty women who had previously breastfed began contraception at 42 days postpartum with an estrogen-containing pill (150 mcg of levonorgestrel [LNG] and 30 mcg of ethinylestradiol), the LNG-IUD (Mirena; Bayer Pharmaceuticals, Leverkeusen, Germany), the etonogestrel implant (Implanon; Merck & Co., Whitehouse

Station, NJ), or the copper-containing IUD (ParaGard; Teva Women's Health Inc., North Wales, PA). No difference in the infants' milk intake was noted among groups in this study. A Cochrane Review indicated that evidence from randomized controlled trials on the effect of hormonal contraceptives during lactation is limited and of poor quality: "The evidence is inadequate to make evidence-based recommendations regarding hormonal contraceptive use for lactating women."[45] Until better evidence exists, it is prudent to advise women that hormonal contraceptive methods may decrease milk supply especially in the early postpartum period. Hormonal methods should be discouraged in some circumstances (III):

1. Existing low milk supply or history of lactation failure
2. History of breast surgery
3. Multiple birth (twins, triplets)
4. Preterm birth
5. Compromised health of mother and/or baby

HORMONAL CONTRACEPTIVE METHOD: PROGESTIN-ONLY OPTIONS

There is theoretical concern related to milk supply when progesterone options are initiated in the initial 48 hours after delivery[23] as a drop in progesterone levels after birth is necessary for secretory differentiation/lactogenesis II to occur. Progestin-containing contraceptives include the progestogen-only pill ("minipill") as well as contraceptive implants such as Nexplanon (Merck & Co.), DepoProvera (depot medroxyprogesterone acetate [DMPA]; Pfizer, New York, NY), and the Mirena intrauterine system. A 2010 systematic review of the effects of progestin-only contraceptive options when initiated after the initial postpartum period found five randomized controlled trials and 38 observational trials addressing the topic.[20] No adverse effects on breastfeeding through 12 months of age, infant immunoglobulins, or infant sex hormones were noted. Research regarding the clinical implications of progestin contraceptive administration in the early postpartum period is contradictory.

Particularly controversial in clinical practice is the effect of DMPA. Prior studies of DMPA did not account for infant weight, milk supply, and the amount of supplement used. A systematic review of prospective studies on the effects of early postpartum DMPA use in lactating mothers by Brownell et al.[5] found all studies to be of low quality with inadequate control of confounders. Another study of low-income new mothers found that of the 31.3% who received DMPA, 62.6% received it prior to hospital discharge,[10] indicating that early postpartum use is common in some settings. This study team quantified the association between postpartum DMPA and early breastfeeding cessation among 183 women and concluded that if there is a causal effect of DMPA on breastfeeding duration, it is minimal. A prospective case control study of 150 women receiving DMPA after initiation of lactation but prior to hospital discharge (days 2 to 10) compared with 100 women not receiving hormonal contraception followed up for 6 months found no difference in satisfaction with their breastfeeding experience or infant growth, although it is unclear how the breastfeeding patterns compared.[39]

A study by Brito et al.[4] compared either insertion of an etonogestrel-releasing implant within 1 to 2 days after delivery or DMPA given at 6 weeks postpartum. Forty women were then followed up through 12 weeks postpartum. Newborns of those in the implant group had a trend toward more weight gain in the first 6 weeks, but the overall duration of exclusive breastfeeding was not statistically different. Gurtcheff et al.[30] similarly studied early (1 to 3 days) versus delayed (4 to 8 weeks) insertion of the contraceptive implant. This noninferiority study found no difference in breastfeeding failure rates with early insertion compared with the delayed group.

ESTROGEN-CONTAINING COMBINED HORMONAL OPTIONS

Estrogen-containing options include combination oral contraceptive (COC) pills (taken daily using monthly cyclic, extended cyclic, or continuous options), transdermal patch (weekly), or combined contraceptive vaginal rings (monthly). Estrogen-containing options are not ideal for early postpartum breastfeeding mothers because of the potential adverse impact on milk supply. The potential for estrogen to cause milk suppression is exemplified by the historical use of large estrogen doses immediately postpartum for lactation suppression prior to our understanding of the elevated thrombogenic risk during that time period. A Cochrane Review on methods of lactation suppression noted seven trials using four different estrogen preparations and found a significant reduction in lactation within 7 days postpartum; of note is that the doses and estrogen preparations used differ from those currently used in hormonal contraceptives.[31]

A 2010 systematic review on COCs and breastfeeding found only three randomized controlled trials and four observational studies; the three randomized controlled trials found a decreased mean breastfeeding duration in COC users and an increased use of supplement.[19] No other documented adverse effects on infant health were noted.

If an estrogen-containing contraceptive is chosen, it is prudent to start the lowest estrogen-containing options as late as possible and after milk supply and lactation are well established. (III) Additionally, estrogen-containing options should not be initiated in the first few weeks postpartum because of the elevated risk of deep venous thrombosis and pulmonary embolism. Absolute and relative contraindications are otherwise the same for lactating women as for nonlactating women.

Contemporary COCs have estrogen doses ranging from 10 to 35 mcg daily. No significant difference in contraceptive efficacy has been found in a Cochrane Review of COCs containing <20 mcg of estrogen compared with those with >20 mcg.[13] This information should provide reassurance regarding anticipated efficacy when choosing lower estrogen dose options in a breastfeeding mother to minimize potential adverse effects.

DIRECT COMPARISON OF PROGESTIN-ONLY PILLS AND COCs

A WHO task force study done in the 1980s found a 41.9% decrease in milk supply in women using COCs within 6 weeks of initiation.[40] However, a recent randomized controlled trial compared 63 women using a 35-mcg progestin-only pill (POP) with 64 women using a COC containing 35 mcg of ethinylestradiol from 2 through 8 weeks postpartum; the authors found no difference in continued breastfeeding at 8 weeks (63.5% POP vs. 64.1% COC).[11] Forty-four percent of those in the POP group stopped breastfeeding because of perceived insufficient milk supply compared with 55% in the COC group. Twenty-three percent of women who stopped their pills in the POP group and 21% in the COC groups reported that they did so because of a perceived negative impact on milk supply.

EMERGENCY CONTRACEPTION

Emergency contraception is most effective when initiated within 72 hours after unprotected sexual intercourse, although it is still useful up to 120 hours. Postcoital copper IUD placement, mifepristone, COC, and progesterone options (LNG) are potentially available choices. Postcoital copper IUD placement would be unlikely to impact lactation (see section on IUDs) and has the advantage of providing continued contraception. LNG options are slightly more effective than the COC and also are less likely to cause significant nausea and vomiting.[7] Furthermore, in theory, LNG options would be less likely to impact lactation. A pharmacologic study of 12 breastfeeding mothers found the estimated infant exposure to the maternal treatment of 1.5 mg of LNG was 1.6 mcg on the day of therapy.[12] A single observational study comparing progestin-only with estrogen-containing options for postcoital contraception found that an adverse effect on breastfeeding was uncommon and similar in both groups.[35] Based on similar efficacy, less propensity to nausea, and the absence of exposure to estrogen, it appears that the use of LNG is likely the preferred option over a COC in a breastfeeding mother. There are limited data on mifepristone and ulipristal in lactation. The use of postcoital mifepristone (an antiprogesterone) is similar to or superior in efficacy to LNG depending on dosage. Based on a small study, mifepristone transfers into milk in low levels (relative infant doses 1.5%) and would not be anticipated to have adverse effects on the breastfeeding infant.[38] Ulipristal is a selective progesterone receptor modulator. There are currently no data available on its use in breastfeeding mothers.

Postcoital contraception has also been evaluated as a backup to lactational amenorrhea. Although this may not be a practical option, one study found a lower pregnancy rate for the group that was provided with a postcoital contraceptive during counseling regarding lactational amenorrhea at the postpartum visit.[37]

BARRIER METHODS

There are no known adverse effects on lactation with the use of barrier methods of contraception. Patients should be counseled regarding the reduced efficacy of these methods compared with other hormonal, intrauterine, or permanent options.

IUDS

The IUD is one of the most frequently used contraceptives in the world. Prevalence rates range from 6% in the United States and in other countries up to 80% of contraceptive users.[18,41] Hormonal and nonhormonal IUDs are available and have different side effect profiles.

Progestin-releasing IUDs are associated with reduced menstrual blood flow, although around the time of insertion, women frequently experience irregular bleeding. This side effect is most pronounced during the initial 6 months and typically improves with time. Other progestin-related side effects are also possible. The copper IUD is associated with increased dysmenorrhea and menorrhagia.

In a study comparing breastfeeding outcomes in women randomized to receive a copper or progestin IUD at 6 to 8 weeks postpartum, the authors found

no difference in full breastfeeding duration, infant growth, or development through 1 year postpartum.[38] However, in a secondary analysis of a randomized controlled trial comparing women who had an LNG-IUD placed immediately postpartum versus 6 to 8 weeks postpartum, early LNG-IUD placement was associated with lower breastfeeding rates;[6] in the delayed placement group, four women received DMPA prior to their 6-week visit. Studies of the copper-containing IUD have found no change in milk or serum copper levels.[36]

Complications related to the device itself include uterine perforation, failure (pregnancy), inability to visualize strings, vaginal discharge, infection, pain, the partner feeling the strings, malpositioning (which may require a surgical procedure to remove the IUD), and expulsion (2% to 10% within the first year). Data do suggest that there is an increased risk of perforation when either IUD is inserted in breastfeeding women.[16] A recent systematic review suggested that IUDs remain a long-acting reversible contraceptive option for breastfeeding women with cesarean birth.[14]

IRREVERSIBLE OPTIONS (STERILIZATION)

Multiple methods of surgical sterilization are available, including male vasectomy, postpartum tubal ligation, laparoscopic tubal ligation, and hysteroscopic tubal occlusion. These procedures involve different technologies, surgical techniques, anesthesia, and procedural settings.

Important considerations for breastfeeding dyads include the potential to impact early maternal-infant interaction. Ideally, procedures should not be performed during the initial hours postpartum to allow skin-to-skin contact between the mother and infant and initiation of breastfeeding. Early maternal-infant contact should not, however, prevent breastfeeding mothers from undergoing postpartum tubal ligation. To minimize disruption, the infant should be kept skin-to-skin with the mother in the preoperative area and be reunited with her as soon as the mother is awake and alert in the recovery room. This interruption should be managed in a breastfeeding-supportive way, and the provider should remain cognizant of the implications of anesthesia and analgesia on the breastfeeding dyad.[30]

Unfortunately, women who do not have the postpartum tubal sterilization procedure performed during their maternity stay are at risk for ultimately not having the procedure performed and subsequent pregnancy.[8,48,44] This risk should be considered. Such considerations may warrant early maternal-infant separation for the procedure to be completed prior to discharge.

The Medical Eligibility Criteria

Criteria provide guidance on the level of safety of contraception in relation to specific medical conditions and other demographic variables. Risks are divided into four categories as outlined in Table J-16, although the categories are sometimes divided into two categories: generally use and generally do not use. The current recommendations from WHO and the Centers for Disease Control and Prevention (CDC) differ. Table J-17 shows the categories for the use of several methods during lactation as presented by WHO and revised by CDC. CDC recently revised recommendations to include reducing the postpartum period from 6 weeks to 4 weeks and no longer contraindicating immediate postpartum use of progesterone-only contraception.

There are limited data from well-conducted scientific studies that adequately take into consideration the effect on the infant of exclusive breastfeeding, especially in the immediate postpartum period when the establishment of lactation and adequate milk production is essential. (III) Moreover, exclusively breastfeeding women are very unlikely to become pregnant in the first 6 weeks after birth as described above. In this setting, hormonal contraception has minimal benefit, and early initiation may derail a woman's exclusive breastfeeding intentions. Unless the risk of unplanned pregnancy or loss to follow-up is high, early initiation of hormonal contraception in breastfeeding women is not recommended.

Future Research

There is need for more detailed prospective research regarding the impact of all hormonal contraception on breastfeeding and on the potential long-term impact on the infant due to exposure to exogenous hormones. Such information will enable women to make informed decisions regarding the risk of unplanned pregnancy versus the risks of disrupted breastfeeding. Prior research has often

TABLE J-16	Medical Eligibility Criteria	
WHO Category	With Clinical Judgment	With Limited Clinical Judgment
1	Use the method in any circumstances	Use the method
2	Generally use the method	Use the method
3	Use of the method not usually recommended unless other, more appropriate methods are not available or acceptable	Do not use the method
4	Method not to be used	Do not use the method

Where a doctor or nurse is not available to make clinical judgments, the four categories can be simplified into a two-category system (third column) by combining World Health Organization (WHO) Categories 1 with 2 and 3 with 4.

TABLE J-17	World Health Organization and Centers for Disease Control and Prevention Medical Eligibility Categories				
		WHO		CDC	
		Timing Postpartum	MEC Level	Timing Postpartum	MEC Level
Combined oral contraceptive		0-6 weeks	4	<1 month	3
		6 weeks to 6 months	3	≥1 month	2
		>6 months	2		
Progestin-only contraceptive (oral and implants)		0-6 weeks	3	<1 month	2
		6 weeks to 6 months	1	≥1 month	1
		>6 months	1		
LNG-IUD		<48 h	3	<10 min	2
		48 h to 4 weeks	3	10 min to <4 weeks	2
		>4 weeks	1	≥4 weeks	1
Cu-IUD		<48 h	1	<10 minutes	1
		48 h to 4 weeks	3	10 min to <4 weeks	2
		>4 weeks	1	≥4 weeks	1

IUD, Intrauterine device; LNG, levonorgestrel.
Adapted from the World Health Organization (WHO) Medical Eligibility Criteria (MEC) and the Centers for Disease Control and Prevention (CDC) Summary Chart of U.S. Medical Eligibility Criteria for Contraceptive Use Updated June 2012 (www.cdc.gov/reproductivehealth/unintendedpregnancy/USMEC.htm). See Table 3 for MEC categories.

not adequately accounted for maternal breastfeeding goals, the importance of breastfeeding exclusivity, and amount of supplement used. Until research has addressed these concerns and focused on women's intentions to exclusively breastfeed, it is not possible to exclude adverse potential effects on milk supply, on long-term breastfeeding success, or on the infant, especially if any of these is a rare occurrence. This is particularly true when initiating hormonal contraception in the initial postpartum period. Research is needed to evaluate the impact of contemporary contraceptive options, which include lower estrogen doses and progestin-only agents, on both breastfeeding in the short term and on the infant in the long term. Further research is also needed on the effectiveness of LAM given the widespread availability of breast pumps and the growing number of mothers who are choosing to exclusively express and feed their infants expressed breastmilk. In sum, rare or long-term adverse outcomes are often not detected, and method efficacy has not been evaluated under a wide variety of conditions. Both of these issues demand study of large populations over time. For the individual breastfeeding family, this lack of sufficient data regarding the impact of hormonal contraception may have significant negative consequences.

Conclusions

Every woman should be offered full information and support about contraception options so she can make an optimal decision for her individual situation. Physicians and other health care providers should not "pre-decide" which method is most appropriate; rather, in discussion with the patient, clinicians should discuss the risks, benefits, availability, and affordability of all methods. This discussion should address contraceptive efficacy and possible impact on breastfeeding outcomes, within the context of each woman's desire to breastfeed, risk of breastfeeding difficulties, and risk of unplanned pregnancy.

Acknowledgments

This work was supported in part by a grant from the Maternal and Child Health Bureau, U.S. Department of Health and Human Services, and through the resources of the Carolina Global Breastfeeding Institute.

The Academy of Breastfeeding Medicine Protocol Committee
Kathleen A. Marinelli, MD, FABM, Chairperson
Maya Bunik, MD, MSPH, FABM, Co-Chairperson
Larry Noble, MD, FABM, Translations Chairperson
Nancy Brent, MD
Amy E. Grawey, MD
Ruth A. Lawrence, MD, FABM
Sarah Reece-Stremtan, MD
Tomoko Seo, MD, FABM
Michal Young, MD

REFERENCES[1]

1. Appendix A Task Force Ratings: *Guide to clinical preventive services: report of the U.S. preventive services task force*, ed 2. www.ncbi.nlm.nih.gov/books/, NBK15430. Accessed December 19, 2014.
2. Bahamondes L, Bahamondes MV, Modesto W, et al: Effect of hormonal contraceptives during breastfeeding on infant's milk ingestion and growth, *Fertil Steril* 100:445–450, 2013.
3. Bouchard T, Fehring RJ, Schneider M: Efficacy of a new postpartum transition protocol for avoiding pregnancy, *J Am Board Fam Med* 26:35–44, 2013. (ABM Protocol 9).
4. Brito MB, Ferriani RA, Quintana SM, et al: Safety of the etonogestrel-releasing implant during the immediate postpartum period: a pilot study, *Contraception* 80:519–526, 2009.
5. Brownell EA, Fernandez ID, Howard CR, et al: A systematic review of early postpartum medroxyprogesterone receipt and early breastfeeding cessation: evaluating the methodological rigor of the evidence, *Breastfeed Med* 7:10–18, 2012. (Erratum in *Breastfeed Med* 7:129, 2012).
6. Chen BA, Reeves MF, Creinin MD, et al: Postplacental or delayed levonorgestrel intrauterine device insertion and breast-feeding duration, *Contraception* 84:499–504, 2011.
7. Cheng L, Che Y, Gulmezoglu AM: Interventions for emergency contraception, *Cochrane Database Syst Rev* 8:CD001324, 2012.
8. Committee on Health Care for Underserved Women: Committee opinion no. 530: access to postpartum sterilization, *Obstet Gynecol* 120:212–215, 2012.
9. Cooney KA, Nyirabukeye T, Labbok MH, et al: An assessment of the nine-month lactational amenorrhea method (MAMA-9) in Rwanda, *Stud Fam Plann* 27:102–171, 1996.
10. Dozier AM, Nelson A, Brownell EA, et al: Patterns of postpartum depot medroxyprogesterone administration among low-income mothers, *J Womens Health (Larchmt)* 23:224–230, 2014.
11. Espey E, Ogburn T, Leeman L, et al: Effect of progestin compared with combined oral contraceptive pills on lactation: a randomized controlled trial, *Obstet Gynecol* 119:5–13, 2012.
12. Gainer E, Massai R, Lillo S, et al: Levonorgestrel pharmacokinetics in plasma and milk of lactating women who take 1.5 mg for emergency contraception, *Hum Reprod* 22:1578–1584, 2001.
13. Gallo MF, Grimes DA, Lopez LM, et al: Combination injectable contraceptives for contraception, *Cochrane Database Syst Rev* 4:CD004568, 2008.
14. Goldstuck ND, Steyn PS: Intrauterine contraception after cesarean section and during lactation: a systematic review, *Int J Womens Health* 5:811–818, 2013.
15. Hatcher RA, Trussell J, Stewart F, et al: *Contraceptive technology*, ed 17, New York, 2011, Contraceptive Technology Communications Inc., Ardent Media Inc.

---

[1]ABM protocols expire 5 years from the date of publication. Evidence-based revisions are made within 5 years or sooner if there are significant changes in the evidence.

16. Heinemann K, Westhoff CL, Grimes DA, et al: Intrauterine devices and the risk of uterine perforations: final results from the EURAS-IUD Study, *Obstet Gynecol* 123(Suppl 1):3S, 2014.

17. Hight-Laukaran V, Labbok M, Peterson A, et al: Multicenter study of the lactational amenorrhea method (LAM). II. Acceptability, utility, and policy implications, *Contraception* 55:337–346, 1997.

18. Jones J, Mosher WD, Daniels K: Current contraceptive use in the United States, 2006-2010, and changes in patterns of use since 1995, *Natl Health Stat Rep* 60:1–25, 2012. Available at: www.cdc.gov/nchs/data/nhsr/nhsr060.pdf. Accessed March 20, 2013.

19. Kapp N, Curtis KM: Combined oral contraceptive use among breastfeeding women: a systematic review, *Contraception* 82:10–16, 2010.

20. Kapp N, Curtis K, Nanda K: Progestogen-only contraceptive use among breastfeeding women: a systematic review, *Contraception* 82:17–37, 2010.

21. Kazi A, Kennedy KI, Visness CM, et al: Effectiveness of the lactational amenorrhea method in Pakistan, *Fertil Steril* 64:717–723, 1995.

22. Kennedy KI: Efficacy and effectiveness of LAM, *Adv Exp Med Biol* 503:207–216, 2002.

23. Kennedy KI, Short RV, Tully MR: Premature introduction of progestin-only contraceptive methods during lactation, *Contraception* 55:347–350, 1997.

24. Koetsawang S: The effects of contraceptive methods on the quality and quantity of breast milk, *Int J Gynaecol Obstet* 25 (Suppl):115–127, 1987.

25. Labbok M, Hight-Laukaran V, Peterson A, et al: Multicenter study of the lactational amenorrhea method (LAM). I. Efficacy, duration, and implications for clinical application, *Contraception* 55:327–336, 1997.

26. Labbok M, Krasovec K: Towards consistency in breastfeeding definitions, *Stud Fam Plann* 21:226–230, 1990.

27. Labbok M, Perez A, Valdes V, et al: The lactational amenorrhea method: a new postpartum introductory family planning method with program and policy implications, *Adv Contraception* 10:93–109, 1994.

28. Labbok MH, Starling A: Definitions of breastfeeding: call for the development and use of consistent definitions in research and peer-reviewed literature, *Breastfeed Med* 7: 397–402, 2012.

29. Labbok MH, Stallings RY, Shah F, et al: Ovulation method use during breastfeeding: is there increased risk of unplanned pregnancy? *Am J Obstet Gynecol* 165:2031–2036, 1991.

30. Montgomery A, Hale T: Academy of Breastfeeding Medicine. ABM Clinical Protocol #15: analgesia and anesthesia for the breastfeeding mother, revised 2012, *Breastfeed Med* 7:547–553, 2012.

31. Oladapo OT, Fawole B: Treatments for suppression of lactation, *Cochrane Database Syst Rev* 9:CD005937, 2012.

32. Perez A, Labbok M, Queenan J: A clinical study of the lactational amenorrhea method for family planning, *Lancet* 339:968–970, 1992.

33. Perez A, Vela P, Masnick GS, et al: First ovulation after childbirth: the effect of breast-feeding, *Am J Obstet Gynecol* 114:1041–1047, 1972.

34. Peterson AE, Perez-Escamilla R, Labbok MH, et al: Multicenter study of the lactational amenorrhea method (LAM). III: effectiveness, duration, and satisfaction with reduced client-provider contact, *Contraception* 62:221–230, 2000.

35. Polakow-Farkash S, Gilad O, Merlob P, et al: Levonorgestrel used for emergency contraception during lactation—a prospective observational cohort study on maternal and infant safety, *J Matern Fetal Neonatal Med* 26:219–221, 2013.

36. Rodrigues da Cunha AC, Dorea JG, Cantuaria AA: Intrauterine device and maternal copper metabolism during lactation, *Contraception* 63:37–39, 2001.

37. Shaaban OM, Hassen SG, Nour SA, et al: Emergency contraceptive pills as a backup for lactational amenorrhea method (LAM) of contraception: a randomized controlled trial, *Contraception* 87:363–369, 2013.

38. Shaamash AH, Sayed GH, Hussien MM, et al: A comparative study of the levonorgestrel-releasing intrauterine system Mirena versus the Copper T380A intrauterine device during lactation: breast-feeding performance, infant growth and infant development, *Contraception* 72:346–351, 2005.

39. Singhal S, Sarda N, Gupta S, et al: Impact of injectable progestogen contraception in early puerperium on lactation and infant health, *J Clin Diagn Res* 8:69–72, 2014.

40. Tankeyoon M, Dusitsin N, Chalapati S, et al: Effects of hormonal contraceptives on milk volumes and infant growth. WHO Special Programme of Research, Development and Research Training in Human Reproduction Task Force on oral contraceptives, *Contraception* 30:505–522, 1984.

41. The ESHRE Capri Workshop Group: Intrauterine devices and intrauterine systems, *Hum Reprod Update* 14:197–208, 2008.

42. The World Health Organization: Multinational study of breast-feeding and lactational amenorrhea. III. Pregnancy during breast-feeding. World Health Organization Task Force on Methods for the Natural Regulation of Fertility, *Fertil Steril* 72:431–440, 1999.

43. The World Health Organization: Multinational study of breast-feeding and lactational amenorrhea. IV. Postpartum bleeding and lochia in breast-feeding women. World Health Organization Task Force on Methods for the Natural Regulation of Fertility, *Fertil Steril* 72:441–447, 1999.

44. Thurman AR, Janecek T: One-year follow-up of women with unfulfilled postpartum sterilization requests, *Obstet Gynecol* 116:1071–1077, 2010.

45. Truitt ST, Fraser AB, Grimes DA, et al: Combined hormonal versus nonhormonal versus progestin-only contraception in lactation, *Cochrane Database Syst Rev* 2: CD003988, 2003.

46. Valde's V, Labbok MH, Pugin E, et al: The efficacy of the lactational amenorrhea method (LAM) among working women, *Contraception* 62:217–219, 2000.

47. Van der Wijden C, Kleijnen J, Van den Berk T: Lactational amenorrhea for family planning, *Cochrane Database Syst Rev* 4: CD001329, 2003.

48. Zite N, Wuellner S, Gilliam M: Failure to obtain desired postpartum sterilization: risk and predictors, *Obstet Gynecol* 105:794–799, 2005.

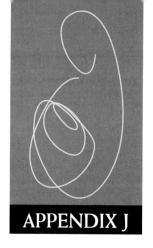

Protocol 14: Breastfeeding-Friendly Physician's Office, Part 1: Optimizing Care for Infants and Children

Definitions

Breastfeeding-friendly physician's office: A physician's practice that enthusiastically promotes, supports, and protects breastfeeding through a warm office environment and education of health care professionals and families.

Breastmilk substitutes: Infant formula, glucose water.

Background

Prenatal intention to breastfeed is influenced to a great extent by health care providers' opinion and support.[4,17] Ongoing parental support through in-person visits and phone contacts with health care providers results in increased breastfeeding duration.[24] Pediatric health care providers are in a unique position to contribute to the initial and ongoing support of the breastfeeding dyad.[21,5] Practices that employ a health care professional trained in lactation have significantly higher breastfeeding initiation and maintenance rates, with mothers experiencing fewer problems related to breastfeeding.[16,15] The World Health Organization's Baby Friendly Hospital Initiative describes Ten Steps for Successful Breastfeeding.[23] These 10 steps are based on scientific evidence and the experience of respected authorities. The scientific basis of many of these recommendations can be extended to outpatient pediatric practices.[5,20] Initiating incremental changes to improving breastfeeding support is of value because there is a dose-response relationship between the number of steps achieved and breastfeeding outcomes.[6]

Recommendations

1. Establish a written breastfeeding-friendly office policy.[23] Collaborate with colleagues and office staff during development. Inform all new staff about policy. Provide copies of your practice's policy to hospitals and physicians covering for you.

2. Encourage breastfeeding mothers to feed newborns only breastmilk and avoid offering supplemental formula or glucose water unless medically indicated.[2] Instruct mother to not offer bottles or a pacifier until breastfeeding is well established.[13]

3. Offer culturally and ethnically competent care.[2] Understand that families may follow cultural practices regarding infant colostrum consumption and maternal diet during lactation. Provide access to a multilingual staff, translators, and ethnically diverse educational material.

4. Offer a prenatal visit and show your commitment to breastfeeding during this visit.[19] If providing antenatal care to the mother, broach the subject of infant feeding in the first trimester and continue to express your support of breastfeeding throughout the course of the pregnancy. Inquire about a feeding plan and previous breastfeeding experience. Provide educational material that highlights the many ways in which breastfeeding is superior to formula feeding. Direct education and educational material to all family members involved in child care (father, grandparents, etc.).[4,2,14] Encourage attendance of both parents at prenatal breastfeeding classes before parents decide about the feeding plan. Identify patients with lactation risk factors (e.g., flat or inverted nipples, history of breast surgery, no increase in breast size during pregnancy, previous unsuccessful breastfeeding experience).

5. Collaborate with local hospitals and maternity care professionals in the community.[2] Convey to delivery rooms and newborn units your office policies on breastfeeding initiation. Leave orders in the hospital not to give formula/sterile water/glucose water to the baby without orders and not to dispense commercial discharge bags containing infant formula and/or feeding bottles to mothers.[7,22] Show support for breastfeeding during hospital rounds. Facilitate breastfeeding within 1 hour of an infant's birth. Help mothers initiate and continue breastfeeding. Counsel mothers to follow the infant's hunger and satiety cues and ensure that the infant breastfeeds 8 to 12 times in 24 hours. Encourage rooming-in and breastfeeding on demand.

6. Schedule a first follow-up visit for the infant 48 to 72 hours after hospital discharge[1] or earlier if there are breastfeeding-related problems, such as excessive weight loss (>7%) or jaundice present at the time of hospital discharge.[2,19,1] Ensure access to a lactation consultant/educator or other health care professional trained to address breastfeeding questions or concerns during this visit. Provide comfortable seating and a nursing pillow for the breastfeeding dyad to facilitate adequate evaluation. Assess latch and successful and adequate breastfeeding at the early follow-up visit. Identify lactation risk factors and assess the infant's weight, hydration, jaundice, feeding

activity, and output. Provide medical help for women with sore nipples or other maternal health problems that impact breastfeeding. Begin by asking parents open-ended questions and then focus on their concerns. Take the time to address the many questions that a mother may have, especially if it is her first nursing experience. Provide close follow-up until the infant is doing well with adequate weight gain and parents feel confident.

7. Ensure availability of appropriate educational resources for parents. Educational material should not be commercial and not advertise breastmilk substitutes, bottles, or nipples.[12] Educational resources may be in the form of handouts, visual aids, books, and videos. Recommended topics for educational material are growth patterns, feeding, and sleep patterns of breastfed babies; management of growth spurts; recognition of hunger and satiety cues; latch-on and positioning; management of sore nipples; mastitis; low supply; blocked ducts; engorgement; reflux; normal stooling and voiding patterns; maintaining lactation when separated from the infant (e.g., during illness, prematurity, return to work); postpartum depression; maternal medication use; and maternal illness during breastfeeding.

8. Do not interrupt or discourage breastfeeding in the office. Allow and encourage breastfeeding in the waiting room. Display signs in the waiting area encouraging mothers to breastfeed. Provide a comfortable private area to breastfeed for those mothers who prefer privacy.[19]

9. Ensure an office environment that demonstrates breastfeeding promotion and support. Eliminate the practice of distribution of free formula and baby items from formula companies to parents.[12] Store formula supplies out of view of parents. Display posters, pamphlets, pictures, and photographs of breastfeeding mothers in your office.[19] Do not display images of infants bottle feeding. Do not accept gifts (including writing pads, pens, or calendars) or personal samples from companies manufacturing infant formula, feeding bottles, or pacifiers. Specifically target material to populations with low breastfeeding rates.

10. Develop and follow telephone triage protocols to address breastfeeding concerns and problems.[19] Conduct follow-up phone calls to assist breastfeeding mothers. Provide readily accessible resources such as books and protocols to triage nurses.

11. Commend breastfeeding mothers during each visit for choosing and continuing breastfeeding. Provide breastfeeding anticipatory guidance in routine periodic health maintenance

---

[1]In cultures or medical situations in which the dyad has remained hospitalized for long enough that weight gain and parental confidence are established prior to hospital discharge, follow-up may be deferred until the initial well child care visit at 1 to 2 weeks of age if otherwise appropriate.

visits. Encourage fathers of infants to accompany mother and baby to office visits.[14,25]

12. Encourage mothers to exclusively breastfeed for 6 months and continue breastfeeding with complementary foods until at least 24 months and thereafter as long as mutually desired.[26] Discuss introduction of solid food at 6 months of age, emphasizing the need for high-iron solids, and assess the need for vitamin D supplementation.[2]

13. Set an example for your patients and community. Have a written breastfeeding policy and provide a lactation room with supplies for your employees who breastfeed or express breast-milk at work.

14. Acquire or maintain a list of community resources (e.g., breast pump rental locations) and be knowledgeable about referral procedures. Refer expectant and new parents to community support and resource groups. Identify local breastfeeding specialists, know their background and training, and develop working relationships for additional assistance. Support local breastfeeding support groups.[9]

15. Work with insurance companies to encourage coverage of breast pump costs and lactation support services.[2] Bill lactation support codes.[3]

16. Encourage community employers and day care providers to support breastfeeding.[2,18]

The following website provides material to help motivate and guide employers in providing lactation support in the workplace[10]: http://www.hmhbwa.org/forprof/materials/BCW_packet.htm.

17. All clinical physicians should receive education regarding breastfeeding.[19,8] Areas of suggested education include the benefits of breastfeeding, physiology of lactation, management of common breastfeeding problems, and medical contraindications to breastfeeding. Make educational resources available for quick reference by health care professionals in your practice (books, protocols, etc.). Staff education and training should be provided to the front office staff, nurses, and medical assistants. Identify one or more breastfeeding resource personnel on staff. Consider employing a lactation consultant or nurse trained in lactation.[16,15]

18. Volunteer to let medical students and residents rotate in your practice. Participate in medical student and resident physician education.[8,11] Encourage establishment of formal training programs in lactation for future and current health care providers.[2]

19. Track breastfeeding initiation and duration rates in your practice and learn about breastfeeding rates in your community.

Recommendations for Future Research

1. There are currently no studies demonstrating the effectiveness of specific educational interventions related to breastfeeding (e.g., distribution of handouts, counseling by the primary care provider, group counseling, counseling by nurse) during pediatric preventative care visits.

2. More studies are needed about specific office practices and their effects on breastfeeding initiation, exclusivity, and maintenance.

3. More studies on the short- and long-term effectiveness of educational programs for physicians would be helpful.

4. Research on specific challenges to providing support in the outpatient setting is needed.

5. Studies regarding the cost-effectiveness of steps related to making an outpatient practice breastfeeding-friendly are needed.

Acknowledgment

This work was supported in part by a grant from the Maternal and Child Health Bureau, U.S. Department of Health and Human Services.

Protocol Committee
Caroline J. Chantry, MD, FABM, Co-Chairperson
Cynthia R. Howard, MD, MPH, FABM, Co-Chairperson
Ruth A. Lawrence, MD, FABM
Nancy G. Powers, MD, Contributor
Ulfat Shaikh, MD, MPH
University of California Davis Medical Center
Sacramento, CA

REFERENCES

1. American Academy of Pediatrics Subcommittee on Hyperbilirubinemia: Management of hyperbilirubinemia in the newborn infant 35 or more weeks of gestation, *Pediatrics* 114:297–316, 2004.

2. American Academy of Pediatrics Section on Breast-Feeding: Breastfeeding and the use of human milk, *Pediatrics* 115(2): 496–506, 2005.

3. American Academy of Pediatrics Section on Breast-feeding and Committee on Coding and Nomenclature: *Supporting breastfeeding and lactation: the primary care pediatrician's guide to getting paid.* Available at: www.aap.org/breastfeeding/PDF/coding.pdf. Accessed February 9, 2006.

4. Bentley M, Caulfield L, Gross S, et al: Sources of influence on intention to breastfeed among African-American women at entry to WIC, *J Hum Lact* 15(1):27–34, 1999.

5. de Oliveira M, Camacho L, Tedstone A: A method for the evaluation of primary health care units' practice in the promotion, protection, and support of breast-feeding: results

from the state of Rio de Janeiro, Brazil, *J Hum Lact* 19 (4):365–373, 2003.

6. DiGirolamo A, Grummer-Strawn L, Fein S: Maternity care practices: implications for breastfeeding, *Birth* 28 (2):94–100, 2001.

7. Donnelly A, Snowden H, Renfrew M, et al: Commercial hospital discharge packs for breastfeeding women, *Cochrane Database Syst Rev* 2:2000. CD002075.

8. Freed G, Clark S, Sorenson J, et al: National assessment of physicians' breast-feeding knowledge, attitudes, training, and experience, *JAMA* 273(6):472–476, 1995.

9. Grummer-Strawn L, Rice S, Dugas K, et al: An evaluation of breastfeeding promotion through peer counseling in Mississippi WIC clinics, *Matern Child Health J* 1(1):35–42, 1997.

10. Healthy Mothers Healthy Babies Coalition of Washington State: *Working and breastfeeding.* Available at: www.hmhbwa.org/forprof/materials/BCW_packet.htm. Accessed November 24, 2005.

11. Hillenbrand K, Larsen P: Effect of an educational intervention about breastfeeding on the knowledge, confidence, and behaviors of pediatric resident physicians, *Pediatrics* 110(5) 2002. e59.

12. Howard C, Howard F, Lawrence R, et al: Office prenatal formula advertising and its effect on breast-feeding patterns, *Obstet Gynecol* 95(2):296–303, 2000.

13. Howard C, Howard F, Lanphear B, et al: Randomized clinical trial of pacifier use and bottle-feeding or cup feeding and their effect on breastfeeding, *Pediatrics* 111(3):511–518, 2003.

14. Ingram J, Johnson D: A feasibility study of an intervention to enhance family support for breast feeding in a deprived area in Bristol, UK, *Midwifery* 20(4):367–379, 2004.

15. Jones D, West R: Effect of a lactation nurse on the success of breast-feeding: a randomized controlled trial, *J Epidemiol Community Health* 40(1):45–49, 1986.

16. Lawlor-Smith C, McIntyre E, Bruce J: Effective breastfeeding support in a general practice, *Aust Fam Physician* 26 (5):573–575, 1997.

17. Lu M: Provider encouragement of breastfeeding: evidence from a national survey, *Obstet Gynecol* 97:290–295, 2001.

18. Ortiz J, McGilligan K, Kelly P: Duration of breast milk expression among working mothers enrolled in an employer-sponsored lactation program, *Pediatr Nurs* 30 (2):111–119, 2004.

19. Section on Breastfeeding: *Ten steps to support parents' choice to breastfeed their baby,* Elk Grove Village, Ill., 2003, American Academy of Pediatrics.

20. Shariff F, Levitt C, Kaczorowski J, et al: Workshop to implement the baby-friendly office initiative. Effect on community physicians' offices, *Can Fam Physician* 46:1090–1097, 2000.

21. Sikorski J, Renfrew M, Pindoria S, et al: Support for breastfeeding mothers: a systematic review, *Paediatr Perinatal Epidemiol* 17(4):407–417, 2003.

22. Snell B, Krantz M, Keeton R, et al: The association of formula samples given at hospital discharge with the early duration of breastfeeding, *J Hum Lact* 8(2):67–72, 1992.

23. UNICEF Breastfeeding Initiatives Exchange: *The baby friendly hospital initiative.* Available at: www.unicef.org/programme/breastfeeding. Accessed November 24, 2005.

24. U.S. Preventative Services Task Force: *Behavioral interventions to promote breastfeeding: recommendations and rationale,* Rockville, Md., 2003, Agency for Healthcare Research and Quality.

25. Wolfberg A, Michels K, Shields W, et al: Dads as breastfeeding advocates: results from a randomized controlled trial of an educational intervention, *Am J Obstet Gynecol* 191 (3):708–712, 2004.

26. World Health Assembly: *The global strategy for infant and young child feeding,* Geneva, Switzerland, 2003, World Health Organization. Available at: www.who.int/nutrition/publications/gs_infant_feeding_text_eng.pdf. Accessed May 13, 2006.

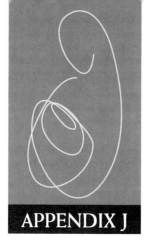

APPENDIX J

Protocol 15: Analgesia and Anesthesia for the Breastfeeding Mother

Anne Montgomery, Thomas W. Hale, and the Academy of Breastfeeding Medicine Protocol Committee

Purpose

Labor, birth, and breastfeeding initiation comprise a normal, continuous process. Oxytocin, endorphins, and adrenaline produced in response to the normal pain of labor may play significant roles in maternal and neonatal response to birth and early breastfeeding.[23] Use of pharmacologic agents for pain relief in labor and postpartum may improve outcomes by relieving suffering during labor and allowing mothers to recover from birth, especially cesarean birth, with minimal interference from pain. However, these methods also may affect the course of labor and the neurobehavioral state of the neonate and have adverse effects on breastfeeding initiation. Unfortunately, the literature in this area has not addressed the whole integrated process. Very few studies directly address breastfeeding outcomes of various approaches to labor pain management. Randomized controlled trials are rare and subject to a great deal of crossover, which confounds results. The technology of epidural analgesia in particular is evolving quickly, so studies that are even a few years old may not reflect current practices. This protocol examines the evidence currently available and makes recommendations for prudent practice.

There is even less information in the scientific literature about anesthesia for other surgery in breastfeeding mothers. Recommendations in this area focus on pharmacologic properties of anesthetic agents and limited studies of milk levels and infant effects.

Analgesia and Anesthesia for Labor

Maternity care providers should initiate an informed consent discussion for pain management in labor during the prenatal period before the onset of labor. Risk discussion should include what is known about the effects of various modalities on the progress of labor, risk of instrumented and cesarean delivery, effect on the newborn, and possible breastfeeding effects.

Unmedicated, spontaneous vaginal birth with immediate, uninterrupted skin-to-skin contact leads to the highest likelihood of baby-led breastfeeding initiation.[35] Longer labors, instrumented deliveries, cesarean section, and separation of mother and baby after birth may lead to higher risks of difficulty with breastfeeding initiation.[32,41,31] Labor pain management strategies may affect these labor outcomes and secondarily affect breastfeeding initiation in addition to any direct effects of the medications themselves.[19]

Women have differing levels of pain tolerance. Pain that exceeds a woman's ability to cope, or pain magnified by fear and anxiety, may produce suffering in labor. Suffering in labor may lead to dysfunctional labors, poorer psychologic outcomes, and increased risk of postpartum depression, all of which may have a negative effect on breastfeeding.[9]

Continuous support in labor, ideally by a trained doula, reduces the need for pharmacologic pain management in labor, decreases instrumented delivery and cesarean section, and leads to improved breastfeeding outcomes both in the immediate postpartum period and several weeks after birth.[18]

Nonpharmacologic methods for pain management in labor such as hypnosis, psychoprophylaxis (e.g., Lamaze), intradermal or subcutaneous water injections for back pain, and so on, appear to be safe, have no known adverse neonatal effects, and may reduce the need for pharmacologic pain management. More study of breastfeeding outcomes is needed for these modalities.[38,39]

Evidence suggests that breastfeeding success is affected by the behavior of the newborn. Depressed or delayed suckling, which can be caused by medications given to mothers, can lead to delayed or suppressed lactogenesis and risk of excess infant weight loss.[29,6]

Intravenous opiates for labor may block the newborn's normal reflexes to seek the breast, root, and suckle within the first hour after birth.[33,30]

1. Shorter-acting opiates such as fentanyl are preferred. Remifentanil is potent and has rapid onset and offset but can be associated with a high incidence of maternal apnea, requiring increased monitoring. Its transfer in utero to the fetus is minimal.
2. Meperidine/pethidine generally should not be used except in small doses less than 1 hour before anticipated delivery because of greater incidence and duration of neonatal depression, cyanosis, and bradycardia.
3. Nalbuphine, butorphanol, and pentazocine may be used for patients with certain opioid allergies or at increased risk of difficult airway management or respiratory depression. However, these medications may interfere with fetal heart rate monitoring interpretation. Observe the mother and infant for psychotomimetic reactions (3%).
4. Multiple doses of intravenous analgesic and their timing of administration may lead to greater neonatal effects. For example, fentanyl administration within 1 hour of delivery or meperidine administration between 1 and 4 hours before delivery is associated with more profound neonatal effects.
5. When a mother has received intravenous narcotics for labor, mother and baby should be given more skin-to-skin time to encourage early breastfeeding.[30]

There is little evidence regarding the effects of epidural analgesia on breastfeeding and the available data are inconclusive. Early studies of epidural analgesia for labor showed neonatal neurobehavioral effects and labor effects that may have had a significant impact on breastfeeding. The few studies that have looked directly at breastfeeding outcomes have suggested poorer outcomes in women who had epidural analgesia.[43,45,15,2] These results must be interpreted with caution, however, as most of these studies have been problematic with poor control groups and much crossover between study groups. Furthermore, it is difficult to ascertain whether the effects were caused by the epidural per se, or epidural use was a marker for abnormal labor with adverse effects not directly attributable to the epidural. Epidural analgesia also may affect labor outcomes, for example, increasing instrumented delivery, which may secondarily affect breastfeeding outcomes.[41,31] One study has suggested that when epidural analgesia is commonplace in a hospital supportive of breastfeeding, longer-term breastfeeding outcomes are not adversely affected by epidural analgesia.[13] A recent randomized, double-blind study showed that epidural analgesia with fentanyl in low to moderate doses, along with bupivacaine, did not have any effect on breastfeeding outcomes compared to epidural analgesia using bupivacaine alone. Higher doses of fentanyl (>150 mg total dose) may have had a small negative effect on maternal perception of breastfeeding at 24 hours and breastfeeding continuation at 6 weeks.[3]

1. If epidural anesthesia is chosen, methods that minimize the dose of medication and minimize motor block should be used. Longer durations of epidural analgesia should be avoided if possible,[36] and administration should be delayed until necessary to minimize the effect on labor outcomes that may secondarily affect breastfeeding. Combined spinal-epidural analgesia and patient-controlled epidural analgesia may be preferable.
2. Infants lose more weight in the first postpartum days when labor medications are used.[6] Some of this weight loss may be a result of mothers receiving an intravenous (IV) fluid load for epidural analgesia. One report notes babies are slightly heavier on average and lose more weight in the first days postpartum when epidural analgesia is used.[28] In addition, the use of large volumes of intrapartum IV fluids has been associated with a decrease in plasma oncotic pressure,[4] which may then increase breast engorgement and interfere with subsequent milk production and/or transfer. Conservative use of fluids may mitigate this effect. Definitive studies of these

interrelationships are needed to better assess first-week weight loss in individual newborns.

3. When epidural analgesia has been used for labor, particular care to provide mothers with good breastfeeding support and close follow-up after postpartum hospitalization should be taken.

There are minimal data concerning the pediatric effects of other labor anesthesia, including inhaled nitrous oxide, paracervical block, pudendal block, and local perineal anesthesia.[27,40] These modalities do not usually expose the infant to significant quantities of medication. In some situations, these may serve as alternatives to intravenous narcotics or epidural analgesia for labor. However, their use is limited by several factors, including lack of efficacy, technical difficulties, and a high rate of complications.

Anesthesia for Cesarean Section

Regional anesthesia (epidural or intrathecal/spinal) is preferred over general anesthesia.[22,21] Separation of the mother and baby should be minimized and breastfeeding initiated as soon as feasible. In fact, the baby may go to the breast in the operating room during abdominal closure with assistance to support the infant on the mother's chest. If breastfeeding is initiated in the recovery room, there is the added advantage that the incision is often still under the influence of the anesthetic.

A mother may breastfeed postoperatively as soon as she is alert enough to hold the baby.

Postpartum Anesthesia

NONOPIOID ANALGESICS

Nonopioid analgesics generally should be the first choice for pain management in breastfeeding postpartum women as they do not impact maternal or infant alertness.

1. Acetaminophen and ibuprofen are safe and effective for analgesia in postpartum mothers.
2. Parenteral ketorolac may be used in mothers not subject to hemorrhage and with no history of gastritis, aspirin allergy, or renal insufficiency.
3. Diclofenac suppositories are available in some countries and commonly used for postpartum analgesia. Milk levels are extremely low.
4. COX-2 inhibitors such as celecoxib may have some theoretic advantages if maternal bleeding is a concern. This must be balanced with higher cost and possible cardiovascular risks, which should be minimal with short-term use in healthy young women.

Both pain and opioid analgesia can have a negative impact on breastfeeding outcomes; thus mothers should be encouraged to control their pain with the lowest medication dose that is fully effective. Opioid analgesia postpartum may affect babies' alertness and suckling vigor. However, when maternal pain is adequately treated, breastfeeding outcomes improve.[16] Especially after cesarean birth or severe perineal trauma requiring repair, mothers should be encouraged to adequately control their pain.

INTRAVENOUS MEDICATIONS

1. Meperidine should be avoided because of reported neonatal sedation when given to breastfeeding mothers postpartum,[48] in addition to the concerns of cyanosis, bradycardia, and risk of apnea, which have been noted with intrapartum administration.[14,17]
2. The administration of moderate to low doses of IV or IM morphine is preferred as its passage to milk and oral bioavailability in the infant are least with this agent.[48,8]
3. When patient-controlled IV analgesia (PCA) is chosen after cesarean section, morphine or fentanyl is preferred to meperidine.[47]
4. Although there are no data on the transfer of nalbuphine, butorphanol, and pentazocine into milk, there have been numerous anecdotal reports of a psychotomimetic effect when these agents are used in labor. They may be suitable in individuals with certain opioid allergies or other conditions described in the preceding section on labor.[47]
5. Hydromorphone (approximately 7 to 11 times as potent as morphine), is sometimes used for extreme pain in a PCA, IM, IV, or orally. Following a 2-mg intranasal dose, levels in milk were quite low, with a relative infant dose of about 0.67%.[7] This correlates with about 2.2 mg/day via milk. This dose is probably too low to affect a breastfeeding infant, but this is a strong opioid and some caution is recommended.

ORAL MEDICATIONS

1. Hydrocodone and codeine have been used worldwide in millions of breastfeeding mothers. This suggests they are suitable choices even though there are no data reporting their transfer into milk. Higher doses (10 mg hydrocodone) and frequent use may lead to some sedation in the infant.

EPIDURAL/SPINAL MEDICATIONS

1. Single-dose opioid medications (e.g., neuraxial morphine) should have minimal effects on breastfeeding because of the negligible maternal plasma levels achieved. Extremely low doses of morphine are effective.
2. Continuous postcesarean epidural infusion may be an effective form of pain relief that minimizes opioid exposure. A randomized study that compared spinal anesthesia for elective cesarean with or without the use of postoperative extradural continuous bupivacaine found that the continuous group had lower pain scores and a higher volume of milk fed to their infants.[16]

Anesthesia for Surgery in Breastfeeding Mothers

The implications of drugs used in anesthesia in postpartum mothers depends on numerous factors, including the age of the infant, stability of the infant, stage of lactation (early or late stage), and ability of the infant to handle the clearance of small quantities of anesthetic medications.[11] Anesthetic agents will have little or no effect on older infants but could cause problems in newborn infants, particularly those who are premature or suffer from apnea.

The ability of the infant to clear small amounts of these medications is of primary concern before returning to breastfeeding. Infants subject to apnea, hypotension, or weakness probably should be protected by a few more hours of interruption from breastfeeding before resuming (12 to 24 hours) nursing.

Mothers with normal term or older infants generally can resume breastfeeding as soon as they are awake, stable, and alert. Resumption of normal mentation is a hallmark that these medications have left the plasma compartment (and thus the milk compartment) and entered adipose and muscle tissue where they are slowly released. A single pumping and discarding of the mother's milk following surgery will significantly eliminate any drug retained in milk fat, although this is seldom necessary and not generally recommended. For women who undergo postpartum tubal ligation, breastfeeding interruption is not indicated, as the volume of colostrum is small.[34] In addition, the levels of medication in the maternal plasma and milk are low once mothers resume normal mentation. Regional anesthesia is recommended for this procedure in preference to general anesthetic for maternal safety.

Mothers who have undergone dental extractions or other procedures requiring the use of single doses of medication for sedation and analgesia can breastfeed as soon as they are awake and stable. Although shorter-acting agents such as fentanyl and midazolam may be preferred, single doses of meperidine or diazepam are unlikely to affect the breastfeeding infant.[11]

Mothers who have undergone plastic surgery, such as liposuction, in which large doses of local anesthetics (lidocaine) have been used probably should pump and discard their milk for 12 hours before resuming breastfeeding.

Specific Agents Used for Anesthesia and Analgesia

ANESTHETICS

Drugs used for induction such as propofol, midazolam, etomidate, or thiopental enter the milk compartment only minimally, as they have extraordinarily brief plasma distribution phases (only minutes) and hence their transport to milk is low to nil.[1,26,5,37]

Little or nothing has been reported about the use of anesthetic gases in breastfeeding mothers. However, they too have brief plasma distribution phases and milk levels are likely nil.

The use of ketamine in breastfeeding mothers is unreported. Because of its high rate of psychotomimetic effect, including hallucinations and dissociative anesthesia (catalepsy, nystagmus), ketamine is probably not an ideal anesthetic agent for breastfeeding mothers.

ANALGESICS/OPIOID ANALGESICS

1. Morphine is still considered an ideal analgesic for breastfeeding mothers because of its limited transport to milk and poor oral bioavailability in infants.[48,47]
2. The transfer of meperidine into breast milk is documented, although it is somewhat low (1.7% to 3.5% of maternal dose). However, the administration of meperidine and its metabolite (normeperidine) is consistently associated with neonatal sedation, which is dose related. Transfer into milk and neonatal sedation have been documented for up to 36 hours after the dose.[48] Meperidine should be avoided during labor and in postpartum analgesia (except, perhaps, within 1 hour before delivery). Infants of mothers who have been exposed to repeated doses of meperidine should be closely monitored for sedation, cyanosis, bradycardia, and possibly seizures.

3. Although there are no published data on remifentanil, this esterase-metabolized opioid has a brief half-life even in infants ($\leq$10 minutes) and has been documented to produce no fetal sedation even in utero. Although its duration of action is limited, it could be used safely, and indeed may be ideal in breastfeeding mothers for short painful procedures.

4. Fentanyl levels in breast milk have been studied and are extremely low to below the limit of detection.[24,25]

5. Sufentanil transfer into milk has not been published, but it should be similar to fentanyl.

6. Nalbuphine, butorphanol, and pentazocine levels in breast milk have not been published. At this time they would only be indicated in the specific situations mentioned previously.[47] If these agents are used, observe the mother and infant for psychotomimetic reactions (3%).

7. Hydrocodone and codeine have been used in millions of breastfeeding mothers. Occasional cases of neonatal sedation have been documented, but these are rare and generally dose related. Doses in breastfeeding mothers should be kept at the minimum necessary to control pain. Routine, consistent dosing throughout the day may lead to sedative effects in the breastfed infant.

NSAID ANALGESICS

1. Ibuprofen is considered an ideal, moderately effective analgesic. Its transfer to milk is low to nil.[42,44]

2. Ketorolac is considered an ideal and potent analgesic in breastfeeding mothers. The transfer of ketorolac into milk is extremely low.[46] However, its use in patients with hemorrhage is risky as it inhibits platelet function. Other contraindications are noted in the preceding section on postpartum anesthesia.[47]

3. Celecoxib transfer into milk is extraordinarily low ($\leq$0.3% of the maternal dose).[12] Its short-term use is safe.

4. Naproxen transfer into milk is low, but gastrointestinal disturbances have been reported in some infants after prolonged therapy. Short-term use (1 week) probably is safe.[10,20]

Recommendations for Future Research

Studies of labor analgesia and labor anesthesia should specifically study breastfeeding outcomes.

Specific data are needed about the use of intravenous fluid loading during labor, such as for epidural anesthesia, and its effects on infant birth weight, breast engorgement, milk supply, and neonatal weight loss to more appropriately assess early infant feeding and weight loss in these babies.

More study is required of the special needs of premature and unstable babies, including how their ability to clear maternal anesthetic and analgesic drugs may differ from healthy term babies.

Acknowledgment

This work was supported in part by a grant from the Maternal and Child Health Bureau, U.S. Department of Health and Human Services.

Contributors
Anne Montgomery, MD
Department of Family Medicine
University of Washington, Seattle, Washington
Thomas W. Hale, PhD
Texas Tech University School of Medicine
Amarillo, Texas
Protocol Committee
Caroline J. Chantry, MD, FABM,
Co-Chairperson
Cynthia R. Howard, MD, MPH, FABM,
Co-Chairperson
Ruth A. Lawrence, MD, FABM
Kathleen A. Marinelli, MD, FABM,
Co-Chairperson
Nancy G. Powers, MD, FABM

REFERENCES

1. Andersen LW, Qvist T, Hertz J, et al: Concentrations of thiopentone in mature breast milk and colostrum following an induction dose, *Acta Anaesthesiol Scand* 31:30–32, 1987.

2. Baumgarder DJ, Muehl P, Fischer M, et al: Effect of labor epidural anesthesia on breast-feeding of healthy full-term newborns delivered vaginally, *J Am Board Fam Pract* 16:7–13, 2003.

3. Beilin Y, Boida CA, Weiser J, et al: Effect of labor epidural analgesia with and without fentanyl on infant breast-feeding, *Anesthesiology* 103:1211–1217, 2005.

4. Cotterman KJ: Reverse pressure softening: a simple tool to prepare areola for easier latching during engorgement, *J Hum Lact* 20:227–237, 2004.

5. Dailland P, Cockshott ID, Lirzin JD, et al: Intravenous propofol during cesarean section: placental transfer, concentrations in breast milk, and neonatal effects. A preliminary study, *Anesthesiology* 71:827–834, 1989.

6. Dewey KG, Nommsen-Rivers LA, Heinig MJ, et al: Risk factors for suboptimal infant breastfeeding behavior, delayed onset of lactation, and excess neonatal weight loss, *Pediatrics* 112:607–618, 2003.

7. Edwards JE, Rudy AC, Wermeling DP, et al: Hydromorphone transfer into breast milk after intranasal administration, *Pharmacotherapy* 23:153–158, 2003.

8. Feilberg VL, Rosenborg D, Broen CC, et al: Excretion of morphine in human breast milk, *Acta Anaesthesiol Scand* 33:426–428, 1989.

9. Ferber SG, Ganot M, Zimmer EZ: Catastrophizing labor pain compromised later maternity adjustments, *Am J Obstet Gynecol* 192:826–831, 2005.

10. Fidalgo I, Correa R, Gomez Carrasco JA, et al: Acute anemia, rectal bleeding and hematuria associated with naproxen ingestion, *An Esp Pediatr* 30:317–319, 1989.

11. Hale TW: Anesthetic medications in breastfeeding mothers, *J Hum Lact* 15:185–194, 1999.

12. Hale TW, McDonald R, Boger J: Transfer of celecoxib into human milk, *J Hum Lact* 20:397–403, 2004.

13. Halpern SH, Levine T, Wilson DB, et al: Effect of labor analgesia on breastfeeding success, *Birth* 26:83–88, 1999.

14. Hamza J, Benlabed M, Orhant E, et al: Neonatal pattern of breathing during active and quiet sleep after maternal administration of meperidine, *Pediatr Res* 3:412–416, 1992.

15. Henderson J, Dickinson JE, Evans SF, et al: Impact of intrapartum epidural analgesia on breast-feeding duration, *Aust N Z J Obstet Gynaecol* 43:372–377, 2003.

16. Hirose M, Hara Y, Hosokawa T, et al: The effect of postoperative analgesia with continuous epidural bupivacaine after cesarean section on the amount of breast feeding and infant weight gain, *Anesth Analg* 82:1166–1169, 1996.

17. Hodgkinson R, Bhatt M, Grewal G, et al: Neonatal neurobehavior in the first 48 hours of life: effect of the administration of meperidine with and without naloxone in the mother, *Pediatrics* 62:294–298, 1978.

18. Hodnett ED, Gates S, Hofmeyr GJ, et al: Continuous support for women during childbirth, *Cochrane Database Syst Rev* (3), 2003, Art. No.: CD003766.

19. C.J. Howell: Epidural versus non-epidural analgesia for pain relief in labour, *Cochrane Database Syst Rev* (4), 2006, Art. No.: CD003521.

20. Jamali F, Stevens DR: Naproxen excretion in milk and its uptake by the infant, *Drug Intell Clin Pharm* 1:910–911, 1983.

21. Kangas-Saarel T, Kovivist M, Jouppila R, et al: Comparison of the effects of general and epidural anaesthesia for cesarean section on the neurobehavioural responses of newborn infants, *Acta Anaesthesiol Scand* 33:313–319, 1989.

22. Krishnan L, Gunaskearan N, Bhaskaranan N: Anesthesia for cesarean section and immediate neonatal outcome, *Indian J Pediatr* 62:219–223, 1995.

23. Kroeger M, Smith L: *Impact of birthing practices on breastfeeding: protecting the mother and baby continuum*, Sudbury, MA, 2004, Jones and Bartlett.

24. Leuschen MP, Wolf LJ, Rayburn WF: Fentanyl excretion in breast milk, *Clin Pharmacol* 9:336–337, 1990.

25. Madej TH, Strunin L: Comparison of epidural fentanyl with sufentanil. Analgesia and side effects after a single bolus dose during elective caesarean section, *Anaesthesia* 42:1156–1161, 1987.

26. Matheson I, Lunde PK, Bredesen JE: Midazolam and nitrazepam in the maternity ward: milk concentrations and clinical effects, *Br J Clin Pharmacol* 30:787–793, 1990.

27. Merkow AJ, McGuinness GA, Erenberg A, et al: The neonatal neurobehavioral effects of bupivacaine, mepivacaine, and 2-chloroprocaine used for pudendal block, *Anesthesiology* 52:309–312, 1980.

28. Merry II, Montgomery A: Do babies whose mothers have labor epidurals lose more weight in the newborn period? *ABM News Views* 6:3, 2000.

29. Mizuno K, Fujimaki K, Sawada M: Sucking behavior at breast during the early newborn period affects later breast-feeding rate and duration of breast-feeding, *Pediatr Int* 46:15–20, 2004.

30. Nissen E, Lilja G, Matthiesen A-S, et al: Effects of maternal pethidine on infants' developing breast feeding behaviour, *Acta Paediatr* 84:140–145, 1995.

31. Patel RR, Liegling RE, Murphy DJ: Effect of operative delivery in the second stage of labor on breastfeeding success, *Birth* 30:255–260, 2003.

32. Rajan L: The impact of obstetric procedures and analgesia/anaesthesia during labour and delivery on breast feeding, *Midwifery* 10:87–103, 1994.

33. Ransjo-Arvidson AB, Matthiesen SA, Lilja G, et al: Maternal analgesia during labor disturbs newborn behavior: effects on breastfeeding, temperature, and crying, *Birth* 28:5–12, 2001.

34. Rathmell JP, Viscomi CM, Ashburn MA: Management of nonobstetric pain during pregnancy and lactation, *Anesth Analg* 85:1074–1087, 1997.

35. Righard L, Alade MO: Effect of delivery room routines on success of first breast-feed, *Lancet* 336:1105–1107, 1990.

36. Rosen AR, Lawrence RA: The effect of epidural anesthesia on infant feeding, *JURMC* 6:3–7, 1994.

37. Schmitt JP, Schwoerer D, Diemunsch P, et al: Passage of propofol in the colostrum. Preliminary data, *Ann Fr Anesth Reanim* 6:267–268, 1987.

38. Simkin PP, O'Hara MA: Nonpharmacologic relief of pain during labor: systematic reviews of five methods, *Am J Obstet Gynecol* 186:S131–S159, 2002.

39. Smith CA, Collins CT, Cyna AM, et al: Complementary and alternative therapies for pain management in labour, *Cochrane Database Syst Rev* (2), 2003, Art. No.: CD003521.

40. Stefani SJ, Hughes SC, Shnider SM, et al: Neonatal neurobehavioral effects of inhalation analgesia for vaginal delivery, *Anesthesiology* 56:351–355, 1982.

41. Tamminen T, Verronen P, Saarikoski S, et al: The influence of perinatal factors on breast feeding, *Acta Paediatr Scand* 72:9–12, 1983.

42. Townsend RJ, Benedetti TJ, Erickson SH, et al: Excretion of ibuprofen into breast milk, *Am J Obstet Gynecol* 14:184–186, 1984.

43. Volmanen P, Valanne J, Alahuhta S: Breast-feeding problems after epidural analgesia for labour: a retrospective cohort study of pain, obstetrical procedures and breastfeeding practices, *Int J Obstet Anesth* 13:25–29, 2004.

44. Weibert RT, Townsend RJ, Kaiser DG, et al: Lack of ibuprofen secretion into human milk, *Clin Pharmacol* 1:457–458, 1982.

45. Wiener PC, Hogg MI, Rosen M: Neonatal respiration, feeding and neurobehavioural state: effects of intrapartum bupivacaine, pethidine, and pethidine reversed by naloxone, *Anaesthesia* 34:996–1004, 1979.

46. Wischnik A, Manth SM, Lloyd J, et al: The excretion of ketorolac tromethamine into breast milk after multiple oral dosing, *Eur J Clin Pharmacol* 36:521–524, 1989.

47. Wittels B, Glosten B, Faure E, et al: Postcesarean analgesia with both epidural morphine and intravenous patient-controlled analgesia: neurobehavioral outcomes among nursing neonates, *Anesth Analg* 85:600–606, 1997.

48. Wittels C, Scott DT, Sinatra RS: Exogenous opioids in human breast milk and acute neonatal neurobehavior: a preliminary study, *Anesthesiology* 73:864–869, 1990.

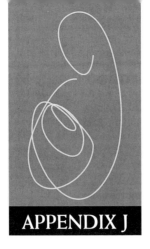

Protocol 16: Breastfeeding the Hypotonic Infant

Goal

To promote, support, and sustain breastfeeding in children with hypotonia.

Definition

Hypotonia, a condition of diminished muscle tone, is also referred to as "floppy infant syndrome" and may occur with or without muscle weakness. There are diverse etiologies including abnormalities of the central or peripheral nervous system, neuromuscular junction, or muscle; metabolic, endocrine, or nutritional disorders; connective tissue diseases; and chromosomal abnormalities. Perinatal hypoxia, hypotonic cerebral palsy, and nonspecific mental deficiency may all result in central hypotonia. There is also a condition referred to as benign congenital hypotonia, which is a diagnosis of exclusion, and improves or disappears entirely with age.[33] Preterm infants as well will have age-appropriate hypotonia. Hypotonic babies often have feeding problems that result from abnormal or underdeveloped control of the oropharyngeal structures, contributing to an uncoordinated and/or weak suck.

Background

One of the more common causes of hypotonia, which we shall use as an example, is Down syndrome. Down syndrome is a genetic disorder caused by a trisomy of chromosome 21 resulting in hypotonia in more than 90% of cases. Associated oral abnormalities characteristically include malocclusion and a small mouth with a relatively large, protruding tongue, which when coupled to the hypotonia, result in significant associated feeding difficulties in some, but not all, of these children.[4]

The Academy of Breastfeeding Medicine, American Academy of Pediatrics, World Health Organization, and other international organizations have recommended that all children should be breastfed, unless there is a medical contraindication.[1] It is particularly important that Down syndrome and other hypotonic children be breastfed to minimize the risk of morbidities associated with artificial feedings, many of which they are at increased risk from by virtue of their condition. For example, in addition to the oral abnormalities and malocclusion, children with Down syndrome have developmental delay; are more susceptible to ear, respiratory, and other infections; and have an increased incidence of other congenital anomalies such as heart and gastrointestinal malformations. In looking at the effects of breastfeeding on these problems in a healthy population, approximately 44% of dental malocclusion can be attributed to lack of or short duration of breastfeeding,[17] suggesting that breastfeeding promotes oral motor strength, a potential benefit to those children with Down syndrome and other causes of hypotonia.[4] Breastfeeding helps with normal mouth and tongue coordination. Breastfeeding has also been shown to be protective against the development of ear and respiratory infections.[17,34,29,28,8] Studies indicate that there is a positive neurocognitive advantage of breastfeeding,[3,2,12,14] which is most pronounced in

907

low birth weight and small for gestational age children[38,27,32,2,37] who may score as many as eight points higher on intelligence tests than their formula-fed counterparts. As hypotonic babies may have disorders associated with neurocognitive impairment, the benefit of human milk feedings could make an important difference to their long-term outcome. Children with congenital heart disease who breastfeed have better growth, shorter hospital stays, and higher oxygen saturations than children with congenital heart disease who are formula fed.[20] Again, this may suggest potential benefit to hypotonic infants with heart disease, seen in a significant proportion of babies with Down syndrome. Thus although children with Down syndrome and other forms of hypotonia have not been specifically studied, based on the wealth of information available from studies in the general population, they may be expected to benefit from breastfeeding and/or expressed breast milk.

Some mothers of children with Down syndrome express anxiety and fear at the time of their child's diagnosis. Many express feeling "helpless"[36] or frustrated that they were not able to breastfeed or felt as if they were not given support for breastfeeding.[30] The ability to breastfeed their babies may empower these mothers.

Challenges to breastfeeding the hypotonic child exist, but many can successfully feed at the breast. No evidence exists that Down syndrome or other hypotonic infants feed better with the bottle than at the breast.[18] Further, no evidence suggests that these children need to feed from a bottle before going to breast.[2] Breastfeeding should be actively promoted and supported in these infants.

Sucking behavior, specifically in Down syndrome, has been documented to be less efficient than in normal-term infants with multiple parameters affected, including sucking pressure, frequency, and duration, as well as a deficiency in the smooth peristaltic tongue movement.[23] When followed longitudinally over the first year, sucking pressure increased significantly by 4 months and again by 8 months. Frequency increased by 4 months. Duration did not increase over time, and peristalsis only normalized in the minority of infants who were restudied at 8 months. However, the overall result was improvement in sucking efficiency over the first year. Mothers tended to report that feeding problems were substantially improved by 3 to 4 months of age. Understanding this time frame allows practitioners to effectively support these mothers and babies to improve breastfeeding skills, and reach and maintain a sufficient milk supply that may enable them to ultimately successfully breastfeed, even with the presence of significant difficulties at the beginning.

Procedures

EDUCATION

1. All mothers should be educated about the benefits of breastfeeding for themselves and their infants. A significant percentage of hypotonic infants can feed at the breast without difficulty.
2. All babies should be followed closely both before and after discharge from the hospital for assessment of further needs.

FACILITATION AND ASSESSMENT OF FEEDING AT THE BREAST IN THE IMMEDIATE POSTPARTUM PERIOD

1. The first feeding should be initiated as soon as the baby is stable. There is no reason this cannot occur as early as the delivery room if the baby is physiologically stable.
2. Kangaroo (skin-to-skin) care should be strongly encouraged. If the baby does not feed well, the touching may be stimulating, so that the baby is easier to arouse for feedings. Skin-to-skin care has also been shown to help increase mother's milk supply,[13] and it can assist with bonding, which may be especially important for these families.
3. Assess the baby's ability to latch, suck, and transfer milk. This assessment should involve personnel specifically trained in breastfeeding evaluation and management.
4. Skin-to-skin contact will facilitate frequent attempts at the breast. For those attempts, particular attention should be given to providing good head and body support as the baby needs to spend effort sucking, not supporting body position. Use of a sling or pillows to support the infant in a flexed position allows the mother to use her hands to support both her breast and the infant's jaw simultaneously.
5. The "dancer hand" position (see Figure 14-1) may be helpful to the mother to try because it supports both her breast and her baby's chin and jaw while the baby is nursing. This involves cupping her breast in the palm of her hand (holding her breast from below), with the third, fourth, and fifth fingers curling up towards the side of her breast to support it, while simultaneously allowing the baby's chin to rest on the web space between her thumb and index finger (see Figure 14-1). The thumb and index finger can then give gentle pressure to the masseter muscle, which stabilizes the jaw.[21,7] Additionally, pulling the jaw slightly forward may allow the infant to better grasp the breast and form a seal. The other hand is

free to be used to support the baby's neck and shoulders.

6. Other strategies to help the infant latch and transfer milk may also be effective. Some mothers facilitate milk transfer with the technique of breastfeeding used in conjunction with hand compression. Instead of placing the thumb and index finger on the baby's jaw for support (dancer position), the fingers are kept proximal to the areola, and milk is hand expressed as the baby suckles. A thin silicon nipple shield may be useful, if production is generous (>500 mL/day) and mothers learn how to keep the reservoir filled by synchronizing breastfeeding with hand compression or using a nursing supplementation device simultaneously inside the shield.[24] By making the mother aware of various techniques, aids, and ideas, she is empowered to experiment and discover the best repertoire to fit her and her baby's individual needs.

7. The mother, and family who is supporting her, should be counseled that more time may be necessary in the early weeks to complete a feeding. They should also know that in many cases the baby's ability to feed will improve over the first weeks to months.

8. Trained personnel must reassess the baby frequently (a minimum of once every 8 hours) because these babies must be considered high (breastfeeding) risk, similarly to the near-term baby (see ABM Protocol #10 Breastfeeding the Near-Term Baby).[5] Encourage frequent nursing throughout the day as the ability to sustain suck may be impaired. Infants should go to breast as often as possible, aiming for at least 8 to 12 times per 24 hours. Prolonged periods of skin-to-skin contact will facilitate these frequent attempts at the breast. Assessments should include state of hydration and jaundice as possible complications of poor intake.

9. Once transitional milk is present, test weighing with an appropriate digital scale may be an option to judge adequate milk transfer. Infants are weighed immediately prior to the feed on an electronic scale with accuracy at minimum 0.5 g, and then reweighed immediately after the feed with the exact same diaper, clothing, blankets, and so on, worn during the prefeed weight. Intake during the feed is reflected by weight gain, 1 g = 1 mL. Term infants with Down syndrome gain weight more slowly than normal full-term infants,[6] so this must be taken into consideration during the early weeks and months. Growth charts specific for Down syndrome are found at http://www.growthcharts.com/charts/DS/charts.htm (last accessed 21 Jan. 2007).

10. Consider alternative modes of feeding if the baby is unable to nurse at the breast or sustain adequate suckling, including the use of a cup,[19] a spoon, or a wide-based silicone bottle. The use of a nursing supplementation aid alone (without a nipple shield—Section B6) may not be as helpful, as it works best with a baby who has an effective latch, the lack of which is often one of the significant problems of hypotonic infants.

11. If supplementation is necessary, please see Academy of Breastfeeding Medicine Protocol #3 (Hospital Guidelines for the Use of Supplementary Feedings in the Healthy Term Breastfed Infant).[31] If the baby is attempting to suckle, following each breastfeeding encounter with breast milk expression (see later), followed by spoon or cup feeding of the expressed milk to the baby, provides more stimulation to the breasts and more milk to the baby.

PREVENTATIVE MEASURES TO PROTECT A MILK SUPPLY

1. If the infant is unable to successfully and fully breastfeed, or if the mother is separated from her infant (e.g., neonatal intensive care unit admission), lactation must be initiated and/or maintained through pumping or hand expression. Anticipating the initial difficulty a hypotonic infant will likely have with sustaining frequent and effective milk removal, insufficient milk production may be prevented by encouraging mothers to express milk shortly after delivery, ideally within 2 hours (certainly within the first 6 hours as is recommended with preterm mothers),[11] and approximately every 3 hours thereafter. Aim to remove milk at least eight times in a 24-hour period, mimicking the stimulation of a vigorous term breastfeeding baby. Even if the baby shows some ability to go to breast, latch, and transfer milk, the mother will likely need to express or pump extra milk in the early weeks in order to build and maintain her milk supply at the higher level. A plentiful milk supply will enhance letdown for these less vigorous babies, and facilitate their feeding effort.

2. Most of the research on initiating and maintaining milk supply by expressing milk has been done on mothers of preterm infants. The strongest determinant of duration and exclusivity of breastfeeding the preterm infant is the volume of milk produced by the pump-dependent mother, while insufficient milk production is the most common reason for cessation of efforts to provide milk for these infants.[35,16,9] As the baby begins to improve with milk transfer,

developing rhythms, and showing feeding cues, pumping times can be led by these cues (i.e., breast emptying by expression after each attempt at the breast). This pattern should continue until the couplet is reunited and/or the infant is able to sustain successful breastfeeding. It is critical that mothers be instructed on effective pumping, including both the use of a hospital-grade electric pump if available and manual expression.

3. Extrapolating from preterm research for guidance in the hypotonic baby, the production of 500 mL/day is commonly cited as the minimum volume enabling premature babies <1500 g to transition from tube or bottle feeding to successful, exclusive breastfeeding.[23] Until studies are done in the hypotonic infant population, this is a minimum volume from which to start and can be adjusted based on calculations of intake necessary for growth.

4. Simultaneous pumping of both breasts with a hospital-grade pump has been shown to be more effective than single pumping. Recent research suggests manually assisted pumping improves effective emptying and production in pump-dependent women. In contrast to the usual practice of passively depending on the pump to suction milk from the breast, manual techniques, used in conjunction with pumping, enable mothers to enhance emptying by using their hands for breast compression, massage, and expression.[15]

5. A pumping/feeding diary or log to enable health care providers to track maternal milk supply and intervene when needed can consist simply of a piece of paper with columns for date, time started pumping, time ended pumping, amount of milk expressed, and comments (such as where pumped, unusual stressors, etc.), or one can be ordered or used as a model from various websites, including: http://www.cpqcc.org/Documents/NutritionToolkit/NutritionToolkit.pdf, appendix "O" (last accessed 21 Jan. 2007).

AT DISCHARGE AND IN THE NEONATAL PERIOD

1. If the baby will remain hospitalized, the mother's milk supply should be assessed daily including pumping frequency, 24-hour milk total, and any signs of breast discomfort. Carefully monitor the baby's weight gain and consider supplementation as necessary.

2. Inform mothers that sucking efficiency frequently continues to improve over the first year, such that the breastfeeding experience may "normalize" and may not continue to require interventions initially necessary for their own

infant; for example, supplementation, pumping, more frequent nursing, and so forth.

3. Provide information about local support groups for breastfeeding and for specific diagnoses such as Down syndrome families. Support and encouragement are particularly important for these mothers and families with the additional patience and time that is sometimes required to breastfeed these infants.

4. Maternal milk supply is affected by ineffective or infrequent pumping/expressing. Although stress, fatigue, and pain are frequently cited as determinants of slow milk supply, recent evidence refutes this.[10] However, it is not unreasonable to encourage maternal rest and analgesics as needed. Review and optimize breast milk expression frequency, schedule, and type of pump used, if necessary. A pumping diary/log (see earlier) can be useful.

5. If maternal milk supply does not equal or exceed the infant's needs or begins to slow despite optimal pumping, the use of galactogogues to enhance maternal milk supply may be considered. Please see Academy of Breastfeeding Medicine Protocol #9 (Use of Galactogogues in Initiating or Augmenting Maternal Milk Supply).[26]

6. In the presence of significant cardiac, gastrointestinal, or renal complications, it is sometimes necessary to increase the caloric density of breastmilk with extra fat, carbohydrate, or protein. If the mother's milk supply is greater than the baby's needs, a trial of feeding hindmilk (higher fat content, therefore more fat calories), either by expressing some of the foremilk before putting the baby to breast or, if supplements are being used, by pumping off a small volume of milk first (foremilk) and then in a separate container pumping the rest of the milk present (hindmilk) and feeding the baby only the hindmilk.

Further Research

This protocol was developed for the Academy of Breastfeeding Medicine to give clinicians guidance based on the expert opinion of practitioners who have worked extensively with this population. There is little scientific evidence upon which to base recommendations. Specific areas recommended for further research include:

1. Methods of optimizing the hypotonic infant's suck and milk transfer need further study.

2. Use of pacifiers in premature infants as "practice" oral feeding during gavage feeds has assisted with the transition to breast and merits evaluation in hypotonic infants.[22]

3. Comparison of autonomic stability between breast- and bottle-fed infants with Down syndrome or other etiologies of hypotonia may be helpful.
4. Evaluation of weight gain in breastfed versus formula-fed hypotonic infants, once breastfeeding has been established.
5. Evaluation of different methods available to supplement hypotonic babies (cup, bottle, spoon) to determine efficacy and best practice.
6. Modifiable factors that may compound or ameliorate the difficulties with breastfeeding in these infants in particular, for example, labor analgesia/anesthesia, skin-to-skin contact perinatally, and others.

Acknowledgment

This work was supported in part by a grant from the Maternal and Child Health Bureau, U.S. Department of Health and Human Services.

Contributors
Jennifer Thomas, MD
Department of Family Medicine and Pediatrics
Medical College of Wisconsin
Wheaton Franciscan Healthcare—All Saints Medical Group, Racine, Wisconsin
Kathleen A. Marinelli, MD
Pediatrics, University of Connecticut School of Medicine, Connecticut Children's Medical Center, Hartford, Connecticut
Margaret Hennessy, MD
Wheaton Franciscan Healthcare—All Saints Medical Group, Racine, Wisconsin
Protocol Committee
Caroline J. Chantry, MD, FABM, Co-Chairperson
Cynthia R. Howard, MD, MPH, FABM, Co-Chairperson
Ruth A. Lawrence, MD, FABM
Kathleen A. Marinelli, MD, FABM
Nancy G. Powers, MD, FABM

REFERENCES

1. American Academy of Pediatrics Section on Breastfeeding: Breastfeeding and the use of human milk, *Pediatrics* 115:496–506, 2005.
2. Anderson JW, Johnstone BM, Remley DT: Breast-feeding and cognitive development: a meta-analysis, *Am J Clin Nutr* 70:525–535, 1999.
3. Aniansson G, Alm B, Andersson B, et al: A prospective cohort study on breast-feeding and otitis media in Swedish infants, *Pediatr Infect Dis J* 13:183–188, 1994.
4. Aumonier ME, Cunningham CC: Breast feeding in infants with Down's syndrome, *Child Care Health Dev* 9:247–255, 1983.
5. Boies E, Vaucher Y, Protocol Committee Academy of Breastfeeding Medicine: *Clinical protocol number 10: breastfeeding the near-term infant (35–37 weeks)*, 2004: 2004, Academy of Breastfeeding Medicine www.bfmed.org (Accessed 21.01.07).
6. Crong C, Crocker AC, Puesschel SM: Growth charts for children with Down syndrome: 1 month to 18 years of age, *Pediatrics* 81:102–110, 1988.
7. Danner SC: Breastfeeding the neurologically impaired infant, *NAACOGS Clin Issu Perinat Womens Health Nurs* 3:640–646, 1992.
8. Duncan B, Ey J, Holberg CJ: Exclusive breast-feeding for at least 4 months protects against otitis media, *Pediatrics* 91:867–872, 1993.
9. Furman L, Minich N, Hack M: Correlates of lactation in mothers of very low birth weight infants, *Pediatrics* 109:e57, 2002.
10. Hill PD, Aldag JC, Chatterton RT, et al: Psychological distress and milk volume in lactating mothers, *West J Nurs Res* 27:676–693, 2005.
11. Hill PD, Brown LP, Harker TL: Initiation and frequency of breast expression in breastfeeding mothers of LBW and VLBW infants, *Nurs Res* 44:353–355, 1995.
12. Horwood LJ, Fergusson DM: Breastfeeding and later cognitive and academic outcomes, *Pediatrics* 101:E9, 1998.
13. Hurst NM, Valentine CJ, Renfro L, et al: Skin to skin holding in the neonatal intensive care unit influences maternal milk volume, *J Perionatol* 17:213–217, 1997.
14. Jacobson SW, Chiodo LM, Jacobson JL: Breastfeeding effects on intelligence quotient in 4- and 11-year-old children, *Pediatrics* 103:E71, 1999.
15. Jones E, Dimmock PW, Spencer SA: A randomized controlled trial to compare methods of milk expression after preterm delivery, *Arch Dis Child Fetal Neonat Ed* 85:F91–F95, 2001.
16. Killersreiter B, Grimmer I, Buhrer C, et al: Early cessation of breastmilk feedings in very low birth weight infants, *Early Hum Dev* 60:193–205, 2001.
17. Labbok M, Hendershot G: Does breastfeeding protect against malocclusion? An analysis of the 1981 child health supplement to the national health interview survey, *Am J Prev Med* 3:227–232, 1987.
18. Lawrence R, Lawrence R: *Breastfeeding: a guide for the medical profession*, ed 6, St. Louis, 2005, Mosby.
19. Marinelli K, Burke G, Dodd V: A comparison of the safety of cup feedings and bottle feedings in premature infants whose mothers intend to breastfeed, *J Perinatol* 21:350–355, 2001.
20. Marino BL, O'Brien P, LoRe H: Oxygen saturation during breast and bottle feeding in infants with congenital heart disease, *J Pediatr Nurs* 10:360–364, 1995.
21. McBride MC, Danner SC: Sucking disorders in neurologically impaired infants: assessment and facilitation of breastfeeding, *Clin Perinatol* 14:109–130, 1987.
22. McCain GC, Gartside PS, Greenberg JM, et al: A feeding protocol for healthy preterm infants that shortens time to oral feeding, *J Pediatr* 139:374–379, 2001.
23. Meier PP: Supporting lactation in mothers with very low birth weight infants, *Pediatr Ann* 32:317–325, 2003.
24. Meier PP, Brown LP, Hurst NM, et al: Nipple shields for preterm infants: effects on milk transfer and duration of breastfeeding, *J Hum Lact* 16:106–114, 2000.
25. Mizuno K, Ueda A: Development of sucking behavior in infants with Down's syndrome, *Acta Paediatr* 90:1384–1388, 2001.
26. Montgomery A, Wight N, Protocol Committee Academy of Breastfeeding Medicine: *Clinical protocol number 9: use of galactagogues in initiating or maintaining maternal milk supply*, 2004, Academy of Breastfeeding Medicine. www.bfmed.org (Accessed 21.01.07).
27. Mortensen EL, Michaelsen KF, Sanders SA, et al: The association between duration of breastfeeding and adult intelligence, *JAMA* 287:2365–2371, 2002.

28. Oddy WH, Sly PD, de Klerk NH, et al: Breast feeding and respiratory morbidity in infancy: a birth cohort study, *Arch Dis Child* 88:224–228, 2003.

29. Owen MJ, Baldwin CD, Swank PR, et al: Relation of infant feeding practices, cigarette smoke exposure, and group child care to the onset and duration of otitis media with effusion in the first two years of life, *J Pediatr* 123: 702–711, 1993.

30. Pisacane A, Toscano E, Pirri I, et al: Down syndrome and breastfeeding, *Acta Paediatr* 92:1479–1481, 2003.

31. Protocol Committee Academy of Breastfeeding Medicine: *Clinical protocol number 3: hospital guidelines for the use of supplementary feedings in the healthy term breastfed infant*, 2002, Academy of Breastfeeding Medicine www.bfmed.org (Accessed 21.01.07).

32. Rao MR, Hediger ML, Levine RJ, et al: Effect of breastfeeding on cognitive development of infants born small for gestational age, *Acta Paediatr* 91:267–274, 2002.

33. Rudolph CD, Rudolph AM, Hostetter MK, et al: *Rudolph's pediatrics*, ed 21, New York, 2003, McGraw-Hill.

34. Saarinen UM: Prolonged breast feeding as prophylaxis for recurrent otitis media, *Acta Paediatr Scand* 71:567–571, 1982.

35. Sisk PM, Lovelady CA, Dillard RG, et al: Lactation counseling for mothers of very low birth weight infants: effect on maternal anxiety and infant intake of human milk, *Pediatrics* 117:e67–e75, 2006.

36. Skotko B: Mothers of children with Down syndrome reflect on their postnatal support, *Pediatrics* 115:64–77, 2005.

37. Slykerman RF, Thompson JM, Becroft DM, et al: Breastfeeding and intelligence of preschool children, *Acta Paediatr* 94:832–837, 2005.

38. Vohr BR, Poindexter BB, Dusick AM, et al: Beneficial effects of breastmilk in the neonatal intensive care unit on the developmental outcomes of extremely low birth weight infants at 18 months of age, *Pediatrics* 118: e115–e123, 2006.

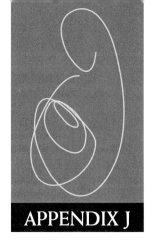

Protocol 17: Guidelines for Breastfeeding Infants with Cleft Lip, Cleft Palate, or Cleft Lip and Palate

Sheena Reilly, Julie Reid, Jemma Skeat, Petrea Cahir, Christina Mei, Maya Bunik, and the Academy of Breastfeeding Medicine

When a cleft lip (CL) occurs, the lip is not contiguous, and when a cleft palate (CP) occurs, there is communication between the oral and nasal cavities.[44] Clefts can range in severity from a simple notch in the upper lip to a complete opening in the lip extending into the floor of the nasal cavity and involving the alveolus to the incisive foramen.[43] Similarly, CP may involve just the soft palate or extend partially or completely through the hard and soft palates.[44] In CP, the alveolus remains intact. A CP may be submucous and not immediately detected if there are subtle or no corresponding clinical signs or symptoms.[44]

Background

INCIDENCE

The worldwide prevalence of CL and/or CP (CL/P) ranges from 0.8 to 2.7 cases per 1000 live births.[14] There are differences in incidence rates across racial groups, with the lowest reported incidence among African-American populations (approximately 0.5 per 1000)[15,33] and white populations (approximately 1 per 1000 births)[14] and higher incidence among Native American (approximately 3.5 per 1000)[12] and Asian (approximately 1.7 per 1000)[51] populations.

Although reports vary considerably, it is estimated that out of the total number of infants with CL/P, approximately 50% have combined cleft lip and palate (CLP), whereas 30% have isolated CP, and 20% have isolated CL; CL extending to include the alveolus occurs in approximately 5% of cases.[32] Clefts are usually unilateral (Figure J-4); however, in approximately 10% of cases, clefts are bilateral.[49]

BREASTFEEDING AND CL/P

In these guidelines, *breastfeeding* refers to direct placement of the baby to the breast for feeding, and *breastmilk feeding* refers to delivery of breastmilk to the baby via bottle, cup, spoon, or any other means except the breast. Babies use both suction and compression to breastfeed successfully. The ability to generate suction is necessary for attachment to the breast, maintenance of a stable feeding position, and, together with the letdown reflex, milk extraction. Normally, when a baby is feeding, his or her lips flange firmly against the areola, sealing the oral cavity anteriorly.

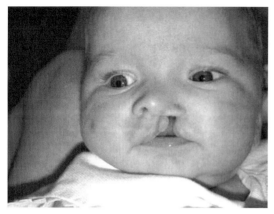

Figure J-4. Unilateral cleft lip. Photo courtesy of John A. Girotto, MD.

The soft palate rises up and back to contact the pharyngeal walls and seal the oral cavity posteriorly. As the tongue and jaw drop during sucking, the oral cavity increases in size, and suction is generated, drawing milk from the breast.[8] Compression occurs when the baby presses the breast between the tongue and jaw. Suction and compression help milk transfer delivery during breastfeeding.[8,47,40]

There is a relationship between the amount of oral pressure generated during feeding and the size/type of cleft and maturity of the baby.[41] For this reason, babies with CL are more likely to breastfeed than those with CP and CLP.[42] Some babies with small clefts of the soft palate generate suction,[28] but others with larger clefts of the soft and/or hard palate may not generate suction.[28,31] Newborns and premature babies generate lower suction pressures compared with older babies.[41,30,9] Babies with CP or CLP have difficulty creating suction[45] because the oral cavity cannot be adequately separated from the nasal cavity during feeding. For these infants, negative consequences may include fatigue during breastfeeding, prolonged feeding times, and impaired growth and nutrition.

The literature describing breastfeeding outcomes is limited, and the evidence is anecdotal and contradictory, making the recommendations that follow challenging.[39]

Recommendations

Quality of evidence (levels of evidence I, II-1, II-2, II-3, and III) for each recommendation, as defined in the U.S. Preventive Services Task Force Appendix A Task Force Ratings,[46] is noted in parentheses.

Summary of Recommendations for Clinical Practice

Based on the reviewed evidence, the following recommendations are made:

1. Mothers should be encouraged to provide the protective benefits of breastmilk. Evidence suggests that breastfeeding protects against otitis media, which is highly prevalent in this population[2,21] (II-2). Breastmilk feeding (via cup, spoon, bottle, etc.) should be promoted in preference to artificial milk feeding. Additionally, there is speculative information regarding possible benefits of breastfeeding versus bottle feeding on the development of the oral cavity.

2. At the same time, mothers should be counseled about likely breastfeeding success. Where direct breastfeeding is unlikely to be the sole feeding method, the need for breastmilk feeding should be encouraged, and, when appropriate, possible delayed transitioning to breastfeeding should be discussed.

3. Babies with CL/P should be evaluated for breastfeeding on an individual basis. In particular, it is important to take into account the size and location of the baby's CL/P as well as the mother's wishes and previous experience with breastfeeding. There is moderate evidence to suggest that infants with CL are able to generate suction[45] (III), and descriptive reports suggest that these infants are often able to breastfeed successfully[18] (III). There is moderate evidence that infants with CP or CLP have difficulty generating suction[28] (I) and have inefficient sucking patterns[31] (I) compared with normal infants. The success rates for breastfeeding infants with CP or CLP are observed to be lower than for infants with CL or no cleft[42,18] (III) (Appendix J, Protocol 3).

4. As in normal breastfeeding, knowledgeable support is important. Mothers who wish to breastfeed should be given immediate access to a lactation specialist to assist with positioning, management of milk supply, and expressing milk for supplemental feeds. Several studies have suggested that there is a need for and benefit from having access to a health professional who specializes in CL/P, such as a clinical nurse specialist, during the newborn/infant periods for specialized advice on feeding a baby with CL/P as well as referrals to appropriate services.[10] Surveys of parents with a child with CL, CLP, or CP indicated a desire

for more instruction on feeding challenges as early as possible[34] (III).

5. Families may benefit from peer support around breastmilk feeding or breastfeeding found through associations like Wild Smile[48] in addition to routine referral to breastfeeding support groups.

6. Monitoring of a baby's hydration and weight gain is important while a feeding method is being established. If inadequate, supplemental feeding should be implemented or increased. (See "ABM clinical protocol #3: Hospital guidelines for the use of supplementary feedings in the healthy term breastfed neonate, revised 2009."[1]) Infants with CL/P may require supplemental feeds for adequate growth and nutrition[18] (III). There is one study that demonstrated that additional maternal support by a clinical nurse specialist can both improve weight gain outcomes and also facilitate referral to appropriate services[5] (III).

7. Modification to breastfeeding positions may increase the efficiency and effectiveness of breastfeeding. Positioning recommendations that have been made on the basis of weak evidence (clinical experience or expert opinion) and that should be evaluated for success are:

   a. For infants with CL:
      i. The infant should be held so that the CL is oriented toward the top of the breast[16,7] (for example, an infant with a [right] CL may feed more efficiently in a cross-cradle position at the right breast and a football/twin style position at the left breast) (III).
      ii. The mother may occlude the CL with her thumb or finger[7,24] and/or support the infant's cheeks to decrease the width of the cleft and increase closure around the nipple[4] (III).
      iii. For bilateral CL, a "face on" straddle position may be more effective than other breastfeeding positions[7] (III).

   b. For infants with CP or CLP:
      i. Positioning should be semiupright to reduce nasal regurgitation and reflux of breastmilk into the eustachian tubes[7,24,3,22,19] (III).
      ii. A football hold/twin position (the body of the infant positioned alongside the mother, rather than across the mother's lap, and with the infant's shoulders higher than his or her body) may be more effective than a cross-cradle position[19] (III).

      iii. For infants with CP it may also be useful to position the breast toward the "greater segment"—the side of the palate that has the most intact bone. This may facilitate better compression and stop the nipple being pushed into the cleft site[29] (III).
      iv. Some experts suggest supporting the infant's chin to stabilize the jaw during sucking[24] and/or supporting the breast so that it remains in the infant's mouth[4,26] (III).
      v. If the cleft is large, some experts suggest that the breast be tipped downward to stop the nipple being pushed into the cleft[16] (III).
      vi. Mothers may need to manually express breastmilk into the baby's mouth to compensate for absent suction and compression and to stimulate the letdown reflex[26] (III).

8. If a prosthesis is used for orthopedic alignment prior to surgery, caution should be used in advising parents to use such devices to facilitate breastfeeding, as there is strong evidence that they do not significantly increase feeding efficiency or effectiveness[27,38] (III).

9. Evidence suggests that breastfeeding can commence/recommence immediately following CL repair and that breastfeeding may be slightly more advantageous than spoon feeding[13,6] (I). Breastfeeding can commence/recommence 1 day after CP repair without complication to the wound.[13] In a survey of CP surgeons regarding postoperative care after palatoplasty, two thirds of surgeons allowed mothers to breastfeed immediately after surgery[25] (III).

10. Assessment of the potential for breastfeeding of infants with CL/P as part of a syndrome/sequence should be made on a case-by-case basis, taking into account the additional features of the syndrome that may have an impact on breastfeeding success.

Recommendations for Future Research

The most pressing issue for health care professionals working with mothers who wish to breastfeed their infants with CL/P is the lack of evidence on which to base clinical decisions. Well-designed, data-driven investigations that document feeding success rates, management strategies, and outcomes for infants with CL/P are imperative. Furthermore, investigators must clearly describe their sample of infants and intervention techniques so that the research outcomes are able to be generalized.

Appendix: Frequently Asked Questions

BREASTFEEDING INFANTS WITH CL, CP, OR CLP

Except where noted, the literature reviewed relates to infants with nonsyndromic clefts of the lip and/or palate.

1. Can infants with CL breastfeed successfully?

    There is no strong evidence with regard to breastfeeding of infants with CL. There was moderate (II-2) evidence that babies with CL create suction during feeding.[28,45] Descriptive (III) studies have demonstrated successful breastfeeding at rates approaching the normal population.[21] Expert opinion (III) suggests that infants with CL may find breastfeeding relatively easier than bottle feeding because the breast tissue molds to the cleft and occludes the defect more successfully than an artificial nipple.[17,11,23] Expert opinion suggests that modifications to positioning can facilitate breastfeeding for these infants.[16,7,24,4]

2. Can infants with CP breastfeed successfully?

    There is no strong evidence with regard to breastfeeding infants with CP. There was moderate (II-2) evidence that infants with CP do not create suction when bottle feeding.[28,45] Although infants with clefts of the soft palate may be able to create suction, this is not usually the case.[41,28] Descriptive studies indicate that breastfeeding success for infants with CP is much lower than for infants with CL.[10,7] There was weak (III) evidence to suggest that partial breastfeeding (with supplementation) can be achieved and that the size and location of the cleft are determining factors for breastfeeding success.[22,19,11] As with infants with CL, modifications to positioning are reported to increase breastfeeding success[16,7,3,22,19] (III).

3. Can infants with CLP breastfeed successfully?

    There is no strong evidence with regard to breastfeeding infants with CLP. There was moderate (II-2) evidence that infants with CLP are unable to create suction when measured using a bottle[41,28,45] and moderate to weak evidence that infants with CLP are sometimes able to breastfeed successfully.[34] Descriptive studies suggest breastfeeding success rates ranging from 0% to 40%.[2,21] Modifications to positioning to increase breastfeeding success are recommended by experts[5,16,24,22,19,26] (III).

4. Is there evidence to guide assessment and management of breastfeeding in infants with CL/P?

    Aside from strong evidence regarding the use of palatal obturators (considered separately), there was moderate evidence (II-3) that lactation education is important to facilitate feeding efficiency in infants with CL/P.[23] The remaining evidence is weak (III) and focuses on (a) areas for monitoring and (b) recommendations for supplementation.

5. Is there evidence that palatal obturators facilitate breastfeeding success with infants with CLP or CP?

    Breastfeeding outcomes may be affected by the use of feeding plates (which obturate some of the cleft and attempt to "normalize" the oral cavity for feeding)[27] or presurgical orthopedics (prosthesis to reposition the cleft segments prior to surgery). These are collectively referred to as "obturators" for this report. There was strong (I) evidence that obturators do not facilitate feeding or weight gain in breastfed babies with CLP[27] and that they do not improve the infant's rate of bottle feeding.[38] There was moderate (II-2) evidence that obturators do not facilitate suction during bottle feeding.[9] This is because obturators do not facilitate complete closure of the soft palate against the walls of the throat during feeding. Contradictory evidence exists supporting the use of obturators to facilitate breastfeeding in infants with CP or CLP, but it is from much weaker sources[5,17,23] (II-2, III).

6. Is there evidence for additional benefits of breastfeeding for infants with CL/P compared with the normal population?

    Several moderate to weak (II-2) studies exist, with the majority of evidence representing expert opinion (III). It is well accepted that breastfeeding and breastmilk feeding convey positive benefits to both mother and baby. With regard to babies with CP, there was moderate to weak evidence that feeding with breastmilk protects against otitis media in infants with CP.[2,35] These babies are more prone to otitis media than the general population because of the abnormal soft palate musculature.[35] There was moderate to weak evidence that breastmilk can promote intellectual development and school outcomes in babies with clefts.[20] Antibacterial agents in breastmilk promote postsurgical healing and reduce irritation of mucosa (compared with artificial milk)[50] (III). Additionally, experts have suggested that breastfeeding facilitates the development of oral facial musculature,[5] speech,[5,19] bonding,[19] and pacifying infants post surgery.[5,11]

7. Is there evidence to indicate when it is safe to commence/recommence breastfeeding following surgery for cleft lip or palate?

CL repair (cheiloplasty) is generally carried out within a few months of birth,[51] and CP repair (palatoplasty) often takes place between 6 and 12 months of age. There are several studies that have yielded strong evidence to inform this area (I, II-2). There is moderate to strong evidence (I, II-2) that it is safe to commence/recommence breastfeeding immediately following CL repair,[13,6] and there is moderate evidence (II-2) for initiating breastfeeding 1 day after CP repair.[13] There is strong evidence (I) that breastfeeding immediately following surgery is more effective for weight gain, with lower hospital costs, than spoon feeding.[13] Contradictory evidence exists, but it is from weaker sources (III) and is divided as to recommendations.[24,4,3]

8. Is there evidence to indicate whether infants with CP as part of a syndrome/sequence are able to breastfeed?

There are over 340 syndromes in which CL/P appears.[22] It is beyond the scope of this protocol to review and make recommendations for them all in detail. However, some key data are presented to guide breastfeeding practice. Moderate to weak evidence suggests that, as well as the cleft, the additional oral facial anomalies associated with these syndromes (e.g., hypotonia, micrognathia, glossoptosis) impact feeding success.[22,37,36] It is important to examine the influence of all anomalies on feeding and design treatment with this in mind.

Acknowledgments

This work was supported in part by a grant from the Maternal and Child Health Bureau, U.S. Department of Health and Human Services.

REFERENCES[1]

1. Academy of Breastfeeding Medicine Protocol Committee: ABM clinical protocol #3: hospital guidelines for the use of supplementary feedings in the healthy term breastfed neonate, revised 2009, *Breastfeed Med* 4:175–182, 2009.
2. Aniansson G, Svensson H, Becker M, et al: Otitis media and feeding with breastmilk of children with cleft palate, *Scand J Plast Reconstr Surg Hand Surg* 36:9–15, 2002.
3. Arvedson JC: Feeding with craniofacial anomalies. In Arvedson JC, Brodsky LB, editors: *Pediatric swallowing and feeding: assessment and management*, ed 2, Albany, NY, 2002, Singular Publishing Group, pp 527–561.

---

[1]ABM protocols expire 5 years from the date of publication. Evidence-based revisions are made within 5 years or sooner if there are significant changes in the evidence.

4. Bardach J, Morris HL: *Multidisciplinary management of cleft lip and palate*, Philadelphia, 1990, WB Saunders.
5. Beaumont D: A study into weight gain in infants with cleft lip/palate, *Paediatr Nurs* 20:20–23, 2008.
6. Bessell A, Hooper L, Shaw WC, et al: Feeding interventions for growth and development in infants with cleft lip, cleft palate or cleft lip and palate, *Cochrane Database Syst Rev* (2) 2011. Art. No.: CD003315.
7. Biancuzzo M: Clinical focus on clefts. Yes! Infants with clefts can breastfeed, *AWHONN Lifelines* 2:45–49, 1998.
8. Brake S, Fifer WP, Alfasi G, et al: The first nutritive sucking responses of premature newborns, *Infant Behav Dev* 11:1–9, 1988.
9. Choi BH, Kleinheinz J, Joos U, et al: Sucking efficiency of early orthopaedic plate and teats in infants with cleft lip and palate, *Int J Oral Maxillofac Surg* 20:167–169, 1991.
10. Chuacharoen R, Ritthagol W, Hunsrisakhun J, et al: Felt needs of parents who have a 0- to 3-month-old child with a cleft lip and palate, *Cleft Palate Craniofac J* 46:252–257, 2009.
11. Cleft Lip and Palate Association: *Breastfeeding a baby with cleft lip and/or palate*, www.clapa.com/antenatal/faq/184, 2009. (Accessed 26.04.13).
12. Cleft Lip and Palate Association of Ireland: *The incidence of clefts*, www.cleft.ie/what-is-a-cleft/incidence-of-clefts, 2003 (Accessed 26.04.13).
13. Cohen M, Marschall MA, Schafer ME: Immediate unrestricted feeding of infants following cleft lip and palate repair, *J Craniofac Surg* 3:30–32, 1992.
14. Conway H, Wagner KJ: Incidence of clefts in New York City, *Cleft Palate Craniofac J* 33:284–290, 1996.
15. Croen LA, Shaw GM, Wasserman CR, et al: Racial and ethnic variations in the prevalence of orofacial clefts in California, 1983–1992, *Am J Med Genet* 79:42–47, 1998.
16. Danner SC: Breastfeeding the infant with a cleft defect, *NAACOGS Clin Issu Perinat Womens Health Nurs* 3:634–639, 1992.
17. Darzi MA, Chowdri NA, Bhat AN: Breastfeeding or spoon feeding after cleft lip repair: a prospective, randomised study, *Br J Plast Surg* 49:24–26, 1996.
18. da Silva Dalben G, Costa B, Gomide MR, et al: Breastfeeding and sugar intake in babies with cleft lip and palate, *Cleft Palate Craniofac J* 40:84–87, 2003.
19. Dunning Y: Child nutrition. Feeding babies with cleft lip and palate, *Nurs Times* 82:46–47, 1986.
20. Erkkila AT, Isotalo E, Pulkkinen J, et al: Association between school performance, breastmilk intake and fatty acid profile of serum lipids in ten-year-old cleft children, *J Craniofac Surg* 16:764–769, 2005.
21. Garcez LW, Giuliani ER: Population-based study on the practice of breastfeeding in children born with cleft lip and palate, *Cleft Palate Craniofac J* 42:687–693, 2005.
22. Glass RP, Wolf LS: Feeding management of infants with cleft lip and palate and micrognathia, *Infants Young Child* 12:70–81, 1999.
23. Gopinath VK, Muda WA: Assessment of growth and feeding practices in children with cleft lip and palate, *Southeast Asian J Trop Med Public Health* 36:254–258, 2005.
24. Helsing E, King FS: Breastfeeding under special conditions, *Nurs J India* 76:46–47, 1985.
25. Katzel EB, Basile P, Koltz PF, et al: Current surgical practices in cleft care: cleft palate repair techniques and postoperative care, *Plast Reconstr Surg* 124:899–906, 2009.
26. Lebair-Yenchik J: Cleft palates, *AWHONN Lifelines* 2:11–12, 1998.
27. Masarei AG: *An investigation of the effects of pre-surgical orthopaedics on feeding in infants with cleft lip and/or palate* (Ph.D. thesis), London, 2003, University College.
28. Maserai AG, Sell D, Habel A, et al: The nature of feeding in infants with unrepaired cleft lip and/or palate compared with healthy noncleft infants, *Cleft Palate Craniofac J* 44:321–328, 2007.

29. McKinstry RE: Presurgical management of cleft lip and palate patients. In McKinstry RE, editor: *Cleft palate dentistry*, Arlington, VA, 1998, ABI Professional Publications, pp 33–66.

30. Mizuno K, Ueda A: Development of sucking behavior in infants who have not been fed for 2 months after birth, *Pediatr Int* 43:251–255, 2001.

31. Mizuno K, Ueda A, Kani K, et al: Feeding behaviour of infants with cleft lip and palate, *Acta Paediatr* 91:1227–1232, 2002.

32. Mulliken JB: Repair of bilateral complete cleft lip and nasal deformity—State of the art, *Cleft Palate Craniofac J* 37:342–347, 2000.

33. Niswander JD, Barrow MV, Bingle GJ: Congenital malformations in the American Indian, *Soc Biol* 22:203–215, 1975.

34. Owens J: Parents' experiences of feeding a baby with cleft lip and palate, *Br J Midwifery* 16:778–784, 2008.

35. Pandya AN, Boorman JG: Failure to thrive in babies with cleft lip and palate, *Br J Plast Surg* 54:471–475, 2001.

36. Paradise JL, Elster BA, Tan L: Evidence in infants with cleft palate that breastmilk protects against otitis media, *Pediatrics* 94:853–860, 1994.

37. Pierre Robin Network: *Feeding your child*, www.pierrerobin.org, 2012(Accessed 26.04.13).

38. Prahl C, Kuijpers-Jagtman AM, van't Hof MA, et al: Infant orthopedics in UCLP: effect on feeding, weight, and length—a randomized clinical trial (Dutchcleft), *Cleft Palate Craniofac J* 42:171–177, 2005.

39. Reid J: A review of feeding interventions for infants with cleft palate, *Cleft Palate Craniofac J* 41:268–278, 2004.

40. Reid JA: *Feeding difficulties in babies with cleft lip and/or palate: an overrated problem or a neglected aspect of care?* (Ph.D. thesis) Melbourne, 2004, La Trobe University.

41. Reid JA, Reilly S, Kilpatrick NM: Breastmilk consumption in babies with clefts. Presentedat the 63rd annual meeting of the American Cleft Palate-Craniofacial Association, Vancouver, BC, Canada 2006.

42. Reid J, Reilly S, Kilpatrick N: Sucking performance of babies with cleft conditions, *Cleft Palate Craniofac J* 44:312–320, 2007.

43. Shah CP, Wong D: Management of children with cleft lip and palate, *Can Med Assoc J* 122:19–24, 1980.

44. Shprintzen RJ, Bardach J: *Cleft palate speech management: a multidisciplinary approach*, St. Louis, 1995, Mosby.

45. Smedegaard L, Dorthe Marxen MJ, Glassou EN, et al: Hospitalization, breast-milk feeding, and growth in infants with cleft palate and cleft lip and palate born in Denmark, *Cleft Palate Craniofac J* 45:628–632, 1998.

46. U.S. Preventive Services Task Force: Appendix A task force ratings. www.ncbi.nlm.nih.gov/books/NBK15430, 2014 (Accessed 26.04.13).

47. Weber F, Wooldridge MW, Baum JD: An ultrasonographic study of the organization of sucking and swallowing by newborn infants, *Dev Med Child Neurol* 28:19–24, 1986.

48. Wide Smiles. www.widesmiles2.org, 1996 (Accessed 26.04.13).

49. Wolf LS, Glass RP: *Feeding and swallowing disorders in infancy: assessment and management*, Tucson, AZ, 1992, Therapy Skill Builders.

50. World Health Organization Health: Factors which may interfere with breastfeeding, *Bull World Health Organ* 67 (Suppl):41–54, 1989.

51. Young G: *Cleft lip and palate*, 1998, UTMB Department of Otolaryngology Grand Rounds. www.utmb.edu/otoref/Grnds/Cleft-lip-palate-9801/Cleft-lip-palate-9801.htm (Accessed 26.04.13).

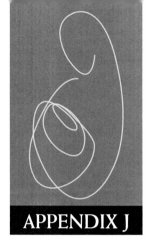

Protocol 18: Use of Antidepressants in Breastfeeding Mothers

N.K. Sriraman, K. Melvin, S. Meltzer-Brody, and the Academy of Breastfeeding Medicine

IIIIIIIIIIIIIIIIIIIIIIIIIIIIIIIIIIIIIIIIIIIIIIIIIIIIIIIIIIIIIIIIIIIIIIIIII

Background

Postpartum depression (PPD) (sometimes referred to as pregnancy-related mood disorder) is one of the most common and serious postpartum conditions, affecting 10% to 20% of mothers within the first year of childbirth.[35] Studies have found that up to 50% of women with PPD are undiagnosed.[17] Risk factors include a prior history of depression (approximately 25% to 30% risk of recurrence),[90,53] including PPD and depression during pregnancy. Other risk factors include recent stressful life events, lack of social support, and unintended pregnancy.[70] Women who are economically stressed, disadvantaged, low income, or black are at a higher risk of PPD, as well.[22] Moreover, studies of economically disadvantaged families have shown that approximately 25% of women will have ongoing depressive symptoms that last well beyond the initial postpartum year.[28]

Treatment approaches include nonpharmacological therapies, such as interpersonal psychotherapy or cognitive behavioral therapy, pharmacological therapies, or a combination of both. Antidepressant medications are one of the most commonly prescribed pharmacologic treatments of PPD. The mother and her provider should work together to make an individually tailored choice. Breastfeeding mothers may be concerned about continuing and/or starting medication for PPD. Some providers are reluctant to prescribe for lactating mothers, due to lack of information about antidepressants and breastfeeding. The risks of untreated depression, the risks of the medication to the breastfeeding dyad, and the benefits of treatment must be fully considered when making treatment decisions.

This protocol will discuss the spectrum of disease, emphasize the importance of screening, and provide evidence-based information recommendations for treatment of PPD in breastfeeding mothers.

SPECTRUM OF DISEASE

There has been controversy about whether PPD is a distinct entity. In the *Diagnostic and Statistical Manual of Mental Disorders*, fourth and fifth editions (DSM-IV and V, respectively), PPD is considered a subtype of major depression, and there is an associated specifier to denote onset in the postpartum period.[57] The newer DSM-V expanded the definition of PPD to include onset of symptoms during pregnancy through 4 weeks postpartum.[3] Diagnosis may be further complicated by other comorbid conditions, including anxiety and bipolar disorder. Postpartum mood disorders are common in the postpartum period. However, they differ according to timing and severity of symptoms and encompass a wide range of disorders.[17,57,78] "Postpartum blues" is a condition characterized by emotional changes, insomnia, appetite loss, and feelings of being overwhelmed that can affect 30% to 80% of women.[28,57] It is a transient condition that usually peaks on postpartum day 5 and resolves by day 10. Unlike PPD, postpartum blues does not adversely affect infant care.

"PPD" is a major depressive episode that impairs social and occupational functioning. Symptoms cause significant distress and can include suicidal ideation. If untreated, symptoms may persist beyond 14 days and can last several months to a year.

"Postpartum psychosis" is a psychiatric emergency and is characterized by paranoia, hallucinations, delusions, and suicidal ideation, with the potential risk of suicide and/or infanticide. It can occur in one to three of every 1000 deliveries and usually has a rapid onset (within hours to a few weeks) after delivery.[28,57] Women with postpartum psychosis may have a prior history of postpartum psychosis or bipolar disorder, but in some women there is no prior psychiatric history.[76,14] Approximately 25% to 50% of women with bipolar disorder are at risk of developing postpartum psychosis.[47]

"Postpartum intrusive thoughts" and "obsessive compulsive disorder" commonly occur in women. With a wide range of severity of symptoms, they are concerns for postpartum women. Intrusive or obsessive thoughts are unwelcome and involuntary thoughts, images, or unpleasant ideas that may become obsessions. These thoughts are usually upsetting or distressing to the woman, and they can be difficult to manage or eliminate.[1,74]

SCREENING FOR PPD

Research confirms that most mothers (80%) are comfortable with the idea of being screened for depression.[35] Internationally, guidelines and authorities recommend screening for PPD.[61-62]

Although definitive evidence of benefit is limited, the American College of Obstetricians and Gynecologists recommends that clinicians screen patients at least once during the perinatal period for depression and anxiety symptoms using a standardized, validated tool.[18] For the first time, a large U.S. multicenter study of screening and follow-up care for PPD in a family practice setting has shown improved maternal outcomes at 12 months.[94] (I) (Quality of evidence [levels of evidence I, II-1, II-2, II-3, and III] is based on the U.S. Preventive Services Task Force Appendix A Task Force Ratings[85] and is noted throughout this protocol in parentheses.)

Most physicians and maternal/child health care providers recognize the detrimental effects of PPD and agree that screening new mothers is within the scope of their practice.[69,16] The American Academy of Pediatrics and the U.S. Surgeon General's Office recognize and call for the early identification and treatment of mental health disorders, including PPD.[84,19] It is important that screening for PPD be done systematically on a global scale, as detection and treatment have been shown to be beneficial in many countries.[60] (I)

SCREENING INSTRUMENTS

The screening instrument that has been most studied throughout the world is the Edinburgh Postnatal Depression Scale (EPDS).[28,20] The EPDS is free and considered to be in the public domain. It is available in many languages and has cross-cultural validity. It has 10 questions to be completed by the mother based on symptoms over the past 7 days and takes approximately 5 minutes to complete.[20] There are multiple points of contact in which screening can occur. In well-child-care visits, EPDS screening could occur during the 1-, 2-, 4-, and 6-month visits.[28,61-62,37-33] The cesarean section incision check at 2 weeks and the postpartum visit at 4 to 8 weeks are also important screening opportunities. The EPDS can be readily administered and has demonstrated validity to detect postpartum mood disorders at as early as 4 to 8 weeks postpartum.[33,26] (II-3) A score of 10 or higher or a positive response to Question 10 about suicidal thoughts is considered positive and indicates that the mother may be suffering from a depressive illness of varying severity.[46] (II-3) Providers caring for the infant must refer a mother with a positive screen for appropriate care.

EFFECTS OF PPD

In addition to the obvious adverse effects on the mother, PPD affects the child, spouse and/or partner, and other family members. It can cause family dysfunction, prevent effective mother-baby bonding, lead to early cessation of breastfeeding, and adversely affect infant growth and brain development.[28,86-48] Rates of paternal depression are higher when the mother has PPD, which can compound the negative effects of depression on children. Infants of depressed mothers show less engagement and eye contact with their mother and are at risk for failure to thrive, attachment disorder, and development delay.[17]

A shared neuroendocrine mechanism among maternal mood, oxytocin levels, and maternal affect during breastfeeding has been demonstrated.[81] This strengthens the position that women with depression would benefit from early and sustained support with breastfeeding. Likewise, women with negative early breastfeeding experiences may be more likely to have depressive symptoms at 2 months postpartum; thus women experiencing breastfeeding difficulties should be screened for depressive symptoms.[86]

Clinical Approach to Treating PPD

Once a woman is identified as being at risk for PPD, treatment choices must be considered and offered to her. For mild to moderate depression in the breastfeeding mother, psychology/cognitive behavioral therapy, if available, should be considered as first-line therapy.[67] (II-2)

Treatment

NONPHARMACOLOGICAL
Psychological Therapy

Psychological therapy is effective for the treatment of major depressive disorder in the postpartum period, and different types of therapies seem equally effective.[25–21] (I) There are three approaches to the administration of psychological therapy in the postpartum period, including interpersonal therapy, cognitive behavioral therapy, and psychodynamic psychotherapy (nondirective therapy).[25–36] Nonpharmacological treatment is not harmful to the infant and is often acceptable to mothers with PPD.

Infant Feeding Considerations

Breastfeeding difficulties and perinatal depression symptoms often present together, and management of depression should include a discussion of the mother's experience of breastfeeding. Some mothers with depression find that breastfeeding enhances bonding and improves their mood, whereas others find breastfeeding to be difficult. For dyads struggling with milk production and latch issues, efforts should be undertaken to simplify feeding plans to ensure that mother and infant have time to enjoy one another. The demands of nighttime breastfeeding can be challenging for mothers for whom interruption of sleep is a major trigger for mood symptoms. In these cases, it may be helpful to arrange for another caregiver to feed the infant once at night, allowing the mother to receive 5 to 6 hours of uninterrupted sleep. A caregiver may also bring the infant to the mother to feed at the breast and then assume responsibility for settling the baby back to sleep, thereby minimizing maternal sleep disruption. (III)

MEDICATIONS

If psychological/cognitive behavioral therapy is unavailable, symptoms are severe, or mothers refuse this therapy, antidepressants are an effective option. Many factors must be considered when choosing an antidepressant during breastfeeding. All antidepressants are present in human milk to some extent. Data to inform clinical decisions are derived primarily from case reports or case series. Therefore the initial treatment choice should be based on an informed clinical approach that takes into account the patient's previous treatments for depression, especially use during the pregnancy, the targeted symptoms, family history of depression, and their experiences with antidepressants, current and past medical disorders, current medications, allergies, side effects of the medications, and maternal wishes. An individualized risk-benefit analysis of the treatments must be conducted (Table J-18).[12] (I)

Clinical Factors Affecting Antidepressant Choice

- Obtain a psychiatric history with a focus on previous episodes of mood and anxiety disorders and effective treatment interventions. If psychotropic medications were used, determine what treatments were effective with a tolerable side effect profile. Past treatment response is often the best predictor of future response.[12] (II-2)
- Obtain a family history of psychiatric illness and treatment response. An immediate family member's history may be indicative of the mother's treatment response.[12] (II-2)
- Consider the primary symptoms that the medication will be targeting and its potential side effect profile.
- Choose psychotropic medications with an evidence base in lactating women. Older medications with available data are preferred over newer antidepressants with limited safety information.

Choosing an Antidepressant During Lactation

When considering the use of any medication in a lactating woman, providers must consider both maternal and infant safety factors. The medication must be both efficacious for the mother and safe for the infant. Although infant serum levels of psychotropic medications are the most accurate measures of infant exposure, it is often difficult to measure

TABLE J-18 Specific Antidepressants

Class	Drug	Dosage per Day	Indications	Maternal Side Effects	Infant Exposure Effects	Comments
SSRIs	Citalopram[40,75] Escitalopram[7,11] Fluoxetine[11,64] Fluvoxamine[4,93] Paroxetine[42,56,54] Sertraline[42,29,27*]	10–60 mg 10–20 mg 10–80 mg 50–300 mg 10–60 mg 25–200 mg (usually a daily dose). Start at 25 mg for 5–7 days, then increase to 50 mg	Depressive or anxiety disorders; may be prescribed for fibromyalgia, neuropathic pain, or premenstrual symptoms and disorders	Gastrointestinal distress, headaches, sexual dysfunction, nervousness, and sedation	All SSRIs have been detected in human milk. Paroxetine[56,79] and sertraline[29,27] have not exceeded the recommended 10% maternal level and are usually undetectable in infant serum.[80] Fluoxetine[49,82] and citalopram[40,51] have exceeded the 10% maternal level.[45] The infant adverse events reported include uneasy sleep, colic, irritability, poor feeding, and drowsiness.[11,13,64,68,72] The FDA indicated that fluoxetine should not be used by nursing mothers[64]	Sertraline is the most likely SSRI to be prescribed. It's low to undetectable in milk and has a relative safety profile in pregnancy. Long-term effects on neurobehavior and development from exposure to any SSRI during pregnancy and lactation have a limited evidence base, but more recent studies are relatively reassuring[11,13,68,5]
SNRIs	Venlafaxine[58,44] Duloxetine[8] Desvenlafaxine[72]	37.5–225 mg 20–120 mg 50–100 mg	Depression	Galactorrhea	Venlafaxine and its active metabolite are in milk, and its metabolite can be found in the plasma of most breastfed infants, but no proved drug-related side effects. Monitor for sedation and adequate weight gain	Sporadic case reports for these medications.[7,8] Limited number to report significant outcomes for nursing infants
Other antidepressants (norepinephrine/ dopamine/ serotonin reuptake blockers)	Bupropion[6,23]	150–450 mg	Depression	Dose-dependent drowsiness, dry mouth, increased appetite, weight gain, and dizziness	Very limited data, ranging from asymptomatic with undetectable infant serum levels to concerns with irritability and seizures	Use is not a reason to discontinue breastfeeding. However, another drug may be preferred
	Mirtazapine[2]	15–30 mg			Limited infant data; no adverse side effects noted	

Class	Medication	Dose	Indications	Side effects	Infant notes	Comments
TCAs/heterocyclics	Amitriptyline, amoxapine, clomipramine, desipramine, doxepin, maprotiline, nortriptyline, protriptyline, and trimipramine	Nortriptyline, 30-50 mg/day, in 3-4 divided doses, or the total daily dosage may be given once a day	Depression and anxiety disorders; often used in low doses for sleep and chronic pain	Hypotension, sedation, dry mouth, urinary retention, weight gain, sexual dysfunction, and constipation. In an overdose, these medications can cause cardiac arrhythmias and death	Only nortriptyline has a sufficient number of reported cases to comment on its use during lactation: it is generally undetectable in infant serum; no adverse events have been reported.[91,89] Use of doxepin is often cautioned because of a case report of hypotonia, poor feeding, emesis, and sedation in a breastfeeding infant that resolved after discontinuation of nursing[34]	One of the older classes
Herbal/natural	St. John's wort (Hypericum perforatum) contains hypericin and hyperforin as well as flavonoids such as quercetin	300 mg	Depression	One study found a slightly increased frequency of colic, drowsiness, and lethargy among breastfed infants but none required treatment[50]	Both hypericin and hyperforin are poorly excreted into human milk	Has been used for the treatment of mild to moderate depression for many years, especially in Europe. Its use as a treatment for depression is controversial in the United States
	Omega-3 fatty acids		Depression during pregnancy and the postpartum period[32]	Appears to be of little risk to mothers and infants. The primary negative side effect is the "fishy smell"		Lack of sufficient evidence at this time to consider it a treatment for depression
Antipsychotic	Quetiapine	Start at 25 mg, titrate. Maximum dose, 600 mg	Bipolar disorder, schizophrenia	Sedation	Sedation	
Mood stabilizer	Lithium	Start at 300 mg, titrate as per LI levels. Maximum dose, 900-1200 mg		Diarrhea, vomiting	Elevated TSH	Dosing is dictated by lithium blood levels in the mother, which need to be regularly checked

FDA, Food and Drug Administration; LI, lithium; SNRI, serotonin-norepinephrine reuptake inhibitors; TCA, tricyclic antidepressant; TSH, thyroid-stimulating hormone.
*Best safety profile of selective serotonin reuptake inhibitors (SSRIs) in lactation.

infant serum levels in routine clinical practice. However, factors affecting the passage of medication into human milk must be considered, including the following:

1. Route of drug administration and pharmacokinetics[39]:
   - absorption rate
   - half-life and peak serum time
   - dissociation constant
   - volume of distribution
   - molecular size
   - degree of ionization
   - pH of plasma (7.4) and milk (6.8)
   - solubility of the drug in water and in lipids
   - binding to plasma protein
2. Amount of drug received by the infant in human milk[39]:
   - milk yield
   - colostrum versus mature milk
   - concentration of the drug in the milk
   - how well the breast was emptied during the previous feeding
   - the infant's ability to absorb, detoxify, and excrete the drug

Up-to-date information about medication use during lactation is easily available from the Internet on TOXNET LACTMED (http://toxnet.nlm.nih.gov/newtoxnet/lactmed.htm) (available in English) and e-lactancia (http://e-lactancia.org/) (available in both English and Spanish).

Most antidepressant studies provide milk levels, or a milk to mother's plasma ratio, that are not constant and depend on factors such as dose, frequency, duration of dosing, maternal variation in drug disposition, drug interactions, and genetic background. Few studies provide infant serum levels, although they are the best measure of infant exposure.[39]

Specific Antidepressants

Data from a recent meta-analysis indicated that all antidepressants were detected in milk, but that not all were found in infant serum.[87] Infant serum levels of nortriptyline, paroxetine, and sertraline were undetectable in most cases. Infant serum levels of citalopram and fluoxetine exceeded the recommended 10% maternal level in 17% and 22% of cases, respectively. Few adverse outcomes were reported for any of the antidepressants. Conclusions could not be drawn for other antidepressants due to an insufficient number of cases. There is little or no evidence that ethnic or regional "medicines" are safe or effective; thus their use by health care providers is strongly cautioned. (II-2) For specific antidepressant medications, see Table J-18.

Recommendations for Antidepressant Treatment in Lactating Women

- Current evidence suggests that untreated maternal depression can have serious and long-term effects on mothers and infants and that treatment may improve outcomes for mothers and infants. Therefore treatment is strongly preferred. (II-2)
- However, it is important not to label mothers who are only suffering from mild cases of postpartum blues as "depressed." We must make a distinction. For women with mild symptoms who are in the first 2 weeks postpartum, close follow-up, rather than initiation of antidepressant medication, is suggested. (II-2)
- When available and when symptoms are in the mild to moderate range, psychological/cognitive behavioral therapy is the first line of treatment for lactating women, as it carries no known risk for the infant. Mothers must be monitored and reevaluated. If they are not improving or their symptoms are worsening, antidepressant drug treatment should be considered. (II-2)
- Both psychological/cognitive behavioral therapy and antidepressant medication are recommended for women with moderate to severe symptoms or for whom there are current stressors or interpersonal issues that psychological therapy may help address. Maternal lactation status should not delay treatment. (II-2)
- Women with moderate to severe symptoms may require only antidepressant drug treatment. In the setting of moderate to severe depression, the benefits of treatment likely outweigh the risks of the medication to the mother or infant.
- There is no widely accepted algorithm for antidepressant medication treatment of depression in lactating women. An individualized risk-benefit analysis must be conducted in each situation and take into account the mother's clinical history and response to treatment, the risks of untreated depression, the risks and benefits of breastfeeding, the benefits of treatment, the known and unknown risks of the medication to the infant, and the mother's wishes.
- If a mother has no history of antidepressant treatment, an antidepressant such as sertraline that has evidence of lower levels in human milk and infant serum and few side effects is an appropriate first choice. (II-2) Sertraline has the best safety profile during lactation. The

recommended starting dose is 25 mg for 5 to 7 days to avoid side effects, which then can be increased to 50 mg/day.

- If a mother has been successfully treated with a particular selective serotonin reuptake inhibitor, tricyclic antidepressant, or serotonin-norepinephrine uptake inhibitor in the past, the data regarding this particular antidepressant should be reviewed. It should be considered as a first line of treatment if there are no contraindications.
- Mothers who were being treated with a selective serotonin reuptake inhibitor, tricyclic antidepressant, or serotonin-norepinephrine uptake inhibitor during pregnancy with good symptom control should continue on the same agent during breastfeeding. It is important to reassure the mother that exposure to the antidepressant in breast milk is far less than exposure to the antidepressant during pregnancy. Moreover, ongoing treatment of the mood disorder is critical for the health of both mother and baby. Mothers should be provided with information regarding the known and unknown risks and benefits of the treatment to make an informed decision.
- Mothers should be monitored carefully in the initial stages of treatment for changes in symptoms, including worsening of symptoms. Specifically, women with histories of bipolar disorder, which may be undiagnosed, are at increased risk of developing an episode of depression, mania, or psychosis in the postpartum period. Although this situation is rare, mothers and partners should be made aware of the symptoms to watch for, such as increased insomnia, delusions, hallucinations, racing thoughts, and talking/moving fast. Women experiencing such symptoms should contact their mental health provider immediately.
- The mother's provider should communicate with the infant's provider to facilitate monitoring and follow-up. Infants should be monitored carefully by the physician/health care worker. Growth, in particular, should be carefully followed. Serum levels are not indicated on a regular basis without a clinical indication or concern. In addition, in most cases, the serum level would not provide helpful information unless it is a psychotropic that has a documented therapeutic window and laboratory norms (i.e., tricyclic antidepressants).
- A strategy that may be used to decrease infant exposure based on breastfeeding pharmacokinetic reports is medication administration immediately after feedings. (III)
- There are several Web-based and book references available for professionals and mothers

to assist in gaining knowledge and help regarding these issues (Table J-19).

Conclusions and Suggestions for Future Research

Despite many publications about antidepressants and breastfeeding, the scientific literature continues to lack the depth of robust large-scale studies for clinicians and mothers to make confident decisions about individual medications. Multiple reviews of the literature broadly suggest tricyclic antidepressants and selective serotonin reuptake inhibitors are relatively safe, and all recommend individual risk-benefit assessments.[58]

Future research that would help guide clinical practice includes:

1. Randomized clinical trials in lactating women for any class of antidepressant that include the following:
   a. sufficient control for level of depression;
   b. provision of drug, information on infant serum levels, the amount detected in human milk, maternal serum levels, and the timing of sampling;
   c. information on infant consumption of the milk;
   d. information on infant behavioral outcomes; and
   e. evaluation of impact of continued breastfeeding on mitigating infant withdrawal symptoms for those mothers treated antenatally.
2. Studies of reasons mothers and clinicians elect to defer treatment in lactating mothers and follow-up behavioral outcomes of these infants.

Acknowledgments

Contributors
    Academy of Breastfeeding Medicine Protocol Committee
    Kathleen A. Marinelli, MD, FABM, Chairperson
    Maya Bunik, MD, MSPH, FABM, Co-Chairperson
    Larry Noble, MD, FABM, Translations Chairperson
    Nancy Brent, MD
    Ruth A. Lawrence, MD, FABM
    Sarah Reece-Stremtan, MD
    Casey Rosen-Carole, MD
    Tomoko Seo, MD, FABM
    Rose St. Fleur, MD
    Michal Young, MD
    For correspondence: abm@bfmed.org

TABLE J-19   Resources for Women's Mental Health and PPD Help

Resource	Description	URL
Websites		
International Marcé Society for Perinatal Mental Health	Primarily a multidisciplinary group of health care providers interested in promoting, facilitating, and communicating about research in all aspects of the mental health of women, their infants, and partners around the time of childbirth	www.marcesociety.com
Maternal and Child Health Bureau, U.S. Health Resources and Services Administration	Handbook entitled "Depression During and After Pregnancy: A Resource for Women, Their Families, and Friends"	www.mchb.hrsa.gov/pregnancyandbeyond/depression
National Suicide Prevention Lifeline, U.S. Substance Abuse and Mental Health Services Administration	1-800-273-TALK (8255)	www.suicidepreventionlifeline.org
Postpartum Support International	Information and resources on postpartum depression for providers, mothers, fathers, and families. Includes live chats and help for new parents. Access help according to state. PSI Warmline (weekdays only) 800-944-4PPD (4773)	www.postpartum.net
Postpartum Depression Online Support Group	A privately funded online support group that offers information, support, and assistance to those dealing with postpartum mood disorders and their families, friends, physicians, and counselors	www.ppdsupportpage.com
Mental Health America	The nonprofit Mental Health America is concerned with fathers' mental health as well as mothers	www.mentalhealthamerica.net/conditions/postpartumdisorders
Beyond Blue	A national initiative in Australia to raise awareness of anxiety and depression, providing resources for recovery, management, and resilience	www.beyondblue.org.au

Books

Bennett SS, Indman P: *Beyond the blues: understanding and treating prenatal and postpartum depression & anxiety*, San Jose, CA, 2011, Moodswings.

Cooper PJ, Murray L, editors: *Postpartum depression and child development*, New York, 1999, Guilford.

Kendall-Tackett KA: *A breastfeeding-friendly approach to postpartum depression*, Amarillo, TX, 2015, Praeclarus Press.

Kendall-Tackett KA: *Depression in new mothers*, ed 2, London, 2010, Routledge.

Kleiman K: *Therapy and the postpartum woman: notes on healing postpartum depression for clinicians and the women who seek their help*, Abingdon, 2008, Routledge.

Kleiman KR: *The postpartum husband: practical solutions for living with postpartum depression*, Bloomington, IN, 2001, Xlibris.

Shields B: *Down came the rain: my journey through postpartum depression*, New York, 2006, Hyperion.

Wiegartz PS, Gyoerkoe KL, Miller LJ: *The pregnancy and postpartum anxiety workbook: practical skills to help you overcome anxiety, worry, panic attacks, obsessions, and compulsions*, Oakland, CA, 2009, New Harbinger Publications.

REFERENCES[1]

1. Abramowitz JS, Meltzer-Brody S, Leserman J, et al: Obsessional thoughts and compulsive behaviors in a sample of women with postpartum mood symptoms, *Arch Womens Ment Health* 13:523–530, 2010.
2. Aichhorn WMD, Whitworth ABM, Weiss UMD, et al: Mirtazapine and breast-feeding, *Am J Psychiatry* 161:2325, 2004.
3. American Psychiatric Association: *Diagnostic and statistical manual of mental disorders (DSM-V)*, Arlington, VA, 2013, American Psychiatric Publishing.
4. Arnold LM, Suckow RF, Lichtenstein PK: Fluvoxamine concentrations in breast milk and in maternal and infant sera, *J Clin Psychopharmacol* 20:491–493, 2000.
5. Austin MP, Karatas JC, Mishra P, et al: Infant neurodevelopment following in utero exposure to antidepressant medication, *Acta Paediatr* 102:1054–1059, 2013.
6. Baab SW, Peindl KS, Piontek CM, et al: Serum bupropion levels in two breastfeeding mother-infant pairs, *J Clin Psychiatry* 63:910–911, 2002.
7. Bellantuono C, Bozzi F, Orsolini L, et al: The safety of escitalopram during pregnancy and breastfeeding: a comprehensive review, *Hum Psychopharmacol* 27:534–539, 2012.
8. Boyce PM, Hackett LP, Ilett KF: Duloxetine transfer across the placenta during pregnancy and into milk during lactation, *Arch Womens Ment Health* 14:169–172, 2011.
9. Brandon AR, Ceccotti N, Hynan LS, et al: Proof of concept: partner-assisted interpersonal psychotherapy for perinatal depression, *Arch Womens Ment Health* 15:469–480, 2012.

[1]ABM protocols expire 5 years from the date of publication. Evidence-based revisions are made within 5 years or sooner, if there are significant changes in the evidence.

10. Brandon AR, Freeman MP: When she says "no" to medication: psychotherapy for antepartum depression, *Curr Psychiatry Rep* 13:459–466, 2011.

11. Brent NB, Wisner KL: Fluoxetine and carbamazepine concentrations in a nursing mother/infant pair, *Clin Pediatr (Phila)* 37:41–44, 1998.

12. Burt VK, Suri R, Altshuler L, et al: The use of psychotropic medications during breast-feeding, *Am J Psychiatry* 158:1001–1009, 2001.

13. Chambers CD, Anderson PO, Thomas RG, et al: Weight gain in infants whose mothers take fluoxetine, *Pediatrics* 104:e61, 1999.

14. Chaudron LH, Pies RW: The relationship between postpartum psychosis and bipolar disorder: a review, *J Clin Psychiatry* 64:1284–1292, 2003.

15. Chaudron LH, Schoenecker CJ: Bupropion and breastfeeding: a case of a possible infant seizure, *J Clin Psychiatry* 65:881–882, 2004.

16. Chaudron LH, Szilagyi PG, Campbell AT, et al: Legal and ethical considerations: risks and benefits of postpartum depressions screening at well-child visits, *Pediatrics* 119:123–128, 2007.

17. Chaudron LH, Szilagyi PG, Tang W, et al: Accuracy of depression screening tools for identifying postpartum depression among urban mothers, *Pediatrics* 125:e609–e617, 2010.

18. Committee on Obstetric Practice: Committee opinion no. 630: screening for perinatal depression, *Obstet Gynecol* 125:1268–1271, 2015. www.acog.org/Resources-And-Publications/Committee-Opinions/Committee-on-Obstetric-Practice/Screening-for-Perinatal-Depression (Accessed 01.06.15).

19. Committee on the Psychosocial Aspects of Child and Family Health and Task Force on Mental Health: Policy statement—the future of pediatrics: mental health competencies for pediatric primary care, *Pediatrics* 124:410–421, 2009.

20. Cox JL, Holden JM, Sagovsky R: Detection of postnatal depression. Development of the 10-item Edinburgh Postnatal Depression Scale, *Br J Psychiatry* 150:782–786, 1987. http://pesnc.org/wp-content/uploads/EPDS.pdf (Accessed 27.05.15).

21. Cuijpers P, Brannmark JG, van Straten A: Psychological treatment of postpartum depression: a meta-analysis, *J Clin Psychol* 64:103–118, 2008.

22. Cutler CB, Legano LA, Dreyer BP, et al: Screening for maternal depression in a low education population using a two item questionnaire, *Arch Womens Ment Health* 10:277–283, 2007.

23. Davis MF, Miller HS, Nolan PE Jr: Bupropion levels in breast milk for four mother-infant pairs: more answers to lingering questions, *J Clin Psychiatry* 70:297–298, 2009.

24. Dekker JJ, Koelen JA, Van HL, et al: Speed of action: the relative efficacy of short psychodynamic supportive psychotherapy and pharmacotherapy in the first 8 weeks of a treatment algorithm for depression, *J Affect Disord* 109:183–188, 2008.

25. Dennis CL, Ross LE, Grigoriadis S: Psychosocial and psychological interventions for treating antenatal depression, *Cochrane Database Syst Rev* 3, 2007. Art. No.: CD006309.

26. Dennis CL: Can we identify mothers at risk for postpartum depression in the immediate postpartum period using the Edinburgh Postnatal Depression Scale? *J Affect Disord* 78:163–169, 2004.

27. Dodd S, Stocky A, Buist A, et al: Sertraline analysis in the plasma of breast-fed infants, *Aust N Z J Psychiatry* 35:545–546, 2001.

28. Earls MF, Committee on Psychosocial Aspects of Child and Family Health American Academy of Pediatrics: Incorporating recognition and management of perinatal and postpartum depression into pediatric practice, *Pediatrics* 126:1032–1039, 2010.

29. Epperson CN, Anderson GM, McDougle CJ: Sertraline and breast-feeding, *N Engl J Med* 336:1189–1190, 1997.

30. Epperson CN, Jatlow PI, Czarkowski K, et al: Maternal fluoxetine treatment in the postpartum period: effects on platelet serotonin and plasma drug levels in breastfeeding mother-infant pairs, *Pediatrics* 112:e425, 2003.

31. Epperson N, Czarkowski KA, Ward-O'Brien D, et al: Maternal sertraline treatment and serotonin transport in breast-feeding mother-infant pairs, *Am J Psychiatry* 158:1631–1637, 2001.

32. Freeman MP, Hibbeln JR, Wisner KL, et al: Randomized dose-ranging pilot trial of omega-3 fatty acids for postpartum depression, *Acta Psychiatr Scand* 113:31–35, 2006.

33. Freeman MP, Wright R, Watchman M, et al: Postpartum depression assessments at well-baby visits: screening feasibility, prevalence, and risk factors, *J Womens Health (Larchmt)* 14:929–935, 2005.

34. Frey OR, Scheidt P, von Brenndorff AI: Adverse effects in a newborn infant breast-fed by a mother treated with doxepin, *Ann Pharmacother* 33:690–693, 1999.

35. Gjerdingen DK, Yawn BP: Postpartum depression screening: importance, methods, barriers, and recommendations for practice, *J Am Board Fam Med* 20:280–288, 2007.

36. Grote NK, Swartz HA, Geibel SL, et al: A randomized controlled trial of culturally relevant, brief interpersonal psychotherapy for perinatal depression, *Psychiatr Serv* 60:313–321, 2009.

37. Hagan JF Jr, Shaw JS, Duncan P, editors: *Bright futures: guidelines for health supervision of infants, children, and adolescents*, 3 ed. Elk Grove Village, IL, 2008, American Academy of Pediatrics.

38. Hagg S, Granberg K, Carleborg L: Excretion of fluvoxamine into breast milk, *Br J Clin Pharmacol* 49.286–288, 2000.

39. Hale T: *Medications and mothers milk*, ed 16, Plano, TX, 2014, Hale Publishing.

40. Heikkinen T, Ekblad U, Kero P, et al: Citalopram in pregnancy and lactation, *Clin Pharmacol Ther* 2:184–191, 2002.

41. Heikkinen T, Ekblad U, Palo P, et al: Pharmacokinetics of fluoxetine and norfluoxetine in pregnancy and lactation, *Clin Pharmacol Ther* 73:330–337, 2003.

42. Hendrick V, Fukuchi A, Altshuler L, et al: Use of sertraline, paroxetine and fluvoxamine by nursing women, *Br J Psychiatry* 179:163–166, 2001.

43. Hendrick V, Stowe ZN, Altshuler LL, et al: Fluoxetine and norfluoxetine concentrations in nursing infants and breast milk, *Biol Psychiatry* 50:775–782, 2001.

44. Ilett KF, Kristensen JH, Hackett LP, et al: Distribution of venlafaxine and its O-desmethyl metabolite in human milk and their effects in breastfed infants, *Br J Clin Pharmacol* 53:17–22, 2002.

45. Ito S, Koren G: Antidepressants and breast-feeding, *Am J Psychiatry* 154:1174, 1997.

46. Jardri R, Pelta J, Maron M, et al: Predictive validation study of the Edinburgh Postnatal Depression Scale in the first week after delivery and risk analysis for postnatal depression, *J Affect Disord* 93:169–176, 2006.

47. Jones I, Craddock N: Familiarity of the puerperal trigger in bipolar disorder: results of a family study, *Am J Psychiatry* 158:913–917, 2001.

48. Kavanaugh M, Halterman JS, Montes G, et al: Maternal depressive symptoms are adversely associated with prevention practice and parenting behaviors for preschool children, *Ambul Pediatr* 6:32–37, 2006.

49. Kristensen JH, Ilett KF, Hackett LP, et al: Distribution and excretion of fluoxetine and norfluoxetine in human milk, *Br J Clin Pharmacol* 48:521–527, 1999.

50. Lee A, Minhas R, Matsuda N, et al: The safety of St. John's wort (*Hypericum perforatum*) during breast-feeding, *J Clin Psychiatry* 64:966–968, 2003.

51. Lee A, Woo J, Ito S: Frequency of infant adverse events that are associated with citalopram use during breastfeeding, *Am J Obstet Gynecol* 190:218–221, 2004.

52. Lester BM, Cucca J, Andreozzi L, et al: Possible association between fluoxetine hydrochloride and colic in an infant, *J Am Acad Child Psychiatry* 32:1253–1255, 1993.

53. Marcus SM: Depression during pregnancy: rates, risks, and consequences—motherisk update 2008, *Can J Clin Pharmacol* 16:e15–e22, 2009.

54. Merlob P, Stahl B, Sulkes J: Paroxetine during breastfeeding: Infant weight gain and maternal adherence to counsel, *Eur J Pediatr* 163:135–139, 2004.

55. Minkovitz CS, O'Campo PJ, Chen YH, et al: Associations between maternal and child health status and patterns of medical care use, *Ambul Pediatr* 2:85–92, 2002.

56. Misery S, Kim J, Riggs KW, et al: Protein levels in postpartum depressed women, breast milk, and infant serum, *J Clin Psychiatry* 61:828–832, 2000.

57. Mishina H, Takayama JI: Screening for maternal depression in primary care pediatrics, *Curr Opin Pediatr* 21:789–793, 2009.

58. Molyneaux E, Howard LM, McGeown HR, et al: Antidepressant treatment for postnatal depression, *Cochrane Database Syst Rev* 9, 2014. Art. No.: CD002018.

59. Mulcahy R, Reay RE, Wilkinson RB, et al: A randomized control trial for the effectiveness of group interpersonal psychotherapy for postnatal depression, *Arch Womens Ment Health* 13:125–139, 2010.

60. Myers ER, Aubuchon-Endsley N, Bastian LA, et al: *Efficacy and safety of screening for postpartum depression. Comparative effectiveness reviews, no. 106,* Rockville, MD, 2013, Agency for Healthcare Research and Quality www.ncbi.nlm.nih.gov/books/NBK137724/ (Accessed 27.05.15).

61. National Institute for Health and Clinical Excellence: *Postnatal care: routine postnatal care of women and their babies (CG37),* London, 2006, National Institute for Health and Clinical Excellence.

62. Network SIG: *Management of perinatal mood disorder,* Edinburgh, 2012, Scottish Intercollegiate Guidelines Network.

63. Neuman G, Colantonio D, Delaney S, et al: Bupropion and escitalopram during lactation, *Ann Pharmacother* 48:928–931, 2014.

64. Nightingale SL: Fluoxetine labeling revised to identify phenytoin interaction and to recommend against use in nursing mothers, *JAMA* 271:106, 1994.

65. O'Hara MW, Schlechte JA, Lewis DA, et al: Prospective study of postpartum blues. Biologic and psychosocial factors, *Arch Gen Psychiatry* 48:801–806, 1991.

66. O'Hara MW, Stuart S, Gorman LL, et al: Efficacy of interpersonal psychotherapy for postpartum depression, *Arch Gen Psychiatry* 57:1039–1045, 2000.

67. Office of Disease Prevention and Health Promotion, U.S. Department of Health and Human Services: Healthy people 2020. Maternal, infant, and child health, http://healthypeople.gov/2020/topicsobjectives2020/overview.aspx?topicid=26 (Accessed 27.05.15).

68. Olivier JD, Akerud H, Kaihola H, et al: The effects of maternal depression and maternal selective serotonin reuptake inhibitor exposure on offspring, *Front Cell Neurosci* 7:73, 2013.

69. Olson AL, Kemper KJ, Kelleher KJ, et al: Primary care pediatricians' roles and perceived responsibilities in the identification and management of maternal depression, *Pediatrics* 110:1169–1176, 2002.

70. Oppo A, Mauri M, Ramacciotti D, et al: Risk factors for postpartum depression: the role of the postpartum depression predictors inventory-revised (PDPI-R). Results from the perinatal depression-research and screening unit (PNDReScU) study, *Arch Womens Ment Health* 12:239–249, 2009.

71. Piontek CM, Wisner KL, Perel JM, et al: Serum fluvoxamine levels in breastfed infants, *J Clin Psychiatry* 62:111–113, 2001.

72. Rampono J, Teoh S, Hackett LP, et al: Estimation of desvenlafaxine transfer into milk and infant exposure during its use in lactating women with postnatal depression, *Arch Womens Ment Health* 14:49–53, 2011.

73. Royal Australian College of General Practitioners: *Guidelines for preventive activities in general practice,* East Melbourne, 2012, Royal Australian College of General Practitioners.

74. Russell EJ, Fawcett JM, Mazmanian D: Risk of obsessive compulsive disorder in pregnant and postpartum women: a meta-analysis, *J Clin Psychiatry* 74:377–385, 2013.

75. Schmidt K, Olesen OV, Jensen PN: Citalopram and breastfeeding: serum concentration and side effects in the infant, *Biol Psychiatry* 47:164–165, 2000.

76. Sharma V: Treatment of postpartum psychosis: challenges and opportunities, *Curr Drug Saf* 3:76–81, 2008.

77. Sheeder J, Kabir K, Stafford B: Screening for postpartum depression at well-child visits: is once enough during the first 6 months of life? *Pediatrics* 123:e982–e988, 2009.

78. Sriraman NK: Postpartum depression: why pediatricians should screen new moms, *Cont Pediatr* 29:40–46, 2012.

79. Stowe ZN, Cohen LS, Hostettler A, et al: Paroxetine in human breast milk and nursing infants, *Am J Psychiatry* 157:185–189, 2000.

80. Stowe ZN, Owens MJ, Landry JC, et al: Sertraline and desmethylsertraline in human breast milk and nursing infants, *Am J Psychiatry* 154:1255–1260, 1997.

81. Stuebe AM, Grewen K, Meltzer-Brody S: Association between maternal mood and oxytocin response to breastfeeding, *J Womens Health (Larchmt)* 22:352–361, 2013.

82. Suri R, Stowe ZN, Hendrick V, et al: Estimates of nursing infant daily dose of fluoxetine through breast milk, *Biol Psychiatry* 52:446–451, 2002.

83. Trapolini T, McMahon CA, Ungerer JA: The effect of maternal depression and marital adjustment on young children's internalizing and externalizing behaviour problems, *Child Care Health Dev* 33:794–803, 2007.

84. U.S. Public Health Service: *Report of the surgeon general's conference on children's mental health: a national action agenda,* Washington, DC, 2000, U.S. Department of Health and Human Services. www.ncbi.nlm.nih.gov/books/NBK44233/ (Accessed 27.05.15).

85. U.S. Preventive Services Task Force: Appendix A task force ratings, *Guide to clinical preventive services: report of the U.S. preventive services task force,* ed 2, Baltimore, MD, 1996, Williams & Wilkins. www.ncbi.nlm.nih.gov/books/NBK15430/ (Accessed 27.05.15).

86. Watkins S, Meltzer-Brody S, Zolnoun D, et al: Early breastfeeding experiences and postpartum depression, *Obstet Gynecol* 118:214–221, 2011.

87. Weissman AM, Levy BT, Hartz AJ, et al: Pooled analysis of antidepressant levels in lactating mothers, breast milk, and nursing infants, *Am J Psychiatry* 161:1066–1078, 2004.

88. Wisner KL, Perel JM, Blumer J: Serum sertraline and N-desmethylsertraline levels in breast-feeding mother-infant pairs, *Am J Psychiatry* 155:690–692, 1998.

89. Wisner KL, Perel JM, Findling RL, et al: Nortriptyline and its hydroxymetabolites in breastfeeding mothers and newborns, *Psychopharmacol Bull* 33:249–251, 1997.

90. Wisner KL, Perel JM, Peindl KS, et al: Prevention of recurrent postpartum depression: a randomized clinical trial, *J Clin Psychiatry* 62:82–86, 2001.

91. Wisner KL, Perel JM: Nortriptyline treatment of breastfeeding women, *Am J Psychiatry* 153:295, 1996.

92. Wisner KL, Perel JM: Serum nortriptyline levels in nursing mothers and their infants, *Am J Psychiatry* 148:1234–1236, 1991.

93. Wright S, Dawling S, Ashford JJ: Excretion of fluvoxamine in breast milk, *Br J Clin Pharmacol* 31:209, 1991.

94. Yawn BP, Dietrich AJ, Wollan P, et al: TRIPPD: a practice-based network effectiveness study of postpartum depression screening and management, *Ann Fam Med* 10:320–329, 2012.

95. Yoshida K, Smith B, Kumar RC: Fluvoxamine in breastmilk and infant development, *Br J Clin Pharmacol* 44:210–211, 1997.

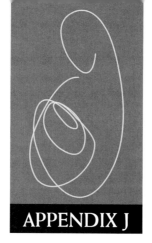

Protocol 19: Breastfeeding Promotion in the Prenatal Setting

Background

Breastfeeding provides ideal infant nutrition and is the physiologic norm for mothers and children.[3,1] Mothers often make a decision regarding breastfeeding early in prenatal care, and many have already decided whether to breastfeed prior to conception.[14] Encouragement and education from health care providers result in increased breastfeeding initiation and duration.[17,19,16] In addition, ongoing educational and support programs can improve initiation and duration of breastfeeding.[17]

Recommendations

1. Create a breastfeeding-friendly office.
   - Staff must be educated and committed to promote, protect, and support breastfeeding.
   - The primary clinician should be involved, but he or she does not need to do each of the following steps. Tasks may be assigned to multiple office staff members (nurses, medical assistants, lactation consultants, health and breastfeeding educators) if adequate training and support are provided for them.
   - Offices providing prenatal care should have a written breastfeeding policy to facilitate such support.[19]
   - Literature and samples provided by artificial formula companies should not be used because this advertising has been demonstrated to decrease breastfeeding initiation and shorten duration rates.[9]
   - Information regarding the mother's intention to breastfeed should be included as part of all transfer-of-care materials, including prenatal records and hospital and birth center discharge summaries.

2. Integrate breastfeeding promotion, education, and support throughout prenatal care.
   - Actively state support of breastfeeding early in prenatal care and acknowledge that breastfeeding is superior to artificial feeding. Consider a statement such as, "As your doctor, I want you to know that I support breastfeeding. It is important for mothers and babies."
   - It is also helpful to let the prenatal patient know that her physician will actively help her, with statements such as, "I like to spend time helping my patients get the information, skills, and support they need to breastfeed successfully."

3. Take a detailed breastfeeding history as a part of the prenatal history.[2]
   - For each previous child, ask about breastfeeding initiation, duration of exclusive breastfeeding, total breastfeeding duration, who provided breastfeeding support, perceived benefits of breastfeeding, breastfeeding challenges, and reason(s) for weaning.
   - For women who did not breastfeed, consider asking about the perceived advantages of artificial feeding, as well as the perceived disadvantages. Inquire about what may have helped her breastfeed previous children.
   - It is also important to determine any family medical history that may make breastfeeding especially helpful for this child, such as asthma, eczema, diabetes, and obesity.[1,3,11]

4. Consider the culture of individual women, families, and communities.
   - Learn about the family structure of patients. In some cultures, enlisting the cooperation of a pivotal family member may greatly assist in the promotion of breastfeeding, whereas in others, the participation of a particular family member may be inappropriate.
   - Understand the partner's perspectives and beliefs that may affect breastfeeding success, and educate where appropriate.
   - Ensure that parents from diverse cultures understand the importance of breastfeeding to their children's growth and development.
   - Respect cultural traditions and taboos associated with lactation, adapting cultural beliefs to facilitate optimal breastfeeding, while sensitively educating about traditions that may be detrimental to breastfeeding.
   - Provide all information and instruction, wherever possible, in the mother's native language, and assess for literacy level when appropriate.
   - Understand the specific financial, work, and time obstacles to breastfeeding and work with families to overcome them.
   - Be aware of the role of the physician's own personal cultural attitudes when interacting with patients.[1]
5. Incorporate breastfeeding as an important component of the initial prenatal breast examination.[12]
   - Observe for appropriate breast development, surgical scars, and nipple contour.
   - Perform areolar compression if nipples are flat or inverted.
   - Review the physiologic changes of pregnancy, such as volume growth and leakage of colostrum.
   - Consider repeating the breast examination in the third trimester, as breast anatomy will change throughout pregnancy.
   - Assure the expectant mother that her anatomy is sufficient for successful breastfeeding, or discuss the availability of support and assistance if suggested by physical exam.
   - If the history and or physical exam findings suggest that the woman is at high risk for breastfeeding problems, consider a prenatal lactation referral or early lactation support.
6. Discuss breastfeeding at each prenatal visit,
   - Breastfeeding can be addressed by clinicians and/or health care staff.
   - Consider use of the Best Start 3-Step Counseling Strategy[12] by:
     - Encouraging open dialog about breastfeeding by beginning with open-ended questions.
     - Affirming the patient's feelings.
     - Providing targeted education.[20,10]

   - Address concerns and dispel misconceptions at each visit.

   During the first trimester
   - Incorporate and educate partners, parents, and friends about the benefits of breastfeeding for mothers and babies.[13]
   - Address known common barriers such as lack of self-confidence, embarrassment, time and social constraints, dietary and health concerns, lack of social support, employment and child care concerns, and fear of pain.[12,8]
   - Continue to ask open-ended questions.

   During the second trimester
   - Encourage women to identify breastfeeding role models by talking with family, friends, and colleagues who have breastfed successfully.
   - Recommend attending a formal breastfeeding course for the patient and her partner in addition to office education.[18]
   - Encourage participation in a breastfeeding peer support group. Provide a list of local educational options and breastfeeding resources for patients.[4,5]
   - The second trimester visits often provide time for discussion of breastfeeding basics such as the importance of exclusive breastfeeding and supply/demand, feeding on demand, frequency of feedings, feeding cues, how to know an infant is getting enough to eat, avoiding artificial nipples until the infant is nursing well, and the importance of a good latch.
   - The mother working outside the home should be encouraged to begin thinking about if and when she will return to work after the baby is born. If she is planning on returning to work, encourage the woman to consider what facilities are available for pumping and storage of breast milk, how much time she will take for maternity leave, and what company policies and legislation are available to support her.

   During the third trimester
   - At the 28-, 30-, or 32-week visits have the prenatal patient and her support persons use props such as dolls, balls, and balloons. Demonstrate how to hold the breast and positions of the baby such as the cradle, cross-cradle, and clutch holds.[7]
   - Discuss what will happen in the delivery room under normal conditions. What will the mother do? What will the doctor do?
   - Review the physiology of breastfeeding initiation and the impact of supplementation.
   - Repeat the breast and nipple examination.
   - Recommend the purchase of properly fitting nursing bras.

- Encourage another visit to a breastfeeding support group as the mother's interest and goals of attending may be different from when she attended early in the pregnancy.[6]
- Recommend the mother discuss plans for infant health care and breastfeeding support with her pediatric care provider.[15]

7. Empower women and their families to have the birth experience most conducive to breastfeeding.
- Confirm postpartum follow-up plans.
- Assure the mother has an adequate support system in place during the postpartum period.
- Recommend the infant see a health care provider within 48 hours of discharge from the hospital to assure well-being and optimal breastfeeding.
- Assure that the patient has information on how to get breastfeeding help.
- Provide anticipatory guidance on topics such as engorgement, growth spurts, and nighttime feedings.
- Inform patients about the Ten Steps to Successful Breastfeeding and how to advocate for breastfeeding-friendly hospital care.[15]
- Discuss support of breastfeeding in the event of a cesarean section.

Recommendations for Further Research

1. There are currently no studies examining only physician interaction in support of breastfeeding during prenatal visits and its effect on initiation, exclusivity, and maintenance.
2. Studies are needed that examine prenatal interventions alone and in combination and their effects on initiation, exclusivity, and duration of breastfeeding.
3. Studies examining the cost-effectiveness of making an outpatient practice breastfeeding-friendly are needed.
4. Research on specific challenges to providing support for breastfeeding during prenatal care (e.g., lack of community resources, cultural barriers, etc.) is needed.
5. Additional research is needed on the effect of varying prenatal breastfeeding interventions on multiple populations, including with women of different socioeconomic status and cultural backgrounds.

Acknowledgments

This work was supported in part by a grant from the Maternal and Child Health Bureau, U.S. Department of Health and Human Services. The authors gratefully acknowledge the contributions of Jane Wilson, MD, MPH, for her assistance on the annotated bibliography.
Contributors
Julie Wood, MD, FABM
Elizabeth Hineman, MD
David Meyers, MD
Protocol Committee
Caroline J. Chantry, MD, FABM, Co-Chairperson
Cynthia R. Howard, MD, MPH, FABM, Co-Chairperson
Ruth A. Lawrence, MD, FABM
Kathleen A. Marinelli, MD, FABM, Co-Chairperson
Nancy G. Powers, MD, FABM

REFERENCES

1. American Academy of Family Physicians: *Family physicians supporting breastfeeding (position paper)*, http://www.aafp.org/online/en/home/policy/policies/b/breastfeedingpositionpaper.html, 2008 (Accessed 08.02.09).
2. American Academy of Pediatrics, American College of Obstetricians and Gynecologists: Breastfeeding: management before and after conception. In Schanler RJ Sr., editor: *Breastfeeding handbook for physicians*, Elk Grove Village, Ill., 2006, American Academy of Pediatrics, pp 55–65. (chapter 5).
3. American Academy of Pediatrics Section on Breastfeeding: Breastfeeding and the use of human milk, *Pediatrics* 115: 496–506, 2005.
4. Chapman DJ, Damio G, Perez-Escamilla R: Differential response to breastfeeding peer counseling within a low-income, predominantly Latina population, *J Hum Lact* 20: 389–396, 2004.
5. Chapman DJ, Damio G, Young S, et al: Effectiveness of breastfeeding peer counseling in a low-income, predominantly Latina population: a randomized controlled trial, *Arch Pediatr Adolesc Med* 158:897–902, 2004.
6. De Oliveira MI, Camacho LA, Tedstone AE: Extending breastfeeding duration through primary care: a systematic review of prenatal and postnatal interventions, *J Hum Lact* 17:326–343, 2001.
7. Duffy EP, Percival P, Kershaw E: Positive effects of an antenatal group teaching session on postnatal nipple pain, nipple trauma and breastfeeding rates, *Midwifery* 13:189–196, 1997.
8. Hartley BM, O'Connor ME: Evaluation of the "Best Start" breast-feeding education program *Arch Pediatr Adolesc Med* 150:868–871, 1996.
9. Howard CR, Howard FM, Lawrence RA, et al: The effect on breastfeeding of physicians' office-based prenatal formula advertising, *Obstet Gynecol* 95:296–303, 2000.
10. Humenick SS, Hill PD, Spiegelberg PL: Breastfeeding and health professional encouragement, *J Hum Lact* 14: 305–310, 1998.
11. Ip S, Chung M, Raman G, et al: Evidence report/technology assessment no. 153: breastfeeding and maternal and infant health outcomes in developed countries. In *AHRQ publication number 07-E007*, Rockville, Md., 2007, Agency for Healthcare Research and Quality.
12. Issler H, de Sa MB, Senna DM: Knowledge of newborn healthcare among pregnant women: basis for promotional and educational programs on breastfeeding, *Sao Paulo Med J* 119:7–9, 2001.
13. Ingram J, Johnson D: A feasibility study of an intervention to enhance family support for breastfeeding in a deprived area in Bristol, UK, *Midwifery* 20:367–379, 2004.

938 | Breastfeeding: A Guide for the Medical Profession

making breastfeeding an even more complicated choice, as breastfeeding may not be recommended for women taking some psychotropic medications.

Despite the myriad factors that may make breastfeeding a difficult choice for women with substance use disorders, drug-exposed infants, who are at a high risk for an array of medical, psychological, and developmental issues, as well as their mothers, stand to benefit significantly from breastfeeding. Although many of the factors listed earlier may pose a risk to the infant, the documented benefits of human milk and breastfeeding must be carefully and thoughtfully weighed against the risks associated with the substance that the infant may be exposed to during lactation. Confounding many efforts to examine longer-term developmental outcomes in infants exposed to some substances is the lack of data evaluating infants who were not exposed during pregnancy but only during lactation.

Ideally, women with substance use disorders delivering an infant and desiring to breastfeed are engaged in comprehensive health care and substance abuse treatment during pregnancy, but this is not always the case. Substance abuse treatment for these women is often not available, not gender specific, and not comprehensive, forcing the mother's health care provider during and after pregnancy to rely on maternal self-report and a "best guess" at adequacy of services, compliance to treatment, length of "clean" time, community support systems, and so forth. In a recent retrospective study in the United Kingdom, significantly lower rates of breastfeeding initiation occurred in mothers who used illicit substances or opioid maintenance therapy during pregnancy (14% vs. 50% of the general population).[17] In Norway, among opioid-dependent women on opioid maintenance therapy, 77% (compared with 98% in the general population) initiated breastfeeding after delivery.[53]

The specific terms used to describe use and misuse of various legal and illegal substances continue to evolve and may vary from country to country and among different organizations. The fifth edition of the *Diagnostic and Statistical Manual of Mental Disorders* combines the previous categories of substance abuse and substance dependence into the category single substance use disorder, which is measured on a continuum from mild to severe.[14]

We would like to make it clear that drugs of any type should be avoided in pregnant and breastfeeding women, unless prescribed for specific medical conditions. The casual use of drugs—legal, illegal, illicit, dose appropriate or not—still may have ramifications for the developing fetus and infant that we have yet to determine; hence, in general, drugs of all types should be avoided unless medically necessary.

Specific Substances

Perhaps the most critical challenge facing the health care provider for the woman with a substance use disorder who wishes to breastfeed is the lack of research leading to evidence-based guidelines. Table J-20 gives two online websites, one in English and one in both English and Spanish, that are kept updated and are easily accessible for current information on drugs and breastfeeding. There have been several comprehensive reviews of breastfeeding among substance-using women, essentially concluding that breastfeeding is generally contraindicated in mothers who use illegal drugs.[12,48,47,16] (III) (Quality of evidence [levels of evidence I, II-1, II-2, II-3, and III] is based on the U.S. Preventive Services Task Force Appendix A Task Force Ratings[4] and is noted throughout this protocol in parentheses.) Yet, research on individual drugs of abuse remains lacking and difficult to perform. Pharmacokinetic data for most drugs of abuse in lactating women are sparse and based on small numbers of subjects and case reports.[47] Most illicit drugs are found in human milk, with varying degrees of oral bioavailability.[47] Phencyclidine hydrochloride has been detected in human milk in high concentrations,[30] as has cocaine,[54] leading to infant intoxication.[11] There is little to no evidence to describe the effects of even small amounts of other drugs of abuse and/or their metabolites in human milk on infant development aside from those discussed later.

TABLE J-20	Online Websites with Updated Breastfeeding and Drug Information	
Website	**URL**	**Language**
U.S. National Library of Health, National Institute of Health, U.S. Department of Health and Human Services, "LactMed"	http://toxnet.nlm.nih.gov/newtoxnet/lactmed.htm	English
e-Lactancia	http://e-lactancia.org/	English
Association for Promotion and Cultural and Scientific Research of Breastfeeding Under a Creative Commons International License	(Also contains medical prescriptions, phytotherapy, homeopathy and other alternative products, cosmetic and medical procedures, contaminants, maternal and infant diseases, and more)	Spanish

METHADONE

For pregnant and postpartum women with opioid dependence in treatment, methadone maintenance has been the treatment of choice in the United States, Canada,[56] and many other countries. In contrast to other substances, concentrations of methadone in human milk and the effects on the infant have been studied. The concentrations of methadone found in human milk are low, and all authors have concluded that women on stable doses of methadone maintenance should be encouraged to breastfeed if desired, irrespective of maternal methadone dose.* (II-1, II-2, II-3) Previously, no apparent effects of methadone exposure prenatally and in human milk were reported on infant neurobehavior at 30 days.[27] Recently an ongoing longitudinal follow-up study of methadone-exposed infants with 200 methadone-exposed and nonexposed, demographically matched families has shown neurocognitive delays in methadone-exposed 1-month-old infants compared with nonexposed infants. When retested at 7 months, methadone-exposed infants were similar to nonexposed, comparison infants. At 9 months of age, 37.5% of this sample of methadone-exposed infants showed clinically significant motor delays (± 1.5 standard deviation) compared with low but typical development in the comparison group.[36] Exposed infants typically have high environmental risk profiles, which continue at birth, posing ongoing risk to the developing child.

The current thought is that environmental risk factors combine with prenatal exposures to promote epigenetic changes in gene expression and methylation patterns that have both immediate and long-term implications related to developmental programming.[28] Note that these findings relate to infants exposed to methadone both prenatally and after birth via breastfeeding, and there is little information available on infants with chronic methadone exposure via breastfeeding alone.

In addition, about 70% of infants born to women prescribed methadone during pregnancy will experience neonatal abstinence syndrome (NAS),[32] the constellation of signs and symptoms often presenting following in utero opioid exposure. Infants with significant NAS can experience difficulties with attaching and sucking/swallowing during breastfeeding that can impact their ability to breastfeed. However, given that there is increasing evidence supporting the conclusion that there is a reduction in the severity and duration of treatment of NAS when mothers on methadone maintenance therapy breastfeed, breastfeeding for these dyads should be encouraged.[53,7,1,27] (II-1, II-3) Unfortunately, the rate

of breastfeeding initiation in this cohort is generally low, less than half that reported in the U.S. general population.[52] A small recent qualitative study demonstrated that lack of support from the health care community and misinformation about the dangers of breastfeeding while on methadone therapy are significant, yet modifiable, barriers to breastfeeding success in these women.[13] Given the benefits to these mothers and infants to remain on methadone maintenance therapy and breastfeed, it is important for us to provide robust ongoing support for this vulnerable group.

BUPRENORPHINE

Buprenorphine is a partial opioid agonist used for treatment of opioid dependency during pregnancy in some countries and increasingly in the United States. Multiple small case series have examined maternal buprenorphine concentrations in human milk. All concur that the amounts of buprenorphine in human milk are small and are unlikely to have short-term negative effects on the developing infant.[26,19,38,29,18,43] In one study, 76% of 85 maternal-infant pairs breastfed, with 66% still breastfeeding 6 to 8 weeks postpartum. The breastfed infants had less severe NAS and were less likely to require pharmacological intervention than the formula-fed infants, similar to methadone discussed earlier, although this did not reach statistical significance with the size of the sample studied.[43]

OTHER OPIOIDS

Use of opioids in the United States has increased substantially over the past decade. A retrospective cross-sectional analysis of NAS in hospital births in the years from 2000 to 2009 found an increase in incidence from 1.2 to 3.39 per 1000 births. Antepartum maternal opioid use was also found to have risen from 1.19 to 5.63 per 1000 hospital births from 2000 to 2009; any use of opioids was included in data collection.[44] A recent Centers for Disease Control and Prevention Morbidity and Mortality Weekly Report highlighted data demonstrating that approximately one third of women of reproductive age filled a prescription for opioids each year between 2008 and 2012.[10]

When use of narcotics during pregnancy is determined to be consistent with an opioid use disorder rather than a modality for short-term pain relief, consideration of initiation of maintenance methadone or buprenorphine as previously discussed is strongly encouraged,[56,2,57] and these mothers should be supported in breastfeeding initiation. (III) Short courses of most other low-dose prescription opioids can be safely used by a breastfeeding mother,[41,22] but caution is urged with

---

*Refs. 53,55,39,6,7,1,27,40,36,28.

codeine, as CYP2D6 ultra-rapid metabolizers may experience high morphine (metabolite) blood levels, and there has been a single case report of a breastfeeding neonatal death after maternal use.[37] (III) Information is lacking on the safety of breastfeeding when moderate to high doses of opioids are used for long periods of time. There is also a lack of information available about transitioning mothers from short-acting opioids to opioid maintenance therapy while breastfeeding rather than during pregnancy.

MARIJUANA

Uniform guidelines regarding the varied use of marijuana by breastfeeding mothers are difficult to create and cannot hope to cover all situations. The legality of possessing and using marijuana varies greatly from country to country; in the United States, there are increasing numbers of states where it is legal for "medicinal use" with a prescription, and a few states where it is legal for "recreational use," but under federal law, it remains illegal in all states. Therefore, basing recommendations on marijuana use and concurrent breastfeeding from a purely legal standpoint becomes inherently complex, problematic, and impossible to apply uniformly across all settings and jurisdictions. As laws shift and marijuana use becomes even more common in some areas, it becomes increasingly important to carefully weigh the risks of initiation and continuation of breastfeeding while using marijuana with the risks of not breastfeeding while also considering the wide range of occasional, to regular medical, to heavy exposure to marijuana.

In addition to the potential legal risk, the health risks to the infant from the mother's marijuana use must be carefully considered. Δ9-Tetrahydrocannabinol (THC), the main compound in marijuana, is present in human milk up to eight times that of maternal plasma levels, and metabolites are found in infant feces, indicating that THC is absorbed and metabolized by the infant.[45] It is rapidly distributed to the brain and adipose tissue and stored in fat tissues for weeks to months. It has a long half-life (25 to 57 hours) and stays positive in the urine for 2 to 3 weeks,[21] making it impossible to determine who is an occasional versus a chronic user at the time of delivery by urine toxicology screening. Evidence regarding the effects of THC exposure on infant development via breastfeeding alone is sparse and conflicting,[5,49] and there are no data evaluating neurodevelopmental outcomes beyond the age of 1 year in infants who are only exposed after birth. Also notable in this discussion of risk is that the potency of marijuana has been steadily increasing, from about 3% in the 1980s to 12% in 2012, so data from previous studies may no longer even be relevant.[51] Additionally, current concern over marijuana use during lactation stems from possible infant sedation and maternal inability to safely care for her infant while directly under its influence; however, this remains a theoretical problem and has not been well established in the literature.[24]

Human and animal evidence examining the behavioral and neurobiological effects of exposure to cannabinoids during pregnancy and lactation shows that the endocannabinoid system plays a crucial role in the ontogeny of the central nervous system and its activation, during brain development. As Campolongo et al.[8] concluded, cannabinoid exposure during critical periods of brain development can induce subtle and long-lasting neurofunctional alterations. Several preclinical studies highlight how even low to moderate doses during particular periods of brain development can have profound consequences for brain maturation, potentially leading to long-lasting alterations in cognitive functions and emotional behaviors.[8] Exposure to second-hand marijuana smoke by infants has been associated with an independent two times possible risk of sudden infant death syndrome (SIDS)[31] (III); because breastfeeding reduces the risk of SIDS, this needs to be additionally considered. Thus careful contemplation of these issues should be fully incorporated into the care plans of the lactating woman in the setting of THC use. Breastfeeding mothers should be counseled to reduce or eliminate their use of marijuana to avoid exposing their infants to this substance and advised of the possible long-term neurobehavioral effects from continued use. (III)

ALCOHOL

Use of alcohol during pregnancy is strongly discouraged, as it can cause fetal alcohol syndrome, birth defects, spontaneous abortion, and premature births, among other serious problems.[3,9] (III) Many women who significantly decrease or eliminate their alcohol intake during pregnancy may choose to resume consuming alcohol after giving birth, with approximately half of breastfeeding women in Western countries reported to consume alcohol at least occasionally.[20] Alcohol interferes with the milk ejection reflex, which may ultimately reduce milk production through inadequate breast emptying.[34] (III) Human milk alcohol levels generally parallel maternal blood alcohol levels, and studies evaluating infant effects of maternal alcohol consumption have been mostly mixed, with some mild effects seen in infant sleep patterns, amount of milk consumed during breastfeeding sessions, and early psychomotor development.[34] (III) Possible long-term effects of alcohol in maternal milk remain unknown. Most sources advise limiting alcohol intake to the equivalent of 8 oz of wine or two beers, and waiting 2 hours after drinking to resume breastfeeding.[12,48,47,57] (III) To ensure complete elimination of alcohol from breastmilk, mothers may consult a normogram devised by the Canadian Motherisk program to determine length of time needed based on maternal weight and amount consumed.[33] (III)

TOBACCO

Approximately two thirds as many pregnant women as nonpregnant women smoke tobacco, with decreasing numbers of women smoking as pregnancy progresses.[46] Many mothers quit during pregnancy, but postpartum relapse is common, with about 50% resuming tobacco use in the first few months after birth.[58,35,50] Data on the epidemiology of breastfeeding mothers who smoke cigarettes remains complex, and smoking in many series has been found to be associated with reduced rates of breastfeeding.[25,42] Nicotine and other compounds are known to transfer to the infant via milk, and considerable transfer of chemicals via second-hand smoke also occurs when infants are exposed to environmental tobacco smoke. Increases in the incidence of respiratory allergy in infants and in SIDS are just two significant well-known risks of infant exposure to environmental tobacco smoke.[16] (III) Most sources endorse promotion of breastfeeding in the setting of maternal smoking while vigorously supporting smoking cessation.[15] (III) Some smoking cessation modalities (nicotine patch, nicotine gum, and possibly buprorion) are compatible with breastfeeding and can be encouraged in many circumstances.[48,47,23] (III)

Recommendations

GENERAL (CIRCUMSTANCES FAVORABLE WITH CONSIDERATION)

Infants of women with substance use disorders, at risk for multiple health and developmental difficulties, stand to benefit substantially from breastfeeding and human milk, as do their mothers. A prenatal plan preparing the mother for parenting, breastfeeding, and substance abuse treatment should be formulated through individualized, patient-centered discussions with each woman. This care plan should include instruction in the consequences of relapse to drug or excessive alcohol use during lactation, as well as teaching regarding potential for donor milk, formula preparation, and bottle handling and cleaning should breastfeeding be or become contraindicated. In the perinatal period each mother-infant dyad should be carefully and individually counseled on breastfeeding prior to discharge from maternity care. This evaluation must consider several factors, including (III)

- drug use and substance abuse treatment histories, including medication-assisted treatment with methadone or buprenorphine;
- medical and psychiatric status;
- other maternal medication needs;
- infant health status (to include ongoing evaluation for NAS and impact on ability to breastfeed);
- the presence or absence and adequacy of maternal family and community support systems; and
- plans for postpartum care and substance abuse treatment for the mother and pediatric care for the child.

Optimally, the woman with a substance use disorder who presents a desire to breastfeed should be engaged in treatment pre- and postnatally. Maternal written consent for communication with her substance abuse treatment provider should be obtained prior to delivery if possible. (III)

Any discussion with mothers who use substances with sedating effects should include counseling on safely caring for her infant and instruction on safe sleep practices. (III)

Encourage women under the following circumstances to breastfeed their infants (III):

- Engaged in substance abuse treatment; provision of maternal consent to discuss progress in treatment and plans for postpartum treatment with substance abuse treatment counselor; counselor recommendation for breastfeeding.
- Plans to continue in substance abuse treatment in the postpartum period.
- Abstinence from drug use for 90 days prior to delivery; ability to maintain sobriety demonstrated in an outpatient setting.
- Toxicology testing of maternal urine negative at delivery.
- Engaged in prenatal care and compliant.

OPIOIDS/NARCOTICS

- Encourage stable methadone- or buprenorphine-maintained women to breastfeed regardless of dose.
- Management of mothers who use chronic opioid therapy for pain should be closely supervised by a chronic pain physician who is familiar with pregnancy and breastfeeding (III):
  a. Length of time on these medications, total dose, and whether the medications were used during pregnancy should all help inform the

decision of whether breastfeeding may be safely undertaken in certain cases.

b. Judicious amounts of oral narcotic pain medication, when used in a time-limited situation for an acute pain problem, are generally compatible with continued breastfeeding if supervision and monitoring of the breastfeeding infant are adequate.[41,22]

- Rapidly increasing narcotic dosing in a breastfeeding mother should prompt further evaluation and reconsideration of the safety of continued breastfeeding.

NICOTINE

- Counsel mothers who smoke cigarettes after giving birth to reduce their intake as much as possible, and not to smoke around their infant, to reduce infant exposure to second-hand smoke. Smoking cessation and nicotine replacement modalities such as nicotine patches and gum may be useful for some mothers. (III)
- Give mothers who smoke tobacco additional support, as maternal smoking appears to be an independent and associated risk factor for noninitiation and early cessation of breastfeeding, to help ensure its success. (III)

ALCOHOL

- Counsel mothers who wish to drink occasional alcohol that alcohol easily transfers into human milk. Recommendations from the American Academy of Pediatrics, the World Health Organization, and others advise waiting 90 to 120 minutes after ingesting alcohol before breastfeeding, or expressing and discarding milk within that time frame.[12,48,47,57] (III)

CANNABIS (THC)

- Information regarding the long-term effects of marijuana use by the breastfeeding mother on the infant remains insufficient to recommend complete abstention from breastfeeding initiation or continuation based on the scientific evidence at this time. However, extrapolation from in utero exposure and the limited data available helps to inform the following recommendations (III):

a. Counsel mothers who admit to occasional or rare use to avoid further use or reduce their use as much as possible while breastfeeding, advise them as to its possible long-term neurobehavioral effects, and instruct them to avoid direct exposure of the infant to marijuana and its smoke.

b. Strongly advise mothers found with a positive urine screen for THC to discontinue exposure while breastfeeding and counsel them as to its possible long-term neurobehavioral effects.

c. When advising mothers on the medicinal use of marijuana during lactation, one must take into careful consideration and counsel on the potential risks of exposure of marijuana and benefits of breastfeeding to the infant.

d. The lack of long-term follow-up data on infants exposed to varying amounts of marijuana via human milk, coupled with concerns over negative neurodevelopmental outcomes in children with in utero exposure, should prompt extremely careful consideration of the risks versus the benefits of breastfeeding in the setting of moderate or chronic marijuana use. A recommendation of abstaining from any marijuana use is warranted.

e. At this time, although the data are not strong enough to recommend not breastfeeding with any marijuana use, we urge caution.

GENERAL (CIRCUMSTANCES CONTRAINDICATED OR REQUIRING MORE CAUTION)

Counsel women under any of the following circumstances not to breastfeed (III):

- Not engaged in substance abuse treatment or engaged in treatment and failure to provide consent for contact with counselor.
- Not engaged in prenatal care.
- Positive maternal urine toxicology screen for substances other than marijuana at delivery [see (b) in the preceding list].
- No plans for postpartum substance abuse treatment or pediatric care.
- Women relapsing to illicit drug use or legal substance misuse in the 30-day period prior to delivery.
- Any behavioral or other indicators that the woman is actively abusing substances.
- Chronic alcohol use.

Evaluate carefully women under the following circumstances, and determine appropriate advice for breastfeeding by discussion and coordination among the mother, maternal care providers, and substance abuse treatment providers (III):

- Relapse to illicit substance use or legal substance misuse in the 90- to 30-day period prior to delivery.
- Concomitant use of other prescription medications deemed to be incompatible with lactation.
- Engaged later (after the second trimester) in prenatal care and/or substance abuse treatment.

- Attained drug and/or alcohol sobriety only in an inpatient setting.
- Lack of appropriate maternal family and community support systems.
- Report that they desire to breastfeed their infant to either retain custody or maintain their sobriety in the postpartum period.

In the United States, women who have established breastfeeding and subsequently relapse to illegal drug use are counseled not to breastfeed, even if milk is discarded during the time period surrounding relapse. There are no known pharmacokinetic data to establish the presence and/or concentrations of most illicit substances and/or their metabolites in human milk and effects on the infant, and this research is unlikely to occur given the ethical dilemmas it presents. The lack of pharmacokinetic data for most drugs of abuse in recently postpartum women with substance use disorders precludes the establishment of a "safe" interval after use when breastfeeding can be reestablished for individual drugs of abuse. Additionally, women using illicit substances in the postnatal period may exhibit impaired judgment and secondary behavioral changes that may interfere with the ability of the mother to care for her infant or to breastfeed adequately. Passive drug exposures may pose additional risks to the infant. Therefore, any woman relapsing to illicit drug use or legal substance misuse after the establishment of lactation should be provided an appropriate human milk substitute (donor milk, formula) and intensified drug treatment, along with guidance on how to taper milk production to prevent mastitis. (III)

The woman with a substance use disorder who has successfully initiated breastfeeding should be carefully monitored, along with her infant, in the postpartum period. Ongoing substance abuse treatment, postpartum care, psychiatric care when warranted, and pediatric care are important for women with substance use disorders. Lactation support is particularly important for infants experiencing NAS and their mothers. Communication among all care providers involved with the health, welfare, and substance abuse support of the mother and the child should provide an interactive network of supportive care for the dyad. (III)

Recommendations for Future Research

1. Long-term randomized controlled trials or paired cohort evaluations of infants exposed to methadone or buprenorphine via human milk, including infant developmental assessments.
2. Further evaluations of maternal milk and plasma and infant plasma pharmacokinetic data regarding prescription opioids and lactation, especially for mothers who were on chronic high-dose medications during pregnancy that are continued when breastfeeding.
3. Long-term controlled evaluations of infants exposed to marijuana via human milk, to include infants and later neurodevelopmental outcomes, including those exposed to marijuana in a controlled manner, such as with legalized medical marijuana.
4. Evaluation of nicotine replacement patches, gum, and vaporized cigarettes as substitutes for tobacco smoking in pregnant and lactating women, to determine if these can or should be widely recommended in place of tobacco products.

Acknowledgments

This work was supported in part by a grant from the Maternal and Child Health Bureau, U.S. Department of Health and Human Services.

Academy of Breastfeeding Medicine Protocol Committee
Kathleen A. Marinelli, MD, FABM, Chairperson
Larry Noble, MD, FABM, Translations Chairperson
Nancy Brent, MD
Ruth A. Lawrence, MD, FABM
Sarah Reece-Stremtan, MD
Casey Rosen-Carole, MD
Tomoko Seo, MD, FABM
Rose St. Fleur, MD
Michal Young, MD

REFERENCES[1]

1. Abdel-Latif ME, Pinner J, Clews S, et al: Effects of breast milk on the severity and outcome of NAS among infants of drug-dependent mothers, *Pediatrics* 117:1163–1169, 2006.
2. ACOG Committee on Health Care for Underserved Women, American Society of Addiction Medicine: ACOG committee opinion no. 524: opioid abuse, dependence, and addiction in pregnancy, *Obstet Gynecol* 119:1070–1076, 2012.
3. American Academy of Pediatrics: *Joint call to action on alcohol and pregnancy,* www.aap.org/en-us/advocacy-and-policy/aap-health-initiatives/fetalcohol-spectrum-disorders-toolkit/Pages/Joint-Call-toAction-on-Alcohol-and-Pregnancy.aspx 2012 (Accessed 18.02.15).
4. US Preventive Services Task Force: *Guide to clinical preventive services: report of the U.S. preventive services task force,* Appendix A task force ratings, ed 2, Baltimore, MD, 1996, Williams & Wilkins, www.ncbi.nlm.nih.gov/books/NBK15430/ (Accessed 27.02.15).

---

[1]ABM protocols expire 5 years from the date of publication. Evidence-based revisions are made within 5 years or sooner if there are significant changes in the evidence.

5. Astley SJ, Little RE: Maternal marijuana use during lactation and infant development at one year, *Neurotoxicol Teratol* 12:161–168, 1990.

6. Begg EJ, Malpas TJ, Hackett LP, et al: Distribution of R- and S-methadone into human milk during multiple, medium to high oral dosing, *Br J Clin Pharmacol* 52:681–685, 2001.

7. Bogen DL, Perel JM, Helsel JC, et al: Estimated infant exposure to enantiomer-specific methadone levels in breastmilk, *Breastfeed Med* 6:377–384, 2011.

8. Campolongo P, Trezza V, Palmery M, et al: Developmental exposure to cannabinoids causes subtle and enduring neurofunctional alterations, *Int Rev Neurobiol* 85:117–133, 2009.

9. Carson G, Cox LV, Crane J, et al: Alcohol use and pregnancy consensus clinical guidelines, *J Obstet Gynaecol Can* 32(8 Suppl 3):S1–S32, 2010.

10. Centers for Disease Control and Prevention: *Opioid pain killers widely prescribed among reproductive age women* (press release). www.cdc.gov/media/releases/2015/p0122-pregnancy-opioids.html. January 2015 (Accessed 23.02.15).

11. Chasnoff I, Lewis DE, Squires L: Cocaine intoxication in a breast fed infant, *Pediatrics* 80:836–838, 1987.

12. D'Apolito K: Breastfeeding and substance abuse, *Clin Obstet Gynecol* 56:202–211, 2013.

13. Demirci JR, Bogen DL, Klionsky Y: Breastfeeding and methadone therapy: the maternal experience, *Subst Abus* 36(2):203–208. 2015. http://dx.doi.org/10.1080/08897077.2014.902417.

14. American Psychiatric Association: *Diagnostic and statistical manual of mental disorders*, ed 5, Washington, DC, 2013, American Psychiatric Association.

15. Dorea JG: Maternal smoking and infant feeding: breastfeeding is better and safer, *Matern Child Health J* 11:287–291, 2007.

16. Eidelman AI, Schanler R, Section on Breastfeeding: Breastfeeding and the use of human milk, *Pediatrics* 129:e827–e841, 2012.

17. Goel N, Beasley D, Rajkumar V, et al: Perinatal outcome of illicit substance use in pregnancy—comparative and contemporary socio-clinical profile in the UK, *Eur J Pediatr* 170:199–205, 2011.

18. Gower S, Bartu A, Ilett KF, et al: The wellbeing of infants exposed to buprenorphine via breast milk at 4 weeks of age, *J Hum Lact* 30:217–223, 2014.

19. Grimm D, Pauly E, Poschl J, et al: Buprenorphine and norbuprenorphine concentrations in human breastmilk samples determined by liquid chromatography-tandem mass spectrometry, *Ther Drug Monit* 27:526–530, 2005.

20. Haastrup MB, Pottegard A, Damkier P: Alcohol and breastfeeding, *Basic Clin Pharmacol Toxicol* 114:168–173, 2014.

21. Hale TW, Rowe HE: *Medications and mothers' milk*, ed 16, Plano, TX, 2014, Hale Publishing LP.

22. Hendrickson RG, McKeown NJ: Is maternal opioid use hazardous to breast-fed infants? *J Toxicol* 50:1–14, 2012.

23. Heydari G, Masjedi M, Ahmady AE, et al: A comparative study on tobacco cessation methods: a quantitative systematic review, *Int J Prev Med* 5:673–678, 2014.

24. Hill M, Reed K: Pregnancy, breast-feeding, and marijuana: a review article, *Obstet Gynecol Surv* 68:710–718, 2013.

25. Horta BL, Victora CG, Menezes AM, et al: Environmental tobacco smoke and breastfeeding duration, *Am J Epidemiol* 146:128–133, 1997.

26. Ilett KF, Hackett LP, Gower S, et al: Estimated dose exposure of the neonate to buprenorphine and its metabolite norbuprenorphine via breastmilk during maternal buprenorphine substitution treatment, *Breastfeed Med* 7:269–274, 2012.

27. Jansson LM, Choo R, Velez ML, et al: Methadone maintenance and breastfeeding in the neonatal period, *Pediatrics* 121:106–114, 2008.

28. Jansson LM, Choo R, Velez ML, et al: Methadone maintenance and long-term lactation, *Breastfeed Med* 3:34–37, 2008.

29. Johnson RE, Jones HE, Jasinski DR, et al: Buprenorphine treatment of pregnant opioid dependent women: maternal and neonatal outcomes, *Drug Alcohol Depend* 63:97–103, 2001.

30. Kaufman R, Petrucha RA, Pitts FN, et al: PCP in amniotic fluid and breast milk: case report, *J Clin Psychiatry* 44:269–270, 1983.

31. Klonoff-Cohen H, Lam-Kruglick P: Maternal and paternal recreational drug use and sudden infant death syndrome, *Arch Pediatr Adolesc Med* 155:765–770, 2001.

32. Kocherlakota P: Neonatal abstinence syndrome, *Pediatrics* 134:e547–e561, 2014.

33. Koren G: Drinking alcohol while breastfeeding. Will it harm my baby? *Can Fam Physician* 48:39–41, 2002.

34. Lactmed: *Alcohol monograph*, http://toxnet.nlm.nih.gov/ (Accessed 11.02.15).

35. Levitt C, Shaw E, Wong S, et al: Systematic review of the literature on postpartum care: effectiveness of interventions for smoking relapse prevention, cessation, and reduction in postpartum women, *Birth* 34:341–347, 2007.

36. Logan BA, Brown MS, Hayes MJ: Neonatal abstinence syndrome: treatment and pediatric outcomes, *Clin Obstet Gynecol* 56:186–192, 2013.

37. Madadi P, Koren G, Cairns J, et al: Safety of codeine during breastfeeding. Fatal morphine poisoning in the breastfed neonate of a mother prescribed codeine, *Can Fam Physician* 53:33–35, 2007.

38. Marquet P, Chevral J, Lavignasse P, et al: Buprenorphine withdrawal syndrome in a newborn, *Clin Pharmacol Ther* 62:569–571, 1997.

39. McCarthy JJ, Posey BL: Methadone levels in human milk, *J Hum Lact* 16:115–120, 2000.

40. McQueen KA, Murphy-Oikonen J, Gerlach K, et al: The impact of infant feeding method on neonatal abstinence scores of methadone-exposed infants, *Adv Neonatal Care* 11:282–290, 2011.

41. Montgomery A, Hale TW, the Academy of Breastfeeding Medicine: ABM clinical protocol #15: analgesia and anesthesia for the breastfeeding mother, revised 2012, *Breastfeed Med* 7:547–553, 2012.

42. Myr R: Promoting, protecting, and supporting breastfeeding in a community with a high rate of tobacco use, *J Hum Lact* 20:415–416, 2014.

43. O'Connor AB, Collett A, Alto WA, et al: Breastfeeding rates and the relationship between breastfeeding and neonatal abstinence syndrome in women maintained on buprenorphine during pregnancy, *J Midwifery Womens Health* 58:383–388, 2013.

44. Patrick SW, Schumacher RE, Benneyworth BD, et al: Neonatal abstinence syndrome and associated health care expenditures, *JAMA* 307:1934–1940, 2012.

45. Perez-Reyes M, Wall ME: Presence of δ9-tetrahydrocannabinol in human milk, *N Engl J Med* 307:819–820, 1982.

46. Substance Abuse and Mental Health Services Administration: Results from the 2013 national survey on drug use and health: summary of national findings, In *NSDUH series H-48, HHS publication no. (SMA) 14-4863*, Rockville, MD, 2014, Substance Abuse and Mental Health Services Administration, www.samhsa.gov/data/sites/default/files/NSDUHresultsPDFWHTML2013/Web/NSDUHresults2013.pdf (Accessed 18.02.15).

47. Rowe H, Baker T, Hale TW: Maternal medication, drug use, and breastfeeding, *Pediatr Clin North Am* 60:275–294, 2013.

48. Sachs HC, American Academy of Pediatrics Committee on Drugs: The transfer of drugs and therapeutics into human breast milk: an update on selected topics, *Pediatrics* 132:e796–e809, 2013.

49. Tennes K, Avitable N, Blackard C, et al: Marijuana: prenatal and postnatal exposure in the human, *NIDA Res Monogr* 59:48–60, 1985.

50. Texas Tech University Health Sciences Center, Infant Risk Center: Tobacco use, www.infantrisk.com/content/tobacco-use (Accessed 20.02.15).

51. Volkow ND, Baler RD, Compton WM, et al: Adverse health effects of marijuana use, *N Engl J Med* 370:2219–2227, 2014.

52. Wachman EM, Byun J, Philipp BL: Breastfeeding rates among mothers of infants with neonatal abstinence syndrome, *Breastfeed Med* 5:159–164, 2010.

53. Welle-Strand GK, Skurtveit S, Jansson LM, et al: Breastfeeding reduces the need for withdrawal treatment in opioid-exposed infants, *Acta Paediatr* 102:1060–1066, 2013.

54. Winecker RE, Goldberger BA, Tebbett IR, et al: Detection of cocaine and its metabolites in breast milk, *J Forensic Sci* 46:1221–1223, 2001.

55. Wojnar-Horton RE, Kristensen JH, Yapp P, et al: Methadone distribution and excretion into breast milk of clients in a methadone maintenance programme, *Br J Clin Pharmacol* 44:543–547, 1997.

56. Wong S, Ordean A, Kahan M, et al: Substance use in pregnancy, *J Obstet Gynaecol Can* 33:367–384, 2011.

57. World Health Organization: *Guidelines for the identification and management of substance use and substance use disorders in pregnancy*, www.who.int/substance_abuse/publications/pregnancy_guidelines/en/. 2014 (Accessed 18.02.15).

58. Yang I, Hall L: Smoking cessation and relapse challenges reported by postpartum women, *MCN Am J Matern Child Nurs* 39:375–380, 2004.

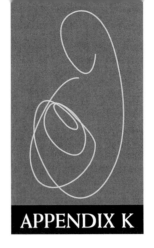

APPENDIX K

Medical Education for Basic Proficiency in Breastfeeding

C.B. Rosen-Carole

Despite the large body of evidence concerning practices and behaviors that support breastfeeding and the positive effect of residency and primary care curricula on breastfeeding rates,[1-12] there remains no information concerning the appropriate and complete education of medical students. It is imperative to ensure that every health care provider graduates medical school with a basic understanding of breastfeeding. The following guide was created in order to support the development of such a curriculum:

Learning objective/transfer goal

By the end of medical school, medical students should have a basic understanding of the histology, anatomy, physiology, pathology, pharmacology, public health and clinical issues surrounding breastfeeding; be able to understand relevance of this knowledge to clinical scenarios; and begin to apply this knowledge in clinical decision-making (see Chapter 23).

(C.B. ROSEN-CAROLE)

The following topics should be included:

1. *Histology*: The histology of the breast, including the acinar cells, ductal cells, and hormonal stimuli of milk release. Impact of breast milk on the newborn gut cells.
2. *Anatomy*: Location of the milk ducts, their proximity to surgical incision sites. Surgeries and surgical sites with varying impacts on breastfeeding. Suspension ligaments. NO lactiferous sinuses. Role of the interstitial spaces that fill with fluid during engorgement to prevent release ("let down") of milk.
3. *Physiology*: Seeing the newborn and mother as a "dyad" biophysically during the first year of life. Normal hormonal stimulation of milk ejection, mechanisms of milk expression by mechanics of neonatal tongue, and differences with milk ejection by artificial methods (hand expression and pumps). Impact of breast milk on the newborn gut, biomes, hormones, and digestion.
4. *Pathology*: Mastitis causes and prevention, and appropriate management of breast abscess while not interrupting ductal tissue. Few contraindications to breastfeeding. Infant malformations associated with difficulty breastfeeding. Diseases impacted by breastfeeding. Genetic and epigenetic influences of breast milk.
5. *Pharmacology*: Impact of artificial infant formula on newborn gut, especially premature gut. Risks of artificial infant formula and proposed mechanisms (e.g., changed microbiota leading to increased inflammation, increased permeability of mucosal membranes, decreased host defenses, and increased infection). Breast milk fortifiers and their role in growth and nutrition of premature babies (both human- and cow-milk-based fortifiers). Considerations of the transfer of medications into human milk. Determining the safety of medications for breastfeeding. Role of certain medications in decreasing breast milk production.
6. *Nutrition and immunology*: Nutritional impact of breastfeeding and breastmilk as species-specific. Co-factors for absorption, presence of cells, and

immunoglobulins for immunologic support. Colostrum as first nutrition and first vaccine.

7. *Public health*: Breastfeeding as a health disparities and access issue. Low rates of breastfeeding and impact on cost of health care and burden of disease.

8. *Primary care clerkship preparation*: How to discuss breastfeeding in a supportive manner with families, the importance of breastfeeding education and physician recommendation. The basics of a good latch and positioning.

Curriculum design considerations:

- Material included should meet the highest standards of evidence-based medicine. Involving a physician with advanced training in breastfeeding medicine is recommended, if available, for this process.
- Curricula should be designed by a multidisciplinary team, including basic science and clinical faculty (obstetric, pediatric, family medicine, surgical, etc.), medical student leaders, patients, and administrators. This is likely to improve buy-in, humanism, and applicability to all parts of the curriculum.
- Each phase of the medical school curriculum should include some information on breastfeeding: basic science, preclinical, and clinical years.
- Material should be considered for inclusion in an integrated manner with other course topics (e.g., a discussion of the role of breastfeeding in breast cancer prevention could be included in a problem-based-learning cancer case or in a traditional lecture on breast cancer).
- Dedicated sessions on breastfeeding should be considered to focus on the clinical skills necessary for the clinical years (e.g., latch, positioning, motivational interviewing).
- In schools that utilize a systems-based integrative model, or modular, problem-based learning, a case/unit on breastfeeding should be strongly

considered or should be included as a teaching point of a related case (e.g., bronchiolitis, diabetes, etc.).

REFERENCES

1. Feldman-Winter L, Barone L, Milcarek B, et al: Residency curriculum improves breastfeeding care, *Pediatrics* 126 (2):289–297, 2010.
2. Feldman-Winter LB, Schanler RJ, O'Connor KG, Lawrence RA: Pediatricians and the promotion and support of breastfeeding, *Arch Pediatr Adolesc Med* 162(12):1142–1149, 2008.
3. Freed GL, Clark SJ, Cefalo RC, Sorenson JR: Breast-feeding education of obstetrics-gynecology residents and practitioners, *Am J Obstet Gynecol* 173(5):1607–1613, 1995.
4. Freed GL, Clark SJ, Curtis P, Sorenson JR: Breast-feeding education and practice in family medicine, *J Fam Pract* 40(3):263–269, 1995.
5. Freed GL, Clark SJ, Lohr JA, Sorenson JR: Pediatrician involvement in breast-feeding promotion: a national study of residents and practitioners, *Pediatrics* 96(3 Pt 1):490–494, 1995.
6. Guise JM, Palda V, Westhoff C, Chan BK, et al: The effectiveness of primary care-based interventions to promote breastfeeding: systematic evidence review and meta-analysis for the US preventive services task force, *Ann Fam Med* 1(2):70–78, 2003.
7. Holmes AV, McLeod AY, Thesing C, et al: Physician breastfeeding education leads to practice changes and improved clinical outcomes, *Breastfeed Med* 7(6):403–408, 2012.
8. Lu MC, Lange L, Slusser W, et al: Provider encouragement of breast-feeding: evidence from a national survey, *Obstet Gynecol* 97(2):290–295, 2001.
9. Renfrew MJ, McCormick FM, Wade A, et al: Support for healthy breastfeeding mothers with healthy term babies, *Cochrane Database Syst Rev* 5:2012, CD001141.
10. Taveras EM, Capra AM, Braveman PA, et al: Clinician support and psychosocial risk factors associated with breastfeeding discontinuation, *Pediatrics* 112(1 Pt 1):108–115, 2003.
11. Taveras EM, Li R, Grummer-Strawn L, et al: Opinions and practices of clinicians associated with continuation of exclusive breastfeeding, *Pediatrics* 113(4):e283–e290, 2004.
12. U.S. Department of Health Human Services: *The surgeon general's call to action to support breastfeeding*, Washington, DC, 2011, Department of Health and Human Services.

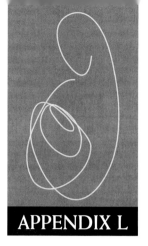

Glossary

A

Acinus The tube leading to the smallest lobule of a compound gland; it is characterized by a narrow lumen.

ACNM American College of Nurse-Midwives.

ACOG American Congress of Obstetricians and Gynecologists.

ACOP American College of Osteopathic Pediatricians.

Adipose tissue See *Panniculus adiposus*.

Afferent Conducting inward to, or toward, the center of an organ, gland, or other structure or area. Applies to sensory nerves, arteries, and lymph vessels.

AHRQ See DHHS/Agency for Healthcare Research and Quality.

Alactogenesis Familial puerperal alactogenesis is a genetically transmitted, isolated prolactin deficiency.

ALPP Academy of Lactation Policy & Practice.

Alveolus A glandular acinus or terminal portion of the alveolar gland, where milk is secreted and stored, that measures 0.12 mm in diameter. From 10 to 100 alveoli, or tubulosaccular secretory units, make up a lobulus.

Ankyloglossia A tight lingual frenulum (the membrane attaching the tongue to the bottom of the mouth). This condition is also referred to as *tongue-tie*. When the frenulum is tight, it can restrict the movement of the tongue, resulting in breastfeeding problems for some mothers and babies.

Ampulla Elastic portion of the duct, just proximal to the nipple, that expands as milk fills the breast.

Apocrine A term descriptive of a gland cell that loses part of its protoplasmic substance.

Apt test A test, named after its developer, performed on fresh blood to distinguish between adult and fetal hemoglobin. The blood is suspended in saline, and an equal amount of 10% sodium hydroxide (NaOH) is added and mixed; adult hemoglobin turns brown, and fetal hemoglobin remains red. A control sample of known adult blood should also be tested for comparison.

Arborization Development of a branched arrangement or structure.

Areola mammae Areola. The pigmented area surrounding the papilla mammae, or nipple.

Australian posture or position A breastfeeding position where the baby is above the mother (or the mother is "down under" the baby—the reason for the name of the posture.

Autophagic vacuole Autophagosome. A membrane-bound body within a cell containing degenerating cell organelles.

B

BALT Bronchus-associated immunocompetent lymphoid tissue, to which the mammary gland may act as an extension. See *GALT* and *MALT*.

Basal lamina The layer of material, 50 to 80 mm thick, that lies adjacent to the plasma membrane of the basal surfaces of epithelial cells. It contains collagen and certain carbohydrates. It is often called the *basement* membrane.

Block nursing Nursing on the same breast for two or more feedings without nursing or otherwise releasing milk from the other breast. This strategy is often used to decrease an overly abundant milk supply.

C

Casein A derivative of caseinogen. The fraction of milk protein that forms the tough curd in cow's milk.

CGBI   Carolina Global Breastfeeding Institute.

CLC   Certified Lactation Counselor. Breastfeeding care provider who has completed a course of study resulting in certification as a lactation counselor.

Cluster feeding   The tendency of young babies to have a cycle of short, closely spaced feedings interspersed with periods of rest or sleep.

Colostrum   The first milk. This yellow, sticky fluid is secreted during the first few days postpartum and provides nutrition and protection against infectious disease with its high level of immune globulins. It contains more protein, less sugar, and much less fat than mature breast milk.

Columnar secretory cell   A type of secretory cell in the shape of a hexagonal prism; it appears rectangular when sectioned across the long axis, the length being considerably greater than the width.

Cooper's ligaments   Triangular ligaments stretching between the mammary gland, the skin, the retinacula cutis, the pectineal ligament, and the chorda obliqua. These ligaments underlie and support the breasts.

Corpus mammae   The mammary gland; breast mass after freeing breast from deep attachments and removal of skin, subcutaneous connective tissue, and fat.

Creamatocrit   Measurement for estimating the fat content and therefore the caloric content of a milk sample. A microhematocrit tube is filled with milk (usually a mix of foremilk and hindmilk) and spun in a microcentrifuge for 15 min. The layer of fat is measured as a percentage, as one measures a blood hematocrit.

Cross nursing   When a lactating woman breastfeeds a baby who is not her own, often temporarily, in the role of a child care arrangement.

Cuboidal secretory cell   A secretory cell that has similar height and breadth measurements.

Cytokines   A generic term for nonantibody proteins that are part of the immune system; examples include interferon-γ and interleukin 6.

Cytosol   Cell fluid.

D

Doula   An individual who surrounds, interacts with, and aids the mother at any time within the period that includes pregnancy, birth, and lactation; this may be a relative, friend, or neighbor and is usually, but not necessarily, female. One who gives psychological encouragement and physical assistance to a new mother. These are lay individuals who train to assist the mother during labor and delivery.

E

Efferent   Carrying impulses away from a nerve center.

Ejection reflex   A reflex initiated by the suckling of the infant at the breast, which triggers the pituitary gland to release oxytocin into the bloodstream. The oxytocin causes the myoepithelial cells to contract and eject the milk from the collecting ductules. Also called *let-down reflex* or *draught*.

Engorgement   The swelling and distention of the breasts, usually in the early days of initiation of lactation, caused by vascular dilatation as well as the arrival of the early milk.

Eosinophil   A granular leukocyte possessing large conspicuous granules in the cytoplasm and containing a bilobed nucleus.

F

Finger feeding   Stimulation of an infant's tongue with a finger to initiate sucking. A feeding tube attached to a syringe of milk along the finger will provide milk to the infant when suckling is correct.

Foremilk   The first milk obtained at the onset of suckling or expression. It contains less fat than later milk of that feeding (i.e., the hindmilk).

G

Galactocele   A cystic tumor in the ducts of the breast that contains a milky fluid.

Galactagogue   A material or action that stimulates the production of milk.

Galactopoiesis   The development of milk in the mammary gland. The maintenance of established lactation.

Galactorrhea   Abnormal or inappropriate lactation.

Galactose   ($C_6H_{12}O_6$). A simple sugar that is a component of the disaccharide lactose, or milk sugar.

Galactosemia   A congenital metabolic disorder in which there is an inability to metabolize galactose because of a deficiency of the enzyme galactose-1-phosphate uridyltransferase. It causes failure to thrive, hepatomegaly, and splenomegaly.

GALT   Gut-associated lymphoid tissue to which the mammary gland may act as an extension. See *BALT* and *MALT*.

Gigantomastia   The excessive enlargement of the breast beyond physiologic needs during pregnancy and lactation, usually of unknown cause. When it occurs in association with medications that cause galactorrhea (calcium-channel blockers), it can be reversed by stopping the drug.

Glandular hypoplasia   Lack of breast growth during pregnancy. Nipples point downward, and there is a tubular shape to the breast, and little palpable glandular tissue. This occurs with failure of lactogenesis.

Golgi apparatus A specialized region of the cytoplasm, often close to the nucleus, that is composed of flattened cisternae, numerous vesicles, and some larger vacuoles. In secretory cells, it is concerned with packaging the secretory product. It is also probably concerned with the secretion of polysaccharides in some cells, but its full range of functions has not yet been elucidated.

H

Heterophagic vacuole Heterophagosome. A membrane-bound body within a cell, containing ingested material.

Hindmilk Milk obtained later during the nursing period, that is, the end of the feeding. This milk is usually high in fat and probably controls appetite.

Homocystinuria A rare inborn error of amino acid metabolism characterized by mental deficiency, epilepsy, dislocation of the lens, growth disturbance, thromboses, and defective hair growth.

Hyperadenia The existence of mammary tissue without nipples.

Hypergalactia The excessive, uncontrolled production of milk over and above the needs of a suckling infant.

Hyperlactation An oversupply of milk beyond the needs or capacity of the infant.

Hypermastia The existence of accessory mammary glands.

Hyperthelia The existence of abundant, more or less developed nipples without accompanying mammary tissue.

I

Immunoglobulin The protein fraction of globulin, which has been demonstrated to have immunologic properties. Immunoglobulins include IgA, IgG, and IgM. They are factors in breast milk that protect against infection.

Induced lactation Process by which a nonpuerperal female (or male) is stimulated to lactate.

K

Kosher Food that is considered ritually fit according to Jewish law (concerning both the source and preparation of the food).

L

Lactiferous ducts The main ducts of the mammary gland, which number from 15 to 30 and open onto the nipple. They carry milk to the nipple and are very elastic.

Lactobacillus bifidus Organism of the intestinal tract of breastfed infants.

Lactocele Cystic tumor of the breast caused by the dilatation and obstruction of a milk duct that is usually filled with milk.

Lacto-engineering The process of enhancing the nutrient value of human milk by adding nutrients obtained by drying and separating out specific nutrients, such as protein, from pooled human milk.

Lactoferrin An iron-binding protein of external secretions, including human milk. It inhibits the growth of iron-dependent microorganisms in the gut.

Lactogenesis Initiation of milk secretion.

Let-down reflex See *Ejection reflex.*

Ligand A low-molecular-weight substance that binds trace elements loosely for ready availability (e.g., zinc ligands in human milk).

Lobulus A subunit of the parenchymal structure of the breast made up of 10 to 100 alveoli, or tubulosaccular secretory units. From 20 to 40 lobuli make up a lobus.

Lobus A subunit of the parenchymal structure of the breast made up of 20 to 40 lobuli. From 15 to 25 lobi are arranged like the spokes of a wheel with the nipple as the central point.

Lymphocyte A mature leukocyte derived through the intermediate stage of lymphoblast from the reticuloendothelium found in lymphatic tissue.

Lyophilization The process of rapidly freeze-drying a fluid in a vacuum, resulting in a solid.

M

MALT Mucosal-associated lymphoid tissue, which includes gut, lung, mammary gland, salivary and lacrimal glands, and genital tract. There is traffic of cells between secretory sites. Immunization at one site may be an effective means of producing immunity at distant sites. See *GALT* and *BALT.*

Mamilla The nipple; any teatlike structure.

Mammogenesis Growth of the mammary gland.

Mastalgia Painful breasts.

Mastitis Inflammation of the breast, including cellulitis and, occasionally, abscess formation.

Matrescence The state of becoming a mother or motherhood as a new event in an individual's life.

Megaloblastic anemia Defective red blood cell formation caused by megaloblastic hyperplasia of the marrow; there are often megaloblasts, or primitive nucleated red blood cells, in the peripheral blood.

Merocrine Pertaining to the type of secretion in which the active cell remains intact while forming and discharging the secretory product.

Mesencephalon The midbrain.

Methylmalonic aciduria The condition of the urine being acidic from an accumulation of methylmalonic acid caused by an inborn error of metabolism.

Milk fever A syndrome of fever and general malaise associated with early engorgement of the breasts or with sudden weaning from the breast.

Mitogen A substance capable of stimulating cells to enter mitosis.

Montgomery glands Small prominences, sebaceous glands in the areola of the breast, which become more marked in pregnancy and lactation. They number 20 to 24 and secrete a fluid that lubricates the nipple and areola.

Morgagni's tubercle Small sinuses into which the miniature ducts of the Montgomery glands open in the epidermis of the areola.

Myoepithelial cell An epithelial cell, usually around a glandular acinus, in which part of the cytoplasm has contractile properties, serving to empty the sinus of its secretion.

N

Nonnutritive sucking The act of suckling the breast with little or no secretion of milk. Infant may suckle when distressed or to be calmed or quieted.

Nonpuerperal lactation The production of milk in a woman who has not given birth.

Nucleotides Compounds derived from nucleic acid by hydrolysis and consisting of phosphoric acid combined with a sugar and a purine or pyrimidine derivative. The milk nucleotides are secreted from glandular epithelial cells.

O

Opsonic Belonging to or characterized by opsonin, a substance in mammalian blood that has the power to render microorganisms and blood cells easier to absorb by phagocytes.

Oxytocin An octapeptide that is synthesized in the cell bodies of neurons, located mainly in the paraventricular nucleus and, in smaller amounts, in the supraoptic nucleus of the hypothalamus. Oxytocin stimulates the ejection reflex by the stimulation of the myoepithelial cells in the mammary gland.

P

Panniculus adiposus Adipose tissue. The superficial fascia, which contains fatty pellicles.

Papilla mammae Mamilla. The nipple of the breast.

Pareve (parve) Food that does not include any meat or dairy derivatives. This includes milk from any mammal except human. Rabbis have defined human milk as pareve but have prohibited the mixing of human milk with other foods.

Perinatal Around birth. The time from conception through birth, delivery, lactation, and at least 28 days postpartum.

Plasma cell Cell derived from the B cell series, which manufactures and secretes antibodies.

Prolactin A hormone present in both males and females and at all ages. During pregnancy, it stimulates and prepares the mammary alveolar epithelium for secretory activity. During lactation, it stimulates synthesis and secretion of milk. At other ages and in the male, it interacts with other steroids.

R

Rachitic Relating to, characterized by, or affected by rickets.

Relactation Process by which a woman who has given birth but did not initially breastfeed is stimulated to lactate (also applies to reinstituting lactation after it has been discontinued).

S

Squamous epithelium A sheet of flattened, scalelike epithelium adhering edge to edge.

Stroma The connective tissue basis or framework of an organ.

Suck training A special technique developed to help an infant who cannot coordinate the undulating (peristaltic) motion of the tongue. See *Finger feeding*.

Switch nursing Nursing in which the mother moves the baby from one breast to the other and back again during the feeding with the hope that this will stimulate the milk supply.

T

Tail of Spence The axillary tail of the breast that can reach the axilla.

Transitional milk The milk produced early in the postpartum period as the colostrum diminishes and the mature milk develops.

Tubuloalveolar Having both tubular and alveolar qualities.

Tubulosaccular Having both tubular and saccular character.

Turgescence The swelling up of a part. The unusual turgid feeling that results from swelling with fluid.

W

Whey protein Protein remaining when the curds of casein have been removed. The mixture of proteins present is complex and includes β-lactoglobulin and α-lactalbumin and enzymes.

Witch's milk Product of neonatal galactorrhea or neonatal breast secretion caused by placental prolactin in the infant's circulation.

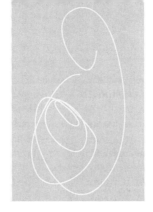

Index

|||||||||||||||||||||||||||||||||||||||||||||||||||||||||||||||||

A

Abrupt weaning, 326
  milk fever and, 330
Abscesses, breast, 776*t*
  brucellosis, 415
  mastitis and, 567, 568*f*, 842
Abstinence method of contraception,
  702*t*, 704, 889*t*
Abuse, 208
  child, 224
  drug, 225*t*, 226
  sexual, 706–707
Academy of Breastfeeding Medicine
  (ABM), 806–807
  educational objectives of, 759
  guidelines of
    for analgesia and anesthesia for
      breastfeeding mother, 901–906
    for ankyloglossia, 874–878, 875*t*,
      877*f*
    for antidepressants for
      breastfeeding mothers, 919–928
    for breastfeeding-friendly
      physician's office, 897–900
    for cleft lip and/or palate, 913–918
    for contraception, 886–896, 887*t*,
      888*f*, 889*t*, 894*t*
    for co-sleeping, 198–199, 199*b*,
      851–855
    for engorgement, 933–936
    for galactogogues, 864–868
    for glucose monitoring and
      hypoglycemia treatment,
      817–824, 818–821*t*
    for hospital discharge of newborn
      and mother, 825–830, 826–827*t*
    for human milk storage, 794
    for hyperbilirubinemia, 504
    for hypotonic infant, 907–912
    for mastitis, 840–844
    for milk storage, 861–863
    for near-term infant, 869–873
    for peripartum breastfeeding
      management, 845–850

Academy of Breastfeeding Medicine
  (ABM) (*Continued*)
    for prenatal breastfeeding
      promotion, 929–932
    for substance use/or substance use
      disorder, 937–945
    for supplementary feedings, 831,
      832–834*t*, 836*t*
    for transitioning premature infant
      from NICU to home, 879–885,
      880*t*, 884*f*
  model breastfeeding policy of,
    856–860
Academy of Family Physicians, 845
Acanthosis nigricans, 589
Accessory breast, 39*b*
Acetylsalicylic acid, in milk,
  374–375
Acid maltase deficiency, 494
Acidemias, organic, 493–494
Aconite, 388*t*
Acquired immunodeficiency syndrome
  (AIDS). *See* Human
    immunodeficiency virus (HIV).
Acrodermatitis enteropathica, 496
Active transport mechanism, on human
  milk, 368–369
Adenomas, breast, 610
Adenoviruses, 776*t*
Adrenal hyperplasia, 498
  congenital, 492
Adrenocorticotropic hormone (ACTH),
  57*b*, 59
Aedes aegypti, 432
African hemorrhagic fever, 776*t*
Aganglionic megacolon, congenital, 514
Age
  comparison of, 322*f*
  natural, at weaning, 322*f*
Ainsworth "strange situation," validated
  techniques, 655
Airborne precautions, 409
Albumin
  in infant serum, 768–769

Albumin (*Continued*)
  in milk, 163*t*
Albuterol, 380
Alcohol, 380–381, 940–942
  milk-ejection reflex and, 262
  oxytocin and, 352
Alfalfa, 770–775
Alfentanil, 605
Alkaline phosphatase, in infant serum,
  768–769
Allergic protective properties, 184–185
Allergies
  cow milk, 633
    acute reactions to, 642–643
    clinical disease in, 641–642
    colitis in, 488
  early feeding and, 644–645
  immunologic aspects of, 639–640,
    640*t*
  intestinal flora in, role of, 640–641
  latex, 617
  management of, 645–646,
    646*f*, 646*t*
  maternal diet for, 309
  natural history of, 633
  prophylaxis of, 217, 634–637,
    635–636*t*, 636*f*
    AAP recommendations for,
      638–639
    long-term effects of, 637–639, 637*t*,
      638*f*
  to solid foods, 643–644
Allografts, renal, 597
Aloe vera, 388*t*, 770–775
Alveolar buds, 36, 51
Alveolar epithelial membrane
  permeability, 85*t*
Alveolar gland, 40, 51
Alveolar lymphangiomas, 519
Alveoli, 40
  of lactating breast, 54
Amastia, 39*b*
Amazia, 39, 39*b*
Amebiasis, 776*t*

Note: Page numbers followed by *b* indicate boxes, *f* indicate figures and *t* indicate tables.

Amenorrhea, 888
American Academy of Pediatrics (AAP),
    1, 324, 651–653
  drug classification by, 374
  guidelines of
    for allergy prophylaxis, 638–639
    for breastfeeding and solid foods,
        201, 342
    for breastfeeding duration,
        148–149
    for hyperbilirubinemia, 504
    for sudden infant death syndrome,
        219
American Academy of Pediatrics
    Committee on Nutrition, 873
American College of Obstetricians and
    Gynecologists (ACOG),
    651–654, 845
Amino acids
  metabolic disorders of, 492
  in milk, 306t, 765–767
    maternal phenylketonuria and, 591,
        591t
  for premature infant, 532
Aminoglycosides, in milk, 376
Ammehjelpen International
    Group, 744
Amphotericin B, for candidal infections,
    468
Ampulla, 43–44
Amylase, 135–136, 137t
  in milk, 135–136, 137t
Analgesia
  for breastfeeding mother, 901–906
  intrapartum, on breastfeeding, 846
  for labor, 901–903
  for mastitis, 841
  purpose of, 901
  recommendations for future research,
    905
  specific agents used for, 904–905
Analgesics, 374–376
  nonopioid, 903
  opioid, 904–905
Anaphylactoid reaction, 641
Anaphylaxis, food, 641
Anesthesia
  for breastfeeding mother, 901–906
  for cesarean section, 903
  for infant surgery, 517
  for labor, 901–903
  postpartum, 903–904
  purpose of, 901
  recommendations for future research,
    905
  specific agents used for, 904–905
  for surgery in breastfeeding mothers,
    904
Anesthetics, 904
Anger, 210–211
Angiotensin-converting enzyme (ACE)
    inhibitors, 674t
Ankyloglossia, 271, 271b, 272f,
    874–878
  assessment of, 875
  definition of, 874
  feeding problems in, 519
  future research for, 877
  management of, 877, 877f
  recommendations for, 876

Anovulation, hyperandrogenic,
    588–589
Anthrax, 413–414, 776t
Antibiotics, 376–377
  on infant, 372
  for mastitis, 567, 569t, 841–842
    bacterial, 378t
  in milk, 372–373
  pseudomembranous colitis and, 488
Antibodies. See also Immunoglobulins.
  allergy and, 636, 636f, 639
  in milk, 98
Antibody-based protein arrays, 169
Anticholinergics, 377
Anticoagulants, 378–379, 566–567
  for epilepsy, 600, 600t
Anticonvulsant, in milk, 393t
Antidepressants, for breastfeeding
    mothers, 919–928
Antihypertensive drugs, for induced
    lactation, 674t
Antiinfective agents in milk. See also
    Antibiotics.
  antibacterial, 163t
  nonimmunoglobulin, 166t
Antiinflammatory drugs, 594–595
Antiinflammatory properties of milk,
    182–184, 183b
Antimicrobial properties, of milk,
    preterm, 545–548, 546–547f,
    546b, 546t, 548t
Antimicrobial prophylaxis, intrapartum,
    421, 422f
Antioxidants, 98, 100
Antiprotozoan factors, 182, 183t
Antiretroviral prophylaxis, 449–450
Antithyroid drugs, 379, 586
α_1-Antitrypsin deficiency, 495
Anus, imperforate, 515–516
Anxiety, 210
Apgar scores, low, 483–485, 484–485f
Apocrine secretion, 54
Apocrine secretory mechanism, for
    lipids, 81f
Apoptosis, mammary, 56–57, 87
Apt test, 516
Arboviruses, 428–429, 776t
Arcanobacterium haemolyticus, 776t
Arching reflex, 508
Arenaviruses, 429
Areola
  engorgement of, 250–251
  examination of, 240, 240f
Areola mammae, 41–44, 41f
  innervation of, 47
Argentine hemorrhagic fever,
    429, 776t
Arnold Steam Sterilizer advertisement, 8f
Arteries, of breast, 44, 46f
Arthritis, rheumatoid, 594–595
Artificial feeding, 1. See also Bottle
    feeding; Formula.
  history of, 743
  morbidity and mortality studies in,
    26–29, 27t
Ascaris lumbricoides, 776t
Ash in milk, 121–122, 122t
  colostrum, 96–98
Asparagus, 770–775
Aspartame, 315

Aspergillosis, 776t
Asphyxiation, 851–852
Asthma, 633
  maternal, 605
  prophylaxis of, 217, 634–637, 635t,
    638f
Astroviruses, 776t
Atenolol, 392
Atherosclerosis, 355
Atopic disease
  natural history of, 633
  prevention of, 635t
  prophylaxis of, 634–637
Attachment
  mother-infant, 195, 207, 655
  to sucking object, 201–202
Attitudes toward breastfeeding, 26
Augmentation mammoplasty, 614–615
Australia, workplace kit for, 662–663, 663f
Australian Breastfeeding Association
    (ABA), 805
Autoimmune thrombocytopenic
    purpura, 594
Autonomic nerves, of breast, 47
Azithromycin, 378t, 570t

B

B lymphocytes, 149–150, 149b, 153
Babesiosis, 776t
Baby Friendly, USA, 5, 14t, 805
Baby Friendly Hospital Initiative, 4–5,
    5b, 745
  steps for successful breastfeeding, 873t
Baby Milk Action Group, 805
Bacillus anthracis, 413, 776t
Bacillus cereus, 776t
Bacteria
  antibodies for, 160–162, 161t
  intestinal, 176–177, 640–641
  in milk
    cultures for, 409–410, 411b, 720,
        720t
    growth of, 725f
    probiotic, 294
    raw donor, 721
    treatment temperature and, 722t
  probiotic, 175–177
Bacterial infections. See also specific
    infection.
  dermatitis from, 616–617
  mastitis from, 567–571, 568f, 568t
  transmission of, 413–415
    anthrax, 413–414
    botulism, 414
    brucellosis, 414–415
    chlamydial, 415
    diphtheria, 415
    gonococcal, 415–417
    Haemophilus influenzae, 416
    leprosy, 416
    listeriosis, 416–417
    meningococcal, 417
    pertussis, 417
    staphylococcal, 417–421
    streptococcal, 421–428
    tuberculosis, 424–428, 424f, 426f,
        427t
Bailey Medical Engineering, 806
Banking of milk. See Milk bank.

Barbiturates, infant and, 372
Barracudas, 257
Barrier methods of contraception, 698, 702t, 889t, 893
Bathing, in breast preparation, 241
B-cell system, 151f, 155
Bed sharing
  breastfeeding and, 853
  co-sleeping and, 851–852
Best Start, 9, 211, 747
Beta blockers, 595
  lactation and, 674t
Bicycle horn pump, 731–733
Bifidobacterium bifidum, 162
Bifidus factor, 162–163
Bile salts, 141
Bilirubin, 500. *See also* Hyperbilirubinemia and jaundice.
  production of, 500
  safe levels of, 501–502
  stool passage and, 502
Bilirubin encephalopathy, 500
Billings ovulation method, natural family planning and, 891
Bioactive agents, in human milk, 527f
Bioactive factors, 147t, 150
  bifidus factor, 162–163
  complement, 165
  cytokines, 168–173, 168b
  glycans, 165–167
  interferon, 165
  interleukins, 167–168, 167t
  lactoferrin, 164–165
  lysozyme, 158f, 163, 163t
  nucleotides, 169–173
  oligosaccharides, 165–167
  resistance factor, 163
  vitamin B_{12}-binding protein, 165
Bioavailability, oral, of drugs, 373
Biochemical monitoring, for premature infants, 880, 880t
Biochemistry of human milk, 91–145
Biotin
  maternal requirements for, 295t, 300
  in milk, 300t, 306t, 541t, 765–767
  recommended daily dietary allowances for infants, 130t
Birth control. *See* Contraception.
Birth interval, breastfeeding and, 693–694, 694t
Black cohosh, 770–775
Black milk, 316
Blastocystis hominis, 776t
Blastomyces dermatitidis, 776t
Bleeding, gastrointestinal, 516
Blessed thistle, 770–775
Blood glucose monitoring, in neonates, 817–824, 818–821t
Blood pressure, 596
  of breastfed infants, 356
Blood supply, to breast, 44–46, 46f
Bloody nipple discharge, 609–610
Blue cohosh, 770–775
  lactation and, 386
Body composition, infant, 558f
  drugs and, 370, 370f
Body contact, cultural tradition and, 197–199, 198f

Body mass index (BMI), 358f, 797–802
  obesity and, 357
  weight classification for, 358t
Bonding, mother-infant, 195–197, 196f, 207
Bone mineral density, maternal, 220, 708
Bone mineralization, in premature infant, 530f, 533–534, 540, 544
Borage, 770–775
Bordetella pertussis, 417, 776t
Borrelia burgdorferi, 462, 776t
Borrelia spp., 776t
Bottle feeding, 835. *See also* Formula.
  breastfeeding vs., growth of, 340
  caries and, 519
  commercial discharge packs and, 22
  feeding frequency in, 267
  tongue action in, 234, 235f
  vs. breastfeeding, 657
    psychological differences in, 199–200, 200f
    psychophysiologic response in, 204
  by working mothers, 659
Bottle-feeding jaundice, 503–504
Botulism, 414, 770–775, 776t
Brain development, 107–108
  head circumference and, 339–340
Brain growth, in premature infant, 535–537
Breast biopsy, 605
Breast cancer, 592–594
  apoptosis in, 57
  breastfeeding and risk for, 221–224, 223t
  radiation therapy and, 223–224
  tumor virus and, 456–458
Breast cysts, 611
Breast implants, 614, 614f
Breast measurement, computerized, 94–95
Breast milk. *See also* Colostrum; Human milk.
  fat in, suckling and, 236–237
  manual expression of, 792–793
  protective effect of, 148
Breast milk jaundice, 505–506
  early, 505
  late diagnosis of, 507–508
Breast pumps, 730–740, 732t
  electric, 718f, 731–732t, 733–740, 734t, 738t
  manual, 730–731, 731–732t, 738t
Breast shells, 242, 242f
Breastfeeding, 1, 913–914
  to 24 months of age, 17t
  ABM guideline on, 851–855
  advantages of, 448
  antiretroviral prophylaxis with, 449–450
  application of, 859
  attitudes toward, 26, 210
  away from home activities and, 650–666
  barriers, 1
  and bed sharing, 853
  benefits for infants, 214–229, 220b
  benefits for mother, 220–224, 220b
  breathing and sucking and, 237
  cesarean delivery and, 238

Breastfeeding (*Continued*)
  cineradiographic study on, 233
  cleft lip and/or palate and, 913–914
  commercial discharge packs and, 22–26
  comparison of, 652f
  conditions and symptoms in, 231t
  contraception during, 886–896
  contraindications to, 224–226, 225t
  counseling, for working mothers, 659–660
  curriculum for medical students, 758
  curriculum for nurses' training for, 759–762
  definitions of, 20–21, 21f, 148b, 201
  demographic factors for, 13–16, 21f, 23–24t
  disadvantages of, 226–227
  duration of, 17–22, 24–25t, 149
    employment and, 651–652, 656, 658
    recommendations for, 323t
    sociodemographic characteristics of mothers for, 331t
  early cessation of, 842
  effect of stopping, 16f
  employment and, 650–666
  ethnic factors for, 10–13, 12f
  evidence-based data, 1
  exceptions to, 859
  exclusive, 274
    definition of, 856
  failure at, 202, 210–211
  frequency of, 9–10
  history of, 5–9
  and HIV transmission, 446–447
    prevention of, 447–448
  human immunodeficiency virus and, 661
  impact of curriculum on, 759t
  infants, with problems, 483–523
  infectious disease, transmission of, 407–482
  jaundice, failure to thrive in, 348
  medical education for basic proficiency in, 946–948
  mismanagement of, 328
  model policy for, 856–860
  morbidity and mortality studies in, 26–29, 27t
  national trends in rate of, 3f, 20f
  for near-term infant, 869–873, 873t
    goals of, 869
    principles of care for, 870–873
    purpose of, 869
  obstetrician, role in, 653–654
  palmar grasp in, 245, 245f
  papal support on, 31
  peer counselor for, 750
  peripartum, management of, 231–232
  plasma cholesterol and, 356, 356f
  positions for, 6, 6f, 484, 484–485f
  precautions and recommendations in, 776–791
Pregnancy Risk Assessment Monitoring System (PRAMS) on, 329
  premature infants and, 524–562
  problems in, 755
    diagnosing, 247–253, 249–250f

Breastfeeding (*Continued*)
  prolonged, 342
  promotion of, 9
    federal activities for, 5*f*
    key elements for, 4*b*
    national campaign for, 31–32
    in prenatal setting, 929–932
  psychological impact of, 194–213
  rates by state, 12*t*, 14*t*
  reasons women stop, 330*t*
  rejection of, 209–210, 336
  savings and costs associated with, 25*t*
  scissor grasp in, 245, 245*f*
  screening form, 279*b*
  steps for successful, 856, 858, 873*t*
  token, 200–201
  tongue action in, 234, 235*f*
  unrestricted, 17, 200
  viral hepatitis associated with, 436*t*
  vs. bottle feeding, 657
  women, support for, 31
  World Alliance of Breastfeeding
    Actions on, 664
Breastfeeding and Human Lactation
    Study Center, 748–749, 758
  on human milk, 374
Breastfeeding Association of South
    Africa, 744
"Breastfeeding Basics", 762
Breastfeeding dyad
  assessment of, 875–876
  complications in, neonatal
    ankyloglossia and, 874–878
Breastfeeding health supervision,
    808–816
Breastfeeding management. *See also*
    Feedings.
  immediate postpartum, 244–247,
    846–847
    diagnosing problems in, 247–253,
      249–250*f*
    engorgement in, 250–252
    first physician visit in, 253–257
    hospital days in, 246–247
    hospital-to-home transition in, 253
    key points in, 246, 246*b*
    nursing at delivery in, 244–246
  for near-term infant, 553
  office practice of, 280–281
  peripartum, ABM protocol for, 845–850
  postnatal, 265, 265–266*t*
    breast rejection in, 270
    carrying and holding in, 274
    colic and crying in, 274–280
    colicky behavior in, management
      of, 276–277
    exclusive breastfeeding in, 274
    feeding frequency in, 266–267, 266*t*
    insufficient milk syndrome in,
      278–279, 279*t*
    maternal diet in, influence of cow
      milk in, 275–276
    maternal rest in, 268
    milk expression in, 273
    one-breast/two-breast feedings in,
      267–268
    oversupply of milk in, 279–280
    pacifiers in, 277–278
    sleeping in, 274
    solid foods in, 274

Breastfeeding management (*Continued*)
    stool patterns in, 278, 278*t*
    supplementary feedings in, 272–273
  prenatal, 239–241, 240*f*, 845–846
    breast preparation in, 241–242
    hand expression in, 243
    nipple preparation in, 242, 242*f*
    nipple stimulation in, 242–243
    surgical correction in, 243
  problems and complications in,
    847–848
Breastfeeding Medicine, 1–2
Breastfeeding Promotion Consortium,
    21, 201
Breastfeeding-friendly physician's office,
    897–900
  background of, 897
  definitions of, 897
  recommendations for, 897–899
Breastmilk feeding, 913–914
Breasts. *See also* Nipples.
  abscesses of, 415, 567, 568*f*, 776*t*, 842
  acquired abnormalities, 40
  anatomy of, 34–55
  apoptosis in, 56–57, 87
  asymmetric, 614–615*f*
  breastfeeding conditions and
    symptoms in, 231*t*
  dermatitis of, 616–618
  eczema in, 271–272, 618
  engorgement of, 250–252
  fat necrosis of, 611
  fibrocystic disease of, 610–611
  fullness and engorgement,
    management of, 843
  galactography of, 569*f*, 611
  gigantomastia of, 611–613, 612–613*f*
  gross anatomy of, 34
    abnormalities in, 39–40, 40*b*
    anatomic location in, 38–39, 38*f*
    blood supply in, 44–46
    developmental stage and, 35*t*, 37*t*,
      57, 57*t*
    embryonic development in, 34–35,
      35*t*, 58–59
    fetal and prepubertal development
      in, 35–37, 37*f*
    innervation in, 47–49, 48*f*
    lymphatic drainage in, 47, 47*f*
    nipple and areola in, 41–44,
      42–46*f*
    pubertal development in, 36*f*, 37–38
  growth of, 59–60
    excessive. *See also* Gigantomastia
    menstrual cycle and, 60
    placental growth and, 66*f*
    pregnancy and, 60–62, 62*f*
    prepubertal, 59–60
    pubertal, 60
  hematomas of, 611
  herpes of, 440, 617*f*
  hypertrophy of, 611–613, 612*f*
  inflammation of. *See* Mastitis.
  inflammatory breast symptoms, 569*t*
  lactating, mammography of, 270*f*
  lipomas, 611
  lumps in, 610
  mammography of, 269–270*f*
  manual expression of, position for,
    250–251, 251*f*

Breasts (*Continued*)
  measurement system for,
    computerized, 263, 263*f*
  microscopic anatomy of, 49–51,
    51*f*
    lactating mammary gland in, 53–54,
      53*f*
    mammary gland in pregnancy,
      52–53, 52*f*
    mature mammary gland in,
      51–52
    postlactation regression and, 54
  neonatal, 499
  pain, other causes of, 271–274
  palmar grasp on, during breastfeeding,
    245, 245*f*
  postlactation involution of, 615, 615*f*
  preparation of
    in breastfeeding management,
      241–242
    in induced lactation, 669
  radiation therapy to, 223–224
  scissor grasp on, during breastfeeding,
    245, 245*f*
  as sex object, 8
  sore, 268–269
  storage capacity of, 351
  suckling on
    radiographic interpretation
      of, 234*b*
    ultrasound interpretation of, 234*b*
  texture, palpation of, 239–240, 240*f*
  volume of, 76*f*
Bromocriptine, 682
Brucella melitensis, 414–415, 776*t*
Brucellosis, 414–415, 776*t*
"Bubble palate", 508
Bulimia nervosa, 209
Bunyaviridae, 428
Bupivacaine
  for delivery, 564
  for labor, 238
  for surgery, 564
Buprenorphine, 939
Bupropion, 604
Burkitt lymphoma, Epstein-Barr virus
    associated with, 432
Burping, ritual of, 6
Buserelin, 700–701
Business Case for Breastfeeding, 650,
    663–664, 748
Butaconazole, for mucocutaneous
    candidiasis, 468
Butorphanol, 902–903, 905

C

Cabbage leaves, for breast engorgement,
    252–253
Cabergoline, 578
Caffeine, 379–380
Calcium
  in foods, 597
  infant requirements for, 533*t*
  in infant serum, 768–769
  maternal requirements for, 297*t*
  in milk, 306*t*, 765–767
    colostrum, 98–99
    fortified, 540, 542*t*
    maternal diet and, 303

Calcium (*Continued*)
    preterm, 531
Calcium channel blockers, lactation and, 674*t*
Calcium/phosphorus ratio, 122–123
Calciviruses, 776*t*
Caloric needs
    maternal, 293, 293*f*
    of small-for-gestational-age (SGA) infants, 347
Campylobacter spp., 776*t*
Canadian Pediatric Society, on weaning, 323
Cancer. *See also* Breast cancer.
    ovarian, 221
Candida albicans, 467
Candida infection, maternal
    of breast, 581–582, 842–843
    transmission of, 467–469
Candidiasis, 776*t*
Cannabis, 604, 770–775, 942
Capsaicin, 770–775
Carbamazepine, 393
Carbimazole, 588
Carbohydrates, 83–84
    maternal requirements for, 296*t*, 298*t*
    in milk, 117–119, 118*f*, 306*t*, 541*t*
    in milk fortifiers, 542*t*
Cardiovascular disease
    maternal, 595–596
    risk for, 220–221
Caries, dental, 519
Carnitine, 110
β-Carotene, 128
    in milk, 765–767
Carotenoids, 128, 306*t*
Carpal tunnel syndrome, 601
Carrying infants, 198
Casein in milk, 112, 306*t*, 765–767
    mature, 101
β-Casomorphins, 138
Caspofungin, for candidal infections, 468
Cat-scratch disease, 776*t*
CD4+ and CD8+ cells, 154
CDC. *See* Centers for Disease Control and Prevention (CDC).
Celecoxib, 905
Celiac disease, 489–491
Cell-mediated immunity, defects in, 149*b*
Cellular components, 86
    of lactating breast, 81–86, 82*f*
    in milk
        immunologically active, 147*t*, 151–155
        stem cells, 155–156
        survival of, 155–156
Center for Science in the Public Interest, 805
Centers for Disease Control and Prevention (CDC), 2, 10, 340, 408
Central nervous system malformations, 516–517
Cephalexin, 378*t*, 570*t*
Cephalgia, 619
Cephalosporins, 377

Cerebrocortical neuronal membrane glycerophospholipids, 108
Cervical caps, 701, 702*t*
Cervical mucus, in natural family planning, 697*f*, 698
Cesarean delivery, 563–565
    anesthesia for, 903
    breastfeeding and, 238
Chamomile, 388*t*, 770–775
Chastetree, lactation and, 387
Cheiloplasty, 917
Chew-swallow reflex, introduction of solid and, 323
Chiari-Frommel syndrome, 575–576, 576*t*
Chickenpox, after exposure of, prevention of, 459*t*
Child abuse and neglect, 224
Children, optimizing care for, 897–900
Child-to-breastfeeding woman transmission (CBWT), HIV, 450–465
Chin, receding, 509, 509*f*
Chlamydial infections, 415, 776*t*
Chloramphenicol, on infant, 372, 376
Chloride (chlorine)
    maternal requirements for, 297*t*
    in milk, 121, 306*t*, 368–369, 765–767
        colostrum, 121
        maternal diet and, 303–304
        prepartum, 95, 96*f*, 96*t*
        preterm, 531, 541*t*
Chloride deficiency syndrome, 354–355
Chlorpromazine, 394, 866
    in induced lactation, 670, 671*t*
    lactation and, 353
Cholesterol, 288–291
    breast milk and, 215
    in infant serum, 768–769
    in milk, 108–109, 306*t*, 765–767
        colostrum, 98
    plasma, breastfeeding and, 356, 356*f*
ChooseMyPlate, 292*f*
Chromium
    infant requirements for, 534
    maternal requirements for, 297*t*
    in milk, 305, 765–767
Chronic fatigue syndrome, Epstein-Barr virus associated with, 432
Chylothorax, congenital, 514–515, 514–515*t*
Ciclopirox, for mucocutaneous candidiasis, 468
Cimetidine (Tagamet), 377
Ciprofloxacin, 377
Circadian variations, in milk composition, 93, 94*f*, 103–104
Circulus venosis, 44
Citrate in milk
    colostrum, 95, 99*f*
    secretion of, 86
Clearinghouse on Infant Feeding and Maternal Nutrition, 804
Cleft lip and/or palate, 509, 510*f*, 511*t*, 913–918
    breastfeeding and, 913–914
    frequently asked questions in, 916–917
    incidence of, 913
    recommendations, 914

Cleft lip and/or palate (*Continued*)
    for clinical practice, 914–915
    for future research, 915–916
    unilateral, 914*f*
Clindamycin, 378*t*, 570*t*
Clonidine, 369*t*
Closet nursing, 334–335
Clostridium botulinum, 414, 776*t*
Clostridium difficile, 776*t*
Clostridium perfringens, 776*t*
Clotrimazole, for mucocutaneous candidiasis, 468
Clove cigarettes, 604
Coach role, 207
Coagulase-negative *Staphylococcus*, 420–421
Cobalt, in milk, 765–767
Cocaine, 938
Coccidioides immitis, 776*t*
Codeine, 903
    milk and, 374
Co-feeding, 685–686
Cognitive development, 342–343, 219. *See also* Intelligence.
Cohosh, black and blue, 770–775
Colic, 274–280
    esophageal reflux and, 277
    smoking and, 603
Colitis, 488–489
Colon, disorders of, 514
Colostrum, 95–100, 99*f*, 100*f*. *See also* Human milk.
    antibacterial factors in, 163*t*
    bioactive factors in, 147*t*
    cellular components of, 151–155
    composition of, 95, 98*t*, 99*f*, 765–767
    preterm, 545, 546*t*
    secretion of, 75–76
    storage of, 719
    in tandem nursing, 708
Comfrey, 385–386, 388*t*, 770–775
Commercial discharge packs, 22–26
Community resources, 743–753
Complement
    defects of, 149–150, 149*b*
    in milk, 165
Complementary feedings, 831
Complementary foods, 341. *See also* Solid foods.
Computer data bank, 806
Computerized breast measurement (CBM), 79, 94–95
Condoms, 701, 702*t*
Conduct disorders, 206, 343
Congenital adrenal hyperplasia, 492
Congenital aganglionic megacolon, 514
Congenital chylothorax, 514–515, 514–515*t*
Congenital heart disease, 518
Congenital hip dislocation, 516
Congenital tuberculosis, 424
Conjunctivitis, 776*t*
Connective tissue disorders, 594–595
Contact, definition of, 455
Contact dermatitis of breast, 617–618
Contact precautions, 409
Containers
    milk collection and storage, 719
    storage, 861

Contraception, 694–704, 886–896
  advantages and disadvantages of, 886, 887t
  algorithms for, 695f, 701f
  emergency, 892–893
  issues in, 886
  medical eligibility criteria of, 894, 894t
  methods of, 887–889, 889t
    abstinence, 704
    barrier, 698, 702t, 704, 893
    effectiveness of, 887t
    hormonal, 699, 891
    implants and injections, 699–701, 700t
    intrauterine and other, 701–704
    IUDs, 893
    lactational amenorrhea, 693f, 695–697, 695–697f, 696t, 887–889, 888f
    milk yield, infant development, and, 700t
    natural family planning, 697–699, 697f, 891–893
    oral, 699
    transitioning to other, 889
  principles of, 887t
  research needs for, 894–895
  touch sensitivity and, 699
Contraceptives
  hormonal, 699, 702t, 889t, 891
    effectiveness of, 887t
  in induced lactation, 669
  oral, lactation and, 699
Contrast agent, 566
Copper
  infant requirements for, 534
  maternal requirements for, 297–298t
  in milk, 306t, 765–767
    fortified, 541–542t
    maternal diet and, 304–305
Corium, of areola, 42–43
Coronavirus
  Middle East respiratory syndrome, 455
  SARS-associated, 454–455, 776t
Corpus mammae, 38–41
  innervation of, 47
Corynebacterium diphtheriae, 415, 776t
Co-sleeping
  ABM guideline on, 199b, 851–855
  cultural tradition and, 198, 199b
  sudden infant death syndrome and, 30–31
Coumarins, 386
Counseling, 751
Covidien, 807
Cow milk
  allergies to, 633
    acute reactions to, 642–643
    clinical disease associated with, 641–642
    colitis and, 488–489
    immunologic aspects of, 639–640
  contamination of human milk with, 729
  diabetes and exposure to, 585
  influence of, in maternal diet, 275–276
C-reactive protein, 571
Creamatocrit, 551, 727
Creamatocrit Plus, 727
Creatine, in milk, 765–767

Creighton model system, natural family planning and, 891
Crohn disease, 489–491, 599–600
Cross-cradle position, 247, 247f
Cross-nursing, 685–686
Crying, 196
Cryptococcus neoformans, 776t
Cryptosporidiosis, 776t
Culture
  body contact and, 197–199, 198f
  breastfeeding duration and, 21–22
  co-sleeping and, 852
  rites of passage in, 743
Culturing breast milk, 409–410, 411b
  for mastitis, 571
Cup feeding, 484, 558–559
Cylindric breast pumps, 733f
Cystic fibrosis, 494–495, 495t, 589–590, 590t
Cysts, breast, 611
Cytokines, 168–173
  in milk, 167t
  nomenclature for, 168b
Cytologic examination of nipple discharge, 608
Cytomegalovirus (CMV), 776t
  transmission of, 412, 429–432
Cytosol, 82

D

Danbolt-Closs syndrome, 496
"Dancer hand" position, 908
"Dancer hold", 484, 484f, 511
DARLING (Davis Area Research on Lactation, Infant Nutrition, and Growth) Study, 111–112
Daycare, 661
Decision, of nursing during pregnancy, 709–710
Dehydration, 353–355
  hypernatremic, 354
Del Castillo syndrome, 576, 576t
Delivery
  cesarean, 563–565
    anesthesia for, 903
  labor and, 846
  mother-infant interaction at, 195, 196f
  nursing at, 244–246
Demographic factors, 13–16, 19t, 23–24t
Dengue fever, 432, 776t
Dental caries, 519
Depot medroxyprogesterone acetate (DMPA), 699, 700t
Depression, mothers experience of dimensions of, 209t
Dermatitis, 809–815
Developing countries, breastfeeding in, 10, 16–17t
Development. See also Growth.
  breastfeeding and, 205–206
  with feeding measure and risk ratio range, 30t
  weaning and, 322–323
Diabetes mellitus
  diet for, 580, 580f
  maternal, 578–580
    adjustment for, 581–585

Diabetes mellitus (Continued)
    breastfeeding and onset of, 582–585, 583–584t, 585f
Diaper candidiasis, 467
Diaphragm, contraceptive, 701, 702t
Diarrhea, 30t
  failure to thrive in, 348
  maternal, 776t
  protracted, management of, 489
  weanlings with, 332
Diathesis, hemorrhagic, coumarins and, 386
Diazepam, 374, 600t
Dicloxacillin, 378t, 570t
Diet, maternal, milk production and, 351–352
Dieting while breastfeeding, 313–314. See also Maternal nutrition.
Diffusion, of drug
  facilitated, 368
  passive, passage of drug and, 365
Digitalis, 392
Diphtheria, 415, 776t
Discharge packs, commercial, 22–26
Discharge planning, 880–882, 880t
Disease, with feeding measure and risk ratio range, 30t
Disease prevention objectives, 2t
Dissociation constant (pK$_a$), drug, 366, 367t
Diuretics
  for hypertension, 612
  lactation and, 674t
Docosahexaenoic (DHA), 102
Domperidone, 389, 865–866
  to enhance lactation, 486
  in induced lactation, 671t, 679
  for lactation, 264
  on milk production, 353
Donor human milk bank, 794, 796
Donor milk, 796, 411–412. See also Human milk, storage of; Milk bank.
  donor qualification for, 717–718, 717b
  frozen/thawed, 722t
  from milk bank, 715
  pasteurization of, 721
  for premature infant, 535b, 536, 538
  raw, standards for, 720–721
  reasons for prescribing, 794–795
Dopamine, 65, 690–691
Dose
  drug, in infant, 372
  schedule, for analgesics, 374–375
Dose-response relationship for milk, 148–149, 148b
Doulas, 207
  breastfeeding and, 231–232
  in labor and delivery, 846
Down syndrome, 497–498, 907
Doxycycline, 462–463
Drip milk, 536
Droplet precautions, 409
Drug abuse, 225t, 226
  milk and, 380–381
Drug-enhanced lactation, 264–265
Drugs. See also specific drug or drug class.
  anticholinergic, 377
  anticoagulant, 378–379
  antithyroid, 379

Drugs (*Continued*)
  caffeine and other methylxanthines, 379–380
  cardiovascular, 392–393
  for central nervous system, 393–394
  characteristics of, 365–369
  cholesterol-lowering, 393
  classification systems for, 374
  contraindicated for breastfeeding, 225t
  data, evaluating, 371–372
  diuretic, 392–393
  effect on nursing infant, 369–371, 370f
  food interactions with, 373
  galactorrhea from, 575
  gastrointestinal, 377–378
  groups, 374–402
  herbal, 381–388, 382t
  hyperprolactinemia from, 563
  to induce relactation, 682–683, 683t
  ionization of, 366, 367t
  for labor and delivery, 563
  mechanisms of transport of, 367
  in milk, 364–365
  milk/plasma ratio for, 367t, 371
  minimizing effect of, on maternal medication, 373
  molecular weight of, 367
  oral bioavailability of, 373
  prolactin secretion and, 65
  protein binding of, 365–369, 366f
  psychotherapeutic, 394–396
  safety of
    in infant, 372
    in pregnancy and lactation, 373
  schedule, for induced lactation, 669–675
  sensitization, 372–373
  solubility of, 367, 367t
  tocolytic, engorgement and, 563
  transdermal, 368–369, 369t
Ductal infection, 809–815
Dummies, 201–202, 201t
Dyphylline, 379–380
Dyspareunia, 705–706
Dysphoric milk ejection reflex, 626

E

Early Childhood Longitudinal Study-Birth Cohort, 659
Early Childhood Longitudinal Survey, Birth Cohort (ECLS-B), 11t
Early-onset GBS disease (EOD), 421
Eating disorders, 209
Ebola virus, 433, 776t
Echinacea, 382t, 386–387, 388t, 770–775
Econazole, for mucocutaneous candidiasis, 468
Eczema
  of breast, 271–272
  management of, 645–646
  prophylaxis of, 634–637, 635t, 638f
Edinburgh Postnatal Depression Scale (EPDS), 625b
Education on breastfeeding, 845–846
Ehrlichiosis, 776t
Eicosapentaenoic acid, 109–110

Ejection reflex
  failure of, psychological stress on, 352–353
  neuroendocrine control of, 70f
  oxytocin and, 72
Electric breast pumps, 718f, 731–732t, 733–740, 734t
Electrolytes, 354
Elimination diets, 642
Embryogenesis, 58–59
Embryonic development
  of breast, 34–35, 58–59
  gastrointestinal tract, 525, 526f
Emergency admission, maternal, 604–606
Emergency weaning, 330
Employment, breastfeeding and, 650–666
Empowerment, 220
Encephalitis, 776t
Endometritis, 776t
Energy supplementation, maternal, 287
Energy value of milk, 765–767, 306t. *See also* Caloric needs.
  colostrum, 95
  preterm, 531
Engorgement, 250–252, 933–936
  areolar, 250–251
  assessment of, 933
  cabbage leaves for, 252–253
  drug-associated, 563
  manual expressions in, 252
  peripheral, 251–252, 251f
  plugged duct or mastitis *vs.*, 568t
  prevention and treatment of, 934–935
  recommendations for future research, 935
Enterobacteriaceae infections, 776t
Enterocolitis, necrotizing. *See* Necrotizing enterocolitis (NEC).
Enteroviruses, 776t
Environmental contaminants, breastfeeding contraindications for, 225t
Enzyme therapy, for engorgement, 934
Enzymes, 135–140, 136t
  pancreatic, use of, 646–647
Ephedra, 382t, 388t
Epidermal growth factor (EGF), 141–142, 147t, 167t, 168–169
Epidural anesthesia, suckling ability and, 237–238
Epidural morphine, for cesarean delivery, 564
Epidural/spinal medications, 904
Epigenetics, genetics and, 178–180
Epilepsy, 600, 600t
Epithelial cells, in milk, 152
Epstein-Barr virus (EBV), 432–433, 776t
Ergot, 65
Ergot alkaloids, prolactin and, 674t
Erythema infectiosum, 776t
Erythrocyte rosette-forming cells, 152f, 154
Erythromycin, 376, 378t
  for mastitis, 570t
Escherichia coli
  maternal infection by, 776t
  microwave effect on, 729t

Escherichia coli (*Continued*)
  sIgA antibodies to, 154, 161t
Esophageal reflux, 277
  metoclopramide for, 673
Estradiol
  lactational infertility and, 689f, 690
  transdermal, 369t
Estradiol/norelgestromin, 369t
Estrogen-containing combined hormonal options, 889t, 892
Estrogens
  breast cancer and, 223
  in breast development
    embryogenesis in, 58
    mammogenesis in, 59–60
  contraceptives with, 700
  in induced lactation, 669–670
  lactogenesis and, 65
  maternal behavior and, 203
  prolactin release and, 52
Ethambutol, for tuberculosis, 424
Ethinyl estradiol, 670
Ethnic factors, 10–13, 12f. *See also* Culture.
Ethosuximide, 600t
Evening primrose, 601, 770–775
Excited ineffectives, 257
Exclusive breastfeeding, 10, 16t, 147t
  atopic disease and, 638
  on blood pressure, 358
  definition of, 645, 856
  duration of, 342
  failure to thrive in, 350
  HIV infection and, 448
  prolonged, 350
Excretion, drug, in milk, 369
Exercise, 311–313, 313f
Expertise issues, 758–759
Extremely low-birth-weight (ELBW) infants, 879, 525, 527–528. *See also* Low-birth-weight (LBW) infants.

F

"Face on" straddle position, 915
Facilitated diffusion, drug transport and, 368
Failure to thrive
  anatomic causes of, 350–351
  definition of, 344–350, 344t, 346f
  dehydration, hypernatremia, or hypochloremia in, 353–355
  diagnosis of, 345
  evaluation of, 346–349, 347b
  maternal causes of, 350, 351f
  no obvious cause of, 353
  observation of nursing process in, 349–350
  prolonged exclusive breastfeeding and, 350
  psychosocial, 350–355
  slow gaining *vs.*, 345–346, 345b
Fair Labor Standards Act (FLSA), 650
Family
  impact of, 205
  nuclear, 743
Family planning. *See* Contraception.
Family practitioners, 26

Fat, 84. *See also* Lipids.
  in American diet, 105
  body, of infant, 370
  distribution in milk, 98t
  mammary, 40–41, 41f
  maternal requirements for, 296t
  in milk, 765–767
    circadian variations in, 103–104
    colostrum, 98
    intake, failure to thrive and, 351
    maternal diet and, 288–291
    mature, 108
    preterm, 531, 537t
    switch-nursing and, 345–346
  in milk fortifiers, 541–542t
  for premature infant, 532
Fat necrosis, of breast, 611
Fathers
  breastfeeding and, 227
  impact of breastfeeding on, 206–207
  lactation induction in, 676
Fatigue, 657, 660
  on milk supply, 352
Fatty acids
  in fortifiers, 540
  in milk, 306t, 765–767
    maternal diet and, 288–291
    mature, 109–110
    pasteurization and, 722t
  N-3, 109–110
  omega-3, 108, 532
Fear of failure, 210
Federation of American Societies for
    Experimental Biology, 762
Feedback inhibitor of lactation
    (FIL), 78
Feeding Infants and Toddlers Study
    (FITS), 324–325
Feeding skills disorder, 347
Feedings. *See also* Artificial feeding; Bottle
    feeding; Nursing; Suckling;
    Supplementary feedings.
  cup, 484, 558–559
  early, impact of, 644–645
  frequency of, 266–267
  one-breast/two-breast, 267–268, 351
  for small-for-gestational-age infant,
    347
  supplementary, 272–273
  tube, 555, 557–558, 557f
Feminism, 207
Fennel, 770–775
Fentanyl, 369t
  for labor, 238, 902
  postpartum use of, 903
Fentanyl citrate, 375
Fenugreek, 390, 770–775, 866–867
  allergies to, 643
  in induced lactation, 671t
Fertility, 688–694
  birth interval and, 693–694, 694t
  conception possibility and, 692, 692t
  lactational, 688–690, 689–690f
  menses return in, 691–692
  milk composition and, 692–693
  prolactin, dopamine and, 690–691
Fetal alcohol syndrome, 940–941
Fetal development
  of breast, 35–37
  of gastrointestinal tract, 525–526, 537t

Fetal development (*Continued*)
    weight gain and nutrients in, 534t
Fetal distress, 483–485, 484–485f
Fever, milk, 330–332
Feverfew, 388t, 770–775
Fiber, dietary, 296t
Fibroadenomas, of breast, 611
Fibrocystic disease, 610–611
Filoviridae, 433–434
Financial aspects, of milk banks, 729–730
Finger sucking, 201t
First-arch disorders, 509, 509f
Fish, 291–292
Fish oil supplements, 109, 646
Flagyl, 376
Flaviviridae, 428
Fluconazole, 572
  for candidal infections, 468
Fluoride (fluorine), 125t, 126–127
  maternal requirements for, 297t
  in milk, 305, 306t, 765–767
Fluoroquinolones, 377
Fluticasone, 380
Flutter sucking, 349
Folacin, 131–132t, 134–135
Folic acid (folate)
  maternal requirements for,
    295t, 298t
  in milk, 300t, 306t, 765–767
    maternal diet and, 300
Food additives, 315
Food adverse reaction, 641
Food allergies, 641
  prophylaxis of, 635t, 638f
  symptoms of, 641
Food anaphylaxis, 641
Food and Consumer Service
    (FCS), 9
Food and Nutrition Information Center,
    803
Food intolerance, 641
Food toxicity (poisoning), 641, 776t
Food-drug interactions, 373
Foods, solid. *See* Solid foods.
"Football hold", 484, 915
Forbes-Albright syndrome, 576, 576t
Foremilk, 315
Formula. *See also* Artificial feeding; Bottle
    feeding.
  advertising of, 1, 24–25
  for atopic disease, 639
  for cystic fibrosis, 494–495, 495t
  human milk *vs.*, 751t
  policy on, 3
  probiotic bacteria in, 175–177
Formula-fed infants, obesity in, 355
Fortifiers, milk
  artificial, 540–543, 541–542t, 542f
  composition of, 541t
  human milk, 543, 544t
Freezing milk, 724
  effect of, 725t
  nutritional consequences of, 725–726
Frenotomy, 874–877, 877f
Fresh-frozen milk, 796
Fresh-raw milk, 796
Frozen milk, 862
Fruit juice excess, failure to thrive and, 350
Fucose intolerance, 488
Full breastfeeding, 148–149, 148b

Fungi, antibodies for, 160–162, 176–177
  Candida infections, 467–469
Furosemide, 392

G

Gadolinium, 401–402
Galactocele, 269
Galactogogues, 388–391, 770–775,
    864–868, 872
  to enhance lactation, 485–486
  herbal/natural, 866–867
  indications for, 864
  in induced lactation, 670
  mother's milk tea as, 385, 385t
  natural, 866–867
  procedure for, 864–865
  specific, 865–867
Galactography, 569f, 611, 611f
Galactopoiesis, 62
  lactation maintenance in, 70, 70f
  mammary gland in, 53
Galactorrhea, 574–575, 668
  drug-associated, 563
  induced lactation *vs.*, 668
  milk composition in, 675, 675t
  neonatal, 499
Galactosemia, 492, 591
  failure to thrive in, 348
GALT (gut-associated lymphoid tissue),
    150, 151f
Gangliosides, 165, 166t
Garlic, 314–315, 382t, 770–775
  infant's first flavor and, 325
Gastric by-pass surgery, 616
Gastric emptying, 526, 526b
Gastroesophageal reflux (GER), 512–513
Gastrointestinal commensal organisms,
    177–178, 177b
Gastrointestinal diseases
  bleeding, 516
  celiac, Crohn's, and inflammatory
    bowel disease, 489–491
  colitis, 488–489
  lactose intolerance, 489
Gastrointestinal medications, 377–378
Gastrointestinal tract, infant
  drug absorption from, 369–371
  premature, 537–538, 537t
    development of, 525–526, 526b,
      526–527f
    priming, 526–528, 527–529b, 529t,
      529f, 554–555
Gender Equality Index, 650
Genetic tests, buccal smears for, 487
Genetics and epigenetics, 178–180
Gentian violet, 572
Gestational diabetes, 582
Giardia lamblia, 463–464
Giardiasis, 463–464, 776t
Gigantomastia, 611–613, 612–613f, 934
Ginkgo, 382t, 386, 770–775
Ginseng, 382t, 387, 770–775
Gliadin, 643
Globulins, in infant serum, 768–769
Glomerular disease, 597
Glucose. *See also* Hypoglycemia.
  in milk, 306t
Glucose monitoring, in neonates,
    817–824, 818–821t

Glucose-6-phosphate dehydrogenase, 137
Glucose-6-phosphate dehydrogenase deficiency, 500–501
Gluten, 489–490, 643
Glycans, 165–167, 166t
Glycoconjugates, in human milk, 118–119
Glycogen storage disease type II, 494
Glycolipids, 165
Goat's rue, 770–775, 867
Goldenseal, 388t
Gonococcal infections, 415–417
Gonorrhea, 415–416, 776t
Gourmets, 257
Government agencies, 803–804
Government organizations, 746–747
Gradual weaning, 332–333, 333t
  vs. abrupt, 333
Granulomatous mastitis, idiopathic, 574
Grape seed, 770–775
Grapefruit seed extract, 770–775
Graves disease, 585, 588t
Green milk, 316
Grief, 210–211
Group A Streptococcus (GAS), 421, 776t
Group B Streptococcus (GBS), 421–423, 422f, 776t
Growth
  brain, 339–340, 535–537
  of breastfed infant, 340
    charts for measurement of, 797–802
    cognitive and motor development in, 342–343
    international growth charts for, 340–341
    maternal smoking and, 603, 603f
    prolonged breastfeeding and, 342
    small-for-gestational age and, 342
    weaning foods and, 341–342
  failure of. See Failure to thrive.
  fortified milk and, 540, 541t
  long-term follow-up of, 543–545, 545b
  milk and, hormones in, 360t
  normal, 338–343
  optimal, 530, 530f, 531t
  postdischarge assessment of, 559, 559t
  of premature infant, 530, 879–880, 880t
  requirements for, 532–535, 533–534t, 533b
Growth hormone (GH), 866
  concentrations, in postpartum women, 261f
  embryogenesis of breast and, 58
  to enhance lactation, 485–486
  in induced lactation, 670, 671t, 674t
  mammogenesis and, 59–60
  prolactin and, 69
Guanarito virus, 429
Guilt, 1, 194–195, 210–211
Gut-associated lymphoid tissue (GALT), 150, 151f

H
Haemophilus influenzae, 416, 776t
Hammurabi's Code, 6
Hand expression. See Manual expression.

Hand pumps, 731–733, 735–736t, 738t
Hantavirus, 776t
Hazelbaker scale, assessment tool for ankyloglossia, 875, 875t
Head circumference, 797–802
  of infant, 339–340
Headache, lactational, 619
Health care professionals. See also specific profession.
  attitudes of, 26, 653–654, 654t
Health care team
  lactation specialist in, 749
  peer counselor in, 750
Health Education Associates, 804
Healthy Children, 5
Healthy People 2010, 754
Healthy People 2020 goals, 2, 2t
Healthy start, 663
Heart disease, congenital, 518
Heart transplantation, 596
Heat-processed milk, 796
  immunoglobulins in, 162
Height measurement, 797–802
Hematomas, of breast, 611
Hemoglobin, 163t
Hemorrhagic fevers, 429, 776t
Heparin, 378, 566–567
Hepatitis
  differential diagnosis of, 434
  maternal, 434–441, 434b, 435f, 436t, 776t
    diagnostic approach to, 435f
    types of, 436t
  misadministration of milk and, 412–413
  terminology for, 434b
  TT virus and, 456
Hepatitis A, 434–435, 434b, 435f, 436t
Hepatitis B, 434b, 435f, 436–437, 436t
Hepatitis C, 434b, 435f, 436t, 437–439
  transmission, mechanisms of, 438
Hepatitis D, 434b, 435f, 436t, 439
Hepatitis E, 434b, 435f, 436t, 439
Hepatitis G, 434b, 436t, 439–440
Hepatocyte growth and scatter factor (HGF/SF), 59, 59f
Herbal preparation, in breast milk, 364–406
Herbs and herbal teas, 381–388, 382–383t, 385b, 770–775
  for engorgement, 935
  in induced lactation, 669
  mother's milk tea, 385, 385t
Heredity in atopic disease, 634
Heregulin, 59, 59f
Heroin, milk and, 374
Herpes gestationis, 617
Herpes simplex virus, 440, 617, 776t
Herpes viruses, 776t
  Herpes simplex virus, 440
  Herpes Herpesvirus 6 and Human Herpesvirus 7, 440–441
  Herpes Zoster, 617
Highly active antiretroviral therapy (HAART), 449
High-temperature short-time (HTST) pasteurization, 721–722, 723t
  donor milk and, 411
  stability of immunoglobulins, 162

Hindmilk, 315
Hip dislocation, congenital, 516
Hirschsprung's disease, 514
Histone modification, 179
Histoplasmosis, 776t
HIV. See Human immunodeficiency virus (HIV).
Holder pasteurization, 162, 721–722
  donor milk and, 411
Holding infants, 484, 484f
Hollister Incorporated, 807
Honey, botulism and, 414
Hookworm infection, 464
Hormonal contraceptive method, 891
  progestin-only pills vs. COCs, 892
Hormones, 138–140, 139t, 139t. See also Contraceptives, hormonal; specific hormone.
  galactopoiesis and, 70
  gastrointestinal trophic, 526–527
  in induced lactation, 669
  lactation control by, 57–58, 57t, 64f
    embryogenesis and, 58
    lactogenesis and, 62, 63f
    mammogenesis and, 59–60
    prolactin and oxytocin in, 71–72, 71f
  lactational infertility and, 688, 689f
  maternal behaviors and, 203
  in milk, 360t
    bioactive, 147t
    protein, 138–140, 139t
Hospitalization, maternal, 604–607
Hospitals
  baby-friendly initiative for, 4–5, 5b, 745
  breastfeeding policies for, 760b
  childbirth training in, 745
  detrimental routines, 26
  discharge from, 825–830, 826–827t
  guidelines for use of supplementary feeding for, 831–839, 832–834t, 836t
  transitioning premature infant to home from, 556–557
Hot flashes, 705
Human chorionic gonadotropin (hCG), 62f
Human growth hormone. See Growth hormone (GH).
Human herpesvirus 6, 440–441, 776t
Human herpesvirus 7, 440–441
Human immunodeficiency virus (HIV)
  child-to-breastfeeding woman transmission, 450–465
  formula distribution for, 3
  hepatitis C and, 437–439
  maternal, 450, 776t
  misadministration of milk and, 412–413
  standard precautions for, 408
  type 1, 446–450
    antiretroviral prophylaxis for, 449–450
    breastfeeding with, 447–448
    early weaning and, 448–449
    maternal health and, 450
    transmission of, 446–447

Human immunodeficiency virus (HIV)
(*Continued*)
type 2, 452
Human mammary tumor virus (HMTV),
457
Human milk, 1. *See also* Colostrum;
Donor milk.
active transport mechanism in, 368
analysis of, 726–727
antibiotics in, 376–377
benefits of, 8
allergy prophylaxis, 217
evidence-based systematic reviews
of, 218–219, 218–219t
immunologic benefits, 146–148
immunologic protection, 217
infection protection, 216–217
nutritional, 214–215
psychological/cognitive, 217–220
species specificity, 214
"best practice guidance" and, 422–423
bioactive, 147t, 150
biochemistry of, 91–145
chloride ions and, 368–369
collection of, 712–742
technique for, 718–719
color of, 315–316
comparison of formula and, 92f
components of, 91–145, 765–767
see also specific component.
bioactive, 527f
cellular, 151–155
gradual weaning and, 332–333, 333t
heat treatment and, 721–722
induced lactation and, 675–676,
675–676f, 675t
in ovulatory menstrual cycle,
692–693
storage container type and, 720t
storage temperature and, 726t
thermal destruction and, 726t
in transitional milk, 100–101
constituents of, 6, 306t
contraceptive agents and, 700
culturing, 409–410, 411b
data on, 1
from days 1 through 36 postpartum,
98t
drug concentrations in, 368
distribution ratios of, 367t
effectiveness of, in controlling
infection, 180–182
expression of. *See* Milk expression.
factors in, passage of drugs, 365
formula *vs.*, 751t
free amino acid concentrations in, 111f
herbal preparations in, 364–406
historical perspective on, 712–714
host-resistance factors and
immunologic significance,
146–193, 147t
immunoglobulin stability and, 162
infectious disease, transmission of,
407–482
lactation cycle and, 94–95, 95f
mammalian milk *vs.*, 101
maternal diet and. *See* Maternal
nutrition.
mature, 101–110, 765–767
lipids in, 102–108

Human milk (*Continued*)
medications in, 364–406
misadministration of, 412–413
natural products in, 364–406
nonantibody, antiviral, and
antiprotozoan factors in, 182t
normal variations in, 92–94, 93–94f
passage of drugs in, steps in, 369
for premature infants, 538
fortification of, 540–543, 541–542t,
542f
LBW or SGA, 552–553
production of, 549–552, 551f, 552b
supplementation of, 538–540
preterm
composition of, 541t
properties of, 530–537, 530b, 531f,
545–548, 546–547f, 546b, 546t,
548t
production of
improving, 557. *See also*
Galactogogues.
maternal diet and, 286–307, 288t
prolactin, 80
as prophylaxis, 633–649
regulation of, 67
sharing of, 715
smoking and, 603f
storage of, 712–742, 794–796, 795t
ABM protocol for, 861–863
containers for, 719, 720t, 861
cow milk contamination in, 729
creamatocrit and, 727
environmental conditions in, 724
general guidelines for, 861–862
heat treatment for, 721
lyophilization and freezing in, 724,
725t
microwave effects on, 728,
728–729t
nutritional consequences of,
725–726, 726t
raw donor, standards for, 720–721
sour milk following, 729
specialty milks and, 728–729
testing of samples in, 720
ultrasonic homogenization for,
727–728
viruses in, 723–724, 724t
supply of
protection of, 909–910
stress and, 657
synthesis of, 79–81, 79f
in transitional milk, 100–101
tumor virus in, 456–458
volume of, 737f
changes in, 93, 93f
colostrum and, 95
maternal diet and, 286
water in, 101, 102t
Human milk bank, 794
Human Milk Banking Association of
North America (HMBANA),
713, 794
Human milk oligosaccharides (HMO),
453
Human milk storage information,
861–863
Human papillomavirus, 441–450, 776t
Human parvovirus B19, 443–444, 776t

Human placental lactogen,
mammogenesis and, 69–70
Human serum prolactin (hPRL) levels,
737f
Human T-cell leukemia virus type I
(HTLV-I)
breastfeeding with, 225t, 226
transmission of, 444–446, 445t
Human T-cell leukemia virus type II
(HTLV-II), transmission of, 446
Human T-cell leukemia viruses (HTLV),
maternal infection by, 776t
Humoral factors in milk, 147t, 156–162
Hydrocodone, 903
Hydromorphone, 903
Hygiene, good, maternal, 843
Hyperadenia, 39b, 40
Hyperandrogenic anovulation, 588–589
Hyperbilirubinemia and jaundice,
499–508
AAP guideline for, 504
bilirubin production in, 500
breast milk-related, 505–506
concern about, 500
determining cause of, 501–502
evaluation and management of,
500–501
kernicterus in, 505–507
risk factors for, 502–504, 502t, 503f
treatment of early, 503–504, 503f,
504b, 504t, 505f, 506b
Hypergalactia, 565
Hyperlipidemia, 220–221
Hyperlipoproteinemia, 108
Hypermastia, 39
Hypernatremia, 353–355, 498–499
breastfed infants and, 354
Hyperplasia, breast, 39–40, 40b
Hyperprolactinemia, 575, 576b
Hypertension, 597
Hyperthelia, 39
Hyperthyroidism
maternal, 587–588, 588t
in neonate, 348
Hypochloremia, failure to thrive and,
353–355
Hypoglycemia
maternal diabetes and, 581
in neonates, 817–818
clinical manifestations of, 819–820,
820t
definition of, 818–819, 818t
documented, management of,
821–822, 821t
general management
recommendation for, 820–822,
820t
maternal diabetes and, 579
physiology of, 817–818
postmature, 483
recommendations for future
research, 822–823
risk factors for, 819, 820t
supporting the mother, 822
testing methods for, 819
small-for-gestational-age, 555–556
Hypomagnesemia, 598–599
Hypomastia, 40
Hypopituitarism, 576–577
Hypoplasia, breast, 39–40, 39–40b

Hypoprolactinemia, 355
Hypothyroidism
  in infants, 498
  maternal, 586–587
Hypotonia, definition of, 907
Hypotonic infant, breastfeeding, 907–912
  assessment of, 908–909
  background of, 907–908
  discharge period, 910
  education in, 908
  facilitation of, 908–909
  goal for, 907
  neonatal period, 910
  procedures of, 908–910
Hypoxia, fetal, 483–485, 484–485f

I

Ibuprofen, 375, 905
Idiopathic granulomatous mastitis, 574
Illnesses. See also Infants, with problems; Maternal complications.
  with feeding measure and risk ratio range, 30t
  life-threatening, breastfeeding and, 226
  maternal, on milk production, 352
  work absenteeism and, 658, 658f
Immune system
  developmental deficiencies in, 149–150, 149b
  enteromammary, 636, 636f
Immunization, 402–403
Immunoglobulin A (IgA, sIgA)
  cow milk allergy and, 640
  in milk, 159f, 161t, 306t, 765–767
    allergy and, 635
    bioactivity of, 150
  in mucosal immune system, 150
  specificity of, 160–162, 161t
Immunoglobulin E (IgE)
  allergy and, 634, 636t
  in milk, 158
Immunoglobulin G (IgG)
  cow milk allergy and, 640
  in milk, 163t, 306t
    bioactivity of, 150
  specificity of, 160–162, 161t
Immunoglobulin M (IgM)
  cow milk allergy and, 640
  in milk, 163t, 306t
    bioactivity of, 150
  specificity of, 160–162, 161t
  in mucosal immune system, 150
Immunoglobulins, 156–160
  in colostrum, 98, 114–115
  developmental deficiencies in, 149–150, 149b
  infection and, 226
  in milk, 161t
    maternal diet and, 308
  specificity of, 160–162, 161t
  stability of, 162
Immunologic benefits of human milk, 146–148
  bioactive factors in, 147t, 150
  cellular components in, 151–155
    B-cell system, 151f, 155
    leukocytes, 152

Immunologic benefits of human milk (Continued)
    lymphocytes, 153
    macrophages, 152–153
    stem cells, 155–156
    survival of, 155–156
    T-cell system, 153–155
  developmental immune deficiencies and, 149–150, 149b
  dose-response relationship in, 148–149, 148b
  humoral factors in, 156–162
    antipathogenic, 166t
    bifidus factor, 162–163
    complement, 165
    glycans and oligosaccharide, 165–167
    immunoglobulins, 156–160, 157–158f, 158t, 160f
    interferon, 165
    interleukins, 167–168, 167t
    lactoferrin, 158f, 164–165
    lysozyme, 158f, 163
    nucleotides, 169–173
    resistance factor, 163
    vitamin B_{12}-binding protein, 165
  maternal nutrition and, 308
  mucosal immune system in, 173–174
    gastrointestinal organisms in, 177–178
    lymphoid tissue in, 174–175
    microbiota, probiotics, and prebiotics in, 175–177
    toll-like receptors in, 175
  overview of, 146–148
  protective effect in, 148
Immunoreactive prolactin, 67f
Imperforate anus, 515–516
Impetigo, 616–617, 776t, 809–815
Implants
  breast, 614
  contraceptive, 699–701, 700t, 702t
Imprinting, 201–202, 201t
Induced lactation, 667–687, 668–679. See also Galactogogues.
  animal studies on, 668
  antihypertensive drugs for, 674t
  co-feeding and, 685–686
  composition of milk in, 675–676, 675t, 675–676f
  cross-nursing and, 685–686
  drug schedules for, 669–675, 671t
  historical perspective on, 667–668
  inappropriate lactation vs., 668
  management of mother and infant in, 676–678
  nutritional supplementation in, 678
  postmenopausal, 678–679
  preparation of breast in, 669
  protocols for, 679
  same-sex couple and, 678
  special devices for, 683–685
  support systems for, 679, 684f
  wet nursing and, 685–686
Infant botulism, 414
Infant Care, 7–8
Infant factors, bed sharing and, 853
Infant Feeding Practices Survey II (IFPSII), 11t, 19t

Infant mortality, 26. See also Sudden infant death syndrome (SIDS).
  bed sharing and, 851–852
  in developing countries, 148
Infant-initiated weaning, 329–330
Infants. See also Neonates; Premature infants.
  ankyloglossia in, 271, 271b, 272f
  aspiration in, clinical signs of potential, 244
  benefits of breastfeeding, 214–229
    abuse/neglect protection, 224
    allergy prophylaxis, 217
    breast cancer risk and, 223
    evidence-based systematic reviews of, 218–219, 218–219t
    immunologic protection, 217
    infection protection, 216–217
    nutritional, 214–215
    psychological/cognitive, 217–220
    species specificity, 214
  body composition of, drugs and, 370, 370f
  bottle-fed, feeding frequency of, 267
  breast rejection by, 270
    unilateral, 271
  breastfed
    and artificially fed, 28
    by birth, cohort and race-ethnicity, 12f, 21f
    cognitive and motor development and, 342–343
    colic in, 275–276
    esophageal reflux in, 277
    growth of, 340
    hypernatremia and, 354
    international growth charts for, 340–341
    normal, 338–343
    prolonged breastfeeding and, 342
    small-for-gestational-age, 342
    stool patterns for, 278, 278t
    total energy intake and, 324
    voiding and stooling in, 260
    vomiting of blood in, 260–265
    weaning foods and, 341–342
  breastfeeding, with cleft lip and/or palate, 916–917
  carrying/holding, 197–198, 274
  by cesarean delivery, breastfeeding on, 238
  chemicals and, 400–401, 400t
  colic and crying in, 274–280
  colicky behavior in, management of, 276–277
    sleep tight method in, 277
  colicky/crying, 603
  death rate per 100, 27f
  drugs on. See also Drugs.
    ability to detoxify and excrete agent, 370–371, 370f
    effects of, 369–371
    safety for, 372
  esophageal reflux in, 277
  extremely low-birth-weight, 879
  feeding. See also Feedings.
    characteristics of, 257–258
    revolution in, 1–33
  formula-fed, obesity in, 355
  growth of, measurement of, 797–802

Infants (*Continued*)
 health of, nursing in pregnancy and,
  708–709
 hormonal contraceptives and, 700,
  700*t*
 hypothyroidism, 586–587
 hypotonic, 907–912
 immune deficiencies in, 149–150,
  149*b*
 immunization for, 402
 impact of breastfeeding on, 205
 LBW, 528–530
 management of, in induced lactation,
  676–678
 maternal diabetes and, 581–585
 maternal interaction with, 195, 196*f*
 milk storage for, 795*b*
 near-term, breastfeeding, 869–873,
  873*t*
 need, for weaning, 320–322
 neurologically impaired, 496
 nursing bottle caries in, 519
 nutrition for, 1, 214–215
 obesity in, 355–361, 359*t*
 optimizing care for, 897–900
 oral health in, 519
 pacifiers for, 277–278
 percentage of, 27*f*
 peripartum breastfeeding management
  for, 845–850
 premature, 524–525
  breastfeeding mothers of, support
   for, 883–884
  growth of, 879–880, 880*t*
  NICU to home transition for,
   879–885, 880*t*, 884*f*
  nutritional assessment, optimal *vs.*
   suboptimal, 880
 with problems, 483–523 *see also*
   specific problem.
  acrodermatitis enteropathica, 496
  adrenal hyperplasia, 498
  α_1-antitrypsin deficiency, 495
  buccal smears for, 487
  central nervous system
   malformations, 516–517
  congenital heart disease, 518
  congenital hip dislocation, 516
  cystic fibrosis, 494–495, 495*t*
  Down syndrome, 497–498
  fetal distress, hypoxia and low
   Apgar scores, 483–485, 484–485*f*
  full-term, 487–494
  gastrointestinal disease, 487–488
  hyperbilirubinemia and jaundice,
   499–508, 502*t*, 503*f*, 504*b*, 504*t*,
   505*f*, 506*b*, 507*f*
  hypernatremia, 498–499
  hypothyroidism, 498
  mastitis, 499
  medical, 487–494
  metabolic, 492, 494–508
  neonatal breasts and nipple
   discharge, 499
  oral defects, 511–512
  otitis media, 491–492, 516
  postmaturity and, 483–486
  requiring surgery, 508–518
  respiratory illness, 491–492
  suckling, 508

Infants (*Continued*)
  sudden infant death syndrome and,
   518–519
   twins and triplets, 486–487, 486*f*
 serum values for, 768–769
 signs of hunger in, 246*b*
 sleeping by, 199*b*
 small-for-gestational-age, growth of,
  342
 of smoking mother, 602–604
 supplementation of, 311
 weaning. *See* Weaning.
 weight loss in, 258–260, 258*t*, 259*f*
 weight of. *See* Weight.
Infection control, 408–412
 for clinical syndromes and conditions,
  413
 culturing breast milk for, 409–410,
  411*b*
 for misadministration of milk,
  412–413
Infections
 acute, failure to thrive and, 348
 chronic, failure to thrive and, 348
 on milk production, 352
Infectious disease
 breastfeeding contraindications for,
  224–226, 225*t*
 protection against, 5–6, 177*b*, 180,
  181–182*t*, 185–186, 216–217
  preterm milk and, 545
 transmission of, 407–482
  bacterial, 413–415
  candidal, 467–469
  chlamydial, 415
  gonococcal, 415–417
  meningococcal, 417
  parasitic, 463–465
  spirochetal, 462–463
  staphylococcal, 417
  streptococcal, 421–428
  viral, 428–434
Infectious mononucleosis, 776*t*
Infertility. *See* Fertility.
Inflammation, protection against, 150
Inflammatory bowel disease, 489–491
Influenza, 776*t*
Injections, contraceptive, 699–701, 700*t*,
  702*t*
Innervation, of breast, 47–49
Innocenti Declaration, 747–748
Insufficient milk syndrome, 278–279,
  279*t*
Insulin, for maternal diabetes, 578
Insulin-like growth factor 1, in breast
  development, 58
Integrins, 59–60
Intelligence
 breastfeeding and, 218, 342
 phenylketonuria and, 494*f*
 premature infant and, 535–537
Interagency Group for Action on
  Breastfeeding, 20–21
Intercellular junctions, lactation
  and, 366
Intercostal nerves, 47
Interferon, 165
Interleukins, 167–168, 167*t*
International Board Certified Lactation
  Consultant (IBCLC), 749

International Board of Lactation
  Consultant Examiners (IBLCE),
  749, 807
International Childbirth Education
  Association (ICEA), 8, 744, 804
International Lactation Consultants
  Association, 661–662, 749, 804
International Nutrition Communication
  Service, 803
International Society for Research
  in Human Milk and
  Lactation, 762
Intestinal flora
 allergy and, 640–641
 bifid bacteria in, 162
Intestinal permeability, 538, 641–642
Intimacy, 207–208
Intrauterine devices (IUDs), 701–704,
  702*t*, 889*t*, 893
Intravenous medications, 903
Inverted nipple, 240, 240*f*, 242
 surgical correction in, 243
Involution
 postlactation mammary, 615, 615*f*
 postlactation regression of mammary
  gland, 54
Iodine (iodide), 127, 592
 infant requirements for, 534
 maternal requirements for,
  297–298*t*
 in milk, 306*t*, 765–767
  maternal diet and, 305
 milk and, 379
Ionization, drug, 366, 367*t*
Ions and water, 85–86
Iron
 in human milk, 121–122*t*, 123–124
 infant requirements for, 534
 lactoferrin and, 164
 maternal requirements for, 297–298*t*
 in milk, 306*t*, 765–767
  fortified, 541*t*
  maternal diet and, 304
 in weaning foods, 341
Isoniazid, 424–425

J

Jackson, Edith, 8, 743
Jaundice. *See also* Hyperbilirubinemia and
  jaundice.
 in failure to thrive, 347–348
John Paul II, Pope, 31
Junin virus, 429, 776*t*
Juvenile rheumatoid arthritis, 30*t*

K

Kanamycin, 376
Kangaroo care, 485, 549, 549*f*, 908
 and skin to skin, 548–549, 549*b*
Kava, 382*t*, 770–775
Kernicterus, 500
Ketamine, 904
Ketoconazole, for candidal infections,
  468
Ketorolac, 905
Ketorolac tromethamine, 376
"Knock-out mouse", 31
Koop, C. Everett, 2–3, 746

L

La Leche League International, Inc., 804
Labor
  analgesia and anesthesia for, 901–903
  breastfeeding management at, 846
  induced, nipple stimulation to,
      242–243
  medications during, 237–238
  preterm, 563
  risk of, 709
Labor force, working mothers and, 650,
      651–652f
Lact-Aid International, Inc., 804, 807
Lact-Aid Nursing Trainer System, 669,
      684f
Lact-Aid supplementer, 354
Lactalbumin, 113–114
α-Lactalbumin
  lactogenesis and, 62
  in milk, 306t, 765–767
Lactase, 489
Lactation, 888. *See also* Induced lactation;
      Relactation.
  alcohol and, 380
  anthropometric changes in, 289t
  breast in, 56, 57t
    apoptosis of, 56–57, 87
    hemodynamic changes in, 72–75,
      73–74f
    involution after, 80, 615, 615f
    size and weight, 38
  contraceptive methods during, 889t
  curriculum
    for medical students, 758
    for nurses' training, 759–762
  cycles of, 94–95, 95f
  delay in, 79
  dermatologic medication and, 402
  drug-enhanced, 264–265. *See also*
      Galactogogues.
  drugs in
    distribution pathways for, 366f
    safety of, 373
  failure of, 350–351, 355, 566
  fundamental mammary unit, 72f
  glomerular disease and, 597
  herbal teas, safe during, 385b
  hormonal control of, 57–58, 57t, 64f
    embryogenesis and, 58–59, 59f
    feedback inhibitor in, 57b, 76f, 78
    galactopoiesis and, 70, 70f
    lactogenesis and, 62–63, 63f
    mammogenesis and, 59–60
    oxytocin level in milk and, 70
    prostaglandins and, 77–78
  hypomagnesemia in, 598–599
  inappropriate, 668
  induced, 667–687, 668–679. *See also*
      Induced lactation.
  intracellular hormonal signaling in the
      lactocyte during, 81f
  maternal adaptation to, 78–79
  metoclopramide for, 353
  "milk coming in" sense in, 75–76
  milk synthesis in, 79–81, 79f
    carbohydrates in, 83–84
    cellular components in, 86
    enzymes in, 86
    fat in, 84
    ions and water, 85–86

Lactation (*Continued*)
    protein in, 84–85
    secretory cells in, 80
  milk volumes in, 87, 88f
  physiology of, 56–90
  reproductive function in, 688–711
  suckling effects on, 76–77, 76f
  suppression, 391–392
  thyrotropin-releasing hormone (TRH)
      effects on, 353
Lactation consultants, 749
  examination and certification
      of, 807
  physician working with, 752
  postgraduate learning opportunities
      for, 761
Lactation management self-study
      modules, 761b
Lactation problems
  infant risk factors for, 827t
  maternal risk factors for, 826t
Lactation specialist, of health care team,
      749
Lactation Study Center, 488, 806
Lactation supplementer, 556, 559
Lactation support, 14t
Lactational amenorrhea method (LAM),
      693f, 695–697, 695–697f, 696t,
      887–889, 888f, 889t
  efficacy of, 888
  management issues of, 888–889
  method of, 887–888, 888f
  use of, definitions for, 888
Lactational infertility, 688–690,
      689–690f
  breastfeeding, birth interval and,
      693–694
  conception risk during, 692, 692t
  prolactin and dopamine in,
      690–691
Lactic and malic acid dehydrogenases,
      137–138
Lactiferous ducts, 41f
  development of, 72
  plugging of, 568t
  ramification of, 38f
Lactiferous sinuses, 36, 43–44
LactMed, on drugs, used during
      lactation, 364
Lacto engineering, 539
Lactobacillus, 162–163
Lactobacillus acidophilus, 468–469
Lactoferrin
  bioactivity of, 163t
  biologic role of, 164
  concentration of, 164
  in milk, 114, 158t, 306t, 765–767
    colostrum, 96–98
  stability of, 162
Lactogenesis, 70
  changes in mammary gland function
      during, 88f
  delay in the onset of, 79
  delayed or inhibited, 279t
  galactopoiesis in, 70, 70f
  mammary gland development in, 53
  milk composition during, 99
  placental lactogen and growth
      hormone in, 69–70
  prolactin in, 63–65, 63f, 65t

Lactogenesis (*Continued*)
  prolactin-inhibiting factor in, 65–69
  sodium as predictor of, 100
  stages of, 58f, 62–63
Lactogenic hormone complex, 56
Lactogogues, 864
Lactose
  circadian variation in, 94f
  excretion of, into urine and
      prolactin, 66f
  malabsorption of, colic and, 275–276
  in milk, 306t, 765–767
    circadian variation in, 93
    colostrum, 95, 96f, 96t
    maternal diet and, 292
    prepartum, 95
    preterm, 531
    progesterone and, 95, 95f
Lactose intolerance, 489
Lactose synthetase, 138
Lactosuria, 579
Lamivudine, 449
Lanolin, breast preparation and, 241
Lansinoh, 255
Lassa fever, 429, 776t
Latch-on response, 248f
Late-onset GBS disease (LOD), 421–422
Late-onset neonatal infection (LONI),
      422–423
Latex allergy, 617
L-Dopa, prolactin and, 674t
Lead, in milk, 398–399, 398t, 399f
Leadership issues, 758–759
Legal issues, for weaning, 335
Legionnaires' disease, 776t
Legislation on breastfeeding, for working
      mothers, 650
Length, infant, measurement of, 797–802
Leprosy, 416, 776t
Leptin, in infant serum, 768–769
Leptospirosis, 776t
Let-down reflex
  breastfeeding and, 260–262, 261f
  milk duct and, 262f
  oxytocin nasal spray on, 353
  phantom, 265
  poor release of milk and, 352–353
  psychophysiologic reaction to,
      203–204, 203f
  side effects associated with, 265
Leukemia, T-cell, 444–446
Leukocytes
  maternal diet and, 308
  in milk, immunologic activity of, 152,
      152f
Levonorgestrel, 700, 702t
Licorice, 386
  root, 770–775
Lidocaine, 369t
Ligaments of Cooper, 44
Lingual frenulum function, Hazelbaker
      assessment tool for, 875t
Linoleic acid, 296t
Lip, cleft, 509, 510f, 511t, 913–918
  breastfeeding infants with, 916–917
  repair of, 917
  unilateral, 914f
Lipases, 136–137, 137t, 532
Lipids. *See also* Fat.
  mature, 102–108, 103–106t

Lipids (*Continued*)
  in milk, 306*t*
    brain development and, 107–108
    mature, 290*t*
Lipomas, breast, 611
Listeria monocytogenes, 776*t*
Listeriosis, 416–417
Lithium, 394
Liver, drug metabolism in, 370–371
Liver transplantation, 596
Lobuloalveolar development, in
      pregnancy, 42
Lobulus (lobuli), 40
Lobus (lobi), 40
Long-term nursing, positive
      consequences, 24*t*
Low-birth-weight (LBW) infants, 524,
      525, 528–530. *See also* Premature
      infants.
    gastrointestinal tract of, 525–526
    human milk for, 552–553
    nutritional needs for, 525
Low-molecular-weight (LMW) heparin,
      378
Low-temperature short-time
      pasteurization, 721
Lutein, 128
Luteinizing hormone-releasing hormone
      agonist, 700–701
Lyme disease, 462–463, 776*t*
Lymphatic drainage of breast, 47, 570*f*
Lymphocytes, bioactivity of, 153
Lymphocytic choriomeningitis, 776*t*
Lymphocytic choriomeningitis virus,
      429
Lymphoid tissue, mucosal-associated,
      174–175
Lymphoma
    non-Hodgkin, 573–574
    T-cell, 444–445
Lyophilization, 724, 725*t*
Lysozyme, 114, 138
    in milk, 158*t*, 160*f*
      bioactivity of, 147*t*, 150
      stability of, 162

M

Machupo virus, 429
Macroglossia, 508
Macrophages, 152–153
Magnesium
    infant requirements for, 532
    in infant serum, 768–769
    maternal requirements for, 297–298*t*
    in milk, 304–305, 306*t*, 765–767
      colostrum, 98–99
      maternal diet and, 304–305
      preterm, 531, 533*t*
    in milk fortifiers, 541–542*t*
    and other salts, 122*t*, 123
Magnesium sulfate, 565
Maimonides, 634
Malaria, 464–465, 776*t*
Malnutrition, 286, 309, 332
MALT (mucosal-associated lymphoid
      tissue), 150, 151*f*
Mammalian species
    composition of milk in, 266*t*
    induced lactation in, 668

Mammals, lactation in, 232
Mammary epithelial cell, 31
Mammary gland, 31, 34. *See also* Breast.
    innervation of, 48*f*
    intermediary metabolism of,
      83, 83*f*
    secretory cell of, 82*f*
Mammary pit, 34–35
Mammary stem cells (MaSCs),
      155–156
Mammogenesis, 57*t*
    breast development in, 94
    hormonal control of, 57
    mammary gland development in, 53
    menstrual cycle and, 60
    prepubertal phase of, 59
    pubertal phase of, 59
Mammoplasty
    augmentation, 614–615, 614*f*
    reduction, 616
Manganese
    infant requirements for, 534
    maternal requirements for, 297*t*
    in milk, 306*t*, 765–767
      preterm and fortified, 541*t*
Manual expression, 792–793. *See also*
      Milk expression.
    for engorgement, 252, 935
    in induced lactation, 669
    position for, 250–251, 251*f*
    technique and procedure for,
      792–793, 793*f*
Marburg virus, 434, 776*t*
Marijuana, 770–775, 940, 604. *See also*
      Cannabis; Tetrahydrocannabinol
      (THC).
Marquette method, natural family
      planning and, 891
Mastitis, 567–571, 568*f*, 568*t*, 809–815,
      840–844
    abscess formation in, 567, 568*f*
    antibiotic for, 378*t*
    bilateral, 573–574
    brucellosis, 415
    candidal, 467–469
    complications of, 842–843
    definition and diagnosis, 840
    diabetes and, 578
    engorgement *vs.*, 934
      and plugged duct, 568*t*
    follow-up for, 842
    laboratory findings in, 573
    laboratory investigations for, 840
    management of, 570–571, 570*t*, 570*f*,
      841–842
    methicillin-resistant *S. aureus* and, 571
    neonatal, 499
    precautions and recommendations for,
      776*t*
    predisposing factors for, 840
    prevention of, 843
    radiation therapy, 223
    recommendations for further research,
      843
    recurrent or chronic, 571–573
    staphylococcal, 418–419
    streptococcal, 421–428
    tuberculous, 425
Mastocytosis, 617
Mastopexy, 614

Maternal and Child Health Bureau
      (MCHB), 663
Maternal behaviors, hormonal control
      of, 203
Maternal complications. *See also* specific
      disorder.
    anaphylaxis, 618–620
    breast cancer, 592–594
    breast cysts, 611
    candidal infection, 571–573
    cephalgia and lactational headache,
      619
    Chiari-Frommel syndrome, 575–576,
      576*t*
    Crohn disease and ulcerative colitis,
      599–600
    cystic fibrosis, 589–590, 590*t*
    Del Castillo syndrome, 576, 576*t*
    dermatitis involving breast, 616–618
    diabetes mellitus, 578–580
    epilepsy, 600, 600*t*
    fat necrosis, 611
    fibrocystic disease, 610–611
    Forbes-Albright syndrome, 576, 576*t*
    galactography, 610–611, 611*f*
    galactorrhea, 574–575
    gigantomastia, 611–613, 612*f*
    glomerular disease, 597
    hematomas, 611
    hospitalization for, 604–607
    hyperactive let-down reflex, 578
    hypergalactia, 565
    hyperprolactinemia, 575, 576*b*
    hypomagnesemia in, 598–599
    lipomas, 611
    lumps in breast, 610
    mastitis, 567–571, 568*f*, 568*t*
    medical, 563–632
      abscess formation, 567, 568*f*
      autoimmune thrombocytopenic
        purpura, 594
    methicillin-resistant *S. aureus* and, 571
    multiple sclerosis, 619–620
    neuropathies, 600
    nipple discharge, 609
    nipple pain, 618
    obstetric, 563–567
      cesarean delivery, 563–565
      engorgement and galactorrhea, 563
      retained placenta and lactation
        failure, 566
      toxemia, 565
      venous thrombosis and pulmonary
        embolism, 566
    osteoporosis, 597–598, 598*b*
    Paget disease, 610
    polycystic ovarian syndrome,
      588–589
    postlactation breast involution, 615,
      615*f*
    psychological, hospitalization for, 606
    radiation exposure and, 591–592
    Raynaud phenomenon, 601–602
    rheumatoid arthritis and connective
      tissue disorders, 594–595
    Sheehan syndrome and
      hypopituitarism, 576–577
    smoking and, 602–604, 603*f*
    surgical, 613–614
      gastric by-pass, 616

Maternal complications (*Continued*)
hospitalization for, 604–607
thyroid disease, 585–586, 586*f*
Maternal Concepts, 807
Maternal illness, on milk production, 352
Maternal milk cells, survival of, 155–156
Maternal nutrition, 285–319
foods to avoid in, 314–315
immunologic substances and leukocyte activity in, 308
infant allergy and, 638, 642
lactational amenorrhea and, 693
milk color and, 315–316
milk content and, 92–93
antibacterial factors in, 163*t*
immunologic factors in, 159–160
lipids in, 102–108
milk production and, 286–307, 288*t*
energy supplementation in, 287
fat, cholesterol, and omega-3 fatty acids in, 288–291, 290*t*
fish consumption in, 291–292
kilocalories in, 293–294, 293–294*f*, 295–299*t*
lactose in, 292
minerals in, 303–307
prebiotics and probiotics in, 294
protein in, 287–288, 288–289*t*
vitamins in, 294–303, 300–301*t*, 302*b*
volume of, 286
water in, 292–293
supplementation of, 309
for allergy, 309
dietary reference intake for, 295–298*t*, 314*t*
for dieting, 313–314, 314*t*
for exercise, 311–313, 313*f*
for malnutrition, 309
for vegetarian diet, 309–311, 310*t*
Maternity leaves, 656–657, 656*f*
Maternity Practices in Infant Nutrition and Care (MPINC), 10
"Maternity Protection at Work", 664
Matrescence, 743
Mature milk, 765–767
lactogenesis of, 62
lipids in, 102–108
Measles, 442, 443*t*, 776*t*
Meconium ileus, 514
Meconium plug syndrome, 514
Medela, 807
Medical education, for basic proficiency in breastfeeding, 946–948
Medical problems. *See* Infants, with problems; Maternal complications.
Medical profession, impact of, 205
Medical professional, educating and training, 754–764
continuing efforts, 754–755
curriculum for medical students, 757–759
curriculum for nurses, 759–762
expertise and leadership issues in, 758–759
postgraduate, 761–762
problem in, 755–757, 756*f*
solution for, 757

Medical professional, educating and training (*Continued*)
Wellstart program for, 759, 759*t*, 760–761*b*
Medical students, curriculum for, 757–759
Medications. *See also* Drugs.
in breast milk, 364–406
breastfeeding and, 225*t*, 226
Medroxyprogesterone (Depo-Provera), 670
Mefloquine, 465
Men, lactation induction in, 676
Meningitis, 776*t*
Meningococcal infections, 417
Menopause, lactation after, 678–679
Menses, return of, 691–692
Menstrual cycle
breast changes in, 37–38
milk composition in ovulatory, 692–693
morphologic criteria for phase assignment in, 50*t*
Menstrual cycle growth, 60
Menstruation, lactation and, 321
Mental problems. *See* Psychological problems.
Meperidine
for labor, 902
in milk, 374
postpartum use of, 903
Merocrine glands, 54
Mesenchyma, dense, 49
Metabolic disorders, 492, 494–508
Metabolic screen, 348, 494
Metals, milk and, 398–399, 398*t*
Methadone, 939
maintenance of, 396, 397*t*
Methicillin-resistant *Staphylococcus aureus* (MRSA), 776*t*
mastitis and, 571, 842
transmission of, 417–418
Methimazole, 379
for hyperthyroidism, 588
Methionine/cysteine ratio, 112
Methylation, 179
Methyldopa, 595
Methylergonovine, 365
Methylphenidate, 369*t*
Methylxanthines, 379–380
Metoclopramide, 388–389, 865
in induced lactation, 671*t*, 673, 674*t*, 682, 683*t*
for lactation, 264, 353, 485
Metoprolol, 392
Metronidazole, 376, 464, 466
Miconazole, 572
for mucocutaneous candidiasis, 468
Microbiota, probiotics, and prebiotics, 175–177
MicroRNA (miRNA), 179
Microsomal fraction, 82, 82*f*
Middle East respiratory syndrome (MERS-CoV), 455
Migraine headaches, 619
Milk. *See also* Cow milk; Human milk.
average volume outputs of, 97*t*
composition of, 92*t*
in mammalian species, 266*t*
constituents of, 93*t*

Milk (*Continued*)
hormones in, growth and, 360*t*
mammalian, 93*t*, 101, 102*t*
oversupply of, 279–280
poor release of, 352–353
production of
domperidone for, 353
factors influencing, 267
poor, 351–353
thyrotropin-releasing hormone (TRH) on, 353
sodium and, 354
storage guidelines, 862
supply of
fatigue on, 352
maternal illness on, 352
thawing or warming, 862
transitional, 100–101
witch's, 36, 499
Milk bank
donor milk from, 715
location of, 716*f*
structure of, 715–716, 717*f*
Milk Club, 762
"Milk coming in", 75–76
Milk ducts, 232, 232*f*
let-down reflex and, 262*f*
Milk ejectors, role of prostaglandins, 77–78
Milk enzymes, 86
Milk expression, 739*t*. *See also* Manual expression.
for culture, 409–410, 411*b*
for engorgement, 935
for hypotonic infant, 909
in workplace, 657
Milk fever, 330–332
Milk flow
mother-infant pattern of, 233, 234*f*
suckling rate and, 233
Milk line or ridge, 34
Milk stasis, 843
Milk streak, 34, 39
Milk synthesis, pathway of, 83*f*
Milk thistle, 770–775, 867
as galactogogue, 391
Milk-ejection reflex
neurohypophysis and, 232–233
practical aspects of, 262–264, 263*t*
Milk/plasma (M/P) ratio, for drugs, 367*t*, 371
Milky discharge, of nipple, 608
Minerals
infant requirements for, 532–534, 533*t*, 542–543
maternal requirements for, 297*t*
in milk, 119–123, 120–121*t*, 306*t*, 765–767
colostrum, 96–98
maternal diet and, 303–307
neonatal reserve of, 100
Minipill, 699–700, 700*t*
Mitochondrial proliferation, 82
Model breastfeeding policy, 856–860
application of, 859
exceptions for, 859
forms for, 859
purpose of, 856
responsibility, 859
statements of, 856–859

Moffat, Thomas, 6–7
Molecular weight, of drug, 367
Molybdenum
    infant requirements for, 534
    maternal requirements for, 297–298t
Monkeypox, 456
Mononucleosis, infectious, 776t
Montgomery glands, 34, 41f, 42
Montgomery tubercles, 42, 43f
Mood, breastfeeding and, 199, 202
Morphine, 904
    epidural, 564
    postpartum use of, 903
    for surgery, 605
Mother-infant dyads, 329
Mother-infant nursing couple, practical
        management of, 230–284
Mothers. *See also* Maternal entries;
        Working mothers.
    attitudes toward breastfeeding, 226
    benefits of breastfeeding for, 220–224
        breast cancer and, 221–224, 223t
        cardiovascular disease and, 220–221
        empowerment and, 220
        evidence-based systematic reviews
                of, 218–219t
        osteoporosis and, 220
        ovarian cancer, 221
        postpartum recovery, 220
    drugs for. *See* Drugs.
    hospital discharge guidelines for,
            825–830, 826–827t
    infant interaction with, 195, 196f
    management of, in induced lactation,
            676–678
    medical complications of, 563–632
    milk supply of, fatigue on, 352
    nursing, immunization for, 402–403
    peer counselor role on, 752
    personality differences in, 202
    rights of, 325
    sociodemographic characteristics of,
            331t
    support group, development of,
            744–745
    "telephone", 744
    weaning decision of, 326, 326–328t
Mother's milk. *See also* Human milk.
    breastfeeding, 713f
        prevalence of breast milk expression
                in, 713f
    for healthy infant, 714
    pasteurizing, 714–715
    for sick infant, 715
Mother's milk tea, 385, 385t
Motilium, for milk production, 353
Motor development, 342–343
Motor problems, oral, 347, 508
Mouth problems, 519
Mouthers, 257
MRSA. *See* Methicillin-resistant
        Staphylococcus aureus (MRSA).
Mucins, 165, 166t
Mucosal immune system, 173–174
Mucosal immunity, 150–151, 151f
Mucosal-associated lymphoid tissue,
        174–175
Mulging, 674–675
Multicolored and sticky discharge,
        608–609

Multiple sclerosis, 619–620
Mumps, 442–443, 776t
Mycobacterium leprae, 416, 776t
Mycobacterium tuberculosis, 776t
Mycoplasma pneumoniae, 776t
Myelin-specific messenger ribonucleic
        acid, 107
Myoepithelial cells
    contraction of, 48
    microscopic anatomy of, 49
MyPyramid, 292f

N

Nadolol, 392
Nalbuphine, 902–903, 905
Naproxen, 905
Narcotics, 941–942
    use of, during pregnancy, 939–940
Nasopharyngeal carcinoma, Epstein-Barr
        virus associated with, 432
National Alliance for Breastfeeding
        Advocacy (NABA), 747–748
National Business Group on Health,
        663–664
National Childbirth Trust, 744, 806
National Health and Nutrition
        Examination Survey
        (NHANES), 11t
National Health Information Center,
        803
National health promotion, 2t
National Immunization Survey
        (NIS), 11t
National Institutes of Health (NIH), 2
National Natality Surveys (NNS), 10
National Organization for Rare
        Disorders (NORD), 494
National Survey of Children's Health
        (NSCH), 11t
National Survey of Early Childhood
        Health (NSECH), 11t
National Survey of Family Growth
        (NSFG), 11t, 19t
    breastfeeding behaviors and, 336
Natural family planning, 697–699, 697f,
        891–893
Natural products, 770–775. *See also* Herbs
        and herbal teas.
    in breast milk, 364–406
Near-term infant
    definition of, 869
    follow-up for, 873
    principles of care, 870–873
        in inpatient, 870–872
        in outpatient, 872–873
Necrotizing enterocolitis (NEC), 515
    in premature infant, 526, 546–547,
            546f
        enteral (oral) intake and, risk factors
                associated with, 546b
Neglect, 208
    child, 224
Neisseria gonorrhoeae, 415–416, 776t
Neisseria meningitidis, 409, 776t
Neonatal abstinence syndrome (NAS),
        methadone and, 939
Neonatal intensive care unit (NICU),
        transitioning premature infant to
        home from, 879–885, 880t, 884f

Neonatal mortality, initiation timing of
        breastfeeding and, 525t
Neonates. *See also* Infants.
    ankyloglossia evaluation and
            management in, 874–878, 875t,
            877f
    antiepileptic drugs in, 600, 600t
    bilirubin production in, 500
    breasts and nipple discharge in, 499
    developmental immune deficiencies
            in, 149–150, 149b
    digestion and absorption in, 537t
    glucose monitoring and hypoglycemia
            treatment in, 817–824,
            818 821t
    guidelines for supplementary feeding
            in, 831–839, 832–834t, 836t
    hospital discharge of term, 825–830,
            826–827t
    hyperbilirubinemia and jaundice in,
            499–508, 502t, 503f, 504b, 504t,
            505f, 506b, 507f, 509t
    loss of, 709
    mastitis in, 499
    weight loss in, 832
Nerves, of breast, 47
Neural disorders, suckling problems in,
        508
Neuroendocrine control of milk
        ejection, 70f
Neurohypophysis
    milk-ejection reflex and, 232–233
    oxytocin and, 233
Neuropathies, 600
Neuropeptides, 150
Neutrophils, 153
Nevirapine (NVP), 449
Newborns. *See also* Neonates.
    administration of vitamin K to, 302b
    physiology of, 832
    Wellstart breastfeeding policies for,
            760b
Newman-Goldfarb protocols, on
        induced lactation, 679
Niacin, 131–132t, 134
    maternal requirements for, 295t, 298t
    in milk, 300t, 306t, 765–767
        maternal diet and, 299
        preterm and fortified, 541t
Nickel
    in animals, 126
    maternal requirements for, 297t
    in milk, 765–767
Nicotine, 369t, 942, 602. *See also*
        Smoking.
Nicotine therapies, 604b
NICU. *See* Neonatal intensive care unit
        (NICU).
Nifedipine, 601
Nipple cups, 737f
Nipple discharge, 609
    diagnosis of, 607–608
    evaluation of, 607–610
    milky discharge, 608
    multicolored and sticky discharge,
            608–609
    neonatal, 499
    painful, 618
    purulent discharge, 609
    types of, 615f

Nipple discharge (*Continued*)
  watery, serous, serosanguineous, and bloody discharges, 609–610
Nipple shields, 255–256, 256*f*
Nipple stimulation
  in induced lactation, 677
  milk ejection and, 68*f*, 70
  oxytocin release and, 71
  prolactin level and, 71
Nipples, 41–44. *See also* Areola mammae.
  accessory, 39
  bi-fed or double, 611*f*
  blanching of, 272
  cracked, 254*f*, 256–257
    management of, 256*b*
  duct anatomy, digital model of, 45*f*
  ectopic, 39*f*
  eczema in, 272
  embryonic development of, 34
  erection of, 42–43
  evolution of, 36*f*
  examination of, 240, 240*f*
  flat, 256
  imprinting on, 201, 201*t*
  innervation of, 47
  inverted, 240, 240*f*, 242
    surgical correction for, 243
  large, 256
  latex, suckling and, 236
  ointments for, 255
  painful, 253–255, 254*f*
    management of, 256*b*
    other causes of, 271–274
  in pregnancy, 52
  preparation of, in breastfeeding management, 242, 242*f*
  Raynaud phenomenon and, 601
  small, 256
  stimulation of, induce labor and, 242–243
  supernumerary, 39, 39*b*, 39*f*
  white bleb in, 269–270
Nitrogen in milk, 306*t*, 765–767
  variation in, 93
Nitroglycerin, 369*t*, 601
Non-A, non-B hepatitis (NANBH), hepatitis C and, 437–438
Non-Hodgkin lymphoma, 573–574
Nonimmunoglobulins, in milk, 114
Noninherited maternal antigens (NIMA), 156
Nonnutritive sucking
  imprinting in, 201–202, 201*t*
  for premature infants, 553–554
Nonopioid analgesics, 903
Nonprotein nitrogen in milk, 115–116, 115*t*, 306*t*, 765–767
  levels and significance of, 115*t*
  measurement of, 94
Nonsteroidal antiinflammatory drugs (NSAIDs), 594–595
Norepinephrine, 47
Norethindrone, 670
Norethindrone enanthate, 700, 700*t*
Normal Pregnancy Virtual Patient program, 759
Norwalk agent, 776*t*
NSAID analgesics, 905
Nuclear family, 743

Nucleotides in milk, 116–117, 116*t*
  bioactivity of, 147*t*, 150, 170–171*f*, 172*t*
Nucleus, 81
Nurses
  attitudes of, 26
  curriculum for, 759–762
  postgraduate learning opportunities for, 761
  public health, 745
Nursing. *See also* Feedings; Suckling.
  closet, 334–335
  comfort, 323
  cross, 685–686
  in delivery, 244–246
  immediate, obstacles in, 244
  mother-infant, practical management of, 230–284
  observation of, 349–350
  during pregnancy, 707–708
  psychophysiologic reactions to, 202–203
  refusal of, 332
  success of, 230
  switch, 345–346
  tandem, 682, 707–708
  wet, 685–686
Nursing bottle caries, 519
Nursing Mothers' Association, 744
Nursing Mothers Counsel, Inc., 804
"Nursing strike", 332
Nursing supplementer, 558
Nut allergies, 643
Nutrient density, of milk, 333*t*
Nutritional screening assessment, 559*t*
Nutritional supplements. *See also* Infants, nutrition for; Maternal nutrition; Supplementary feedings.
  for mother, 285–319
Nystatin, 572
  for mucocutaneous candidiasis, 468

O

Obesity
  asthma and, 636–637
  gastric by-pass, 616
  in infants, 355–361, 359*t*
Obstetric complications
  cesarean delivery, 563–565
  engorgement and galactorrhea, 563
  retained placenta and lactation failure, 566
  toxemia, 565
  venous thrombosis and pulmonary embolism, 566
Obstetricians, 26
  in breastfeeding, 653–654
Office of Women's Health (OWH), 31–32
Ointments, for nipples, 255
Oligosaccharides, in milk, 165–167, 306*t*
  colostrum, 96–98, 118–119
Omega-3 fatty acids, 108, 288–291, 532
One-breast *vs.* two-breast feeding, 351
Ophthalmia neonatorum, 415–416
Opioids, 939–942
Opportunistic infections, 776*t*
Optimal feeders, 324

Optimal nutritional status, suboptimal nutritional *vs.*, 880
Oral bioavailability, of drug, 373
Oral defects, 511–512
Oral health, 519
Oral medications, 903
Oral motor problems, 347, 508
Oral searching reflex, definition of, 237, 248*f*
Oral tactile hypersensitivity, 508
Organic acidemias, 493–494
Organizations supporting breastfeeding, 803–807
Organogenesis, 37–38, 59–60
Orgasmic cephalgia, 619
Ornithine transcarbamylase deficiency, 494
Orthostatic reflex tachycardia, 596
Osmolarity
  of colostrum, 98–99
  human milk, 127
Osteoporosis, 220, 597–598, 598*b*
Otitis media, 491–492, 516
  protection against, 216–217
  risk for, 28, 29*f*
Ovarian cancer, 221
Ovaries, polycystic, 588–589
Ovulation
  lactation and return of, 692, 692*t*
  touch sensitivity and, 699
Ovulation method of contraception, 697, 702*t*
Ovulatory menstrual cycle, milk composition in, 692–693
Oxacillin-resistant *Staphylococcus aureus* (ORSA), 573. *See also* methicillin-resistant *Staphylococcus aureus* (MRSA)
Oxybutynin, 369*t*
Oxytocin, 326, 737*t*
  alcohol and, 352, 380
  in induced lactation, 670
  for lactation, 264
  let-down reflex and, 203, 203*f*, 353
  levels of, after delivery, 244
  in milk, concentrations of, 77
  suckling and, 704–705

P

Pacifiers, 30, 201–202, 201*t*, 277–278, 857
  in neonatal period, 847
Paget disease, 610
Pain
  breast, 809–815
  nipple, 618, 809–815
Palate
  abnormal, 508
  cleft, 509–518, 510*f*, 511*t*, 913–918
    breastfeeding infants with, 916–917
  high arched, 512
Palmar grasp, in breastfeeding, 245, 245*f*
Palpation, of breast texture, 239–240, 240*f*
Panada, 7
Pancreatic enzymes, 488–489, 495*t*
Pantothenic acid, 134
  maternal requirements for, 295*t*
  in milk, 300*t*, 306*t*, 765–767

Pantothenic acid (*Continued*)
  maternal diet and, 299–300
  preterm and fortified, 541*t*
  recommended daily dietary
      allowances for infants, 130*t*
Papilloma, intraductal, 609–610
Papillomaviruses, 441–450, 776*t*
Paracrine factor, 58
Parainfluenza viruses, 776*t*
Parasites, 463–465
Parenchyma, 40
Parental factors, bed sharing and, 853
Parents magazine, 7–8, 22–23
Parity, milk composition and, 101*f*, 108
Partial breastfeeding, 28, 148–149, 148*b*
Parvovirus, 443–444
Parvovirus B19, 776*t*
Passive diffusion, on passage of drug, 365
Pasteurization of milk
  immunoglobulins after, 162
  nutritional consequences of, 725–726
  standards for, 721
Patient Protection and Affordable Care
      Act, 650
Peanut allergy, 643
Pectoral fascia, 44
Pediatric incunabulum, 6–7
Pediatric Nutrition Surveillance System
      (PedNSS), 10, 11–12*t*, 12*f*, 14*t*
Pediatricians
  AAP recommendation for, 762
  attitude of, 26
Peer counseling, 749–752, 751*t*
Peer counselor, 750
Pelvic inflammatory disease, 776*t*
Pennyroyal, 388*t*
Pentazocine, 902–903, 905
Peppermint, 618
Perioral stimulation, 485
Peripartum breastfeeding, management
      of, 231–232
  maternal, 845–850
Personality
  infant, 206
  maternal, 202
Pertussis, 417, 776*t*
Pesticides, pollutants and, 396–398
Pewter pap spoon, 7*f*
Peyer patches, 151*f*, 174
pH
  drug ionization and, 366
  human milk, 127
Phagocytes, defects in, 149*b*
Phantom let-down, 265
Pharmacokinetics, 365
Pharmacologic food reaction, 641
Phencyclidine hydrochloride, 938
Phenobarbital, 600*t*
  on infant, 372, 393
  in milk, 371
  newborn and, 600*t*
  for toxemia, 600
Phenylalanine, 492
Phenylketonuria (PKU), 492–494
Phenytoin, 393, 600*t*
Phosphatases, 138
Phospholipids in milk, 306*t*
  colostrum, 98
Phosphorus
  infant requirements for, 532, 533*t*

Phosphorus (*Continued*)
  in infant serum, 768–769
  maternal requirements for, 297–298*t*
  in milk, 306*t*, 765–767
    fortified, 540, 542*t*
    maternal diet and, 304–305
    preterm, 531
Phototherapy
  for breast milk jaundice, 506–507,
      507*f*
  for early hyperbilirubinemia, 503
Physicians
  attitude of, 26
  as consultants, 657
  education for, 755
    curriculum in, 757–759
    expertise and leadership issues in,
        758–759
    postgraduate learning opportunities
        for, 761–762
    problem in, 755–757, 756*f*
    solution for, 757
  international organization for, 806
  lactation consultant working with, 752
  peer counselor with, 750
  role of
    breastfeeding promotion, 205
    working mothers and, 654
  weaning, 333–334
  who breastfeed, 762
Physician's office, breastfeeding-
      friendly, 897–900
Pierre Robin syndrome, 510, 511*t*
Pigmentation, areolar, 42, 52
Pink or pink-orange milk, 315
Pinocytosis, 365–369
Pitocin, on let-down reflex, 353
Pituitary disorders, 574–575
Placenta
  antibody transfer via, 150
  retained, 566
    lactation failure and, 350–351
Plasma glucose levels, operational
      thresholds for treatment of, 819*t*
Plasma prolactin, 64, 67*f*
Plasmodium spp., 464
Pleat-seat baby carrier, 484, 485*f*
Pneumocystis jiroveci, 776*t*
Pneumonia, 776*t*
  risk for, 28, 29*f*
Poison ivy, 617–618
Poland syndrome, 39–40, 40*b*
Poliomyelitis, 776*t*
Polioviruses, 444
Pollutants, pesticides and, 396–398
Polyamines, 114–115
Polychlorinated biphenyls (PCBs),
      396–397
Polycystic ovarian syndrome, 588–589
Polymorphonuclear leukocytes, 151*f*, 153
Polythelia, 39, 39*b*, 39*f*
Polyunsaturated fatty acids (PUFAs)
  brain development and, 107–108
  in milk, 102–103, 765–767
Pompe disease, 494
Pooled milk, 796, 538–540. *See also*
      Donor milk.
Positive pressure, on milk-ejection reflex,
      232–233
Postmature infants, 483–486

Postmenopausal lactation, 678–679
Postnatal period, breastfeeding
      management in, 265, 265–266*t*
  breast rejection in, 270
    unilateral, 271
  carrying and holding in, 274
  colic and crying in, 274–280
  colicky behavior in, management of,
      276–277
    sleep tight method in, 277
  exclusive breastfeeding in, 274
  feeding frequency in, 266–267, 266*t*
  insufficient milk syndrome in,
      278–279, 279*t*
  maternal diet in, influence of cow milk
      in, 275–276
  maternal rest in, 268
  milk expression in, 273
  one-breast/two-breast feedings in,
      267–268
  oversupply of milk in, 279–280
  pacifiers in, 277–278
  sleeping in, 274
  solid foods in, 274
  stool patterns in, 278, 278*t*
  supplementary feedings in, 272–273
Postnatal rubella, 454
Postpartum anesthesia, 903–904
Postpartum depression, 622*f*
  early weaning and, 206
  thyroiditis *vs.*, 622–626
Postpartum recovery, 220
Post-traumatic stress disorder, 208, 626
Postural orthostatic tachycardia
      syndrome, 596
Potassium
  maternal requirements for, 297*t*
  in milk, 119–121, 121*t*, 306*t*,
      765–767
    colostrum, 96–98
    maternal diet and, 303–304
    prepartum, 95, 96*f*, 96*t*
    preterm and fortified, 541*t*
Prebiotics, 294
  microbiota, probiotics and, 175–177
Pregnancy
  breast in, development of, 52
  breastfeeding promotion in, 929–932
  components of, 531*t*
  drug safety in, 373
  growth during, 60–62, 61–62*f*
  hypertrophy of, 611–613, 612–613*f*
  maternal-infant bonding in, 197
  nursing during, 707–708
  postpartum possibility of, 692
  prevention of. *See* Contraception.
  prolactin in, 60
  toxemia, 565
Pregnancy Nutrition Surveillance
      System (PNSS), 11*t*
Pregnancy Risk Assessment Monitoring
      System (PRAMS), 11*t*, 329, 852
Premature infants, 524–525
  body composition of, 558*f*
  brain growth and intelligence in,
      535–537
  breastfeeding, 524–562
    for extremely premature infant,
        554–555
    for near-term infant, 553

Premature infants (*Continued*)
  breastfeeding mothers of, support for, 883–884
  gastrointestinal tract of, 537–538, 537t
    development of, 525–526, 526b, 526–527f
    priming, 526–528, 527–529b, 529t, 529f
  growth of, 879–880, 880t
    long-term follow-up of, 543–545
    optimal, 530
    requirements for, 532–535, 533–534t, 533b
  hospital to home transition for, 556–557
  human milk for, 528, 538
    antimicrobial properties of, 545–548, 546–547f, 546b, 546t, 548t
    feeding schedule for, 545b
    fortification of, 540–543, 541–542t, 542f, 544t
    LBW or SGA infant and, 552–553
    maternal production of, 549–552, 551f, 552b
    preterm, properties of, 530–537, 530b, 531f
    supplementation of, 538–540, 539b
  kangaroo care for, 549, 549f
  kernicterus in, 505–507
  LBW, 528–530, 530b
  NICU to home transition for, 879–885, 880t, 884f
  nutritional assessment, optimal *vs.* suboptimal, 880
  recommendations for, 557–559, 557–558f, 559t
  relactation in, 679, 680f
  SGA, 555–556
  twins and triplets, 486, 486f
Premature weaning, 328t
Prenatal period, breastfeeding management in, 239–241, 240f
  breast preparation in, 241–242
  hand expression in, 243
  nipple preparation in, 242, 242f
  nipple stimulation in, 242–243
  surgical correction in, 243
Prenatal setting, breastfeeding promotion in, 929–932
Prepartum milk, 95, 96f, 96t
  composition of, 96t
Prepubertal breast development, 35–37, 59–60
Prepubertal growth, 59–60
Preterm Infant Breastfeeding Behavior Scale (PIBBS), 555t
Preterm milk, 796
  composition of, 541t
  properties of, 530–537, 530b, 531f, 545–548, 546–547f, 546b, 546t, 548t
Primaquine, 465
Primidone, 600t
Private organizations, 804–805
Probiotics, 294
  microbiota, and prebiotics, 175–177
Procrastinators, 257

Progesterone
  breast development and
    embryogenesis in, 58–59
    mammogenesis in, 59–60
  contraceptives with, 699, 700t
  in induced lactation, 669–670
  lactational infertility and, 690, 690f
  lactogenesis and, 62
  maternal behavior and, 203
Progestin, 699, 700t, 702t
Progestin-only options, in hormonal contraceptive method, 889t, 891–892
Program on Breastfeeding in Pediatric Offices, 762
Prolac Inc., 807
Prolact CR®, 534f, 535b
Prolactin, 63–65, 690–691, 737f
  breast development and
    embryogenesis in, 58
    mammogenesis in, 59, 63f
  concentrations, in postpartum women, 261f
  drugs affecting, 669–670
  exercise and, 313f
  factors affecting, 65
  in induced lactation, 670, 673
  lactational infertility and, 690
  lactogenesis and, 78
  maternal behavior and, 203
  molecular sizes of, 575
  in pregnancy, 52
  secretion of, influence of drugs in, 674t
  sucking stimulus and, 238–239
  thyrotropin-releasing hormone (TRH) on, 353
Prolactinemic disorders, 574–575, 576b, 576t
Prolactin-inhibiting factor (PIF), 52, 65–69
  hormonal regulation of, 61
  lactogenesis and, 66
  mammogenesis and, 66
Prolactin-releasing factors, 69, 71f
Proline, in milk, 765–767
Propranolol, 392, 595
Propylthiouracil (PTU), 379
Prostaglandins, 140–141, 140f
  let-down reflex and, 262
Proteases and antiproteases, 138
Protein binding, of drugs, 365–369, 366f
Protein nitrogen, 765–767
Proteins, 84–85
  human milk and, 675–676, 675–676f
  increase in, 330
  infant requirements for, 528, 531t, 540, 541t, 542–543, 543b
  in infant serum, 768–769
  maternal requirements for, 296t, 298t
  in milk
    bioactive, 150
    changes in, 110–114
    colostrum, 96–98
    fortified, 532, 540, 542t
    human and bovine, 111f
    maternal diet and, 287–288
    mature, 105t, 110–114, 111t
    preterm, 530b, 531, 531f
    total, 306t, 539
  synthesis of, 83f, 84–85

Proteins (*Continued*)
  total, 159f
    in milk, 765–767
  in weaning foods, 341
Protracted diarrhea, management of, 489
Pseudoephedrine, 391
Pseudomembranous colitis, 488
Psychoactive substances, in herbal teas, 383t
Psychological factors, in relactation, 680–682, 681t
Psychological impact, of breastfeeding, 194–213
  abuse and neglect, 208
  body contact and cultural tradition in, 197–199, 198f, 199b
  bottle feeding *vs.*, 199–200, 200f
  failure at breastfeeding and, 210–211, 211t
  mother-infant interaction in, 195, 196f
  personality differences and, 202
  psychophysiologic reactions and, 202–203
  psychosocial risk factors and, 208–209
  rejection of breastfeeding and, 209–210
  society, medical profession, and family in, 204–208
Psychological problems, 620–626, 621t
  hospitalization for, 606
Psychophysiologic reactions, 202–203
Psychosis, postpartum, 606
Psychosocial failure to thrive, 350–355
Psychosocial risk factors, and early weaning, 208–209
Pubertal growth, 60
Public education, 3
Public health nurses, 745
Pulmonary embolism, 566
Pumping. See also Breast pumps; Manual expression.
  in induced lactation, 669, 678
PUPP syndrome, 617
Puronyx, Inc., 807
Pyloric stenosis, 513
Pyridoxine therapy, for tuberculosis, 424
Pyrrolizidine alkaloids, 385–386

Q
Q fever, 776t
Quaternary anticholinergics, 377

R
Rabies, 452–453, 776t
Radiation exposure, 591–592, 592f
Radiation therapy, 223–224
Radioactive materials, milk and, 401
Raspberry root, 770–775
Rat-bite fever, 776t
Raynaud phenomenon, 601–602, 809–815
Reactive attachment disorder, 350
Red Book: Report of the Committee on Infectious Disease, 409
Reduction mammoplasty, 616
Regional anesthesia, 903

Relactation, 667–687, 680f, 680t
  drugs to induce, 682–683
  history of, 667
  psychological factors in, 680–682, 681t
  tandem nursing and, 682
Relapsing fever, 776t
Relative infant dose (RID), 372
Relaxin, 141
Remifentanil, 902
Renal transplantation, 596
Reoviridae, 428
Reproductive function. See also Contraception; Pregnancy.
  contraception in, 694–704
  in fertility, 688–694
  during lactation, 688–711
  sex in, 704–707
Reserpine, 595
Residency training programs, 762, 763t
Resistance factor, 163
Respiratory illness, 28
  in infant, 491–492
    protection against, 216
    smoking and, 603
Respiratory syncytial virus (RSV), 776t
  antibodies against, 491–492
  transmission of, 453
Rest, maternal, 843
Resters, 258
Retinol, 306t
Retroviruses, 444–450, 445t, 451b, 776t
Reverse pinocytosis, 366–369
Reverse pressure softening technique, 934
Reverse pump, sodium and, 368–369
Rh immune globulin, immunization, 402
Rheumatoid arthritis, 594–595
Ribavirin, 429, 453
Riboflavin
  maternal requirements for, 295t, 298t
  in milk, 300t, 306t, 765–767
    maternal diet and, 299
    preterm and fortified, 541t
Rice allergy, 643
Rickets, 532
Rickettsial disease, 776t
Rickettsial pox, 776t
Rifampin, for tuberculosis, 424
Rites of passage, 743
Ritodrine, 563
Rocky Mountain spotted fever, 776t
Ross Laboratories Mothers Survey MR77-48, 9
Rotarix, 454
RotaTeq, 454
Rotaviruses, 453–454, 776t
Rotigotine, 369t
Roundworm infections, 465
Rubber nipple, 201–202
Rubella, immunization, 403
Rubella virus, 454, 776t
Rural health issues, 747
Rusty pipe syndrome, 260

S
Sabia virus, 429
Sage, 770–775

Salazosulfapyridine (SASP), 599
Salmonella infection, 776t
SARS-associated coronavirus (SARS-CoV), 454–455
Sassafras, 386
Satcher, David, 2–3
Scissor grasp, in breastfeeding, 245, 245f
Scopolamine, 369t
Screening
  metabolic, 348
  nutritional, 559t
Sebaceous gland, 34, 41, 43f
Secretory cells, cycle of, 82f
Secretory differentiation and activation, 56, 63f, 76
Seizures, 600, 600t
Selective serotonin reuptake inhibitors (SSRI), 395b
Selegiline, 369t
Selenium
  infant requirements for, 534
  maternal requirements for, 297–298t
  in milk, 306t, 765–767
    maternal diet, 305
"Self-weaning", 329–330
Sensitive periods, 197
Sensitization, drug, 372–373
Sensory nerves, of breast, 47
Serotonin, 71
Serous or serosanguineous nipple discharge, 609–610
Serrapeptase®, for engorgement, 934
Severe acute respiratory syndrome (SARS), 454–455, 776t
Sexual abuse, 706–707
Sexual activity, 705–706
Sexual arousal, 704–705
Shame, 210–211
Sheehan syndrome, 576–577
Shigella, 776t
Siblings, breastfeeding and, 207
Silicone, in breast implants, 614, 614f
Silymarin, in induced lactation, 671t
Sleeping
  co-sleeping
    ABM guideline on, 851–855
    sudden infant death syndrome and, 30–31
  safe environment for, 199b
Sling baby carrier, 484, 485f
Small intestine, disorders of, 513–514
Small-for-gestational-age (SGA) infants, 555–556. See also Premature infants.
  catch-up growth in, 342
  failure to thrive in, 347
  human milk for, 524–525, 552–553
Smallpox, 455–456, 776t
  immunization, 402
Smoking, 602–604
  clove cigarette, 604
  let-down reflex and, 352
  marijuana, 604
  milk production and, 603f
  Raynaud phenomenon and, 601
  sudden infant death syndrome and, 852
Social marketing, 747
Society, impact on breastfeeding, 204–205

Sodium
  infant requirements for, 541t
  as lactogenesis predictor, 100
  maternal requirements for, 297t
  in milk, 119–121, 121t, 306t, 354, 765–767
    colostrum, 95
    fortified, 541–542t
    maternal diet and, 303–304
    preterm, 530b, 531
Solid foods, 274
  AAP recommendations for, 201
  allergies to, 643–644
  growth and, 341
  percentage of infants first introduced to, 331t
  poor intake of, 350
  weaning to, 323–325
Solids, total milk, 765–767
Solubility, drug, 367, 367t
Somatostatin, 603
Specialty milks, 728–729
Specific gravity of milk, 95
Spermicides, 702t, 704
Spinal defects, 516–517
Spinal/epidural medications, 904
Spirochetes, 462–463
St. John's wort, 382t, 387–388, 770–775
Standard precautions, 408
Staphylococcal enterotoxin F, 420
Staphylococcal infections, 417–421
  coagulase-negative, 420–421
  resistance factor for, 163
  toxin-mediated, 420
Staphylococcal scalded skin syndrome, 420
Staphylococcus aureus, 417, 776t
  methicillin-resistant, 417–418, 571, 776t, 842
  oxacillin-resistant, 573
Staphylococcus epidermidis, 420–421, 776t
Starvation, hyperbilirubinemia and, 502–503
State, breastfeeding rates by, 12t, 14t, 20f
Stem cells, mammary, 56, 155–156
Sterilization, surgical, 702t, 889t, 893
Steroids, for rheumatoid arthritis, 595
Stools, bilirubin level and passage of, 502
Storage capacity, of breast, 351
Storage containers, milk, 719, 861
Streptococcal infections, 421–428, 776t
  group A, 421
  group B, 421–423, 422f
Streptococcus agalactiae, 421
Streptococcus pneumoniae, 776t
Streptococcus pyogenes, 420, 776t
Stress
  breastfeeding and perceived, 199
  early weaning and, 208
  milk supply and, 657
  psychological, on ejection reflex, 352–353
Stroma, 40, 49
Strongyloides, 465–466
Strongyloides stercoralis, 465
Submammary space, 38
Substance use disorder, guidelines for breastfeeding and, 937–945
  contraindications for, 942–943
  future research, 943

Substance use disorder, guidelines for breastfeeding and (*Continued*)
  purpose of, 937
  recommendations for, 941–943
  specific substances in, 938–941, 938t
Sucking
  definition of, 233–234, 237
  disorders of, 347b
  nonnutritive, 201–202, 201t, 553–554
  stimulus, 238–239
  suckling and, 674–675
  swallowing and, 349
Suckling. *See also* Feedings; Nursing.
  definition of, 233
  factors influencing, 236
  fat content and, 236–237
  lactational infertility and, 688, 689f
  maternal effects of, 76–77
  mechanism of, 247–248, 248f
  patterns, as indicators of problems or pathology, 237, 238f
  problems with, anatomic and neural, 508
  process of, 234
  prolactin levels after, 66f
  radiographic interpretation of, 234b
  rate, milk flow and, 233
  science of, 232–237
  sexual arousal and, 704–705
  sucking and, 674–675
  swallowing and, coordination of, 235–236
  ultrasound interpretation of, 234b
  uterine contractions and, 261–262
Sudden infant death syndrome (SIDS), 29–31, 518–519
  bed sharing and risk of, 851
    ethnic diversity and, 852
    infant factors of, 853
    laboratory studies of, 853
    parental factors of, 853
    prevention of, 852
    recommendations for future research, 854
    risk of, 852
  breastfeeding and, 219–220
  marijuana and, 940
  smoking and, 603
  tobacco and, 941
Sufentanil, 905
Sulfacetamide, 366
Sulfamethoxazole, 378t
Sulfanilamide, 366
Sulfapyridine, 377–378
Sulfasalazine, 377–378
Sulfonamides, 366, 367t
Sulfur, in milk, 765–767
Sulpiride, 389, 866
  in induced lactation, 671t, 674t
Supernumerary glands, 39
Supernumerary nipple, 39, 39b, 39f
Supplemental nursing system, 669, 684f
Supplementary feedings, 272–273, 831–839
  background of, 831–833
  breastfeeding and, 847
  choice of, 834
  definition of, 831
  inappropriate reasons for, 832, 836t
  indications for, 832–833t
  methods of providing, 835

Supplementary feedings (*Continued*)
  recommendations for, 833–834
  research needs for, 835
  volume of, 834
Supplementation
  of human milk, 538–540
  for infant, 285–319
  for mother, 285–319
Support
  for induced lactation, 679
  organizations providing, 803–807
Support groups, 8, 743–753
Supraclavicular nerves, 48, 48f
Surgeon General's Workshop on Breastfeeding and Human Lactation, 662, 746, 754
Surgery
  in breastfeeding mothers, anesthesia for, 904
  herbal medicines and, 382t
  infants, 508–518
    neonatal, 517–518
  maternal, hospitalization for, 604–607
Swallowing
  disorders of, 347b
  sucking and, 349
  suckling and, coordination of, 235–236
Switch-nursing process, in breastfeeding, 345–346
Symmastia, 39, 39b
Symptothermal method
  of contraception, 698, 702t
  natural family planning and, 891
Syntocinon, for lactation, 264
Syphilis, 463, 776t

T
T lymphocytes, 154
Tactile hypersensitivity, oral, 508
Tagamet, 377
Tail of Spence, 38, 38f
Tandem nursing, 682, 707–708
Taurine, 112–113
T-cell leukemia/lymphoma, 444–445
T-cell system, 151f, 153–155
Tea, herbal, 381–388, 385b
  psychoactive substances used in, 383t
Tea tree oil, 388t
"Telephone mothers", 744
Ten Steps to Successful Breastfeeding, 856, 858
Tennis elbow, 601
Terconazole, for mucocutaneous candidiasis, 468
Terminal end buds, 36, 51, 51f
Testosterone, 369t
Tetanus, 776t
Tetracycline, on infants, 376
Tetrahydrocannabinol (THC), 940
Thawing milk, 862
The Womanly Art of Breastfeeding, 744
Theobromine, 380
Theophylline, 379
  in induced lactation, 673
  prolactin and, 673, 674t
Thiamin
  maternal requirements for, 295t, 298t
  in milk, 300t, 306t, 765–767
    maternal diet and, 299
    preterm and fortified, 541t

Thiopental sodium, 605
Thiouracil, 379
Thorazine. *See* Chlorpromazine.
Thread-leafed groundsel, venoocclusive disease and, 385–386
Thrombocytopenic purpura, autoimmune, 594
Thrush, 467
Thumb sucking, 201t, 202
Thymosin, 153–154
Thyroid disease, maternal, 585–586, 586f. *See also* Hypothyroidism.
Thyroiditis, postpartum, 586, 587f
Thyroid-stimulating hormone (TSH), 59
Thyroliberin, for relactation, 682
Thyrotropin-releasing hormone (TRH), 866
  engorgement and, 563
  in induced lactation, 671t, 674t
  on lactation, 353
  prolactin and, 65
Thyroxine (T_4), 498
Tinea, 776t
Tobacco, 941, 602. *See also* Smoking.
Togaviridae, 428
Token breastfeeding, 20, 148–149, 148b, 200–201
Toll-like receptors, 175
Tongue-tie, 271, 271b, 874
Topiramate, 600t
Total parenteral nutrition (TPN), 514–515
Toxemia of pregnancy, 565
Toxic shock syndrome (TSS), 420, 776t
Toxin, psychological impact of, 401
Toxin-mediated illness, 776t
Toxin-mediated staphylococcus disease, 420
Toxoplasmosis, 465–466, 776t
Trace elements, 122t, 123–142
  in milk, 765–767
Trace minerals, infant requirements for, 534
Tracheoesophageal fistula, 512, 512f
Transdermal drug delivery system (TDDS), 368–369, 369t
Transferrin, 164
Transforming growth factor beta (TGF-β), mammogenesis and, 59
Transitional milk, 65, 100–101
Transplantation, organ, 596
Transport, mechanism of, drug, 367
Transpyloric tube feeding, in VLBW infants, 555
Treponema pallidum, 462, 776t
Triacylglycerols, 98t, 102–103
Trichinosis, 776t
Trichomonas vaginalis, 466, 776t
Triglycerides
  in infant serum, 768–769
  in milk, 98, 306t
Triiodothyronine (T_3), 498
Trimethoprim, 378t
Trimethoprim/sulfamethoxazole, 570t
Triplets and twins, 186–187, 186f
Trypanosoma cruzi, 467
Trypanosomiasis, 776t
TT virus (TTV), 434b, 436t, 456, 776t
Tubal ligation, 605, 702t

Tube feedings, 536, 555, 557–558, 557*f*
Tuberculin skin test (TS), 424, 424*f*
Tuberculosis, 409, 424–428, 424*f*, 426*f*, 427*t*
Tuberculous mastitis, 425
Tubuloalveolar glands, 40–41
Tularemia, 776*t*
Tumor necrosis factor alpha (TNF-α), 168*b*
Tumor virus, 456–458
Twin position, 915
Twins and triplets, 486–487, 486*f*
Typhus, 776*t*
Tyrosinemia, 492

U

Ulcerative colitis, 491, 599–600
Ultrasonic homogenization, 727–728
Ultrasound examination of breast lumps, 610
Unilateral cleft lip, 914*f*
United Nations Children's Fund, 4–5, 5*b*
United Nations International Children's Education Fund (UNICEF), 745
United States Breastfeeding Committee (USBC), 21, 32, 664, 747–748
Unrestricted breastfeeding, 17, 200
Urea
    in colostrum, 98–99
    in milk, 765–767
Urea nitrogen, in infant serum, 768–769
Ureaplasma urealyticum, 776*t*
Urinary tract infection, 776*t*
U.S. Breastfeeding Committee, for working mothers, 662
U.S. Consumer Product Safety Commission (USCPSC), 851–852
U.S. Department of Agriculture (USDA), 9
U.S. Department of Health and Human Services (HHS), 663

V

Vaginal rings, 700*t*, 702*t*
Vaginitis, 776*t*
Valerian, 382*t*
    root, 770–775
Valium, infants and, 374
Valproic acid, 393, 600*t*
"Value of Natural Feeding" poster, 28*f*
Varicella-zoster virus, 458–459, 459*t*, 776*t*
Varicose veins, 566
Vasectomy, 702*t*, 889*t*
Vegetarian diet, 309–311, 310*t*
Veins, from breast, 44
Venoocclusive disease, comfrey and, 385
Venous thrombosis, 566
Very low-birth-weight (VLBW) infants, 528–529. *See also* Low-birth-weight (LBW) infants.
    growth parameters in, long-term follow-up of, 543–545, 545*b*
    gut of, biology of, 527*b*
Very-low-density lipoprotein (VLDL), 356–357, 357*f*
Vibrio cholerae, 776*t*

Viral infections. *See also* specific infection.
    dermatitis of breast from, 617
    transmission of, 428–434
        arboviruses, 428–429
        arenaviruses, 429
        cytomegalovirus, 429–432
        dengue disease, 432
        Epstein-Barr virus, 432–433
        Filoviridae, 433–434
        hepatitis, 434–441
        herpes simplex virus, 440
        human herpesvirus 6 and 7, 440–441
        human papillomavirus, 441–450
        measles, 442, 443*t*
        misadministration of milk and, 412–413
        mumps, 442–443
        parvovirus, 443–444
        polioviruses, 444
        rabies virus, 452–453
        respiratory syncytial virus, 453
        retroviruses, 444–450
        rotaviruses, 453–454
        rubella virus, 454
        severe acute respiratory syndrome, 454–455
        smallpox, 455–456
        TT virus, 456
        tumor virus, 456–458
        varicella-zoster virus, 458–459, 459*t*
        West Nile virus, 460–461
        yellow fever virus, 461–462
Viruses
    antibodies for, 160–162
    in human milk, 723–724, 724*t*
Visiting Nurses Association, 745
Vitamin A, 128, 129*t*
    in colostrum, 100
    maternal requirements for, 295*t*
    in milk, 128, 128–129*t*, 300–301, 301*t*, 306*t*, 765–767
        maternal diet and, 300–301
        preterm and fortified, 541*t*
Vitamin B complex, 131–135
Vitamin B₁, 131–134, 131–132*t*
Vitamin B₂, 131–132*t*, 134
Vitamin B₆, 131–132*t*, 134
    maternal requirements for, 295*t*, 298*t*
    in milk, 300*t*, 306*t*, 765–767
        maternal diet and, 299
Vitamin B₁₂, 131–132*t*, 135
    maternal requirements for, 295*t*, 298*t*
    in milk, 300*t*, 306*t*, 765–767
        maternal diet and, 309–310
        preterm and fortified, 541*t*
Vitamin B₁₂-binding protein, 165
Vitamin C, 129*t*, 131, 131–132*t*
    infant requirements for, 535
    maternal requirements for, 295*t*, 298*t*
    in milk, 300*t*, 306*t*
        maternal diet and, 296
        preterm and fortified, 541*t*
Vitamin D, 762
    in human milk, 128–130, 129*t*
    infant requirements for, 533
    maternal requirements for, 295*t*
    in milk, 301*t*, 306*t*, 765–767
        maternal diet and, 301–302

Vitamin D (*Continued*)
    in milk fortifier, 541*t*
Vitamin E, 128*t*, 130
    infant requirements for, 532
    maternal requirements for, 295*t*, 298*t*
    in milk, 128*t*, 130, 301*t*, 306*t*, 765–767
        colostrum, 100
        fortified, 541*t*
        preterm, 540
Vitamin K
    in human milk, 128*t*, 130–131
    maternal requirements for, 295*t*
    in milk, 301*t*, 306*t*, 765–767
        maternal diet and, 302–303
        preterm and fortified, 541*t*
    for newborns, 302*b*
    recommended daily dietary allowances for infants, 130*t*
Vitamins, 128–131
    maternal requirements for, 295*t*
    in milk, 306*t*, 765–767
        colostrum, 96–98
        fortified, 541*t*
        maternal diet and, 294–303, 300–301*t*
        pasteurization and, 722*t*
    neonatal reserve of, 100
    for premature infant, 533, 533*b*
Volume of distribution (V_d), of drug, 367
Vomiting, failure to thrive and, 348
Voriconazole, for candidal infections, 468
Vulvovaginitis, candidal, 467

W

War on Want, 806
Warfarin, 566–567
    milk and, 378–379
Warming milk, 862
Water
    in body, 370, 370*f*
    maternal intake of, 292–293
    maternal requirements for, 296*t*
    in milk, 101, 102*t*
Watery nipple discharge, 609–610
Weaning, 320
    closet nursing, 334–335
    culture and, 21–22, 198
    to a cup, 325
    at delivery, 334
    diarrhea and malnutrition in, 332
    emergency, 330
    gradual *vs.* abrupt, 333
    HIV infection and, 448–449, 451–452
    infant-initiated, 329–330
    infant's need for, 320–322, 322*f*, 323*t*
    introduction of solids in, 323–325
    legal issues for, 335
    lipase activities during, 333
    milk composition during, 332–333, 333*t*
    mother initiated, 335
    mother's rights regarding, 325
    motivation for, 334
    phenylketonuria and, 493
    physician's role in, 333–334
    during pregnancy, 707
    premature, 328*t*
    process of, 325–328, 326–328*t*

Weaning (*Continued*)
  psychosocial risk factors and, 208–209
  reasons for, 326–328*t*, 328–329
  refusal to breastfeed and, 332
  role of development in initiation of,
      322–323
  timing and techniques in, 320
  types of methods of, 326*t*
  working mothers and, 335
Weaning age, 321
Weaning foods, on growth, 341–342.
      See also Solid foods.
Weaning/gestation ratio, 321
Weanling, 320
Weanling diarrhea, 332
Weight
  infant, 797–802
    bilirubin level and, 501
    body composition and, 370, 370*f*,
        558*f*
    failure to thrive and, 344, 344*t*
    return to pregnancy, 220, 313–314,
        314*t*
Weight gain. *See also* Obesity.
  induced lactation and, 677
  infant, 340
    median daily, 344*t*
    premature, 534*t*
Weight loss
  in infants, 258–260, 258*t*, 259*f*, 340
  in newborn, 832
Welfare-to-work program, 657–658
Well water, 399–400
Wellstart International, 748, 754, 805
Wellstart program, 759, 759*t*, 760–761*b*
West Nile virus, 412, 460–461, 776*t*
Wet nursing, 685–686, 712
Wheezing, 637, 637*t*
Whey, 113
Whey proteins, 111*f*, 113–114, 113*t*,
    306*t*
  premature infant growth and, 532

White River Concepts, 807
Whittlestone, 807
Whooping cough, 776*t*
WIC Participant and Program
      Characteristics (WPPC), 11*t*
Witch's milk, 36, 499
Women, Infants, and Children (WIC)
      program, 8, 9*t*, 324, 657, 746–747
  peer counseling and, 750
Work Group on Breastfeeding, 762
Working mothers, 650, 651*t*, 651–652*f*
  breastfeeding by, 655–665, 656*f*
    benefits of, 664
    business case for breastfeeding on,
        663–664
    comparison of, 652*f*
    considerations for, 660–661
    counseling for, 659–660
    daycare, 661
    physician's role in, 664–665
    rates for, 655
    resources for parents on, 661–662
    stress, milk supply and, 657
    Surgeon General's Workshop on,
        662
    vs. bottle feeding, 657
    workplace and, 657–659, 658*f*
    workplace kit for, 662–663, 663*f*
  employer and employees, attitudes
      toward, 654
  health care professionals, attitudes
      toward, 653–654, 654*t*, 659
  historical perspective on, 652–653
  labor force and, 650, 651–652*f*
  outcome for children and, 654–655
  U.S. Breastfeeding Committee for,
      662
  weaning and, 335
Workplace, maternal support at,
      657–659, 658*f*
World Alliance for Breastfeeding Action
      (WABA), 805

World Health Organization (WHO),
      803
  Baby Friendly Hospital Initiative of,
      4–5, 5*b*, 745
  code for infant feeding, 3
  exclusive breastfeeding and, 342
  growth charts of, 340–341
  guidelines from, 451*b*
  on mastitis, 840
  Medical Eligibility Criteria of,
      694–695
  statistics, 16–17*t*
  on weaning, 323
WW Kellogg Foundation, 746

X

Xanthine oxidase, 138

Y

Yeast, 809–815
Yellow fever, 776*t*
Yellow fever virus, 461–462
Yersinia enterocolitica, 776*t*
Yersinia pseudotuberculosis, 776*t*
Young Women's Christian Association
      (YWCA), 745

Z

Zidovudine (ZDV), 448
Zinc
  deficiency of, 496
  infant requirements for, 534
  maternal requirements for, 297*t*
  in milk, 124–126, 125*t*, 304–305, 306*t*,
      765–767
  in milk, preterm, 531, 542*t*
  in milk fortifiers, 541–542*t*
  in weaning foods, 341